D0188370

Heidi Ridley - studying at Sheffield Hallam University 2004.

47.2 Phoenix Court
133 Rockingham street
Sheffield
S1 4EE

14 Painswick Road
Hall Green
Birmingham
B28 0HH

Walter and Miller's
Textbook of Radiotherapy

Senior Commissioning Editor: Sarena Wolfaard
Project Development Manager: Dinah Thom
Project Manager: Jane Dingwall
Designer: Judith Wright

Walter and Miller's Textbook of Radiotherapy

Radiation Physics, Therapy and Oncology

C. K. Bomford BSc MPhil FIPEM
Formerly Head of Radiation Physics, Central Sheffield University Hospital Trust;
Honorary Lecturer, University of Sheffield; Visiting Lecturer, Sheffield Hallam University, UK

I. H. Kunkler MA MB BChir FRCR DMRT FRCPE FRSA
Consultant and Senior Lecturer in Clinical Oncology, Western General Hospital, Edinburgh, UK

Foreword by

B. W. Hancock MD FRCP FRCR DCH
Professor of Clinical Oncology, University of Sheffield, Weston Park Hospital, Sheffield, UK

SIXTH EDITION

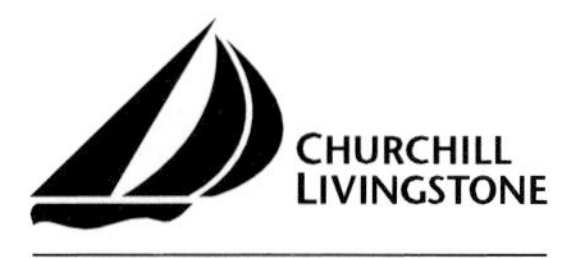

EDINBURGH LONDON NEW YORK OXFORD PHILADELPHIA ST LOUIS SYDNEY TORONTO 2003

CHURCHILL LIVINGSTONE
An imprint of Elsevier Limited

© Elsevier Limited 1959. All rights reserved.

No part of this publication may be reproduced, stored in a retrieval system, or transmitted in any form or by any means, electronic, mechanical, photocopying, recording or otherwise, without either the prior permission of the publishers or a licence permitting restricted copying in the United Kingdom issued by the Copyright Licensing Agency Ltd, 90 Tottenham Court Road, London, W1T 4LP. Permissions may be sought directly from Elsevier's Health Sciences Rights Department in Philadelphia, USA: phone: (+1) 215 238 7869, fax: (+1) 215 238 2239, e-mail: healthpermissions@elsevier.com. You may also complete your request on-line via the Elsevier Science homepage (http://www.elsevier.com), by selecting 'Customer Support' and then 'Obtaining Permissions'.

First edition 1950
Second edition 1959
Third edition 1969
Fourth edition 1979
Fifth edition 1993
Sixth edition 2003
Reprinted 2003, 2004

ISBN 0 443 06201 3

British Library Cataloguing in Publication Data
A catalogue record for this book is available from the British Library.

Library of Congress Cataloging in Publication Data
A catalog record for this book is available from the Library of Congress.

Note
Medical knowledge is constantly changing. As new information becomes available, changes in treatment, procedures, equipment and the use of drugs become necessary. The authors, contributors and publishers have taken care to ensure that the information given in this text is accurate and up to date. However, readers are strongly advised to confirm that the information, especially with regard to drug usage, complies with the latest legislation and standards of practice.

Where material has been borrowed from other sources, every effort has been made to contact the copyright owners to get their permission. However, should any copyright owners come forward and claim that permission was not granted for the use of their material, we will arrange for a settlement to be made.

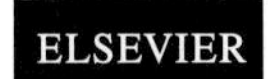

your source for books, journals and multimedia in the health sciences
www.elsevierhealth.com

The publisher's policy is to use **paper manufactured from sustainable forests**

Printed in China
N/03

Contents

Contributors

Robert Coleman MD FRCP
Professor of Medical Oncology, Cancer Research Centre, YCR Department of Clinical Oncology, Weston Park Hospital, Sheffield, UK

Martin Errington MB ChB MA FRCR MRCP
Consultant Radiologist, Imaging Directorate, Western General Hospital, Edinburgh, UK

John R. Goepel MB ChB FRCPath
Consultant Histopathologist, Royal Hallamshire Hospital, Sheffield Teaching Hospitals NHS Trust; Honorary Clinical Senior Lecturer, University of Sheffield, Sheffield, UK

B. W. Hancock MD FRCP FRCR DCH
Professor of Clinical Oncology, University of Sheffield, Weston Park Hospital, Sheffield, UK

Duncan McLaren BSc MB BS MRCP FRCR
Consultant Clinical Oncologist, Western General Hospital, Edinburgh, UK

Trevor J. McMillan BSc PhD HonMRCP
Peel Professor of Cancer Biology; Dean, Institute of Environmental and Natural Sciences, Lancaster University, UK

David Radstone BA DipDroit Compare-Solicitor of the Supreme Court MB BS DHRT FRCR
Consultant in Clinical Oncology, Weston Park Hospital, Sheffield; Honorary Senior Lecturer in Medicine, University of Sheffield, Sheffield, UK

Martin Robinson MD FRCP FRCR
Senior Lecturer Clinical Oncology, Department of Clinical Oncology, Weston Park Hospital, Sheffield, UK

Roger E. Taylor MA FRCP FRCPE FRCR
Consultant Clinical Oncologist, Cookridge Hospital, Leeds Teaching Hospitals, West Yorkshire, UK

Foreword

I am delighted to be asked to write the foreword for the 6th edition of this internationally respected textbook which first appeared in 1950 as a *Short Textbook of Radiotherapy for Technicians and Students*. The fact that this further edition is now with us represents a major tribute to the late Dr Joseph Walter and Professor Harold Miller, the original co-authors.

Though the main emphasis of the text remains the principles and practice of conventional radiotherapy, a knowledge of research and development into novel and potentially improved ways in which therapy may be planned and delivered is essential; this new edition aims to provide such knowledge against the background of improved multidisciplinary care. The potential audience still comprises those training for therapeutic radiography, or in technical or medical radiotherapeutic disciplines. The broadened coverage of treatment approaches (incorporating chemotherapy and supportive care) also commends the text to medical oncology trainees and chemotherapy nurses so that they may gain insight into the major role of radiotherapy in the management of cancer.

The editors are to be congratulated on this excellent revised version of the *Short Textbook of Radiotherapy* which I'm sure will remain indispensable for anyone requiring up-to-date information on the treatment of patients with cancer.

B. W. H.

Preface

Joseph Walter and Harold Miller would never have dreamt that their scribbling on the back of an envelope while on the train between Lincoln and Sheffield over 50 years ago would outline a book of such universal acclaim and now in its sixth edition. It has become affectionately known around the world simply as *Walter and Miller*, and in recognition of this affection, the authors readily agreed to incorporate their names into the title of the fifth edition. And so it remains.

This sixth edition, as with the previous five, has as its primary aim to provide an introductory text for cancer professionals and, in particular, those seeking to qualify as therapy radiographers and clinical oncologists preparing for postgraduate qualifications in radiation/clinical oncology such as the FRCR. It will also be of interest to trainees in medical oncology seeking a basic understanding of radiotherapy and the relevant radiation physics; to palliative care physicians and cancer nurses and to clinical physicists and medical technologists.

Over the years, training needs have, of course, changed. For example, in the UK, the therapy radiographer's training has changed from a 2-year in-house to a 3-year university degree course and the latter rightly includes material beyond the scope of this book. It would be invidious to suggest that any one text could provide all the resources for the undergraduate. This we do not claim but the references and bibliography will enable the student to study further.

Part 1 has been completely rewritten to reflect the major changes in radiotherapy practice over the last 10 years, such as multileaf collimation and virtual simulation, while recognising that it can neither do them justice in the space available nor be fully up-to-date in such rapidly changing areas of technology. For reasons such as these, references to currently available literature have been included, so that students can follow up particular lines of enquiry. The authors have resisted the temptation to include sample examination questions at the end of each chapter in the interests of cost and space.

The reordered chapters in Part 1 should enable the first-time reader to get a better grasp of the subject while allowing easier access to particular areas of interest when a quick reference is required. The authors have sought to maintain a balance between establishing a sound understanding of the basic physics while radically reducing, or eliminating altogether, references to outmoded technologies. For example, less space is now given to cobalt-60 but in recognition of its universal acceptance as a baseline for comparisons and of its continued use in some parts of the world, some basic data remain. The two chapters on imaging seek to focus on their applications in radiotherapy while providing the reader with a basic understanding of the technologies involved.

The chapters in Part 2 follow the pattern of the previous edition based on each cancer site. This seeks to fit in with the increasing trend towards cancer site-specific specialisation among cancer professionals. Developments in molecular biology are covered in the Biological and Pathological Introduction and in the section on Radiobiology. New contributors provide chapters on Radiobiology, Paediatric Oncology, Sarcomas, gynaecological and haematological malignancy. While this textbook has always had a strong emphasis on the technical aspects of radiotherapy, we have included substantial text on modern aspects of systemic therapy.

Every effort has been made by the authors to ensure the accuracy of the treatment regimes recommended. However, practice will vary from centre to centre and it is not possible to include all the alternative treatment regimes that may be safe and effective. It remains the responsibility of the individual clinician to check that treatments they prescribe are in keeping with locally agreed protocols and national guidelines. If in doubt, expert advice should always be sought before treatment is undertaken.

C. K. B.
I. H. K.

Acknowledgements

As always one is indebted to one's colleagues who, over the years, have contributed invaluably to one's education and experience and it would be invidious to try to mention them all. I, CKB, had the privilege of working with both Walter and Miller for many years before their well-earned retirements. Without them I should not have contributed to the last three editions of this text. For the current edition, I must acknowledge the considerable help and advice of Dr John Conway, currently Head of Radiotherapy Physics at Weston Park Hospital, Sheffield, and David Ramsden and Sue Otter of the Impression Suite and Planning sections of that Department; also Dr Lee Walton of the Radiosurgery Unit at the Royal Hallamshire Hospital. I am indebted to Dr Martin Errington for contributing the chapter on Nuclear Medicine Imaging at relatively short notice, without which this text would not be complete, and to Dr Sue Sherriff for allowing us to make use of her text from the fifth edition. We are grateful to many who have assisted in the drafting stages of the text and in the provision of illustrations in this as in the previous edition. In particular, we are grateful to Dr David Cameron, Dr Catriona Maclean and Mr Michael Dixon and acknowledge with gratitude the excellent Medical Illustration services of Mr Ronnie Robertson.

Our thanks are due to Elsevier Science in particular to Sarena Wolfaard and Dinah Thom, for their patience, guidance and encouragement in the preparation of this book. Finally, we should like to thank our families who have supported us during the long hours working on this new edition.

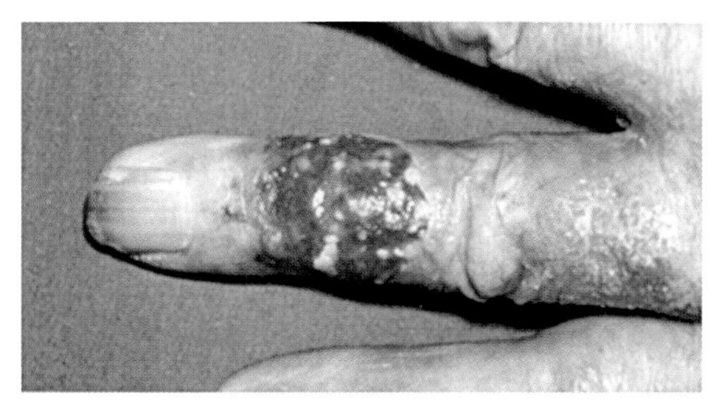

Plate 1.1 The fingers of a pioneer radiation worker; note the ridged finger nails as well as the soft tissue damage (p. 70).

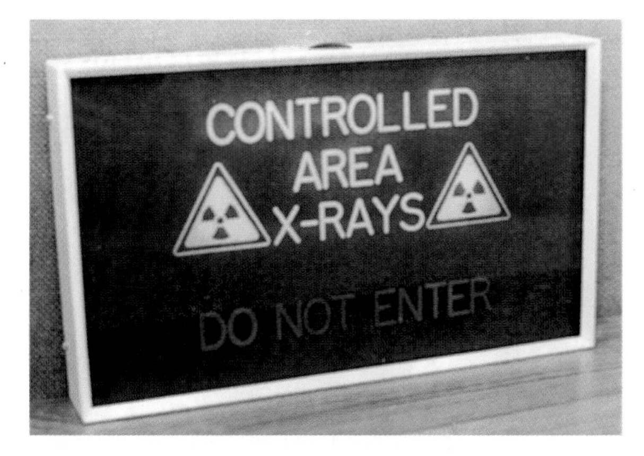

Plate 1.2 An electrically operated controlled area warning sign for an X-ray generator; the legends are not visible when the sign is switched off (p. 77).

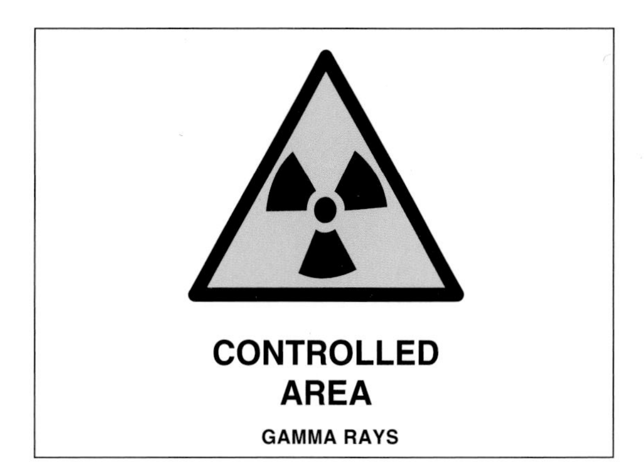

Plate 1.3 A controlled area warning sign for a radioisotope source for permanent display on the door of a gamma beam or remote afterloading unit or for temporary display on the door and/or bed of a brachytherapy patient (p. 77).

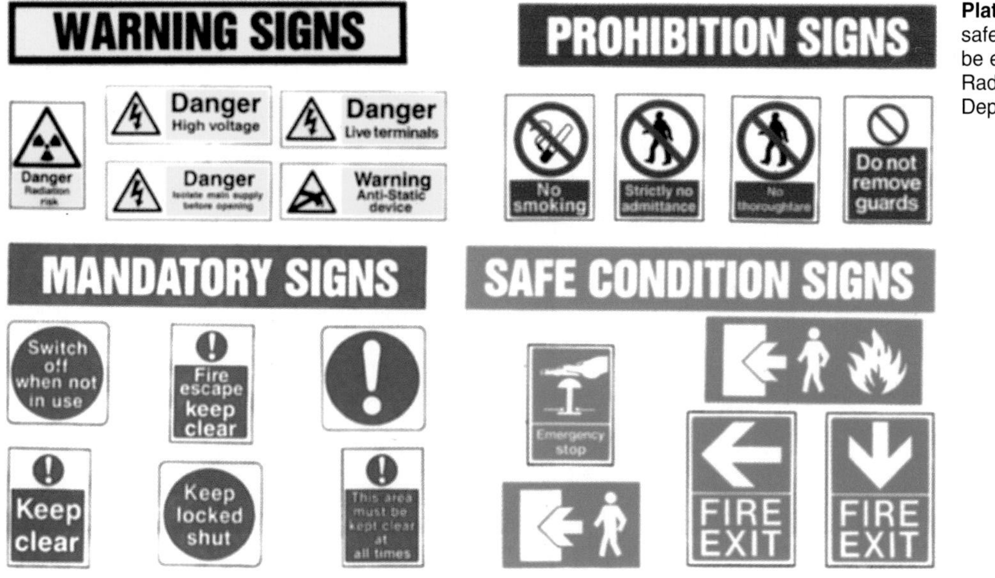

Plate 1.4 Some safety signs likely to be encountered in the Radiotherapy Department (p. 86).

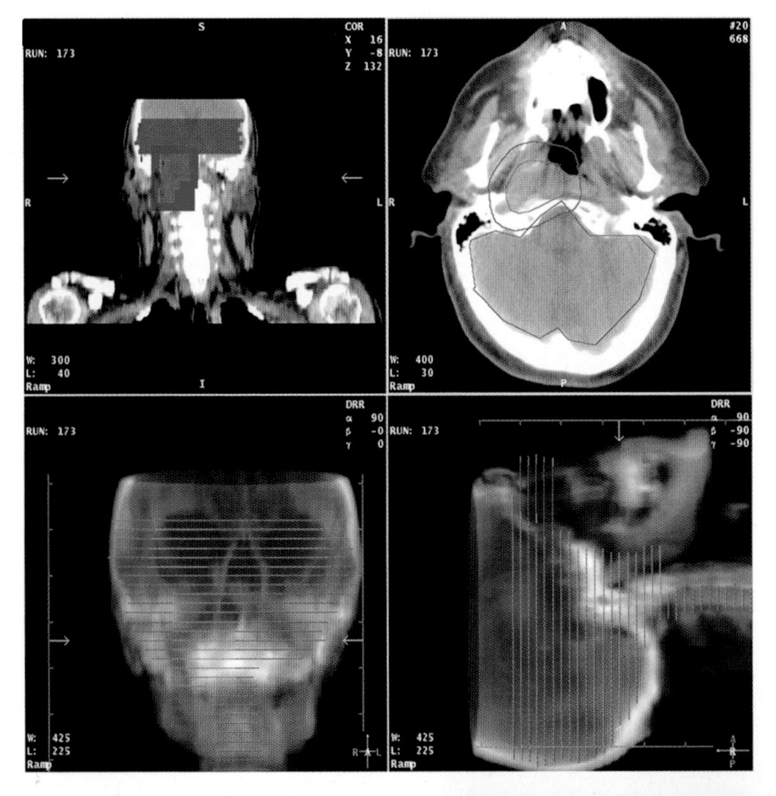

Plate 1.5 The localisation screen of the Picker virtual simulator showing the anatomy and planning contours on three orthogonal planes; note the contours of the eyes on the lower images (p. 108).

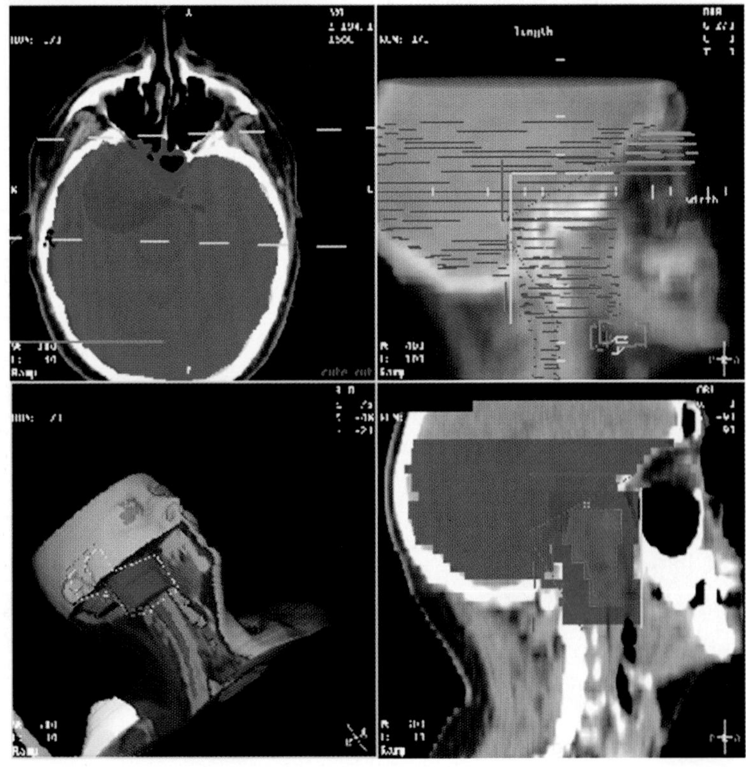

Plate 1.6 The virtual simulation screen of the Picker virtual simulator showing the field positioning and size superimposed on the digitally reconstructed radiograph (DRR) (top right); note the outline of the local shielding. The solid colour on the CT image (bottom right) hides some of the anatomical detail (p. 108).

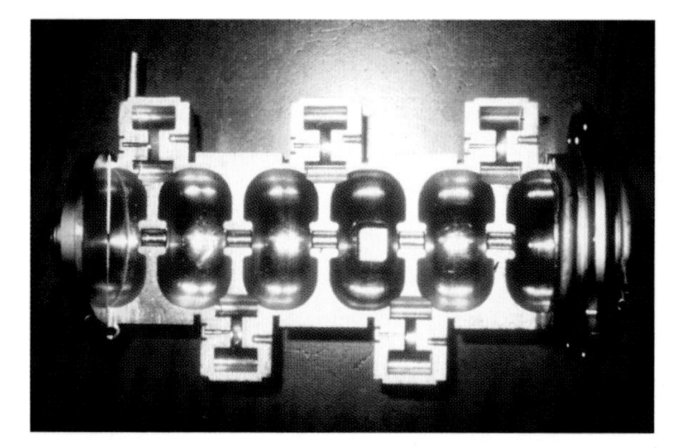

Plate 1.7 A section through a side-coupled waveguide (p. 165). (Courtesy of Varian Medical Systems UK Ltd.)

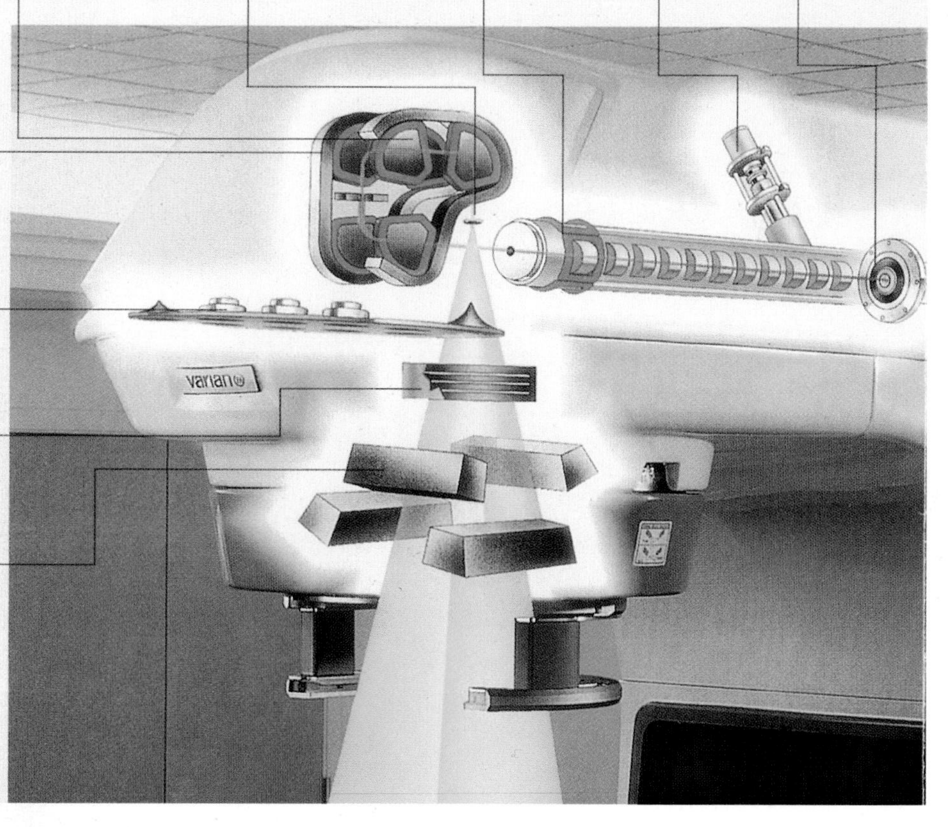

Plate 1.8 A standing wave accelerator showing the principal components (p. 166). (Courtesy of Varian Medical Systems UK Ltd.)

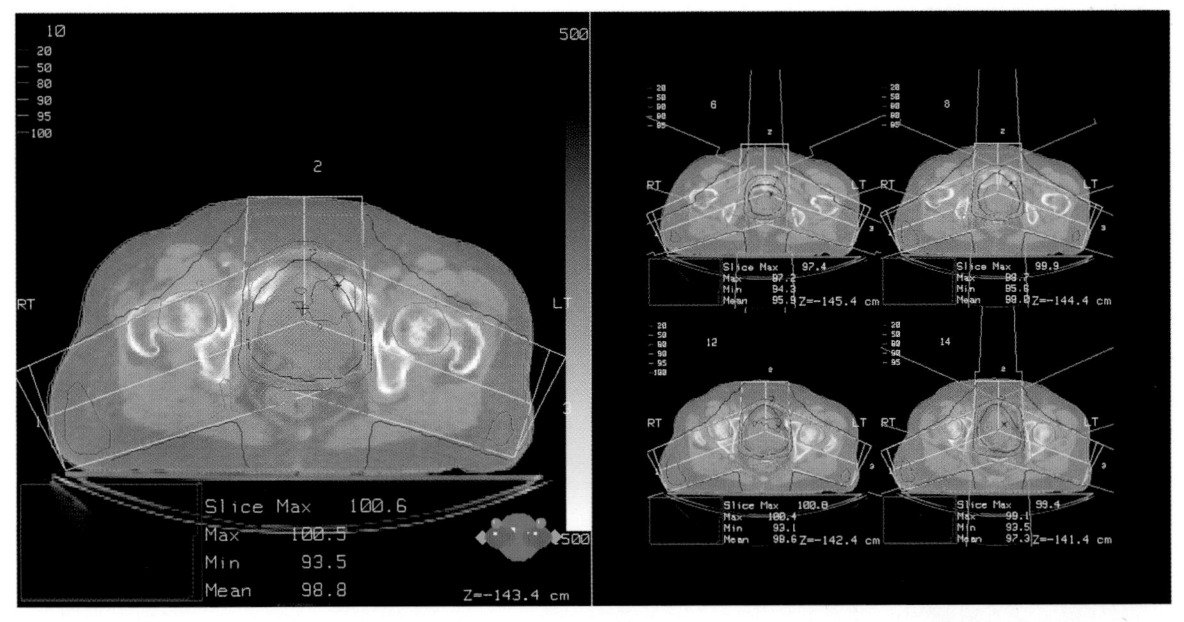

Plate 1.9 A three-field bladder dose distribution in the midplane (main) and in two planes above and below the midplane. Two 15° wedged posterior oblique beams at 110° to the midline and one non-wedged anterior beam have been used (p. 210).

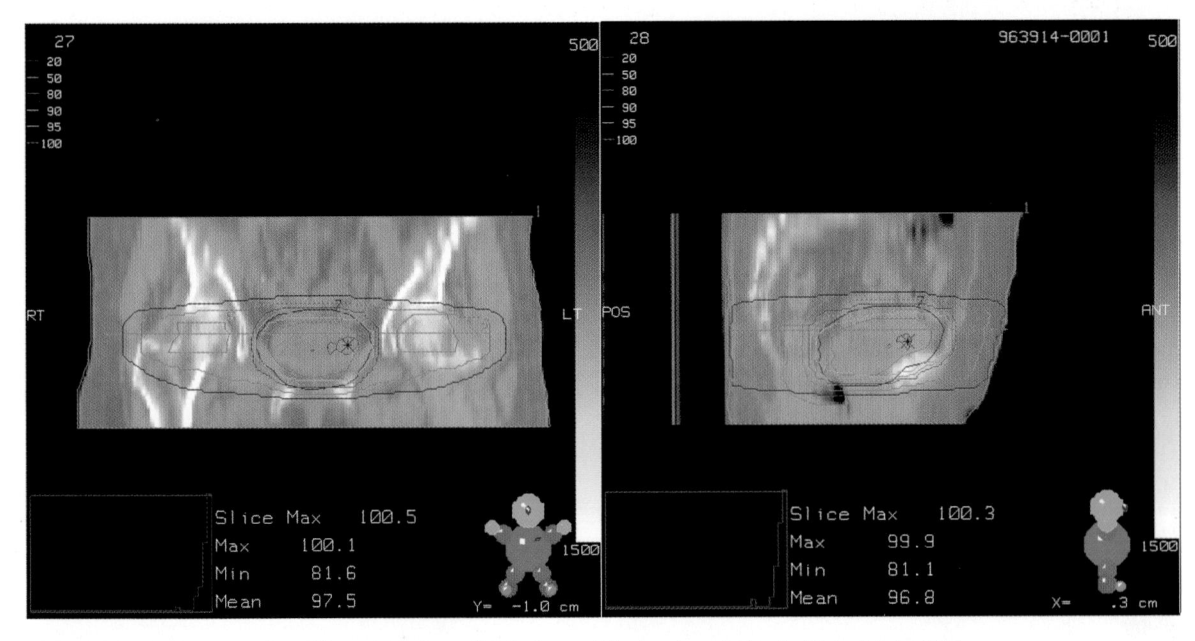

Plate 1.10 **A** The coronal and **B** sagittal plane distributions of the treatment plan in Plate 1.9 (p. 210).

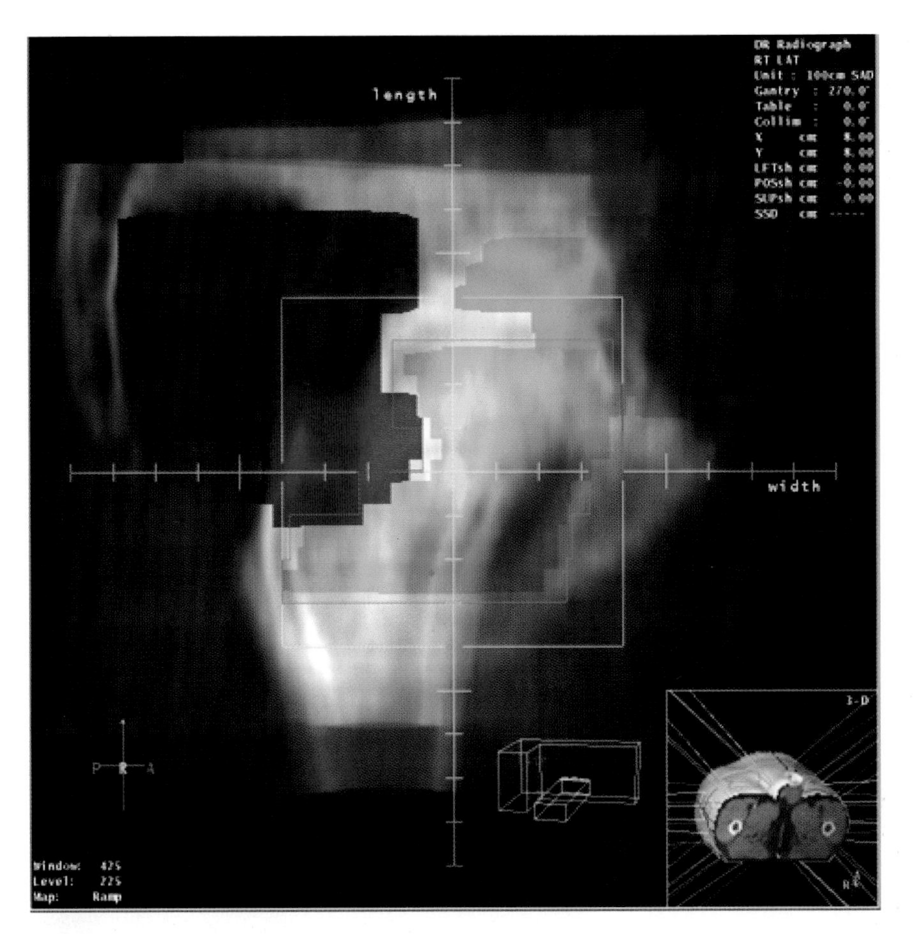

Plate 1.11 Six-field prostate plan using conformal fields. Beam's eye view (BEV) with MLC leaf positions overlaid on a DRR of the lateral field (p. 210).

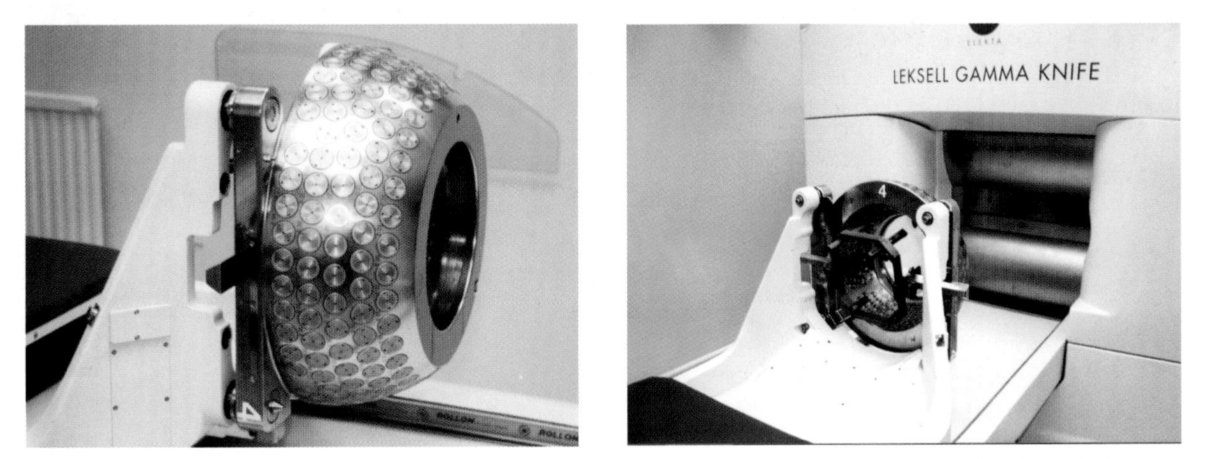

Plate 1.12 The Sheffield stereotactic radiosurgery unit showing: **A** the 4 mm collimator helmet mounted on the end of the patient couch; **B** the helmet and headframe and shielding doors (p. 218).

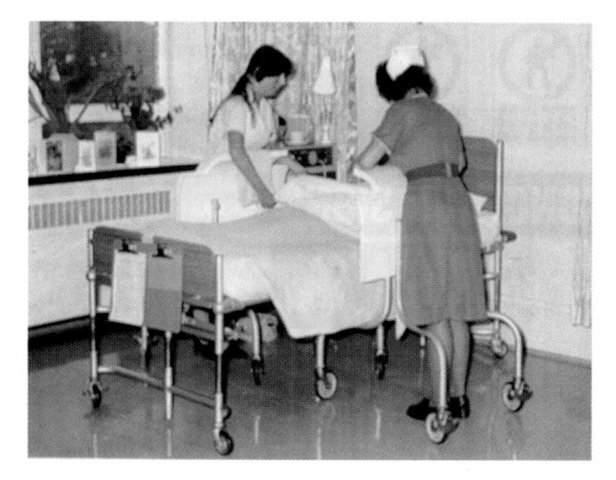

Plate 1.13 The use of mobile lead screens to protect the Nursing Staff tending the brachytherapy patient, a third screen at the foot of the bed is to be recommended (p. 229).

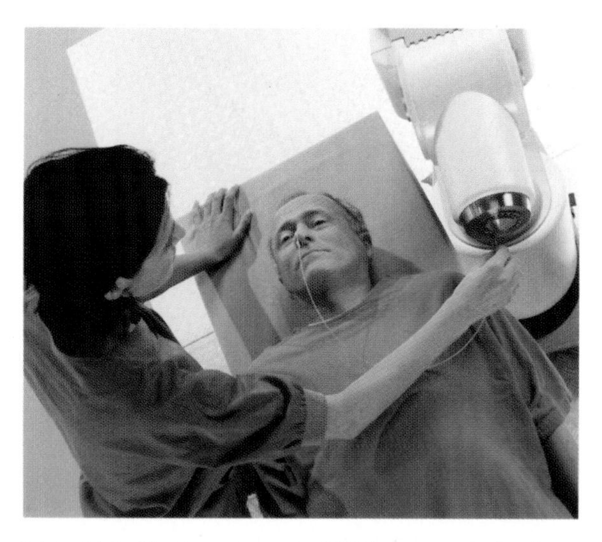

Plate 1.14 The high-dose-rate (HDR) remote afterloading unit (p. 230). (Courtesy of Nucletron Trading Co., Chester.)

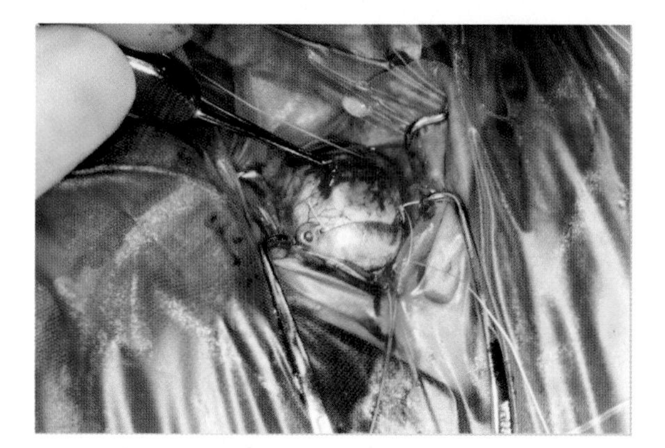

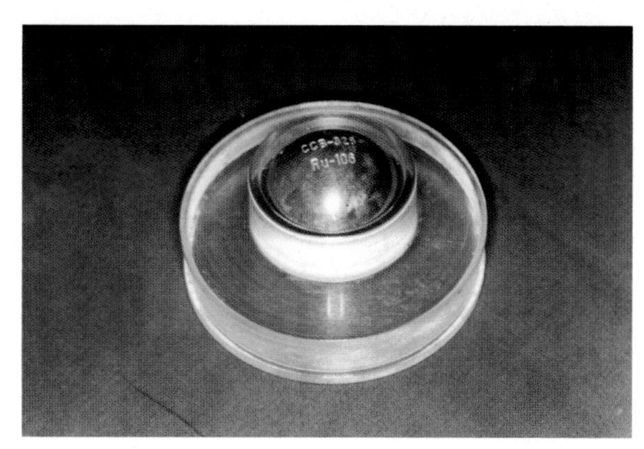

Plate 1.15 **A** A ruthenium plaque insertion and **B** the plaque (p. 239).

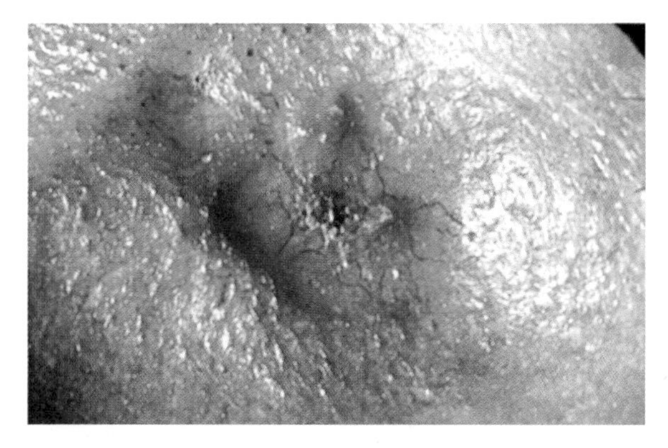

Plate 2.1 Basal carcinoma on the nose, showing pearly edge, telangiectasia over the surface and central ulceration (p. 325).

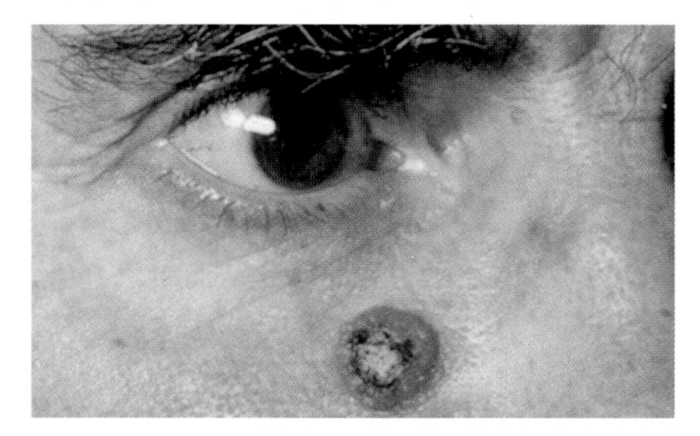

Plate 2.2 Squamous carcinoma of the skin (p. 326). (Courtesy of Dr D Gawkrodger, Sheffield.)

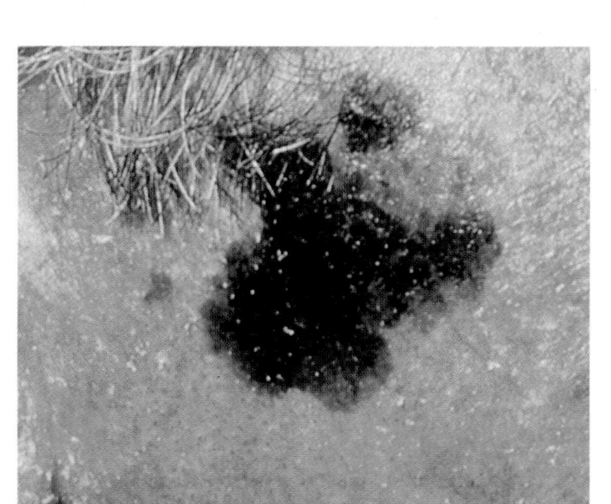

Plate 2.3 Skin melanoma (lentigo maligna) (p. 332). (Courtesy of Dr M Kesseler, Rotherham.)

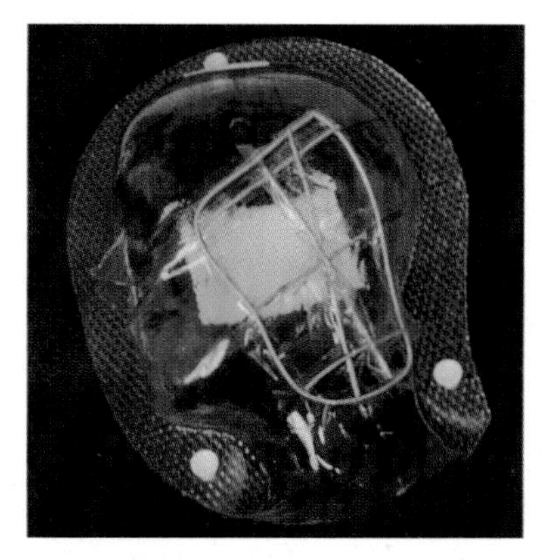

Plate 2.4 Mould for treating carcinoma of the parotid with anterior and posterior oblique wedged pair of fields. Catheters on the surface showing the oblique plane for CT reconstruction of 'beam's eye' view (p. 377). (Courtesy of Dr I Manifold and Dr J Conway Sheffield.)

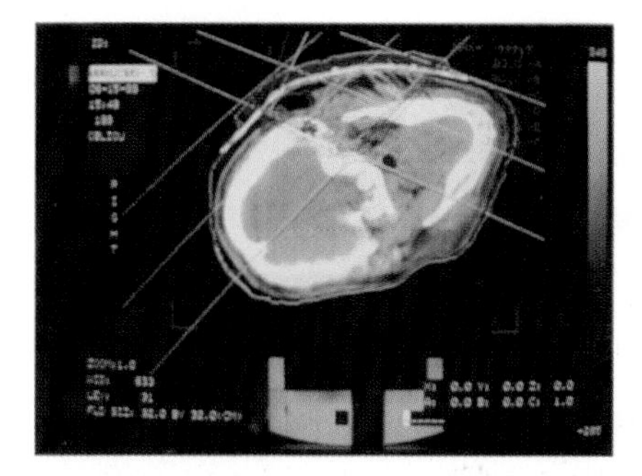

Plate 2.5 CT reconstruction of oblique plane. The catheter on the upper surface is the central catheter seen in Plate 2.4, the correct obliquity of the reconstruction (p. 377). (Courtesy of Dr I Manifold and Dr J Conway Sheffield.)

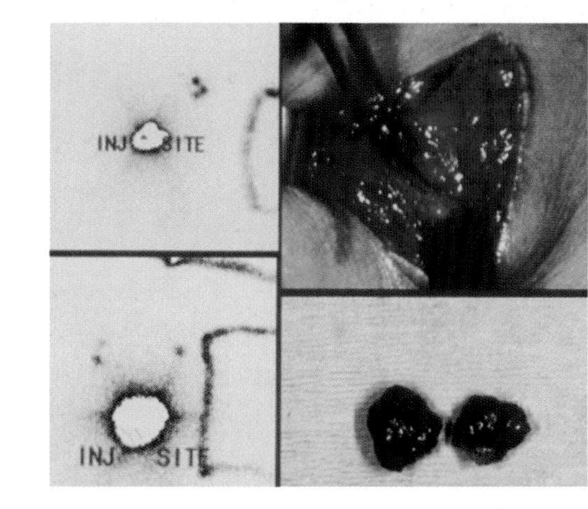

Plate 2.6 Scintigram (left) showing drainage of technetium-99m-labelled albumin to multiple sentinel axillary nodes and (right) blue dye in sentinel axillary node following injection around primary breast tumour (p. 442). (Courtesy of Mr J M Dixon, Edinburgh Breast Unit.)

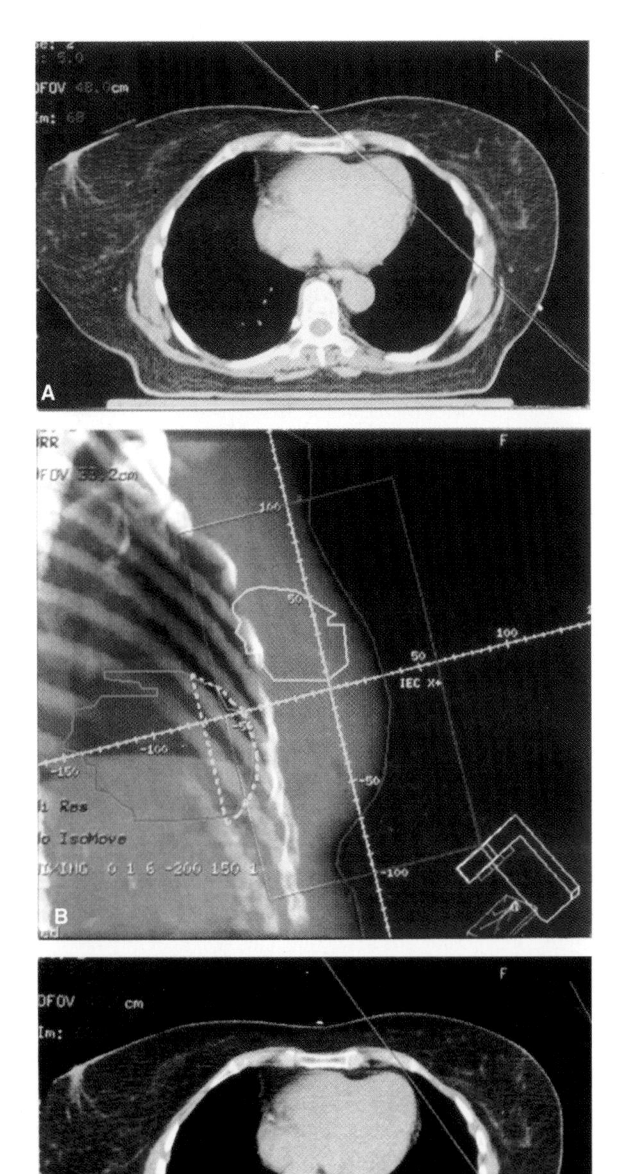

Plate 2.7 CT-based radiotherapy treatment planning to minimise volume of heart irradiated (p. 445). **A** Standard tangential radiotherapy beams. **B** Beams'-eye-view of the tangential beam with boost PTV (planning target volume) outlined (solid yellow) and a cardiac block (dotted yellow). **C** Modified tangential beams to minimise cardiac volume included. The medial field border no longer extends to the midline; however, this beam arrangement was considered acceptable in this patient with an upper, outer quadrant tumour. (Reproduced with permission from Elsevier Science, The Lancet Oncology 2001; 2: 14.)

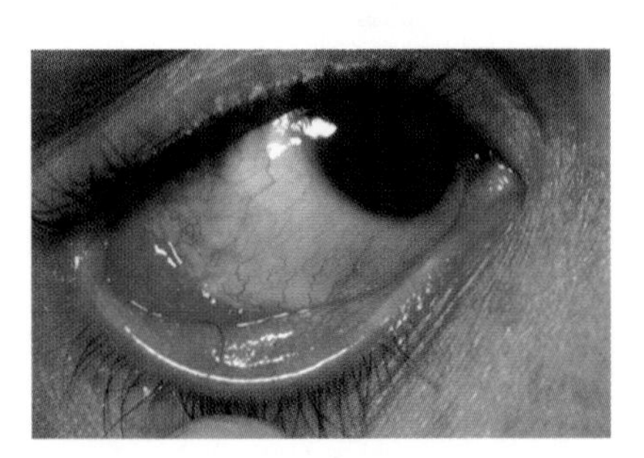

Plate 2.8 Pink fleshy deposits of non-Hodgkin lymphoma of the conjunctiva (p. 523). (Courtesy of Mr I Rennie, Sheffield.)

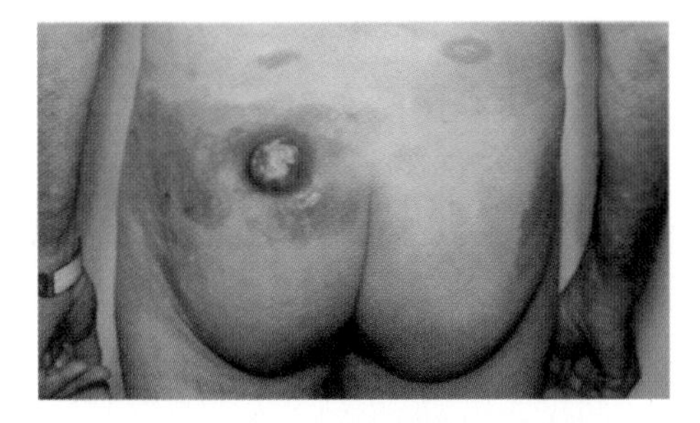

Plate 2.9 Typical eczematous lesions of classical early mycosis fungoides (p. 524). (Courtesy of Dr M Kesseler, Rotherham.)

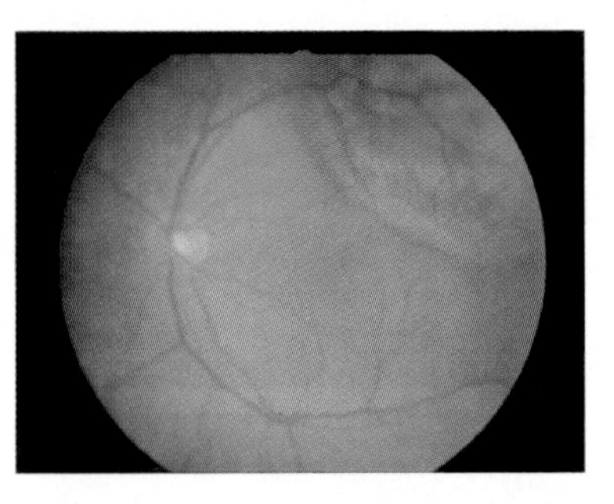

Plate 2.10 Choroidal melanoma (p. 560). (Courtesy of Mr I Rennie, Sheffield.)

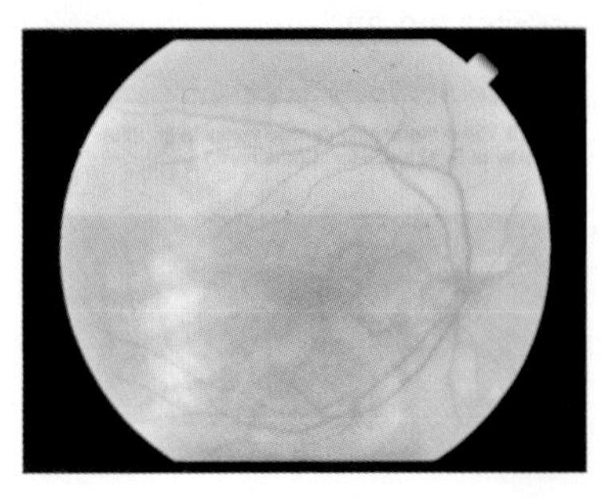

Plate 2.11 Choroidal metastases, showing typical honeycomb pattern of fundus (p. 563). (Courtesy of Mr I Rennie, Sheffield.)

PART 1

Radiation physics

PART CONTENTS

CHAPTER CONTENTS

1

Some basic physics

Keith Bomford

INTRODUCTION

This chapter is a general introduction to quality assurance, a subject that will be addressed throughout the book in more detail in the context of each chapter. In the subsequent sections of this chapter we restate some of the fundamental concepts of physics with which the reader will probably be already familiar, but are essential to an understanding of the rest of the book.

Quality assurance

Quality assurance (QA) has been practised in radiotherapy for over half a century insofar as the output of X-ray generators has been checked on a regular basis. In more recent years, QA has become more thorough and more widespread to the extent that today all data must be doubly checked in accordance with a written procedure document and/or traceable to an accepted standard. Many radiotherapy departments have sought and obtained accreditation under a recognised standard which demands a quality system in which any failure or error is fully investigated and the lessons learned are fed into a revision of the procedure documents. The accreditation is subject to annual review.

Increasingly, bodies such as the Institute of Physicists and Engineers in Medicine (IPEMB 1996a,b,c, IPSM 1988a), the World Health Organization (WHO 1988) and the European Communities (EC 1997) are publishing protocols and procedures in an effort to establish a standard across the country. These are widely adopted—to neglect them would be hard to justify in the event of an untoward incident—although, however carefully worded, they may be open to interpretation or, at worse, to ambiguity. To overcome such problems, interdepartmental discussion is invaluable.

In addition to such a system, the radiotherapy physics departments throughout the UK have been grouped on an informal basis whereby, on a regular programme, each department sends an experienced radiotherapy physicist to another department in the group to carry out a spot check on a range of parameters and procedures (Thwaites et al 1992). Although initially aimed at confirming the calibration of output dose (rate) from megavoltage radiation generators, the visit may also include checks on depth doses and wedge factors, kilovoltage generators, assay of brachytherapy sources and questions on procedure and practice.

To reflect its importance, matters of quality assurance are addressed throughout this book. In some cases, the reader's attention is drawn to established practices, and in others, the authors make suggestions based on their own experience, which the reader may accept or reject. The authors offer their experience to promote quality and good practice, but cannot accept any responsibility for the reader's interpretation of that experience. In all QA work, it must be emphasised that all reports, data and records must be fully documented, signed and dated.

GENERAL PROPERTIES OF MATTER

Atoms and molecules

The smallest identifiable quantity of an element is the *atom*. There are 90 naturally occurring elements and an additional 14 artificially produced elements. Combinations of elements form *compounds* and these may be organic or inorganic. The organic compounds found in living matter are mainly composed of carbon, nitrogen, oxygen and hydrogen together with traces of other elements. The smallest unit of a compound is a *molecule*. Organic molecules are very complex and contain very many atoms.

Solid matter is made up of atoms or molecules arranged in a regular pattern (or lattice). The forces which hold the atoms or molecules together in the lattice are very strong and give solid matter its hardness and rigidity.

If a solid is heated, the heat energy is transferred to the atoms or molecules, they vibrate more vigorously and the solid *expands*. Further heating causes the partial breakdown of these forces and, at a defined temperature, the solid melts, i.e. at its *melting point*. In the liquid state the interatomic forces remain strong, but relative movement between the atoms or molecules is possible, the stronger these forces are the greater the *viscosity* of the liquid. Some super-cooled liquids are so viscous they appear to be solid, e.g. glass.

The further application of heat reduces the forces between the atoms or molecules until there is a free and random movement between them and matter takes the form of a gas. Their constant movement inevitably means there are collisions between them and between them and the containing walls. This bombardment of the walls constitutes the *gas pressure*. A solid heated in a vacuum may evaporate without passing through the liquid state, a process which may occur in a kilovoltage X-ray target (p. 144).

Subatomic particles

All atoms are made up of three subatomic particles, the negatively charged *electron*, the positively charged *proton* and the *neutron*, which carries no electrical charge. (There is an electrostatic force of attraction between unlike charges, and therefore protons and electrons will move towards each other; conversely the like charges of two electrons or of two protons tend to force them apart—the force of repulsion.) Normally an atom contains an equal number of protons and electrons and is therefore electrically neutral. The forces holding the atoms and molecules together are electrostatic. If the atom is electrically charged by the addition or removal of an electron, it is called an *ion*. If this process results in free or loosely bound electrons, the matter will conduct electricity when a potential difference is applied. If the electrons are not free to move, even under the pressure of an applied potential difference, then we have an insulator. There are a few elements which exhibit both the properties of *conduction* and *insulation*. When a crystal of one of these *semiconductor* materials is placed in contact with a conductor, the junction allows a free flow of electrons in one direction but not in the other, i.e. the junction behaves like a diode valve or *rectifier*. These *solid state rectifiers* have largely replaced the vacuum diode valves in rectification circuits (p. 148) but because an X-ray tube is, to all intents and purposes, electrically the same as a vacuum diode valve, some understanding of its method of operation is important (p. 6).

Electricity and magnetism

Direct current electricity

In direct current (DC) electricity, *Ohm's law* states that: 'The current flowing through a conductor is proportional to the potential difference which exists across it provided other physical conditions (e.g. the temperature of the conductor) remain constant, $I \propto V$'. The law is often written as $V = IR$, where the constant of proportionality, R, is called *resistance*; it is measured in ohms, Ω, when the potential difference, V, is in volts and the current, I, in amps (or amperes, abbreviated, A). One application, where this is relevant, is in the high-tension (HT) cables of an X-ray generator. Some of the generated voltage will be used in pushing the tube current, I, through the resistance, R, of the cables, reducing the potential difference available to the X-ray tube; this is sometimes referred to as *voltage drop*.

Electrical power is measured in watts, $W = I^2R$ or VI (watts = volts × amps). In the kilovoltage X-ray generator, the electrical power, I^2R, dissipated within the HT cable will be demonstrated in the form of heat which, ultimately, will harden and damage the insulation (p. 148). Linear accelerators use tens of kilowatts while electronic circuits may use milliwatts of power.

Electromagnetism

An electric current flowing through a conductor will create a magnetic field around that conductor—the field would cause a unit north pole to move clockwise as the (conventional) current flows away from the observer. (Note: 'Conventional' current flow is opposite to the actual flow of the electrons.) Through a loop or a series of loops of wire (a solenoid), the magnetic field is stronger down the axis, and stronger still in the presence of a soft iron core. This is the basis of the electromagnetic switch we call a *relay*—the magnetic field resulting from the current through the coil of the relay causes the contacts of a switch to operate in an otherwise totally independent circuit. For example, a low-voltage circuit in the control desk may be used to switch on the high-tension circuit to generate the X-ray beam (p. 145).

The motor principle is a corollary of this same phenomenon, namely that a current-carrying conductor will experience a mechanical force when placed within a magnetic field—the direction of the force is at right angles to both the current and the magnetic field and may be predicted by *Fleming's left hand rule*: holding the thuMb, First and seCond fingers mutually at right angles, they point in the directions of Motion, Field and Current, respectively. (Fleming's right hand rule must be used if working with electron flow rather than conventional current.) The motor principle, as the name implies, is fundamental to all electric motors, of which there are many in radiotherapy equipment, and to moving-coil meters although these have largely been replaced by digital displays or visual display units in microprocessor-controlled equipment.

The same principle is at work in the electromagnet used in a linear accelerator to 'bend' the electron beam prior to it striking the X-ray target (p. 166). Here, there is no conductor as such, but the effect of the magnetic field on the flow of electrons is to cause them to move along a circular path.

Alternating current electricity

If a second conductor is wound round the same soft iron core as the first, then it is found that when the (direct) current is switched in the first conductor, an electromotive force (e.m.f., or potential difference) appears momentarily between the ends of the second conductor—a phenomenon known as *mutual induction*. However, if the current in the first is continuously changing, as in an alternating current (AC), the e.m.f. in the second alternates at the same frequency with a magnitude in proportion to the ratio of the numbers of turns on the two windings. This is the *transformer*. The ratio of the primary (input)/secondary (output) voltages, V_P/V_S, is the same as the ratio of the number of turns, n_P/n_S. The transformer is known as a step-up transformer if V_S is the greater, or a step-down transformer if V_P is the greater. Again, the kilovoltage X-ray generator uses both, e.g. a step-up transformer to generate the anode voltage and a step-down transformer to supply the filament in the X-ray tube (p. 147). Unlike the X-ray tube, the transformer can be made to be very efficient, close to 100%, although the so-called copper losses (due to the electrical resistance and therefore the heating of the two windings) can never be completely eliminated.

Electrons

The electron is a small negatively charged particle. Its charge (1.602×10^{-19} coulombs) approximates to that of a proton but is opposite in sign. Its mass (9×10^{-31} kg) is considerably smaller than the mass of the proton (1.673×10^{-27} kg) or neutron (1.675×10^{-27} kg). Electrons may be released from a metal by heating in a vacuum or from a gas by applying a voltage between two electrodes in a partially evacuated discharge tube.

Thermionic emission

Electrons may be produced by a process known as *thermionic emission*. When a substance is heated, but before the melting point is reached, the vibration of the surface electrons may be sufficient to cause them to leave the surface. They leave the surface positively charged and are consequently pulled back by the force of electrostatic attraction. If, however, the heated surface is in a vacuum together with a second positively charged electrode (or anode), the electrons released by the heated surface may be attracted to that electrode and a stream of electrons will flow from the heated *cathode* to the positive *anode*. (Note: this electron flow is in the opposite direction to 'conventional' electric current.) Providing the anode remains cold there will be no electron flow in the reverse direction. With the gas pressure being much lower than in a discharge tube, there are too few gas molecules to produce the fluorescence associated with the cathode rays in a vacuum tube.

Thermionic diode valve. Figure 1.1A shows a simple (vacuum tube) diode consisting of a heated wire filament (the cathode) surrounded by a cylindrical anode contained in a sealed evacuated glass envelope. The filament is heated by passing an electric current through it (Fig. 1.1B). The anode voltage, V_a, or potential difference between the anode and the cathode, may be at about + 100 volts and the anode current, I_a, through the diode about 1 mA. (By definition, an anode is always positive with respect to the cathode.) Since the number of electrons leaving the filament depends on the filament temperature, the maximum anode current is determined by the value of the filament voltage, V_f. The actual value of the anode current will also depend upon whether the anode voltage is sufficient to draw all the electrons released from the filament across the vacuum to the anode. A graph of this variation of anode current with anode voltage is known as the *characteristic curve* of the diode and is shown in Figure 1.1C. At lower anode voltages, a cloud of electrons—the *space charge*—forms around the filament and, being negatively charged, encourages the recapture of the electrons released by the filament. As the anode voltage increases, the effect of the space charge is reduced and the anode current increases in what is known as the *space charge limited region* of the characteristic curve. Under *saturation* conditions, a further increase in V_a does not increase the anode current because all the available electrons are being collected on the anode. This saturation (anode) current may only be increased by raising the temperature of the filament (by increasing V_f) to release more electrons—the kilovoltage X-ray tube operates under saturation conditions and the tube current is controlled by adjusting the filament voltage (p. 147).

The number of electrons leaving a metal surface at a given temperature is also dependent on the surface conditions. Metal surfaces coated with the oxides of calcium or barium release electrons freely and are used in thermionic valves and in the electron gun of some linear accelerators (p. 163), where they are described as having *oxide-coated cathodes*. Such cathodes are usually heated indirectly, that is, by a filament in close proximity behind the coated surface.

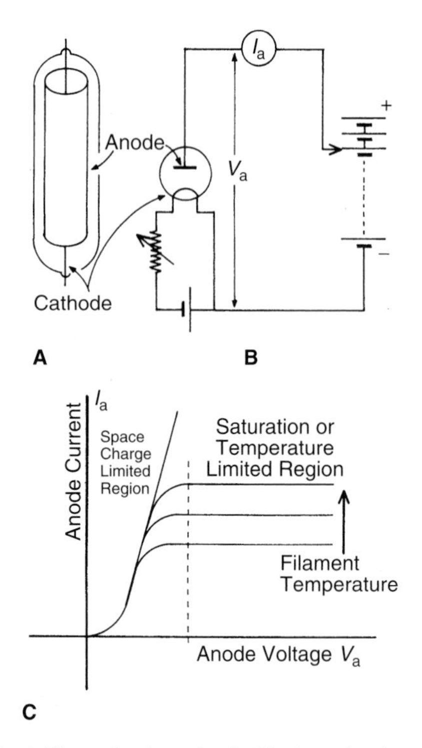

Fig. 1.1 **A** The cathode and cylindrical anode of a thermionic diode valve and **B** a simple diode in circuit to measure **C** the characteristic curves of the diode.

The photoelectric cell. The *photoelectric cell* (Fig. 1.2) is similar to the diode in its operation. Two electrodes are enclosed in an evacuated glass container and a positive potential applied to the anode. The cathode is not heated, but made of a metal which will release its surface electrons when exposed to light of a suitable wavelength. This is the *photoelectric* effect. Visible light, especially ultraviolet light, gives up its energy to the electrons on the surface of the (photo) cathode and releases them from the surface. The anode attracts and absorbs these electrons under the influence of its positive potential and causes the photocell to pass an electric current. The photoelectric cell may therefore be used as a switch operated by a beam of light—for example, to terminate the exposure of a therapy machine if a radiographer inadvertently interrupts the light beam guarding the maze entrance to the treatment room (p. 180). A semiconductor known as a *photodiode* may also be used in a similar manner.

Cathode rays

Dry air at normal atmospheric pressure (760 mmHg or 101.3 kPa) is a good insulator and only breaks down

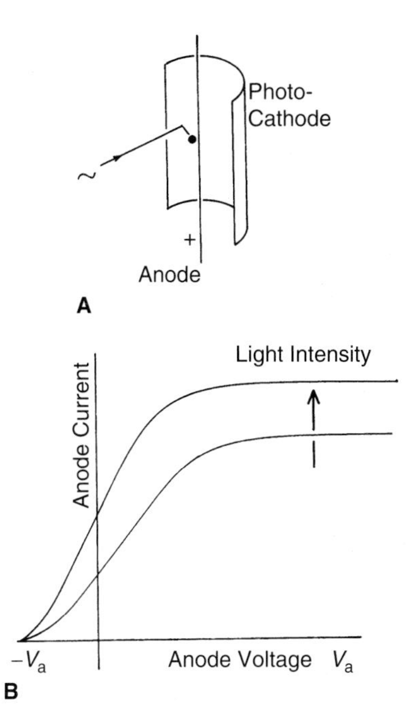

Fig. 1.2 **A** The photoelectric cell and **B** its characteristic curves for two levels of light intensity.

with a violent spark in very high electric fields. At 10 mmHg pressure, a gas will conduct electricity smoothly and this is accompanied by the emission of light, the colour of which is characteristic of the gas, e.g. neon. At 0.01 mmHg pressure, the emission is confined to streamers from the cathode to a point where the streamers strike the walls of the glass vacuum container. These streamers appear to come from the cathode but in fact trace the paths of the electrons which cause the gas to fluoresce. These electron streams are called *cathode rays*.

Cathode rays generated in a vacuum tube form the basis of the television set, video display unit (VDU) and the cathode ray oscilloscope (CRO). Their principal properties are:

- They travel in straight lines in a vacuum. Cathode rays are emitted at right angles to the surface of the cathode and may be focused using a concave cathode.
- They carry electrical charge. Electrons carry negative charges and therefore their path may be deflected by the application of either an electrostatic field or a magnetic field. The deflection is along the electrostatic field towards the positive electrode, the mutual force of attraction; or at right angles to the magnetic field, following Fleming's left hand rule.
- They carry energy. They can cause suitable light objects to move. Their energy is proportional to the accelerating voltage and their velocity is proportional to the square root of the accelerating voltage. They will penetrate thin metal foils, but if stopped in a metal target they produce heat and/or X-rays. When they strike glass or certain other crystals (e.g. zinc sulphide) they cause fluorescence (p. 100).

The cathode ray tube. The arrangement of the electrodes may enable the cathode rays to bombard a fluorescent screen, thereby producing a spot of light (Fig. 1.3). If a variable electrostatic or magnetic field is applied across the tube, the spot of light can be made to move over the fluorescent screen as in a *cathode ray oscilloscope* (CRO). The waveform of a voltage which varies with time may be displayed by applying two signals at right angles: the voltage connected to the Y plates to cause a vertical deflection on the screen and a time signal to the X electrodes to cause a horizontal deflection. A *television* picture is produced on a CRO tube by applying time signals both vertically and horizontally so that a raster covers the screen; the picture, in different shades of grey from black to white, is then produced by varying the anode current as the spot moves over the screen. (A colour television uses three spots of light, each contributing one of the primary colours, which mix to make up the full spectrum of colour on the screen.) Television systems are widely used in the radiotherapy department—as a means of observing the patient in the treatment room through a closed-circuit television, as an output device for the images off a simulator, CT scanner, MR scanner or gamma camera. The video display from the treatment planning computer or other computer-controlled equipment is simply a television with a special screen format.

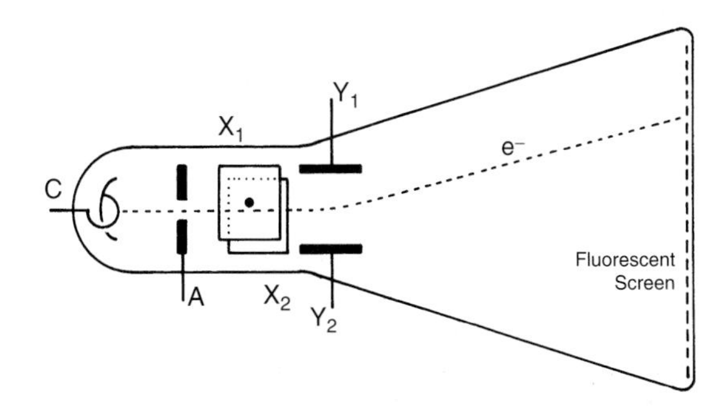

Fig. 1.3 The cathode ray tube—the electron stream is deflected by two fields between plates X and Y before reaching the fluorescent screen.

SECTION 1

Physics of radiation

SECTION CONTENTS

CHAPTER CONTENTS

2

The atom and the production of X-rays

Keith Bomford

ATOMIC STRUCTURE

The atom is a miniature solar system consisting largely of empty space. At the centre of the system is the nucleus (approx. 10^{-15} m diameter) and around that centre the electrons move in orbits (approx. 10^{-11} m diameter). The simplest atom, hydrogen, consists of one positively charged particle (a proton) and one electron in orbit.

The number of protons, positive charges, in the nucleus is called the *atomic number*, *Z*, and equals to the number of orbiting electrons in the neutral atom. Since a proton is some 1840 times heavier than an electron, practically all the mass of the atom lies in the nucleus. For each element, except hydrogen, the nucleus contains both protons and neutrons. These occur in almost equal numbers, except for the higher values of *Z* (Ch. 3).

Atomic mass, weight and size

Three scales of atomic mass are recognised:

- The absolute scale, related to the kilogram
- The physical scale measured in atomic mass units (a.m.u.)
- The chemical scale or atomic weight which takes into account the normal isotopic mix of the element.

The *atomic mass unit* has been defined by setting the mass of one atom of the nuclide carbon-12 equal to 12.000 a.m.u. Carbon-12 has six protons and six neutrons (Fig. 2.1) and since protons and neutrons have nearly the same mass each elemental particle on this scale has a mass of nearly 1. For example, hydrogen, with one proton in its nucleus and one orbiting electron, has a mass of 1.008 a.m.u., while bismuth, with 83 protons, 125 neutrons and 83 electrons, has a mass of 208.98 a.m.u.

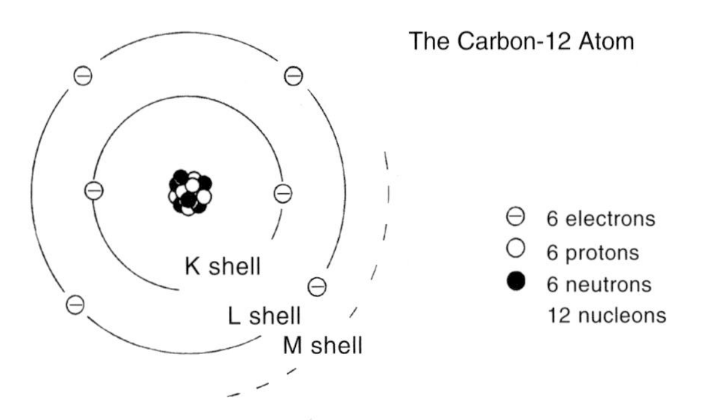

Fig. 2.1 The carbon-12 atom ($Z = 6$).

Atomic weights, as used in chemistry, are usually different from the atomic masses because most naturally occurring elements have a number of stable isotopes. For example, chlorine consists of a mixture of two isotopes, chlorine-34 and chlorine-36. They occur with an abundance of 75.5% and 24.6% respectively, giving an atomic weight of 35.46.

A relationship between the absolute scale and the physical scale can be obtained with the aid of *Avogadro's number*. Avogadro's number (or constant) is 6.0225×10^{23} and is the number of atoms in one mole of a substance. In the case of carbon-12, one mole is that amount of substance which contains as many elementary parts as there are in 0.012 kg, i.e. 6.0225×10^{23} atoms. But by definition, 1 a.m.u. is one-twelfth of the mass of a carbon-12 atom. Therefore:

$$1 \text{ a.m.u.} = 1 \times 10^{-3}/6.0225 \times 10^{23} \text{ kg} = 1.66 \times 10^{-27} \text{ kg}$$

The mass of the electron is only 1/1840 that of a proton or neutron so a good estimate of the mass of an atom can be obtained by multiplying the number of nucleons or the atomic number by 1.66×10^{-27} kg.

Since the number of neutrons is approximately the same as the number of protons, the number of electrons per unit mass, the *electron density* (e/g), for hydrogen is almost twice that for any other element (a fact we shall come back to in Chapters 12 and 13).

Yet another physical aspect of an atom is its size. The radius of a proton or neutron is 1.45×10^{-15} m, and that of an electron 2.82×10^{-15} m. If we assume the nucleus to be a sphere then the radii of nuclei vary from 1.45×10^{-15} m for the hydrogen nucleus, mass number 1, to 9×10^{-15} m for nuclei with mass number 257. The radius of the atom is much greater, varying from 0.9×10^{-10} to 1.6×10^{-10} m. This means that the nucleus, whilst containing most of the mass, occupies only one part in 3×10^{13} of the total volume of the atom. The extranuclear space is occupied by the electrons. These electrons must be widely spaced because electrons are about the same size as a nucleon. The properties of various particles are given in Table 2.1.

If the atom is pictured as being as large as a sports stadium then the nucleus in the centre of the stadium is about as big as a fly. This picture helps us to understand how the atomic radiations can penetrate many layers of atoms without undergoing any interaction.

Electron shells

The electrons around the nucleus are located in a few specific *orbits* or *shells*, the nearest to the nucleus is labelled the K orbit and subsequent ones are given the labels L, M, N, etc. (Note: We often use the words *orbit* and *shell* interchangeably. The atom is a three-dimensional solar system and each electron orbit is in a different plane—it is only for convenience that the orbits are depicted as concentric circles.) The K orbit is the one with the least energy but the greatest *binding energy*. Each orbit can hold only a limited number of electrons, the maximum number in the *n*th orbit is $2n^2$ (e.g. the M shell is the third and can only have up to 18 electrons). In general, the electrons occupy the innermost orbits but the outermost shell will never have more than eight electrons, before the next outer shell starts to fill (Table 2.2).

This rather simple picture of the atom, referred to as the *Rutherford–Bohr* model, helps to explain the similar chemical properties of different elements, e.g. the six

Table 2.1 Properties of the elemental particles

Particle	Symbol	Rest mass (kg)	Rest energy		Charge*	Radius (m)
			(a.m.u.)	(MeV)		
Proton	p	1.673×10^{-27}	1.0073	938.2	1	1.45×10^{-15}
Neutron	n	1.675×10^{-27}	1.0087	939.2	0	1.45×10^{-15}
Electron	e^- or β^-	9.108×10^{-31}	0.00055	0.511	−1	2.82×10^{-15}
Positron	e^+ or β^+	9.108×10^{-31}	0.00055	0.511	+1	2.82×10^{-15}
Neutrino	ν	1.000×10^{-34}	1.0×10^{-6}	0.001	0	0
Gamma ray	γ	—	—	—	0	0

* The unit of charge, $+1 = +1.6 \times 10^{-19}$ coulombs

Table 2.2 The atomic structure of selected atoms

Element	Symbol	Atomic no. Z	Nuclear charge	Number of electrons in shell			
				K	L	M	N
Hydrogen	H	1	+1	1			
Helium	He	2	+2	2			
Lithium	Li	3	+3	2	1		
Neon	Ne	10	+10	2	8		
Sodium	Na	11	+11	2	8	1	
Calcium	Ca	20	+20	2	8	8	2

inert gases (the radioactive gases *radon* and *xenon* among them) are those elements whose outermost orbits have their full complement of eight electrons, and the four halogen gases—fluorine, chlorine, bromine and iodine—all have only one vacancy in their outer shell. Elements in which there are one or two loosely bound electrons in the outer shell are good electrical conductors, whereas those with a few vacancies in the outer shell are good insulators. This extranuclear region is where chemical bonding takes place. It is also where the majority of interactions between radiation and matter take place (Ch. 4).

Equivalence of mass and energy

In 1905, Albert Einstein put forward his famous *theory of relativity*. The most important concept of Einstein's theory is that mass is a form of energy, the two being related by the simple formula:

$$E = mc^2$$

where c is the velocity of light in metres per second (in free space), m is the rest mass in kilograms and E is the energy measured in joules. If 1 g of matter is converted into energy, the energy released will be:

$$E = (1 \times 10^{-3}) \times (3 \times 10^{8})^2 = 9 \times 10^{13}\ \text{J}$$

This is an enormous amount of energy, sufficient to supply the daily power requirement of over a million homes. A more convenient unit of energy in this context is the *electron volt*, which is equivalent to 1.6×10^{-19} J. The rest mass of an electron is 9.1×10^{-31} kg and therefore has an equivalent energy value of:

$$9.1 \times 10^{-31} \times (3 \times 10^{8})^2 / 1.6 \times 10^{-19} = 0.511\ \text{MeV}$$

similarly, 1 a.m.u. = 931 MeV.

Energy and mass can be considered as two manifestations of the same entity and in certain circumstances are interchangeable. For example, as we shall see in Chapter 4, a photon of energy greater than 1.022 MeV may interact with the electric field around the nucleus and disappear while simultaneously creating two particles of matter, one negative electron and one positive electron or positron. This process is known as *pair production*. Conversely when the positron is brought to rest in matter it combines with a neighbouring 'free' electron, the two charges neutralise and the mass of the two electrons is converted back into energy appearing as two photons of electromagnetic radiation, each of 0.511 MeV energy, this is *annihilation radiation*.

Ionisation and excitation

If an atom or a molecule has a surfeit of electrons, it is called a negative ion. A positive ion is an atom or molecule with a shortage of electrons. Ions may be produced by a variety of external agents. A solution of sodium chloride (NaCl) in water will conduct an electric current because it readily ionises into Na^+ and Cl^- ions. Gas at normal pressures will conduct electricity when the gas is ionised by irradiation with X-rays (p. 51).

At the atomic level, the atom is said to be ionised when an electron is completely removed from the electrostatic field around the nucleus, and the process is known as ionisation (Fig. 2.2A). If the electron is only partially removed, i.e. moved from one orbit to a more distant orbit, the atom is said to be in an excited state, and the process is known as excitation (Fig. 2.2B). The ionised or excited atom will resume its stable state by

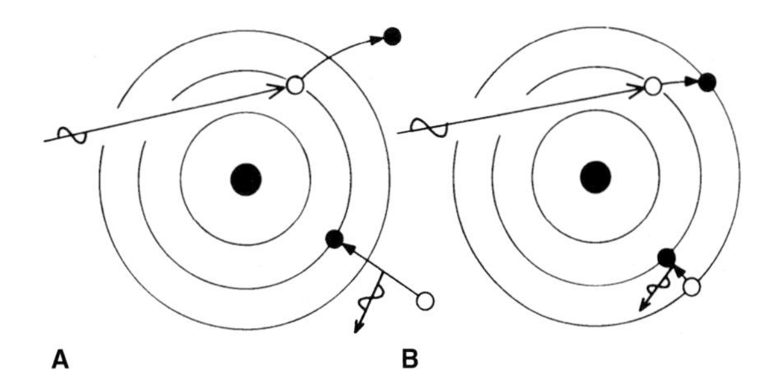

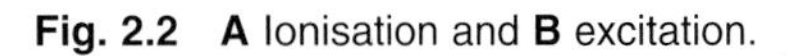
Fig. 2.2 **A** Ionisation and **B** excitation.

attracting an electron into the vacant space in the orbit concerned. This inward movement of the electron through the shell structure is accompanied by the emission of electromagnetic radiation which may be visible, as fluorescence in the discharge tube, or invisible X-radiation depending on the difference in the binding energies of the two orbits. Excitation and ionisation may be initiated by high-energy particles or by electromagnetic radiations (Ch. 4).

Binding energy

In our solar system, there are gravitational forces of attraction pulling the planets towards the sun exactly compensated by the centrifugal forces due to the rotation of the planets round the sun. The exact orbit a planet takes round the sun is determined by this balance which may be affected, to a greater or lesser degree, by the other planets in the system; for this reason the orbits are not circular. The same applies to the atom.

Electrons in a given shell of a particular nuclide experience a specific *binding energy*. The electrons in the K shell have the greatest binding energy and are tightly bound to the nucleus; those on the periphery of the atom are more loosely bound electrons. The magnitude of the electron binding energy is dependent on the atomic number of the nuclide and the electron shell location. The binding energy is equivalent to the amount of energy necessary to remove that electron from that atom. Examples of binding energy are given in Table 2.3.

If we imagine two ions in isolation, a single positive charge and a single negative charge separated by an infinite distance, the force of attraction is zero and the total energy of the system is zero. (The force is proportional to the product of the two charges and to the inverse square of the distance between them and therefore zero when the distance is infinite.) As the distance between the ions is reduced, the force of attraction increases and the two ions accelerate towards each other. The kinetic energy (the energy of movement) is therefore increasing and, providing no energy has been given to or taken from the system, we must assume the potential energy (the energy of position) is decreasing (from zero). This potential energy is therefore negative. At some distance from the positive ion, the negative ion will find the electrostatic force of attraction is balanced by its centrifugal force due to its rotation round the positive ion (the nucleus), thereby fixing the electron in an orbit around the nucleus. Now, having established its orbit, it is clear that the electron is bound to that nucleus with an energy. We call it the electron *binding energy* for, to move the electron to an orbit further from the nucleus, we must add energy to the system and if we are to remove the electron completely we must add an amount of energy equal to or in excess of its binding energy. Any energy surplus after overcoming the binding energy will be given to the electron in the form of kinetic energy. Conversely, if the electron moves to an orbit closer to the nucleus, its surplus energy is released in the form of electromagnetic radiation.

This simple picture is complicated by the fact that different electrons in the same shell will follow slightly different orbits giving rise to slightly different binding energies, K_α, K_β, L_I, L_{II}, L_{III}, etc.

In the single atoms described above the energy levels are discrete, but when the atoms are brought closer together, as in solid material, the energy levels of each orbit are influenced by the proximity of others. This results in the broadening out of the discrete levels into energy bands (Fig. 2.3). The outermost band normally occupied by electrons is known as the *valence band*. The next outer band which may be occupied is the *conduction band*. In a conductor (e.g. copper) the valence band and the conduction band overlap and electrons move freely between them, whereas in an insulator there is a broad *forbidden zone* between them preventing, under normal circumstances, the valence electrons from entering the conduction band. (Remember these are energy bands and any forbidden zone may be crossed if an electron is given sufficient

Table 2.3 Binding energies of the electrons in the K, L and M shells for various elements

Element	Z	Chemical symbol	Binding energy (keV)		
			K	L	M
Copper	29	Cu	9.0	1.1	0.12
Iodine	53	I	33.2	5.1	1.07
Lead	82	Pb	88.0	15.9	3.8

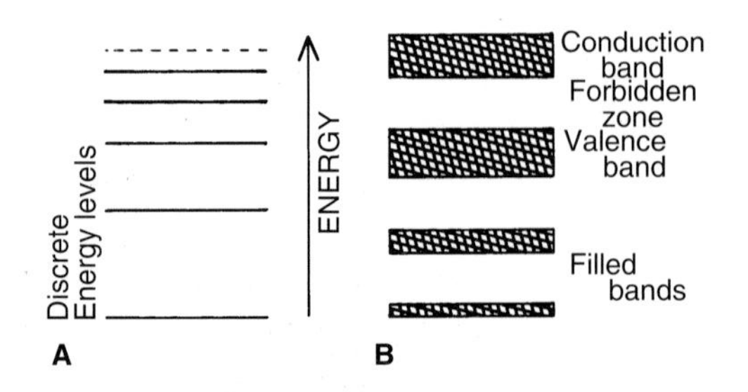

Fig. 2.3 **A** Electron energy levels in an atom and **B** electron energy bands in a solid.

energy to cross it.) Once in the conduction band an electron can move freely through the material. In semiconductors, the forbidden zone is quite narrow.

Solid state rectifiers

The semiconductor elements of silicon and germanium are quadrivalent having four electrons in their outer shell, making them both poor conductors and poor insulators. N-type silicon is pure silicon to which a small quantity of an impurity has been added, the impurity being pentavalent, i.e. having five outer electrons (e.g. phosphorus). The impurity therefore donates a spare electron which can be readily released into the *conduction band* (Fig. 2.3) and take part in electrical conduction. (This donation of a negatively charged particle gives the silicon the name of N-type.) Conversely, P-type silicon carries a small trivalent impurity leaving the crystalline structure short of electrons and is therefore rich in holes ready to accept any free electrons from the surrounding silicon. A *P–N junction diode* may be made by fusing together P-type silicon with N-type silicon. The fusion results in the surplus electrons crossing the barrier from the N-type silicon to occupy the holes in the P-type silicon, thereby leaving a *depletion layer* between the two materials in which there are no surplus electrons and no surplus holes. When a potential difference is applied to the junction a current will flow when the P-type is at a higher potential than the N-type. If the polarity is reversed, no current will flow because it increases the potential barrier across the junction and extends the depletion layer. The P–N junction therefore passes current only in one direction. This *solid state rectifier* is very rugged in operation, smaller in size than the thermionic diode and does not require a filament supply (Fig. 1.1). Solid state rectifiers are widely used in electronic circuitry as well as in kilovoltage X-ray generators.

THE WAVE THEORY

Both *X-rays* and *gamma rays* are electromagnetic radiations and as such may be considered either as waves or particles (photons or quanta, a quantum is a discrete quantity of energy). An X-ray photon is indistinguishable from a gamma ray photon of the same energy unless its source is known. The former results from the deceleration of an electron, as in the target of an X-ray tube, whereas the latter results from the spontaneous disintegration of an unstable (radioactive) nucleus.

A wave is a progressive disturbance in a medium by which energy is transferred through the medium without any transfer of the medium. Ripples on an otherwise still water surface are *transverse waves* because the oscillation of the water is at right angles to the direction of travel. Sound waves on the other hand are called *longitudinal* or *compression* waves because their oscillations are along the direction of travel, as in the vibrations of a drum. The general properties of waves are summarised in Figure 2.4. The *frequency* of the wave is the number of oscillations of an element of the medium in one second, e.g. middle C in music is a sound wave of frequency of 256 Hz (hertz or cycles per second). The *wavelength* is the distance, measured in the direction of travel, between two successive peaks. A helium–neon laser emits a beam of red light of 632.8 nm wavelength (1 nm = 1 *nanometre* = 10^{-9} m). The velocity, c, is the rate at which the disturbance is transmitted through the medium and related to frequency (n) and wavelength (λ) by the formula: $c = n\lambda$. The *amplitude* of the wave is the maximum value of the disturbance from its equilibrium value. This point of maximum disturbance is referred to as the *antinode*

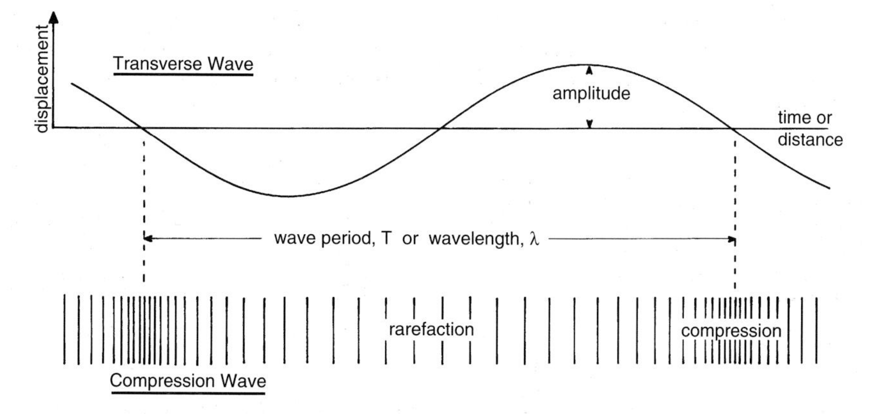

Fig. 2.4 Transverse and longitudinal waves.

whereas the point of zero disturbance is called the *node*.

A single wave will have a unique wavelength and frequency, but many waves of different wavelengths may coexist in a *spectrum*. For example, sunlight contains all the colours of the rainbow, but the individual colours only become evident when the wavelengths are separated out (or dispersed) within the raindrops. White light is a *continuous spectrum* of all the wavelengths from approximately 400 nm (violet) to 800 nm (red). In the laboratory, a prism will demonstrate that white light is only a small part of a much wider spectrum of wavelengths spreading from even shorter wavelengths (ultraviolet) to longer wavelengths (infrared). Other light sources may emit only one wavelength, like the helium–neon laser mentioned above, or several discrete wavelengths which then make up a *line spectrum*. In fact, the electromagnetic spectrum extends from wavelengths of many kilometres (10^3 m) to less than a picometre (10^{-12} m), these invisible waves being called radiowaves and X-rays respectively (Fig. 2.5). Radiations of wavelength less

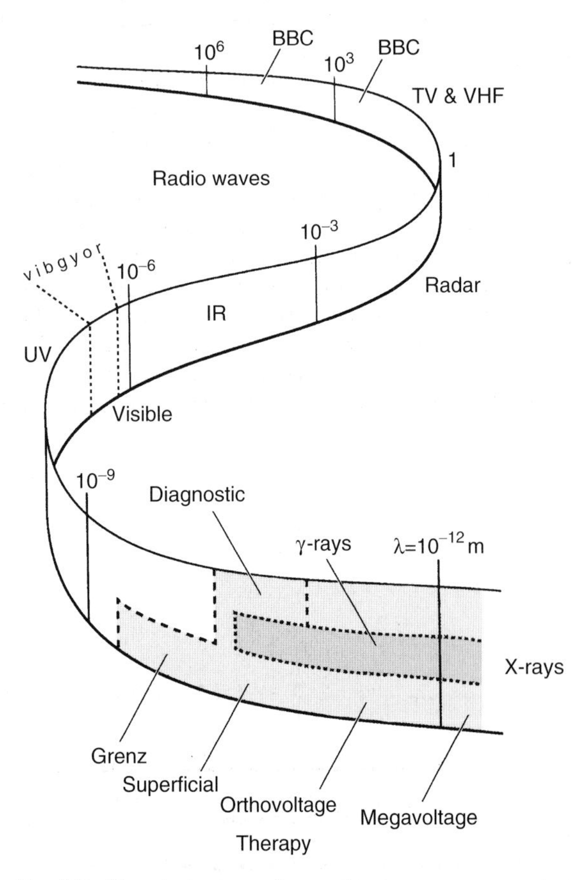

Fig. 2.5 The electromagnetic spectrum.

than 100 nm (3×10^{15} Hz) are referred to as *ionising radiations*. All these electromagnetic waves travel in straight lines in free space with the *velocity of light*, $c = 2.998 \times 10^8$ m s^{-1}.

Waves penetrate matter to a degree which varies in a complex manner with the wavelength and the nature of the matter. Long (radio) waves can penetrate non-conducting materials, such as brick walls, but are reflected by electrical conductors, such as overhead power lines. Radiations in or near the visible spectrum penetrate optically transparent materials like glass. X- and gamma rays have penetrating powers which increase with decreasing wavelength (p. 153).

THE QUANTUM THEORY

When considering the properties of atoms it is sometimes more convenient to think of radiation as small packets of energy—called photons or quanta. The energy of each quantum (or photon) is proportional to the frequency.

$$\text{Quantum energy, } E = h\nu$$

where h is Planck's constant ($h = 6.626 \times 10^{-34}$ J s). The *electron volt* (eV) is the unit of energy of an electron in motion, or a quantum of radiation, and equal to the energy acquired by an electron when accelerated through a potential difference of 1 volt (1 eV = 1.602×10^{-19} J); in practice, the MeV (10^6 eV) and keV (10^3 eV) are in common use.

As we have seen, the electrons orbit the nucleus of an atom in precisely defined shells and any transfer of an electron from one shell to another will be accompanied by the absorption or emission of energy equal to the difference in their binding energies. When the energy is emitted, it is lost to a single photon of frequency, ν, where:

$$E_1 - E_2 = h\nu = hc/\lambda$$

Since the energy of each electron shell is unique to the atom, so the emitted wavelengths are characteristic of the element. This effect is demonstrated in the photoelectric cell, as described earlier. In the graph of anode current against anode voltage (Fig. 1.2B), it will be noticed that a small anode current flows when the light is present but the anode voltage is zero and the current is only reduced to zero when a negative (retarding) anode voltage is applied. The electrons are emitted from the cathode with a finite energy and this energy does not change when the intensity of illumination is increased. The change of intensity simply changes the number of electrons emitted.

THE PRODUCTION OF X-RAYS

Continuous radiation spectrum

X-rays are produced whenever high-energy particles are suddenly slowed in a target. This process is unlikely at low particle energies but becomes increasingly more probable at higher energies. The energy lost by the particle appears directly as a photon of *bremsstrahlung* radiation, (from the German: *Bremse* = brake and *Strahlung* = radiation). At the atomic level, this 'braking' results from the interaction between the particle and the electrostatic field near the nucleus. For particles of a given energy the deceleration varies directly with the square of the atomic number, Z, of the absorber and z, the number of unit charges on the particle, and inversely with the mass of the particle, m. Thus the intensity of bremsstrahlung varies between charged particles and materials as: Zz/m. It follows that particles of small mass such as electrons and positrons are much better producers of bremsstrahlung than heavier particles. Similarly materials of high atomic number such as lead and tungsten are more efficient producers of bremsstrahlung than low atomic number materials such as plastic and soft tissue.

In the X-ray tube, the fast electron may lose all its energy in a single interaction with the electric field round the target nucleus. It is more likely, however, that it will lose only a part of its energy in that first interaction and then proceed further, interacting with other target atoms before coming to rest (Fig. 2.6C). It follows that a beam of electrons interacting with the target will produce X-ray photons with energies spread over a range from very small values up to the maximum energy of the electrons in the beam. Different amounts of energy are lost by the particles at each bremsstrahlung event. The maximum energy of the bremsstrahlung will equal the maximum energy of the particle and corresponds to the particle losing all its energy in one interaction. The bremsstrahlung radiation appears as a *continuous spectrum*.

The continuous spectrum has a maximum photon energy (keV) equal to the tube voltage (kV). Photons of maximum photon energy have the minimum wavelength in the spectrum—wavelength is inversely proportional to photon energy. The minimum wavelength may be calculated thus:

$$\text{Minimum wavelength, } \lambda_{min} = hc/(\text{kV}_{max})$$

This equation is known as *Duane–Hunt's law* and may be used to calculate the wavelength of any known photon energy (or vice versa). After incorporating the physical constants, the equation simplifies to:

$$\text{Wavelength, } \lambda = 1.24/(\text{keV}) \text{ nanometres}$$

The spectra shown in Figure 2.7 show but few low-energy photons for the simple reason that they are readily absorbed either within the target, the wall of the X-ray tube, the surrounding insulation and/or the tube housing itself (which together are known as providing the *inherent filtration*) and do not emerge. These low-energy photons may be further reduced by the addition of beam-hardening filters (p. 154) thereby raising the mean photon energy of the useful beam.

The distribution of the relative intensity of the radiations in the continuous spectrum as a function of photon energy is shown in Figure 2.7 for three representative tube voltages in the low-energy X-ray range. In this diagram, the ordinate represents the energy flow per unit interval of energy as expressed by the number of photons with that particular energy multiplied by the energy of those photons. The three curves show the continuous spectrum for tube voltages of

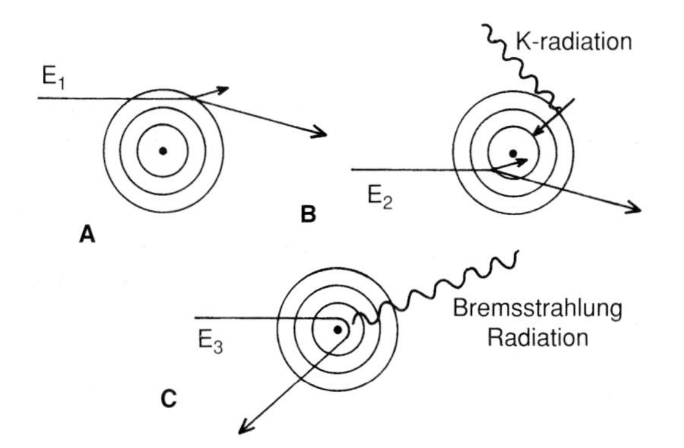

Fig. 2.6 The interactions occurring within an X-ray target: **A** the emission of a delta ray; **B** the emission of an electron and a characteristic photon; and **C** the emission of bremsstrahlung radiation.

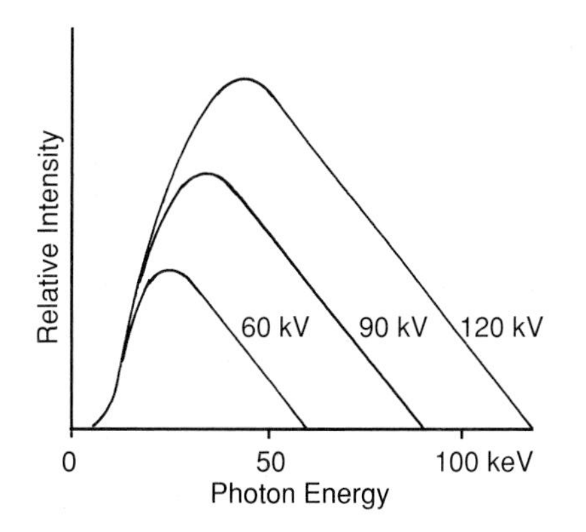

Fig. 2.7 The continuous X-ray spectra for three accelerating voltages (60, 90, 120 kV).

60 kV, 90 kV and 120 kV. (Note that in these curves the characteristic radiations have not been shown, and the beam current is assumed to be the same for all three curves.) Note the following properties of these curves:

- The existence of a maximum photon energy (minimum wavelength) for each tube voltage.
- The existence of a peak in the relative intensity distribution at a photon energy about one-third of the maximum value.
- The low intensity of the lower-energy photons. These low-energy photons have little penetrating power and are readily absorbed within the inherent filtration provided by the target and tube housing.
- An increase in tube voltage increases the intensity of emission at all photon energies as well as introducing higher-energy photons. The total intensity of the radiation is proportional to the area under the curve and the family of curves illustrates that the total emission is approximately proportional to the square of the voltage applied to the tube.
- With the increase in applied voltage the proportion of high-energy photons increases and the peak of the curve moves to higher energies.

Efficiency of X-ray production

The efficiency of X-ray production, that is, the proportion of the total energy of the incident electron beam energy that appears as X-rays, is normally small, the majority of the energy appearing as heat. The efficiency of X-ray production is approximately proportional to both the tube voltage (Fig. 2.8) and the atomic number of the target. A target of high atomic number material therefore is very advantageous and tungsten ($Z = 74$) is generally used in kilovoltage therapy tubes. It is also a suitable material because of its high melting point (3387°C), reasonable heat conductivity and good mechanical properties. For a tungsten target in an X-ray tube at 100 kV, the efficiency of X-ray production is approximately 0.5%—that is, 99.5% of the electron beam energy goes into producing heat. The X-ray production efficiency at 200 kV is approximately 1%. Accelerating voltages of 20–40 million volts (MV) are required before the X-ray production becomes more efficient, at say 60–70%.

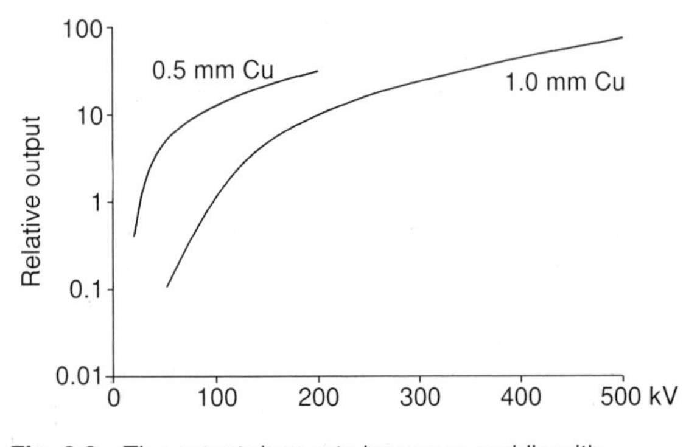

Fig. 2.8 The output dose rate increases rapidly with increasing tube voltage.

The distribution of X-rays round the target

When electrons strike a theoretically *thin* target, X-rays are emitted in all directions. The distribution of that emission depends very much on the tube voltage. For low-energy X-rays, the maximum intensity of emission is approximately at right angles to the electron beam. As the voltage increases, the direction of maximum intensity moves towards that of the bombarding electrons with the result that for megavoltage beams most of the X-ray emission is confined to a narrow cone centred on the *forward direction* of the electron beam. Figure 2.9 illustrates, by polar diagram, the distribution of X-ray energy from a thin target for four representative electron energies. (The curves are such that the radius from the target is proportional to the intensity of the beam in the direction of that radius.) It can be seen that at 100 kV, the X-ray intensity at right angles to the electron stream is greater than in the forward direction, whereas at 20 MV the forward intensity is many times that at right angles.

The actual distribution of X-ray intensity round the *thick* targets of practical X-ray tubes only approximates to that shown in Figure 2.9 because of the self-attenuation of the X-rays in the target material, especially for beams generated at low voltages, but the design of practical targets is influenced by this spatial distribution. At low voltages, it is advantageous to use the X-ray beam coming from the target at right angles to the electron stream, and most diagnostic and therapy X-ray tubes up to 300 kV use a *reflection target* in which the useful beam is taken from the front surface of the angled target. At tube voltages of 1 million or more, however, it is advantageous to use the X-ray beam in the same direction as the incident electron stream in spite of the self-attenuation in the target. Such targets, which are made thick enough to absorb all the bombarding electrons, are known as *transmission targets*.

The variation of X-ray beam intensity with direction means that at low energies the target angle has to be chosen carefully if large fields are to be irradiated uniformly (p. 144) while at megavoltage energies, field flattening filters have to be introduced to compensate

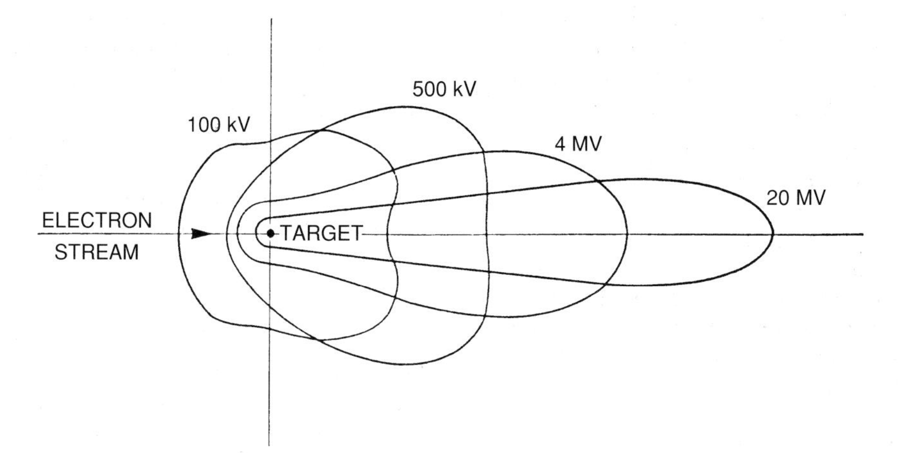

Fig. 2.9 The spatial distribution of X-rays from a thin target. (With permission of Meredith and Massey, from Fundamental Physics of Radiology, Wright, Bristol, 1977.)

for the concentration of the X-ray emission in a very narrow solid angle around the direction of the electron beam (p. 166).

Characteristic radiation spectrum

A second type of interaction also leads to the emission of X-rays. Some of the bombarding electrons interact with the inner orbital K or L electrons of the target and cause ionisation or excitation of the target atoms. The vacant spaces or 'holes' so created in the electron orbits are then filled by electrons transferring from outer orbits or beyond (Fig. 2.6B). This transfer of an electron to an inner orbit results in the emission of a photon of electromagnetic radiation and the energy may be high enough to be in the X-ray region of the electromagnetic spectrum. These photons therefore contribute a *line spectrum* of X-rays characteristic of the target material.

For a tungsten target, the characteristic X-ray photons have an energy of about 69 keV. The resultant characteristic radiation spectrum consists of two photons, K_α and K_β, of nearly the same value and appears as a line spectrum superimposed on the continuous spectrum for all tube voltages above 69 kV. If the target material were of some other element, the voltage needed to dislodge the K electron would be different and the characteristic radiation would have a different wavelength. Figure 2.10 shows the two spectra including both continuous and characteristic radiation for a tungsten (W) target and a tin (Sn) target for the same tube voltage (120 kV) and the same tube current. Note the following points:

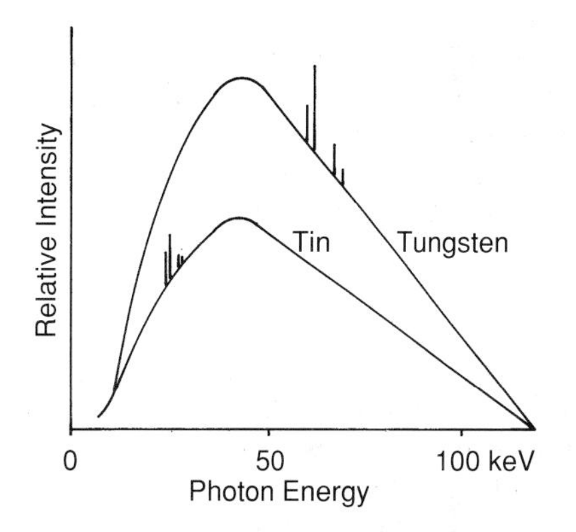

Fig. 2.10 The 120 kV X-ray spectra for tungsten and tin targets—note the characteristic radiations of tin ($Z = 50$) are of lower energy than those for tungsten ($Z = 74$).

- The continuous spectrum from tin ($Z = 50$) is less intense than from tungsten ($Z = 74$)—the total emission being approximately proportional to the atomic number of the target.
- The characteristic radiation from tungsten appears between 57 keV and 69 keV photon energy whenever the tube voltage exceeds 69 keV, while that from the tin target appears between approximately 25 keV and 29 keV and whenever the tube voltage is above 29 kV.
- Note that although the intensity of the lines of the characteristic radiation may be high compared to that of the continuous spectrum, its contribution to the total emission of X-ray energy from the tube is relatively small.
- The characteristic line spectrum of the target material will also include photons of lower energies appropriate to the binding energies of the L orbital electrons, but these are rarely shown as they are

readily absorbed by the target and the inherent filtration of the tube and housing.

Production of heat

We have seen that X-rays are produced whenever fast electrons are rapidly slowed in passing through matter. In a conventional tube, the continuous spectrum of X-rays is produced when the beam of electrons is stopped in a metal target, the anode of an X-ray tube. The line spectrum of X-rays are released through ionisation of the target material.

The third type of interaction between the bombarding electrons and the target atoms is with the outer electrons around the target nuclei before coming to rest (Fig. 2.6A) and at each deflection a little of the electron's energy is transferred to the target material as heat. In these interactions, the orbiting electrons may be removed with sufficient kinetic energy of their own to produce further ionisations and excitations of the target atoms along tracks known as *delta rays*. At accelerating voltages up to 500 kV, most of the energy of the impinging electrons appears as heat in the target and cooling of the target is a major requirement of X-ray tube design (p. 145).

CHAPTER CONTENTS

3

The nucleus and radioactivity

Keith Bomford

THE NUCLEUS

An understanding of radioactivity is possible only if we have some concept of the nucleus as well as the nature of the atom (Ch. 2). We have seen that atoms are classified according to the number of protons, Z, and nucleons, A (i.e. the number of protons and neutrons) in their nuclei. Each different combination of Z and A identifies a distinct species of nuclide, symbolised as ${}^{A}_{Z}X$, where X is the element symbol. Thus hydrogen, which has only a single proton in its nucleus, is expressed as ${}^{1}_{1}H$ while deuterium, which has one proton and one neutron, is expressed as ${}^{2}_{1}H$ and radioactive tritium, ${}^{3}_{1}H$, has one proton and two neutrons. It should be noted that because the element X is identified by its atomic number Z, Z may be omitted from the shorthand notation and the symbol written as ${}^{A}X$ or X-A as in H-3.

Those nuclides with the same atomic number (Z), and therefore the same number of electrons and chemical properties but different neutron (N) and mass (A) numbers, are known as *isotopes* ('same place'). Most elements found in nature have more than one isotope and isotopes may be stable or unstable. For example hydrogen and deuterium, cited above, are both stable but tritium, ${}^{3}_{1}H$, with one proton and two neutrons, is unstable and hence radioactive.

Nuclides with the same mass number, A, but different Z and N are known as *isobars* ('equal weight'), e.g. ${}^{40}_{18}Ar$, ${}^{40}_{19}K$, ${}^{40}_{20}Ca$. There are several sets of triple isobars where the middle one is radioactive, and many stable pairs of isobars in which Z differs by two. This suggests that the stable nucleus favours even numbers of protons and of neutrons. Now, just as a shell model can be used to describe the arrangement of electrons in the extranuclear region of the atom, an analogous model can be used for the arrangement of neutrons and protons in the nucleus. In this case, the shell closures occur at particle numbers 2, 8, 20, 28, 50, 82, 126. These are known as *magic numbers* and apply separately to neutrons and protons. Nuclei with full shells are unusually stable, e.g. $^{208}_{82}Pb$ which has 82 protons and 126 neutrons, that is, it contains two of the magic numbers. Helium ($^{4}_{2}He$), which has two neutrons and two protons, also has a very stable nucleus and it is this feature which explains why it is ejected from the atom as a particle during alpha decay.

Nuclear energy levels

The nucleons occupy definite energy levels in the nucleus. For each nuclide there is one set of energy levels available to the neutrons and a second set available to the protons. A nucleus is in its *ground state* when its lowest energy levels are filled. Occasionally the nucleus may exist in an excited state, that is, a proton or neutron is raised to a higher energy level. *Nuclear excitation* is associated with the configuration and energy of the particles within the nucleus. (It is important to distinguish between nuclear and atomic excitation.) When such a nucleus returns to its stable state, electromagnetic radiation is emitted in the form of *gamma ray* photons. The energy may be released as a single photon or as a cascade of several gamma ray photons.

Two nuclei having the same values for *Z* and *A* but different nuclear configurations are known as *isomers*, e.g. the metastable $^{99m}_{43}Tc$ emits gamma rays as it decays into $^{99}_{43}Tc$. While gamma rays and X-rays are both forms of electromagnetic radiation, gamma rays originate from changes in nuclear energy, whereas the characteristic X-rays arise from changes in electron shell energy.

Nuclear forces

The nucleus is very small and consists of neutrons and protons. Protons have a positive electrical charge and, since 'like charges repel', there must be a large electrostatic force of repulsion resulting from the high density of like charges. We might therefore expect the nucleus to 'explode' but it does not. This can only be explained if there is a force of attraction present which is greater than the electrostatic force of repulsion. This attractive force is known as the *nuclear force* and is some 100 times greater than the electrostatic force.

The nuclear force is greater between neutron and proton than between neutron and neutron which, in turn, is greater than that between proton and proton. This *nuclear binding energy* varies from element to element but the average is approximately 8 MeV per nucleon. The nuclear force is only effective over a very limited range of 0.4×10^{-15} m to 2.4×10^{-15} m, being at its strongest when nucleons are 1×10^{-15} m apart. This is less than the radius of a large nucleus. (In contrast the electrostatic repulsive forces work over a relatively large range.) This means that in heavier atoms, in order to keep the nucleus stable, extra neutrons are required to increase the total attractive force while not altering the repulsive force. This is shown graphically in Figure 3.1 where the number of neutrons has been plotted against the number of protons for all the stable nuclides.

Nuclear binding energy

If we return to our atom of carbon-12 (p. 12) and try to recreate the atom out of its constituent parts as follows:

$$n = 6\ (1.0087\ \text{a.m.u.}) = 6.0522\ \text{a.m.u.}$$
$$p = 6\ (1.0073\ \text{a.m.u.}) = 6.0438\ \text{a.m.u.}$$
$$e^- = 6\ (0.00055\ \text{a.m.u.}) = 0.0033\ \text{a.m.u.}$$
$$\text{we find that the sum} = 12.0993\ \text{a.m.u.}$$

But we have already stated that the nuclide mass of carbon-12 is 12.000 a.m.u., by definition, which is 0.0993 less than the sum of the constituent parts. This is known as the *mass defect* and is not in fact lost but is converted into the nuclear binding energy. The energy equivalent of this mass defect for carbon-12 is:

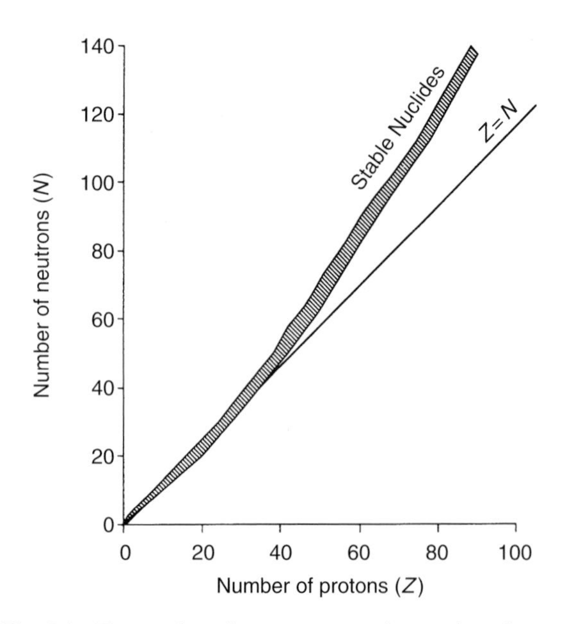

Fig. 3.1 The number of protons versus the number of neutrons with increasing atomic number.

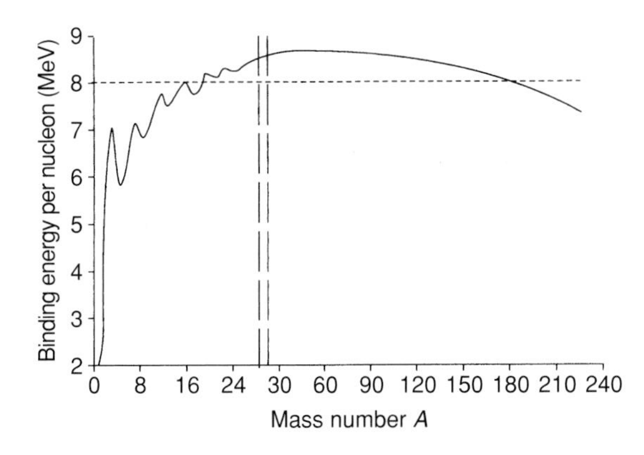

Fig. 3.2 Average nuclear binding energy per nucleon as a function of mass number.

$$0.0993 \text{ a.m.u.} \times 931 \text{ MeV/a.m.u.} = 92.448 \text{ MeV}$$

which gives the nuclear binding energy per nucleon as:

$$\frac{92.448}{12} = 7.7 \text{ MeV/nucleon}$$

The average nuclear binding energy per nucleon for different nuclides is shown plotted as a function of the mass number in Figure 3.2. This demonstrates:

- A rapid increase in nuclear binding energy per nucleon for the lighter nuclei with a notable peak at $A = 4$ (^{4}He)
- Approximately the same nuclear binding energy (7.5–8.8 MeV) for all nuclei with A greater than 16
- The maximum nuclear binding energy per nucleon occurring at about $A = 60$ for iron, nickel and cobalt, and
- A gradual decrease in nuclear binding energy with A greater than 60 to 7.3 MeV/nucleon at $A = 238$.

Nuclear stability

From the previous discussions it is apparent that the requirements for a stable nucleus are that it complies with one or more of the following statements.

- There should be even numbers of neutrons and of protons.
- The shells of the nucleus should be full.
- There should be a slight excess of neutrons.
- The nucleus should have no more than 200 nucleons.

RADIOACTIVITY

Although many elements have several naturally occurring isotopes, the number of stable arrangements of neutrons and protons is rather limited and any other configuration results in an unstable nucleus. Sooner or later such nuclei will spontaneously emit surplus energy in the form of charged particles or gamma rays in order to achieve a more stable proton–neutron configuration. In so doing the atom changes its atomic number and so its chemical identity. This phenomenon is called *radioactive decay*, and the nucleus is said to be *radioactive*. The change from one nuclide, known as the parent, to another nuclide, known as the daughter, is called a *radioactive disintegration*. The new atomic nucleus may be a stable form or it may itself be unstable and radioactive.

The *periodic table* lists the 103 elements, from the lightest to the heaviest, according to the number of electron shells (grouped horizontally) and their chemical properties (grouped vertically, according to the number of electrons in the outermost shell). Both stable and unstable isotopes are known for most elements. The total number of nuclides available is in excess of 1900 but of these only 266 are stable, that is, the elements exist in both non-radioactive and radioactive forms. The radioactive nuclides are those in which the number of neutrons present in the nucleus falls short of, or is in excess of, the number present in the stable nuclides. For example, the element carbon ($Z = 6$) is known to have isotopes with the following mass numbers: 10, 11, 12, 13, 14, 15. Of these, the isotopes of $A = 12$ and 13 are stable and exist in nature with six and seven neutrons respectively in the nuclei. The isotopes $A = 10$ and 11 are neutron deficient and those with $A = 14$ and 15 have a neutron excess; all four are radioactive. For most elements, radioactive isotopes can be produced by various techniques of nuclear bombardment as described later.

Some radioactive nuclides do occur in nature, however, either because their rate of disintegration is extremely slow or because they are being produced continuously by the disintegration of other very slowly disintegrating nuclides. An example of the former is the radioactive isotope of potassium ($Z = 19$, $A = 40$) which occurs as part of the normal naturally occurring element. An example of the latter is the radioactive element radium ($Z = 88$, $A = 226$) which occurs in nature as a radioactive by-product of the slow disintegration of the radioactive element uranium. Furthermore, the slow decay of radium produces the radioactive gas radon ($Z = 86$, $A = 222$). The decay scheme of uranium is discussed further on page 29.

Units of activity

The original definition of the curie was the amount of radiation in equilibrium with 1 g of radium and could, therefore, only be applied to radium-226 and its decay products. The *curie* was subsequently redefined as the rate of decay of 1 g of radium, namely 3.7×10^{10} disintegrations/second. More recently, the curie has been superseded by the SI unit for radioactivity, the becquerel (Bq), where:

$$1 \text{ Bq} = 1 \text{ disintegration/second}$$

Thus 1 curie is equivalent to 37 gigabecquerels (GBq, giga = 10^9); the becquerel is a very small unit. The MBq is the most commonly used multiple.

It will be appreciated that the becquerel is not a measure of the mass of the radioactive material present. In a radionuclide with a slow disintegration rate a large mass of substance will be necessary to provide 37 GBq of activity. As has already been stated, for radium-226 with its half-life of 1600 years, 37 GBq of activity will be provided by 1 g of radium. In a rapidly decaying radionuclide, however, a very much smaller mass of material will be equivalent to 37 GBq of activity. For example 37 GBq of carrier-free iodine-131 with its half-life of 8 days will have a mass of 8×10^{-6} g.

Radioactive decay

Disintegration of radioactive nuclei is spontaneous and random. The break-up of any particular nucleus is not predictable but the proportion of nuclei in any particular radionuclide which disintegrates in unit time depends on the instability of the nucleus. The fraction of the total number of atoms of a particular radionuclide ($\delta N/N$) which disintegrate per unit time is a constant for that nuclide and is known as the *decay constant* or *transformation constant*, λ.

$$\lambda = (\delta N/N)/\delta t$$

It can easily be demonstrated that the disappearance of a constant fraction of the atoms per unit time can be represented mathematically by the exponential law:

$$N = N_0 e^{-\lambda t}$$

where N is the number of atoms remaining after time t, N_0 is the initial number present at time $t = 0$. This is the law of *exponential decay*.

Since the intensity of emission from a radioactive sample is directly proportional to the number of radioactive atoms present, the exponential law of decay can be observed readily by measuring, under fixed geometrical conditions, the variation with time of the number of beta particles emitted per unit time or the gamma ray intensity. Figure 3.3A shows a radioactive decay curve for sodium-24.

If the exponential curve represented by the above equation is plotted logarithmically, that is, if log (intensity) is plotted against time, a straight line of gradient $-\lambda$ results, as shown in Figure 3.3B. This is an important aspect of the curve. If an experimentally determined logarithmic decay curve is not a straight line then it suggests that two or more radionuclides are present which are decaying at different rates.

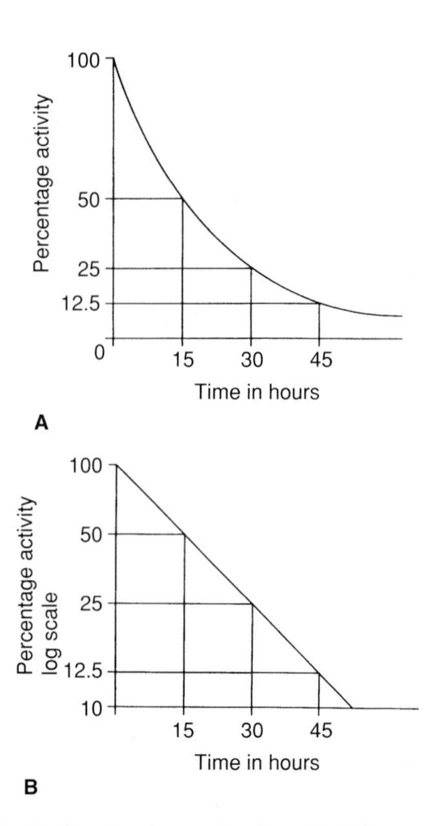

Fig. 3.3 Radioactive decay of sodium-24: **A** linear and **B** logarithmic.

Half-life

The time taken for the activity, i.e. the intensity of the emitted radiation or the number of radioactive atoms present, to be reduced to one-half of the original value is a constant. Physically, this means that any radionuclide has a characteristic transformation constant leading to a fixed time for the number of atoms of the nuclide to be reduced to half the original value, i.e. when $N/N_0 = ½$. This time is the *half-life*. It can be shown that the half-life, $T_{½}$, is related to the transformation constant, λ, by the simple relationship:

$$T_{½} = \frac{0.693}{\lambda}$$

Half-lives of radionuclides vary enormously, corresponding to a wide range of instability of the radioactive nuclei. For example, the isotope sodium-24 has a half-life of 15.0 hours—but extreme values of half-life are represented by potassium-40, 1.3×10^9 years, and polonium-214, 1.6×10^{-4} seconds. It will be seen later that the half-life of a radionuclide has an important bearing on its use in clinical practice.

Mean life

It can be demonstrated mathematically that the law of radioactive decay is a statistical law and radioactive decay is subject to the laws of probability. The average number of atoms disintegrating per second may be N, while the actual number disintegrating will fluctuate around this value. The *mean life* is a measure of the average life-expectancy of the atoms of a radionuclide. Since the decay process is statistical, any single atom could have a lifetime from zero to infinity. Based upon this, the mean life is simply the reciprocal of the decay constant.

$$\text{Mean life} = \frac{1}{\lambda} = \frac{T_{1/2}}{0.693} = 1.44T_{1/2}$$

Mean life is useful for calculating the dose due to 'infinite exposure' resulting from ingested or implanted radioactivity (on the assumption that excretion is negligible).

Radiations from radioactive nuclides

Radioactive nuclei may give off one of four different types of particulate radiation and may at the same time give off photons of electromagnetic radiation. The following particulate radiations will be described below in more detail:

- Alpha particles (α)
- Beta particles (β^-)
- Positrons (β^+)
- Neutrons (n).

Electromagnetic radiation from the nuclei of radioactive atoms is called *gamma radiation*. In a small number of radioactive nuclides only gamma radiation is emitted and, since no charged particle leaves the nucleus, the atomic number, Z, of the disintegrating atom does not change and the resulting atom is of the same chemical element as the initial one and the radioactive process has merely changed the internal energy of the nucleus.

The characteristics of the various decay processes are given in Table 3.1. Each type of disintegration can be indicated by a decay scheme, as shown in Figure 3.4. A decay scheme is a combination of a graph and an energy level diagram. The atomic number of the nuclide is represented by the horizontal scale, while the vertical scale represents the energy involved in the disintegration process. The direction of the arrow to the right or left indicates whether the atomic number of the daughter nuclide has increased or decreased.

Alpha decay

Certain types of radionuclides, with mass number greater than 150, emit positively charged particles called alpha (α) particles. *Alpha particles* consist of two protons and two neutrons tightly bound together and have a mass of 4 on the atomic scale and a positive charge of 2 units. They are the nuclei of helium atoms. For each disintegration, the energy lost by the parent atom can either be carried entirely by the alpha particle as kinetic energy or partly by the alpha particle and partly by an associated gamma ray. In each case the atomic number decreases by 2 and the mass number decreases by 4.

$${}^{A}_{Z}X \rightarrow {}^{A-4}_{Z-2}X + \alpha + Q$$

where Q is the energy released.

Table 3.1 Nuclear disintegration processes

Name	Symbol	Change in nucleus		Radiation emitted*
		Z	A	
Alpha decay	α	−2	−4	α
Isobaric transition				
Beta decay	β^-	+1	0	e^-, ν
Positron decay	β^+	−1	0	e^+, ν, (γ_a)
Electron capture	EC	−1	0	ν, (γ_x, e^-_{Au})
Isomeric transition				
Gamma ray decay	γ	0	0	γ
Internal conversion	IC	0	0	e^-, (γ_x, e^-_{Au})

* ν = neutrino; γ_a = annihilation photons; γ_x = characteristic X-rays; e^-_{Au} = Auger electrons

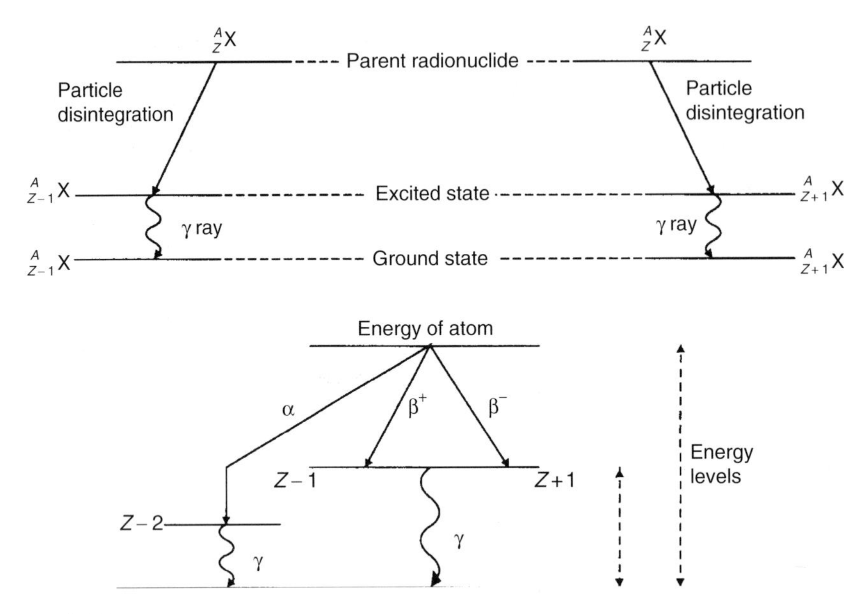

Fig. 3.4 Decay scheme diagrams.

Several of the naturally occurring radionuclides, such as radium-226, are alpha emitters, as are many of the artificially prepared radionuclides of atomic numbers greater than 92, such as plutonium-239. The alpha decay scheme for radium-226 is shown in Figure 3.5A.

Isobaric transitions

Atoms may have an imbalance in the number of protons and neutrons in the nucleus. If the excess energy is less than about 8 MeV, i.e. the binding energy of the nucleons, the nucleus may reach a stable state by changing one of its neutrons into a proton or vice versa which means the mass number stays the same but the atomic number either increases or decreases by one. These are called *isobaric transitions*. Isobaric transitions fall into three groups: beta minus (β^-) or *negatron decay*, beta plus (β^+) or *positron decay* and *electron capture*.

Negatron decay. Negatron or beta (β^-) decay occurs when a neutron changes into a proton with the emission of an *electron–antineutrino pair*.

$$n^0 \rightarrow p^+ + \beta^- + \nu$$

β^- particles are negatively charged particles with the same charge and mass as an electron. They are therefore electrons emitted with kinetic energy from the nucleus of the atom. Negatron decay leaves the mass number the same but the atomic number increases by one. Phosphorus-32 is a radionuclide which decays by this process, as shown in Figure 3.5B.

The beta particle ejected may have any energy from just above zero to a maximum, characteristic of the parent nucleus (Fig. 3.6)—a useful point to remember is that the average energy is approximately one-third the maximum energy. However, the transformation within a given nuclide always results in the loss of the same amount of energy. This is achieved by the ejection of a second particle, the *antineutrino*, ν, simultaneously with the β^- particle. Thus the total energy of the transformation may be shared differently by the two particles. The antineutrino has no electrical charge, almost no rest mass and has very little interaction with matter.

Positron decay. Positron (β^+) decay is analogous to negatron decay but in this case a proton changes into a neutron, which stays in the nucleus, and a *positron–neutrino pair* is emitted.

$$p^+ \rightarrow n^0 + \beta^+ + \nu$$

The positive charge lost by the nucleus is carried off by the positron. In this case the atomic number will decrease by one. Since positron emission decreases the atomic number by one, the number of electrons orbiting the nucleus must also be decreased by one. Thus for positron decay to take place, the difference in the energy between the parent and daughter nuclide must be at least 1.022 MeV (2 × 0.511 MeV).

Positrons are positive electrons, and are the same kind of particles as are produced in the pair production process when very high-energy photons interact

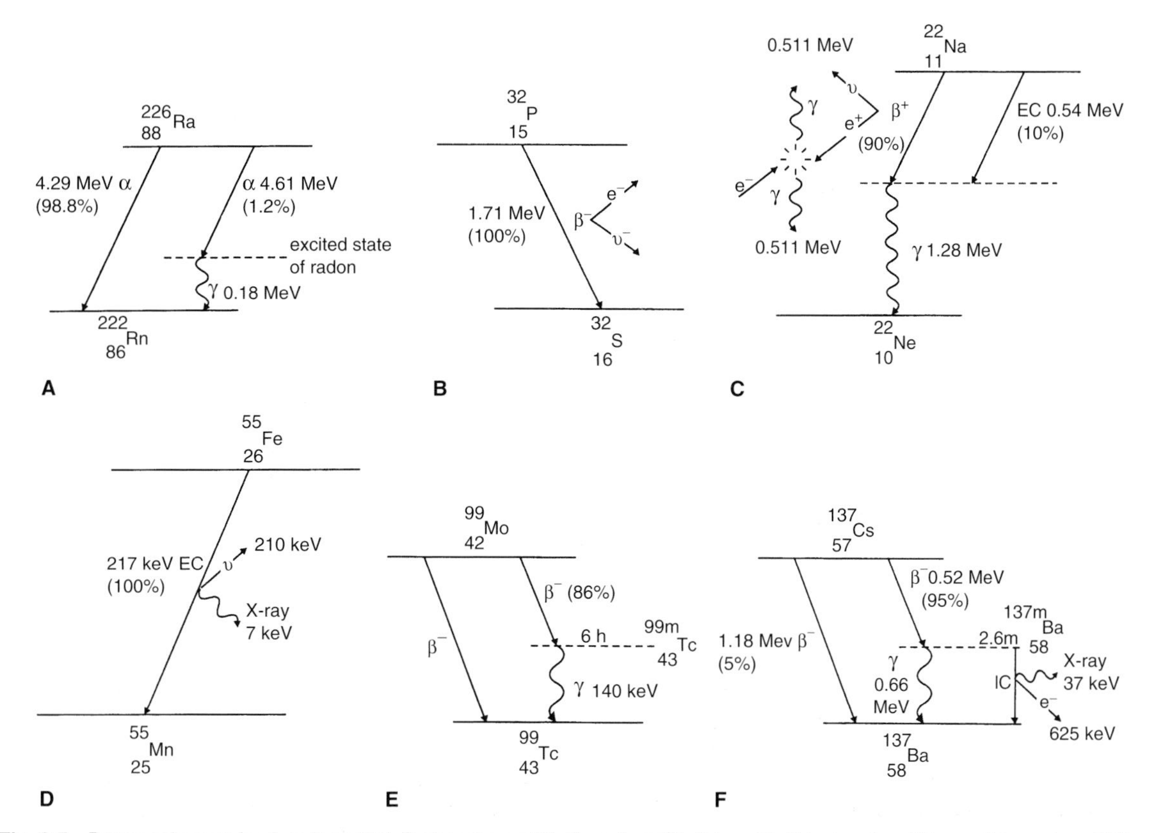

Fig. 3.5 Decay schemes for **A** radium-226, **B** phosphorus-32, **C** sodium-22, **D** iron-55, **E** technetium-99m and **F** caesium-137.

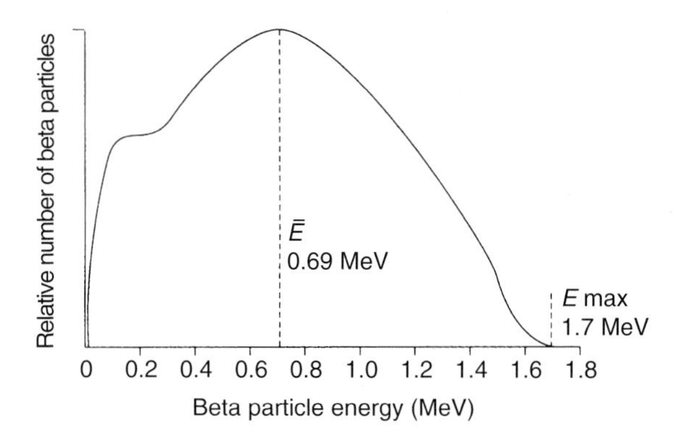

Fig. 3.6 Energy spectrum of beta particles from phosphorus-32.

with matter (Ch. 4). Although the positrons have a very short life they behave in most respects exactly like negative electrons during their passage through matter, losing energy by production of ions. When the energy has been completely lost in this way, the positron combines with a negative electron and the rest mass of the two particles is converted into two photons of electromagnetic radiation, each of energy 0.511 MeV. This is called *annihilation radiation*. A common example of an isotope which undergoes positron decay is sodium-22 (Fig. 3.5C).

Electron capture. If the nuclear energy levels of the parent and daughter of a proton-rich nuclide do not differ by more than 1.022 MeV, *electron capture* takes place. In this case the nucleus captures an electron from one of its orbits, usually the K shell, and the electron and proton combine in the nucleus to form a neutron and a neutrino. The neutrino is ejected from the nucleus, carrying away any excess energy.

$$p^+ + e^- \rightarrow n^0 + \nu$$

If K capture occurs, the 'hole' in the K shell must be filled by another electron. This will give rise to K radiation. An example of such a decay scheme is given in Figure 3.5D.

In many cases both positron decay and electron capture will take place, as was seen in Figure 3.5C for the decay of sodium-22. The higher the atomic number of the nucleus and the closer the K shell is to the nucleus the greater the probability of electron capture.

Isomeric transitions

Following decay by alpha or beta particle emission, the daughter nucleus is often in an excited state and possesses excess energy. *Isomeric transition* is the change of this excited nucleus or isomer to the stable isomer. The residual energy may be emitted as a gamma ray or passed to an orbital electron.

Gamma radiation. The nuclei may be transformed from a high energy level to a low energy level by the emission of one or more quanta of electromagnetic radiation known as gamma rays (Fig. 3.5A and C). Gamma rays are indistinguishable from X-rays, being differentiated only by their origin; that is, gamma rays are emitted from an excited nucleus; X-rays are emitted either as a result of changes in the electron shells (characteristic radiation), or as *bremsstrahlung* radiation. The gamma rays emitted have discrete energies characteristic of the daughter nuclide.

In most cases gamma emission happens virtually instantaneously but occasionally the daughter nuclide can remain in the excited state for several hours. This is known as a *metastable state*. These nuclides are designated by use of the suffix or superscript 'm'. Technetium-99m (^{99m}Tc, $T_{½} = 6$ hours) is an example of such a decay process (Fig. 3.5E). These metastable radionuclides are of great value in nuclear medicine imaging as they only emit gamma rays; there being no particulate radiation, the radiation dose to the patient is lower.

Internal conversion. In heavy atoms the electrons of the subshells, particularly of the K shell, may bombard the large nucleus as they orbit around it; the nucleus may then transfer its excess energy to the electron. This is known as *internal conversion*. The converted electron will be ejected from the atom and travel away with a discrete energy equal to the difference between the energy lost by the nucleus and the binding energy holding the electron to the atom.

The longer the half-life of the excited state, the greater is the probability of internal conversion taking place. Therefore internal conversion is important in metastable decay. Caesium-137 decays to barium-137m, which then decays to barium-137 by a combination of gamma ray emission and internal conversion (Fig. 3.5F).

Auger electrons. Following internal conversion, the atom is left with a vacancy in the K shell which will be filled by an electron from the L shell and an electron cascade will follow until the outer shell captures a free electron. These transfers will be accompanied by the emission of characteristic electromagnetic radiation. Not all the X-rays produced during internal conversion are emitted from the atom; some transfer their energy to an outer electron, ejecting it from the atom as an *Auger electron*. The kinetic energy of the Auger electron is low, being the difference between the energy of the X-ray photon and the binding energy of the orbital electron.

Neutrons

The emission of neutrons during radioactive decay is quite rare. However, some radionuclides, such as the artificially prepared californium-252, emit neutrons of considerable energy during their disintegration. Neutrons have no charge and are not themselves ionising radiations, being able to pass freely through the charged electron structure of the atoms of an absorbing medium. Their ionising potential arises from the collision of the neutron with the nuclei of the atoms of the medium, producing an efficient transfer of energy to these nuclei. Since the nuclei are both charged and heavy they produce intense ionisation along their tracks. Californium-252 has been used as an implantable neutron source, but with mixed results and is not considered further in this text.

Radioactive equilibrium

A radioactive disintegration process involving the emission of a charged particle generally results in the production of a new non-radioactive nuclide of a different element. Sometimes, however, the nuclide formed by the disintegration is itself an unstable nuclide and undergoes a further radioactive transformation. This can be represented by the following decay scheme:

$$N_1 \xrightarrow{\lambda_1} N_2 \xrightarrow{\lambda_2} N_3$$

where N_1 and N_2 are the parent and daughter radionuclides respectively and N_3 is stable; λ_1 and λ_2 are the decay constants of the parent and daughter nuclides. At radioactive equilibrium, the weight of each nuclide present is inversely proportional to the half-life of the nuclide. An example of such a transformation is the decay of strontium-90, which disintegrates with the emission of a negative beta particle, forming an isotope of the element yttrium:

$$^{90}_{38}\mathrm{Sr} \xrightarrow[T_{½} = 28 \text{ years}]{\lambda_1 = 0.0000028\ \mathrm{h}^{-1}} {}^{90}_{39}\mathrm{Y} \xrightarrow[T_{½} = 64\ \mathrm{h}]{\lambda_2 = 0.0108\ \mathrm{h}^{-1}} {}^{90}_{40}\mathrm{Zr}$$

Yttrium-90 is itself radioactive and emits a further negative beta particle, the final product of this second disintegration process being a stable isotope of the element zirconium (Zr-90). Strontium-90 has a relatively long half-life of 28 years but its daughter product, yttrium-90, is much more unstable energetically and has a half-life of 64 hours. In a pure sample of strontium-90 the radionuclide yttrium-90 formed from the parent element will accumulate. The amount of yttrium-90 will grow until the number of yttrium-90 atoms breaking up per second ($\lambda_2 N_2$) equals the number being formed per second by disintegration of the parent element ($\lambda_1 N_1$). A state of *radioactive equilibrium* is then said to exist between the parent and daughter radionuclides. In this case the parent nuclide (strontium-90) and the daughter nuclide (yttrium-90) then decay at the same rate ($\lambda_1 N_1 = \lambda_2 N_2$), that is, at the decay rate of the parent element ($T_{½}$ = 28 years). It can be shown that the growth of the daughter product in the mixture is exponential and is governed by the decay rate of the daughter nuclide—that is, it will reach half its full equilibrium value in 64 hours and three-quarters of its equilibrium value in 128 hours, and so on.

The practical importance of this particular example arises from the fact that, though the maximum range of the beta particle from strontium-90 is only 1.2 mm in water, the beta particles from yttrium-90 are much more energetic, with a maximum range in water of 11 mm. An equilibrium mixture of the two radionuclides therefore supplies beta particles of the long range, but with an effective half-life of 28 years. The use of the strontium-90 beta plaque for corneal irradiation is described on page 238.

The phenomenon of radioactive equilibrium is very important in the production of other short-lived radionuclides for use in medical investigations. Several of these short-lived products are available as daughter radioelements, easily separated by elution from longer-lived parent elements (p. 34).

Successive disintegration

The naturally occurring radioactive elements arise from a series of decay processes producing several successive radioactive daughter products. Radioactive equilibrium is established between the primary long-lived radioactive elements—uranium, thorium, actinium—and several generations of daughter products. The most important of these is the *uranium series*.

Radium is one of the radionuclides in the decay chain of the parent nuclide of uranium. It is isolated chemically from uranium ores. Radium ($Z = 88$, $A =$ 226, $T_{½}$ = 1600 years) is an alpha particle emitter. Its immediate daughter product is an inert gas, radon-222, which is also an alpha emitter of short half-life ($T_{½}$ = 3.8 days). Radon, however, is only the first step in a series of *successive disintegrations* leading finally to a stable isotope of the element lead ($Z = 82$, $A = 206$). Figure 3.7 gives a detailed account of the successive transformations of the radium series in which some 10 different radionuclides are involved. If pure radium element is sealed in a container so that the successive radioactive products cannot escape, all the radionuclides of the series accumulate until each is in equilibrium with the others. At equilibrium each nuclide will decay at the same rate, each being produced by the decay of the radionuclide preceding it in the chain and giving rise to the nuclide following it.

The importance of this *radioactive family*, as it is called, is that two of the radioactive nuclides in the series are emitters of penetrating gamma rays: lead-214 or radium-B ($T_{½}$ = 26.8 min) and bismuth-214 or radium-C ($T_{½}$ = 19.7 min) but, in equilibrium with the rest of the chain, they have the same effective half-life as the parent element radium ($T_{½}$ = 1600 years). Radium in a sealed container in equilibrium with its products will therefore act as a long-lived radioactive source emitting a mixture of alpha particles, beta particles and gamma rays. In a container of a suitable thickness to absorb all the particulate radiations (e.g. 0.5 mm of platinum, $Z = 78$, $\rho = 21.5$ g cm^{-3}), it will act as a pure gamma emitter of effectively constant activity, since the half-life is so long as to be considered infinite in clinical work. The gamma spectrum covers the range from 0.2–2.4 MeV.

Because the inert gas *radon* is very different chemically from its parent element radium, it can be separated reasonably easily. If radon is sealed in a suitable container, the successive radioactive products of the radium family would accumulate to equilibrium amounts and would again include the gamma emitters lead-214 and bismuth-214. In this case the container would be an emitter of the same clinically useful penetrating gamma rays but with an effective half-life equal to that of radon ($T_{½}$ = 3.8 days). The gas used to be sealed into thin-walled gold capsules, called *radon seeds*, as small implantable gamma ray sources of short half-life.

The potential escape of radon gas from any leaky container constitutes such a serious hazard that, together with the high-energy component of the spectrum making protective shielding difficult, has lead to the replacement of radium and radon by other artificially produced radionuclides of similar half-life and gamma-emitting properties in brachytherapy (Ch. 14).

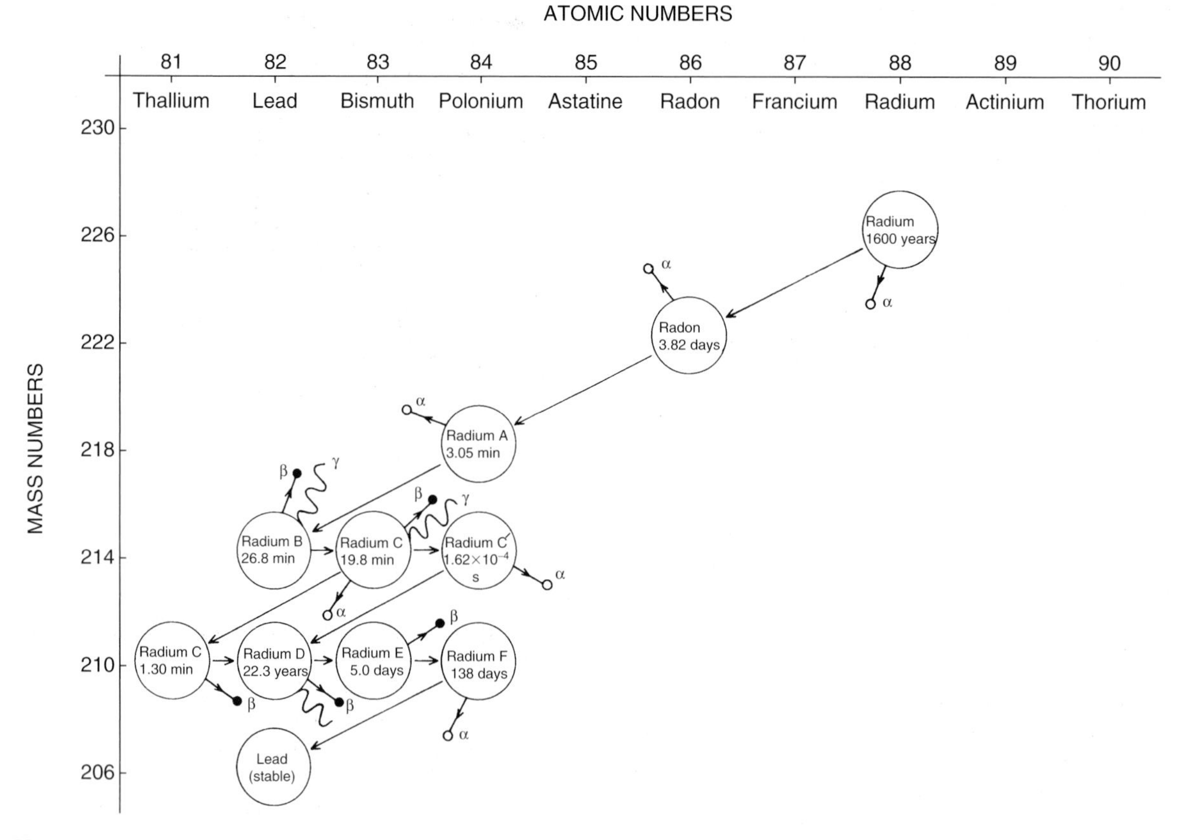

Fig. 3.7 The radium family.

PRODUCTION OF RADIOACTIVE MATERIALS

The production of radioactive materials in forms suitable for use in medicine is an expensive and difficult matter. Amongst the naturally occurring radioactive elements radium was the only one used medically in any major way.

The majority of radioactive isotopes used in medicine are produced artificially by bombarding a stable target nucleus with a suitable particle to produce nuclear reactions. The bombarding particles used can be:

- positively charged, such as protons or alpha particles from a charged particle accelerator, such as a cyclotron; or
- uncharged, such as neutrons in a nuclear reactor.

If charged particles are used they must have energies large enough to overcome the electrostatic repulsion between themselves and the positively charged nucleus of the target atom. Neutrons, on the other hand, can react with the nucleus of an atom without having a high initial energy.

Fission

As we discovered earlier, the very heavy elements having large nuclei tend to be unstable as the electrostatic force of repulsion between the protons overcomes the nuclear force of attraction between the nucleons, and therefore radioactive. Elements with mass number greater than 230 are unstable in a manner different from other nuclei. Under neutron bombardment, these nuclei may capture a neutron and break up into two approximately equal parts. This *nuclear fission* is accompanied by the emission of two or three further neutrons from the broken nucleus. Other nuclei of the same type in the vicinity can be stimulated to undergo further fission by capturing these secondary neutrons. If each nucleus that undergoes fission produces two neutrons and these two are capable of causing fission in two more nuclei, the speed of the fission reaction will increase exponentially and a *chain reaction* is produced. A very large amount of energy is released at each disintegration, corresponding to the conversion of a small part of the mass of the fissionable nucleus into energy (p. 13)—the fundamental processes underlying the release of energy in the atom bomb and in the nuclear reactor.

The nuclear reactor

The nuclear reactor is an important device for releasing energy, mainly in the form of heat, from atomic nuclei. There are many different types of reactor but most are based on the nuclear fission of uranium-235 by neutron bombardment:

$${}^{1}_{0}n + {}^{235}_{92}U \rightarrow {}^{236}_{92}U \rightarrow \begin{cases} \text{fission fragment A} \\ + Q + {}^{1}_{0}n + {}^{1}_{0}n + {}^{1}_{0}n \\ \text{fission fragment B} \end{cases}$$

The fission fragments, A and B, are unstable nuclei of mass number between 70 and 170. They are over-rich in neutrons for their atomic number and will therefore be radioactive. Q is an energy release. The energy release can be qualitatively predicted from Figure 3.2. The nuclear binding energy or mass defect per nucleon is about 7.3 MeV for mass number 240 and 8.4 MeV for mass number 120. Division of the 240 nucleus into two 120 nuclei could result in the release of $(240 \times (8.4 - 7.3)) = 264$ MeV.

On average, 2.4 neutrons are produced for each fission. For a controlled release of energy only one of the neutrons released per fission is needed to cause further fission. The chain reaction is kept to an equilibrium controllable level by neutron-absorbing *control rods* which prevent excessive numbers of neutrons being produced in the uranium bulk.

Natural uranium consists mainly of uranium-238; only 0.7% of the uranium nuclei are uranium-235. Unfortunately uranium-238 is not a suitable nuclide for controlled fission because it is able to capture the *fast neutrons* (energy > 0.5 MeV) produced during the fission of uranium-235 and form plutonium-239. However, the fission of uranium-235 is most efficient when bombarded by *thermal neutrons* (energy ~ 0.025 eV) which do not interact with uranium-238 to the same extent. The slowing-down process is achieved by use of a material of low atomic mass such as graphite, which acts as a *moderator*.

The basic components of a typical reactor are shown in Figure 3.8. The core consists of a block of graphite which acts as the moderator into which are inserted the *fuel rods*. Most thermal reactors use, as fuel, enriched uranium in which the amount of uranium-235 has been artificially raised to 2–3%. Clusters of fuel elements are

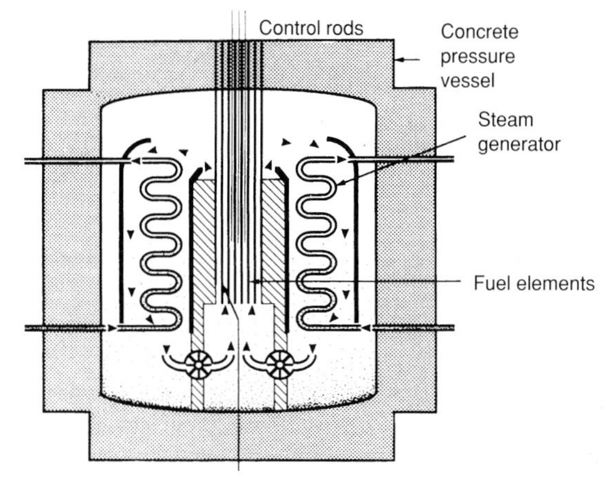

Fig. 3.8 A gas-cooled thermal reactor.

joined together end to end in a *stringer*, and placed in vertical holes in the graphite. Interleaved with the fuel rods are the control rods for absorbing the excess neutrons.

The *control rods* are usually made of boron or cadmium and are inserted further into or withdrawn from the core depending on whether the rate of the fission reaction needs to decrease or increase. As we have already shown, each fission event releases a great deal of energy, mainly in the form of heat. Carbon dioxide gas acts as a coolant by extracting heat as it passes over the fuel in the core. It transfers its heat to water in a steam generator outside the core and the steam can be used to drive turbines coupled to an electric generator.

Around the reactor is a massive concrete shield. This protective screen is necessary to give protection not only from the large neutron emission in the reactor core but also from the beta particles and gamma rays arising from the radioactive materials produced in the core.

Radionuclides produced by nuclear reactors

The fission events in the uranium result in a high neutron flux in the volume surrounding the fuel rods. Radionuclides can be produced in two ways, either by neutron bombardment of a specific target material placed within the region of high neutron flux, or by separation of the products produced by the fission of uranium.

Neutron bombardment. For the production of artificial radioactive isotopes, holes are made through the concrete shield into the core of the reactor to allow for the insertion of the target materials to be irradiated by the neutrons. The neutron enters the nucleus of the target atom, thus raising the energy level of the nucleus to above ground state. The nucleus rearranges and the excess energy is given off either as a gamma photon, or by the ejection of a proton or alpha particle. The shorthand notation for these reactions is:

$$X\ (n,b)\ Y$$

where X is the target nucleus, Y is the final nucleus, n is the bombarding particle (i.e. the neutron), and b is the ejected particle (p or α) or the gamma ray (γ). Two reactions are considered:

(n,γ) reaction. This is the most common nuclear reaction with low-energy (thermal) neutrons. The resultant radionuclide will be an isotope of the target material with the mass number increasing by one and the atomic number staying the same. For example, the bombardment of stable phosphorus-31 with neutrons results in the production of radioactive phosphorus-32:

$$^{31}_{15}P\ (n,\gamma)\ ^{32}_{15}P$$

It is very difficult and too costly to separate the product from the target material to produce a carrier-free radionuclide and hence the specific activity of the radionuclide (i.e. the activity per unit mass of the element) will be low.

These (n,γ) reactions generate radioactive products which decay by beta particle emission or by electron capture, thus creating a daughter which is not an isotope of the target element. This daughter product may itself be radioactive and can be recovered carrier-free. Two important examples are the production of iodine-131 from tellurium-130:

$$^{130}_{52}Te\ (n,\gamma)\ ^{131}_{52}Te \xrightarrow[T_{1/2} = 25\ \text{min}]{\beta^-} {}^{131}_{53}I$$

and the production of technetium-99m from molybdenum-98:

$$^{98}_{42}Mo\ (n,\gamma)\ ^{99}_{42}Mo \xrightarrow[T_{1/2} = 66.6\ \text{h}]{\beta^-} {}^{99m}_{43}Tc \xrightarrow[T_{1/2} = 6\ \text{h}]{\gamma} {}^{99}_{43}Tc$$

The relatively long half-life of molybdenum-99 makes it ideal for use in a generator system to produce the gamma-emitting radionuclide technetium-99m widely used in nuclear imaging.

(n,p) and (n,α) reactions. These are less common reactions and require fast (high-energy) neutrons. In (n,p) reactions, the atomic number decreases by one while the mass number remains the same, e.g. the production of carbon-14 from nitrogen-14:

$$^{14}_{7}N\ (n,p)\ ^{14}_{6}C$$

In (n,α) reactions, the atomic number decreases by two and the mass number by three, e.g. the production of tritium from lithium:

$$^{6}_{3}Li\ (n,\alpha)\ ^{3}_{1}H$$

The product in both these examples is easily separated from the target and hence is carrier-free and has a high specific activity.

Target choice and activity. The choice of target material is obviously dependent on considerations of the final radionuclide, but several other factors also need to be considered. It should be chemically pure and contain a high proportion of the target isotope. It must be able to withstand the high temperatures generated within the nuclear reactor without giving off noxious products. It should be cheap and in a form that can be easily processed chemically to separate it from the product radionuclide.

When a target is bombarded by neutrons, the atoms in the target are steadily changed into radioactive atoms. However, at the same time as production is taking place, some of the newly formed radioactive nuclei will disintegrate and the product material will decay. The activity of the product will therefore depend on the relative rates of these two processes. When the rate of production equals the rate of decay, saturation has been achieved and equilibrium exists. The activity at time t, A_t, is given by:

$$A_t = NF \times \lambda \times S$$

where N is the number of atoms of the target isotope per m^3, F is the incident neutron flux per m^2 , and S is the saturation factor. S is dependent on the decay factor λ of the product material and will equal 1 at equilibrium but will equal $(1 - e^{-\lambda t})$ at any time prior to equilibrium. This is shown in Figure 3.9.

Fission products

As has been discussed already, fission is the process by which a heavy isotope such as uranium-235 splits into isotopes of two lighter elements. For example:

$$^{1}_{0}n + {}^{235}_{92}U \rightarrow {}^{236}_{92}U \rightarrow {}^{131}_{50}Sn + {}^{103}_{42}Mo + 2n$$

Fission of uranium-235 does not always produce tin and molybdenum. A whole range of fission products are formed. Figure 3.10 shows the relative amounts of materials of different mass numbers produced, one product comes from each peak. Most of the fission fragments can be chemically separated to provide carrier-free radionuclides. Like all heavy elements, uranium has considerably more neutrons than protons in its nucleus. The medium mass fission products will therefore have a neutron excess and will decay by beta particle emission.

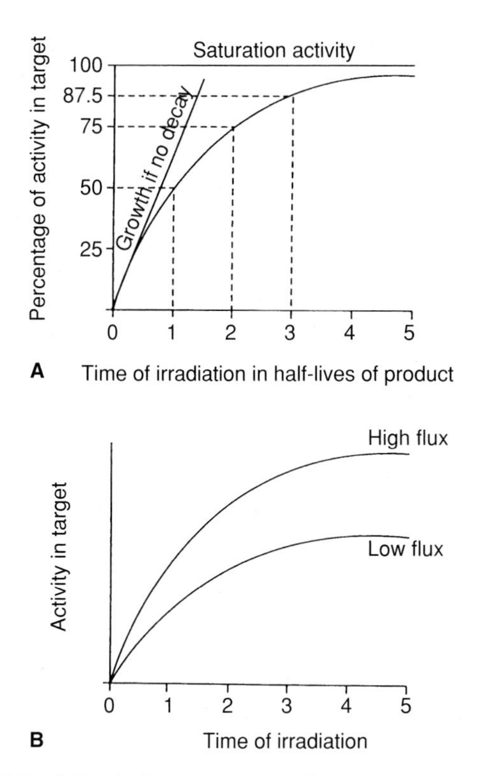

Fig. 3.9 **A** Activity in the target as a function of time. **B** Activity in target at two different levels of neutron flux.

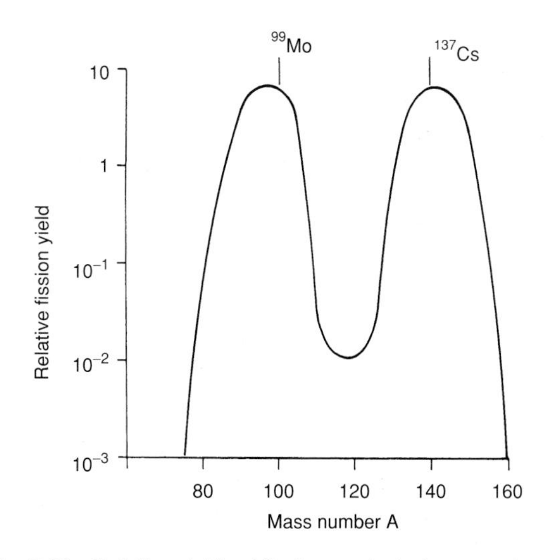

Fig. 3.10 Relative yields of fission products from uranium.

Fission products such as the long-lived caesium-137 are extracted from spent fuel rods. However, the short-lived radionuclides such as molybdenum-99 and the gas xenon-133 are normally obtained by neutron bombardment of a uranium target.

The cyclotron

The cyclotron consists of two hollow semicircular electrodes called *dees* (Fig. 3.11A). The dees, in an evacuated container, are placed between the pole pieces of an electromagnet such that the magnetic field runs perpendicular to the plane of the electrodes (Fig. 3.11B). An alternating electric field is applied between the two electrodes. Positive particles of the kind to be accelerated (e.g. protons) are produced at point A in the centre of the gap between the electrodes (Fig. 3.11C). With the electric field between the electrodes D_1 and D_2 in the right direction (i.e. D_2 negative and D_1 positive) the particles are accelerated towards point B. The charged particles are then under the influence of the magnetic field and any charged particle moving in a magnetic field will have a force exerted on it in a direction perpendicular to the magnetic field and to the direction of motion (Fig. 3.11D). Hence, the particles move in a circular path and arrive at the gap between the electrodes at C. Correct adjustment of the frequency of the electric field between D_1 and D_2 will ensure that the charge on the dees reverses as the particles reach point C (i.e. D_2 becomes positive and D_1 negative). The particles will then be accelerated across the gap into the opposite electrode. They then move again in a circular orbit, arriving at the gap again in time to receive a further acceleration. This is possible because the time taken to travel round the semicircular paths under the influence of the magnetic field remains constant; with increasing velocity of the charged particles

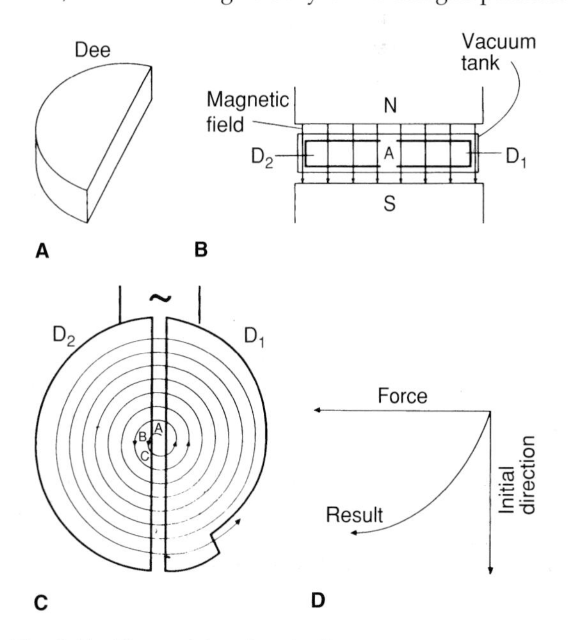

Fig. 3.11 The cyclotron (see text).

only the radius of the path increases. The particles therefore travel on a pseudo-spiral path of gradually increasing radius and are accelerated by the peak potential difference between the electrodes each time they cross the gap. In a typical cyclotron, the peak potential difference between the electrodes might be 20 kV but particles are accelerated across the gap 800 times in electrodes of 75 cm radius, thus producing an energy equivalent to an acceleration by 16 million volts. At the edge of the electrodes the beam is no longer under the influence of the magnetic field and emerges tangentially. The high-energy positive-ion beams produced in the cyclotron can then be used to bombard a suitable target in which nuclear reactions result in the production of radionuclides.

Radionuclides produced by cyclotrons

Beams of protons (p or ^1_1H), deuterons (d or ^2_1H) or alpha (α or ^4_2He) particles are used in the cyclotron. The nomenclature we employed to describe the reactions from neutron bombardment is also used to specify charged particle nuclear reactions. These include the following: (p,n); (p,pn); (p,d); (d,n); (d,p); (d,α); (α,n); (α,pn); (α,2n)—of which three examples are given:

(d,α) reaction. The bombarding particle is a deuteron and an alpha particle is released.

$$^{24}_{12}Mg + ^2_1H \rightarrow ^{22}_{11}Na + ^4_2\alpha$$

or $^{24}Mg\ (d,\alpha)\ ^{22}Na$

(p,pn) reaction. Here a proton is used as the bombarding particle and two particles are released—a proton and a neutron.

$$^{58}_{28}Ni + ^1_1H \xrightarrow{EC} ^{57}_{27}Co + ^1_1p + ^1_0n$$

or $^{58}Ni\ (p,pn)\ ^{57}Co$

(α,2n) reaction. In this case an alpha particle is used as the bombarding particle and two neutrons are released.

$$^{121}_{51}Sb + ^4_2He \rightarrow ^{123}_{53}I + ^1_0n + ^1_0n$$

or $^{121}Sb\ (\alpha,2n)\ ^{123}I$

The two main features of cyclotron-produced radionuclides are:

- the product is a different element from the target and can therefore be separated chemically to produce a high specific activity carrier-free radionuclide, and
- since the bombarding particle always includes at least one proton, most of the radionuclides produced will be proton rich and will therefore decay by positron emission or electron capture.

Radionuclide generators

A generator is a system which contains a long-lived parent radionuclide which decays to a short-lived daughter radionuclide. The parent and daughter radionuclides are different elements so chemical separation of the two can take place. A number of generator systems have been developed and some of these are listed in Table 3.2.

The activity of the daughter radionuclide, A_2, at any given time depends on several factors:

- The activity of the parent, A_1, at time zero
- The rate of decay of the parent, i.e. the rate of formation of the daughter proportional to the decay constant, λ_1
- The rate of decay of the daughter, proportional to the decay constant, λ_2
- The time since the last elution, t
- The percentage conversion of the parent to the daughter.

If initially there is no daughter product present the daughter activity can be calculated from:

$$A_2 = \frac{A_1\,(e^{-\lambda_1 t} - e^{-\lambda_2 t})\,\lambda_2}{\lambda_2 - \lambda_1}$$

This equation can be used for any parent–daughter relationship. However, in special cases the equation can be simplified, see below.

Secular equilibrium

When the parent half-life is very much greater than the daughter half-life ($\lambda_1 << \lambda_2$), the radionuclides are said to be in *secular equilibrium*, e.g. germanium-68 ($T_{½} = 280$ days) and gallium-68 ($T_{½} = 68$ minutes). The decay of the parent can be ignored relative to the decay of the daughter so the above equation can be simplified to:

$$A_2 = A_1\,(1 - e^{-\lambda_2 t})$$

This is shown graphically in Figure 3.12. As can be seen, if the time t is short compared to the $T_{½}$ of the parent but long, 5 to 6 half-lives, compared to the half-life

Table 3.2 Radionuclide generator systems

Parent	$T_{½}$	Daughter	$T_{½}$	E_γ*	Decay product
^{99}Mo	67 h	^{99m}Tc	6 h	140 keV	^{99}Tc
^{81}Rb	4.7 h	^{81m}Kr	13 s	190 keV	^{81}Kr
^{132}Te	78 h	^{132}I	2.3 h	Several	^{132}Xe
^{68}Ge	280 days	^{68}Ga	68 min	511 keV	^{68}Zn

* E_γ = energy of gamma radiation

of the daughter, then $A_2 = A_1$ and thereafter activity decays with the half-life of the parent.

Transient equilibrium

When the parent half-life is just greater than the daughter half-life, as in the case of molybdenum-99 ($T_{½} = 67$ h) and technetium-99m ($T_{½} = 6$ h), then the radionuclides are said to be in *transient equilibrium*. In this case the time to reach equilibrium is not short compared to the parent half-life so that at equilibrium:

$$A_2 = A_1 \frac{\lambda_1}{\lambda_2 - \lambda_1}$$

and hence from this time on the activity is greater than the parent activity, but once again it decreases with the half-life of the parent (Fig. 3.12).

Technetium generator. The growth and decay of the molybdenum-99–technetium-99m transient equilibrium generator system is shown in Figure 3.13. The maximum activity is present after approximately 24 hours (i.e. 4 daughter half-lives). However, the total activity is not greater than the activity of the parent as

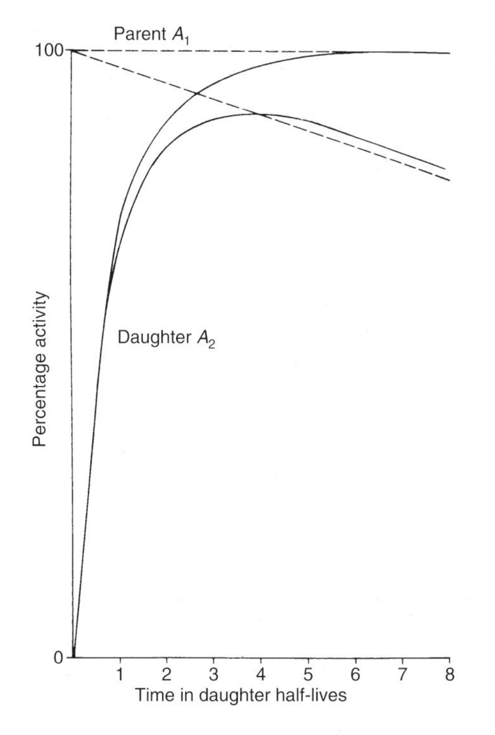

Fig. 3.12 Radioactive equilibrium: (1) secular equilibrium, uppermost curve; (2) transient equilibrium, lower curve. The dashed line represents the activity of the parent radionuclide and the solid line the activity of the daughter radionuclide.

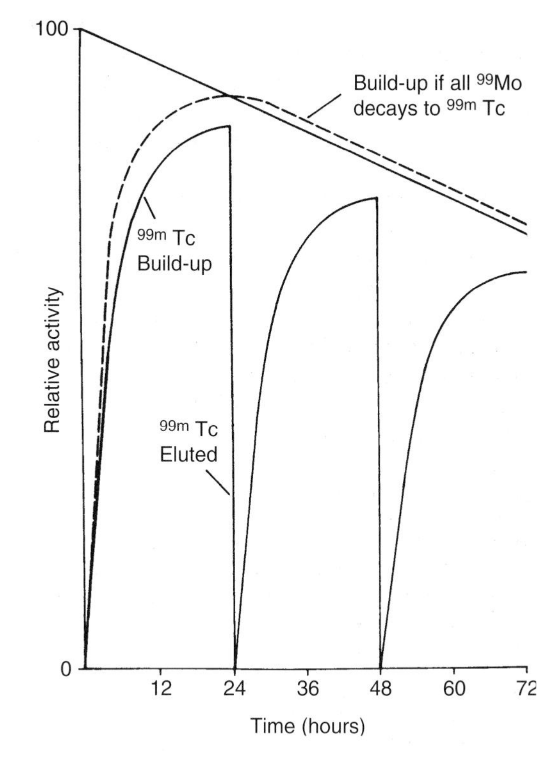

Fig. 3.13 Activity–time curves for a molybdenum-99–technetium-99m generator.

indicated by the dotted line, as we might expect, but is in fact slightly less than the activity of the parent. This is due to the fact that molybdenum-99 is converted to the metastable technetium-99m for approximately 90% of the disintegrations; the other 10% convert straight to technetium-99.

Separation of daughter radionuclides. The most common method of separating daughter nuclides from their parents is by *chromatography*. The parent is adsorbed on to some binder substance such as ion exchange resin, alumina or other organic exchanger. The daughter is in a different chemical form to the parent and has less affinity for the binder so it can be separated from the parent by washing the column with a suitable eluting solution. In the case of the molybdenum-99–technetium-99m generator, the molybdenum as ammonium molybdate is adsorbed on to alumina. As the molybdenum-99 decays, technetium-99m is formed as pertechnetate. When saline is passed through the column, ion exchange takes place between the chloride and pertechnetate ions and the technetium-99m is washed off, or eluted from the column as sodium pertechnetate.

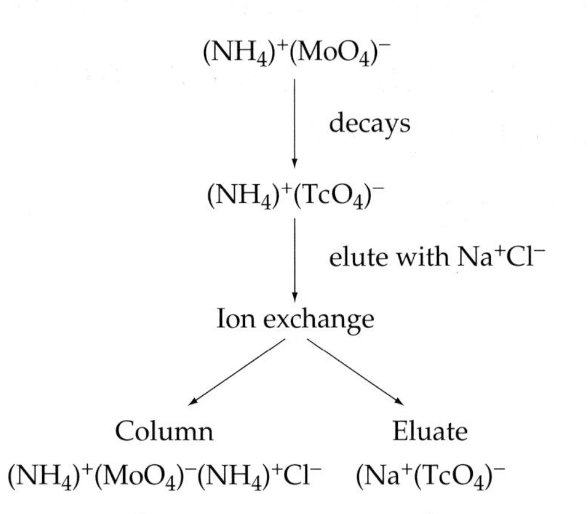

The use of technetium-99m and its pharmaceuticals will be discussed later (Ch. 8).

CHAPTER CONTENTS

4

Radiation interactions with matter

Keith Bomford

INTRODUCTION

All radiations have energy, either kinetic energy as in the case of moving charged particles, or inherent energy as in the case of electromagnetic radiation. When radiation passes through matter it may interact with the material, transferring some or all of its energy to the atoms of that material. A knowledge of the fundamentals of the interaction of radiations with matter is important because it forms the basis of radiobiology, radiation protection, radiation detection and the effective use of safe and appropriate methodologies in both radiodiagnosis and radiotherapy.

The presence of a beam of radiation is only apparent if some of the energy of the beam interacts with, and is transferred to, an absorbing material. If the radiation passes straight through a detector without interacting, then it will not be detected. Similarly, if it passes through tissue without interacting with that tissue then it will not have transferred any of its energy and hence will not have delivered a radiation dose to the tissue—by radiation dose, we mean the absorption of radiation energy. The material with which the radiation interacts, whether it is a detector or tissue, consists of atoms.

At the atomic level, the radiation can interact with the extranuclear region (Ch. 2) or the nuclear region or nuclear field (Ch. 3) or, because of the wide open spaces within the atom, it may pass straight through without interacting. How radiation interacts depends upon many factors including: the mass, energy and electrical charge of the radiation and the atomic number, mass number and density of the absorbing medium.

INTERACTIONS OF CHARGED PARTICLES WITH MATTER

In Chapter 2, we considered the interaction between the high-speed electron and the target of an X-ray tube. We shall not consider that situation again here although there will be similarities. Our concern here is the interaction of charged particles, including the electron, positron and alpha particle with matter such as tissue; we shall not consider the proton here. In Chapter 3, we saw that high-speed charged particles may be ejected from a radioactive material during radioactive decay as negative or positive beta particles, *Auger electrons* or *internal conversion* electrons. High-speed electrons may have been accelerated in a linear accelerator to produce an electron beam or, perhaps more importantly, they may be the secondary electrons resulting from photon interactions. It is these secondary charged particles which are responsible for the tissue damage attributed to X- and gamma rays.

The forces operating between the charged particles and the absorbing material are the electrostatic forces of attraction and repulsion which exist between charged bodies. The negatively charged electron will experience a repulsive force in encounters with the orbiting electrons of the atom, but an attractive force when in the vicinity of the positively charged nucleus. An alpha particle will experience the opposite interactive forces. We will now consider these interactions in more detail.

Excitation and ionisation

The charged particle may excite the atom by moving an orbital electron to a higher orbit or it may ionise the atom to form a positive and negative ion. Each of these processes depletes the energy of the incident charged particle. In Chapter 2, we saw these same two processes initiated by an incident photon (Fig. 2.2). The energy required to excite an atom may be only a few electron volts and hence the energy lost by the colliding incident particle is small and the particle will go on to produce many more interactions. When the excited atom returns to the ground state it will give off the excess energy acquired in the interaction as heat, UV, or visible light. This is the mechanism involved in scintillation counters (Ch. 5). If the incident particle completely removes an orbital electron from the atom then *ionisation* has occurred. The average energy required to form an ion pair in air is about 34 eV. If the ejected electron leaves the atom with a kinetic energy of about 100 eV then it is known as a *delta ray* and that may, in turn, cause further ionisation and excitation (Fig. 2.6A).

Electromagnetic radiation

We have seen in Chapter 2 that high-speed electrons impinging on a target will produce a continuous spectrum of X-rays and, as a result of ionisation of the target atoms, an additional line spectrum characteristic of the target material. It is important to realise now that any high-speed electrons impinging on any absorbing medium will produce similar continuous and line spectra of X-rays regardless of the circumstances. For example, the dependence of bremsstrahlung on Z means that a plastic shield is a more suitable material for protection against pure high-energy beta particle emitters such as phosphorus-32 or ruthenium-106 than the more usual high atomic number lead shields. The electron beam from a linear accelerator will inevitably be contaminated with X-rays generated within the accelerator's ionisation chamber and collimators, in the intervening air and the patient's tissues—in some circumstances, this X-ray dose may significantly affect the patient's response to treatment.

High-energy positrons may interact with the orbiting electrons of the atoms without crashing into them but they will cause excitations and ionisations in much the same way as the negative electrons. Once they have lost most of their kinetic energy and slow down they are attracted to a free electron. The opposite charges of the two particles cancel each other out and the two particles disappear, their mass being converted into energy. The *annihilation* of the two particles results in the production of two photons, each having an energy of 0.511 MeV (Fig. 4.1). We discussed in Chapter 1 that the energy equivalence ($E = mc^2$) of a positron or an electron is 0.511 MeV. The two photons are indistinguishable from gamma rays except in one respect that they leave the site of collision in diametrically opposite directions. This feature is utilised in positron detectors (p. 115).

The alpha particle carries more mass and charge than the positron. Its extra mass means that its path

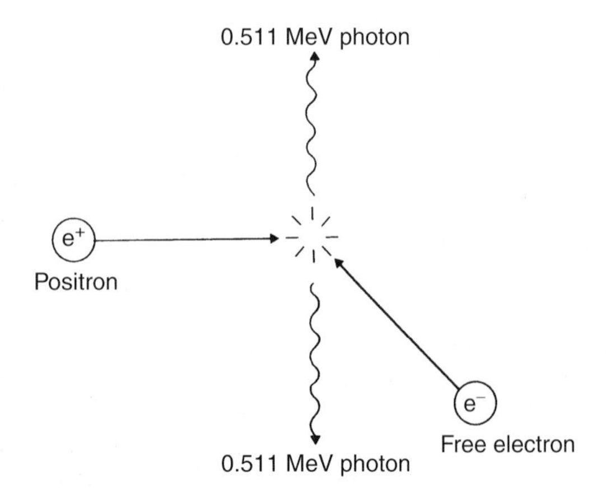

Fig. 4.1 The annihilation of a positron and an electron.

through matter is less tortuous and essentially straight and its extra charge produces more ionisations and excitations. This intense ionisation means that its path is very short and having lost its kinetic energy, the alpha particle—the helium nucleus—will attract two 'free' electrons and become a neutral helium atom.

Linear energy transfer

The energy that a particle dissipates to the absorbing medium per unit length of its path is termed the *linear energy transfer* (LET). It is usually expressed in kilo electron volts per micron (keV μm^{-1}). As a charged particle loses energy in one of the processes described above it will eventually lose all its kinetic energy until it is moving so slowly that it cannot cause further effects. An inverse relationship exists between a particle's velocity and the resulting LET. The higher the velocity or kinetic energy, the lower the LET value. The LET value for a 1 MeV electron in water is 0.25 keV μm^{-1} while at 0.1 MeV it is 0.4 keV μm^{-1}, the LET increases along the track of the particle. The LET value is also dependent upon particle type; the heavy alpha particles move straight through material, dislodging atomic electrons and losing energy very rapidly. The LET of a 1 MeV alpha particle in water is 260 keV μm^{-1} —some 1000 times greater than for the electron.

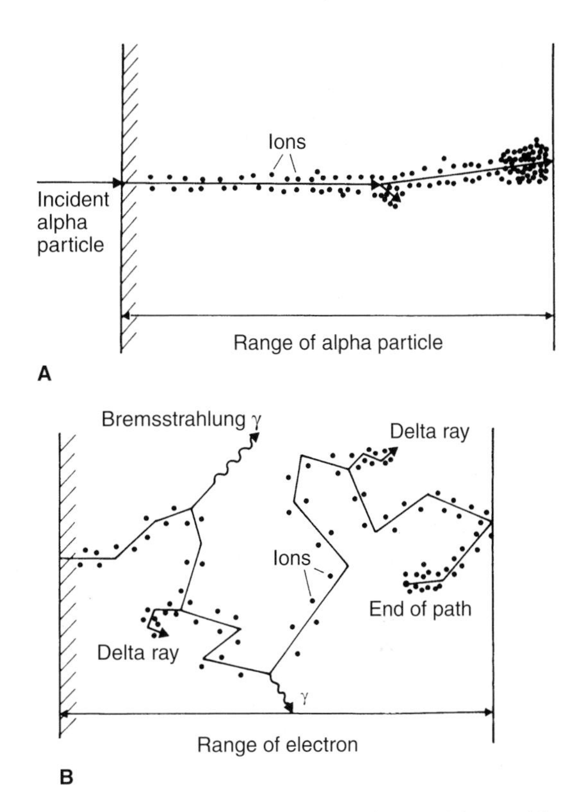

Fig. 4.2 The course through matter of **A** an alpha particle and **B** a beta particle.

Specific ionisation

The number of ion pairs produced per millimetre of path length travelled by the charged particle is called the *specific ionisation* (SI). It is directly related to the length of path along which the particle moves before being stopped and to the electrical charge on the particle and again inversely proportional to the velocity of the charged particle. Alpha particles relative to other particulate radiations are quite massive. They are not easily deflected by interactions with electrons and travel in straight lines (Fig. 4.2A). They posses a double positive electrical charge and so are highly ionising. The atomic electrons are pulled out of their orbits by the attractive force of the heavy alpha particle as it passes close by. An 8 MeV alpha particle has a range in air of 8 cm and has a specific ionisation value of about 2000 ion pairs per millimetre at the beginning of its path, rising to about 7000 ion pairs per millimetre at the end of its track. As it slows down it literally spends more time electrically influencing the atoms along its path. This is illustrated in Figure 4.3B.

Positrons and electrons carry a single electrical charge and are relatively light, having the same mass as the atomic electrons. They are easily deflected and their path through matter is tortuous (Fig. 4.2B). For these reasons their specific ionisation is much less than for an alpha particle.

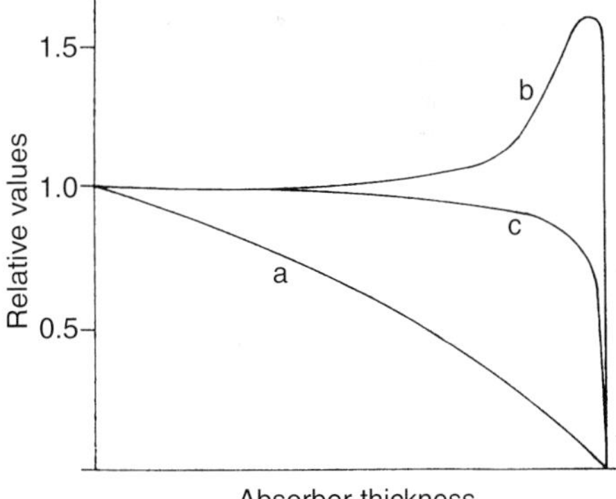

Fig. 4.3 Composite diagram of alpha particle interaction with matter: (a) particle velocity, (b) specific ionisation and (c) range.

Particle range

The furthest distance penetrated by a charged particle from its point of origin to the position at which it no

Table 4.1 The range of some alpha and beta particles in water and in tissue

Particle	Energy (MeV)	Range in air (mm)	Range in water (mm)
Alpha	1	5.0×10^0	7.0×10^{-3}
	8	7.3×10^1	1.0×10^{-1}
Beta	1	3.5×10^3	4.2×10^0
	8	3.4×10^4	4.1×10^1

longer interacts with the material is known as the *range*. The ranges of some alpha and beta particles (electrons) in air and in water are given in Table 4.1. Alpha particles have a maximum range in tissue that is always less than 0.1 mm and do not therefore constitute an external radiation hazard. However, if alpha-emitting nuclides are ingested and deposited in tissues, the alpha particles, which have high specific ionisation and LET values, will cause significant radiation damage to the tissue.

The range of an electron or positron is much greater than the range of an alpha particle of the same energy. The specific ionisation is less and hence the local radiation damage to tissue is also less than for an alpha particle. However, because of the very convoluted and tortuous path taken by the beta particle, the straight line distance between the beginning and end of the beta particle track, i.e. the range, may be only half its path length.

INTERACTIONS OF X- AND GAMMA RAYS WITH MATTER

Photons (X- and gamma rays) react with matter in a very different way from charged particles. They do not experience long-range electrostatic forces and interact only in direct collision processes. Hence the behaviour of a beam of photons differs from the behaviour of a beam of particles. Charged particles have a definite range in matter but photons are much more penetrating; having no definite range they demonstrate *exponential absorption*.

Intensity

The intensity of a beam of electromagnetic radiation is the amount of energy per unit time crossing a unit area perpendicular to the beam. For example, if 1 joule of energy passes through an area of 1 square metre every second then the intensity, I, equals 1 watt per square metre: $I = \text{W m}^{-2}$ (watts = joules/second).

Inverse square law

When a photon beam diverges from its point of production, its intensity is reduced as the distance from the source increases in a manner determined by the inverse square law. This law indicates that for radiation spreading from a point source, in a non-absorbing medium, the intensity varies inversely with the square of the distance from the source to the point of measurement.

From an uncollimated point source, the electromagnetic radiation radiates in all directions (i.e. isotropically) and each photon has an equal opportunity to pass through any chosen surface area of a sphere of radius, r, centred on the point source (Fig. 4.4). Provided there is no absorption or scattering of the beam, all the photons leaving the source will pass through the surface of the sphere. The area of the surface of any sphere is given by $4\pi r^2$. Therefore the intensity, I, at any given distance r from the source S is given by:

$$I = \frac{S}{4\pi r^2}$$

and since S and 4π are constants the intensity, I, is varying by $1/r^2$. If the power of the point source is 2012 W and we measure the intensity at distances of 2, 4 and 8 metres from the source then we find intensity values of 40, 10 and 2.5 W m^{-2} respectively.

The inverse square law holds for all electromagnetic radiations from a point source, provided there is no attenuation by absorption or scattering, whether it is collimated in a narrow beam or irradiating in all directions.

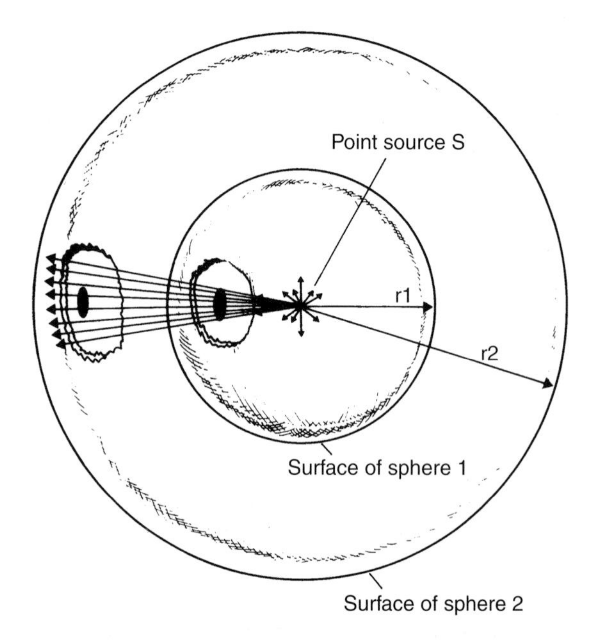

Fig. 4.4 The inverse square law.

Attenuation

When describing the attenuation of electromagnetic radiations with matter, we must consider the radiations as *waves* when describing their reflection and refraction, and as *corpuscular* when considering their origin and interactions. They carry discrete quanta (pl. of *quantum*) or packets of kinetic energy, travel at the speed of light (in vacuo), can exert forces on impact with certain objects and carry momentum. However, they have no mass and therefore can only interact with the electrical fields around electrons and positrons and the electrostatic field of the atomic nucleus. On passing through matter, photons may pass straight through without interacting with the atoms of the medium, or:

- they may be totally absorbed by the medium (photoelectric absorption), or
- they may be scattered from their original path without being absorbed (classical scattering), or
- they may be scattered and partially absorbed (Compton scattering), or
- they may be scattered and partially or completely absorbed (pair production).

Removal of radiation energy from the beam either by scattering or absorption is called *attenuation*. Attenuation of homogeneous radiation, i.e. monochromatic radiation or radiation of one wavelength, follows an exponential law, namely:

> Equal thicknesses of the same attenuating material remove equal fractions of the incident radiation intensity and that fractional reduction of intensity per unit thickness of attenuator is constant.

This law gives rise to an exponential attenuation curve (Fig. 4.5) and can be expressed by the mathematical equation:

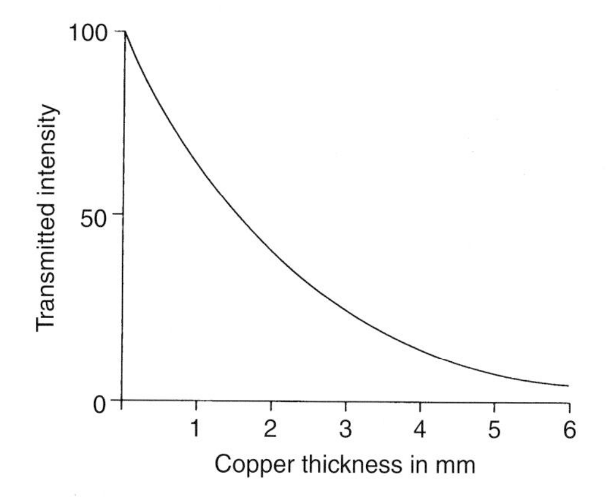

Fig. 4.5 Attenuation curve in copper for homogeneous 100 keV X-rays.

$$I_t = I_0 e^{-\mu t}$$

where I_t is the intensity transmitted through an attenuator of thickness t, I_0 is the intensity with no attenuator present, e is the mathematical constant (= 2.718) and μ is a constant for a given material and a given photon energy. μ is called the *total linear attenuation coefficient* and is defined as the fractional reduction of intensity per unit thickness of attenuator (for small thicknesses of attenuator). The product μt is the probability that a photon will be absorbed or scattered by a very thin absorber t. The attenuation of inhomogeneous beams of radiation is complicated by the fact that the value of μ is dependent on the photon energy.

The probability of a photon of electromagnetic radiation interacting with a single atom is very low. However, in a solid there is a high concentration of atoms in a small volume. In any thin layer, a proportion of its area is occupied by atoms which may block the transmission of the photons. Each atom offers a *cross-section area*, a, to the photon. The larger the value of a the greater is the chance of an interaction occurring. Figure 4.6 shows a very thin section of attenuating material having an area A and thickness δt, containing N atoms each of cross-sectional area a. The total area blocking the transmission of the photons is $aNA\delta t$. The product of the cross-section of each interaction centre (a) and the number of interaction centres (N) for a unit volume ($A\delta t$) of the target material is denoted by the symbol μ. The cross-section per unit volume, μ, varies with photon energy and atomic number, as will be seen later in this chapter. You will have noticed that cross-section per unit volume and total linear attenuation coefficient refer to the same physical quantity and are usually measured in mm^{-1}. These two terms may be used interchangeably.

The mathematical form of the attenuation curve for homogeneous beams is the same as the mathematical form of the exponential decay curve of a single radioactive material (Ch. 3). The exponential attenuation curve similarly has two characteristic properties. First, if plotted logarithmically, i.e. if log (I_t/I_0) is

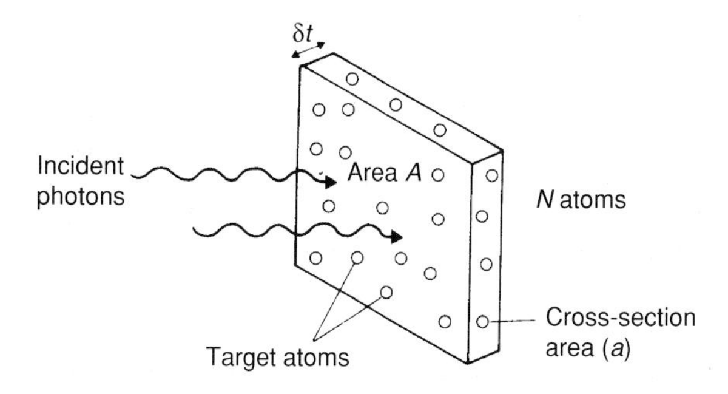

Fig. 4.6 The concept of 'cross-section' of target atoms.

plotted against t, a straight line is obtained whose slope is $-\mu$, where μ is the attenuation coefficient. Second, there is a constant value of thickness of attenuator which reduces the incident intensity to half its initial value. This is called the *half value layer* (HVL). It will be seen that the attenuation curve of Figure 4.5 corresponds to an HVL of 1.5 mm of copper. It can easily be shown that there is a simple relationship between the HVL (mm) of a homogeneous beam and the attenuation coefficient $\mu(\text{mm}^{-1})$ for a specified absorbing material, e.g. copper, namely:

$$\text{HVL} = \frac{0.693}{\mu}$$

The quantity μ, the attenuation coefficient, is a constant for a particular photon energy of the beam and for a particular attenuating material. It increases with the density and the atomic number of the attenuator and decreases with increasing photon energy of the beam.

In protective shielding and radiation dosimetry we may refer to the tenth value layer (TVL), i.e. the thickness of absorbing material which will reduce the radiation to one-tenth of its unattenuated value. This is given by: $\text{TVL} = 2.3/\mu$. A selection of HVL and TVL values are given in Table 6.4.

Mass attenuation coefficient

In Figure 4.6, the absorber of thickness δt reduces the intensity of the radiation via interactions between the photons and the electrons and atoms in the absorber. The attenuation produced will depend upon the number of atoms in the layer. If the layer could be compressed to half its thickness it would still contain the same number of atoms and hence still attenuate the same number of photons. However, the linear attenuation coefficient (attenuation per mm) would be doubled. Linear attenuation is therefore dependent on the density of the material. If the constant μ is divided by the density ρ of the attenuating material, a quantity (μ/ρ) is obtained which is independent of the density of the attenuator. This is known as the *total mass attenuation coefficient* and gives the fractional reduction of intensity if the beam passes through an attenuating layer of thickness 1 g mm^{-2}. The significance of the word 'total' in these definitions of attenuation coefficients will be explained later (p. 47).

The total mass attenuation coefficient changes rapidly with the photon energy of the beam and the atomic number of the attenuator but the relation is a complicated one. This is because attenuation, i.e. the loss of energy from the beam, arises from a number of different interaction processes. A rough guide, however, is as follows. For the low-photon-energy, long-wavelength, region of the X-ray spectrum (for diagnostic X-rays, for example), μ/ρ is roughly proportional to Z^3 and $1/(h\nu)^3$. In the high-photon-energy, short-wavelength, region of the spectrum (for high-energy radiotherapy beams) μ/ρ is roughly proportional to $1/h\nu$ and is largely independent of Z. We now look at these processes in turn.

Classical scattering

For long-wavelength low-energy radiations, that is soft diagnostic X-rays, and in materials of high atomic numbers such as metals when the energy of the photon will be much less than the binding energy of the electrons in the absorbing medium, then the photon may be scattered without loss of energy. This radiation is therefore of the same wavelength as the incident radiation. This scattering phenomenon is similar to the scattering of light from dust particles. Since it can be explained by well-established theories which treat X-rays as a wave propagation, it is often referred to as *classical scattering* or, alternatively, as elastic, unmodified or coherent scattering. It does not contribute any real absorption of energy to an attenuator since no fast electrons are liberated from the attenuating atoms. This type of scattering is relatively unimportant in health care since such low-energy X-ray beams and high atomic number attenuators are not generally used together.

Compton scattering

In practice, it is found that when more energetic radiation beams are used to irradiate materials of lower atomic number, such as tissue, the electromagnetic radiation interacts with the *free electrons* in the attenuating medium. A collision-like process occurs in which the incident photon gives up some of its energy to the electron, to be known as a *recoil* or *Compton electron*, and the remainder appears as a scattered photon of lower energy. The energy of the incident photon, therefore, is shared between the scattered photon of longer wavelength and the recoil electron. In addition, the greater the angle through which the photon is scattered the longer is the wavelength of the scattered radiation. This scattered radiation is therefore called *modified scatter* and the process is referred to as inelastic scattering or *Compton scattering* and the change in wavelength is known as the *Compton shift*.

This interaction process is represented diagrammatically in Figure 4.7. The incident photon of energy $h\nu_1$

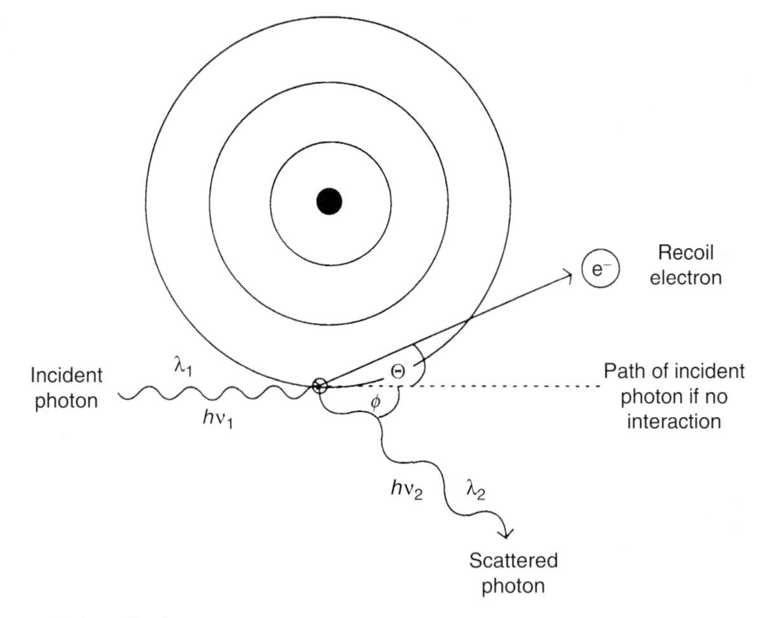

Fig. 4.7 The Compton scattering effect.

and wavelength λ_1 collides with the free electron and produces a recoil electron with kinetic energy E_e at an angle θ and a scattered photon of reduced energy $h\nu_2$ and longer wavelength λ_2 at an angle ø. Since total energy is always conserved, $h\nu_1 = h\nu_2 + E_e$, the energy of the electron and the energy of the scattered photon depend upon the original energy of the incident photon and the angle of scatter as follows:

$$h\nu_2 = \frac{h\nu_1}{1 + \frac{h\nu_1}{mc^2}(1 - \cos\phi)}$$

where mc^2 is the rest energy of the electron, 0.511 MeV. A range of energies from a maximum to a minimum are possible for the scattered photon and the recoil electron; however, their values are inversely related as the total energy must remain the same as the energy of the incident photon. The minimum scattered photon energy occurs when the incident photon makes a direct hit, ejecting the electron straight forward ($\theta = 0$) and scattering the Compton photon backwards through 180° (cos 180° = –1 and hence (1 – cos ø) = +2). Conversely, the maximum scattered photon energy occurs when the incident photon makes only a glancing collision with the electron ejecting it with an angle θ of ~0° and scattering the Compton photon with an angle of *0°* (cos *0°* = +1 and hence (1 – cos ø = 0). Any intermediate values are possible and Table 4.2 gives values of the energies of the scattered photon and the recoil electron for a selection of incident photon energies and scattering angles.

It is worth noting that the change in photon wavelength—the so-called Compton shift—is solely dependent on the angle of scatter, ø, and independent of the incident photon energy and the absorber:

$$\lambda_2 - \lambda_1 = 0.024\ (1 - \cos ø)$$

Table 4.2 Energies of Compton scattered photons and recoil electrons

Incident photon energy (MeV)	Angle ø of scattered photon: 30°		90°		120°		180°	
	$h\nu_2$	E_e	$h\nu_2$	E_e	$h\nu_2$	E_e	$h\nu_2$	E_e
0.05	0.049	0.001	0.046	0.004	0.044	0.006	0.042	0.008
0.10	0.097	0.003	0.084	0.016	0.077	0.023	0.072	0.028
0.50	0.442	0.058	0.253	0.247	0.202	0.298	0.169	0.331
1.00	0.792	0.208	0.338	0.662	0.254	0.746	0.204	0.796

It can be seen from Table 4.2 that low-energy photons do not lose much energy upon scattering. The 50 keV photon loses at maximum only 8 keV. On the other hand the higher-energy 1 MeV photon loses 796 keV of energy upon 180° scattering. The proportion of photons scattered in different directions varies with the energy of the incident photon; low-energy photons are scattered in all directions with almost equal probability, whilst high-energy photons, greater than about 1 MeV, are scattered principally in the forward direction (i.e. $ø < 90°$). (θ is always $<90°$ and both ø and θ tend to zero as the incident photon energy increases.)

The *recoil electron* behaves the same as any electron, it is so named to indicate its origin. Since the recoil electron has been given kinetic energy it can now undergo the various types of electron particle interactions described earlier in this chapter. It is the recoil electron resulting from the Compton collision which causes the radiation damage to the tissue, not the initial photon interaction which has created only one ion directly.

We stated that the photons interact with *free electrons*. The term 'free' refers to those electrons whose binding energy is negligibly small compared to the energy of the incident photon. The binding energy of the outer electrons in light elements, such as the primary building blocks of soft tissue, is only a few electron volts (eV). This is quite small compared to the energy of a diagnostic X-ray photon—which is generally more than 50 kV—and very small compared with the megavoltage photons used in radiotherapy.

Mass absorption and scatter coefficients

The Compton effect occurs with free electrons so the cross-section σ can be expressed in terms of target area per electron. Therefore, with the exception of hydrogen, the Compton effect is independent of atomic number. This is because:

- all electrons have the same cross-section for interaction with photons of a given energy, and
- the ratio of neutrons to protons is similar for all elements and hence all elements contain approximately the same number of electrons per gram ($\sim 3 \times 10^{23}$).

Hydrogen is an exception to this as it contains no neutrons and the number of electrons per gram is twice that of other elements ($\sim 6 \times 10^{23}$). The significance of this is discussed in Chapter 12. It follows that for the Compton process and for any given photon energy, the attenuation per gram and the mass attenuation coefficient σ/ρ is the same for all materials except hydrogen (and hydrogen compounds) and inversely proportional to the photon energy. The mass attenuation, absorption and scattering coefficients for different incident photon energies are depicted graphically in Figure 4.8. These three coefficients, assuming the recoil electron does not produce significant bremsstrahlung radiation, are related as follows:

$$\sigma/\rho = \sigma_a/\rho + \sigma_s/\rho$$

The mass absorption coefficient for Compton scattering, σ_a/ρ, represents the energy transferred to the recoil electron, and hence deposited in the absorbing medium. It increases with increasing energy up to about 1 MeV and then decreases again, whilst the mass scattering coefficient, σ_s/ρ, representing the proportion of the energy removed by the scattered photon, decreases with increasing incident energy. The two curves intersect at about 1.5 MeV; this is the point at which the scattered photon and the recoil electron carry away equal amounts of energy. At energies below 1.5 MeV, the greater fraction is removed by the scattered photon. Above 1.5 MeV the greater fraction is removed by the recoil electron. The higher the incident photon energy, the greater is the proportion of that energy which is given up to the electron.

Summary of the Compton process

- The wavelength of the scattered radiation increases with the angle of scattering relative to the incident beam increases.
- The energy of the incident beam is shared between recoil electrons in the attenuator and scattered photons of longer wavelength. If the photon energy

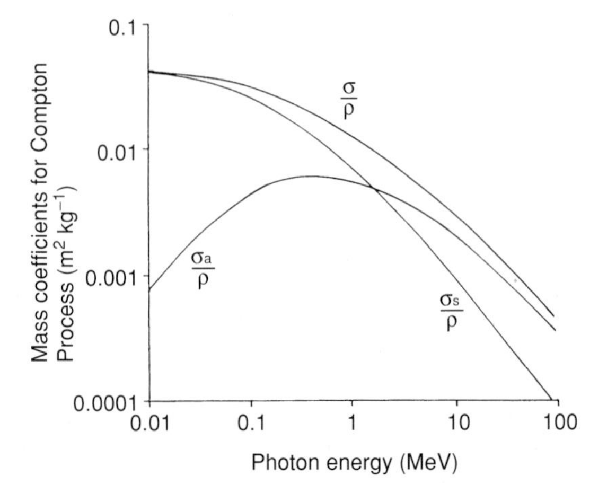

Fig. 4.8 The mass attenuation (σ/ρ), absorption (σ_a/ρ) and scattering (σ_s/ρ) coefficients for Compton scattering.

of the incident beam is low, the proportion of the energy appearing as scattered radiation is high, but for incident beams of high photon energy the majority of the energy lost from the beam appears as kinetic energy of recoil electrons.

- As the incident photon energy increases, the scattered radiation is concentrated more and more in the forward direction.
- The recoil electrons are emitted in the forward direction and are increasingly concentrated in the direction of the incident beam as the energy of the incident photons increases.
- The total attenuation of a beam produced by the Compton process is independent of the atomic number of the attenuator (except for hydrogen) but decreases as the photon energy of the radiation increases.

Photoelectric absorption

The photoelectric process involves an interaction between an incident photon and a *bound electron*. We saw earlier that if the incident photon had low energy compared to the binding energy then classical scattering occurs. If, however, the incident photon has an energy just greater than the binding energy of the electron the photon is totally absorbed and a complete transfer of the photon energy to the electron occurs. This is shown schematically in Figure 4.9. If a photon of energy $h\nu$ ejects, say, a K shell electron of binding energy BE_K, the electron escapes from the atom with a kinetic energy E_e equal to that of the incident photon minus the energy required to release it from its orbit.

$$E_e = h\nu - BE_K$$

There is no scattered photon; the incident photon is completely absorbed and all its energy has been transferred to the electron, known as a *photoelectron*. By definition, E_e is small and the track length of the photoelectron is very short (Table 4.3). Interactions of this kind may take place with electrons in the K, L, M and N shells.

The probability of a photoelectric process occurring depends upon the incident photon energy. Figure 4.10 shows the mass attenuation coefficient for the photoelectric process, τ/ρ, plotted against incident photon energy for two materials, lead and water (tissue equivalent). For water, the graph is a rapidly falling straight line, the mass attenuation coefficient is approximately inversely proportional to the cube of the photon energy: $\tau/\rho \propto 1/(h\nu)^3$.

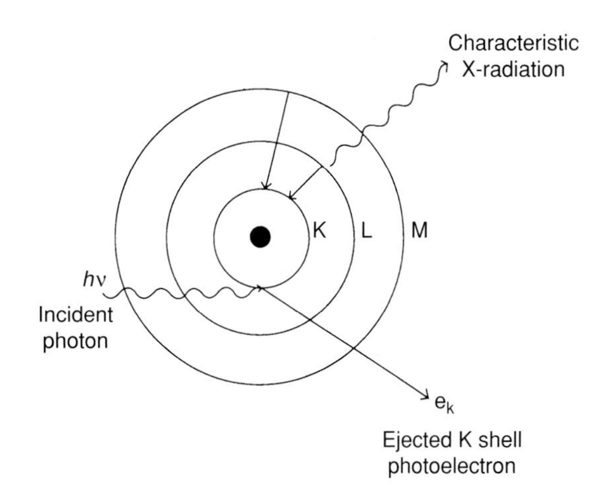

Fig. 4.9 Photoelectric absorption and the emission of a photoelectron with the subsequent emission of characteristic X-rays.

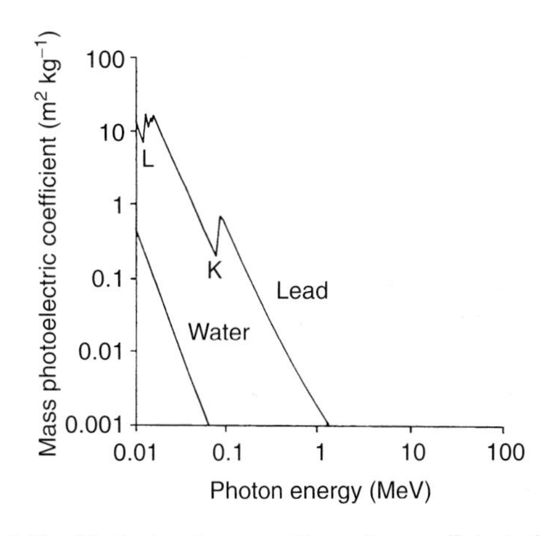

Fig. 4.10 Photoelectric mass attenuation coefficients for water and lead.

Table 4.3 Some examples of the electron ranges involved in the attenuation processes

Photon energy of incident radiation	Energy of electrons		Range in tissue
50 keV	Photoelectron	50 keV	42 μm
	Recoil electron	4–8 keV	0.5–1.7 μm
250 keV	Recoil electron	50 keV	42 μm
1 MeV	Recoil electron	500 keV	2 mm
8 MeV	Recoil electron	5 MeV	28 mm

For lead, the picture is a little more complicated. The graph shows a series of vertical *absorption edges* with straight portions between them. The probability of a photoelectric interaction occurring is greatest when the photon energy is equal to or just greater than the binding energy of the electron and decreases rapidly thereafter. If the photon has sufficient energy to liberate a K shell electron it will transfer its energy to that electron rather than to one further from the nucleus. The K absorption edge for lead occurs at 88 keV, which is the binding energy of the K shell in lead. At this point the attenuation coefficient increases by a factor of about 5. Thus there is about a 5 : 1 preference for the K shell electrons over the other shells. If the energy of the incident photon is less than the binding energy of the K shell the photon will transfer its energy to a less tightly bound electron, e.g. in the L shell, always preferring the inner to the outer shells. In the straight portions between the edges, the mass attenuation coefficient is again reduced by approximately $1/(h\nu)^3$ as the energy of the incident photon increases. However, this law does not apply at the edges and a high-energy photon may have a higher mass attenuation coefficient than a lower-energy one. Figure 4.10 also demonstrates that the attenuation coefficient in lead may be approximately 1000 times greater than in water.

The mass attenuation coefficient is also approximately proportional to the cube of the atomic number. Hence:

$$\tau/\rho \propto \frac{Z^3}{(h\nu)^3}$$

This is an important factor in producing high contrast between bone and soft tissue and in the use of lead in radiation protection in diagnostic radiography.

Characteristic radiation

Since the photoelectric process ionises the atom of the attenuator, a vacant space is left in that electron shell. A readjustment is made by electrons falling from outer shells into the vacancies producing *characteristic X-rays* and *Auger electrons*. This shell-filling process is the same as that following internal conversion described in Chapter 3; it should also be compared, but not confused, with the emission of characteristic radiation from an X-ray target (Ch. 2).

The photoelectric interaction prevails over Compton scattering for low-energy photons and high-atomic-number absorbing materials. The atom completely absorbs the photon in a photoelectric event and the energy of the photon is converted into electron energy. Once again, it is the secondary photoelectron which transfers the energy to the absorbing material and produces the radiation damage in tissue.

Summary of the photoelectric process

- All of the energy of the incident beam is given up to the photoelectron.
- Characteristic X-rays and Auger electrons may be produced.
- The probability of occurrence increases with the cube of the atomic number of the absorbing medium.
- The probability of occurrence decreases with the cube of the photon energy except when the energy is just greater than the binding energy of the electrons, at which point absorption edges occur.

Pair production

One further interaction process occurs for photons whose energy is greater than 1.022 MeV. Photons of energy greater than this threshold may interact with the electric field around the nucleus. This interaction results in the complete absorption of the photon and the simultaneous creation of two electrons, one positive and one negative (sometimes referred to as a *positron* and a *negatron* respectively), as shown in Figure 4.11. This *pair production* process represents the creation of matter from energy. This has been discussed in Chapter 1 where we saw the energy equivalent to the mass of one electron to be 0.511 MeV. In order to create two electrons, therefore, a minimum energy of 1.022 MeV is necessary. Since the electrons are opposite in charge, no creation of charge is involved. If the energy of the initiating photon $h\nu$ is greater than 1.022 MeV then the excess energy will appear as kinetic energy, E, and be shared between the two particles:

$$h\nu = mc^2 + mc^2 + E^+ + E^-$$

Thus for an 8 MeV photon the sum of the kinetic energies for the two particles will be 8 – 1.022 = 6.978 MeV. The most probable distribution is for this energy to be shared equally between the positron and the electron, but this is not necessarily the case. Just as in the case of Compton scattering and the photoelectric process, the kinetic energy of each particle is then dissipated in the absorbing medium.

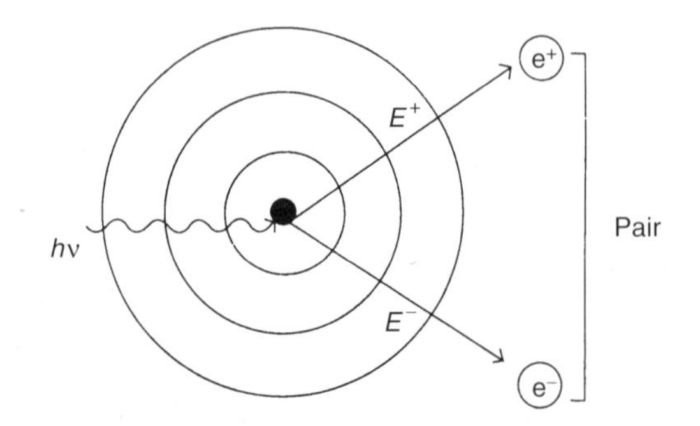

Fig. 4.11 The absorption of photons by pair production.

As we have seen previously, the positive electron does not have an isolated existence for, when it comes to rest, it combines with a neighbouring negative electron. The two charges neutralise each other and the mass of the two electrons is converted back into two photons of electromagnetic radiation, each of 0.511 MeV energy, travelling in opposite directions to each other. This *is annihilation radiation* and was shown in Figure 4.1.

The mass absorption coefficient for pair production is represented by π/ρ. Above the threshold energy of 1.022 MeV, the probability of the process occurring increases rapidly with photon energy but it does not become the dominant process in water below about 30 MeV. The cross-section for the pair production process also increases with increasing atomic number of the attenuator. This is because pair production occurs in the nuclear field, and the electric field around the nucleus increases with increasing Z. Thus:

$$\pi/\rho \propto (h\nu - 1.022)\,Z$$

In practice this process is of little importance in the low-atomic-number elements of soft tissue except above about 20 MeV radiation. In industrial radiography, however, when high-energy beams are used to penetrate metals it can become the major attenuation process.

Summary of the pair production process

- An electron and a positron are produced.
- The photon energy must be at least 1.022 MeV.
- The probability of occurrence increases with increasing energy ($h\nu - 1.022$) and with increasing atomic number.

Summary of interaction processes

All four processes are involved in the loss of energy from a beam of photons passing through an attenuating material. Three of these processes give rise to deposition of energy in the attenuator, via secondary charged particle interactions. They are:

- the photoelectric process
- that part of the Compton process that gives rise to recoil electrons, and
- the pair production process.

The rest of the energy lost to the main beam either escapes from the attenuator as scattered radiation or gives rise to further interactions remote from the first. These include:

- classical scattering of long waves
- the characteristic radiation following the photoelectric process
- the scatter component of the Compton effect, and
- the annihilation radiation arising from the pair production process.

Total mass attenuation coefficient

When a single photon interacts with matter any one of the processes described above may occur. When a beam of photons interacts with matter all of them may occur. The total mass attenuation coefficient discussed at the beginning of this section is composed of contributions from each of the processes. Thus:

μ/ρ	$= \sigma/\rho$	$+ \tau/\rho$	$+ \pi/\rho$
Total	Compton	Photoelectric	Pair production

The total mass attenuation coefficient, being the sum of the three partial attenuation coefficients, varies in a complicated way with both photon energy, $h\nu$, and atomic number, Z. The total mass attenuation coefficient and the relative contribution of the individual coefficients for water and for lead are shown in Figure 4.12. At the lower energies, the rapid variation of the photoelectric effect with $h\nu$ and Z is the dominating influence and the total attenuation curves fall rapidly with increasing energy. The absorption edges are pronounced in the higher atomic number materials. The curves decrease more slowly in the region where the Compton effect is the important influence. The Compton effect is independent of atomic number and is therefore similar for both tissue and lead. Finally the curve rises slightly at high energies owing to pair production. For soft tissue the rise in total coefficient at high energies is negligible as the decrease in Compton effect is matched by the increase in pair production. However, in lead the rise in the curve at high energies is quite marked. Hence, for high-atomic-number materials, increasing the energy of the photon results in a less penetrating beam. Figure 4.13 shows the percentage contribution to the total attenuation of each of the three processes. It can be seen that for water (soft tissue) the Compton process dominates over a wider range of energies (0.03–20 MeV) than for lead where the photoelectric effect and pair production are the more important.

These curves have important implications for the differential absorption of photons in bone and soft tissue and for the choice of absorbing materials in radiation protection. Where photoelectric absorption predominates, the bone will absorb approximately six times as much energy as soft tissue. For diagnostic-

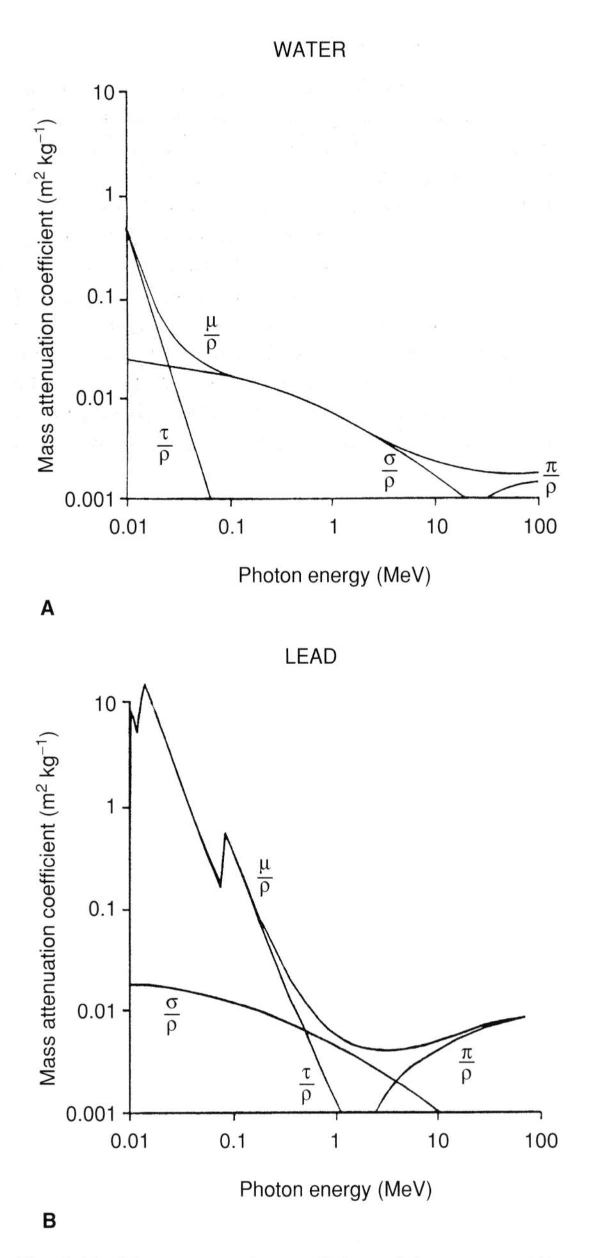

Fig. 4.12 Mass attenuation coefficients **A** for water and **B** for lead.

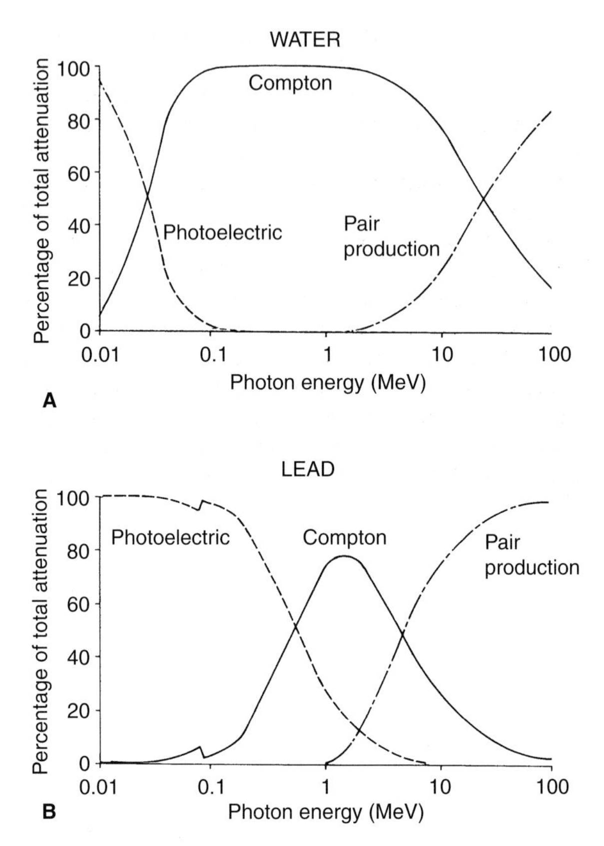

Fig. 4.13 The percentage contribution to the total attenuation from each of the three processes **A** in water and **B** in lead.

X-rays operating between 50 and 150 kV this will give good contrast in the image. When Compton absorption is the dominant process, bone and soft tissue absorb approximately the same amount of energy per gram. This is advantageous in radiotherapy, particularly when treating tumours through, or overlying, bony structures. Pair production is only of importance with very high photon energies when bone will absorb approximately twice as much energy per gram as soft tissue.

Real energy absorption

When a beam of electromagnetic radiation is attenuated in a medium, all the interaction processes involved give rise to some form of electromagnetic radiation as a secondary product. This radiation does not cause the direct deposition of energy to the attenuating medium though, as scattered radiation, it has important effects both in diagnostic radiology and in radiotherapy and is very important from the point of view of radiation hazard control. Energy is only transferred to the attenuating medium through the production of fast electrons which produce ionisation in the medium. Real energy absorption arises therefore from photoelectrons, the recoil electrons of the Compton process and the pair of electrons in the pair production process. In terms of partial attenuation coefficients, therefore, real energy absorption over the main range of photon energies used in radiotherapy can be represented by the coefficients: $\tau/\rho + \sigma_a/\rho$ where τ/ρ is the mass photoelectric attenuation coefficient and σ_a/ρ is the mass attenuation coefficient representing the conversion of the incident photon energy to energy of recoil electrons in the Compton process. We have seen that σ_a/ρ is an increasingly high proportion of the coefficient σ/ρ for the whole Compton attenuation process as the photon energy increases. For very high photon energy beams where the pair production process becomes important, an additional contribution to real energy absorption in the medium will arise from the kinetic energy of the two electrons produced in the interaction. Calculations on the real energy absorbed using these partial attenuation coefficients are relevant to the subject of dose measurement discussed in the next chapter.

Electron ranges in tissue

The ranges of the electrons responsible for the ionisation in the attenuating medium and therefore for the deposition of energy, vary with the incident photon energy (Table 4.3). For X-rays in the diagnostic range the ranges in tissue are very small and the deposition of energy is local. At the high photon energies used in megavoltage radiotherapy, the electron ranges become larger, being of the order of several millimetres, and the deposition of energy may be remote from the primary interaction. They thus become comparable with the size of the coarse structure of the tissues being treated. The range then has profound effects on the distribution of absorbed energy in tissues. This will be dealt with in Chapter 12.

CHAPTER CONTENTS

5 Measurement and detection of X- and gamma rays

Keith Bomford

INTRODUCTION

In this chapter we describe in some detail the methods by which reliable quantitative measurements of X- and gamma rays can be obtained and used in radiotherapy. The primary interaction processes discussed in the last chapter showed that the initial effect of radiation on matter is to produce ionisation. This ionisation precipitates biological damage in living tissues and it is vital that we can measure it with a degree of accuracy consistent with the measure of the damage it can cause. It is possible to seek a quantitative estimate of the total flow of photons through a point in space or in tissue being irradiated by an X- or gamma ray beam by measuring the ionisation produced in air or in an appropriate air cavity within an irradiated medium respectively. The quantity so measured is referred to as *exposure*. On the other hand, energy is only absorbed in an irradiated medium when secondary electrons deposit their kinetic energy. This energy is the absorbed energy and a quantitative estimate of this is referred to as the *absorbed dose*. Both of these concepts of measurement are in use and it is important to distinguish between them.

An illustration might help to clarify the difference. When one moves around the garden in sunlight one is bombarded from all sides by photons of light of a variety of wavelengths (colours). Some of these are the primary photons from the sun and some are scattered photons from the environment. This photon flux is equivalent to exposure. One is exposed to light. However, some of these photons enter the eye and by producing chemical changes on the retina impart visual information, while others enter the skin and produce chemical changes leading to pigmentation. They equate to absorbed dose. Exposure and absorbed dose are clearly related to each other. The second is proportional to the first but the constant of proportionality will depend on a variety of conditions. In tissues being irradiated, the constant of proportionality will depend on the relative magnitudes of the different processes of attenuation and therefore on the photon energy distribution in the irradiating field and on the atomic number of the medium.

The dependence of the absorption coefficients on photon energy and atomic number are seen in this chapter in two forms of *differential absorption*:

- photons of the same energy will be differentially absorbed in different tissues, and
- photons of different energy will be differentially absorbed in the same tissue.

The concept of exposure

(Exposure in this context is a precisely defined technical term and must not be confused with the concept of mAs (p. 98) used in diagnostic radiography.) *Exposure* is a measure of the photon flux (or flow of photons) to which the point of interest (in air) is subjected in a given time. It is a measure of the amount of ionisation (the number of ions) produced in a unit mass of air under standard conditions. The formal definition of *exposure*, adopted by the International Commission on Radiological Units (ICRU 1980), is:

$$X = \Delta Q / \Delta m$$

where ΔQ is the sum of the electrical charge on all the ions of one sign produced in air when all the electrons liberated by *photons* in a volume element of *air* whose mass is Δm are completely stopped in air. (NB: Exposure is only defined in terms of photons in air.) There is no special SI unit for exposure and the units are simply coulombs per kilogram (C/kg) of dry air. Previously, the special unit of exposure was the roentgen (R) and defined as 'that amount of X- or gamma radiation such that the associated corpuscular emission per 0.001293 g of dry air produces, in air, ions carrying one electrostatic unit of charge of either sign'. The density of dry air at standard temperature and pressure is 0.001293 g cm^{-3}. 1 R = 2.58×10^{-4} C/kg. This definition is less precise than the ICRU definition quoted above but it helps to explain the conditions under which measurements of exposure are made—as illustrated by the description of the standard free air ionisation chamber (p. 58).

The concept of kerma

A high-energy recoil electron can travel a considerable distance in air and produces ionisation throughout the length of its track (p. 39). Since the definition of exposure demands that all such electrons liberated by photons are completely stopped in air, the collection of charge could be very remote from the elemental mass of air, Δm, where the electron originated. The roentgen was never defined above about 3 MeV for this reason. However, the number of ionisations produced by a high-speed electron is determined principally by its initial kinetic energy, since the energy required to produce one ionisation in air is constant. This concept of the kinetic energy of the electrons liberated is given the name *kerma*—an acronym for the kinetic energy released per unit mass—and defined by ICRU as:

$$K = \Delta E_{\mathrm{tr}} / \Delta m$$

where ΔE_{tr} is the sum of the initial kinetic energies of all the charged particles liberated by uncharged ionising particles in a material of mass Δm. The suffix denotes the energy transferred to the particles. Since kerma is an energy per unit mass, its units are joules per kilogram or grays. The reader will note that the use of kerma is not confined to photons-in-air as was the case with exposure, but a quantity called *air kerma*, K_{air}, can be defined and related to exposure.

The concept of absorbed dose

While kerma is a measure of the energy *released* by photons in a small mass of absorber, that energy may not be totally *deposited* in the same small mass but carried by the energetic electrons to be deposited in neighbouring masses of the absorber. Our major interest in radiotherapy is the energy actually deposited in a small mass and this we call the *absorbed dose* or simply *dose*. ICRU defines absorbed dose as:

$$D = \Delta E_{\mathrm{d}} / \Delta m$$

where ΔE_{d} is the energy imparted by ionising radiation to the matter in a volume element of mass Δm. Unlike that of exposure, this definition encompasses all absorbing materials and all types of ionising radiation. The special unit of absorbed dose is the *gray*, where 1 Gy = 1 J/kg. The old unit of absorbed dose, the rad (= 0.01 J/kg) has been replaced by the gray, although the centigray (1 cGy = 1 rad) has come into common usage for obvious reasons. The gray is also used as a measure of kerma.

Conversion from exposure to absorbed dose

Absorbed dose in many cases is difficult to measure and is usually calculated from the measurement of exposure and the knowledge of the real mass absorption coefficients of air and tissue. From the definition of mass absorption coefficient (p. 42), we have:

$$(\mu_a/\rho) = \frac{\text{Energy absorbed per unit mass}}{\text{Energy in the beam}}$$

This equation is true for any absorbing medium and, being true for both tissue and air, it follows that:

$$\frac{(\mu_a/\rho)_{tissue}}{(\mu_a/\rho)_{air}} = \frac{\text{Energy absorbed per unit mass of tissue}}{\text{Energy absorbed per unit mass of air}}$$

Now, if the charge on one electron, e, is 1.6×10^{-19} C and the average energy required to produce one ionisation (one electron or one ion pair) in air, W, is 5.44×10^{-18} J, then the energy required to produce one coulomb of charge is $W/e = 5.44 \times 10^{-18}/1.6 \times 10^{-19} = 33.97$ J/C. Therefore:

$$\text{Dose in air (grays), } D_{air} = 33.97X \text{ (J/kg)}$$

and by substitution in the equation above:

$$\text{Dose in tissue (grays), } D_{tissue} = FX \text{ (J/kg)}$$

$$\text{where} \quad F = 33.97 \frac{(\mu_a/\rho)_{tissue}}{(\mu_a/\rho)_{air}} \text{ (J/C)}$$

Although for most purposes, the F-factor will be that for soft tissue and energy dependent (Table 5.1), it is instructive to realise that a different factor will apply to other body tissues—bone and fat, for instance—owing to the differences in their atomic numbers. Bone, for example, has an atomic number ($Z \cong 13.8$) nearly twice that of soft tissue ($Z \cong 7.4$) and a lower hydrogen content. Gram for gram therefore the dose to bone is several times greater than that to soft tissue at low photon energies, while at higher energies it is less (Fig. 5.1). Armed with this information, any measurement of the exposure, X, at a point can be converted into absorbed dose by multiplying by an appropriate F-factor. This is true for the range of photon energies for which exposure can be measured—up to cobalt-60 or 2 MV.

Table 5.1 Typical values of the F-factor for soft tissue

Beam quality	F-factor (J/C)
1 mm Al HVL	34.0
4 mm Al HVL	34.0
2 mm Cu HVL	36.5
Cobalt-60	37.0
4 MV	36.5
6 MV	36.5
10 MV	36.0

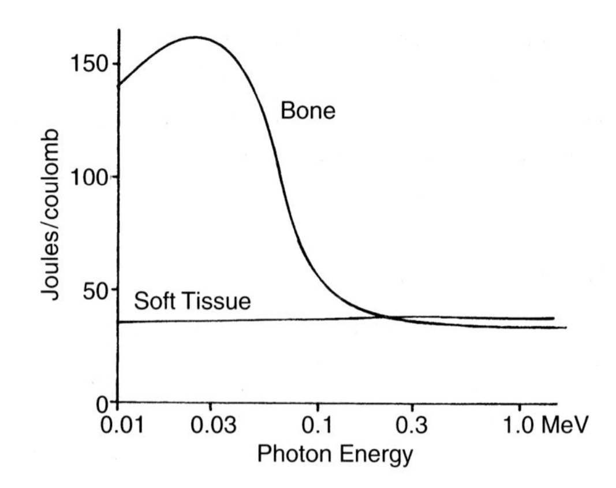

Fig. 5.1 The relative absorption in bone and soft tissue.

Conversion from kerma to absorbed dose

Under conditions of electronic equilibrium, all the kinetic energy released in a unit mass of air may be absorbed in the air and none is lost in bremsstrahlung (X-ray) production in which case:

$$\Delta E_{tr} = \Delta E_d$$

and

$$\text{Dose in air, } D_{air} = K_{air} = 33.97X \text{ J kg}^{-1}$$

but, if the energy liberated, ΔDE_{tr}, is not all absorbed and some is lost to bremsstrahlung production, then

$$\text{Dose in air, } D_{air} = K_{air} \frac{(\mu_a/\rho)_{air}}{(\mu_{tr}/\rho)_{air}}$$

where (μ_a/ρ) is the mass energy absorption coefficient and (μ_{tr}/ρ) is the *mass energy transfer coefficient* and the ratio accounts for the energy lost in bremsstrahlung production. (The ratio increases with energy, being approximately 1.003 for cobalt-60 photons.) It follows that:

$$\text{Dose in soft tissue, } D_{tissue} = K_{air} \frac{(\mu_a/\rho)_{tissue}}{(\mu_{tr}/\rho)_{air}}$$

PRACTICAL IONISATION CHAMBERS

Three aspects of the free air chamber (p. 57) must be applied to practical ionisation chambers, these are:

- The chamber must operate under saturation conditions

- The chamber must have an air (equivalent) wall
- The contained air mass must be known.

The latter requires the chamber to be sealed and contain a fixed mass of air or to be open to atmosphere and of fixed volume.

Thimble chamber

For clinical purposes the exposure at a point can be measured using a thimble ionisation chamber. This term describes an ionisation chamber in which a small volume of air (typically < 1 ml) is enclosed in a thimble-like conducting cap insulated from an axial collecting electrode (Fig. 5.2A). The cap is often made of a unit density material such as graphite, of nylon made conducting on the inner surface by a layer of colloidal graphite, or of Shonka® plastic. The central electrode may be aluminium. The insulator may be amber but Perspex and polythene are often used. When a potential difference (usually a few hundred volts) is maintained between the cap and the collecting electrode and radiation falls on the chamber, the contained air will be ionised and an ionisation current will flow between the two electrodes. The *polarising voltage* must not be so large that it causes ionisation of the air enclosed in the chamber but large enough to prevent ion recombination (p. 56 and Fig. 5.6).

Such a chamber will give an accurate measure of the exposure providing (a) the walls are made of a material with the same atomic number as air and (b) the wall has a thickness greater than the range of the secondary electrons produced in the material. A chamber wall of unit density material 1 mm thick would be equivalent to approximately 75 cm of air. The actual wall thickness required is determined by the energy of the radiation to be measured. For low-energy radiations a very thin-walled chamber is required (e.g. 2 mg cm^{-2}) as the electron range in the material is small and the radiation would be attenuated by a thicker wall before reaching the enclosed air. In practice, because the chamber wall will be of fixed thickness, the calibration factor, N, increases rapidly as the photon energy falls (Fig. 5.2B). On the other hand, as the energy increases, the thickness of the chamber wall may need to be increased to maintain electronic equilibrium. For example, a close-fitting build-up cap of some 4 mm of unit density material will be added to such a chamber to measure cobalt-60 radiation—gross errors result if the build-up cap is omitted!

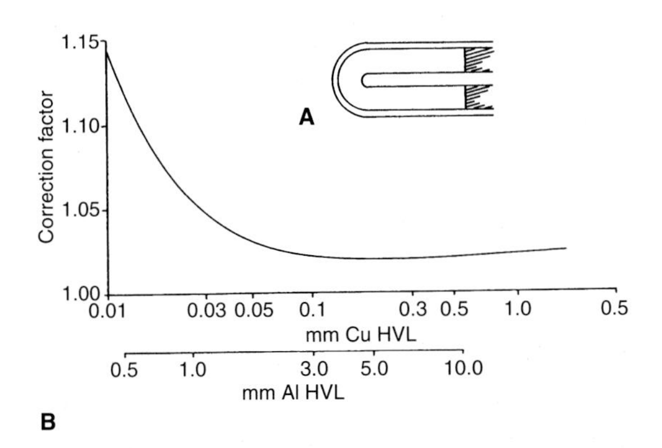

Fig. 5.2 A A thimble ionisation chamber and **B** a typical correction curve for its energy response, the energy is shown here in terms of HVL.

The volume of the chamber required depends on the sensitivity of the measuring system and on the intensity (or exposure rate) of the radiation to be measured. The exposure rate in the useful beam of the therapy unit may be conveniently measured using a chamber volume of approximately 0.5 ml while the leakage radiation through the treatment room walls will require a chamber of 200–1000 ml (Fig. 6.2).

Errors are introduced into the measurement of exposure if the chamber wall material has an atomic number which differs from that of air, especially in measurements at depth in a tissue-equivalent phantom where the low-energy scatter is absorbed via the photoelectric effect. At higher energies discrepancies in atomic number are less pronounced.

The measurement of exposure (rate)

The thimble chamber measures the ionisation at a particular point—usually taken to be the centre of the chamber for photon beams, but forward of centre for electron beams depending on the design of the chamber. The thimble chamber may be used to measure total exposure, X, or to measure exposure rate. From the definitions of exposure and exposure rate, it can be seen that to measure exposure, the total charge released, ΔQ, must be determined, while to measure exposure rate the ionisation current, $\Delta Q/t$, is required. Thus, to measure total exposure, the potential difference developed across a *capacitor* is measured, and to measure exposure rate, the potential difference developed across a *resistor* is measured. It is, of course, possible to determine the exposure rate by measuring the exposure and dividing by the duration of the exposure, but this assumes the exposure rate is constant—an assumption that is not always valid.

The two electrodes separated by a very good insulator which go to make an ionisation chamber may be thought of as an electrical capacitor and a means of storing electrical charge. When such a *capacitor-chamber* is irradiated, the ionisation will cause some of the stored charge to leak away and, providing the polarising voltage is sufficient to maintain saturation, the change in charge will be directly proportional to the total exposure given to the chamber and measured by determining the change in the potential difference across the chamber. This may be interpreted mathematically as follows: If the electrical capacitance of the ionisation chamber is C, then the storage of a charge Q will produce a potential difference (the polarising voltage) across the capacitor of V where $V = Q/C$. If now an exposure, X, is given to the chamber resulting in an ionisation of ΔQ then the potential difference will fall by ΔV where $\Delta V = \Delta Q/C$. Thus, the exposure, X, will be given by $C\Delta V/m$, where m is the mass of air enclosed in the chamber.

This type of capacitor-chamber has the particular advantage that it is possible to use many chambers with only one charging/measuring instrument as the chambers will not be connected to the instrument during exposure. This system could, therefore, be used to measure the exposure at various points in the beam during a single irradiation.

On the other hand, a permanent connection to the measuring device enables the exposure to be integrated and the polarising voltage to be maintained throughout the irradiation. A simplified circuit of a direct-reading exposure meter, based on the popular Farmer exposure meter, is illustrated in Figure 5.3A. The chamber is connected via a screened flexible cable to the exposure meter. (The purpose of the screen is to counter the effects of external electromagnetic signals.) The polarising voltage causes the ions to flow through the collecting electrode onto the capacitor C, thereby increasing the potential difference across the capacitor. This rise in the grid voltage applied to the (triode) electrometer valve V, causes a change in the anode current and the null meter N, to deflect. This deflection is corrected by adjusting the potentiometer T (the Townsend balance) to lower the grid voltage to its initial value. The voltmeter R then measures the change in the potential difference across the capacitor C and can be calibrated in air kerma or grays depending on whether the chamber is used in air or water respectively. The function of the electrometer valve V is simply to amplify the small change in grid voltage, thereby increasing the sensitivity of the instrument. As mentioned before, the ionisation current in the chamber is very small, $\sim 10^{-10}$ A. A similar circuit using an operational amplifier in place of the electrometer valve is shown in Figure 5.3B.

If the Townsend balance is omitted and the integrating capacitor C in the circuit (Fig. 5.3A) is replaced by a very high resistor (say 10^{10} ohms), then the ionisation current will flow through the resistor and develop a potential difference (Ohm's law) proportional to the exposure rate. The deflection of the meter N is then a measure of the exposure rate.

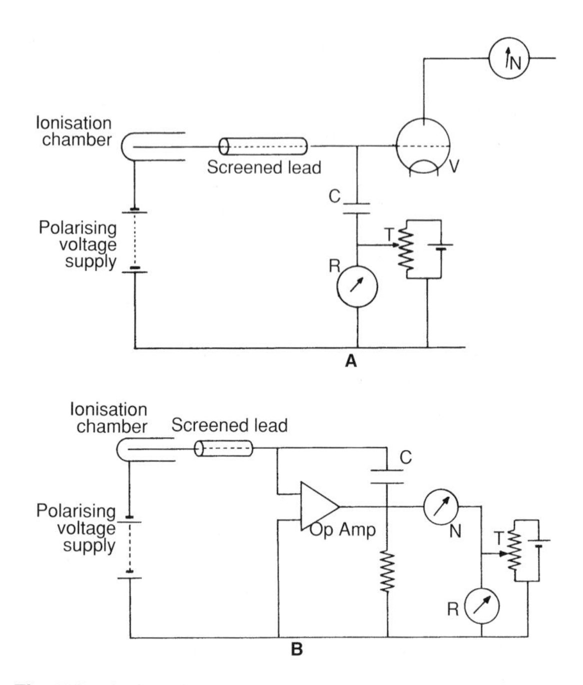

Fig. 5.3 A simplified schematic circuit for an integrating exposure meter **A** using an electrometer (triode) valve, **B** using an operational amplifier.

Air mass correction

Since any measurement of ionisation is dependent on the air mass enclosed within the chamber, it is important that the chamber contains either a fixed mass of air or a fixed volume of air at the ambient atmospheric temperature, pressure and relative humidity. If the chamber is sealed so as to enclose a fixed mass of air, then fluctuations in the ambient temperature and pressure will not affect the air mass and the instrument reading obtained will not require a correction factor to be applied.

If the chamber is unsealed, fluctuations in the ambient conditions will affect the mass of the contained air and the magnitude of the reading obtained, and two correction factors will be required, namely the temperature correction and the pressure correction—together they are referred to as the *air mass correction factor*. The density of air at 0°C and 760 mm mercury (101.3 kPa) is 0.001293 g cm^{-3} but if the temperature rises, the density falls; if the pressure rises, the density also rises. The density of air and, therefore, the reading obtained in the measurement of exposure, has to be corrected by multiplying the instrument reading by:

$$A = \frac{760}{P} \times \frac{(T + 273)}{273}$$

where the ambient temperature is T°C (or T + 273°K) and the atmospheric pressure is P mmHg providing the standard pressure is also quoted in mmHg. The alternative units of kPa or mbar may be used. Standardising laboratories use 20°C as a reference temperature, in which case the air mass factor becomes:

$$A = \frac{760}{P} \times \frac{(T + 273)}{(20 + 273)}$$

Most practical chambers are designed to be unsealed, as a deliberate ventilation hole is less likely to become sealed than the seal on a sealed chamber is likely to fail. The structure of the unsealed chamber must be rigid to guarantee the enclosed volume is the same at all times.

Relative humidity can also affect the reading of an ionisation chamber. The normal relative humidity is taken as 50% and a correction factor of 1.00 may be applied over a specific range, say, from 10–90%; it is the responsibility of the user to ensure the ambient conditions of relative humidity are within the acceptable range specified for the instrument in use.

The parallel-plate ionisation chamber

So far, only a small (cylindrical) thimble chamber has been considered. In fact, provided two insulated electrodes enclose a volume of air, an ionisation chamber can be almost any desired shape, the simplest shape is probably the parallel-plate chamber where two flat electrodes are separated by an annular insulator. The four principal applications of parallel-plate chambers encountered in radiotherapy are:

- To control the exposure on a linear accelerator or kilovoltage generator
- To monitor the output on kilovoltage generators
- To measure very low-energy X-rays, and
- To measure high-energy electron beams.

On a linear accelerator, the chamber is a complex structure and serves to control the delivered dose and to monitor the beam flatness (p. 166) and may be either sealed or unsealed and used in conjunction with temperature and pressure transducers to correct variations in the enclosed air mass. A similar chamber may be used to control the exposure on medium-kilovoltage generators. At low or very low kilovoltage energies, parallel-plate chambers may be used to *monitor* exposure rate and so confirm, or otherwise, the correct operation of kilovoltage beam generators; this practice is highly recommended (Bomford 1976). In all these applications, the electrodes must be sufficiently rigid to enclose a constant volume of air and large enough to extend over the whole of the useful beam defined by the primary collimator. The electrodes will contribute to the added filtration and therefore the HVL (or quality index, QI) and output dose rate must be assessed with the monitoring chamber in situ. The chamber (Fig. 5.4) must be positioned beyond any added (beam-hardening or beam-flattening) filters. The terms 'low energy' and 'very low energy' are defined on page 143.

Very low-energy X-rays will be readily absorbed in the walls of any thimble chamber and the beam spectrum significantly changed by the filtration effect of the wall. Some measurements on low-energy X-ray beams and all measurement of very low-energy X-rays must be made using a thin window ionisation chamber. For this purpose, the parallel-plate chamber will have a Perspex or tissue-equivalent body, a disc-shaped air cavity of less than 0.5 ml volume and a thin (~2 mg cm^{-2}) window. The window is fragile! In practical use, these chambers are mounted in a tissue-equivalent phantom, e.g. solid water, with the window flush with the surface of the phantom (p. 158). High-energy electron beam measurements are also made with chambers of this design.

Strontium reference checks

Most ionisation chambers designed for the absolute measurement of radiation are also designed to fit, in a rigid and reproducible geometrical relationship, with a strontium-90 reference source. Being a high-energy beta-emitting source of long half-life (28.7 years), strontium-90 can be loaded into a small source container and used to irradiate the chamber and check its

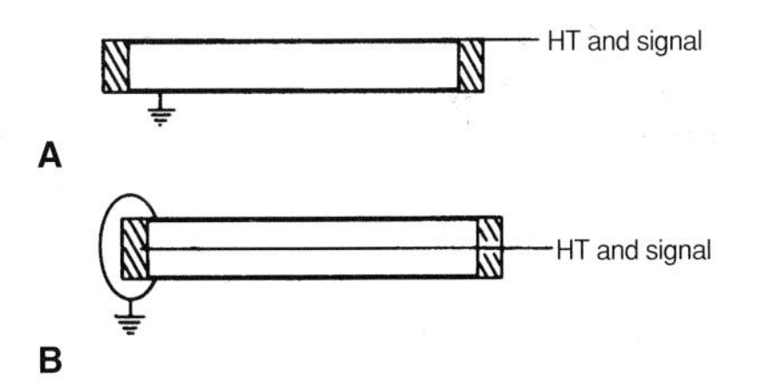

Fig. 5.4 Typical beam monitor chambers used to monitor the output from therapy units.

operation. Such consistency checks need to be repeated at regular intervals (and whenever the chamber is suspect) and the readings corrected for the air mass (if applicable) and for the decay of the strontium source. The consistency should be within a few tenths of 1% and not only from one check to the next but year on year.

Timer error

Timer error is a misnomer insofar as it is a phrase used to describe a phenomenon which is technically unavoidable rather than an avoidable error. For example, where the gamma or kilovoltage beam is controlled by a timer, any quotation of output dose rate assumes that dose rate is constant so that the product of dose rate and time is an accurate estimate of total dose delivered. However, the dose rate is not constant for it rises slowly to its steady state on switch-on and falls to zero on completion of the exposure. It increases from the moment of switch-on as the kV ramps up to its operating value on the X-ray generator or as the shutter/source movement partially exposes the source on the gamma beam generator. It may not fall immediately to zero at the end of the pre-set exposure time. During the switch-on phase, the dose rate is less than the steady-state value; while at switch-off, there may be some extra exposure added after the timer has stopped. The *error* introduced in this way must be measured for each beam generator and at each beam quality (Heales et al 1998).

If the timer error is Δt and a reading R_1 is obtained during a set exposure of time t, then the reading is related to the time by the equation:

$$R_1 = \mathrm{k}\,(t + \Delta t)$$

where k is an unknown constant related to the steady-state dose rate. If the exposure is now repeated except for the fact it is deliberately interrupted once part way through, then a reading R_2 will be obtained where:

$$R_2 = \mathrm{k}\,(t + 2\Delta t)$$

The overall time, t, is the same total exposure time as before but the interruption has introduced a second switch- on/switch-off sequence and therefore the error is $2\Delta t$. Eliminating the unknown, k, by dividing these equations and solving for Δt, we get:

$$\Delta t = \frac{R_2 - R_1}{2R_1 - R_2} \times t$$

Δt is usually negative and the prescribed treatment time must be increased by adding Δt to the prescribed set time (and each and every time the beam is energised after any interruption). The inclusion of Δt in the pre-set treatment time becomes increasingly important the shorter the treatment time. The value of Δt should be checked in the course of the routine quality assurance programme.

Where the delivered dose is controlled by an integrating dose meter, as on a linear accelerator and on some medium-energy X-ray generators, a similar phenomenon may be encountered during the initial switching-on process when the beam is unstable and the beam quality is reduced. While to ignore the effect may be justified, it is wise to check the linearity of the integrating dose meter down to a small number of monitor units.

Saturation and ion recombination

It has been stated above that ionisation chambers should always be used under saturation conditions, i.e. with a polarising voltage sufficiently high to guarantee the collection of all the ions produced within the air volume and to prevent any *ion recombination*. In gamma beam units, the radiation intensity is constant, other than for a slow decline due to the radioactive decay of the source. In kilovoltage equipment, there will be some variation of intensity depending on type of voltage generator (due to slow fluctuations in the electrical supply and to voltage ripple). In both these cases, the radiation is emitted continuously. At the dose rates encountered at kilovoltage energies and on gamma ray beam units, the ion recombination effects are often negligible, providing the polarising voltage on a thimble chamber is a few hundred volts, and accommodated within the calibration factor quoted for the secondary standard dose meter.

In linear accelerators, however, the instantaneous dose rate is significantly higher than the mean dose rate of a few gray per minute because the radiation is emitted in short pulses, e.g. 0.02 cGy per 2 msec. At these instantaneous dose rates, saturation is unlikely to be complete and it is customary to determine an *ion recombination* factor based on the design of the chamber and on the dose per pulse. The mean dose rate on clinical accelerators may be variable but it is varied by changing the pulse repetition frequency leaving the dose per pulse and the ion recombination factor unchanged. The (delivered) dose per pulse will vary, however, with large changes in treating distance, e.g. for total body irradiation (p. 217).

On many *field instruments*, the polarising voltage on the chamber can be varied both in magnitude and in polarity to enable checks to be performed to assess the *ion-collection efficiency* of the chamber under differing conditions. A complete failure in the polarising voltage supply will give rise to almost random readings while a partial failure will underestimate the true value.

STANDARDISATION OF DOSE

Hierarchy of dose meters

There is a hierarchy of instruments for measuring dose to ensure not only the accuracy of the dose measured but also to ensure a consistency of dose between radiotherapy centres (HSE 1998a). This is particularly important where patients are entered into multicentre trials or where the results of treatment are published. As a means of standardising the unit of dose in every radiotherapy centre, *field instruments* have calibrations traceable to *national standard instruments* which, in turn, are compared internationally. These standard instruments are purely laboratory instruments and of no practical value in the radiotherapy department (IPSM 1990). The field instruments are used to calibrate the radiotherapy generators in terms of their output dose rate or the built-in 'dose' meter; the latter measures the dose in terms of *monitor units* (mu) rather than gray as the readings are only numerically equal to dose for one (the reference) field size.

Standard free air ionisation chamber

The standard free air ionisation chamber is the fundamental instrument in the practical interpretation of the definition of exposure (p. 51) enabling measurements to be made of the charge liberated from a known mass of air. It is the basic instrument for the standardisation of the field instruments used routinely in kilovoltage radiotherapy. The measurements are made under strictly standardised conditions.

A narrow and accurately defined beam of radiation is passed between two parallel plates (electrodes) under conditions such that the volume of air where the primary ionisation is taking place is known accurately. The ions produced are collected and measured. The apparatus is illustrated in Figure 5.5. Between the two electrodes, a potential difference is maintained so that ions of one sign are collected on one electrode while ions of the opposite sign travel to the other. The potential difference between these electrodes must be sufficient to collect all the ions liberated—and to prevent any recombination of the (negative) electrons and positive ions—that is, the ion chamber must operate under *saturation conditions*. One electrode consists of two sections, an inner *collecting electrode* and, insulated from it, an annular electrode known as a *guard ring*. The collecting electrode and the guard ring are held at the same potential by an external connection. Isolating the collecting electrode from the guard ring by a narrow insulated region guarantees that, when the potential difference is applied between the electrodes, the electric field will be uniform and, in particular, the lines of force will be straight and perpendicular over the whole area of the collecting electrode. The volume of air of interest is therefore defined by the cross-sectional area of the accurately collimated beam, and the length of the collecting electrode and its mass can be calculated from the known ambient conditions (of atmospheric temperature and pressure). The electric charge liberated is measured directly on the collecting electrode. This charge is small and sensitive instruments are required.

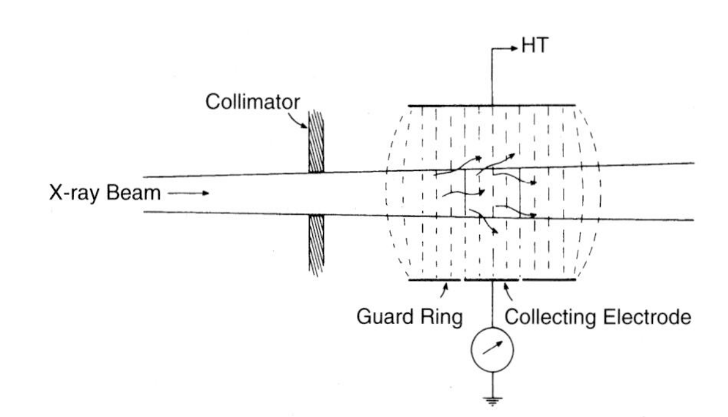

Fig. 5.5 The standard free air ionisation chamber. The guard ring is held at the same potential as the collecting electrode.

In using the free air chamber, care must be taken to ensure that the distance between the plates is large enough that the high-energy electrons produced in the central region of the chamber lose all their kinetic energy in the production of ions before they hit the electrodes. For X-rays generated at 200 kV, the plates will be of the order of 20 cm apart, the separation increasing with photon energy. The overall chamber size is, therefore, large and it is this size which places the rather arbitrary 3 MeV limit on the measurement of exposure.

In addition, the collimating system and the exit port of the chamber must be far enough from the prescribed air volume so that electrons released from them lose all their kinetic energy before reaching that air volume. This isolation of the collection volume from the surrounding components by a wall-of-air of a thickness which is greater than the range of the most energetic electrons, is the reason for describing the chamber as 'free air' and an appreciation of this requirement will assist the reader to understand the need for an *air-equivalent wall* in the more practical chambers described above.

It will be appreciated that photo- and Compton recoil electrons will be released at all points within the beam and not only in the collection volume and that these electrons will follow tortuous paths of considerable length before losing all their kinetic energy by producing further ionisations—each producing several hundred further ionisations. It is inevitable that some electrons originating outside the collection volume will enter that volume and contribute to the collection of charge but, fortunately, the converse is also true, i.e. electrons originating inside the volume will stray outside and the ions these produce will be collected by the guard ring and lost from the measurement; it is a reasonable assumption that what is gained is balanced by what is lost. A state of *electronic equilibrium* is said to exist. It can, therefore, be assumed that the ions collected by the collecting electrode and therefore measured, all originate from the collection volume.

Standard calorimeter

A more direct method of measuring the energy absorbed from an X-ray beam in a medium is to measure the total amount of heat produced in joules, to which the gray is directly related. There are great difficulties in making such a measurement because of the small temperature changes involved—a beam of X-rays giving a soft tissue dose of 5 Gy, for example, causes a temperature rise of only 10^{-3} °C. However, small temperature changes can be measured and the dose in grays calculated as:

$$\text{Dose (Gy)} = 4.18 \times C \times \Delta T$$

where C is the specific heat of the irradiated material in cal kg^{-1} $°C^{-1}$ and ΔT is the change in temperature in degrees centigrade. 4.18 is the conversion from calories to joules.

The early calorimeters were used, for example, to measure the energy in the beam of gamma rays from a cobalt-60 therapy unit. The absorber was a block of lead suspended in a vacuum inside a well-insulated box. The heat-detecting element was a *thermistor*—a semiconducting material whose resistance changes very rapidly with temperature—and its resistance change was detected electrically by using it as one arm of a Wheatstone bridge.

Today, the *calorimeter* is used as an absolute dose meter in the standardising laboratory for the megavoltage range of energies (Burns et al 1988), i.e. those beyond the practical range of the free air chamber. Calorimetry is ideal for pulsed radiations as there are no saturation or recombination effects. The temperature rise is almost simultaneous with the pulse of radiation but falls slowly over time through thermal conduction, enabling both peak and mean dose rates to be measured. For photons, water calorimeters may be used and have the advantage of being tissue equivalent (the temperature change in water is about 0.2×10^{-3} °C per Gy), but in practice, the carbon calorimeter is easier to use (the temperature change is nearer 10^{-3} °C per Gy) together with knowledge of the absorption coefficients to convert dose-in-carbon to dose-in-water. For electrons, a calorimeter-based direct-dose-to-water service has been piloted and will form the basis of a revised protocol in the near future.

Secondary standards

To avoid the need for having every field instrument calibrated directly against the national (primary) standards, there are a limited number of *secondary standard instruments*, usually held by competent physicists in regional centres. In the UK, there are some 25 secondary standard instruments, using a 0.5 ml carbon thimble chamber, and these are calibrated over a range of energies against the primary standards every 3 years. The calibration factors, N_K and N_D, will be supplied in terms of air kerma for kilovoltage X-rays based on the free air chamber and in terms of dose-to-water based on the graphite calorimeter for megavoltage photons respectively. In addition to providing these factors, the standardising laboratory will check the instrument for the linearity of scale and inter-range factors to an accuracy of better than 0.1% and provide a strontium reference check. All the data take the midpoint on the scale as a reference.

The *field* instruments are calibrated, at least every 12 months, against a secondary standard instrument on the same X-ray generator as that on which the field instrument will be deployed and at each beam quality on that generator (HSE 1998a). Each exposure should be made under conditions which are typical of the clinical use of that generator, i.e. beam quality, dose rate and an exposure (in monitor units or time) typical of the clinical practice, usually 2–3 Gy. Where there is a choice, the measurements should be made using the clinical mode rather than in the physics or service mode of operation of the generator. The physical arrangement for the different energy ranges is detailed below. In each case, a series of measurements are made with the two chambers interchanged to iron out the effects of any asymmetry of the beam profile—statistically, four sets of three measurements should be made, interchanging the position of the chambers three times. The mean value of the ratio of secondary standard/field instrument readings, $[M_s/M_f]$, is then calculated. (Note: on the assumption that both chambers are unsealed and at the same ambient temperature and pressure, the air mass correction factors will cancel out in this calculation.) The correction factor, N_{Kf} or N_{Df}, for the field instrument can then be calculated and used for the regular calibrations of output dose (rate) as described in Chapters 9 and 10.

Intercomparisons with secondary standards

Calibration of instruments for megavoltage photons

The secondary standard chamber will be used in the same thin Perspex sheath for the intercomparison measurements as was used in its primary calibration at the standardising laboratory (even when the measurements are made in a Perspex phantom). Megavoltage photons (cobalt-60 gamma and megavoltage X-rays) are measured at depth in a water-equivalent phantom. The depths used vary with the photon energy, but for most clinical purposes a depth of 5 cm is used; the recommended depths are given in Table 5.2.

The axes of the secondary standard and field chambers will be parallel and centred at the recommended depth in a water (equivalent) phantom of not less than $20 \times 20 \times 12$ cm^3, with their centres 3 cm apart and equidistant from the beam axis. The surface of the phantom will be at the normal treating distance and at right angles to the beam axis of a 10×10 cm^2 field. A correction factor for the ion recombination effects (p. 56) based on the dose-per-pulse will have to be applied to the secondary standard chamber.

$$N_{Df} = N_{Ds}\,[M_s/M_f]$$

where the suffixes, s and f, identify the secondary standard and field instruments respectively, M is the instrument reading corrected for air mass (if applicable) and ion recombination and N_D the calibration factor for the radiation quality to convert the corrected instrument reading to absorbed dose in water. The radiation quality is specified in terms of the quality index in the range from 0.57–0.79.

Table 5.2 Recommended calibration depths

Radiation energy	Depth
8–50 kV	Zero
50–160 kV*	
160–300 kV	2 cm
Cobalt-60, 4–10 MV X-rays	5 cm
11 MV–24 MV	7 cm
25 MV–50 MV	10 cm
Electrons	d_{max}

* X-rays in the range 50–60 kV are calibrated 'in-air' and not 'in-phantom' (see text)

Calibration of instruments for electron beams

Field (parallel-plate) electron chambers are not cross-calibrated directly against the secondary standard chamber. An intermediate carbon thimble chamber is calibrated in a low-energy megavoltage (e.g. 6 MV) X-ray beam at 5 cm deep in a phantom as described above. A correction factor for the carbon thimble chamber, N_c, is then calculated:

$$N_{D,air,c} = 0.978\, N_{K,s}\,[M_s/M_c]$$

where $N_{D,air,c}$ is the absorbed dose-to-air factor for the carbon thimble chamber, 0.978 is a perturbation factor, $N_{K,s}$ is the in-air air kerma factor for the secondary standard chamber measured at cobalt-60 or 2 MV X-rays and $[M_s/M_c]$ is the mean ratio of the corrected readings from the intercomparison of the secondary and carbon chambers respectively.

For all practical measurements on electron beams in the department, parallel-plate chambers are preferred. These chambers have disc-shaped air cavities, usually less than 20 mm diameter × 2 mm thick, and mounted so that the electron beam enters through the thin 'window' electrode with the minimal perturbation. Because the high-energy electrons passing through the chamber may themselves contribute to the ionisation current produced within the cavity, the polarity of the chamber voltage is important and the significance of this effect should be checked by reversing the polarity between readings. Ion recombination (p. 56) must also be taken into account. The field (parallel-plate) electron chamber is then calibrated against the carbon thimble chamber at the depth, d_{max}, in a water phantom in each electron beam and at each energy in which it will be deployed.

If a solid water-equivalent phantom is used, steps must be taken to avoid electrostatic charge building up in the phantom under the bombardment of the electrons and thereby distorting the readings from the chamber. Several commercial parallel-plate chambers have been recommended, each with its own characteristics and derived correction factors; these are too numerous to include here and the reader must refer to the chamber data in the light of the original protocol for the relevant correction factors (IPEMB 1996a).

Calibration of instruments for 160–300 kV X-rays

The secondary standard and field chambers will be parallel and centred 2 cm deep in a water (equivalent) phantom of no less than $20 \times 20 \times 12$ cm^3, with their centres 3 cm apart and equidistant from the beam axis. The surface of the phantom will be at the normal treating distance (or in contact with the treatment applicator) and at right angles to the beam axis of a 10×10 cm^2 field (IPEMB 1996b). The chamber correction factor is then calculated as follows:

$$[N_K \, k_{ch}]_f = N_{K,s} \, k_{ch,s} \, [M_s / M_f]$$

where k_{ch} is a correction for the change in the chamber response as it moves from an 'in-air' environment to an 'in-phantom' environment, a factor of about 2% at medium X-ray energies, but the precise value depends on the chamber in use.

Calibration of instruments for 50–160 kV X-rays

The secondary standard and field chambers will be mounted in air, parallel to each other and 3 cm apart, equidistant from and at right angles to the beam axis, but at least 5 cm from the face of the treatment applicator; the field size at the chambers should be approximately 7 cm (square or diameter) giving at least a 2 cm margin around the chambers. (Whether the two chambers should be parallel to or at right angles to the tube axis is not specified, but the orientation should be agreed and specified in the records. The author prefers the latter.) Matter irradiated by the beam beyond the chambers should be sufficiently far away as not to influence the readings. The chamber correction factor is then calculated as follows:

$$N_{K,f} = N_{K,s} \, [M_s / M_f]$$

There being no conversion from air to phantom, k_{ch} is not included in this calculation.

Calibration of instruments for 8–50 kV X-rays

The secondary standard and field chambers should both be of the parallel-plate design and mounted at the surface of a water (equivalent) phantom of more than 5 cm thickness to provide full back scatter. The two chambers should be exposed simultaneously within a beam large enough to give at least a 2 cm margin around both chambers; alternatively, the two chambers may be exposed alternately on the beam axis in a field large enough to give at least a 2 cm margin around the chamber. The front surface of the phantom should be at the normal treating distance and at right angles to the beam axis. At the dose rates encountered at kilovoltage energies, ion recombination effects should be negligible and included in the calibration factor. The chamber correction factor is then calculated as follows:

$$[N_K \, k_{ch}]_f = N_{K,s} \, k_{ch,s} \, [M_s / M_f]$$

where k_{ch} is a correction for the change in the chamber response as it moves from an 'in-air' environment to and 'in-phantom' environment, a factor of unity is recommended for these chambers until more precise values become available.

DETECTION OF RADIATION

Both beta and gamma rays may be detected and measured by the ionisation techniques described above providing they can penetrate the thin window of the chamber and they are of sufficient intensity to produce a measurable ionisation current. Unsealed radioactive materials are, however, generally used in amounts which are too small to make simple ionisation chamber methods very satisfactory and much more sensitive devices are required. The most common of these devices are the Geiger counter and the scintillation counter. These are very sensitive systems in which individual ionising particles or individual photons can be detected. Each beta particle or photon gives rise to a pulse of electrical charge at the output of the detector. The recording system usually records the total number of individual pulses produced in the detector. Hence the use of the word 'counter'. A detector of this type therefore records pulses and counts them. The number of pulses recorded per unit time is a measure of the count rate at which particles or photons arrive at the detector and this is proportional to the disintegration rate of a radioactive material situated in the vicinity of the detector.

Geiger–Muller tubes

The Geiger counter (sometimes referred to as the Geiger–Muller counter after its inventors) is one of the most widely known radiation detectors and is extensively used in radiation protection. It forms the basis of both the personal dosimeters (Ch. 6) and the gamma alarms used to detect the movement of gamma ray sources in brachytherapy (Ch. 14) applications and to monitor the operation of gamma beam generators (Ch. 10). It is essentially a simple ionisation chamber in which the ionisation produced by a single charged particle takes place in a gas at very low pressure and in an electric field high enough to cause multiple secondary ionisations in the gas. In this case, unlike the thimble chamber described above, the current produced is not only saturated but also undergoes an enormous amplification. Figure 5.6 shows the graphical relationship between the current or count rate through the ion chamber or Geiger counter and the voltage applied between the anode and the cathode in a constant radiation field. At low voltages, when the counter is placed in a radiation field, the pulse size increases as the voltage increases until the region of saturation is reached. At this stage the count rate is independent of applied voltage and all the ions produced in the gas are collected as in the ion chamber.

As the applied voltage is increased above the saturation region, the ions are given enough energy to produce further ionisation by collision with the gas atoms, and the pulse size increases as the applied voltage increases. This is known as the proportional region because the pulse size is proportional to the energy liberated by the initial interaction. If the applied voltage is increased still further, a plateau, known as the Geiger region, is reached. In this region the pulse size is almost independent of applied voltage, the maximum possible amplification takes place and all ionising events produce pulses of the same magnitude. Thus a heavily ionising alpha particle or a lightly ionising beta particle produces a pulse of the same size. At voltages above the Geiger region, the intensity of the electric field is itself sufficient to ionise the gas atoms and produce continuous unwanted multiplication. The tube will then break into continuous discharge.

The Geiger counter normally consists of a cylindrical conductor, the cathode, along the axis of which is stretched a fine wire acting as the positive electrode, the anode. This electrode system is often placed in a glass container filled with a gas at a pressure of 100 mmHg (13 kPa) (Fig. 5.7). However, the outer electrode may itself be the container for the gas. Typically the gas is 90% argon and 10% ethanol or 99.9% neon and 0.1% chlorine. These are known as organic or halogen quenched tubes respectively. A high voltage of between 500 and 1000 volts is applied across the electrodes producing an intense electric field around the central wire.

The ions originally produced by the fast charged particle are attracted towards the collecting electrodes under the influence of the high electric field. The positive ions move slowly towards the cathode and the negative ions (electrons) accelerate towards the anode. Because of the intense electric field and the low gas pressure, the path length between each successive collision between the electrons and the un-ionised gas molecules surrounding them is long enough for the electrons to acquire sufficient energy to ionise these molecules. The secondary electrons so produced are also accelerated to an energy level where they too cause ionisation. A cascade process is thus produced which gives rise to an *avalanche* of charged particles being swept to the collecting electrode, giving an amplification of the initial ionisation of several million and a very high charge pulse on the electrode system. The avalanche process involves only the light electrons. It takes only a few microseconds for the avalanche effect to take place and for the electrons to reach the anode. The heavy positive ions, however, migrate more slowly towards the cathode, where upon arrival

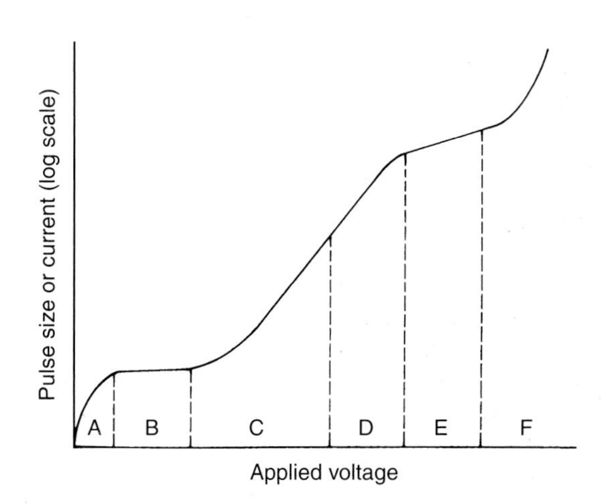

Fig. 5.6 Relationship between pulse size and the voltage applied between anode and cathode: A, recombination; B, ionisation chamber; C, proportional counter; D, transition range; E, Geiger counter; F, discharge.

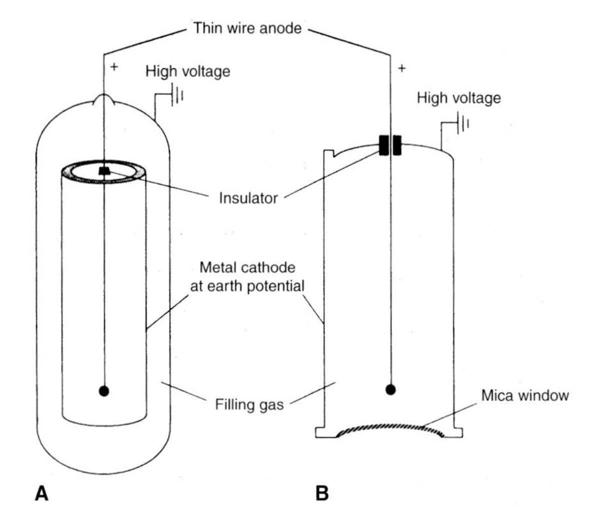

Fig. 5.7 Schematic diagram of two types of Geiger counter: **A** gamma counter; **B** end window beta counter.

they may initiate a further discharge. These spurious discharges will be quenched by dissociation, rather than ionisation, of the molecules of ethanol or halogens in the gas.

Until they have been neutralised at the cathode, the presence of the slowly moving positive ions disables the counter from further detection. This may take several hundred microseconds and is known as the *dead time*. The Geiger counter, therefore, will miss some particles if it is exposed to a radiation field of high intensity. Counting rates of 250 per second, for example, will miss about 5% of the received ionising particles.

Three properties of the Geiger counter are important for its use as a sensitive detector for radiations from radioactive material or X-rays.

- The pulse size is dependent only on the number of ions initiating the discharge. It cannot therefore be used to distinguish, say, an alpha particle from a beta particle, or between photons of different energy. It is in fact a 'trigger' device.
- The detection efficiency for beta particles can be very high, but for X- or gamma rays is low. The response of the counter to X- or gamma rays depends mainly on the interaction of the photons in the walls of the detector and is therefore dependent on the atomic number of the wall material and the energy of the photon. In some Geiger tubes a cathode of very high atomic number, lead for example, is introduced deliberately to enhance the sensitivity for high-energy gamma rays. Even so, the efficiency of Geiger counters for gamma rays is only 1–2%. The Geiger counter therefore is unsuitable for accurate measurement of X- or gamma rays but very suitable for detecting and estimating low intensities of these radiations.
- When the voltage applied to a Geiger tube is too, low the cascade process does not work and, if it is too high, a continuous discharge is set up which damages the electrodes. However, over an intermediate range, the plateau, the counting rate is nearly independent of the voltage for a constant radiation intensity. Under good working conditions, therefore, the counter is relatively insensitive to fluctuations in the voltage supply. It thus becomes a simple and fairly rugged instrument of high sensitivity easily made in a portable form.

Scintillation counters

The scintillation detector makes use of the flashes of light produced in a suitable crystal when it absorbs photons. The device consists of a crystal sealed in a container, usually of aluminium, which is light-tight except on one face. This face is optically coupled by the use of silicone grease, or in some cases a specially constructed light pipe, to the photocathode of a photomultiplier tube (Fig. 5.8).

The crystal material most commonly used is *sodium iodide* activated by the addition of a small amount, 0.1–0.5%, of the element thallium. The addition of the thallium greatly increases the light output. When a photon is absorbed in the crystal by either photoelectric absorption or Compton scattering, some or all of its energy is transferred to a secondary electron, point A in Figure 5.8. This electron moves around the crystal lattice exciting the atoms which in turn produce photons of light of a wavelength characteristic of the crystal.

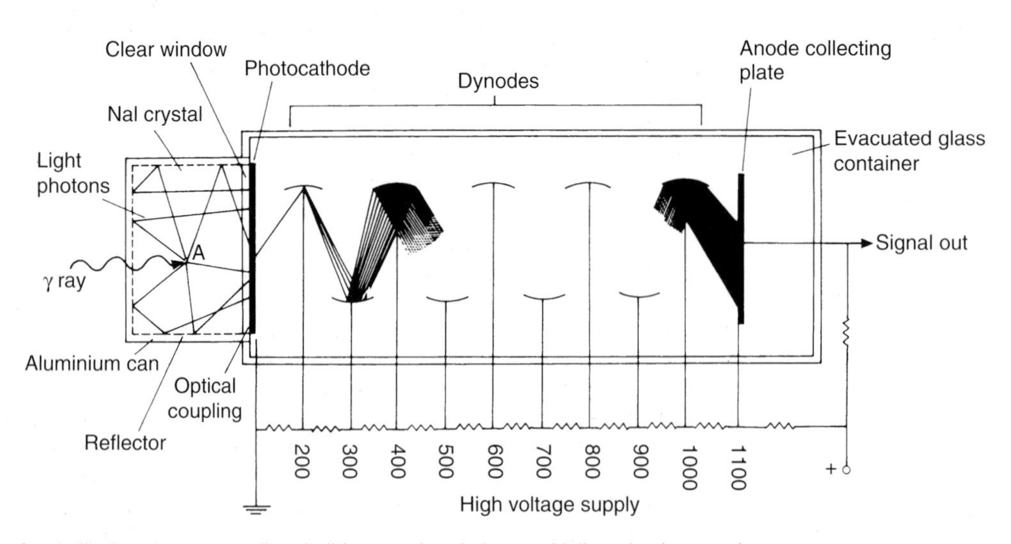

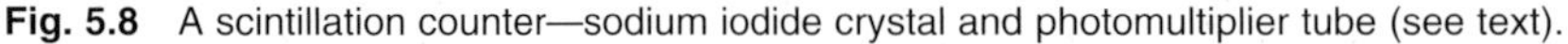

Fig. 5.8 A scintillation counter—sodium iodide crystal and photomultiplier tube (see text).

These photons are emitted in all directions but reflected towards the photomultiplier by the diffuse reflector—of titanium dioxide or magnesium oxide—which lines the container (dashed lines Fig. 5.8).

The *photomultiplier* (PM) tube converts the light photons from the crystal into an electrical pulse. The tube consists of a photocathode, a series of *dynodes* and an anode sealed in an evacuated glass envelope (Fig. 5.8). When light strikes the photoemissive surface of the photocathode, low-energy photoelectrons are ejected. A voltage of approximately +200 volts is applied between the photocathode and the first dynode, and then 100 volts between each successive dynode along the dynode chain. Each electron leaving the photocathode is focused and accelerated towards the first dynode with sufficient energy to release additional electrons, typically about four. These four secondary electrons are in turn accelerated towards the second dynode where each one releases four more electrons. This acceleration and multiplication process takes place along the length of the dynode chain. For a 10-dynode tube releasing four electrons for each incident electron, the electron gain or multiplication is such that, for each one electron released by the photocathode, there will be over one million electrons arriving at the anode. The average number of electrons released at the dynodes depends on the accelerating voltage applied, and on the material coating the dynode. Increasing the applied voltage increases the number of electrons released and hence increases the gain of the PM tube.

A further characteristic of scintillation counting is important. In a crystal, any photon absorption results in a detectable event. A large mass of crystal may therefore be used to detect photons, as long as it is a single optically transparent crystal so that light pulses produced anywhere inside it can reach the photocathode of the multiplier. This makes the scintillation counter very sensitive compared to the Geiger counter.

The most important feature of a scintillation detector is the relationship between the energy of the incident gamma ray and the size of the electrical pulse coming from the detector. If the incident gamma ray photon is completely absorbed within the sodium iodide crystal, then the average number of light photons produced in the crystal is proportional to the energy of the incident gamma ray photon and the average number of electrons ejected from the photocathode. The size of the pulse arriving at the anode is the number of electrons released at the photocathode multiplied by the gain factor of the PM tube. Thus the size of the electrical signal emerging from the detector is, on average, proportional to the energy of the gamma ray absorbed in the crystal. A 300 keV gamma ray would thus produce a pulse twice the size of that from a 150 keV gamma ray. This property is exploited in gamma spectrometry.

Gamma spectrometry

This proportionality property of the scintillation counter can be used to determine the spectrum of the pulses deposited in the crystal when photons are absorbed and hence the energy spectrum of the photon field itself can be explored. The components that make up the gamma spectrometer system are shown in Figure 5.9A. The *pulse height analyser* (PHA) contains a lower level energy discriminator (LLD), which only allows inclusion of pulses greater than a given size, and an upper level energy discriminator (ULD), which rejects signals greater than the predetermined size. Thus the only pulses counted are those which fall within this 'window' (Fig. 5.9B). By adjusting the size and position of the window, the scintillation spectrometer can be made to discriminate between photons of one isotope and those of another. Similarly, it is possible to reject those pulses which arise from general background radiation. By adjusting the size of the pulses selected for counting, the energy spectrum of a gamma ray source may be explored and the assay of two or more gamma-emitting isotopes in one sample becomes possible.

Each gamma-emitting radionuclide has a characteristic spectrum, and the energies are discrete and discontinuous. For example, the emission spectrum of caesium-137 contains a single energy of 662 keV, whereas the iodine-131 spectrum contains photons with five principal energies: 80 keV (2%); 284 keV (6%); 364 keV (80%); 638 keV (9%) and 724 keV (3%) (Fig. 5.10A and B)). The PHA, however, shows these spectra as a series of humps (Fig. 5.10C and D) instead of a series of discrete lines. This is because of statistical variations within the crystal and the photomultiplier—(i) not all the photon's energy appears as light because a variable fraction is turned into heat; (ii) the photocathode is not completely uniform in its sensitivity to light and its photoelectron production; and (iii) there is variable efficiency of multiplication in succeeding dynodes—all of which combine to produce a distribution of pulses about a mean value.

We know both photoelectric and Compton interactions will take place in the crystal. The photoelectric effect gives rise to the bell-shaped peak centred around the photon energy. The Compton recoil electron will be absorbed and the energy of the scintillation will be proportional to the energy of that recoil electron, not the energy of the initiating photon; the Compton

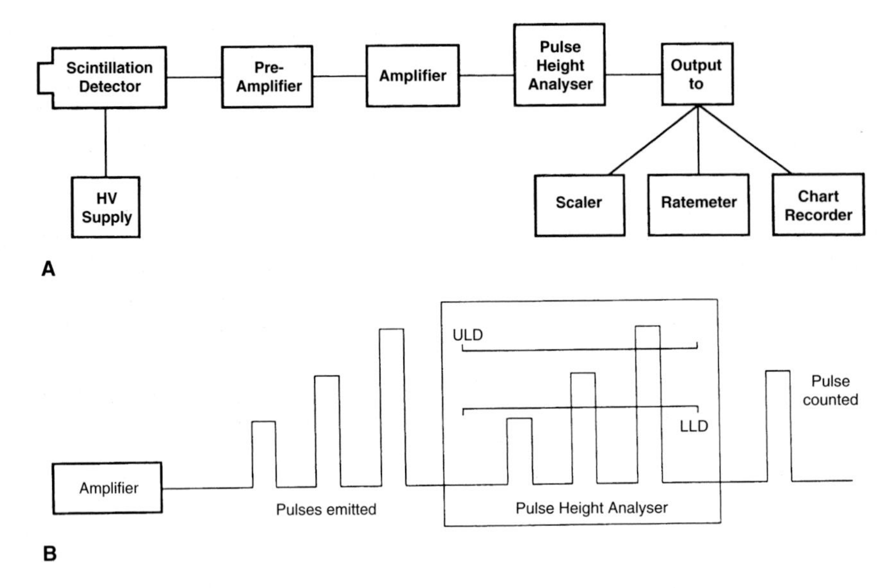

Fig. 5.9 **A** The components of a scintillation spectrometer and **B** pulse height processing.

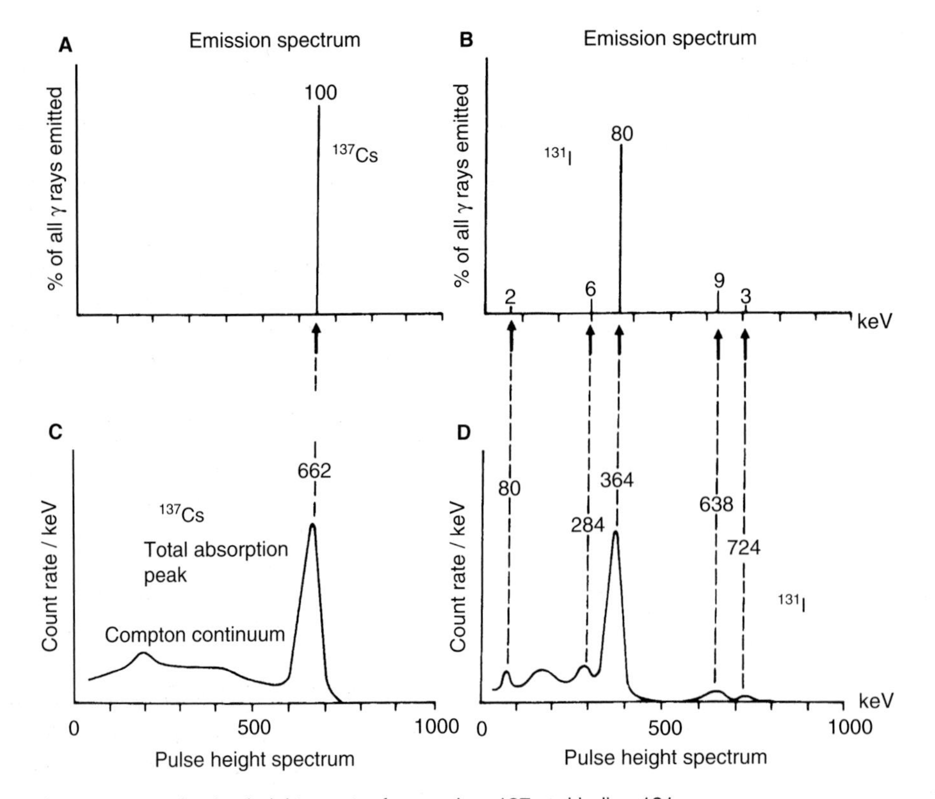

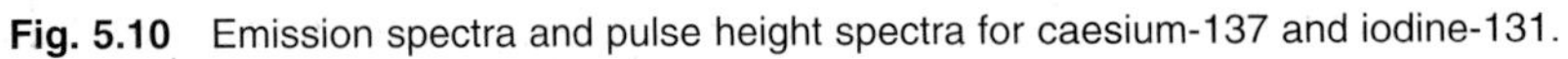
Fig. 5.10 Emission spectra and pulse height spectra for caesium-137 and iodine-131.

scatter may escape from the crystal. As we saw in the last chapter, the recoil electron can have a range of energies depending on the scattering angle. In addition, multiple Compton collisions may occur and the resultant pulse height represents the total energy lost. These events give rise to the region known as the *Compton continuum* (Fig. 5.10C). Multiple Compton interactions may culminate with a photoelectric interaction and hence total absorption of the photon energy. The pulse from these combined scintillations will appear in the total absorption peak of the pulse height spectrum.

Other extraneous events, such as photon scattering, annihilation radiation following pair production, and characteristic X-radiation from interactions within the lead collimators, can all add features to the pulse height spectrum.

Multiple nuclide detection. When two radionuclides are present in the same sample then careful use of the spectrometer window will enable simultaneous measurement of the two nuclides. For example, Figure 5.11 shows the pulse height spectra for chromium-51 and iron-59, two nuclides frequently used together. Two pulse height analyser windows are set, one to encompass the two high-energy absorption peaks from the iron-59, and the other to encompass the lower-energy peak from the chromium-51. It will be seen that the iron-59 can be detected free from contamination by the chromium-51, but the chromium-51 window includes counts, or *cross-talk*, from the Compton continuum of the iron-59. Corrections can be made for this cross-talk to give true chromium-51 counts.

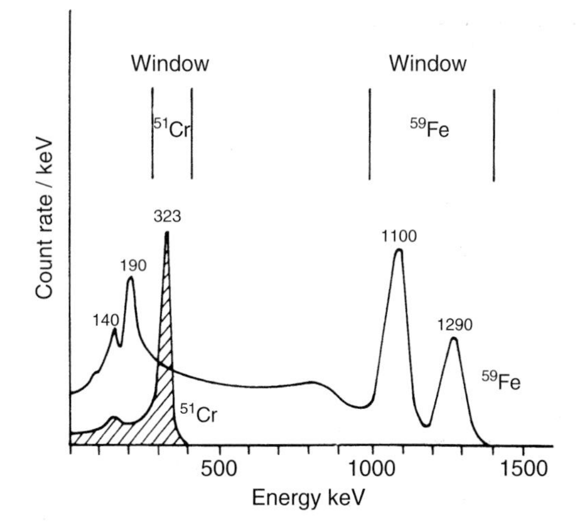

Fig. 5.11 Pulse height spectra and window positions for chromium-51 and iron-59.

Measurement of fluid samples. The assay of low-activity fluid samples is necessary in many procedures involving the use of unsealed sources for therapy, diagnosis and radioimmunoassay. A *well counter* is a scintillation counter with a sodium iodide crystal, say, 6 cm diameter by 6 cm deep into which a cylindrical hole, or well, is drilled. The crystal and photomultiplier tube are mounted inside a substantial lead shield to reduce background radiation, and the small bottle containing the sample is placed in the well. The well counter can measure gamma-emitting samples of less than 1 kBq activity.

ALTERNATIVE METHODS OF MEASUREMENT

The primary effect of the radiations in which we are interested is the production of ionisation and this may be revealed as electrical conductivity in air, a property exploited in the ionisation chambers described above. It may also be revealed in a number of other ways such as physical or chemical effects in solids or liquids. Any of these physical or chemical effects which can be estimated quantitatively can be used as a dose-measuring system and in the past most of them have been tried. A satisfactory dose-measuring system requires, however, that the effect observed does not show too great a variation of sensitivity with photon energy. This is because of the continuous nature of the X-ray spectrum and the presence of scattered radiation which degrades the primary spectrum as it passes through the absorbing medium. For high-energy gamma rays, the beam consists initially of radiation of a single wavelength or of a few discrete wavelengths but scattering again changes the spectral distribution and an energy-independent dosimeter is desirable. The effect observed should also be independent of the prevailing ambient conditions. Some of the methods used in the past have now only a historical interest but others are quite important in radiation protection although none of them should be used to measure the output dose (rate) of a radiotherapy generator, where the thimble ionisation chamber is always recommended. Any measuring device needs to be calibrated in such a way that the measurements are traceable to national standards. A brief account of several different techniques is given below.

Thermoluminescence

The transition of an electron from an outer orbit to an inner orbit and the consequent emission of a characteristic X-ray photon has already been discussed (Chs 2 and 4). Similar transitions take place between the outer orbits with the corresponding emission of characteristic radiation within the longer wavelength parts of the spectrum. In a crystal, these outer orbits are shared by the atoms and again transitions can occur between them. If the emission is in the visible part of the spectrum the phenomenon is known as *luminescence*. For example, sodium iodide produces scintillations under irradiation. In Chapter 7, it will be seen that intensifying screens enhance the photographic action of X-rays by emitting visible light of a wavelength to which X-ray film is particularly sensitive and *fluoroscopy* (or *screening*) is a means of making an X-ray image visible to the human eye. In each of these instances, the visible light emission is an immediate and instantaneous response to the absorption X-rays. This is *fluorescence*. Another form of luminescence of particular interest in radiotherapy (and in radiation protection is that of thermoluminescence.

Certain crystalline materials, such as *lithium fluoride*, can absorb X-ray energy and store that energy at room temperature for a very considerable time, many months in fact. At the atomic level this process can be explained briefly as follows. When X-ray energy is absorbed, secondary electrons are lifted from the outer electron orbits into another orbit which is normally empty in a non-conducting material. Since these electron orbits are not uniquely defined in a solid they are referred to as bands (Fig. 2.3), the normally filled *valence band* and the normally empty *conduction band* respectively with a *forbidden zone* between them, as between any two electron shells in a single atom. In a pure crystal, the electrons will fall back from the conduction band into the holes they left in the valence band. If an impurity is deliberately added to the crystal—*manganese*, for example—some of these electrons will fall into the *impurity traps* which now lie in the forbidden zone. Here the electron is held and its energy stored. This energy is only released when sufficient heat is applied to lift these trapped electrons back into the conduction band from where they may return to the valence band emitting their excess energy in the form of photons of visible light. This is *thermoluminescence*. The intensity of the light output is small but it is proportional to the X-ray energy previously absorbed and hence the value of the technique as a means of measuring radiation dose.

Thermoluminescent dosimeters may be in the form of powder, impregnated plastic discs or of extruded chips or rods, each containing some 50–100 mg of phosphor material. After irradiation, the phosphor is placed in a planchet in the 'TLD Reader' where it is heated to 300°C in an oxygen-free (nitrogen) atmosphere (Fig. 5.12). The light output is measured using a

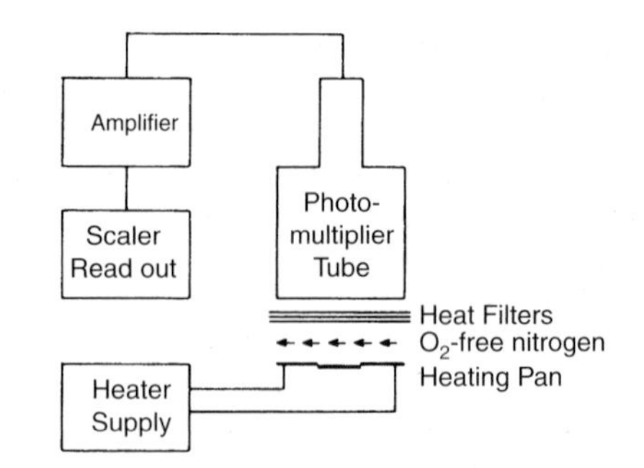

Fig. 5.12 A thermoluminescent dosimeter read-out system.

photomultiplier. The system is essentially a comparator and any measurement of dose relies on the readout of identical dosimeters exposed to known doses of the same quality radiation. Lithium fluoride has an atomic number close to that of soft tissue and therefore its response is almost independent of the photon energies encountered in the radiotherapy department. A wide range of doses may be measured enabling the system to be used for measuring patient doses (in both diagnosis and therapy), doses to sensitive organs outside the treatment beam (Ch. 13) and for personnel monitoring (Ch. 6). Crystals of *lithium borate* and of *calcium fluoride* may be used as alternatives to lithium fluoride.

Solid state detectors

Silicon diode detectors are widely used for the measurement of electron beams and megavoltage photon beams. Their relatively high atomic number ($Z = 14$) makes them unsuitable for lower photon energies. The silicon diode may be thought of as a solid ionisation chamber of very small size (Fig. 5.13)—their small size makes them particularly useful in the measurement of isodose charts. The radiation causes ionisations within the detector and the ions are collected in the same way as in an ionisation chamber. The principal differences

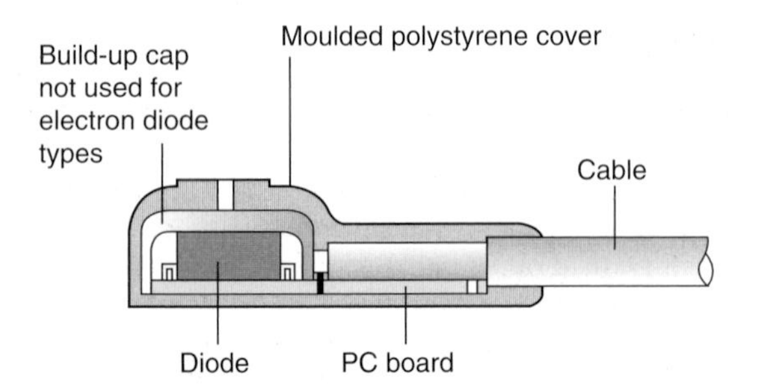

Fig. 5.13 A solid state detector. (Redrawn/adapted courtesy of Nuclear Associates.)

are that the ionisations occur in a material of a much higher density than air—volume for volume, the silicon diode is some 20 000 times more sensitive than the air ionisation chamber—and there is no need for a large polarising voltage because the contact potentials within the diode are sufficient to prevent ion recombination. Their disadvantages are principally their (photon) energy dependence and their ultimate destruction through radiation-induced damage—this is a gradual process which shows in changes in sensitivity to both dose and temperature. Careful use and frequent calibration is required.

The sensitive part of the silicon diode is the junction between the P-type and the N-type silicon (p. 15). The P-type silicon is silicon with a boron ($Z = 5$) or an aluminium ($Z = 13$) impurity which absorbs electrons from the silicon leaving positive (P) 'holes' in the material. On the other side of the junction the phosphorus impurity ($Z = 16$) donates negative (N) electrons to the silicon. This imbalance results in a contact potential being set up at the junction between the dissimilar materials and a mopping up of the 'free' ions creating a depletion layer of only a few microns thick. If the atoms in this depletion layer are ionised by radiation, then the negative ions (electrons) will be attracted to the positively charged phosphorus impurity in the N-type silicon and the positive 'holes' will diffuse towards the boron impurity in the P-type silicon. This flow of ions constitutes an ionisation current proportional to the dose-rate incident on the detector and can be measured on a sensitive ammeter (an electrometer).

Although all these detectors use both N-type and P-type material, some are described as P-type while others are N-type. The label identifies which material forms the larger part of the junction. The junction is very small—a few millimetres square by half a millimetre thick—and encapsulated in a suitable protective sheath. The sheath is usually of a material and thickness to provide full electron build-up in the (megavoltage) photon beam, which means they cannot be used to measure 'skin' or 'lens' dose during radiotherapy, although their small size would make them ideal. Detectors designed for use in a water phantom have a different encapsulation which usually enables the build-up curve to be measured.

It should be noted that where silicon diodes—with build-up material in the encapsulation—are used to monitor the patient entry dose during radiotherapy, there may be a significant spatial error (~2–5%) between the detector and the point at d_{max} where the dose is prescribed. These measurements therefore need careful interpretation in the light of the geometrical set-up and the energy of the radiation (p. 224).

Photographic methods

The effect of X- and gamma rays in producing blackening on a processed photographic film may also be used to estimate dose, especially if the photon energy is high and the amount of blackening is measured with a densitometer. A densitometer causes a pencil beam of (visible) light to pass through an area of the film on to a photocell (p. 6) which measures the intensity of the light transmitted by the film in the form of an electric current, the current being proportional to the intensity. The degree of blackening is expressed as an *optical density*, which is the logarithm (to base 10) of the light intensity transmitted by an unexposed area of the film divided by that transmitted by the exposed part of the film. Thus, an optical density of 1 means that only one-tenth of the light is transmitted, while a density of 2 transmits only one-hundredth. Film saturates at a density of about 5. Over a limited range, density is proportional to dose. The properties of photographic film exposed to ionising radiation are dealt with more fully in Chapter 7 in the context of radiographic imaging.

The photographic method suffers from several disadvantages. It is difficult to obtain reproducible and accurate results even though great care is taken to process films under standard and controlled conditions. For instance, variations of developer strength and temperature and of processing techniques can each make great differences to the density. Films also show great differences in sensitivity to radiation over the photon energy range in which measurements are needed in radiotherapy. Film may be used in a solid phantom to ascertain the distribution of dose from a megavoltage beam (p. 199) or from an array of beams, but the energy sensitivity makes it unsuitable for kilovoltage beam assessment. The principal application of film in radiotherapy is in imaging on the simulator (p. 103) or in portal imaging on the therapy generators (p. 109). It is also used in personal monitoring, because the photographic method of dosimetry is a very sensitive one, particularly if the time involved in the exposure is long and if a high degree of accuracy is not required. These conditions prevail in radiation protection and the use of the film badge is described more fully in Chapter 6.

Chemical method

Following the demise of the 'Pastille Dose' used by the early pioneers, there has been something of a revival of interest in chemical dosimeters, since they can be used under two conditions in which ionisation methods are somewhat unsatisfactory. These are the measurement of very large doses (thousands of grays), such as might be experienced in the neighbourhood of massive radioactive sources and the measurement of extremely high dose rates such as might be experienced in the neighbourhood of a nuclear explosion. They are ideal for use with pulsed radiation sources. They can be used to advantage in radiotherapy as a means of measuring the average absorbed dose over a large or irregularly shaped volume and in the laboratory as a means of comparing the effects of different types of radiation. Chemical dosimeters can be made relatively simply to work under these conditions. The most widely used is the Fricke dosimeter but others are available.

The ability of ionising radiations to promote the oxidation of ferrous compounds has been known for a long time as one of the many chemical effects of radiation. The *Fricke dosimeter* uses a solution of ferr*ous* (Fe^{2+}) sulphate in sulphuric acid. On irradiation, ferr*ic* (Fe^{3+}) sulphate is produced. The quantity produced is estimated by measuring the optical density of a sample before and after the irradiation in a beam of light of suitable wavelength (304 nm) using a *spectrophotometer*. With care, it can be accurate to approximately 2% over a range from 10–350 Gy. The yield varies little over the megavoltage energy range.

Biological method

A biological method of measuring dose was attempted in the early days of radiotherapy using the property of the radiations to produce a reddening of the skin—the *skin erythema*. This biological reaction is described in Chapter 17. In using this reaction as a dose-measuring system, a unit of dose was defined as the amount of radiation which just produced an appreciable reddening of the skin. The method was extremely inaccurate because of the difficulty of determining the threshold erythema and its variability from one person or one site to another. It was abandoned once it was established that different amounts of X-ray energy are necessary to produce the erythema when beams of different effective wavelength are used.

CHAPTER CONTENTS

6

Radiation protection

Keith Bomford

INTRODUCTION

The biological effects of ionising radiation on a single component cell and on a complete organism such as the human body are described briefly in this chapter; there is more detail in Part 2 of this book. Arising from the study of these effects, the levels of radiation which present an acceptable risk in a normal working environment and in the environment as a whole have been specified by authoritative international expert committees, principally the International Commission on Radiological Protection (ICRP) (ICRP 1991). This chapter contains an account of the relevant acceptable dose levels, and the steps which must be taken to keep within these dose levels in practice. However, in order to appreciate the problems involved in establishing adequate control of the radiation hazard, and also to understand the apparently complicated specifications of a dose limit, it is necessary to summarise the available knowledge of the effects produced in human beings by low doses of ionising radiations. Radiation hazards are a matter of great concern to members of the general public. Health care workers are professionally in an important position to help ensure that the public, particularly patients in hospital, have an appreciation of the hazards, of the steps taken to control them, and of the relative dangers of using ionising radiation compared to other activities of normal living.

In later chapters, specific radiation generators are described together with the control of their associated hazards.

BIOLOGICAL EFFECTS OF RADIATION

It is well known that a variety of injuries can result from excessive doses of ionising radiation. The following list illustrates the need to consider a wide variety of possible working conditions and techniques when safety rules are drawn up:

- Injuries to the skin arising from exposure of the epidermis to radiations of quite low penetrating power, such as beta rays or low-energy photons.
- Changes in the blood-forming organs and in the number and nature of the circulating blood cells. These changes will arise from exposure of the bone marrow to penetrating radiations received from external radiation sources or from internally distributed radioactive materials.
- Cancer produced by exposure to radiation arising from either external or internal sources of radiation.
- Cataract formation due to irradiation of the lens of the eye by radiation of low penetrating power.
- Genetic effects arising from the production of mutations by the irradiation of the reproductive system.

To specify levels of radiation exposure so as to avoid these injurious effects, detailed quantitative information is needed to correlate the incidence of the effect with the radiation dose. The information available is not complete but it is sufficient to enable *dose limits* to be incorporated in the various regulations and recommendations published in many countries.

EVIDENCE OF DAMAGE BY LOW DOSES

There are five main sources of information on either the long-term effects of low doses of ionising radiation or the effects of higher doses or dose rates of radiation which may be used to estimate their effects, although the extrapolation to low doses is fraught with difficulty and assumption.

Early history of radiation damage

The radiation damage received by many early workers with X-rays and radium has been studied in detail. It was realised in the early days when the medical use of radiation was growing rapidly that there could be a long time interval, often of many years, between the radiation exposure and the observable damage but it was not realised then that long periods of exposure at low dose rates could be as damaging as shorter periods at higher dose rates. The damage suffered by the early radiologists was predominantly of two types. First, damage to the tissues of the hands resulting from exposure to the direct beam of X-rays (Plate 1.1) or fingering radium sources. (In these early days, radiologists practised both radiodiagnosis and radiotherapy). This damage was often very serious and sometimes fatal. Second, damage to the haemopoietic system—the site of blood cell formation in the bone marrow—by exposure of the whole body to scattered radiation over long periods or the ingestion of radionuclides. Though these two effects have since been recognised, the magnitude of the dose to which the early workers had been subjected years before could never be established accurately.

In the nuclear industry today, some of those occupationally exposed may be receiving doses close to the recommended limits, and the doses may be assessed, but the numbers of workers are small and the exposures too recent, in comparison to the latent period, to correlate the effects accurately.

Evidence from radiation accidents

A great deal of evidence about radiation damage has been obtained from the study of accidental exposures to X-rays and to radionuclides in industrial and research processes and in medical practice. In spite of extreme care, accidental exposures do occur and detailed investigations into such events reveal valuable information of two kinds. First, a consideration of the circumstances which led to the accident may suggest improved techniques for the safe control of the radiation facility. These may become incorporated into the regulations and recommendations in an attempt to avoid any repetition. Second, if it is possible to observe the clinical damage produced and to obtain a reasonable estimate of the dose involved, the information can be valuable in establishing further data on the dose–effect relationships. The Chernobyl disaster of April 1986 has precipitated a great deal of evaluation and investigation in this area of dose and effect which is on-going.

Long-term effects of atomic weapons

The use of the atomic bombs on the Japanese cities of Hiroshima and Nagasaki in 1945 exposed large populations to a sudden acute radiation dose. The immediate effects of these explosions were due mainly to the intense heat and the explosive violence of the event and only in part to the high doses of radiation. However, large numbers of survivors in both cities have been studied continuously since 1945. The incidence of disease amongst these survivors, and the incidence of possible effects on those irradiated in utero or the offspring of irradiated parents, have all been matched carefully against a similar population believed to be unirradiated. The radiation dose which the victims received at the time of the explosion has been estimated in a number of ways including investigations of the position of the subject with respect to the explosion centre. The effects of this single dose of gamma rays and neutrons have been followed for over half a century, and the results have contributed valuable data on which safety levels can be based. A recent re-evaluation of the doses received by the survivors has suggested that earlier estimates were too high and the subsequent injuries were due to lower doses than previously thought. This study played a major part in the decision in the late 1980s to lower the 'acceptable' dose limits (p. 75).

Results of animal experiments

Radiobiology has developed greatly over the last 40 years and much information has been obtained by experimental irradiation of various animals about both the radiation effects and the administered dose. The radiation damage to chromosomes is well established, but a quantitative estimate of the magnitude of these effects could not be observed in human beings. The extrapolation of experimental animal data to humans accounts for the doubt, for example, of the exact radiation dose which would double the naturally occurring mutation rate in humans, though this is estimated to be about 0.5 Gy. There is also some uncertainty about the exact relationship between effect and dose for very low dose rates. Conservative extrapolations are invariably used when deducing appropriate safety standards so as to err on the side of safety.

Evidence from radiotherapy

Finally, a great deal of careful observation and long experience in radiotherapy gives a firm correlation of radiation effects against administered dose for a wide variety of conditions. However, this evidence always relates to dose levels between perhaps 1 gray and (say) 50 Gy to selected tissues. Sadly, there have been a few accidental irradiations to higher levels of dose but again to small selected volumes of tissue. It is doubtful if these data can be extrapolated to estimate the effect of a few milligray on the whole body. The investigations into such accidents invariably result in the revision of the recommendations to improve the safety of the generators themselves or the operating procedures.

RADIATION EFFECTS AT LOW DOSES

There are two facts about the effects of radiation at low dose levels which make precision very difficult:

- The predicted effects cannot be distinguished from the same conditions which occur spontaneously. For example, there is a natural incidence of malignant disease and the incidence rate varies with the type and site of the cancer, and with the environment to which the population is subjected.
- The natural background radiation in the environment, to which all populations down the ages have been exposed, will be responsible, statistically at least, for some malignancies; one estimate suggests a few hundred cancer deaths in the UK per annum.

The addition of man-made sources of ionising radiation to the environmental sources will give rise to an increase, albeit small, in both the incidence of malignant disease and of genetic abnormalities.

The effects of ionising radiation begin with the ionisation of an atom or molecule within a cell. The cell is not necessarily damaged. If it is slightly damaged, the damage may be repaired by the body's defence mechanisms. If it is severely damaged, it may die or it may go on proliferating in a modified form and, after a latent period, produce a cancer. These effects are very much chance effects, starting from the ionisation of a single cell. There is therefore no threshold dose below which one can say it will not happen, but equally no dose above which it is certain to happen. The technical term used to describe these chance effects is *stochastic*, and where the effect is manifest in the person exposed, the effect is said to be *somatic*. Somatic stochastic effects then are those which cannot be clearly ascribed to a particular dose of ionising radiation received by an individual. They can only be detected by observing an increased incidence of a known abnormality in a large group of individuals for whom an increase in radiation exposure has taken place. On the basis that many million million ionisations are produced in the DNA alone every year by the naturally occurring radiations and only one in four deaths is attributable to cancer, then we must conclude that such cell damage is only rarely manifested in the formation of a cancer.

In the event that the cell damage leads to a predictable loss of organ function, as revealed by some pathological conditions, the effect is said to be *deterministic*. In contrast to the stochastic effect, the deterministic effect appears to require a threshold dose (or dose rate) below which the condition will not be observed—unless there are other contributory causes.

Where the damaged cells belong to the reproductive system (germ cells), they may be responsible for passing on incorrect hereditary information to the next generation. Such genetic defects may be trivial or may lead to serious disability or even death. However, these hereditary effects have only been suggested by experiments on plants and animals; there is little evidence in man.

The effects of radiation on an embryo are very dependent on its stage of development. At the early stages, there are few cells involved and exposure to radiation is likely to cause an undetectable death of the embryo rather than result in deterministic or stochastic effects in the live-born. After the third week, radiation may increase the probability of cancer or organ malfunction. Data from Hiroshima and Nagasaki on children exposed in utero suggest there may be a shift downwards in IQ, with the shift increasing with dose. The shift seems to be smaller where the exposure was after the 16th week of pregnancy (other evidence suggests the 8th–15th week is the most sensitive period). The probable mechanism is interruption of nerve cells migrating into the cerebral cortex. Mental retardation has been observed only in a few cases where it amounted to about 30 IQ points per sievert of exposure (the sievert is a large dose in this context).

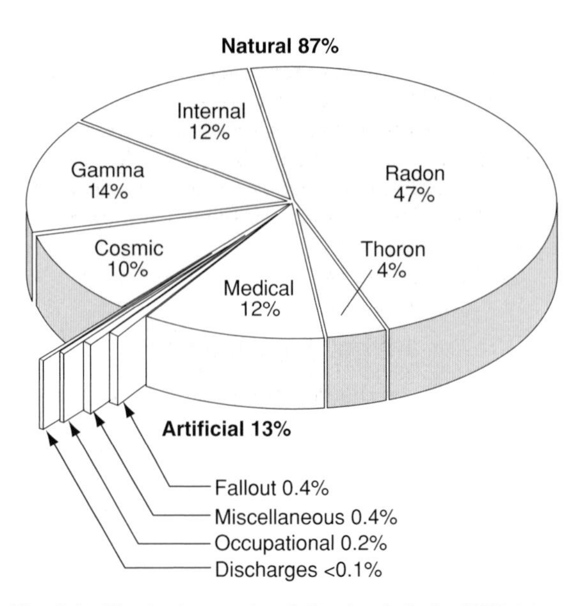

Fig. 6.1 The background radiation levels in the UK total an average of 2.6 mSv per year. (Courtesy of the National Radiological Protection Board.)

Natural background radiation

To put these radiation effects into perspective, it is worth looking at the 'natural' radiations to which we are all exposed, and then at the 'artificial' radiations to which we are all exposed at some time or another.

By *natural* radiations, we mean those radiations within the environment over which we have no control other than to protect ourselves by choosing a particular lifestyle. For example, cosmic radiations bombard the earth from outer space and their intensity will depend on the angle at which they strike the surface of the earth and the degree to which they are absorbed in the atmosphere. Our exposure to cosmic radiation will therefore depend on the altitude at which we live and the time we spend in high-flying aircraft; the crew of supersonic aircraft are at greater risk than most of us. The 'holes' on the ozone layer have a lesser effect on these more penetrating cosmic radiations than on the ultraviolet radiations which contribute to sunburn and the increased incidence of skin cancer.

The major source of 'natural' radiation is the gas *radon* and its close relative *thoron*; together they contribute over half of the average background radiation dose in the UK (Fig. 6.1). Radon permeates through the rocks into the atmosphere. The intensity of radon exposure varies considerably around the world and within the UK it is minimal in the fenlands of Lincolnshire, higher in parts of the Pennines and up to three times the national average in Cornwall. The radon entering our homes will be determined by the design of the foundations and the choice of building materials. Therefore the place we choose to live and the type of dwelling we choose to live in will affect our exposure to radon. Where radon permeates into a well-insulated house, its concentration will be higher. A well-ventilated house with a special membrane incorporated into the foundations will have a lower concentration of the gas. Existing properties may be improved by increasing the under-floor ventilation, thereby diverting the radon before it enters the living quarters; sadly some older properties have been abandoned because of the radon problem. For miners, radon is an occupational hazard and has been well documented over the years, and pot-holers are increasingly aware of the potential hazards of radon.

Small traces of potassium-40, which is a beta emitter of long half-life ($T_{½} = 1.3 \times 10^9$ years), can be found in the human body and it is also present in many fertilisers through which it enters the food chain. All these 'natural' sources contribute an average dose to the UK population of approximately 2.3 mSv per annum, of which about one-half is attributable to radon.

In addition, there is the smaller component from the 'artificial' or 'man-made' sources of radiation amounting, on average in the UK, to about 0.3 mSv per annum. Most of this comes from the diagnostic uses of X-rays. (Although the individual doses are small, large numbers of exposures are performed. On average every member of the UK population has at least one

X-ray examination every year.) A major report (NRPB 1990) on diagnostic medical exposures resulted in some considerable reduction in the diagnostic patient dose by optimising the exposure parameters and the equipment and through the publication of 'diagnostic reference levels' (DRLs) for particular diagnostic procedures. Some 75% of hospitals have now developed conditions whereby their patient doses are below these national guidelines. A further consequence has been a more stringent control over the use of the 'high-dose techniques' such as CT scanning (p. 105). A further review has lead to a proposal to set national DRLs (NRPB 1996). Although the exposure to patients receiving radiotherapy is considerably greater, the relatively small numbers (~0.25%) contribute little to the population average. The other 'artificial' sources of radiation (e.g. the nuclear industry), often highlighted in the media, contribute relatively insignificant levels to the overall background dose, while others (e.g. smoke detectors) are readily accepted because their benefit is considered to outweigh the associated risk.

The UK average background dose is therefore approximately 2.6 mSv per annum and breaks down as shown in the pie chart (Fig. 6.1); it should be remembered that regional variations are quite large, principally due to the radon component. The average in the EU is said to be ~3.5 mSv.

DOSE LIMITATION

Before any use of ionising radiation is put into practice, a formal *risk assessment* must be documented to cover the control measures needed under normal and accident situations and the designation of areas and staff, including pregnant workers. These risk assessments must be kept under review in the light of changes in regulations as well as in procedure and/or practice.

The deleterious effects of radiation are recognised and the aim of radiation protection legislation and practice is to allow the benefits of radiation to be gained, both for the individual and for the population as a whole, with minimal, but acceptable, risk. To this end, the International Commission on Radiological Protection (ICRP 1991) elaborated on the three main features for dose limitation they had laid down previously (ICRP 1977b) for any practice involving ionising radiation. (The extracts that follow together with Tables 6.1, 6.2 and 6.3 are reprinted, with kind permission, from the Annals of the ICRP, Publication 60, H Smith (ed), copyright 1990, International Commission on Radiological Protection.)

- *Justification of a practice*: No practice involving exposures to radiation should be adopted unless it produces sufficient benefit to the exposed individuals or to society to offset the radiation detriment it causes.
- *Optimisation of protection*: In relation to any particular source within a practice, the magnitude of individual doses, the number of people exposed, and the likelihood of incurring exposures where these are not certain to be received should be kept as low as reasonably achievable, economic and social factors being taken into account. This procedure should be constrained by restrictions on the doses to individuals (dose constraints), or the risks to individuals in the case of potential exposures (risk constraints), so as to limit the inequity likely to result from the inherent economic and social judgements.
- *Individual dose and risk limits*: The exposure of individuals resulting from the combination of all the relevant practices should be subject to dose limits, or to some control of risk in the case of potential exposures. These are aimed at ensuring that no individual is exposed to radiation risks that are judged to be unacceptable from these practices in any normal circumstances. Not all sources are susceptible to control by action at the source and it is necessary to specify sources to be included as relevant before selecting a dose limit.

The second of these statements has been widely known as the ALARA principle (as low as reasonably achievable) or ALARP (as low as reasonably practicable). The first two statements apply equally to those occupationally exposed as to those exposed as patients. There are no dose limits laid down for the exposure of patients. Medical practitioners are legally responsible for ensuring their practice is within the national guideline doses for particular procedures. The exposure of patients should be the minimum consistent with the medical benefit to the patient.

Equivalent dose

Absorbed dose, D, has been defined (p. 51) as the energy absorbed per unit mass, and in the context of radiotherapy, the dose-to-water (in gray) is an adequate measure, along with the statement of beam quality, as the dose is given under controlled conditions. Absorbed dose is, however, inadequate as a measure of the deleterious effect resulting from the many sources of radiation which may be encountered and need to be considered in radiation protection. The total effect may result from an accumulation of exposures from different types of radiation and to different tissues of the body, T. The term *equivalent dose*, H_T, is the summation of the absorbed dose averaged over the tissue or organ, D_{TR}, due to radiation R, weighted by W_R, *the radiation weighting factor* (Table 6.1). The equivalent dose is then given by:

$$H_T = \Sigma\, D_{TR}\, W_R$$

where the summation allows for the effects of a range of radiations to be taken into account. In Table 6.3, the dose limits for the lens of the eye, the skin and the hands and feet are equivalent dose limits. Equivalent dose cannot be used to assess the effects of radiotherapy or the early consequences of severe accidental exposures.

Effective dose

The probability of a stochastic effect is dependent not only on the equivalent dose but also on the sensitivity of the organ or tissue receiving that dose. It is therefore necessary to bring the tissue itself into the analysis of risk by applying a *tissue weighting factor*, W_T, to the equivalent dose, H_T. The summation of this product is called the *effective dose*, E, where:

$$E = \Sigma\, H_T\, W_T$$

The recommended values of W_T are given in Table 6.2. In the event of the whole body being uniformly irradiated, the equivalent dose, H_T, is numerically equal to the effective dose, E, because $\Sigma W_T = 1$. Both equivalent dose and effective dose are quoted in sieverts (1 Sv = 1 J/kg) and, where $W_R = 1$ and $W_T = 1$ respectively, they will be numerically equal to the absorbed dose in gray.

Weighting factors are particularly important when radioisotopes may be taken into the body by inhalation or ingestion or through injuries or absorption through the skin. The chemistry of the radionuclide itself, or of the label to which it is attached, will determine where the isotope is likely to be concentrated in the body and which organ or tissue will receive the majority of the dose. The length of the exposure will be determined by the effective half-life taking into account, as it does, the physical half-life of the isotope and its likely excretion rate or biological half-life.

Table 6.1 Radiation weighting factors* (reproduced with permission from ICRP 1991)

Type and energy range	Radiation weighting factor, W_R
Photons, all energies	1
Electrons and muons, all energies	1
Neutrons, energy < 10 keV	5
> 10–100 keV	10
> 100 keV – 2 MeV	20
> 2–20 MeV	10
> 20 MeV	5
Protons, other than recoil protons, energy >2 MeV	5
Alpha particles, fission fragments, heavy nuclei	20

* All values relate to the radiation incident on the body or, for internal sources, emitted from the source.

Table 6.2 Tissue weighting factors* (reproduced with permission from ICRP 1991)

Tissue or organ	Tissue weighting factor, W_T
Gonads	0.20
Bone marrow (red)	0.12
Colon	0.12
Lung	0.12
Stomach	0.12
Bladder	0.05
Breast	0.05
Liver	0.05
Oesophagus	0.05
Thyroid	0.05
Skin	0.01
Bone surface	0.01
Remainder	0.05†‡

* The values have been developed from a reference population of equal numbers of both sexes and a wide range of ages. In the definition of effective dose they apply to workers, to the whole population, and to either sex.

† For purposes of calculation, the remainder is composed of the following additional tissues and organs: adrenals, brain, upper large intestine, small intestine, kidney, muscle, pancreas, spleen, thymus and uterus. The list includes organs which are likely to be selectively irradiated. Some organs in the list are known to be susceptible to cancer induction. If other tissues and organs subsequently become identified as having a significant risk of induced cancer they will then be included either with a specific W_T or in this additional list constituting the remainder. The latter may also include other tissues or organs selectively irradiated.

‡ In those exceptional cases in which a single one of the remainder tissues or organs receives an equivalent dose in excess of the highest dose in any of the 12 organs for which a weighting factor is specified, a weighting factor of 0.025 should be applied to that tissue or organ and a weighting factor of 0.025 to the average dose in the rest of the remainder as defined above.

Effective dose limits

The annual effective (whole body) dose limits have largely remained unchanged over the last 35 years, but how they are applied in practice has changed. At one time, the permitted cumulative dose was limited to $50(n - 18)$ mSv, where n was the age of the individual in years. This was effectively reduced when the formula was abandoned in preference to a limit for the calendar year of 50 mSv, ignoring any previous lower levels of dose. The latest recommendation (ICRP 1991, HSE 1999) is that while the annual limit remains at 50 mSv in special circumstances, the dose averaged over any 5-year period should not exceed 20 mSv per year for those occupationally exposed and over 18 years of age. Women of reproductive capacity at work are subject to the further constraint that the equivalent dose from external radiation averaged throughout the abdomen shall not exceed 13 mSv in any consecutive period of 3 months. Radiation workers under 18 years of age are subject to a limit of 6 mSv in any calendar year; there is a proposal to ban all persons under 16 years of age from working with ionising radiations.

Occupational exposure is that exposure incurred at work to radiations considered to be the responsibility of the management. Occupational exposure therefore generally excludes exposure to the natural background radiation, that is, unless these levels are raised above the average through the nature of the work, e.g. radon in mines or piloting high-flying aircraft; and excludes personal exposures for medical purposes.

All those not occupationally exposed, i.e. other staff, patients, visitors and contractors, etc., are subject to the lower 'public' dose limit of 1 mSv in any calendar year averaged over 5 years subject to a maximum of 5 mSv in 1 year. Special arrangements are made for limiting the dose to healthy volunteers exposed for research purposes. The effective dose limits (Table 6.3) do not apply to patients undergoing medical exposures for diagnostic or therapeutic purposes.

Limits may also be derived from Table 6.3 for the accumulation of radioisotopes in the body by ingestion or inhalation. These dangers may arise from damage to sealed sources but, more frequently, from the use of unsealed sources in the form of solutions, aerosols, gases or powders. Using appropriate assumptions about the way in which the various isotopes are metabolised in the body, it is possible to deduce the concentration of isotopes in the air or in water which can be accepted in the environment. Similar figures may be derived for the total body content of the various isotopes which in time would lead to a given whole-body dose, known as *annual limits of intake* (ALI).

Previously, women of reproductive capacity have been subjected to the same dose limits only on the understanding that the exposure was crudely at a uniform rate. Under the new definitions, no distinction is made between men and women. Once a pregnancy has been confirmed, however, an effective dose limit to the surface of the woman's abdomen of 2 mSv is applied for the remainder of the pregnancy, together with the intake of radionuclides reduced to one-twentieth of the normal annual limit of intake (ALI). (These reduced dose limits cannot be applied retrospectively, and it is the woman's responsibility to formally notify her employer once the pregnancy is confirmed.) In hospitals where good practice is well established, the dose levels reported in recent years are so low that there is rarely any need for changes in routine duties resulting from the declaration of pregnancy on the grounds of radiation dose. The decisions must be based on local circumstances. However, the mutual concern for the welfare of the unborn child is such that staff are often only too willing to change their rosters to minimise any risk, however small it may be.

Table 6.3 Recommended dose limits* (reproduced with permission from ICRP 1991)

Application	Dose limit (mSv)	
	Occupational	Public
Effective dose	20 per year, averaged over defined periods of 5 years†	1 in a year‡
Annual equivalent dose in		
the lens of the eye	150	15
the skin§	500	50
the hands and feet	500	—

* The limits apply to the sum of the relevant doses from external exposure in the specified period and the 50 year committed dose (to age 70 years for children) from intakes in the same period.
† With the further provision that the effective dose should not exceed 50 mSv in any single year. Additional restrictions apply to the occupational exposure of pregnant women.
‡ In special circumstances, a higher value of effective dose could be allowed in a single year, provided that the average over 5 years dose not exceed 1 mSv per year.
§ The limitation on the effective dose provides sufficient protection for the skin against stochastic effects. An additional limit is needed for localised exposures in order to prevent deterministic effects.

Basic principles

The following principles of dose limitation are discussed in isolation, but in practice it is often necessary to consider them together and to come to a compromise as to the most effective means of minimising the radiation hazard in a particular situation.

Time

Total exposure is the product of exposure rate and time and therefore it is important to keep the exposure time as short as possible. In the case of diagnosis or treatment of a patient, the exposure has to be the minimum, but consistent with the desired clinical result as any further reduction may jeopardise the outcome and result in further exposure. The time staff spend in the vicinity of patients with brachytherapy sources in situ or unsealed sources in vivo should be restricted to only performing essential duties and these may be shared with others to keep the individual doses to a minimum. Where patients need little more than a watchful eye, then relatives should be asked to co-operate. Complex procedures should be practised initially with inactive sources until they can be performed efficiently. Fluoroscopy screening times in diagnosis or treatment simulation may be kept short by the use of last frame hold facilities.

Distance

Photons travel in straight lines. The intensity of radiation, and therefore the exposure rate, is reduced with increasing distance from the source, following the inverse square law. Long-handled forceps and the long handles on lead pots and trolleys, etc. all increase the distance—pulling, rather than pushing, a trolley further increases the distance between the source and the operator. Where patients have sources in situ, standing at 3 metres' distance is more than twice as effective as standing at 2 metres. In diagnostic radiology, increasing the focal–patient distance reduces the patient dose (although the exposure factors will have to be increased).

Barriers

Wherever possible, an appropriate protective barrier should be used between the source of radiation and the patient or member of staff. It is important that the shielding is of a material appropriate to the radiation. A simple Perspex shield can be very effective against beta particles (p. 239); a lead rubber apron is totally ineffective against the photons from caesium or iridium. Tungsten syringe shields in nuclear medicine combine attenuation with increased distance to reduce the finger dose by an order of magnitude from the radioactive contents of the syringe. Lead glass spectacles may be usefully employed for screening procedures which require manipulation of the patient, but the hands must be kept well out of the primary beam as lead rubber gloves give limited protection. Lead rubber aprons must be worn and fastened and the use of thyroid shields by staff is to be encouraged to protect them from scattered radiation; lead rubber is ineffective against the primary beam. Gonad shields etc. are of course essential for the patient unless the shields will obscure the diagnostic information being sought. In all these examples, the operator is responsible for seeing that the shields are used correctly on the patient and that their staff colleagues are adequately protected. Elsewhere the careful design of protected walls (p. 239), benches, etc. encourages good practice.

Contamination

Where unsealed sources of radioactivity are used, a further factor has to be considered, namely the possibility of the operator becoming contaminated. As seen above, contamination can occur by inhalation or ingestion of the isotope or by absorption through the skin. Simple protective clothing—theatre clothes, for example—may be all that is necessary in most situations, with the addition of masks, plastic aprons, gloves and overshoes when appropriate. The laundering or disposal of theatre clothes is simpler than of the operator's personal clothing! Where contaminated clothing has to be laundered, it must be laundered separately from other hospital laundry and preferably in a dedicated machine within the nuclear medicine department.

Contamination of floors, benches, furnishings, etc. can be minimised by the use of lipped trays lined with absorbent tissues and the well-disciplined procedures detailed in the Local Rules (p. 78). Floors, benches and other surfaces should be finished with continuous impervious surfaces for ease of decontamination and to minimise the seepage of radioactive material into joints and cracks. These simple precautions will help to reduce the exposure rather than eliminate it altogether.

Respect

The presence of ionising radiation cannot be detected by any of the five human senses and great reliance has to be placed on the use of instruments. Sadly, no one instrument can detect the whole range of ionising radiations and the instrument has to be carefully chosen. Radiation trefoil signs (Plates 1.2 and 1.3) will be displayed in any situation where there might be a radiation hazard or where special precautions are required. It is imperative, therefore, that members of staff heed the warning signs so as not to put themselves, or others, at risk—the 'others' in this context are unlikely to know the meaning of the trefoil sign, making it even more important that members of staff accept their responsibilities in this matter. The misuse of the trefoil sign is a disciplinary matter.

ADMINISTRATIVE STRUCTURE

Designation of areas

All medical X-ray generators and some therapy sources of radiation are large enough to require strict controls to be implemented, both in the construction of the area in which they are to be housed and in their operation, if the dose limits are to be satisfied. (The maximum permitted leakage of radiation from X- and gamma ray beam generators will be discussed in Chs 7, 9 and 10.) Radiation generators should be housed in areas where sufficient protection is afforded so that staff working in adjacent areas need not be regarded as occupationally exposed. ('*Radiation generator*' in this context is an all-inclusive term for radionuclides and electrically powered radiation machines.) Where persons are required to work in or near radiation areas, then engineering controls and design considerations must be used to protect them from the radiation. For example, concrete protective barriers are preferred to moveable lead screens which may or may not be used; an interlock is preferred to an instruction, which may or may not be obeyed.

Under the current ICRP recommendations (ICRP 1991) and UK legislation (HSE 1999), radiation areas must be designated

- as *controlled areas* wherever a person is required to follow special procedures to restrict significant exposure or is likely to receive an effective dose greater than 6 mSv per year or an equivalent dose greater than three-tenths of any relevant dose limit
- as *supervised areas* where it is necessary to keep the conditions of the area under review to determine whether the area should be designated as a controlled area or where any person is likely to receive an effective dose greater than 1 mSv per year or an equivalent dose greater than one-tenth of any relevant dose limit.

At the design stage, locally agreed *dose constraints* may be applied to restrict the radiation exposures to levels below the formal effective dose limits quoted above.

Both controlled and supervised areas are required to be clearly defined, preferably by easily definable boundaries. For example, a permanently controlled area may be 'the treatment room and the maze corridor'; a temporary controlled area may be 'the area within 2 metres of the patient' being X-rayed on a ward. The radiation warning trefoil sign should be clearly displayed together with words on a white or yellow background explaining the designation, the nature of the radiation—gamma rays, X-rays, etc.—and the risks. The warning sign is a black trefoil on a yellow background within a black equilateral triangle, with its point uppermost (Approved Code of Practice, HSE 1985a). Electrically operated signs are ideal for X-ray rooms as the restrictions may be lifted and the sign switched off when the generator is isolated from the electrical supply (Plate 1.2); a permanent sign is required for laboratories and wards where radioisotopes are stored (Plate 1.3). However the area is marked on site, the site must be fully described in the Local Rules. All staff working in the vicinity of radiation areas must be made aware of the meaning of the signs for their own safety and the safety of others. Only four groups of people are allowed to enter a controlled area:

- The patient undergoing medical diagnosis or treatment with radiation or persons participating in research (for whom there are very stringent controls, not considered here).
- Those who are authorised to inspect the areas for compliance with the regulations.
- Those who do not need to be designated as classified workers and who have been issued with a written *system of work* ensuring that they do not receive a dose in excess of any relevant dose limit in any calendar year.
- Classified workers subject to individual dose assessment.

Where classified workers from another undertaking, e.g. servicing company engineers, have to enter a controlled area within the hospital, then the hospital must make an entry, detailing an estimate of the engineers' personal exposure received during the visit, in their personal Radiation Passports (HSE 1993).

Occupationally exposed workers

Just as a controlled area has been defined as one where a person's effective dose might exceed 6 mSv per year or three-tenths of any relevant dose limit, so people who are occupationally exposed are designated as *classified persons* if their personal effective doses might exceed 6 mSv per year or an equivalent dose in excess of three-tenths of any relevant dose limit. In hospitals, there are unlikely to be many staff classified in this way. Those practising manual techniques involving therapeutic activities of caesium-137 or iodine-131, etc.

may be classified. Some of those practising interventional radiology—cardiologists and orthopaedic surgeons—may need to be classified on the basis of their eye dose, assuming their whole body doses are kept low by the adequate use of lead rubber aprons, etc. Those operating radiotherapy beam equipment are unlikely to be classified. Classified workers must be over 18 years of age and regarded as 'fit for the work with ionising radiation which they are to carry out' by the appointed doctor (p. 79). The designation as a classified person may only be withdrawn at the end of a calendar year and that person should be given a 'termination record' of their radiation dose.

A useful aid to maintaining the high standards of radiation safety is to establish local *investigation levels* about the expected radiation exposure of staff for different, but specific, procedures. These will, of course, be less than three-tenths of the relevant dose limits. An example may be where experience of a particular procedure has shown staff rarely exceed 3 mSv per year. The level may be set at 2 mSv per year (or pro rata for each monitoring period). Using this locally agreed level then justifies an enquiry into the circumstances surrounding any dose report suggesting it may be exceeded. These constraints should be revised (downwards) from time to time as the practice improves. At a national level, the UK has an agreed investigation level such that any person on course for an accumulated dose of 75 mSv in 5 years will be subject to a thorough investigation.

Local Rules

It is the employer's duty to draw up Local Rules. The *Local Rules* will contain a description of, and the extent of, each designated area, a list of the named officers responsible for radiation safety, systems of work, contingency plans and the arrangements for personal monitoring. Local Rules are required for each controlled area and, where appropriate, for supervised areas; the employer may choose to provide Local Rules for other areas.

Systems of work

The majority of hospital staff required to enter classified areas will enter under a written system of work. The *systems of work* describe in detail how procedures can be carried out in such a way that the exposure will not exceed three-tenths of any relevant dose limit or locally agreed action level. They may specify the techniques and/or the equipment to be used; they may limit the time spent in the area. They will include the precautions that need to be taken and the location and meaning of warning signs, alarms and the emergency procedures to be followed should anything untoward occur.

Contingency plans

In anticipation of any foreseeable emergency in a designated area, the Local Rules will contain contingency plans, so that those responsible for radiation safety know exactly what to do and who to inform should an emergency arise. Obvious contingency plans include the suspected loss of or damage to a sealed source (p. 242), the failure of the source transfer mechanism on remote afterloading equipment (p. 240), the failure of the shutter mechanism on a gamma ray beam unit (p. 182), the resuscitation of a patient with unsealed or sealed sources in situ (pp. 240, 248), the death of a patient following the administration of a therapeutic dose of iodine-131 (p. 248), etc. Other contingency plans will deal with problems such as the spillage of an unsealed radionuclide (p. 248) or the breakout of fire in the radiotherapy ward or department (p. 87). Where unsealed sources are used or sealed sources are at risk of damage, then an emergency kit should be made available (p. 249). Its contents and recommended procedures for use should be detailed in the Local Rules, so that any contamination can be dealt with promptly and efficiently.

Radiation Protection Supervisor

A *Radiation Protection Supervisor* (RPS) will be appointed, in writing, for each area subject to Local Rules and named in those rules.

- On a day-to-day basis, the RPS is responsible for seeing that the radiation procedures are carried out in accordance with the Local Rules and the regulations, and that high standards of safety are maintained, and for ensuring the effectiveness of both the environmental and personal radiation monitoring.
- The RPS should be someone in a position of authority and familiar with both the work of the Department and the requirements of the regulations governing their uses of radiation, but not necessarily the Head of Department. The Radiation Protection Adviser (RPA; see below) should be consulted about the appointment.
- The RPS should be involved with the writing of the Local Rules, Systems of Work and Contingency Plans to ensure they are both practical and not prohibitive.

- The RPS should ensure the Local Rules are kept under review and assist others in investigating any untoward occurrence.

Operating procedures

Although not strictly a part of the administrative structure for radiation safety, operating procedures play a vital part in ensuring the safety of staff and patients. The operating procedures are more than the operating instructions issued by the suppliers of equipment, although they will be a part. The operating procedures will specify the staffing levels and the responsibilities of each grade involved. They will include the normal operating parameters under which the equipment will be used, what is the acceptable variation in each of those parameters and when the equipment should be taken out of clinical use and by whom. They will include those indicators which warn of malfunction. They will contain the programme of safety checks and their recommended frequency, the need for keeping an up-to-date log of the machine faults (pp. 157, 177) etc. and to whom those faults should be reported and when.

A sign should be clearly displayed at all times to show who is carrying responsibility for each radiation generator—e.g. during clinical use, the radiographers; during servicing, the engineers; during maintenance, the technicians; during quality control, the physicists, etc.—and each of these hand-over procedures needs to be clearly documented.

Radiation Protection Adviser

While the ultimate responsibility for ensuring the recommendations are put into practice lies with the radiation employer, the employer will engage the services of a radiation physicist to act as *Radiation Protection Adviser* (RPA) in relevant areas and provide the necessary information and facilities.

- The RPA must have demonstrated competence in the relevant areas of radiation protection to the satisfaction of a recognised professional body.
- The RPA will advise the employer on the need to identify controlled areas and classified workers and supervise the implementation of the radiation safety legislation.
- The RPA is required to examine all proposals to install new radiation equipment and subsequently to assess and report on how effectively the equipment itself and its accommodation satisfies the recommendations, and periodically carry out such tests as are necessary to restrict the exposure to ionising radiation. In return, he/she needs to be kept informed of any changes of equipment or its use or any changes of use of radiation areas.
- The RPA will be involved in training staff in all aspects, in overseeing the personal monitoring and the investigation of any abnormally high exposures.
- The RPA should also be consulted about the design and content of quality assurance programmes.

Employment Medical Adviser

If classified workers are to be appointed, then an *Appointed Doctor* (appointed by the Health and Safety Executive) or *Employment Medical Adviser* (EMA) should ensure that their physical fitness is appropriate in the first instance and keep it and their annual accumulated dose under review. An entry must be made in the record every year (between 11 and 13 months). The Appointed Doctor will receive training on the regulations (HSE 1999). The EMA will also be responsible for counselling women who are, or may become, pregnant, those who are anxious about their personal exposure record, those reported as receiving an overexposure and those who may volunteer themselves as subjects in radiation research. Medical surveillance records are to be kept for at least 50 years from the date of the last entry or until the person to whom they relate would have attained 75 years of age.

Radiation Safety Committee

Under the regulations (HSE 1999), the employer is held responsible to the Health and Safety Executive for compliance with the regulations. In a large establishment, like a hospital, the employer will set up a *Radiation Safety Committee*, where users, advisers and management can discuss matters relating to radiation safety, receive reports on the overall effectiveness of the measures adopted and reports on any incidents which may have occurred. The RPA and EMA should be ex-officio members of this committee. While radiation is only one of many hazards covered by legislation in a hospital, its technical nature suggests it should be discussed by a committee of specialists, who in turn report to a more general forum on health and safety matters.

BUILDING MATERIALS

Before looking at specific protection problems, it is important to look at the materials available and their properties. The photon interaction processes suggest the atomic number is an important factor at the lower photon energies and density is important over the whole range. The two materials in most common use are lead ($Z = 82$, $\rho = 11\ 350$ kg m^{-3}) and concrete ($\rho = 2350$ kg m^{-3}) and a range of data is given in Table 6.4. Other materials are used in selected areas, but their use must be carefully monitored. For example, clay bricks ($\rho = 1600$–2000 kg m^{-3}) may be adequate in a superficial therapy or diagnostic room, but they can vary both in their construction (density) and in their design (there may be weight-reducing cavities within each brick!). The effectiveness of a wall will also be affected by the cement (mortar) used to bind the bricks together. There are many lightweight building blocks ($\rho \leq 1000$ kg m^{-3}) in modern buildings, but they are totally unsuitable in themselves against radiation.

Where new rooms are planned, solid concrete is preferred for its cheapness and its contribution to the structure of the building, as well as its protection properties. For temporary accommodation or alterations to existing buildings, lead bonded between plywood and secured to a supporting frame is probably the preferred material for diagnostic X-ray, low energy therapy rooms and nuclear medicine laboratories, but barytes plaster ($\rho \sim 2000$ kg m^{-3}) on clay brick may be used. For megavoltage energies (including isotope therapy facilities), lead is too expensive. Large thicknesses of lead are best avoided; being a soft metal, it 'creeps' under its own weight and needs substantial support. Concrete is the preferred material. The addition of barytes to concrete, to increase its density (to ~ 3500 kg m^{-3}) is now prohibitively expensive for most applications. Lapped steel plate can be used in conjunction with concrete for a megavoltage installation where space needs to be conserved, but it is best avoided where neutron activation is likely (e.g. for installations generating photons of more than 10 MV).

The protective material used in or on walls must be continuous and without cracks or perforations. For example, the tie-bars used to hold the shuttering in place whilst concrete is poured to form a wall must not be removed. The fixing of towel holders, pictures, etc. to lead-panelled walls can jeopardise the effectiveness of the protection. (This hazard is even greater when these accessories are removed!) Some perforations in the shielding have to be planned; for example, to admit electricity and water supplies, oxygen and vacuum lines, air conditioning, etc. These should be routed round the maze in a ceiling or floor void wherever possible, but inevitably, some have to pass through an otherwise protective barrier (p. 179). They must not be allowed to pass through a primary barrier. Routes through secondary barriers can be accommodated providing they are designed to adequately trap the scattered photons, either by carefully angling the duct against the radiation or creating angles in the duct, e.g. by taking supplies through a wall below the level of the solid floor. Be wary of suspended floors and ceilings.

Lead equivalence

Table 6.4 gives some thicknesses of lead and concrete to attenuate radiations of different energies to one-half (HVL) and to one-tenth (TVL). For example, at 300 kV,

Table 6.4 The approximate half and tenth value layers in lead and concrete for heavily filtered broad beams of X- and gamma rays

X-ray energy/isotope	HVL mm Pb	TVL mm Pb	HVL mm concrete	TVL mm concrete
50 kV	0.06	0.2	—	—
100 kV	0.30	0.95	—	—
150 kV	0.32	1.04	—	—
200 kV	0.43	1.42	—	—
300 kV	1.33	4.4	29	95
Iridium-192	5.5	20	45	145
Iodine-131	7.2	24	47	160
Caesium-137	6.5	22	50	160
Cobalt-60	11	40	65	205
4 MV	—	—	85	275
6 MV	—	—	105	340
10 MV	—	—	120	390
20 MV	—	—	140	460

NB: These values are for illustration purposes only, the filtration effect of any protective barrier changes the energy spectrum of the radiation and therefore the thickness of the HVL and TVL.

95 mm concrete provides the same attenuation as 4.4 mm Pb, whereas for cobalt-60, 205 mm of concrete has the same effect as 40 mm Pb. Putting these comparisons another way, we could say: 'At 300 kV, 95 mm concrete has a *lead equivalence* of 4.4 mm Pb'; and 'At cobalt-60 energies, 205 mm concrete has a lead equivalence of 40 mm Pb'. The effectiveness of any barrier, of whatever construction, can be stated in '*mm Pb equivalent*' provided the photon energy is known. In practice, barriers are often specified in mm Pb equivalence at the design stage and before the material is decided. Protective barriers should be clearly labelled so that their construction is known and their effectiveness is not subsequently compromised.

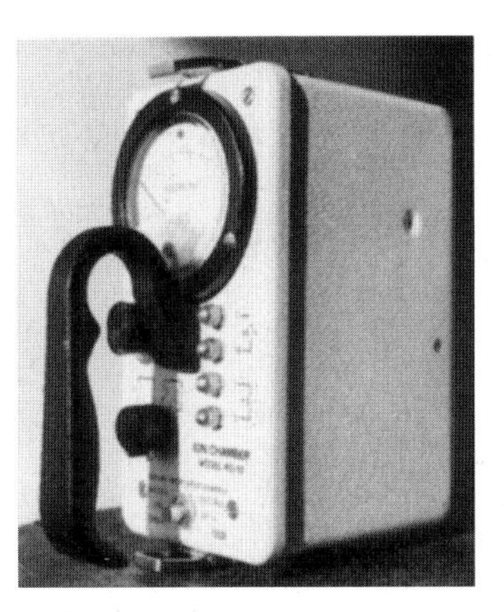

Fig. 6.2 A hand-held survey dose meter incorporating a 200 ml ionisation chamber.

ENVIRONMENTAL MONITORING

The aim of environmental monitoring is to check that the protective measures provide an adequately safe environment for those working in the department, for the members of the general public and for workers from other departments who may be exposed to radiation through their presence in or near the radiological department. It is particularly important to survey any new department and to repeat the survey whenever modifications have been made to the structure of the building, to the equipment or to the working practices. Environmental monitoring will include the measurement of radioactive contamination of surfaces, and air concentrations of radioactivity in areas in which unsealed sources are being processed (p. 138), as well as assessing the effectiveness of permanent and temporary protective barriers in radiation laboratories, wards and rooms. An environmental survey is also often necessary if personnel monitoring reveals excessive doses are being reported, as these may indicate the need for some further modification to the shielding or to the working practice.

Environmental monitoring equipment

Measurements of exposure rates around departments can be made by portable ionisation chamber monitors. The exposure rates likely to be encountered will be in the range from 0.01 mSv h^{-1} to 1 mSv h^{-1} and therefore a large-volume chamber will be required. Hand-held instruments with chamber volumes of 200–1000 ml and battery-driven amplifiers are available (Fig. 6.2), but have the disadvantage that they have a long time constant, i.e. they do not respond quickly to changes in the incident radiation intensity.

Instruments involving Geiger counters or scintillation detectors (Ch. 5) are more sensitive than ionisation chambers, respond more quickly and use detectors of smaller size. They do, however, suffer from the disadvantage that their sensitivity is more dependent on the radiation quality than that of ionisation chamber devices. It is therefore more difficult to rely on an accurate reading of the exposure rate. These instruments are more suited to checking for contamination in the isotope laboratory. Other portable instruments are available to which a number of different detector probes may be attached: scintillation probes, with thin windows, are suitable for the detection of alpha and beta radiations and for the detection of contamination on benches, floors and clothing; end window GM tubes are more robust but not suited to alpha detection.

Mains-operated 'gamma alarm' instruments (preferably with a battery back-up) may be permanently installed at strategic points to give audible and/or visual warning when a radiation level reaches a predetermined level. In laboratories, they can warn of an unsatisfactory increase in the radiation level, due to the accumulation of radioactive waste, for example, in an otherwise satisfactory working environment. Located at the exits from a radiotherapy ward and near sluices, they can monitor for the unauthorised passage of sealed sources and thereby help to prevent the inadvertent movement of sources in waste bins or in the clothing of patients or staff. In the radiotherapy department, they are required to provide independent confirmation that the source(s) on gamma beam generator or remote afterloading unit has returned to the safe position.

PERSONAL MONITORING

The personal monitoring of members of staff who are occupationally exposed to radiation is aimed at ensuring that their individual exposures are within the limits laid down (Table 6.3; ICRP 1982). This differs from the estimates made from environmental monitoring as it will be affected by the distribution of duties at different locations during the working day. A number of different types of dosimeter are available including film badges, thermoluminescent badges, quartz fibre electrometers, solid-state dosimeters and pocket-sized Geiger counter instruments. These must be worn continuously during working hours, but kept away from radiation exposure out of working hours. The dosimeter should be worn on the front of the person between the waist and the shoulder to measure whole-body dose, which in the main arises from scattered radiation and does not differ widely at different parts of the trunk. If a protective apron is being worn, the dosimeter should be worn underneath, since the whole-body radiation exposure to the trunk is the quantity to be measured. Additional dosimeters may be worn to monitor the dose to particular sites, for example on the forehead to monitor the dose to the eyes, or on the cuff to monitor hand dose. A thermoluminescent (TL) dosimeter may be small enough to attach to the finger to measure the extremity dose during brachytherapy or radiopharmaceutical procedures.

The quartz fibre electrometer, the pocket Geiger and solid-state dosimeters permit immediate readings to be obtained. It is usual therefore for these to be worn during particular procedures attended by high exposure risk, such as the loading of new sources into gamma ray beam or remote afterloading units. They may incorporate an alarm to indicate the incident exposure rate. The film and TL badges are more suited to measuring the accumulated dose over longer periods of time, of several weeks for example. Shorter periods are advised where the risks are higher.

Personnel monitoring is obligatory wherever classified workers are employed and their dosimeters must be processed by an *approved dosimetry service* (ADS) and calibrated to a national standard. The ADS will keep the records (for at least 50 years from the date of the last entry or until the person to whom it relates would have attained the age of 75 years) and supply reports annually and at other agreed intervals. For other workers, personnel monitoring provides reassurance that the protective measures in the environment and the working practices are satisfactory.

Personal monitoring for internal radiation hazards, aimed at estimating the radiation dose received by staff through the accidental intake of unsealed radioactive substances, is more difficult than that for external radiation. The body burden of gamma-emitting isotopes can be measured using a whole-body counter or simple counting equipment (p. 62). Information can also be deduced, especially for beta- or gamma-emitting materials, by measuring the excretion of radioactive materials, particularly in the urine. A common example of biological monitoring is checking the accumulation of small quantities of iodine-131 in the thyroid gland of workers handling this isotope (Ch. 8).

Film badges

The use of photographic film for the measurement of radiation dose has been outlined in Chapter 5, and the properties and processing techniques are described in Chapter 7. It is easy to obtain a rough estimate of dose by measuring the blackening produced by development under standard conditions. For a given radiation quality, the film density is roughly proportional to the exposure, if the exposure is small. Figure 7.7 shows the exposure–density relationship for a typical film exposed to gamma rays. The high atomic number of the silver halide in the film emulsion makes the film sensitive to radiation quality and much smaller exposures would be needed to produce the same film densities at say 100 keV. Curve A in Figure 6.3 shows that film is some 24 times more sensitive at 40 keV than it is at high energies. Add to this the fact that in radiation protection, the radiation to be measured is mainly low-energy scatter and the fact that the processing conditions can affect the characteristic curve, it is easy to appreciate that film on its own will not give a very accurate estimate of the incident exposure. In spite of these disadvantages, the photographic film is extremely useful for personnel monitoring. It is relatively cheap, easy to process and provides a permanent record of the exposure.

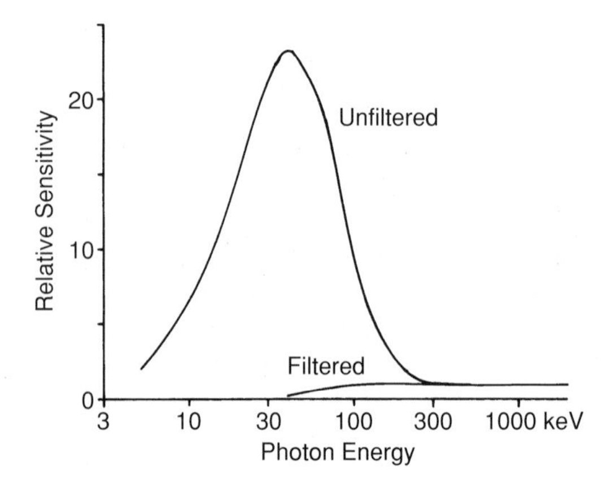

Fig. 6.3 The energy response of photographic film, (A) unfiltered and (B) filtered through the Sn/Pb filter of the AERE/RPS film badge.

In practice, the photographic films used for personnel monitoring are used in a holder or cassette fitted with a variety of metal filters designed to improve the accuracy of the dose estimate. The absorption curve of the filter is designed to match the energy response curve of the film. At high energies, the filter has a negligible attenuation effect and the film is blackened in the normal way. The lower-energy photons, to which the film is more sensitive, are attenuated in the filter leaving fewer to penetrate the emulsion of the film. It is therefore conceivable that, if the degree of attenuation in the filter exactly balances the sensitivity of the film over the whole range of photon energies, then the sensitivity of the film–filter combination would be flat over a wide range of energies; curve B in Figure 6.3 is typical.

A typical badge is illustrated in Figure 6.4. The holder is a moulded polypropylene case into which is fitted a wrapped Kodak Radiation Monitoring (RM) film. The blackening under the different filters is a function of the quality of the radiation to which the whole badge has been exposed. The badge has an open window (4) in the centre through which the identification number stamped on the wrapping can be seen. The effect of the pressure applied in the stamping process enables the number on the film to be read after processing. The window also allows any radiation capable of penetrating the film wrapper, beta rays and very low-energy X-rays, to cause blackening on the film. There are two plastic filters, of 50 mg cm^{-2} (5) and of 300 mg cm^{-2} (6) corresponding to the critical depths of the skin and the lens of the eye respectively. The thinner plastic filter attenuates beta rays and a comparison of the blackening under this filter compared with that under the open window enables beta and very soft X-ray doses to be estimated. The filter composed of 0.028″ tin plus 0.012″ lead (3) is chosen to give a response which is nearly independent of radiation quality from 75 keV to 2 MeV. The filter (1) is an alloy of aluminium and copper 0.040″ thick, chosen to give an estimate of the dose for energies between 15 and 85 keV. Finally, the 0.028″ cadmium plus 0.012″ lead filter (2) may be incorporated to estimate any dose from exposure to neutrons—neutrons interacting with cadmium produce gamma radiation which in turn causes blackening in the film. Where neutrons are unlikely to be encountered, badges have the tin/lead filter extended to replace the cadmium/lead. The 0.012″ lead edge shielding (7) extends round the edge of the tin/lead and the cadmium/lead filters to reduce errors due to the entry of low-energy photons through the edge of the badge, producing blackening under those filters which could be misconstrued as a large high-energy photon exposure. Finally, 0.4 g of indium (8), may be added where appropriate to monitor accidental exposure in nuclear reactors.

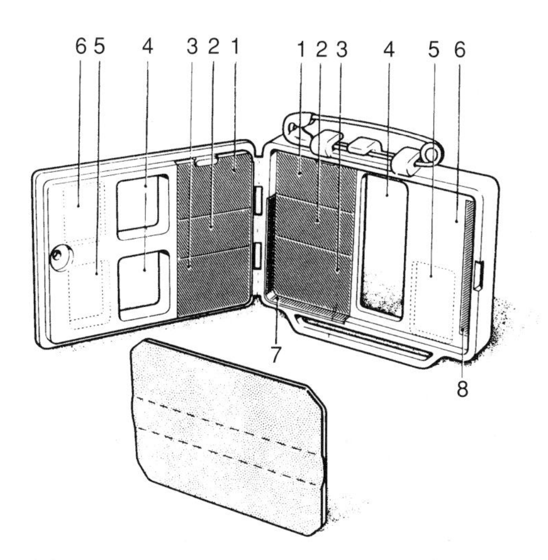

Fig. 6.4 The AERE/RPS film badge. (Courtesy of the Harwell Laboratory.)

The used films are developed with a set of suitable calibration films previously exposed to a range of known doses of gamma rays, together with unexposed films to estimate background and fog effects. A number of empirical methods are adopted by various laboratories to deduce the exposure from the densities measured under the various filters. For handling large numbers of films, an automated densitometer and computer program are used to assess and record the estimated doses. One advantage of the film badge is that the processed film is a permanent record and can be archived for reassessment at a later date should the original dose estimate be challenged.

In order to extend the range of exposure covered by the film, the Kodak RM film has a thick sensitive emulsion coated on one side of the cellulose-acetate base and a thinner, less sensitive coating on the other. In normal use, the density through both emulsions is measured and the doses of a few per cent of the dose limit estimated. High doses make the sensitive emulsion too black for measurement, but it can then be stripped off and a measurement of the density of the thin emulsion alone can be made leading to estimates of up to about 1 Sv.

Thermoluminescent dosimeters

The measurement of exposure by the thermoluminescent effect has already been outlined (Ch. 5). Lithium fluoride powder can be used in a variety of capsules or

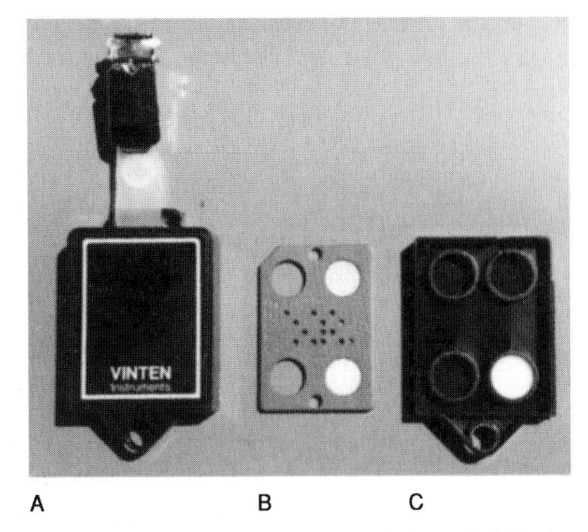

A B C

Fig. 6.5 A TL Badge: **A** the cassette, **B** the coded TL plate and **C** the cassette back.

impregnated into plastic discs for use in cassettes. The advantages of this method of personnel dose monitoring are: (i) freedom from dependence on photon energy because the atomic number of the phosphor is close to that of soft tissue; (ii) the stability of the detector over long periods of time; (iii) a very large dose range (0.1 mSv to 10 Sv) covered by a single dosimeter; (iv) a re-usable dosimeter (there is no permanent record); and (v) ease of automatic processing. The TL badge usually consists of a metal plate carrying a binary coded identification number and housing two lithium fluoride loaded discs (Fig. 6.5). This assembly is loaded into a thin black plastic sheath and fitted into a plastic cassette of a similar size to the film badge. The plastic sheath is to keep the light from the phosphor and to avoid radioactive contamination of the plate; the sheath is monitored for contamination before being removed and the discs are read out. The TL cassette carries only two filters, one thicker than the other, to separate the low-penetration radiations which only contribute to the skin dose from the more penetrating radiations which contribute to the whole-body dose.

Solid state dosimeters

Integrated circuit technology using silicon diode radiation detectors is now available and offers a very robust and compact personal dosimeter, with instantaneous dose or dose rate display and preset dose rate alarm indication. The energy response is similar to the TL badge and film badge for both beta and gamma radiations and covers the range from 1 μSv to 1 Sv.

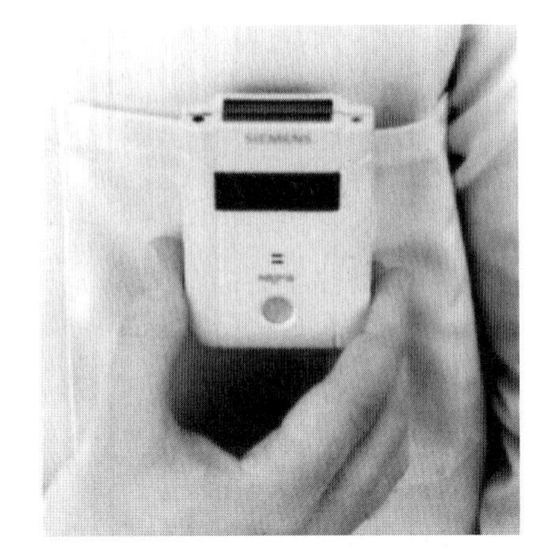

Fig. 6.6 The Siemens/NRPB electronic dose meter. (courtesy of Siemens Plessey Controls, Ltd.)

These instruments (Fig. 6.6) are especially valuable where the risks are relatively unknown.

Quartz fibre electrometer

The pocket-type *quartz fibre electrometer* (QFE) is an instrument in which a direct and immediate reading of the dose can be obtained, and being the size of a pen torch, it is affectionately known as a 'pen monitor'. Its advantage therefore is that the worker can check his or her own exposure at intervals during a particular procedure, instead of having to wait for laboratory processing of the dosimeter, which at best takes a day or two. In this instrument (Fig. 6.7), a metallised quartz fibre is mounted in a small ionisation chamber and illuminated by an external light source shining through one end and viewed by a microscope built into the other end. The fibre system is charged to about 200 volts to bring the position of the fibre to the zero of the scale incorporated in the microscope—the fibre moves away from a fixed fibre by electrostatic repulsion. On exposure to radiation, the ionised air causes the stored charge to leak away and the fibre moves towards the fixed fibre, its shadow on the scale showing an increase in recorded exposure. A selection of sensitivities are available, with different instruments covering full-scale deflections from 2 mSv up to 5000 mSv. The two disadvantages of the instrument are its energy dependence and the fact that doses over and above the full-scale reading are not recorded.

Pocket GM dosimeter/alarms

Microelectronics enable battery-operated Geiger–Muller detectors to be made not much larger than the

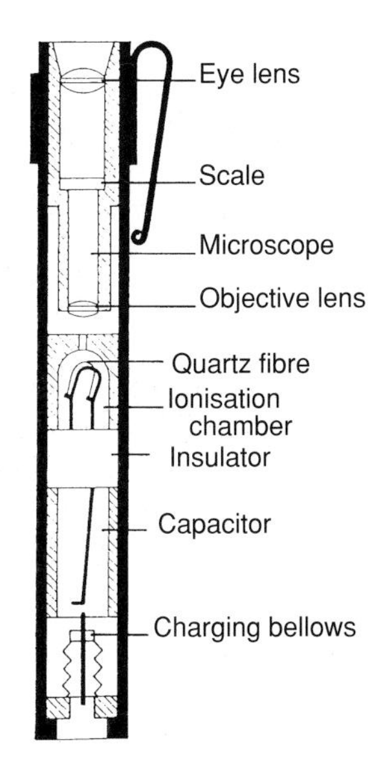

Fig. 6.7 The quartz fibre electrometer. (Courtesy of FAG Kugelfischer Georg Schafer KGaA, Germany.)

QFE and often with more facilities. They may have one of several specifications. The basic device will simply bleep slowly in normal background radiation at, say, one bleep every 20–30 minutes, the rate increasing with radiation level to a continuous tone above about 5 μSv h^{-1}. The second specification will mute the background bleeps below a pre-set threshold level. Neither of these instruments will have an on/off switch or any other operator controls and so continuously monitor their environment. Higher specifications may provide a digital read-out of the total accumulated exposure from the time the instrument was switched on and an alarm signal should the rate exceed one of several pre-settable levels.

DOSE MONITORING RECORDS

Several references have been made to the necessity for keeping appropriate records in order that radiation protection procedures can be adequately controlled and to reduce the risk of accident through changes of working practice not known to the operators. Discipline in this matter is essential and good record keeping is important. The records required fall into two groups, those dealing with personnel and those dealing with equipment.

There are those dealing with the safety of personnel, such as medical records, radiation dose records and records of any unusual exposure or contamination. A separate radiation record has to be kept for each individual classified worker and the recorded doses totalled for each calendar year and for the preceding 5-year period to ensure they are within the dose limits. These records are kept at a central registry, via the approved dosimetry service, so that the record can be maintained even when the worker moves between jobs. Dose records are of great assistance to the EMA in the event of a worker receiving a dose in excess of accepted limits—the EMA must decide whether to carry out a special medical examination and to consider if any rearrangement of the duties of the exposed person is required. The reports of any investigation into a real or suspected overexposure of a member of staff or a patient must be kept for 50 years.

There are records dealing with checks on the safety status of the department, such as the environmental monitoring and contamination monitoring of working areas. These records will include modifications to shields and barriers, to equipment, to controlled areas, warning signs and notices.

Records of daily monitoring for radioactive contamination of personnel and the environment will need to be kept in addition to those of annual inspections of the laboratory/ward areas. The movement, assay, use, leak testing (of sealed sources) and disposal of radioactive sources must be recorded along with the reports of investigations into any suspected loss of, or damage to, sealed sources.

A number of records are required dealing with the care and checking of tools and both radiation-generating and radiation-measuring equipment whose malfunction could lead to a radiation hazard—these will be part of the quality assurance programme—and include the calibration of dosimeters. Full detailed records must be maintained of measurements of output dose rates and any modifications to therapy equipment which may affect the output beam dose rate or beam quality.

Properly organised, record keeping is not an onerous, unnecessary chore but a disciplined activity contributing to a high level of radiation safety in the radiotherapy department. Gross radiation effects, such as that shown in Plate 1.1, should now be a thing of the past.

RELATED SAFETY MATTERS

Safety signs

The radiation hazard is not the only hazard with which the operators of radiation generators need to be familiar. They need to take precautions against the mechanical, electrical, fire and health hazards associated with their equipment. A variety of safety signs will be used around the department and the equipment and these will need to be understood and observed by all members of staff and visitors. In the UK, the four groups of safety signs may be recognised by their shape and colour (Plate 1.4), as follows:

- PROHIBITION signs give instructions about what you are not to do, the symbol is printed in black on a white background within a red circle with a red diagonal line through the symbol.
- WARNING signs warn of risks or dangers, the symbol is printed in black on a yellow background within a black equilateral triangle (point uppermost).
- MANDATORY signs give instructions about what you must do, the symbol is printed in white on a blue circular background.
- SAFE CONDITION signs give a white symbol or lettering on a solid green rectangular background.

These signs may be used singly or in conjunction with others appropriate to the situation and may be supplemented by explanatory wording in black lettering on a white background or on the background colour of the sign itself. They are required to be large enough to be clearly seen from the likely viewing distance.

Acceptance testing

The acceptance tests on a new installation check the equipment's compliance with a previously agreed specification. That specification will detail the operating parameters and the acceptable ranges. In addition, the specification should also include statements requiring the installation to conform to the international and national recommendations on electrical and mechanical performance, on operating temperatures and on the inclusion of materials hazardous to health. Unless these recommendations are cited in the specification, the suppliers may not be legally bound to comply with them. As with radiation protection, internationally agreed recommendations are not necessarily legally adopted at national levels without modification.

Acceptance testing on a new piece of equipment does not guarantee its future performance, and how it does perform will be largely determined by how it is handled and maintained. On-going quality assurance is essential.

Mechanical hazards

The one characteristic which is common to all radiological equipment is the weight. Radiation generators incorporate lead in large quantities making them very heavy. Although the lead is usually supported on a substantial steel framework, the lead can be distorted under its own weight particularly when its movement is stopped suddenly. The overall weight is further increased by the need for counterbalancing the movements.

Where megavoltage equipment is concerned, merely rotating the gantry from one position to another involves the acceleration and retardation of several tonnes. This movement is generally controlled by an electric motor and gearbox. Rapid changes in speed or direction can put considerable strain on that gearbox, increasing the wear and tear, leading to early failure and the need for frequent replacement. The movement of the gantry is easily appreciated, but the same consideration needs to be given to the movement of the collimators, couch, etc.

Kilovoltage therapy tube stands will incorporate either a *counterbalance* weight or a balance spring to counter the weight of the tube housing via a multi-stranded cable or chain. If these are not duplicated as a safeguard against the failure of one, then an automatic brake must be included in the design to arrest the free fall of the tube housing. Any apparent damage to, chafing of or broken strands in the cable, or visual damage to the chain must be reported immediately and attended to as a matter of urgency.

Smaller weights, by comparison, which have to be handled regularly include the kilovoltage applicators and local shielding blocks—all of which are easily damaged if dropped.

All movements lead to wear and tear and the observant operator can report the early signs of damage before accidents occur or expensive repairs become necessary. Arresting movement is most easily achieved by reducing the speed first. The application of brakes should be regarded more as a means of stopping a stationary object from moving rather than a means of bringing a moving object to rest. Brakes rely on the friction between two surfaces and abuse leads to the wearing away of those surfaces, reducing their effectiveness. The observant operator detects this reduction in effectiveness and may recognise the build-up of dust particles from the brake itself.

Plugs and sockets are mechanical devices for making electrical connections and rely on the mechanical pressure between metallic contacts. Inappropriate pulling and twisting of the plug or socket leads to a weakening of the contact pressure, which in turn leads to poor electrical continuity, sparking, oxidation and failure. Equally, they are not designed to support a lot of weight. Heavy cables should be supported independently, high-tension (HT) cables are particularly heavy and need that support.

New HT cables will flex fairly readily. Their inherent electrical resistance and the passage of electric current leads to internal heating of the heavy insulation, which in turn becomes hard and brittle. Unnecessary bending and strain will accelerate this hardening effect leading to the eventual breakdown of the insulation—accompanied by large fluctuations in the displayed tube current and the smell of burning!

Electrical hazards

All electrical equipment is potentially dangerous—even low voltages can cause fatalities. Never operate electrical equipment with wet hands or wet shoes. Residual current detectors (RCD) are recommended.

All major components of any installation should be visibly connected to 'earth' using either a continuous copper tape or a single core wire covered with a green or green and yellow sheath. These connections should all be brought together at a common *earth reference terminal* (ERT). The earthing of a metal frame via the screens of an HT cable is not acceptable. The resistance of each earth connection should be checked regularly. All potentially hazardous electrical and electronic circuitry will be housed in cabinets either behind fixed panels or locked doors. These doors must be kept locked and only opened by authorised personnel after isolating the supply. Furthermore, large capacitors are likely to hold their charge and special precautions need to be taken to discharge them before maintenance work is undertaken. Strict safety procedures must be followed. Maintenance staff must not work alone on electrical equipment (IEC 1998).

The colour codes of indicator and control lamps and cables (Table 6.5.) and the international markings and symbols should be understood.

Reporting of faults

Faults, however trivial they may seem, should be reported in a fault book allocated to that particular equipment and dealt with either immediately or as soon as possible in accordance with the locally agreed protocol. A separate fault book should be kept for each major piece of equipment. The faults recorded will include the failure of warning lights, the fraying or chafing of cables, the stiffness of movements, the ineffectiveness of brakes, the sticking of analogue meter movements, squeaks and rattles, nuts and bolts lost or found, etc., etc. All these are in addition to reporting

Table 6.5 Some colour codes

Coloured indicator lights (e.g. on a control desk)	
RED:	Warning of danger requiring urgent action to terminate an unintended state of operation
YELLOW:	Requiring attention, caution (e.g. radiation on)
YELLOW (flashing):	Sources in transit (e.g. in remote afterloading equipment)
GREEN:	Ready for action
WHITE:	Equipment switched on but further operations required to bring it to the ready state
Coloured cables (single phase mains)	
BROWN:	Live
BLUE:	Neutral
GREEN/YELLOW:	Earth
Coloured cables (three phase mains)	
BROWN/BLUE/YELLOW:	Three live phases
GREEN/YELLOW:	Earth

any deviations from the normal parameters and conditions listed in the operating procedures (p. 79).

Fire hazards

Radiotherapy equipment uses a mixture of high current and high voltages with the consequent potential for fire. In the event of a fire, the mains electrical supply must be switched off immediately—an emergency off control should be available in the treatment room and must be available at the control desk. A second isolator may have to be operated to completely isolate a linear accelerator's ion pump supply. Once isolated from the supply there is no radiation hazard from an X-ray generator (unless there is a risk of neutron activation from > 10 MV photons). Isolating a gamma ray beam unit or remote afterloading unit from the supply should, by design, automatically terminate the exposure and render the sources safe. This must be checked by using a pocket personal alarm or the independent gamma alarm in the treatment room—this is one reason for the instrument being powered independently from the treatment unit. In a major fire, the fire crew must keep the gamma beam unit and/or remote afterloading unit cool.

Water-based fire extinguishers must not be used on electrical equipment of any sort. Carbon dioxide (CO_2) powder may be used on electrical fires.

The radiological department will be designed to permit ready evacuation in the event of a fire. Therapy treatment rooms will rarely have an alternative escape route and the use of combustible materials in the construction or decoration should be minimised, particularly in the maze entrance. Early warning smoke detectors should be fitted either to the ceiling or in the extract air ducting and should be tested regularly, not only to check their operation but also to remind staff of the warning sound they emit, so that it is immediately recognised in the event of an emergency. Consideration and rehearsal of the evacuation of patients from the treatment rooms should include the release from immobilisation devices and the removal of the patient from the maximum height of the couch; bearing in mind that the electrically controlled movements may not be available.

The evacuation of patients with brachytherapy sources in situ or following the administration of unsealed sources should be detailed in the Local Rules. The safety of the patient must take precedence, but the security of long-lived sealed sources must be ensured, whether the policy is to remove the sources before or after the evacuation. Where the source of radiation cannot be removed to a 'safe' position, then alternative safety precautions will need to be implemented. The procedures to be adopted should be agreed with the local Emergency Services in advance.

Ozone is generated wherever intense electron beams are used and, being both corrosive and hazardous to health, adequate air-extraction facilities must be available to minimise the ozone concentration in the atmosphere.

SECTION 2

Imaging with radiation

SECTION CONTENTS

CHAPTER CONTENTS

7

X-ray imaging

Keith Bomford

INTRODUCTION

In previous chapters the word *exposure* has been given to a clearly defined scientific concept, namely the ionisation produced by photons per unit mass of air ($X = \Delta Q/\Delta m$). In this chapter, the word will assume its non-technical meaning of 'being exposed to' unless it is accompanied by the symbol (X).

The most direct method of checking the accuracy of the position of a treatment field is to expose an X-ray film during treatment and so produce a picture of the irradiated tissues. This process is known as *portal imaging* and the film as a *port film* or *check film*. The film should show the entire treatment volume enclosed, thereby confirming that the treatment beam is correct in position, size and shape, and direction. In addition, it is convenient if the film can be left in position for the whole treatment fraction rather than to have to disturb the patient to remove the film before completing the dose.

At orthovoltage X-ray energies, the image quality of the check film is poor but adequate providing the exposure factors and processing combine to produce the maximum contrast. The advent of megavoltage radiotherapy brought several potential improvements in treatment not least:

- Improved penetration (greater depth dose)
- Reduced skin dose (the build-up effect)
- More sharply defined beams (narrow penumbra)
- Reduced bone absorption.

The reduced bone absorption is advantageous to the radiotherapy but not to the portal image. The only significant contrast on a check film taken using megavoltage photon beams results from the difference in density between the tissues and the air passages (Fig. 7.1). The portal imaging technique is discussed later in the chapter (p. 109). One alternative is to have a machine

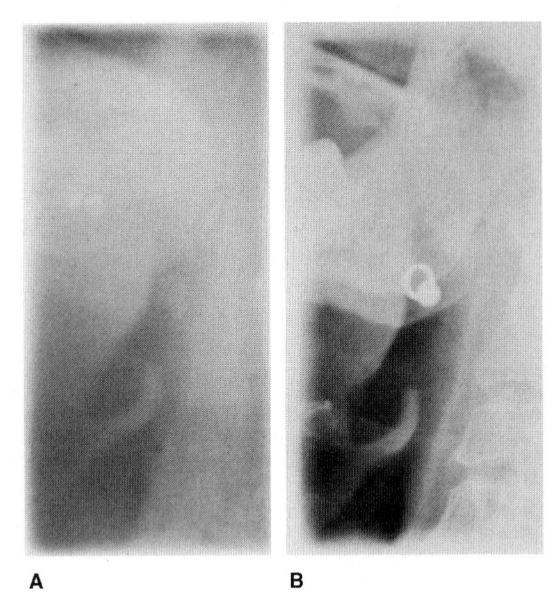

Fig. 7.1 Radiographs of the same patient: **A** note the clarity of the air passages but loss of bone detail at 8 MV; and **B** on the simulator.

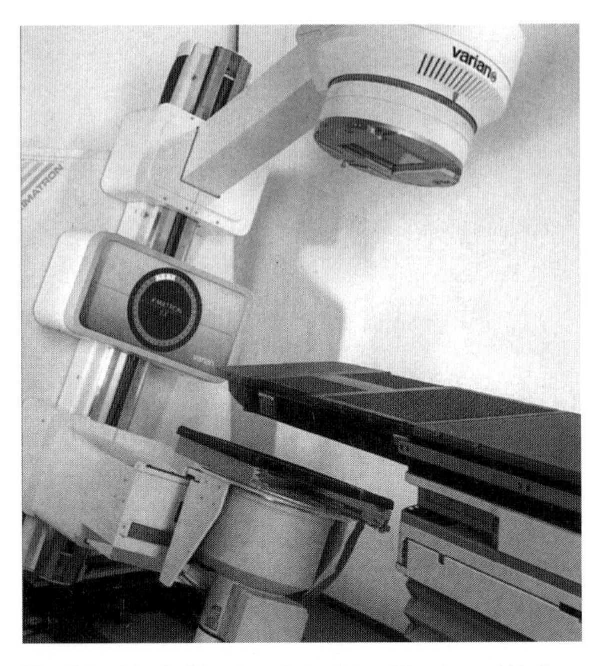

Fig. 7.2 A typical treatment simulator. (Courtesy of Varian Medical Systems UK Ltd.)

which simulates all the movements and geometry of the therapy unit but uses a source of lower-energy X-rays. The *treatment simulator* is, therefore, a unit incorporating a diagnostic X-ray tube in a gantry similar to the treatment unit, particularly in regard to beam collimation and direction and the patient's couch. The simulator (Fig. 7.2) is a sophisticated unit (p. 101) and often considered essential to the planning of any course of radical radiation treatment using megavoltage radiation. A second alternative is to use a CT scanner and to create the simulated geometry within the computer, i.e. a *virtual simulator* (p. 105). Whichever unit is chosen, it is best situated close to the treatment units it simulates but perhaps more important, it should be close to the mould and planning room facilities. In most departments, the simulator will be in the hands of the therapy radiographic staff.

This chapter seeks to introduce those aspects of diagnostic radiology which are relevant to the use of the treatment simulator and of the CT scanner.

PHYSICAL CONSIDERATIONS

Magnification and distortion

Any X-ray image will be a magnified image. Just as an optical shadow is larger than life size, so the X-ray image is larger than the anatomy it portrays. X-rays diverge from a small focal spot and travel in straight lines through the object before reaching the image receptor which may be the radiographic film (p. 94), the input phosphor of an image intensifier (p. 98) or an array of radiation detectors (p. 110). The simple geometry (Fig. 7.3A) shows the *magnification factor* is defined as:

$$m = \frac{XY}{xy} = \frac{f}{s} = \frac{f}{(f-h)}$$

providing both the object and the image are perpendicular to the central ray. If this condition is not satisfied,

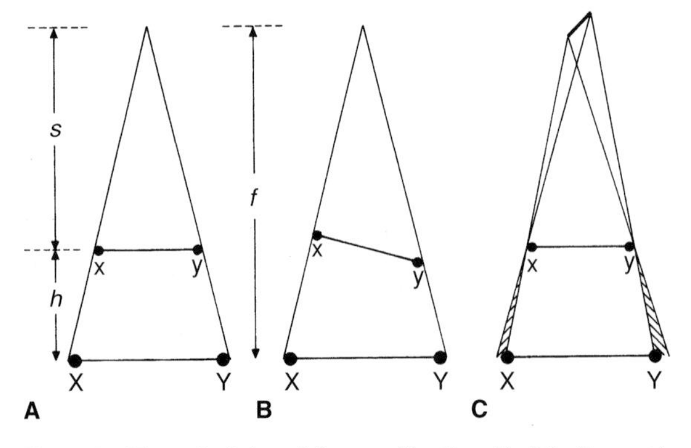

Fig. 7.3 The principles of **A** magnification, **B** distortion and **C** geometric distortion.

the image will suffer distortion in that the magnification at the two extremes will be different (Fig. 7.3B). (It should be noted that *f*, *h* and *s* are normally measured parallel to the beam axis, not along the ray from the focal spot.)

Geometric unsharpness

Diagnostic X-ray tubes usually have the choice of two focal spot sizes, *broad focus* or *fine focus*. The broad focus is several times larger than the fine focus and because the latter is not negligible, all diagnostic images will suffer from some *geometric unsharpness* (analogous to the geometric penumbra of the therapy beam, p. 171). Figure 7.3C shows that the unsharpness at the two ends is different due to the angle of the target. Geometric unsharpness may be reduced by increasing the focal–film distance and/or by reducing the film–object distance, i.e. in the same way as for the therapy beam penumbra.

These effects are simply illustrated when the object is, for example, an iridium pin (e.g. Fig. 7.3). On treatment simulators, the unsharpness is exaggerated in the image of the wire diaphragms used to define the field size (p. 102). The wires are of small diameter, a long distance from the film and cast a large shadow on the film—particularly when a broad focus tube is used (Fig. 7.4B). Note: a double image is sometimes visible from one pair of diaphragm wires but not on the other until the diaphragms are rotated. This is due to the nature of the focal spot. The *focal spot* usually consists of two relatively intense line sources of X-rays separated by an area of lower intensity. When the wire of the diaphragm system is parallel to these line foci, two images of the wire are produced under conditions of large magnification. This effect is not so apparent in the tissues of the patient because the magnification is smaller and the effect reduces to one of simple geometric unsharpness.

The magnified image of more solid objects of a random three dimensional shape will not only exhibit distortion but also suffer from unsharpness. Cylindrical and more complex shapes present different thicknesses to the primary radiation and the transmitted intensity will vary with that thickness. The fine focus should be used to obtain the best geometry wherever the operating parameters of the X-ray tube permit.

Differential absorption

Consider the situation in Figure 7.5 where an inhomogeneity is introduced into an otherwise homogeneous medium. In mathematical terms and considering exponential attenuation only, the intensity transmitted

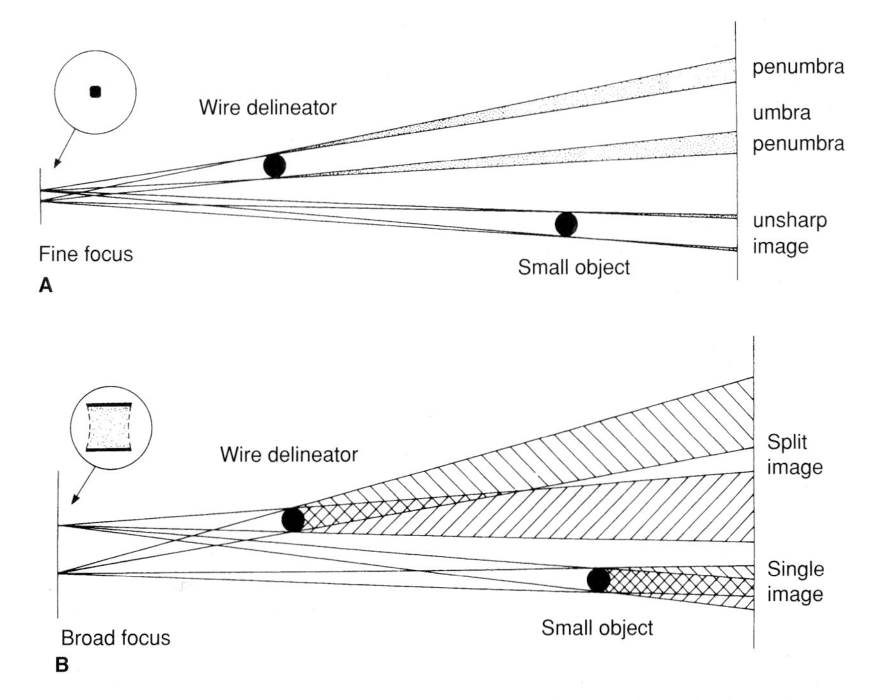

Fig. 7.4 Geometric distortion under **A** fine and **B** broad focus conditions. The split image is due to the non-uniform emission over the broad focus.

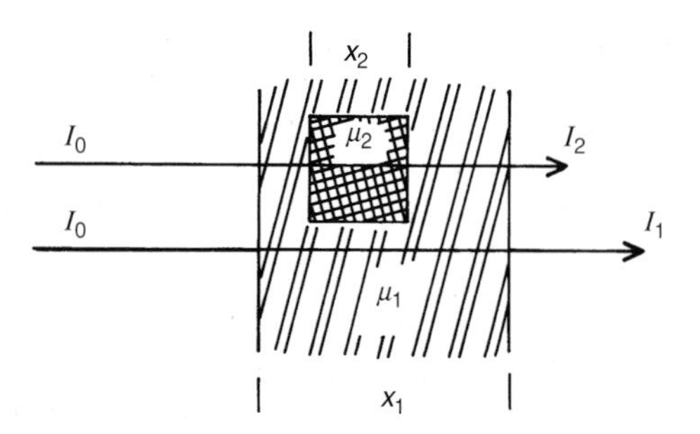

Fig. 7.5 Exponential attenuation through an inhomogeneity in an otherwise homogeneous medium (see text).

by the homogeneous medium, I_1, is given by the equation:

$$I_1 = I_0\, e^{-\mu_1 t_1}$$

while in the shadow of the inhomogeneity, the transmitted intensity, I_2, is given by

$$I_2 = I_0\, e^{-\mu_1 (t_1 - t_2)}\, e^{-\mu_2 t_2}$$

where I_0 is the unattenuated intensity, μ_1 and μ_2 the attenuation coefficients in the media of thickness t_1 and t_2 respectively. Rearranging the terms in the second equation gives:

$$I_2 = I_0\, e^{-\mu_1 t_1}\, e^{-(\mu_1 - \mu_2) t_2}$$

and substituting the first equation gives

$$I_2 = I_1\, e^{(\mu_1 - \mu_2) t_2}$$

Thus the ratio of the transmitted intensities, I_2/I_1, is dependent on the thickness of the inhomogeneity and on the *difference* in the linear attenuation coefficients. The presence of a small inhomogeneity or the thin edge of a larger inhomogeneity will only be detected when I_2 and I_1 are visualised as being different on the radiograph, i.e. when $(\mu_1 - \mu_2)t_2$ is significant. It follows that if vessels are not normally visualised by using X-rays, they may be visualised if they can be filled with a medium with an attenuation coefficient different from their surroundings—i.e. with a suitable *contrast medium*. Contrast media may rely on a higher atomic number, e.g. barium, or a reduced density, e.g. air. Both parameters will profoundly affect the value of $(\mu_1 - \mu_2)$ in the above equation.

Patient movement

Further image unsharpness or *blur* may be caused by patient movement during the exposure. This can be minimised by careful immobilisation of the patient (Ch. 11), by asking the patient to lie still and/or to hold his/her breath. The most effective method is to arrest any movement by the use of short exposure times—providing this is consistent with other factors governing the image quality.

Some movement of the patient can, however, provide important information. It is not physically possible to stop the patient from moving altogether during a treatment fraction of several minutes' duration. During simulation, therefore, it is helpful to ascertain the magnitude of that movement so that an allowance may be made for it in subsequent procedures such as in radiation treatment planning. The rise and fall of the chest wall, for example, may be several centimetres and seriously affect the localisation of the diseased tissues in the thorax unless the point of respiration at which the image is taken is known (Essapen et al 2001).

Quantum mottle

The production of X-rays is a random process involving the bombardment of a target by high-speed electrons. Over a long period of time, the distribution of photons in the X-ray beam is averaged out and can be predicted with some accuracy. However, if the exposure times are very short in order to arrest movement as suggested above, this averaging effect may be incomplete and the distribution of photons less uniform, giving rise to what is called *quantum mottle* on the radiographic film.

THE RADIOGRAPHIC FILM

The radiographic film is a bluish transparent polyester base approximately 0.2 mm thick coated on both sides with a gelatine layer containing silver halide crystals in suspension. Each crystal will be a regular lattice of silver and bromine (Ag^+ and Br^-) ions made sensitive to visible light or X-ray photons by the addition of a small impurity—of silver sulphide. This impurity adds a *sensitivity speck* to each otherwise perfect crystal of silver bromide. Now, when a photon ionises a bromine ion, the negative electron is released leaving an uncharged bromine atom behind, while the electron is temporarily held by the sensitivity speck until a slower moving and positively charged silver ion drifts by and attracts the electron to itself. The electron neutralises the positive charge leaving an uncharged atom of silver. If the exposure of photons was allowed to continue, the number of silver atoms would eventually become visible to the naked eye. However, it is normal to use a much smaller exposure to create an invisible *latent image* which can be developed later using chemicals.

Film processing

The processing of the latent image is in two stages: the *development* of the latent image by chemically accelerating the action already begun during the exposure and the *fixation* of the developed image by the removal of the unaffected silver bromide. During both processes the emulsion swells and is easily damaged making absolute cleanliness and careful handling essential. Automatic processing not only reduces the risk of damage through mishandling but also enables more concentrated chemicals to be used and at higher temperatures, thereby reducing the processing time to typically 90 s. The basic chemistry is common to both but the chemicals are not interchangeable between manual and automatic processing.

The developer is an organic reducing agent containing hydroquinone which reduces the silver halide—affected by the radiation—to base metal silver, a process which depends on both temperature and time. For manual processing, this is typically 5 minutes at 20°C and with occasional agitation to ensure 'fresh' developer is not denied access to the emulsion by the surface build-up of bromine. With the continued use of the same solution over a period of weeks, the solution becomes diluted by the bromine and needs to be replaced by a fresh solution or replenished at regular intervals by the addition of a chemical high in hydroquinone and in the other alkaline elements exhausted by the process. The automatic processor injects the appropriate quantity of *replenisher* solution as required. Overdevelopment slightly increases the effective speed, the gamma and the fog level of the film (p. 96).

Having developed the latent image, the image has to be fixed by removing the remaining silver halides. The fixing agent, sodium thiosulphate or ammonium thiosulphate, clears the film by dissolving the undeveloped silver halide from the emulsion. This fixing agent, or *fixer*, also contains other chemicals to harden the emulsion to make it less prone to damage. The final but important stages in the processing of the film are the washing and the drying. The acid fixer quickly neutralises the alkaline developer but these acids need to be washed out thoroughly. Inadequate washing can result in the clear film appearing greyish-white and the image turning brown after a time. A well-maintained automatic processor avoids many of these processing pitfalls but this does not mean that the careful attention to details of cleanliness can be relaxed, e.g. a filtered water supply, the regular cleaning and the use of fresh chemicals.

The chemicals, particularly for automatic processors, are strong and precautions are necessary to ensure the safety of the staff involved. A well-ventilated atmosphere and the use of protective clothing, goggles and gloves are essential when handling the chemicals. Those with sensitive skins or respiratory problems should be particularly careful. An eyewash bottle should be readily available for use in an emergency.

The automatic processors mentioned above need to be housed in a darkroom so that the film cassette can be unloaded and loaded into the processor manually. The processor will then develop, fix, wash and dry the film and dispense it into a tray ready for collection. In so-called *daylight processing*, the film is processed in total darkness using a machine which automatically unloads the film from special cassettes. These cassettes are both loaded from a film dispenser and unloaded into the processor through light-tight connections. Daylight processing is the preferred option in the busy diagnostic department, whereas the radiotherapy department will require a darkroom to process envelope-wrapped therapy verification film (p. 109) as well as diagnostic film from cassettes.

Silver recovery

The silver dissolved into the fixing solution may be recovered by electrolysis or by metal exchange. Silver can also be recovered from the processed film once the films can be released for disposal; there are strict time limits set for which films must be kept. The quantities of silver recovered are small—0.5% by weight—but silver recovery is commercially viable and environmentally beneficial.

The darkroom

So far as the radiotherapy department is concerned the darkroom should be adjacent to the simulator—a carefully positioned through-the-wall processor can dispense the processed film directly into the simulator control room, thereby minimising the time that staff spend in the darkroom. Some photographic material has to be handled in total darkness but, in general, radiographic film can be handled safely under subdued lighting of the appropriate colour. The film emulsion is sensitive to the green–blue–violet range of the visible spectrum but relatively insensitive to the yellow–red light. Therefore providing the darkroom is well sealed against white light entering through cracks—round the door, for example—it may be lit with *safelights* incorporating yellow–red filters. The precise filter requirements will be given in the film data sheets. When checking for sources of light in the darkroom, it is necessary to stay in the dark for a minimum of 10 minutes simply to let the eyes dilate before making any checks. Once accustomed, the eyes will readily identify any light likely to affect the emulsion on the film. Pieces of unwrapped, unexposed film can be used to check any doubtful sources of light—such as the indicator lights on the processor control panel!

The characteristic curve

The degree of blackness or the *optical density* of the processed film depends, not only on the chemical processing, but on the exposure received by the film, which in turn depends on the intensity of the incident beam and on the thickness and composition of the object being radiographed (Fig. 7.6). The optical density, D, is expressed mathematically as:

$$D = \log_{10} (I_0/I_1)$$

where I_0 is the intensity of the (visible) light incident on the film and I_1 the intensity transmitted. The instrument used to measure optical density is called a *densitometer*.

A graphical representation of the variation of optical density with exposure (X) is called the *characteristic curve*. At very low exposures (X), there is very little

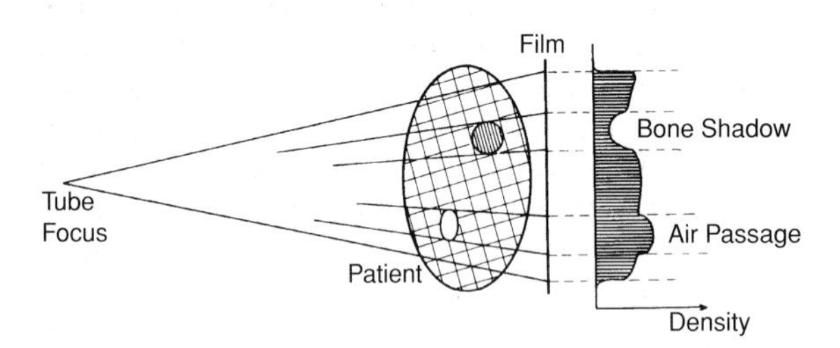

Fig. 7.6 The principle of the radiograph.

density change and the density measured is mostly that of the *fog level* of the film—the inherent density of the polyester base and the gelatine emulsion. At very high exposures (X), any further increase produces no density change and the density measured is that of the silver deposit when all the available silver halide crystals have been reduced—a situation which exists when the film has been grossly *overexposed*. Between these two extremes, there is a region of *correct exposure* (X)—the relatively straight portion of the characteristic curve where the gradient is at a maximum (Fig. 7.7). The correctly exposed film will have a range of densities within this region of the curve, that is, within the range from about 0.4 to 2.0. It is important in producing a radiograph to obtain the maximum difference between the points of interest. The difference in density at two points, A and B, is known as the *contrast*, C, where

$$C = D_A - D_B$$

The human eye under ideal conditions can detect density differences as small as 0.02. Although contrast between two points on the film is the difference in their densities, the *film contrast* at a point is the gradient of the characteristic curve at the point of measurement, D, in Figure 7.7A.

$$\text{Film contrast} = \frac{D_A - D_B}{\log X_A - \log X_B}$$

The slope of the straight portion of the curve is known as the film *gamma* or *contrast index* and represents the region of maximum contrast—usually between the densities of 1 and 3. At densities above 4, the film contrast is reduced as the film becomes saturated.

In any radiograph (Fig. 7.6) a range of densities will be produced and if this range is to be accommodated

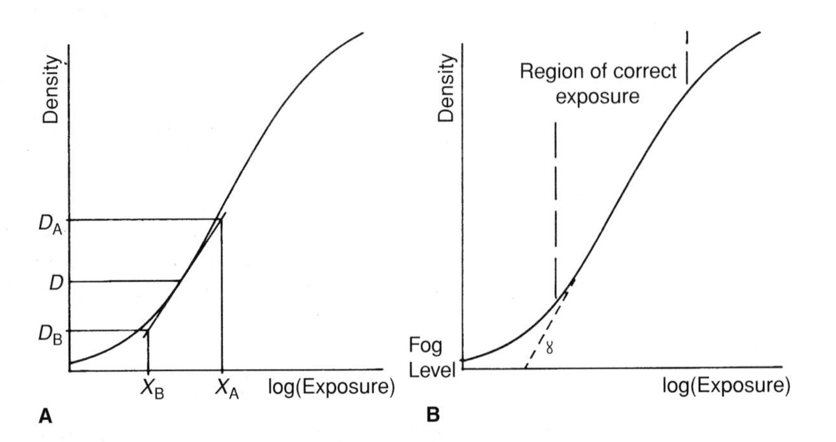

Fig. 7.7 The characteristic curve: **A** film contrast; **B** region of correct exposure for maximum contrast.

within the 'straight' portion of the curve, then the exposure given will have to be carefully chosen. The *latitude* of the film defines its useful dynamic range; the longer the straight portion of the curve, the less critical the exposure for an optimum image. The gamma of the film used has to be chosen to maximise the visual contrast while accommodating the range of X-ray intensities transmitted by the patient. In general, the greater the gamma, the greater the contrast and the more critical the choice of exposure (X).

Another important parameter of the film is its *speed*. If only a small exposure is required to produce a given density, the film is said to be *fast*, whereas a *slow* film requires a longer exposure to produce the same degree of blackening. Film speed is usually quoted in terms of the exposure required to produce a density of 1.6.

Unfortunately, a film is made faster by increasing the size of the silver halide crystals in the emulsion, which also increases the *grain* in the final image, and there is a consequent loss of fine detail. Either a crystal is rendered 'developable' or it is not; either it turns black or it does not. The radiographic image may therefore be considered as being built up with finite-sized black spots or building bricks. The faster the film, the larger the building brick and the less the fine detail that results. The granular appearance may be seen under a magnifying glass.

Intensifying screens

The sensitive emulsion of the film is very thin and the X-ray energy absorbed in that emulsion is small, making the film slow to respond to the radiation. The efficiency of the latent image formation and therefore the speed can be increased by using *intensifying screens*. An intensifying screen is a plastic base coated with a reflective layer and a layer of crystals of a luminescent material. These crystals *fluoresce* under irradiation with X-rays; that is, they emit visible light as an immediate response to the stimulus of the X-ray photons (Fig. 7.8). (*Phosphorescence* or *afterglow* is the name given to a similar response which is delayed or persistent—an undesirable process in intensifying screens.) The brightness of the visible light is proportional to the X-ray stimulus and the wavelength of the visible light is characteristic of the screen material, the consequence of the photoelectric absorption process. The crystals are therefore carefully chosen so that the wavelength of the visible light is near the peak sensitivity of the emulsion of the film—in the blue–green part of the visible spectrum. The once-popular calcium tungstate has largely been replaced by compounds of the rare-earth elements of gadolinium and lanthanum.

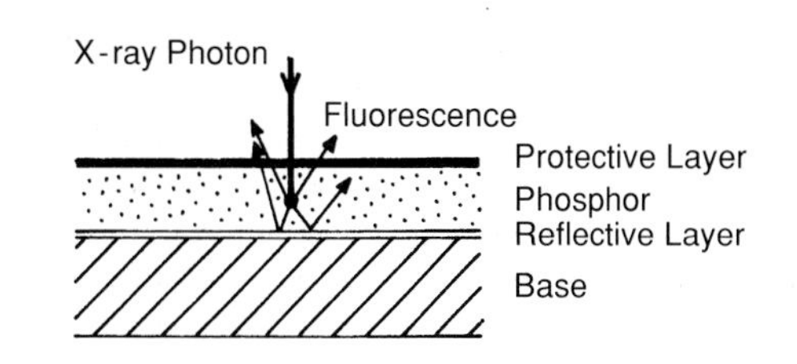

Fig. 7.8 The principle of intensifying screens.

The image is therefore formed in the intensifying screen in visible light and, providing the screen and the film are in very close contact, the light emitted from the screen will enhance the latent image formed in the film emulsion. The crystalline structure of the screen will, however, add to the granular appearance of the radiograph and there will be some further loss of fine detail because the fluorescence is random in direction and not confined to the direction of the primary photon beam. The built-in reflecting layer in the screen redirects some of the light back onto the film. This loss of detail is minimised by keeping the screens scrupulously clean and keeping the screen in close contact with the film emulsion. Particles of dirt can prevent the light reaching the film as well as forming a space between the screen and the film enabling the light to diffuse over a larger area of emulsion. Screens are best cleaned with a proprietary screen cleaner or a cotton cloth moistened with a mild soap solution. Faulty cassettes can prohibit good film–screen contact.

Radiographic emulsion is more sensitive to visible light than to ionising radiation and therefore the exposure required is much reduced when using screens. Screens may be used singly, but more commonly in pairs to enhance the image formation in both emulsions on the film. The front screen is usually thinner than the back screen. The saving in exposure is considerable and is quoted as an intensification factor, IF, where:

$$\text{IF} = \frac{\text{Exposure required to produce a given density when the screens are not used}}{\text{Exposure required to produce the same given density when the screens are used}}$$

In practice, a pair of calcium tungstate (fast) screens had intensification factors of about 30 or 40 while rare-earth screens increase these by a further factor of four or more.

Film holders

The photographic emulsion is sensitive to light and to X-rays and must be stored away from both. It also deteriorates with age, moisture and temperature. Film should therefore be stored in a cool dry place, preferably in a refrigerator well away from the X-ray generator, and dated stocks should be used in strict rotation. Film should be stored vertically to reduce the pressure on the emulsion. Adverse storage conditions result in an increased fog level on the processed film with the consequent loss of contrast.

Films may be individually envelope-wrapped in which case they will be enclosed in a lightproof envelope of plasticised paper to keep out both light and moisture. There will be a loose wrap of yellow or black paper to facilitate handling and there may also be a card stiffener. Envelope-wrapped film is used where extreme fine detail is required or where the increased radiation dose to the patient is of no consequence—intensifying screens cannot be used with envelope-wrapped film. Therapy verification film (p. 109) is often envelope-wrapped.

X-ray film is otherwise supplied unwrapped, separated by thin sheets of paper, and will be supplied in boxes sealed against light and moisture. The boxes must only be opened under the safe conditions of the darkroom. Unwrapped film is designed for use in a cassette firmly sandwiched between two intensifying screens (Fig. 7.9). For this reason the film is sometimes referred to as *screen film*, its thinner emulsion specially prepared to be sensitive to the fluorescence of the screens. The film–screen combination is carefully chosen.

A cassette is essentially a lightproof container consisting of a rigid frame of aluminium or stainless steel with a hinged back and a thin aluminium, carbon fibre or plastic front through which the X-radiation enters. Carbon fibre is the preferred material for the cassette front in that it provides maximum strength and minimal attenuation of the X-radiation. Inside the front will be the front screen. A foam rubber pressure pad is sandwiched between the back screen and the back of the cassette, so that when the cassette is closed pressure is applied evenly over the whole area of the film to ensure good film–screen contact. Care needs to be taken when loading and unloading the cassette so as to prevent the build-up of static electricity which may discharge later emitting flashes of light which, after processing, appear as black spots on the film. Poor handling can damage both the cassette and the film emulsion. The daylight cassette is of similar construction but loading and unloading is automated thereby minimising the ingress of dust and the chance of damage.

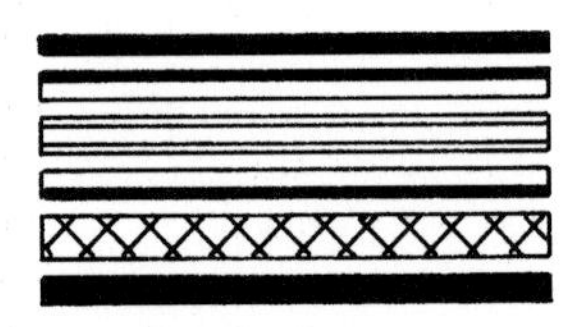

Fig. 7.9 The film cassette.

Loss of contrast

All the attention so far has been on the differential attenuation of the X-rays passing through the patient, reaching the film and causing differential blackening on the film. The contrast produced is the result of the photoelectric attenuation being dependent on the atomic number and the density of the tissues. Inevitably, Compton scatter will be present. This scattered radiation does not reflect the attenuation pattern of the primary radiation, but randomly irradiates the whole film, increasing the fog level and reducing the contrast. Fog may be reduced by:

- Lowering the tube kilovoltage to reduce the scatter generated
- Reducing the field size to reduce the scatter generated
- Preventing the scatter from reaching the film by using a scatter grid or
- Increasing the patient–film distance.

A *grid* (sometimes called a *scatter grid* or *anti-scatter grid*) is a stack of equally spaced lead strips, usually between 20–40 strips per centimetre, such that X-rays travelling from the tube focus can pass unhindered between the strips while scattered radiation, travelling in random directions, will be mostly absorbed in the lead. For most purposes a *parallel grid* is adequate providing the *grid ratio* is not too large, the grid ratio being defined as:

$$\text{Grid ratio} = h / D$$

where h is the height and D the width of the space between the lead strips (Fig. 7.10). If the grid ratio is too large, even the divergent primary radiation from the focus will be absorbed at the edges of large fields. To overcome this, a *focused grid* may be used in which the lead strips are mounted so as to lie along the rays from the focus rather than parallel to the central axis. Focused grids must be used at or close to the stated focal distance. The presence of any grid inevitably means some loss of film speed and an increase in the required exposure.

Radiographic exposure and reciprocity

Several hints have already been given as to the choice of the exposure factors required to produce a good radiograph:

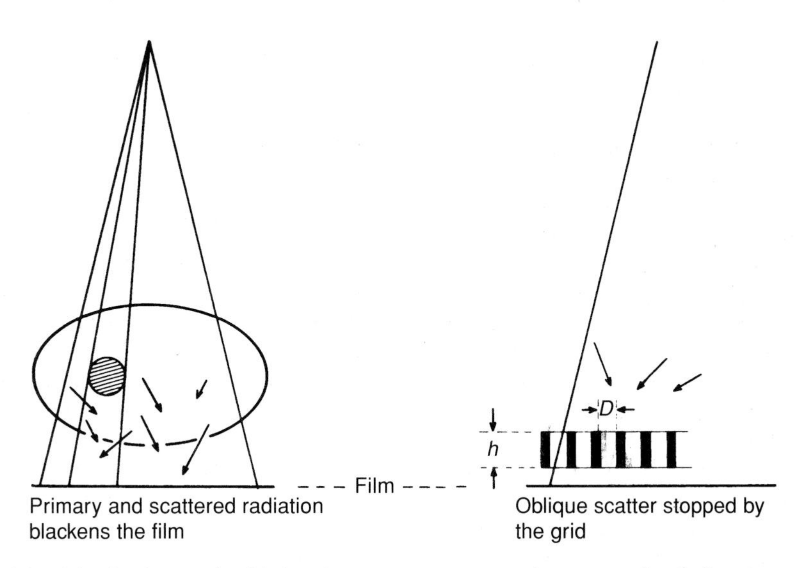

Fig. 7.10 The principle of the (anti-scatter) grid; the short arrows represent the scattered radiation generated within the patient.

- to use a low kV for maximum contrast and minimise scatter generation
- to adjust the total exposure to keep the range of densities within the straight portion of the characteristic curve and maximise contrast
- to use the minimum exposure time to arrest any voluntary or involuntary movement of the patient, and
- to use a fast film–screen combination to minimise the dose to the patient.

The exposure (X) at the surface of the patient is related to the exposure factors as follows:

$$X \propto (\text{kV})^2 \times (\text{mA}) \times (s) / d^2$$

where d is the focal distance, kV the peak voltage of the tube, mA the tube current and s the exposure time. For a given kV and patient–film geometry, the total exposure (X) is proportional to both the tube current and the exposure time; i.e. the film response will be the same whatever combination of these two parameters is chosen providing their product remains constant. This is known as *reciprocity*. It is often convenient therefore to quote the exposure in *mAs* leaving the final choice of tube current and exposure time to the radiographer. An effect known as *reciprocity failure* occurs under certain conditions where the exposure time is very long or very short, but modern equipment usually corrects for this automatically. In general, one chooses the shortest exposure time to arrest the patient movement and maximise the mA. If this necessitates a change of focal spot size—from the fine to broad focus—then other factors, such as geometric unsharpness (p. 93) will need to be considered.

How does the radiographer ascertain the correct mAs in the first place? In any one department, the film–screen–grid combination and the processing chemistry will be decided upon in advance and there will be little or no choice. Secondly, radiographs will have been taken many times before and satisfactory exposure factors will be available based on experience. Published 'Exposure Tables' may be used as an alternative guide, but it must be remembered that on a simulator the source–skin distance (SSD) and the focal– film distance (FFD) may be very different (by up to a factor of 3) from those used in a diagnostic department and the mAs recommended may need to be increased to obtain comparable films. It is for this reason that X-ray generators giving up to 800 mA or even 1000 mA are used on simulators. Once the mAs has proved adequate for a given examination, then patient-to-patient differences will usually be accommodated by small changes in kV.

Unlike the policy adopted in diagnostic X-ray departments, it is often said that in treatment simulation, the patient dose is unimportant in that the dose to be given in the treatment situation will be many times greater than that from the simulator. This is true of the lesion and the adjacent tissues. However, if the patient receives an extensive radiographic examination in regions where subsequently every effort will be taken to minimise the dose received during the treatment (e.g. the lens of the eye), then the radiographic dose to those tissues may become a significant fraction of the whole. Patient dose is minimised by the use of high kV and long SSD. The final choice of kV is therefore a compromise between maximum contrast and minimum patient dose (IPSM 1988b).

IMAGE INTENSIFICATION

So far we have concentrated on the production of the image on film and much of what has been said is true for other imaging technologies. The film image is a static image only made visible after processing. The instantaneous and therefore dynamic image made available using an *image intensifier* is, in many situations, far superior. The dynamic image on the simulator not only enables the operator to watch for patient movement but also enables the simulator movements to be adjusted to the desired positions, quickly and positively.

The image intensifier tube is a highly evacuated glass envelope containing a fluorescent screen. Like the intensifying screens discussed above, the fluorescent screen or *input phosphor* is a layer of crystals (in this situation usually caesium iodide) which absorbs some of the X-ray photons and converts the invisible X-ray image into a visible fluorescent image, albeit of low brightness. In contact with the input phosphor is a *photocathode*, which promptly converts the visible image into an electronic image (Fig. 7.11). This input phosphor and photocathode are usually convex to the incident X-ray beam (flat surfaces implode under vacuum). The electrons emitted from the inner concave surface are accelerated by a high voltage (~25 kV) and focused onto a much smaller *output phosphor*. The acceleration of the electrons increases their energy while the minification of the image concentrates the electron flux onto a smaller area increasing the brightness of the visible image produced in the output phosphor. (The output phosphor is made up of smaller crystals than the input phosphor in order to maintain the fine detail of the image.) This bright image could be viewed by the naked eye—providing sufficient X-ray protective material is available to make it safe to look directly at the output phosphor, which is still in the primary X-ray beam. More commonly, the output phosphor is viewed through a mirror by a built-in television camera and the image displayed on a television monitor. The use of the 45° mirror enables the camera to be positioned outside the X-ray beam and reduces the overall length of the image intensifier assembly—an important factor in simulator design—while protecting the camera from radiation damage.

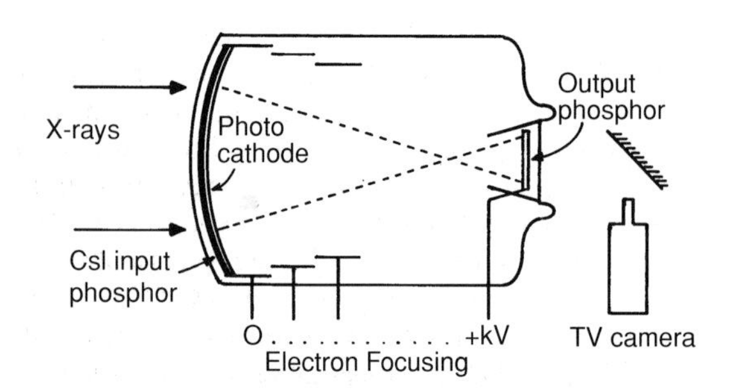

Fig. 7.11 The image intensifier.

The X-ray image contained within the transmitted beam is therefore converted in turn into light, into electrons, into light again and then into the final television viewing system. At each stage there will be some loss of information and the displayed image will be of poorer quality than the original. The image may be further degraded if the X-ray beam penetrates through to the output phosphor, if there is poor focusing of the electrons (this is particularly noticeable at the edges of the image), or if there is stray light or stray magnetic fields (from nearby MRI equipment, for example). These losses of image information are outweighed by the advantages of the visual acuity which results from being able to view the brighter image with cone vision. The gain in brightness is sufficient to allow a reduction in the X-ray beam intensity and therefore in the dose to the patient. The television chain can electronically further enhance the image contrast.

There are several other advantages which result from the use of image intensifiers. The television screen may be viewed in any position in any location—in the case of the simulator, the television monitor will normally be located in the adjacent control room—and the video image can be readily recorded. Under normal operation, the dynamic image is ideal for the positive localisation of anatomical structures and tumours; for example, an oesophageal obstruction during the barium meal examination. However, in many examinations a static picture gives the operator time to absorb more of the detail displayed which would otherwise be lost. A series of static pictures (as in cine photography) may replace the dynamic image. A static picture may be produced by a short exposure to X-rays and displayed for any length of time using a storage display tube or recording the frame on a video disc. Such a picture may be updated manually or triggered automatically at some prescribed frequency. This *flash radiography* helps to reduce the patient dose.

The real value of the immediate television display over the delayed radiographic film will become clear when the use of the simulator is discussed below, but both facilities are required if the simulator is to be used to maximum advantage. The full-sized radiograph is required for the planning of the treatment, and the dynamic television picture is required in the initial localisation and verification procedures. Miniature multiformat pictures may be used for record keeping and follow-up purposes (multiformat images may be produced by photographing a flat video screen onto film through a camera lens in a so-called *multiformat camera* or by scanning the film with a laser controlled directly by the computer in a *laser imager*).

THE TREATMENT SIMULATOR

Having looked in some detail at the formation of the radiographic image, we must now examine the treatment simulator itself (Fig. 7.2). The simulator adds the X-ray system of a diagnostic unit to a gantry–couch system of an isocentric therapy unit and incorporates a unique beam collimating system. The *treatment simulator* is a misnomer insofar as it does not simulate the treatment, it simulates the treatment beam–patient geometry.

Simulator movements

The gantry–couch system of the simulator will reproduce all the movements of the therapy gantry and couch and to the same accuracy or better than the therapy unit. The source–axis distance (SAD) may have to be variable if the unit is to simulate several therapy units but, since the demise of the telecobalt unit, the SAD is invariably 100 cm. The simulator couch will have to offer all the immobilisation devices used on the therapy equipment (Ch. 11) and at the same time be transparent to the diagnostic X-ray beam. The couch top will therefore be both light and strong in construction—carbon fibre perhaps being the best material currently available. All the movements will be available under both local and remote control with fail-safe brakes.

X-ray generator

The X-ray system will comprise a voltage generator, X-ray tube, image intensifier and television monitor. The generator may be of a simple design similar to those described in Chapter 9, but a three-phase generator providing a rectified potential of 6 or 12 pulses per cycle (using six or twelve rectifiers) is more likely—Figure 7.12 shows the secondary circuit of a six-rectifier-six-pulse three-phase generator. The secondary voltages from the three windings of the HT transformer will be 120° out of phase, each one reaching its peak

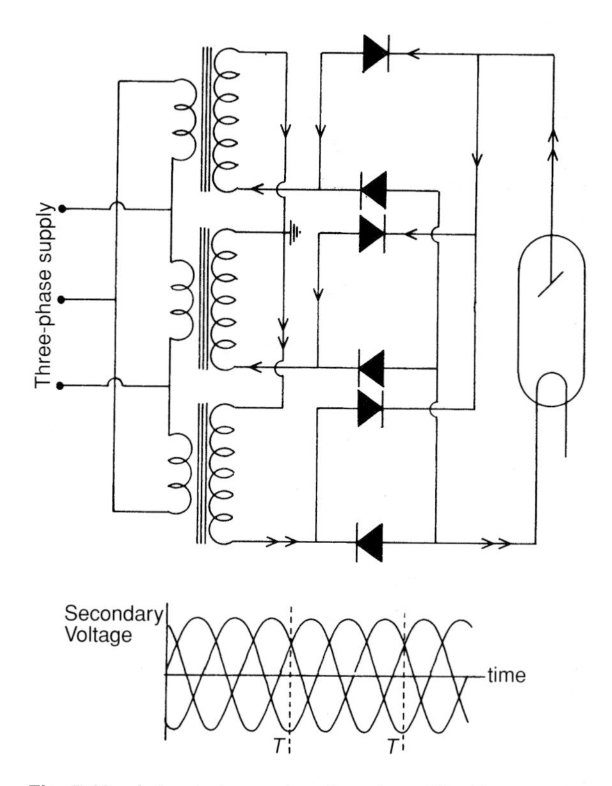

Fig. 7.12 A three-phase, six-pulse, six-rectifier X-ray generator circuit.

value in turn. Thus, in general, one voltage will be increasing when the other two are decreasing or vice versa, which means three of the rectifiers will be conducting and three will not. In the diagram, the electron flow is indicated for the instant in time, T, when two windings are generating half their peak positive potential with respect to earth and the third is at its peak negative potential. The secondary voltage applied to the tube peaks six times during each cycle giving an almost constant potential. The few per cent *voltage ripple* may be further smoothed using capacitors (not shown) as described in Chapter 9. High-frequency generators (p. 148) are being used increasingly in diagnostic radiology.

Rotating anode tube

The diagnostic unit operates at between 50–125 kV but at much higher tube currents than found in therapy units. Tube currents are commonly 300 or 500 mA and may go as high as 1000 mA in the radiography mode, while in fluoroscopy mode the tube current will normally be less than 2 mA. The heat dissipation in the target during radiography is therefore some ten times higher than in a therapy tube—albeit for very short exposure times—and dictates the design of the target. The diagnostic tube insert is usually of the *rotating anode* type (Fig. 7.13). The electrons from the off-axis filament strike the bevelled edge of the anode, which rotates at up to 3000 r.p.m. spreading the heat dissipation over an annulus. The bevelled edge acts as a reflection target (p. 18). The rate at which the target can cool is limited because the heat has to be lost by radiation from the surface—which can reach incandescence. The broad focus results from spreading the electron bombardment over a wider annulus on the rotating anode in order to spread the heat generated by the higher tube currents. (There can be no convection in a vacuum and conduction has to be minimised to prevent the rotor bearings seizing up because of thermal expansion.) The anode will be permanently damaged if repeated exposures are made too frequently. The recommended *tube rating* and *duty cycle* should never be exceeded. The target is usually tungsten mounted on a molybdenum disc and stem (molybdenum is a poor conductor of heat).

The anode is mounted on the rotor of an induction motor within the evacuated envelope. The stator coils are outside the tube insert and, using the three-phase supply, cause a magnetic field to move round the tube at high speed. Fields are induced in the copper cylinder, the rotor, causing it to rotate. The rotation of the anode should be heard to start as soon as the exposure button is pressed to the 'prep' (preparation) position. The recommended pause at 'prep' is to allow the anode rotation to reach its maximum speed before the exposure is made. The rotation should continue for several minutes after the exposure has been completed. This free running of the anode confirms the rotor and its bearings are in good condition; any shortening of the free running time or change in the noise from the bearings is indicative of failure.

Beam collimation

The diaphragm system is unique to the treatment simulator (Fig. 7.14). In addition to the beam-limiting

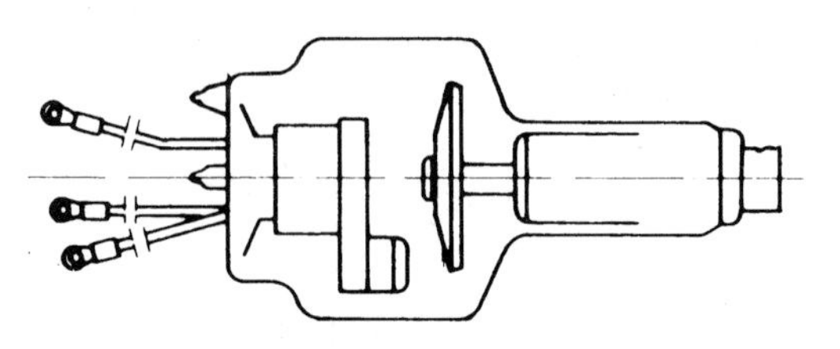

Fig. 7.13 A rotating anode diagnostic tube insert; the stator is not shown. (Courtesy of Elekta Ltd.)

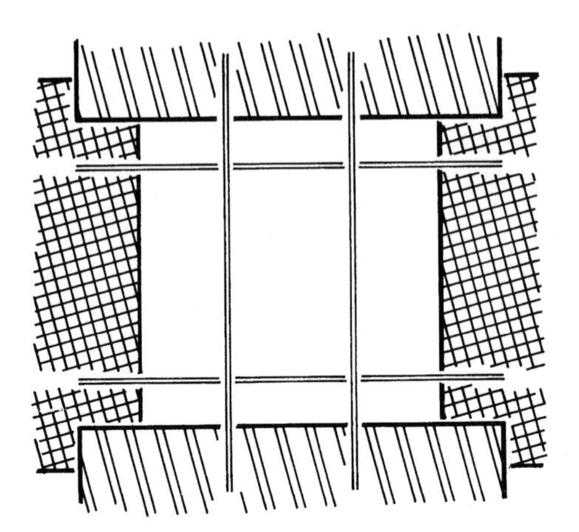

Fig. 7.14 The beam-limiting and field-defining diaphragm system.

diaphragms—similar to those on a diagnostic unit—there are field-defining *wire diaphragms*. The latter are designed to give an accurate indication of the edges of the therapy beam being simulated and to allow the anatomy outside the therapy beam to be visualised. The beam-limiting diaphragms are used to control the amount of tissue irradiated outside the therapy beam size—and to minimise the production of image-degrading scatter. Under computer control these diaphragms can limit the maximum beam to the area covered by the image intensifier or radiographic film and automatically reduce it to a size only slightly greater than that delineated by the wires.

Treatment simulation is primarily the simulation of the therapy beam edges. The correct and reproducible alignment of the wire delineators over the whole range of field sizes is of paramount importance. It is unavoidable that the imaging parameters for the wire delineators are not ideal (Fig. 7.4) with the result that they are not sharply imaged on the image receptor. Their magnification factor is large but their diameter is small compared with the focal spot, giving rise to considerable image unsharpness. However, providing measurements are taken to the centre of their visible image then errors will be small. Unfortunately, the wires give no indication of the penumbra width of the therapy beam, and due allowance must be made for the penumbra when interpreting the simulator image.

The choice of image receptor on the simulator is commonly radiographic film (43×35 cm^2 or 35×35 cm^2) and an image intensifier of 23 or 30 cm diameter. Neither will image the maximum available field size at the isocentre in its entirety. To do so would require a larger image intensifier and the more bulky that becomes the more it restricts the movements of the simulator; a typically difficult situation is illustrated in Figure 7.15. To partially overcome this difficulty, the smaller image intensifier is allowed to move orthogonally in three directions, the X–Y scanning movement enables it to track round the edges of a large field in most situations while the Z movement controls its distance from the isocentre. Within these restrictions the simulator can provide images of the patient with greater geometric accuracy than most diagnostic units and thereby localise the tissues targeted for radiotherapy and verify the proposed treatment plan.

The role of the simulator

Localisation

The treatment simulator is a sophisticated diagnostic X-ray unit with two principal roles in radiotherapy—the *localisation* of the target tissues and the *verification* of the proposed treatment plan. It is not intended as an aid to diagnosis. The diagnosis of the disease and its extent is more readily achieved using the facilities in the Departments of Diagnostic X-ray, Nuclear Medicine, Ultrasound and of Magnetic Resonance. Magnetic resonance imaging is not widely available to the radiotherapy patient, but offers potential advantages for the localisation process over other techniques (Khoo 2000). The results of such tests should be available at the first simulation of the patient. Similarly, if the patient is expected to require an immobilisation device, that too should be made (p. 185) and brought to the first simulation where the sole aim is to localise the target tissues within the patient in relation to external markers attached to the patient or immobilisation shell. During this first simulation, the simulator is used simply as a diagnostic X-ray unit but with a sophisticated and highly accurate gantry. The patient must take up the position to be adopted during treatment. After placing the midpoint of the target volume at the isocentre and indicating the cephalocaudal dimension with the field-defining wires, two orthogonal films are taken of known magnification. These AP and lateral films will provide the localisation information on which the treatment plan will be based. Where possible, the simulator scale readings as well as the exposure factors should be recorded for future reference. (The orthogonal films are usually AP and lateral, but any orthogonal pair may be used providing they can be uniquely related to the patient contour.)

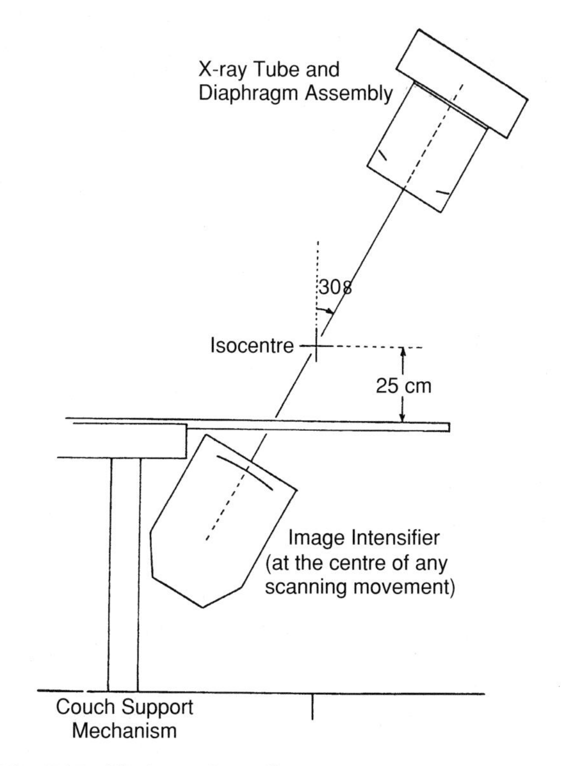

Fig. 7.15 The image intensifier can restrict the movement of the simulator.

The patient contour should be taken through the midplane whilst the patient remains in the same position on the simulator couch so that the contour relates uniquely to the information recorded on the localisation films. Contours in other parallel planes may be taken at the same time to provide three-dimensional data. Alternatively the patient contours could be taken from the patient's shell, providing the shell is not distorted by the weight of the patient. The size and position of the target tissues within the patient contour is determined from the localisation/planning films. Where suitable CT facilities are readily available, a simple scan will give both the external contour and the internal anatomy (p. 108).

Localisation from films

In the following analysis the films will be referred to as AP (suffix 1) and Lateral (suffix 2) (Fig. 7.16).

Under screening conditions, the midpoint of the target tissues is placed at the isocentre, O, and the film–axis distance for each film, F_1O and F_2O, is noted; they may be the same or different. The magnification factors for the target tissues imaged on the two films are therefore:

$$M_{\text{Lat}} = \frac{S_2F_2}{S_2O} = \frac{S_2O + F_2O}{S_2O}$$

and

$$M_{\text{AP}} = \frac{S_1F_1}{S_1O} = \frac{S_1O + F_1O}{S_1O}$$

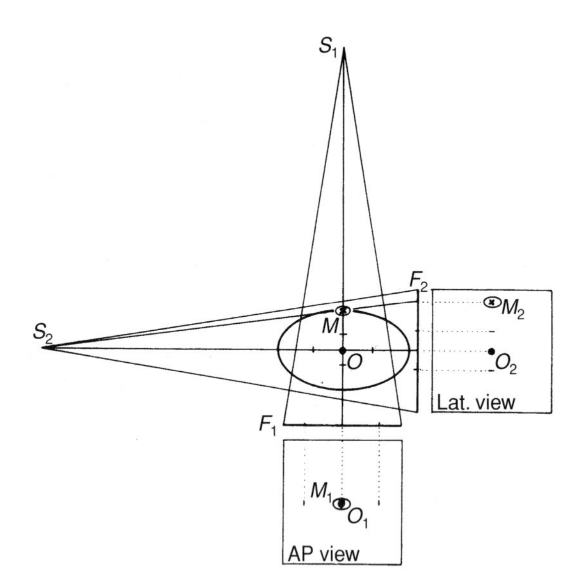

Fig. 7.16 The principle of localisation using orthogonal films.

where S_1O and S_2O are the source–object distances, say 100 cm.

The principal axes of the target volume can therefore be measured off the films and reduced to their actual size by dividing by the appropriate magnification factor. The cephalocaudal dimension can be obtained from either film. Similarly, the depth of the target centre, O, below the marker, M, can be measured on the lateral film and de-magnified.

Some centres prefer to use a ring of known outer diameter, d (say, 5 cm), as a marker and determine magnification factors from its image instead of having to record F_1O and F_2O. The image of the ring will be permanently recorded on each film, and being a ring, the maximum diameter of the image divided by the known diameter gives the magnification of the ring (Fig. 7.17).

For the lateral film in Figure 7.17, the magnification factor is required at the midline and will be that of the ring: $M_{\text{Lat}} = d_2/d$. On the AP film, however, the ring is at a different distance from the focus than the target tissues and therefore d_1/d cannot be applied without modification (Fig. 7.16):

$$M_{\text{AP}} = \frac{S_1F_1}{S_1O} = \frac{S_1M \times (d_1/d)}{S_1O}$$

S_1M is unknown but S_1O is and MO can be calculated from the lateral film, and therefore:

$$M_{\text{AP}} = \frac{(S_1O - MO) \times (d_1/d)}{S_1O}$$

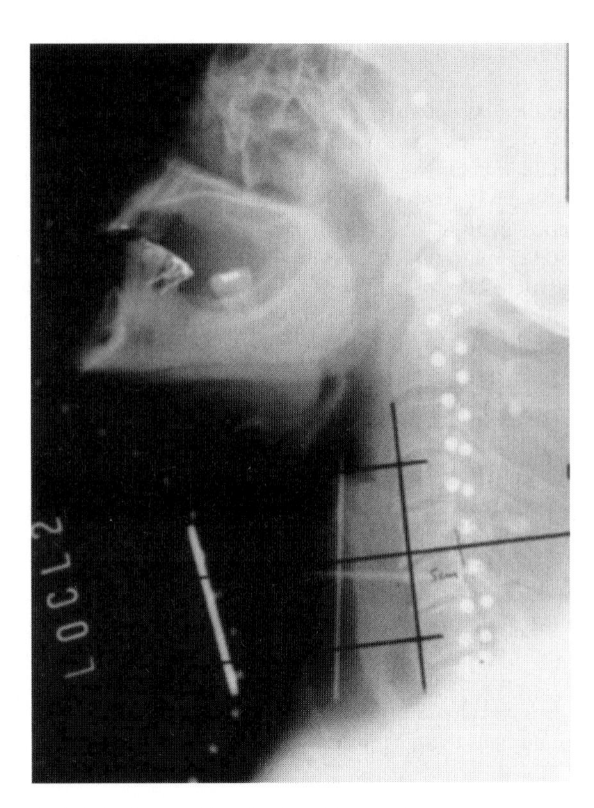

Fig. 7.17 A typical localisation film showing the markers and ring.

In some circumstances, it is more convenient to place the marker M at the isocentre, in which case the relevant magnification factors derived from the diameter of the ring placed at M become:

$$M_{\text{Lat}} = d_2/d \text{ and } M_{\text{AP}} = \frac{S_1M \times (d_1/d)}{S_1M \times MO}$$

The use of the ring is particularly valuable when the planning/simulator films are likely to be archived in a miniature format as the relevant magnification data will be permanently recorded.

Verification

Following the preparation of a treatment plan based on the localisation films and patient contour, a second visit to the simulator will verify that plan prior to the commencement of treatment. The most accurate and reliable means of *verification* is to set the patient up on the simulator couch as prescribed, with the immobilisation devices if any, and then to set up each proposed treatment beam in turn—in position, size, shape and direction—and confirm that the included and excluded tissues are exactly as required. The confirmation may be observed under screening conditions or recorded on film for record purposes. In some instances, however, the small oblique projections of the anatomy displayed on the screen will not be sufficiently familiar to provide this confirmation, and alternative verification techniques will be required. On the other hand, the actual visualisation of each beam in turn, together with the manufactured local shielding blocks attached to the shadow tray, may be the only means of verifying that the beam edges are placed correctly in relation to excluded sensitive tissues.

Where tailor-made shielding blocks or multileaf collimators are to be used, it is essential that each beam is accurately simulated, so that the film can be marked up to show the shape required in relation to the principal axes of the field. The shape may be indicated by skin marks and recorded by attaching marker wires whilst films are taken. Such films may not be required where small areas of local shielding will be achieved by selecting blocks from a standard set.

Once verified, the parameters of each beam and the patient position may be transferred to the therapy generator, preferably through the computer network.

Electron treatment simulation

There is little experience to date in the simulation of electron treatment. It is advantageous if the electron applicators can be attached to the simulator. The positioning of the rather bulky applicator to treat the more difficult site can then be sorted out in the simulator room rather than in the treatment room. Once the position has been determined, the profile of the field-shaping cut-out (to fit the end of the applicator, (p. 169)) can be marked and made ready for casting in low-melting-point alloy. Electron treatment simulation is largely mechanical and does not involve the X-ray imaging facilities unless a verification film is required through the field-shaping cut-out for record purposes.

Where mixed modality treatments, involving both X-ray and electron fields, or two or more electron fields, are planned, then the accuracy of the beam edges becomes critical and simulation is important. It must be remembered, however, that neither the light beam diaphragm nor the diagnostic beam will adequately simulate the penumbra and divergence of the electron therapy beam. Advanced computer planning systems are required to ensure the overlap of divergent beams does not lead to gross over- or under-dosage of the target, or healthy tissues.

Quality assurance

The simulator has the geometry and the movements of a linear accelerator but the tolerances are tighter and the QA needs to be more carefully carried out. The mechanical QA programme (including the isocentre lasers and backpointers) will be similar to that of a linear accelerator (p. 178) for the geometry of the simulator needs to be at least as accurate as the treatment units in every respect.

The radiographic and fluoroscopic image quality on the simulator may not be as good as on the diagnostic X-ray unit, where all the parameters can be optimised to that one end. Image quality is, however, important and steps must be taken to ensure that the image quality is the best possible. The imaging chain QA—including kV, mA, intensifier, TV and film processor—will follow the practices for diagnostic X-ray generators (Moores et al 1987, IPEM et al 1997). The X-ray/optical beam coincidence needs to be repeated under both fine and broad focus conditions, bearing in mind the (therapy) beam-delineating wires are more important than the beam-limiting collimators. The regular use of a test phantom, such as that shown in Figure 7.18 (Bomford et al 1989), enables most of the geometrical and radiographic parameters to be checked on a daily basis. A comparison with the previous record will draw attention to any dramatic changes, whereas a careful study of the records will highlight any gradual deterioration of performance.

THE CT SCANNER

The CT scanner has a small-focus X-ray tube which rotates around the axis of a fixed annulus of 600 or 1200 individually collimated radiation detectors (Fig. 7.19). The patient lies along the same axis and is irradiated by the fan-shaped X-ray beam as the tube rotates round the patient through a full 360°, preferably in a few seconds—in *spiral CT*, the X-ray tube rotates continuously as the couch moves slowly through the annulus of detectors. Each detector is calibrated and measures the intensity of the transmitted X-ray beam and therefore measures the attenuation of the X-rays as they pass through the patient. The radiation is usually pulsed at a rate of (say) 100 pulses per second, each pulse lasting a few milliseconds. During the scan, therefore, some 100 000 measurements are made by the detectors and recorded in the computer. For radiotherapy purposes, it is important that the CT gantry remains vertical with the scan plane at right angles to the longitudinal axis of the couch.

The detectors need to be very reliable and stable in operation, linear in response and, above all, sensitive

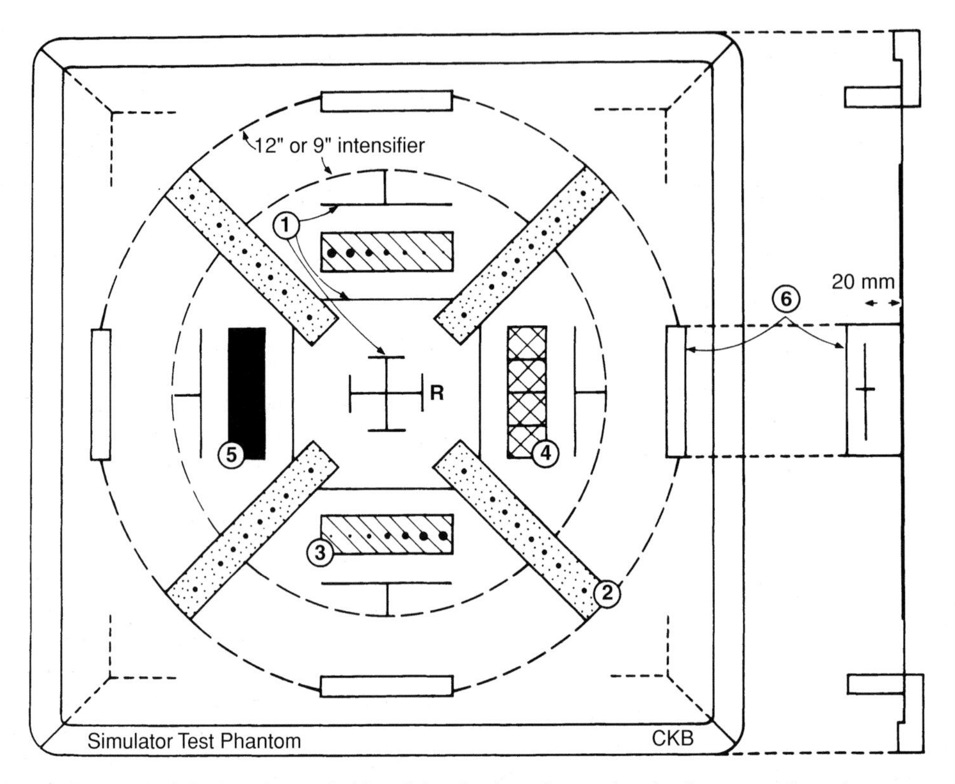

Fig. 7.18 A test phantom to fit in the cassette holder of the simulator for regular checks on a variety of parameters including: 1. field sizes and SSD; 2. uniformity of the image; 3. image resolution; 4. beam quality; 5. image brightness; 6. isocentre projectors and many others.

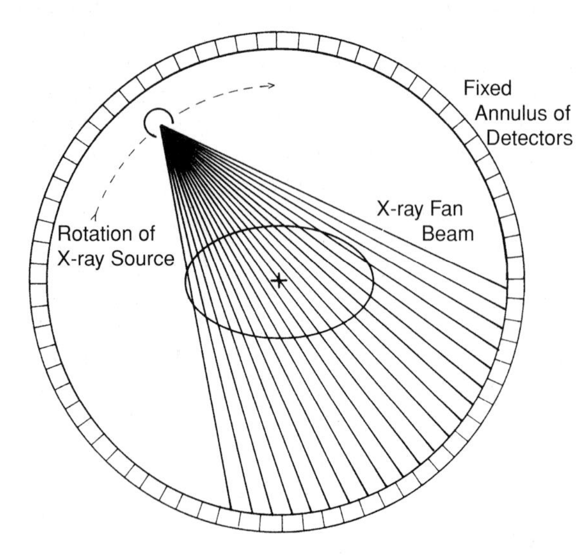

Fig. 7.19 The principal components of the CT scanner.

and respond very quickly while being of small physical size. Thallium-doped caesium iodide crystals—as used in image intensifiers—have been used in conjunction with silicon photodiodes, which together have the added advantage of not requiring a high-voltage power supply. The alternative is to use sealed ionisation chambers. Ionisation chambers usually require large volumes to improve their sensitivity, but increasing the contained air mass by using high-atomic-number gases under pressure, can increase their sensitivity while keeping the volume small. Under saturation conditions, ionisation chambers can be very stable. Whatever the detector system, regular calibration is vital and this is often carried out automatically using the edge of the fan beam which is uninterrupted by the patient.

The number and spacing of the detectors is fundamental to the detail in the computed image—the larger the number of measurements recorded the smaller the pixel size. The thickness of the fan beam determines the thickness of the slice of tissue irradiated, which may be varied up to, say, 15 mm (Fig. 7.20), while for most radiotherapy purposes both the thickness and spacing are set to about 3 mm. (The *pixel* is the two-dimensional picture element derived from the average X-ray attenuation in the three-dimensional *voxel* or

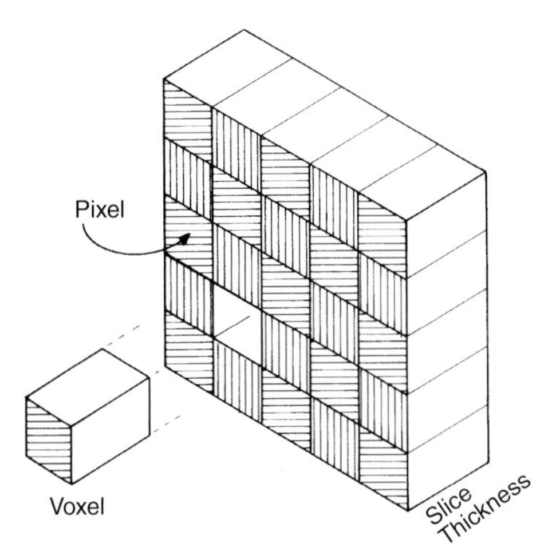

Fig. 7.20 The pixel and the voxel.

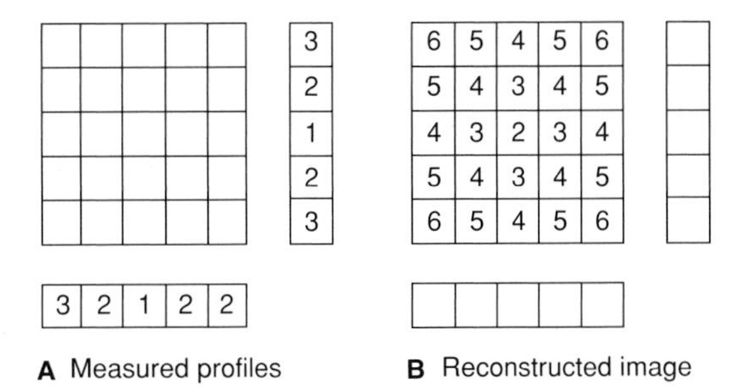

A Measured profiles **B** Reconstructed image

Fig. 7.21 The principle of back projection.

volume element within the patient.) The image will be degraded by the scattered radiation generated in the thicker slice, or by using fewer (larger) detectors. On the other hand, the thinner the slice and the more (smaller) detectors used, the smaller the signal-to-noise ratio. (*Noise*, in this context, is the unwanted signal generated in the electronics of the detector system and is present irrespective of the radiation incident on the detectors. The smaller the signal generated by the radiation, the greater the significance of the noise.) These factors have to be carefully balanced to obtain the optimum image quality.

The X-ray tube requires a small focal spot, say 0.6 mm, and a high output, so, although the applied voltage is pulsed, the target cooling may limit the frequency of the scans. The tube is operated at no more than 120 kV for, above that, the Compton scattering interactions begin to dominate, reducing both the differential absorption in the tissues and effective absorption in the detectors. The higher energy radiation may be more penetrating and reduce the dose to the patient; the image quality deteriorates to an unacceptable level. (The patient dose in CT is some 20–50 times greater than for many other diagnostic X-ray examinations.)

A variety of mathematical algorithms have been used to reconstruct the two-dimensional image from the measured transmission profiles. Let two examples suffice. If the pixels in a square array produce the two transmitted beam profiles shown in Figure 7.21A, then immediately we can expect the centre to produce less attenuation than the periphery because both profiles dip in the centre. If we now use the method of *back projection* and add the profiles together row by row and column by column, the matrix fills as in Figure 7.21B confirming the lower attenuation in the centre. Although this illustrates the technique the actual computation is far more complex!

A second method is known as the *iterative method* where a guess is made and then modified repeatedly until the model fits the measured data. This method is perhaps best illustrated by the party puzzle where one is asked to place the numbers 1 to 25 into a five by five matrix in such a way that each row, column and diagonal adds up to the same value, namely 65. Although there is a logical approach to such a problem, most party-goers use a purely iterative approach!

Whatever method is used to reconstruct the image, a *CT number* is allocated to each pixel as a measure of its attenuation coefficient relative to water. The numbers vary between –1000 for air to +1000 for the densest bone, and these numbers are used to determine the degree of blackness in the final picture. The average video display system can only display about 10 different levels of grey between black and white, but the operator can select the range of CT numbers to be displayed—a wide *CT window* portrays the tissues with grossly different attenuation coefficients and is ideal for obtaining patient contours and principal anatomy for example. A narrow window enables tissues only marginally different in attenuation coefficient to be displayed in different shades of grey. A window width of unity enables the CT number of individual pixels to be identified. Unfortunately it does not follow that one can distinguish malignant tissue from healthy tissue.

CT in treatment planning

Diagnosis

The CT scanner has two distinct roles in radiotherapy—as an aid to diagnosis and as an aid to treatment planning. In general, the patient will be referred to the diagnostic X-ray department for the former. Where the visit is purely for diagnostic purposes, no special arrangements need to be made but if the images produced are likely to be used for assessing the dimensions or position of the target tissues within the contour or to produce the patient contour itself, then the use of a flat-topped couch and the position of the patient become critical.

Localisation

Preparation for treatment planning will require a much longer appointment—up to an hour is common—and the attendance of staff from the Mould Room, the Planning Room and, preferably, the Radiotherapist.

A flat-topped couch insert will be required—to simulate the flat therapy couch—with the appropriate facilities to enable headrests and other patient immobilisation devices to be fitted. It may be advantageous to incorporate markers into the couch insert to facilitate localisation and/or magnification factors to be determined from the CT image. Metals, however, must be avoided as these cause artefacts in the image. Markers of a lower-contrast medium give a clearer mark with the minimum of artefacts—nylon tubing filled with a mixture of barium and silicon cream, for example. They must be continuous line markers and positioned to intersect the scan plane if they are to be recorded on the image. Two parallel lines of known separation laid into the couch top will provide a record of the magnification factor, whereas two divergent straight lines enable the distances between slices to be recorded and measured; a large capital **N** provides information on both magnification and slice separation. Lasers may be fitted to illuminate the transverse section of the patient and to facilitate taking the contour but, as these cannot be in the same plane as the scan, the couch must be moved longitudinally to correct for the off-set before marking the patient and/or taking the contour.

A single scan through the midplane of the proposed treatment will present the patient contour and internal anatomy in the transverse plane to which the planning computer can overlay the two-dimensional dose distribution. The CT number assigned to each tissue type is a measure of the absorption coefficient at the photon energy of the scanner. However, the CT number cannot be used to determine the relative electron density of the tissue and therefore the inhomogeneity coefficient for use in treatment planning (Fig. 12.11; Thomas 1999). Alternatively, manually prepared inhomogeneity factors may be used. The use of CT in treatment planning is dealt with more fully in Chapter 13.

From the data collected from multiple slices, the computer can reconstruct the coronal and sagittal images as well as the transverse images (Plate 1.5), providing the slice width and spacing are small (preferably less than 3 mm). Oblique plane images can be reconstructed from the raw data, albeit with some loss of quality owing to the interpolation process. It must be remembered, however, that all these images are as seen from an infinite distance and do not attempt to portray any effects of beam divergence. Divergence can be taken into account when a more realistic viewing distance is introduced—for example, a beam's eye view (BEV) can be computed once a source–axis distance (SAD) is specified. The BEV assumes the eye is positioned at the radiation source and the near anatomy is seen as larger than the distant anatomy.

Verification

The so-called *virtual simulation* (CT-SIM) is the result of integrating the CT scanner software and the treatment planning software so that the therapy beam parameters—of SSD and field size—and the movements of the treatment simulator may be incorporated into the image reconstruction process. The beam axis may be collated with the CT scans to produce the BEV image while the computer superimposes a delineation of the therapy field size on to the image (Plate 1.6), thereby creating a simulation of the therapy beam without requiring the patient to be present. As with the treatment simulator image, the edges of the therapy beam are delineated by discrete lines rather than the true penumbra edges. This virtual simulation assumes the patient position on the treatment couch will be identical to that when the CT examination was performed and that no changes have taken place in the meantime, e.g. further growth of the tumour. The conventional simulator has the advantage that the dynamic (fluorescent) image shows patient movement over a short period of time.

Not all treatment sites are deemed suitable for virtual simulation (e.g. not all patient positions can be held in the confines of the scanner). Where virtual simulation is appropriate, the overall time between the localisation of the target tissues and the commencement of treatment can be significantly reduced in that the process can be completed without having to bring the patient back for a second appointment. The rate of data transfer between the CT scanner and the simulator workstation is a key factor in the length of the virtual simulation session itself.

Quality assurance

Among the routine QA tests of the CT scanner will be a set of critical tests using a cylindrical tissue-equivalent phantom containing several smaller-diameter inhomogeneities of known size and consistency. Any CT image must be checked for:

- the accuracy of size and shape in the scan plane—several diameters of the image are measured against the known diameters of the phantom to detect any distortion of that image
- the accuracy of size and shape in the longitudinal direction
- the accuracy of CT number—by comparison with the known consistencies of the phantom and its inhomogeneities
- the image quality, resolution, contrast, etc. (Moores et al 1987, IPEM et al 1997).

The virtual simulator will require additional QA checks to cover aspects such as:

- the simulated components of the treatment simulator geometry including the isocentre, gantry, couch and collimator rotations, field size and SSD
- laser alignment with the scan plane
- data transfer to and from the treatment planning computer.

PORTAL IMAGING

The treatment simulator was born out of the need for better-quality images than could be obtained from simple check films on megavoltage therapy units. But portal imaging still has a role in verifying the accuracy of the position and direction and, in the use of local shielding blocks or multileaf collimators, in confirming the shape of the therapy beam. It may be done once for each patient simply to verify the beam set-up; it may be repeated, say, weekly or even daily, to monitor the on-going accuracy of that set-up. Such checks may highlight deficiencies in the practice but are more likely to draw attention to the inevitable and unavoidable variations in patient position which need to be accommodated in prescribing the clinical target volume (CTV) (McKenzie 2001). Various techniques are available but, in general, the image quality remains poor compared with diagnostic images.

Therapy verification film

Therapy verification film is deliberately very slow and can be left in the exit beam throughout the treatment fraction, it requires an incident dose of approximately 1 gray. A conventional scatter grid is of no value in eliminating the effects of scattered radiation in that the scatter is of a similar photon energy to the primary beam and not significantly attenuated in the lead strips. It is, however, advantageous to place the verification film, in its light-proof envelope, in close contact with but behind a 1 mm (up to 6 MV) or 2 mm lead (over 8 MV) sheet. The lead serves two purposes. It is thick enough to attenuate some of the low-energy scatter resulting from the multiple scattering processes but, more importantly, it helps to restore the dose build-up lost in the air gaps between the exit surface of the patient and the surface of the film. The attenuation of the primary radiation in the lead is negligible and therefore the exposure is unaffected by its presence. If a 'cassette' is used to hold the (wrapped) film in close contact with the lead, ensure the radiation passes through the lead before reaching the film. (The lead in a diagnostic film cassette is behind the film to minimise the effects of back-scattered radiation).

Several companies have developed special film–screen–cassette combinations using metal (e.g. stainless steel) intensifying screens, and claim improved image quality.

Inevitably, the quality of the image is poor as it relies on the differential absorption in the tissues due to the Compton scattering process. This differential is dependent on the density and the electron density of the tissues and independent of atomic number. The contrast between tissue and air is therefore much greater than between tissue and bone as has been illustrated in Figure 7.1. The image will be further degraded by the involuntary movements of the patient during the treatment.

An alternative film is available which is about eight times faster than the verification film described above, and therefore requiring a smaller incident dose. This film is used for the *double-exposure technique* of beam verification, where the film is placed in the transmitted therapy beam and given a short exposure with a larger field size, followed by a second exposure with the field collimators closed down to the planned therapy field size. The small gamma of the film should allow reasonable images to be produced despite the 2 : 1 difference in exposure. This double exposure identifies the small therapy field within the adjacent anatomy. It is important that the patient is not allowed to move between the two exposures.

Fluorescent image

Non-film portal imaging may be achieved by attaching a light-proof box to the gantry in which a fluorescent screen is held in the exit beam. The screen is viewed through a mirror by a sensitive (night-vision) video camera mounted in the counterbalance of the gantry and protected from the X-radiation. The video image is then displayed on a television screen. The system has the advantage that the maximum field viewed is only limited by the size of the fluorescent screen and the mirror while, using the zoom lens on the camera, smaller fields can be examined in detail. As with any fluorescent image, it is a dynamic image and patient movements can be observed.

Digital imaging

A second non-film technique is to use a matrix containing a very large number of individual detectors (e.g. silicon diodes or ionisation chambers) as an image receptor. Each detector occupies a unique position in the matrix and provides a signal proportional to the radiation intensity at that point. Processing these signals through the computer can electronically enhance the contrast before displaying a digital image on a remote video display unit. The image needs an exposure of, say, 0.2 Gy, which is similar to the faster therapy verification film described above, but it does mean the image is not a dynamic one. The fine detail is limited by the pixel size (of each detector) and the number of detectors strictly limits the size of the image reproduced; the X–Y movement of the matrix allows larger fields to be covered.

SIMULATOR/CT SUITE

The simulator/CT room with an adjacent control room, should be close to the treatment units, the planning suite and the mould room, as the staff from all three areas will be frequent visitors, and close to the film processor. The wall protection will be lead or concrete of a thickness dependent on the equipment specification, but typically 2 mm Pb equivalent. The primary beam of the CT scanner should be absorbed within the housing itself. The primary beam of the simulator should be absorbed within the image intensifier housing, but this requires the movement controls to be interlocked so that the collimators move with the X–Y–Z movement of the intensifier and places a limit on the maximum field size for radiography. It is advisable to provide for a primary barrier of an additional thickness (as for an accelerator) and to avoid having any door or window in the primary beam. The other features for kilovoltage therapy rooms are otherwise applicable. Insofar as there will usually be more than one entrance door, door interlocks are to be recommended. For a more detailed discussion, see Bomford et al 1989.

The control room will be somewhat larger than for a treatment unit to accommodate the additional staff involved and the 'lead glass' observation window large enough so that several members of staff can use it at the same time. CCTV is less convenient and less satisfactory in this context unless it is used to observe the 'blind side' of the couch when using the remote movement controls. While all the movement controls will be available in the room for setting-up purposes, the radiation controls will only be available in the control room alongside the duplicate set of movement controls.

CHAPTER CONTENTS

8

Nuclear medicine

Martin Errington

INTRODUCTION

Nuclear medicine is the science and clinical application of unsealed radiopharmaceuticals for diagnostic, therapeutic and investigative purposes. By combining a suitable radionuclide or isotope with a pharmaceutical it is possible to monitor the behaviour of the pharmaceutical by measuring the distribution of the radioactivity. The most commonly used radioactivity in diagnostic imaging is the energy of the gamma rays emitted from the decaying isotope nucleus. The gamma ray energy is constant and characteristic for each isotope. Measurement is made with a conventional gamma camera. In cases where there are too many protons in the isotope nucleus, decay may proceed by positron emission. The positron usually travels only a short distance and combines with an electron in an annihilation reaction. When this happens, two photons of 511 keV are emitted simultaneously in opposite directions (p. 26). The radiation of these annihilation photons which escape the patient is detected with a dedicated positron-emission tomography (PET) camera, a single photon emission computed tomography (SPECT) gamma camera with a high-energy collimator or a SPECT gamma camera with coincidence counting.

The procedures routinely performed in nuclear medicine departments can be broken down into four main categories: (1) imaging procedures; (2) in vivo function studies; (3) in vitro tests; and (4) therapeutic applications.

1. Imaging procedures provide diagnostic information about organs or body systems based upon the accumulation or selective exclusion of the radiopharmaceutical. The images are only clinically useful if the disease state under investigation causes the localisation of the tracer in a different manner to normal. Measurement is usually made with a gamma camera, a SPECT gamma camera or a PET camera.

2. In vivo function studies measure the function of a given organ based upon the concentration, dilution, absorption or excretion of a radiopharmaceutical. They do not require an image of the distribution of the radiopharmaceutical but an accurate measurement of the activity present within an organ or body fluid sample.

3. In vitro studies are made on samples such as blood, urine and faeces taken from the patient. They do not involve the administration of a radioactive material to the patient. The sample is subjected to procedures such as radioimmunoassay and becomes radioactive outside the patient.

4. Therapeutic applications involve the administration of a radiopharmaceutical with the intent of selectively destroying diseased tissue. The biological effects of the emitted ionising radiations are maximised to produce local therapeutic results in the tissues in which the radionuclide is deposited. This has therapeutic implications as discussed in Chapter 15.

The required properties of the radiopharmaceutical vary according to the category of work being performed and are discussed below.

GAMMA CAMERAS

Gamma cameras are the devices used to observe the distribution of an isotope in an organ, or in a part of the body. In this device a very large diameter crystal, 50 cm diameter by 1 to 1.3 cm thick, receives the gamma ray photons from the patient through a grid of thousands of holes drilled parallel to each other in a 5 cm thick lead plate. If this multihole collimator is placed near the patient, a distribution of scintillations is produced in the crystal which corresponds to the distribution of isotope in the field of view covered by the crystal and collimator. The scintillations in the crystal are detected by an array of between 37 and 75 photomultiplier tubes, depending upon the size and shape of the crystal. The output pulse from each multiplier corresponding to a particular single flash in the crystal depends on the position of the flash relative to the multiplier. The relative pulse heights from the photomultiplier tubes are compared by pulse arithmetic circuits to give, as an X, Y coordinate, the spatial location of the scintillation. By summing the outputs from all the PM tubes a Z pulse is obtained whose amplitude corresponds to the total energy deposited in the crystal by the gamma ray photon. Provided the Z pulse is accepted by the pulse height analyser then the X and Y signals are applied to the deflection plates of a cathode ray tube (CRT); the electron beam is switched on and produces a brief flash of light on the face of the cathode ray tube. The position of this flash corresponds to the position of the scintillation in the gamma camera crystal and in turn to the position within the patient from which the detected gamma ray originated. Thus a distribution of thousands of dots is built up on the CRT screen corresponding to the activity distribution in the field of view. The eye sees these dots as forming a picture. The more dots there are present (i.e. the greater the number of gamma rays) the better the quality of the picture. The image can be reproduced on to film by photographing the CRT screen or captured digitally for image display.

Figure 8.1 shows a diagram of the detector head of a gamma camera. The crystal, collimator and photomultiplier array are mounted inside a substantial lead shield of considerable weight, which is itself mounted on a stand so that the face of the collimator can be adjusted into any suitable position relative to the patient under investigation.

Performance characteristics

The performance of a gamma camera is characterised by six interrelated parameters:

- Spatial resolution
- Sensitivity
- Uniformity
- Spatial distortion and linearity
- Energy resolution
- Field size.

Spatial resolution. This is the ability to distinguish an object from its surroundings and is a measure of the sharpness of the image. It is affected by the collimator,

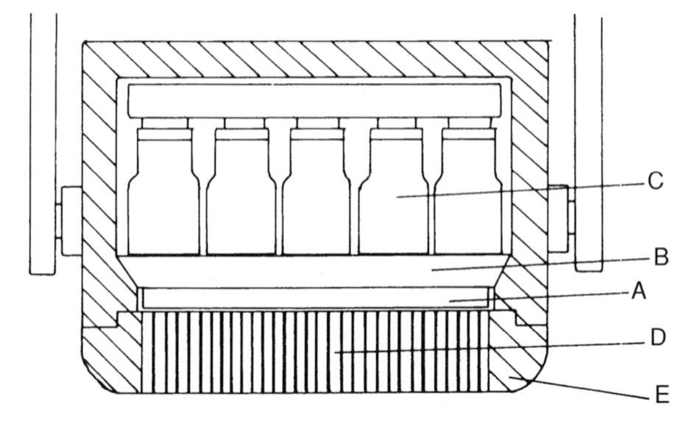

Fig. 8.1 Gamma camera head: A, crystal detector; B, light guide; C, photomultipliers; D, parallel-hole collimator; E, lead shield.

the energy resolution, and the electronic positioning circuitry. It is often specified as the Full Width at Half the Maximum count rate (FWHM) of the counting profile obtained from a single line source. This is shown diagrammatically in Figure 8.2. Two types of spatial resolution are specified: the *intrinsic resolution*, which is the fundamental resolution of the crystal photomultiplier electronics assembly without a collimator applied, and the *system resolution*, which includes the collimator. The intrinsic resolution of a modern gamma camera is about 3 mm.

Sensitivity. This term relates to the counting efficiency of the gamma camera. It is normally quoted as counts per second per megabecquerel. The thickness of the crystal, the width of the pulse height analyser window and the type of collimator in use are all factors which affect sensitivity.

Uniformity. This refers to the variations in count rate across the field of view when the detector is exposed to a uniform source of a gamma ray emitting radionuclide. Variations are caused by such factors as deviations in the sensitivity across the crystal, variability in the responses of the photomultiplier tubes, and mechanical imperfections in the collimator.

Spatial distortion and linearity. These refer to the ability of the gamma camera to translate and accurately reproduce both the spatial and geometric relations of a radioactive distribution beneath the detector and so reproduce a linear activity source as a linear image. Factors influencing distortion include errors in the calculation of the point of interaction within the crystal of the gamma ray and the thickness of the crystal.

Energy resolution. Statistical variations in the detection of gamma rays by the crystal photomultiplier assembly result in a characteristic broadening of the total absorption peak of the energy spectrum. The energy resolution is expressed as the width of the absorption peak at half the maximum count rate observed at the peak. This is analogous with the FWHM concept discussed previously in connection with spatial resolution. Poor energy resolution has an adverse effect upon spatial resolution, sensitivity and uniformity.

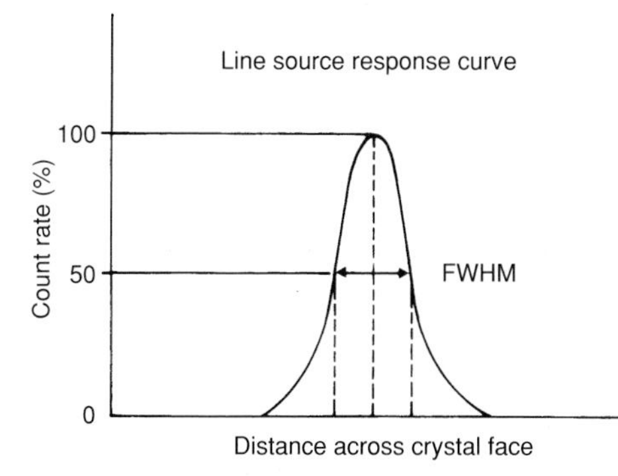

Fig. 8.2 Line source response function and the calculation of full width at half maximum (FWHM).

Field size. This refers to the maximum field of view of the camera. Field sizes vary from 25 to 50 cm.

With the aid of digital microcomputer technology, corrections can be made to overcome some of the non-random defects in camera performance mentioned above. These include corrections for intrinsic non-uniformity and non-linearity.

Collimators

The function of a gamma camera collimator is to project an image of the radioactive distribution beneath the camera face on to the scintillator. This is achieved by stopping gamma rays from entering the crystal by any route other than via the holes in the collimator. Three principal types of collimator are in use: parallel-hole, pin-hole and converging. These are shown schematically in Figure 8.3.

Parallel-hole collimators. These are the most commonly used and consist of a thick lead plate with several thousand small parallel-sided holes penetrating the lead perpendicular to the plane of the plate. For this type of collimator there is a 1 : 1 relationship between the object and its projection on to the crystal. Thus the size of the image is independent of the distance from the subject to the detector face. Similarly, provided the object is completely in the field of view, the sensitivity of the collimator or the count rate remains essentially the same irrespective of the distance in air between the subject and the collimator face. However, the image resolution is best when the subject is close to the collimator face.

Various factors affect the performance of a parallel-hole collimator. These include hole diameter, hole length and septal thickness. Sensitivity and resolution are intimately linked and improvements in one almost inevitably lead to deterioration in the other, as shown in Table 8.1. For example, improving the resolution by

Table 8.1 Factors affecting the performance of parallel-hole collimators

Parameter increases	Resolution	Sensitivity
Hole diameter	Deteriorates	Improves
Hole length	Improves	Deteriorates
Septal thickness	No change	Deteriorates
Object distance	Deteriorates	No change

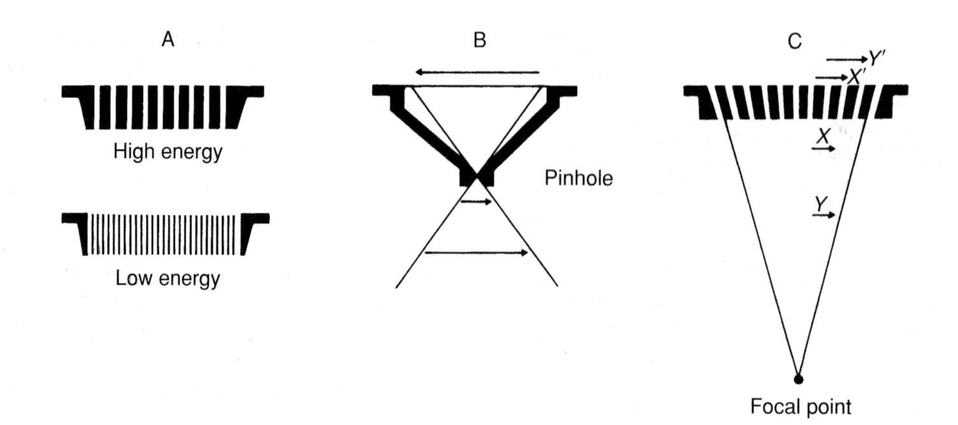

Fig. 8.3 Examples of collimators for a gamma camera. **A** Multihole parallel—high energy having thicker septa than the low energy; **B** pin-hole—objects closest to the hole are imaged with greatest magnification; **C** converging—objects X and Y are displaced and appear as different sizes on the image.

a factor of two by increasing hole length will decrease the sensitivity by a factor of four.

A low-energy collimator has thin septa. If this were to be used with high-energy gamma rays the gamma rays would pass through the septal walls and impinge on the crystal from directions other than those defined by the holes, thus degrading the image. On the other hand, a high-energy collimator has thick septal walls and would appear to be suitable for all gamma ray energies. However, in this case one is unnecessarily sacrificing sensitivity. In practice there is a range of collimators available, as shown in Table 8.2, low, medium and high energy, high resolution–low sensitivity, medium energy–medium sensitivity, and low energy–high sensitivity.

Pin-hole collimators. The pin-hole collimator works in an analogous way to the optical pin-hole camera. It consists of a lead cone with a small hole, a few millimetres in diameter, at the tip of the cone (Fig. 8.3B). Its main use is to give an enlarged image of a small superficial organ such as the thyroid gland. For objects close to the aperture this type of collimator provides the best effective resolution, being close to the inherent resolution of the camera. However, it is very insensitive and, in addition, sensitivity falls off with distance in accordance with the inverse square law. Objects close to the collimator are magnified more than objects further away and objects located off the central axis or at a different depth are imaged obliquely. These factors cause image distortion.

Converging collimators. The converging collimator is a half-way house between the parallel-hole collimator, which has good sensitivity, and the pin-hole collimator, which has good resolution. It is a multihole collimator with the holes converging on a focal spot several centimetres in front of the collimator face (Fig. 8.3C). The resolution improves with distance from the collimator face until the focus is reached. Sensitivity also increases with distance since a larger number of photons from each point within the object can pass through the holes in the collimator. Unfortunately the image is distorted, the back of the object being magnified to a greater extent than the front and the side of the object being seen at a more oblique angle than the

Table 8.2 Examples of types of collimator and their characteristics

Type	Energy limit (keV)	Number of holes	Length (mm)	Size (mm)	Resolution at 10 cm (mm)	Absolute sensitivity (cps MBq^{-1})
Low energy–high sensitivity	160	20 000	22.5	2.5	15.5	405
Low energy–general purpose	170	50 000	22.5	1.5	9.5	158
Low energy–high resolution	190	55 000	27.5	1.5	7.5	101
Medium energy–general purpose	300	10 000	27.5	2.5	14.0	180
High energy–general purpose	400	4 200	57.0	4.5	15.6	180
Pin-hole	400	1	213	3.0	4.8	45

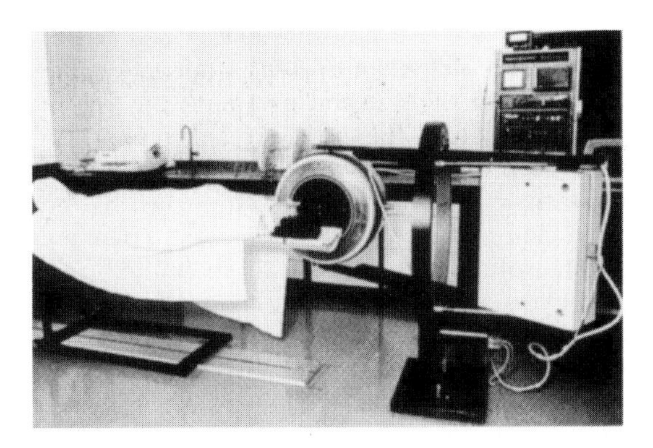

Fig. 8.4 A gamma camera capable of SPECT imaging.

centre. The main use of this type of collimator is brain imaging.

Tomographic gamma cameras

There are two major types of tomography using gamma cameras, single photon emission computed tomography (SPECT) and positron-emission tomography (PET). The first uses a conventional gamma camera with the detector head mounted in such a way that it can rotate around the patient. A photograph of such a system is shown in Figure 8.4.

A series of two-dimensional images, typically 64, are taken and stored on computer as the camera rotates. The data can then be manipulated to produce tomographic sections.

PET CAMERAS

PET scanning uses a special kind of gamma camera to detect isotope decay by positron emission. The positron usually travels only a short distance from the isotope nucleus and combines with an electron in an annihilation reaction. When this happens, two photons of 511 keV are emitted simultaneously in opposite directions. The radiation of these annihilation photons which escape the patient is detected with a dedicated positron-emission tomography (PET) camera, a single photon emission computed tomography (SPECT) gamma camera with a high-energy collimator or a SPECT gamma camera with coincidence counting. Localization of the decay event at the site of origin of the two photons is achieved by taking advantage of the fact that the two photons are emitted simultaneously and travel away from each other at 180 degrees in opposite directions. Two detectors are placed on opposite sides of the patient and are connected to a coincidence circuit designed to register an event only if both detectors detect a photon within a small timing window which is typically nanoseconds. This system only registers simultaneous photons which originate within the volume of the patient between the two detectors. If annihilation originates outside this volume only one of the photons will be detected, this will not satisfy the coincidence condition so the event is rejected. This is therefore *electronic collimation*.

The resolution of a PET camera is mainly dependent on the detector size; the smaller the cross-sectional area, the better the resolution. There are two main inherent limits on the resolution. Firstly, the positron has travelled a few millimetres from the nucleus before annihilating, reducing the localization accuracy for the nucleus. Secondly, the positron and electron are not completely at rest when they annihilate. This results in a slight deviation from the 180 degree angle between the paths of the two resulting photons which further reduces localization accuracy. The minimum resolution of a PET system is therefore typically a few millimetres.

A typical PET scanner consists of multiple radiation detectors housed in a circular ring gantry which surrounds the patient on the imaging table. The most commonly used detectors are bismuth germinate scintillators coupled to photomultiplier tubes. Bismuth germinate detectors are non-hygroscopic, unlike the sodium iodide crystals in gamma cameras, and are more efficient at detecting high-energy photons. Each detector is in coincidence with detectors on the opposite side of the ring. Computerized reconstruction of the PET data is performed to obtain information about the distribution and localization of the isotope within the patient. Current scanners have in-plane resolution of 5 mm and 6.5 mm slice thickness.

When compared with traditional gamma camera nuclear medicine studies, PET studies have higher spatial resolution, higher signal-to-noise ratio, three-dimensional images and they allow quantitative measurement. Unlike SPECT, the spatial resolution and sensitivity of PET are relatively uniform, independent of the location and depth of the event detected.

GAMMA CAMERA RADIOPHARMACEUTICALS

A wide range of radiopharmaceuticals are available to meet the varied needs of the different procedures. The primary route of administration is intravenous, but oral, intramuscular, intracavity and intrathecal routes may also be used. When deciding upon the efficacy of a given radiopharmaceutical, the physical and chemical properties of the radionuclide, together with biochemical, physiological and pharmacological properties of the pharmaceutical, must be considered.

The radionuclide

The various properties which need to be considered when choosing a suitable radionuclide are listed below:

- Type of radiation emitted:
  a. Energy
  b. Abundance
- Half-life
- Specific activity
- Radionuclide purity
- Chemical properties.

It is apparent from the introduction that the desirable requirements of the radionuclide will vary depending upon the type of study being performed. Each of the properties listed above will be considered, firstly as they apply to diagnostic imaging, then as they may be modified for other diagnostic procedures and then as harnessed for therapeutic applications.

Type of radiation

Diagnostic imaging involves external detection of the isotope. The favourable physical characteristics therefore should include the emission of gamma or X-radiation.

The photon energy should be high enough to avoid serious attenuation in tissue, but low enough to allow the photon to be stopped by and interact with the detector and for the detector to be shielded and collimated without using excessive thicknesses of lead. The design characteristics of a standard gamma camera mean that gamma rays with energies between 75 keV and 300 keV are preferred. Positron-emission tomography (PET) cameras, by definition, detect the 511 keV photons released during positron annihilation.

It is also an advantage if the gamma rays are monoenergetic. If more than one gamma ray is emitted then the detector must be collimated against the higher-energy photon, even though it may not be being used for the imaging. Septal penetration by the higher-energy photon results in a loss of image resolution, but increasing the septal thickness to accommodate the high-energy photon reduces the sensitivity of the detector.

A primary aim in diagnostic nuclear medicine is to keep the absorbed radiation dose as low as reasonably achievable (ALARA) while obtaining the required information. It is therefore advantageous if the isotope used is one which gives no significant particulate emissions. This can be accomplished by using radionuclides which decay by isomeric transition or electron capture. Particles will still be emitted (Auger and conversion electrons) but at a much lower rate than from radionuclides decaying by beta or alpha particle emission (Ch. 3).

Radiation dose can also be limited by using radionuclides of high abundance. These are radioactive materials where a high gamma ray yield accompanies the disintegrations. Thus iron-52, which emits 99 photons of 169 keV for every 100 disintegrations, has a higher abundance than chromium-51, which emits only nine photons of 320 keV per 100 disintegrations. In the case of chromium-51, 91 of the disintegrations produce no useful externally detectable gamma ray, but they increase the radiation burden.

Physical half-life

In addition to having an abundant supply of photons of suitable energy the half-life of the radionuclide must be sufficiently long to allow for production, administration, localisation and imaging of the radiopharmaceutical within the organ of interest. At the same time it should be remembered that the radiation dose to the patient is proportional to the half-life of the isotope (p. 25) and the half-life therefore should be as short as possible. In practice it is advantageous to use radionuclides with half-lives about the same as the time over which the test is to be conducted.

Biological half-life

The removal of a radioactive material from a site in the body is determined not only by the physical decay of the radioisotope but also by the metabolic processes to which the isotope, as a chemical material, is subjected. The metabolic activity may result in the elimination of the material at a fast rate or, if the element is absorbed in some particular tissue, it may disappear from the body only slowly. A *biological half-life* can be defined which is the time during which the amount of an element in an organ or in the body falls to half its value by metabolic processes. The biological half-life of a given element is the same for all isotopes of that element no matter what the radioactive physical half-life might be, but it does depend on the chemical state of the element in the body.

In some circumstances the biological half-life of an administered isotope is very important, an example being the biological half-life of iodine in the thyroid gland. In problems of dosimetry and radiation hazard the real or effective rate at which radioactivity disappears from a particular site is a critical factor. The *effective half-life* is a combination of the physical and biological half-lives and is given by the formula:

$$\frac{1}{T_{\text{eff}}} = \frac{1}{T_{\text{biol}}} + \frac{1}{T_{\text{phys}}}$$

where T_{eff}, T_{biol} and T_{phys} are respectively the effective, biological and physical half-lives. Occasionally it is possible to use for human administration isotopes of long physical half-life because in the chemical form used the biological half-life is very short.

Specific activity

The specific activity, that is the ratio per unit mass of radioactive to non-radioactive atoms in the element, should be as high as possible. This will allow very small quantities of the agent to be used and will ensure that the radiolabel does not significantly alter the chemical or biological properties of the pharmaceutical. This is of particular importance when measuring physiological function.

Radionuclide purity

In order to maintain a low radiation dose to the patient and to prevent degradation of the image it is important to control radionuclide purity. Impurities can arise from the manufacturing process (Ch. 3), from daughter radionuclides or from parent radionuclides.

Chemical properties

The chemistry involved in the production of a radiopharmaceutical is very important. Even if the radionuclide has ideal physical properties, it is of little value if it cannot be efficiently attached in an appropriate chemical form to a suitable pharmaceutical to give organ/disease specificity. *Chemical toxicity* is normally not a matter of major concern as radiopharmaceuticals are administered in extremely small quantities. For example a diagnostic dose of 400 kBq of [^{131}I] sodium iodide contains approximately 8×10^{-11} g of iodine. This is only about 1 or 2×10^{-6} of the normal dietary intake of iodine. This amount of the element is well below the amount detectable by normal chemical analytical procedures and also well below the level which can produce physiological effects on the thyroid gland. It is very uncommon for the administration of a radioactive material to a patient to cause any interference with the physiological effects being investigated and it never happens if carrier-free isotopes are used.

The ideal radionuclide for imaging

To summarise, the ideal radionuclide for routine nuclear medicine imaging using a standard gamma camera will be a high-abundancy monoenergetic gamma emitter of energy 75–300 keV. It will decay with a half-life similar to the length of investigation by isomeric transition or electron capture, have low internal conversion and no radioactive daughter products. Technetium-99m comes close to meeting these requirements. It emits a 140 keV photon in 88% of its disintegrations. It decays by isomeric transition with a half- life of 6 hours and is readily 'attached' to a range of pharmaceuticals.

Nevertheless radionuclides which decay by beta particle emission and have a high gamma ray yield can be used for radiopharmaceutical preparation if their chemical and biological properties outweigh any undesirable physical properties. A good example of such a nuclide is iodine-131 which decays by beta particle emission, emits a relatively high energy photon of 364 keV in 82% of disintegrations and has a half-life of 8.1 days. The various radioisotopes of iodine are of physiological importance in thyroid work and are very chemically reactive, allowing them to be attached to many different chemical molecules. This makes them valuable radionuclides in nuclear medicine.

In vivo function studies

In these types of study the radiopharmaceutical must be a true physiological tracer. It is therefore essential that labelling the compound does not interfere with or significantly alter the chemical and biological properties of the compound. Radionuclides iodine-131 or iodine-123 will mimic stable dietary iodide in thyroid function studies. Similarly radioactive cobalt-57 or cobalt-58 can be directly substituted for stable cobalt-59 in cyanocobalamin to study the absorption and excretion of vitamin B_{12}.

The radionuclide properties required are similar to those for imaging, as external detection of the uptake or absorption is desired. However, the detector resolution necessary for good image definition is no longer required. The detectors are more sensitive over a wider range of photon energies. Lower activity levels are used, kilobecquerels rather than megabecquerels; hence the radionuclide requirements are less stringent and the need for a non-particulate emitter is reduced. The half-life must be similar to the length of the investigation. For investigations involving the absorption, utilisation and retention of an element this may be a period of several weeks.

In vitro studies

In vitro studies, unlike all other nuclear medicine procedures, do not involve the administration of a radionuclide to the patient. Therefore all the requirements relating to radiation absorbed dose and external gamma ray detection no longer apply.

Techniques such as saturation analysis and radioimmunoassay, used to measure the concentration of a hormone or chemical in a small sample of blood or urine, require very low levels, becquerels, of activity. The nuclide may be a pure beta emitter, such as carbon-14 which is easily incorporated into many compounds and has a half-life of 5760 years, or it may be a photon emitter such as iodine-125 with X- and gamma radiations of 27 and 36 keV and a half-life of 60 days.

Therapeutic applications

The aim of radionuclide therapy is to maximise the radiation dose to the treatment zone while minimising the dose to normal tissue. It is clearly advantageous to have a radionuclide where a large proportion of the energy emitted per disintegration is in the form of beta particles. Beta particle radiation is completely absorbed by the tissue in which it is lodged and delivers a high localised radiation dose.

A physical half-life of 1 or 2 weeks is desirable. Shorter half-life radionuclides require the administration of high levels of activity to achieve the required dose. Longer half-life nuclides produce a radiation hazard and cause problems with radiation protection.

The pharmaceutical

The desirable factors involved in the choice of pharmaceutical include a high target-to-background ratio; no adverse reactions or unwanted pharmacological responses; and ease of preparation. To image an organ, or to measure the physiological function of an organ or body system, the administered radiopharmaceutical should localise in the target organ with little localisation in other organs or tissues, giving a high target-to-background ratio. A variety of mechanisms affect the localisation and behaviour of the different radiopharmaceuticals available, and some of these are listed below:

- Metabolic accumulation
- Synthesised compounds
- Capillary blockage
- Exclusion
- Drug analogy
- Excretion and secretion
- Compartment localisation
- Antibody–antigen reactions.

Metabolic accumulation

Two elements studied in this way are iodine and iron.

Iodine is an element incorporated into the hormones produced by the thyroid gland, and a study of the metabolic behaviour of iodine in the body gives valuable diagnostic evidence of thyroid function. Radioactive iodine introduced into the body therefore enables iodine metabolism to be studied easily. The concentration of iodine in the thyroid gland also means that therapeutic doses of ionising radiation can be given to the gland from deposited radioactive beta emitters. There are a number of possible iodine isotopes which can be used in these procedures. These include iodine-131 ($T_{½}$ = 8 days; β γ emitter), iodine-125 ($T_{½}$ = 60 days; γ emitter), and iodine-123 ($T_{½}$ = 13 h; γ emitter). In every case, however, the radioactive iodine is supplied and administered as a solution of sodium iodide, though in the body radioactive iodide ion is the entity whose behaviour is of importance.

A study of the metabolism of the element iron is of importance in the clinical diagnosis of blood disorders. The element, again in its ionic form, is built into the haemoglobin of red cells following its absorption from the bloodstream, to which it may be introduced directly or through the processing of food in the alimentary canal. The most useful isotope is iron-59 ($T_{½}$ = 45 days; β γ emitter) and it is administered in the form of a simple iron salt, often ferric citrate, though the precise compound used will depend on the nature of the particular test.

Synthesised compounds

A large number of medically and biologically important compounds are available where a non-radioactive component atom of the molecule has been replaced by a radioactive atom of the same element. These are *synthesised radioactive compounds*. Two examples of clinical interest are vitamin B_{12} and water.

Vitamin B_{12}, of great importance in the study of anaemias, is a compound (cyanocobalamin) containing an atom of cobalt. The compound is synthesised on a large scale by biological processes in which radioactive cobalt is built into the molecule. The most commonly used isotopes are cobalt-57 ($T_{½}$ = 270 days; γ emitter) and cobalt-58 ($T_{½}$ = 71 days; β γ emitter).

Labelled water is available in which one hydrogen atom of the normal molecule is replaced with tritium, the isotope hydrogen-3 ($T_{½}$ = 12.3 years; β emitter). This compound, *tritiated water*, is used, in vivo, to study electrolyte and water absorption problems. The relatively long half-life of tritium is tolerable because the beta ray emission energy is extremely small and the biological half-life of this compound is short, approximately 12 days. A tremendous variety of organic compounds labelled with hydrogen-3 (tritium) or carbon-14 ($T_{½}$ = 5760 years; β emitter) is available.

Capillary blockade

If radioactive particles in the size range 20–50 μm are injected into the vascular system, they will partially occlude the first capillary bed they encounter (size of capillaries 8–10 μm). An intravenous injection of half a million ^{99m}Tc-labelled particles of macroaggregated albumin will block approximately 0.05% of the capillaries of a normal lung, thus permitting the visualisation of the vascular bed of the lungs. A protein such as albumin is chosen for production of the particles as it will be quickly broken down and removed from the lungs.

Exclusion

Pharmaceuticals may be selectively excluded from an organ except in the presence of disease. For example, because of the so-called blood–brain barrier, normal brain tissue is relatively impermeable to substances such as [^{99m}Tc] sodium pertechnetate. Many mass lesions within the brain are more permeable than normal tissue and hence interfere with the blood–brain barrier. This allows the technetium to diffuse across the barrier, accumulate in the lesion and enable visualisation of the lesion.

Drug analogy

A pharmaceutical may be similar either to a substance for which an organ expresses receptors or to a substance that is normally metabolised by an organ and may be used as a substitute to investigate that organ.

The dopamine transporter is expressed exclusively on the presynaptic terminals of dopaminergic neurons in the basal ganglia of the brain. As the degeneration of these terminals proceeds in true Parkinson's disease, the number of dopamine transporters reduces as a direct consequence. The radiopharmaceutical [^{123}I]-ioflupane belongs to the group of compounds derived from cocaine that bind to the dopamine transporter. Specific binding of [^{123}I]-ioflupane is reduced by approximately 50% in symptomatic Parkinsonian individuals relative to controls or patients with essential tremor, thereby facilitating differentiation from the latter group and allowing institution of appropriate therapy.

To some extent the pertechnetate ion (TcO_4) behaves in the thyroid in a similar way to the iodine ion, and the use of technetium-99m for the study of thyroid function is often an advantage since it gives a low-absorbed dose to the gland.

The reticuloendothelial cells in the body have the capacity to ingest bacteria and small particles in the range 0.01–10 μm. This is known as *phagocytosis*. If a radiolabelled colloid is injected intravenously, the phagocytic action of the reticuloendothelial cells, in particular the Kupffer cells in the liver, will remove the colloid from the circulation, enabling the organ to be externally visualised. Areas of non-functioning liver tissue will not remove colloid material.

Thallium-201 is concentrated in muscle tissue in a similar manner to potassium. This can be used to image the heart muscle and detect areas of ischaemic and infarcted myocardium.

Excretion, secretion

Many drugs are excreted or secreted by body organs. These properties can be utilised to both visualise the organ and to quantify its level of physiological function.

The radiopharmaceutical [^{123}I]*o*-iodohippurate is taken up by the kidneys, passes through the tubules into the kidney pelvis, and is then excreted via the ureters into the bladder. The transit of the pharmaceutical through the kidney gives information about function.

[^{99m}Tc] sodium pertechnetate is concentrated in the gastric mucosa and secreted into the lining of the gut. It can be used to visualise sites of ectopic gastric mucosas such as Meckel's diverticulum.

Compartmental localisation

The distribution of certain types of cells and molecules is restricted to particular body compartments. Radiolabelled forms of such cells can be used to visualise the compartment or to measure the volume of that compartment. ^{99m}Tc-labelled red cells, when re-injected into the patient from whom the cells have been withdrawn, will be retained almost exclusively within the vascular compartment. With the application of simple dilution analysis techniques the labelled cells can be used to measure the red cell volume of the compartment, or by ECG gating the data collection they can be used to image the functioning heart.

Antibody–antigen reactions

Antigens are produced in low concentrations by normal tissue but are present in relatively high concentration on the surface of certain tumour cells. Monoclonal antibodies can be raised against specific antigens. If the antibodies are radiolabelled then the sites of antigen–antibody binding can be located.

Sterility and purity of radiopharmaceuticals

The radiopharmaceutical must not produce a pharmacological reaction within the patient. It must be chemically pure, non-toxic and contain only small quantities of chemical carrier and radionuclide.

The preparation of radiopharmaceuticals and the form in which they are made available for use in clinical departments is influenced by the method by which it is intended to introduce the product into the patient. For some tests, oral administration is the preferred method and indeed sometimes the only suitable one. In this case clean, stable, palatable solutions are ideal. For many tests, however, intravenous injections must be used and for some cases intracavity or intrathecal (into spinal fluid) injection is necessary. In these cases great care must be taken to produce a radiopharmaceutical in a sterile solution of the correct pH value and free from pyrogens (foreign proteins arising from previous bacteriological activity).

The details of the necessary procedures are beyond the scope of this text but these requirements do influence the laboratory facilities necessary in hospital departments where radiopharmaceuticals are prepared. In addition to the radiation safety requirements discussed in Chapter 6 and later in this chapter, the needs of good pharmaceutical practice are also important.

The special laboratory facilities and equipment required are described in detail in other publications. Many of the desirable design features necessary for the production of pharmaceuticals are also desirable for radiation safety. However, there is one major area of conflict. For radiation safety, in order to contain any airborne contaminants, rooms where high activity levels are in use are often kept at a lower pressure than the surrounding environment. The requirements for a radiopharmacy are exactly the opposite. The preparation area must be bathed in a pure sterile air at a pressure higher than that of its surroundings so as to avoid leakage inward of non-sterile air and microorganisms.

PET RADIOTRACERS

The radiotracers used for PET are either chemical analogues of natural substrates, such as ^{18}F fluorodeoxyglucose, in which a hydrogen of a glucose molecule is replaced with a positron emitter, or a radioactive-labelled natural substrate, such as ^{15}O-labelled water. The isotopes used in PET are of biologically abundant elements, which is unlike the isotopes used in traditional gamma camera nuclear medicine studies. PET images therefore reveal function rather than structure. They provide information about biochemical and physiological processes that can be complementary to more anatomical imaging modalities such as CT and MRI. The most routinely used isotopes for labelling the radiotracers in PET studies are carbon (^{11}C), nitrogen (^{13}N), oxygen (^{15}O) and fluorine (^{18}F). These elements can be substituted for the stable isotopes in biological molecules without changing the physiological characteristics of the molecule. Of the three most abundant elements in biomolecules (hydrogen, carbon, oxygen), only hydrogen has no positron-emitting isotopes. Fluorine can be substituted for hydrogen in many instances.

Positron emitters have a high specific activity (radioactivity per unit mass) so that only very small amounts need be administered for the study. Radiation dose is also relatively low because of the short physical half-life of these positron emitters. This permits high-quality images and the opportunity to repeat studies frequently with tolerable radiation exposure to the patient.

All of the commonly used positron-emitting isotopes in PET studies have to be produced with a particle accelerator, usually a small cyclotron. Their half-lives are 2.07 minutes for ^{15}O, 9.96 minutes for ^{13}N, 20.4 minutes for ^{11}C and 109.7 minutes for ^{18}F. A radiochemistry laboratory is used to attach the isotopes to the tracer which will be used in the study. The short half-lives of all these isotopes require rapid synthesis of tracer and in the case of ^{11}C, ^{13}N and ^{15}O, close proximity of the cyclotron and radiochemistry laboratory to the PET scanner. The relatively long half life of ^{18}F permits regional distribution to PET scanners away from the cyclotron and ^{18}F studies are becoming the commonest clinically performed.

RADIOPHARMACEUTICALS IN THE BODY

Consideration of the various processes through which the radiopharmaceutical may pass has shown that many of the compounds will at some stage be located in a particular organ or tissue, at least for a time. The localisation of iodine in the thyroid gland or of radioactive albumin particles of appropriate size in the lungs are good examples. This aspect of the behaviour of radioactive materials in the body is important in several ways: it capacitates the use of radionuclides in dilution analysis and metabolic function studies; it permits organ visualisation; it has an impact on radiation dose and the import of critical organs; and it allows for therapeutic applications.

Use for dilution analysis and metabolic function

Dilution analysis

The localisation of the radiopharmaceutical within a space or compartment enables an estimate to be made of the volume of that space within the patient. If a known amount of a radioactive material is introduced into a vessel containing an unknown volume of liquid and thoroughly mixed, it is easy to deduce the unknown volume by measuring the concentration of activity in a sample taken from the mixture.

An important example of the dilution technique is the measurement of the volume of the circulating red cells in the blood. For this purpose a sample of the patient's own red cells are used and the cells are labelled with either chromium-51 or technetium-99m. An accurately known volume of the labelled red cells is then re-injected into the patient and a smaller accurately known volume used to make up a standard. 2–30 minutes after re-injection a venous blood sample is withdrawn from the patient. The radioactive assay consists of comparing the activity of equal volumes of the whole blood and of the standard solution. The red cell volume (RCV) is calculated from the formula:

$$\mathrm{RCV} = \frac{A_\mathrm{s}}{A_\mathrm{b}} \times V \times D \times \frac{H}{100}$$

where A_s and A_b are the count rates from the standard and blood sample, V is the volume of labelled cells re-injected, D is the dilution factor used in preparing the standard and H is the percentage haematocrit of the venous blood sample.

Metabolic function

The investigation of a radioisotope's distribution about the body and the way in which this varies with time provides valuable information about the metabolism of the compound.

As we have mentioned previously, a very common and important metabolic study is that of the element iodine, which is involved in the function of the thyroid gland. Knowledge of iodine metabolism gives diagnostic information about thyroid disease. The normal daily intake of iodine is about 100 µg. When the thyroid gland is functioning normally about half of this iodine is abstracted from the circulating blood by the thyroid gland and about half is abstracted by the kidney and excreted in the urine. The thyroid gland synthesises the thyroid hormones, of which the element iodine is one of the atomic constituents, and the hormones are transported throughout the body in the blood circulation to control the bodily functions influenced by these hormones. Between 150 and 200 kBq of iodine-131 in the form of a solution of sodium iodide is administered orally to the patient. An equal amount is stored in a small bottle for use as a comparison standard. The uptake of the radioiodine in the thyroid gland is observed by means of a collimated scintillation counter. Four measurements are required for an uptake measurement:

1. The activity in the thyroid gland in counts per minute, P.
2. By positioning a lead block between the patient's neck and the detector, a measure of the patient's non-thyroidal background activity, P_{bg}.
3. With the standard placed in a neck phantom underneath the detector, the activity of the standard, S.
4. With the phantom covered with the lead block a phantom background, S_{bg}.

It therefore follows that:

$$\%\ \text{thyroid uptake} = \frac{P - P_{bg}}{S - S_{bg}} \times 100$$

The curves of Figure 8.5 show the variation of uptake in the thyroid gland over 3 days following the administration of the tracer dose. The ordinates represent percentage of the administered dose taken up by the gland, and the three curves A, B, and C represent typical results: A in a patient with normal thyroid function; B in a case of hyperactivity, or thyrotoxicosis of the gland; and C in a case of hypoactivity of the gland leading to myxoedema. It should be noted that during the time of the test, sometimes up to 7 days, there will have been a physical decay of the iodine-131, and in the curves in Figure 8.5 the percentage of administered dose has in each case been corrected for this decay.

Use for organ visualisation

The localisation of a radiopharmaceutical within an organ makes possible the visualisation of that organ.

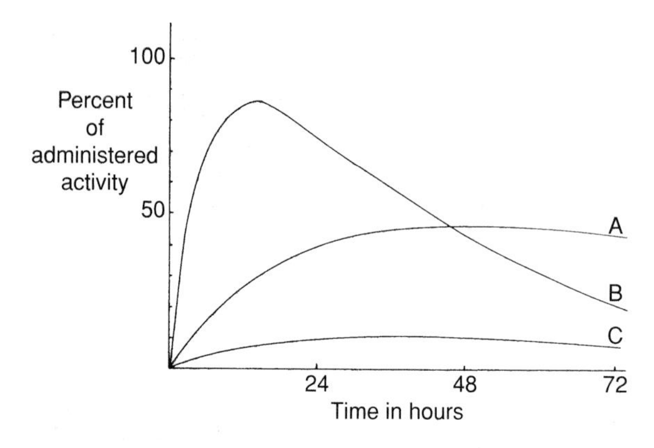

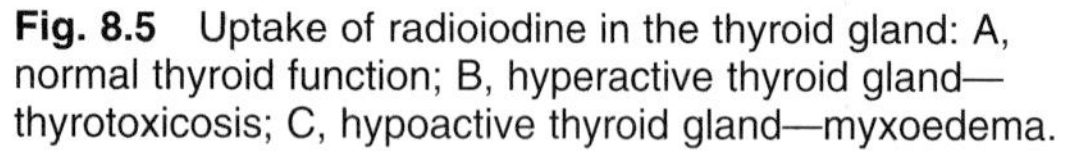
Fig. 8.5 Uptake of radioiodine in the thyroid gland: A, normal thyroid function; B, hyperactive thyroid gland—thyrotoxicosis; C, hypoactive thyroid gland—myxoedema.

Furthermore, if the distribution of the administered isotope in the organ concerned is abnormal, or changes with time, then deductions can be made about the function of the organ. Abnormal isotope distribution may appear as an increase in isotope concentration above the norm, revealing lesions as 'hot spots', or as reduced activity in the visualised pattern, revealing lesions as 'cold spots'.

The main purpose of organ imaging is to investigate the function of system pathology rather than anatomical definition. This may be achieved by the use of either static imaging, both planar and tomographic, or by dynamic imaging, the monitoring of changes in distribution with time. There follows a brief description of some of the more important clinical applications of radionuclide imaging. This is not meant to be a comprehensive list of every conceivable use, but more an introduction to the types of investigation possible.

Skeletal imaging

Bone is made up of collagen and minerals, mainly calcium, phosphates and hydroxides. The minerals form a crystalline lattice known as hydroxyapatite. Following intravenous injection, a bone-seeking agent will be transported to the bone and become adsorbed on to the newly forming hydroxyapatite crystals, thus reflecting the bone-forming activity at a given skeletal site. Hence areas where there is an abnormally high increase in bone turnover will show increased uptake and will appear as 'hot spots' on the image.

All current bone-seeking radiopharmaceuticals are based on phosphate-containing compounds which

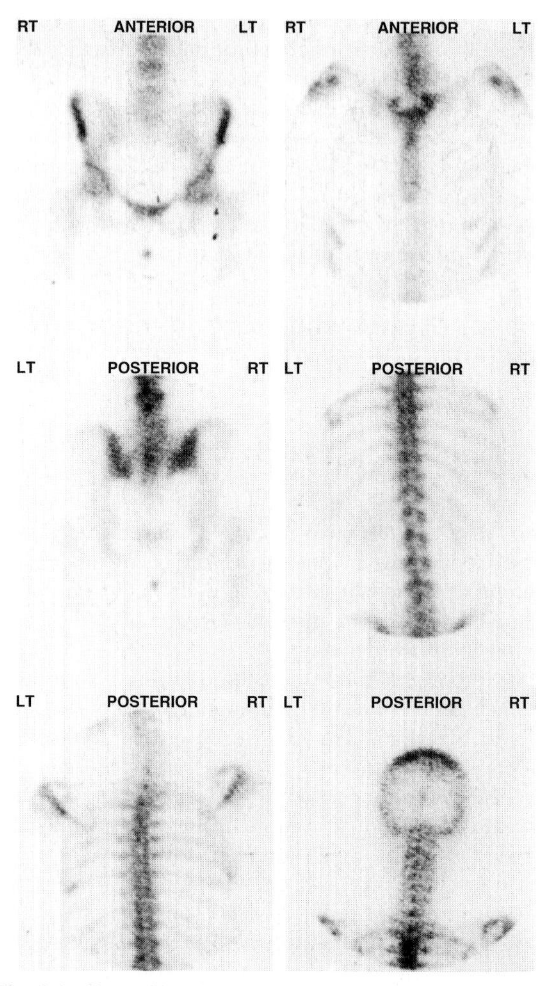

Fig. 8.6 Normal bone scan 4 hours after intravenous injection of [^{99m}Tc]MDP.

can be labelled with technetium-99m. A variety of these analogues are available but the most widely used is methylene diphosphonate (MDP). Typically, 400–600 MBq of [^{99m}Tc]MDP are administered intravenously and after a period of 2–4 hours 50–60% of the injected dose will be localised in the bone, the remainder being excreted via the kidneys. Multiple static views or a combination of a whole body image and selected static views are recorded. The appearances of the normal bone scan are shown in Figure 8.6, where it can be seen that each of the bones is well demonstrated.

Bone scan changes occur when there is increased osteoblastic activity, and increased or decreased blood flow to a lesion. The bone scan is a very sensitive technique for demonstrating bone lesions, but the findings are non-specific. An abnormal distribution of activity

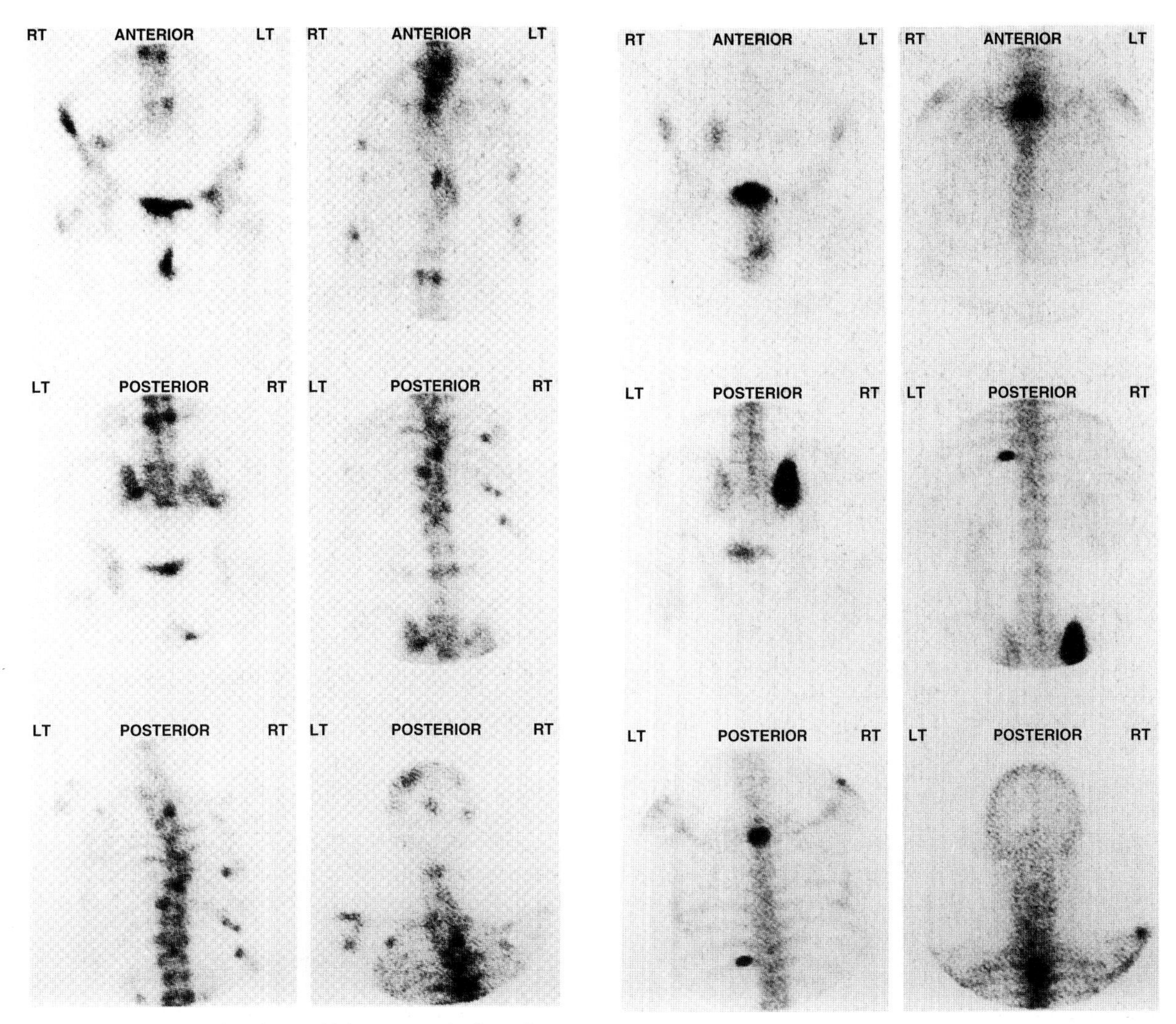

Fig. 8.7 Bone scan showing multiple metastatic deposits from carcinoma of the breast.

Fig. 8.8 Bone scan showing high-activity focal 'hot spots' from prostatic metastases.

must be interpreted together with the relevant clinical history and appropriate X-rays.

Applications of skeletal imaging include those described below.

- The detection of metastases in bone, particularly from breast and prostate tumours. Figure 8.7 shows a patient with extensive metastatic involvement, from a primary breast carcinoma, as demonstrated by the multiple areas of increased uptake. Figure 8.8 shows just three focal 'hot spots', one in the dorsal spine, one posteriorly in a left rib, and the third in the right side of the sacrum. This high activity pattern is typical of metastases from a prostate tumour. Radionuclide bone imaging provides earlier diagnosis of a lesion than X-ray techniques, since for a lesion to be apparent on an X-ray there needs to be about a 50% decrease in calcium content.
- The diagnosis of functional changes caused by metabolic bone disease. These techniques depend on the quantitative estimates of the uptake and clearance of a bone-seeking radiopharmaceutical.
- Monitoring the progression and regression of known active disease or the response of a lesion to treatment.
- Detection of bone infarction or aseptic necrosis, where the lesion will appear as an area of decreased activity, not as a 'hot spot'.

Breast

Breast cancer cells take up [^{99m}]Tc-sestamibi by an active transport mechanism, the [^{99m}]Tc-sestamibi is then stored in mitochondria and cytoplasm. Cancer cells which are more metabolically active than their surrounding normal counterparts will show as areas of increased [^{99m}]Tc-sestamibi activity. There is a role for this nuclear medicine technique as a complementary method of breast imaging to mammography, ultrasound or magnetic resonance imaging in dense breasts, in patients with breast implants, in breasts with previous scarring or therapy and in assessing the extent of multifocal breast cancer.

Thyroid

The normal function of the thyroid gland includes the concentration of iodine from the circulation, and the synthesis and storage of thyroid hormones. Iodine may also be trapped in the salivary glands and the gastric mucosa. Iodine-131 was once the radionuclide of choice for thyroid imaging, but because of the relatively high radiation dose to the patient it has now been superseded by iodine-123 and [^{99m}Tc]pertechnetate. The latter is the most readily available and is trapped in the thyroid gland by an active transport mechanism in the same way as iodine. However, it is not incorporated into the thyroid hormones.

An intravenous injection of 40–80 MBq of [^{99m}Tc]pertechnetate is administered and a static image of the thyroid gland acquired approximately 30 minutes later. Imaging may be performed, with a parallel-hole collimator, on a small field of view mobile gamma camera, or on a conventional gamma camera using either a pin-hole or converging collimator.

The commonest clinical conditions evaluated by this technique are the differentiation between benign and malignant nodules; assessment of the size of the gland in hyperthyroidism; and the localisation of metastatic thyroid cancer. Figure 8.9 shows uniform uptake to a normal bilobed thyroid gland.

A non-functioning 'cold' nodule, corresponding to the visible mass in the patient's neck, is seen in the right lobe of the thyroid gland of Figure 8.10; also visible at the top of the image are the submandibular salivary glands. Thyroid malignancies do not concentrate radioisotopes and appear as cold nodules, but only 20% of the cold nodules detected are malignant.

Medullary carcinoma of the thyroid, arising from the calcitonin-secreting C cells, is rare (only accounting for 5% of all thyroid malignancies) but can be imaged using more specific tumour-imaging agents. Medullary carcinoma can be either sporadic (usually unilateral, not associated with other abnormalities), familial (usually bilateral, not associated with other abnormalities, least malignant) or as a component of the multiple endocrine neoplasia (MEN) syndrome type 2a (usually bilateral, commonly a family history, associated with phaeochromocytoma in approximately half of patients and pseudonodular

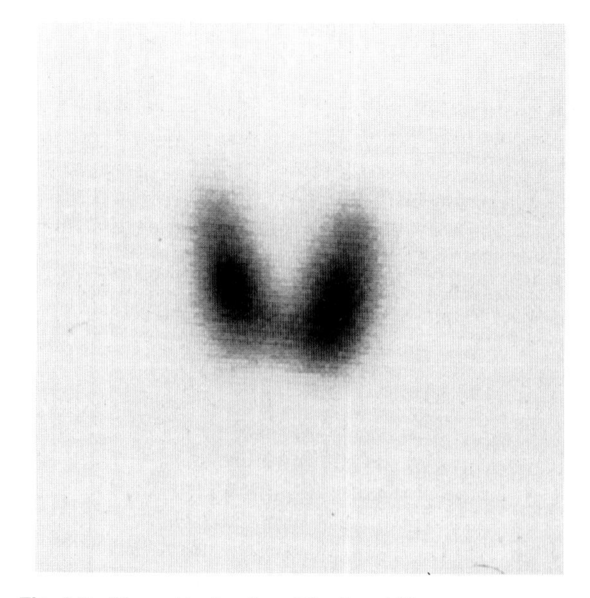

Fig. 8.9 Normal technetium-99m thyroid image.

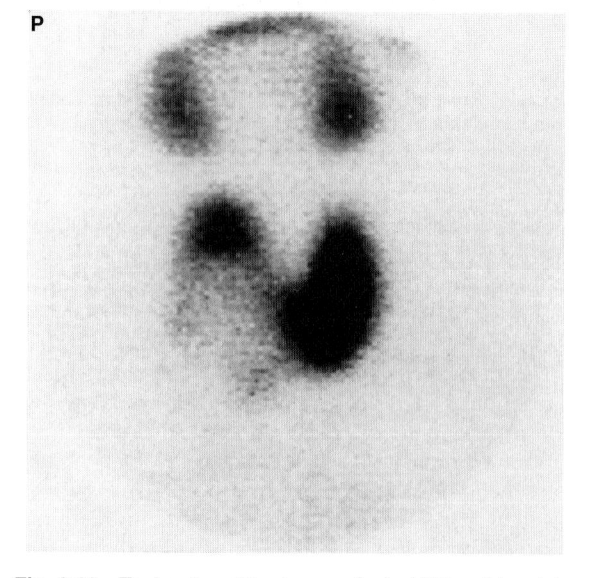

Fig. 8.10 Technetium-99m image of a 'cold' thyroid nodule corresponding to an area of swelling in the neck.

hyperparathyroidism in one-third of patients) and type 2b (usually bilateral, the most malignant form, commonly associated with phaeochromocytoma, mucosal neuromas and ganglion neuromas). The most sensitive diagnostic test is measurement of plasma calcitonin level. However, several radiopharmaceuticals can be used for localization, of which DMSA[V] and pentetreotide have proved most useful. Technetium-DMSA[V] has a sensitivity of 85–95% for detection of medullary carcinoma but is not recommended for localization of phaeochromocytoma, whereas ^{111}In-pentetreotide has the highest sensitivity for detecting both primary and secondary medullary carcinoma and any associated phaeochromocytoma. False positives can occur with pentetreotide in some benign adenomas and in chronic inflammation; the false-negative rate with both DMSA[V] and pentetreotide is 5–15%. As DMSA[V] is substantially less expensive than pentetreotide, it is usually used first, reserving pentetreotide for DMSA[V]-negative patients. Tumour deposits appear as focal accumulations of increased count density.

Parathyroid

The four parathyroid glands, weighing only 35 mg each, are situated at the poles of the thyroid gland. The primary use of parathyroid imaging is the localisation of parathyroid adenomas.

The technique involves the combined injection of 40 MBq of [^{99m}Tc]pertechnetate and 40 MBq of thallium-201 followed by subtraction imaging. Thallium-201 is localised in both the thyroid gland and in parathyroid adenomas. Technetium-99m is localised in the thyroid gland but not the parathyroid glands. Two images are taken and stored on computer, one using the technetium-99m window, the other using the thallium-201 window. The images are then normalised and the technetium-99m image is subtracted from the thallium-201 image. An example of such a procedure is given in Figure 8.11, where, following subtraction, a

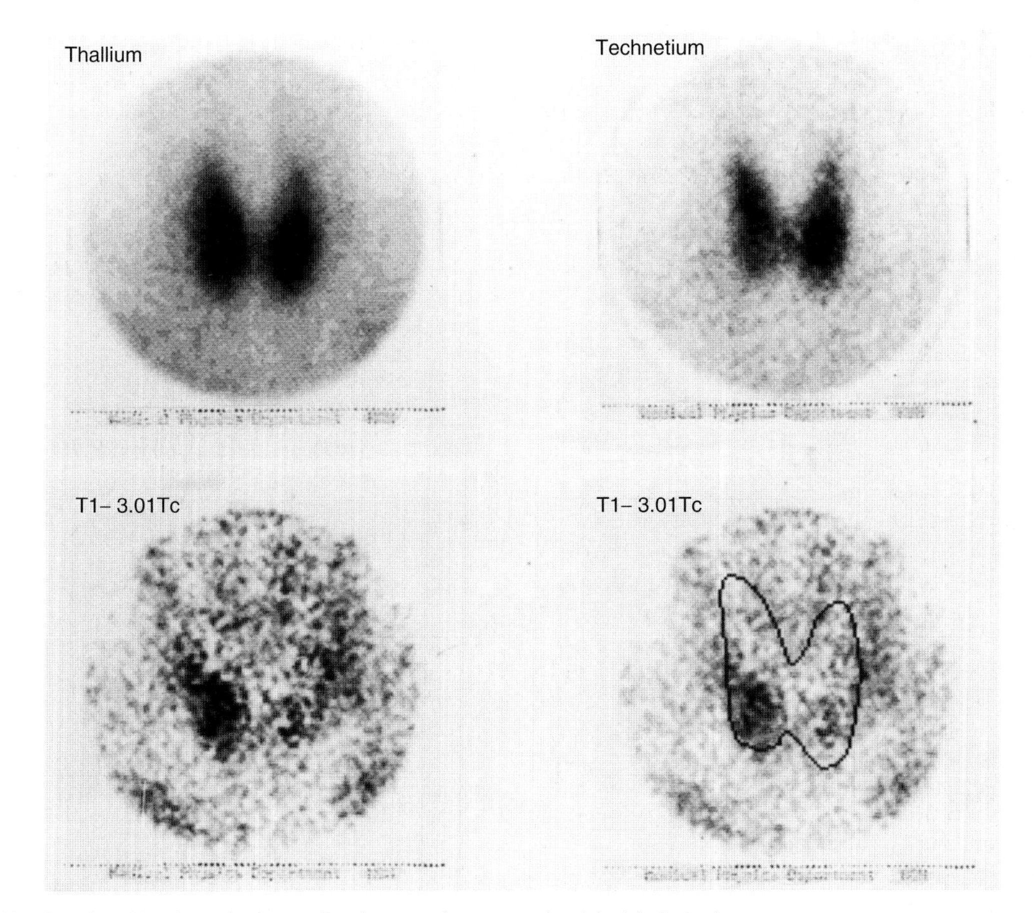

Fig. 8.11 Parathyroid subtraction scan showing an adenoma at the right inferior pole.

parathyroid adenoma is seen at the inferior pole of the right lobe of the thyroid gland.

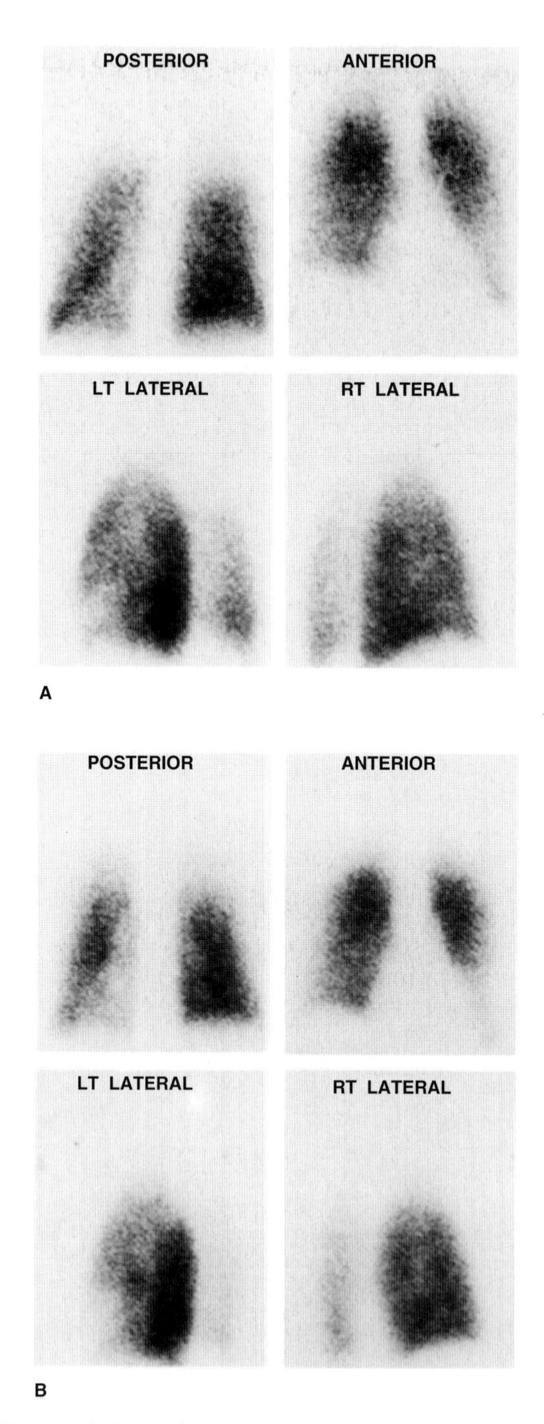

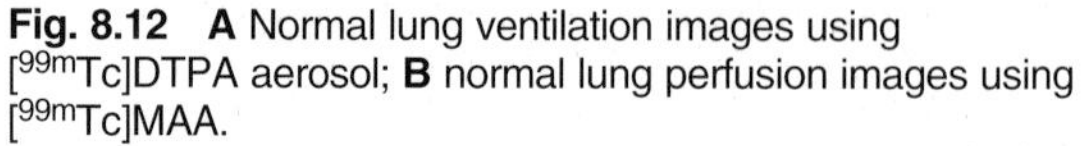

Fig. 8.12 **A** Normal lung ventilation images using [^{99m}Tc]DTPA aerosol; **B** normal lung perfusion images using [^{99m}Tc]MAA.

Lung

The function of the lungs is to exchange gases between the air and the blood. There are therefore two mechanisms to be investigated: the regional perfusion, and the regional ventilation. The main clinical use of these techniques in oncology patients is in the investigation of suspected pulmonary embolus.

Regional perfusion is studied by administering an intravenous injection of 80 MBq of [^{99m}Tc]macro-aggregated albumin. The albumin particles have a diameter of between 10–20 μm and after mixing in the heart will be trapped in the pulmonary arteriolar or capillary bed of the lungs. The resultant image will show the areas of lung which are perfused (Fig. 8.12B).

Lung ventilation is studied by the inhalation of either an inert radioactive gas such as xenon-133 or krypton-81m or a radioactive aerosol such as [^{99m}Tc]DTPA. All have their advantages and disadvantages. Xenon-133 is cheap, readily available and has a long shelf-life. However, it emits a low-energy gamma ray of 80 keV, making it less than ideal for gamma camera imaging because it produces images of low resolution, and it is only possible to take views from one projection for each examination. Krypton-81m is produced from a rubidium-81 generator. It has an ideal gamma ray energy of 190 keV, a half-life of 13 seconds, giving a low radiation dose to the patient, and a full range of views can be obtained. Unfortunately the rubidium-81 in the generator also has a short half-life, has limited availability and is very expensive. [^{99m}Tc]DTPA aerosol can be inhaled by the patient and has all the advantages of any [^{99m}Tc]radiopharmaceutical. The residency time of the activity within the lungs depends on the physiological state, but it is usually possible to obtain at least four views. Figure 8.12A shows a normal ventilation lung scan following inhalation of [^{99m}Tc]DTPA aerosol. The main disadvantage is that the same radionuclide, technetium-99m, is used for both the ventilation and perfusion phase of the study. This means that the ventilation image must be acquired before the perfusion image and, depending on the physiological status, a time gap between the two stages of the investigation may be necessary.

The most common clinical application of lung scanning is the differential diagnosis of pulmonary embolism. Here the ventilation capacity of the lungs is normal, and hence the ventilation image is normal (Fig. 8.13A), while the perfusion pattern is abnormal in the regions occluded by the clot (Fig. 8.13B). These

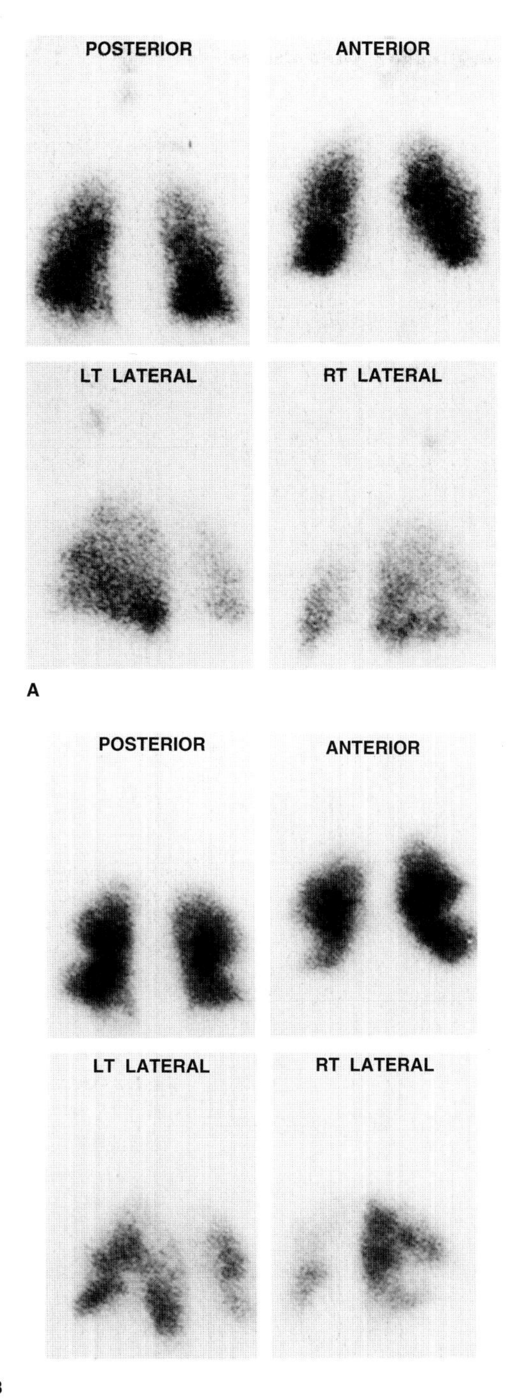

Fig. 8.13 **A** Normal lung ventilation; **B** lung perfusion images showing wedge-shaped filling defects. These are not matched on the ventilation images and are indicative of pulmonary embolism.

normally appear as wedge-shaped or segmental defects on the perfusion image.

Cardiac

In oncology, measuring cardiac function in response to anthracycline chemotherapy is often performed using an isotope technique sometimes referred to as the MUGA (multigated acquisition) scan.

The heart is a muscular organ divided internally by a muscular septum into right and left sides, each side having two chambers. The right and left atria collect the blood returning from the pulmonary and systemic circulations. The right and left ventricles are pumping chambers and are more muscular, particularly the left ventricle, which pumps the blood to the systemic circulation.

The contractions of the left ventricle of the heart are investigated by means of gated blood pool imaging—multigated acquisition (MUGA). 20–30 minutes following a cold injection of pyrophosphate, or stannous fluoride, 400–800 MBq of technetium-99m is administered intravenously and in vivo labelling of the patient's red cells takes place. By using the patient's ECG to gate or control image acquisition, a series of images (16–24) is recorded and stored on computer during each cardiac cycle. Data collection continues for several minutes. High spatial resolution images are then obtained by summing images of identical time segments in consecutive cardiac cycles. The images can be processed to assess regional wall motion, and give ventricular ejection fractions. Functional images of stroke volume and paradoxical motion can be obtained together with phase and amplitude images. Amplitude refers to the actual change in ventricular volume throughout the cardiac cycle, while phase refers to the timing of the contraction. Figure 8.14 shows a patient with a normal ventricular ejection fraction and uniform heart muscle contractions. Figure 8.15 demonstrates an abnormal ejection fraction of 15% and a small area of dyskinesia at the apex of the left ventricle. This can be seen on both the paradoxical image and the phase image.

Renal

The kidney produces urine and disposes of metabolic waste products. It is divided into an outer cortical and an inner medullary region. Urine drains from the medullary region via the renal pelvis into the ureter and thence into the bladder. Several radiopharmaceuticals are available for imaging the kidney and investigating renal function. The choice of pharmaceutical depends on the specific renal function measurements required and the clinical condition being studied. The commonest reason for renal isotope investigation in

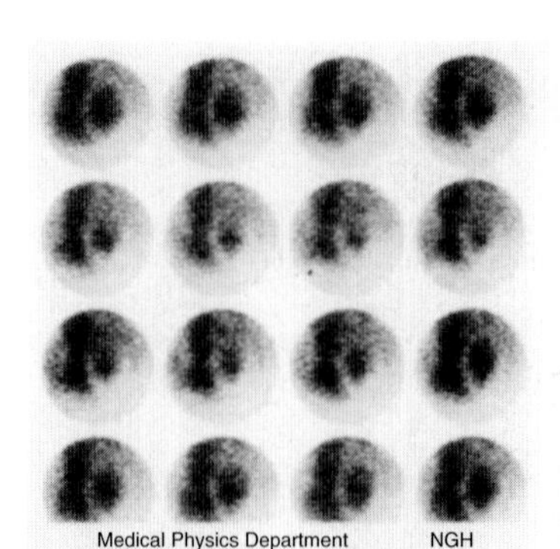

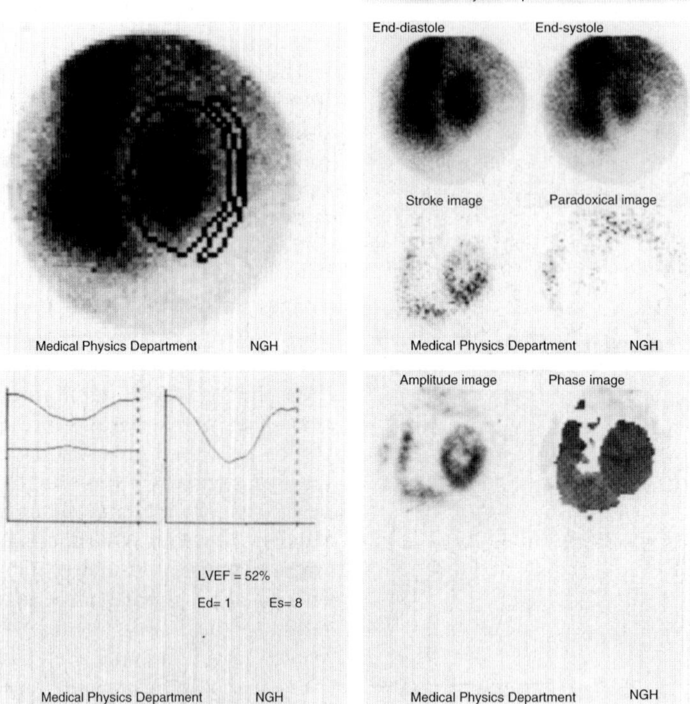

Fig. 8.14 Multigated acquisition study of a normally functioning heart—normal ventricular ejection fraction of >50%, normal contraction of the ventricle in systole, uniform amplitude and phase images.

oncology patients is to investigate suspected obstruction to urine drainage down the ureters caused by primary tumour masses such as gynaecological pelvic malignancy or bladder and prostate carcinomas, or by secondary metastatic disease spread to lymph nodes in the para-aortic or iliac chains, which lie adjacent to the ureters. There follows just one example of a renal investigation.

The most widely used radiopharmaceuticals are [^{99m}Tc]MAG3 and DTPA. They are suitable for the assessment of individual kidney function, and detection of drainage obstruction. With the kidneys, bladder, and if possible the heart, in the field of view of the gamma camera, up to 80 MBq of [^{99m}Tc]MAG3 is injected intravenously. For the following 25–30 minutes a series of images (e.g. 90 20-second frames) are collected and stored on computer. Regions of interest can then be drawn around the kidneys, the bladder and the heart and, after suitable background correction, time–activity curves can be calculated for each region. This is known as a renogram.

Figure 8.16 shows the renogram data from a patient with one normally functioning kidney and one obstructed kidney. The top two pictures show the

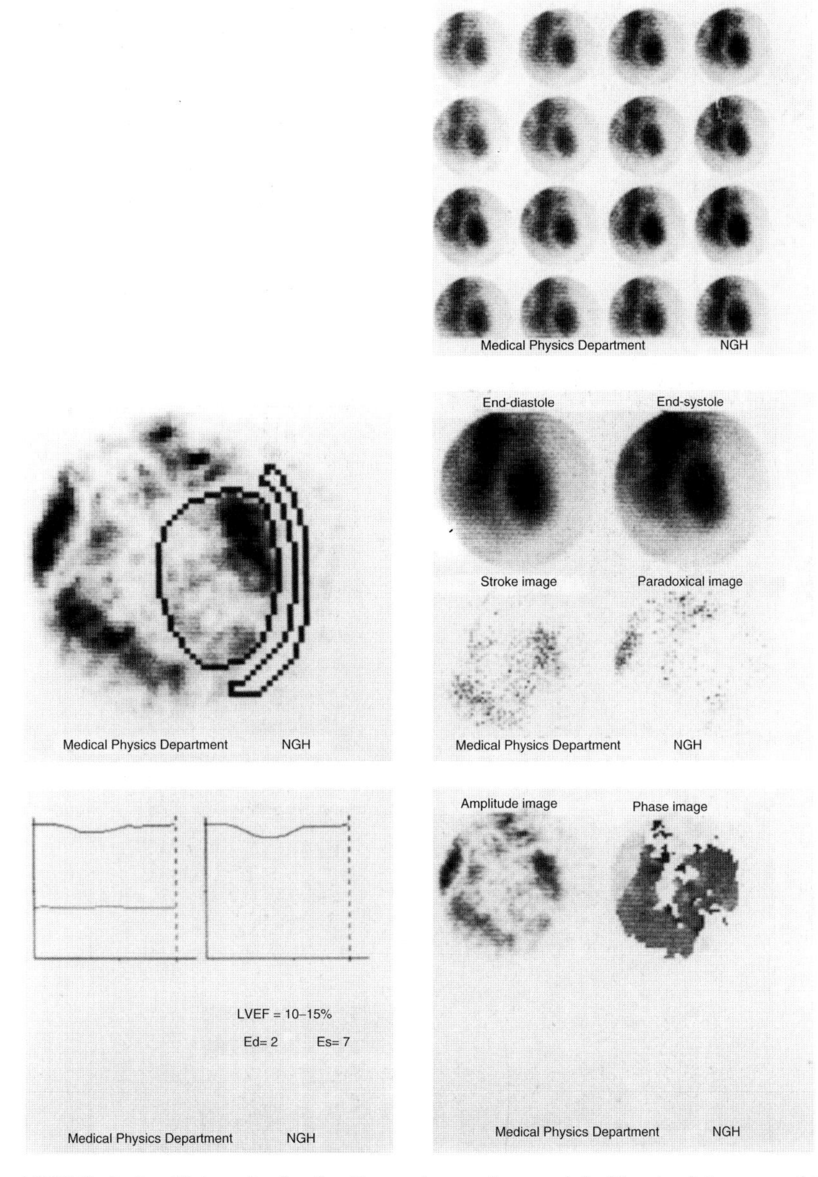

Fig. 8.15 Abnormal MUGA study with low ejection fraction and a small area of dyskinesia at the apex of the left ventricle.

changes in the kidney images with the passage of time. The centre left image shows the regions of interest associated with each kidney. The bottom left image shows the net kidney curves. The renogram from the normal left kidney is seen to contain three phases: a vascular phase denoted by an initial sharp rise; a secretory phase denoted by a slower steadier rise peaking after about 4 minutes; and an excretory phase denoted by the falling slope. An injection of a diuretic, which enhances renal excretion, was administered part-way through the excretory phase and is seen as a rapid fall in the curve. The abnormal right kidney shows pelvic retention on the images and a continuously rising obstructive pattern on the renogram. There is a fall in the curve following administration of the diuretic. Other images show the accumulation of activity in the bladder and the clearance of tracer from the circulation. Values for relative kidney function have been calculated and these are displayed on the centre right picture.

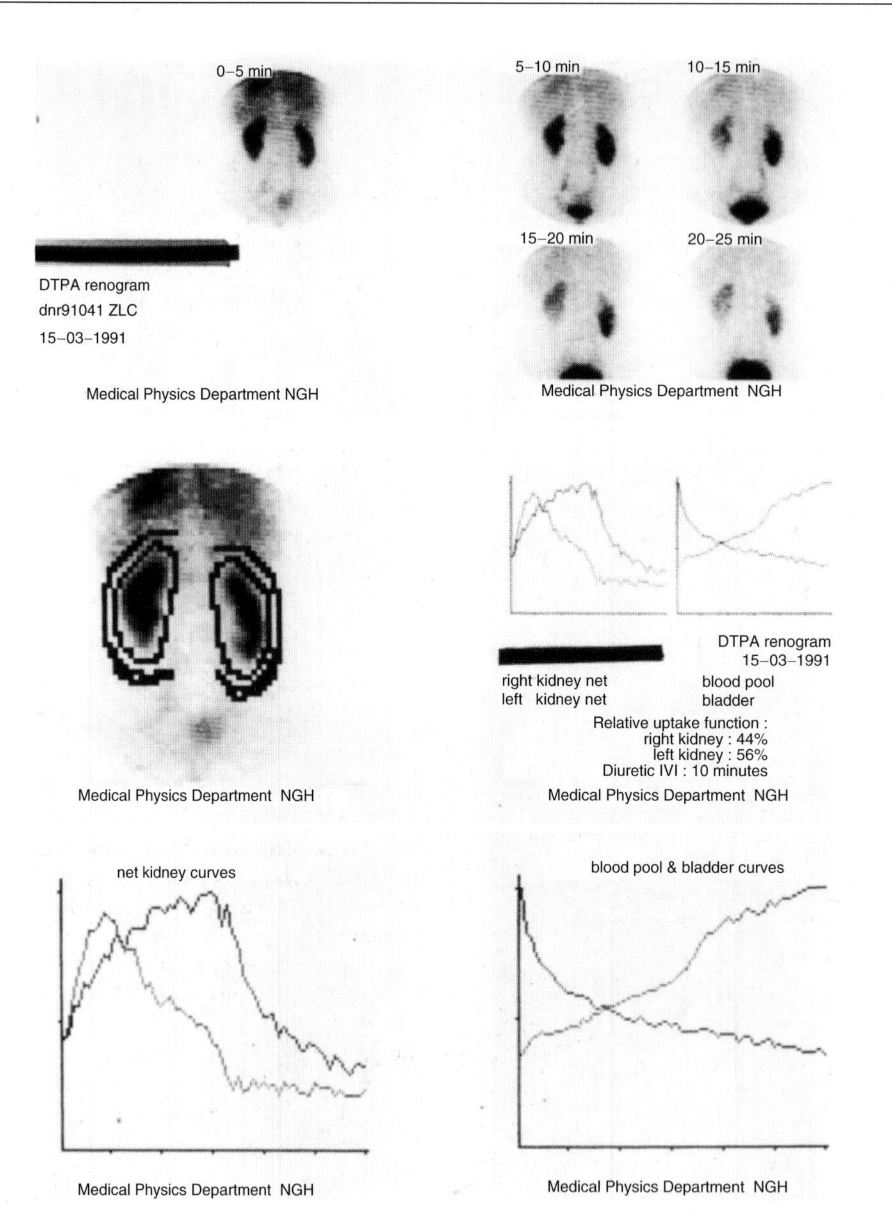

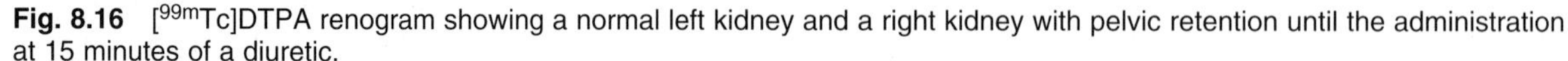

Fig. 8.16 [^{99m}Tc]DTPA renogram showing a normal left kidney and a right kidney with pelvic retention until the administration at 15 minutes of a diuretic.

Adrenal medulla tumours

Tumours arising from this tissue are neuroblastomas of childhood, phaeochromocytomas and paraganglionomas of adults (some regard phaeochromocytomas as secretory and paraganglionomas as non-secretory, while others regard paraganglionomas as a term for all neural crest tumours and phaeochromocytomas as those tumours arising from adrenal glands). Phaeochromocytomas can be sporadic or part of the multiple endocrine neoplasia syndromes types 2a and 2b (see thyroid section above). Normal adrenal medulla tissue and tumours contain neurosecretory granules and mechanisms for uptake, storage, synthesis and reuptake of amine precursors and amines, such as noradrenaline and guanethidine. The specific radiopharmaceutical used is meta-iodobenzyl-guanidine, which is an analogue of noradrenaline (norepinephrine) and guanethidine, labelled with either ^{123}I in children in whom imaging is rarely required beyond 24 hours or ^{131}I in adults, despite the higher radiation dose, because imaging may be required up to 7 days post-administration. Uptake into tumour can be inhibited by many drugs, including tricyclic antidepressants; therefore care must be taken to withdraw any potentially interfering medication well in advance.

Other tumours

Somatostatin receptor imaging is clinically useful in a variety of tumours. Somatostatin is a 14-amino acid peptide found in brain, where it acts as a neurotransmitter, the gastrointestinal tract and the pancreas. Somatostatin receptors, as well as being found in normal pituitary, pancreas and upper gastrointestinal tract from stomach to jejunum, are also found in small cell lung cancer, in tumours of ovary, cervix, endometrium, breast, kidney, larynx, paranasal sinus, salivary gland and some skin tumours, and tumours arising from glial cells in the central nervous system. Octreotide is an eight-residue analogue to which indium-111 is attached via DTPA to form pentetreotide. Sufficient pentetreotide uptake for visualization can occur with many carcinoid tumours, pituitary tumours, gastrointestinal tract endocrine tumours (except insulinomas, of which only about 50% are seen), small cell lung cancer, medullary carcinoma of thyroid, neuroblastoma, phaeochromocytoma, meningioma, Hodgkin's and non-Hodgkin lymphoma. Many of these tumours may be better visualized with CT and MRI but pentetreotide imaging uptake may be used to demonstrate small symptomatic tumours and metastatic spread. Evidence of pentetreotide uptake is a guide for therapy with octreotide, especially with carcinoid tumours, although hepatic metastases are difficult to visualize because of uptake in normal liver.

Somatostatin receptor overexpression has been demonstrated in small cell lung cancer, in the peritumoral veins of a number of human tumours and on some non-small cell lung tumours and cell lines. Therefore physiological imaging of somatostatin receptors makes it possible to diagnose lung tumours. Depreotide is a synthetic peptide that carries a somatostatin-binding domain. Its ability to form complexes with technetium-99m results in higher resolution images and lower cost in comparison to octreotide imaging with ^{111}In-pentetreotide. SPECT images are acquired and a positive study, indicating a high probability of lung neoplasm, has uptake which is abnormally increased compared to surrounding lung tissue. False-positive studies can occur with benign manifestations of previous infection with granuloma-forming organisms such as mycobacteria and histoplasmosis.

It is possible to produce monoclonal antibodies targeted against specific tumour types. The antibodies can be labelled with iodine-131, technetium-99m or indium-111. When injected into the patient the radiolabelled antibodies will seek out the tumour-associated antigens. However, the absolute uptake in the tumour is normally less than 1% and image quality is rather poor. Work in this field to refine the specificity of the antibodies continues.

Table 8.3 gives a list of some commonly used radiopharmaceuticals and includes notes on their more important uses, details of the maximum recommended activity, the absorbed dose to the critical organ and the effective dose equivalent. Table 8.4 gives comparative examples of effective dose equivalent from some common radiopharmaceutical investigations and common radiology investigations.

PET imaging of tumours

There are many established and more emerging roles for PET in oncology. Currently, ^{18}F-fluorodeoxyglucose (^{18}FDG) is the most widely used oncology tracer. Because glucose hypermetabolism has been linked with tumour aggressiveness, the primary role of ^{18}FDG in oncolgy has been in the diagnosis and grading of tumours. The ability to determine regions of hypermetabolism with ^{18}FDG has led to its use in differentiating active tumour from oedema and necrosis. This has led to improvements in the diagnostic yield of biopsies. In addition to fluorine-labelled compounds, several ^{11}C-based tracers have been used at facilities adjacent to cyclotrons. ^{11}C-methionine has been used to study protein synthesis and transport across the blood–brain barrier. It has been found to be superior to ^{18}FDG for differentiating tumour from necrotic tissue, especially in lower-grade, less metabolic tumours. Similar applications are being sought for ^{11}C-tyrosine and ^{11}C-thymidine.

There are generic ways in which PET contributes to the management of oncology patients, namely:

- distinguishing benign from malignant disease, e.g. lung nodules, brain lesions
- establishing the grade of malignancy, e.g. brain tumours, soft tissue masses
- establishing the stage of malignant disease, e.g. lung cancer, lymphoma
- establishing whether there is residual or recurrent disease, e.g. lymphoma, teratoma, seminoma

Table 8.3 Examples of some radiopharmaceuticals in common use

Radionuclide	Chemical form	Clinical use	Max. activity (MBq)	Half-life	Route	Critical organ	Absorbed dose (mGy MBq^{-1})	Effective dose equivalent (mSv MBq^{-1})
Chromium-51	Sodium chromate solution	Labelling red blood cells for RBC volume, survival and splenic sequestration	4.0	27.8 days	i.v.	Spleen	1.6	0.26
Cobalt-57 Cobalt-58	Cyanocobalamin capsules and solution	Diagnosis of pernicious anaemia and vitamin B_{12} malabsorption	0.04	270 days 71 days	p.o.	Liver	24 36	2.7 5.1
Gallium-67	Gallium citrate	Tumour imaging; localisation of inflammatory lesions	150	78.3 h	i.v.	Bone surfaces	0.59	0.12
Indium-111	Indium oxine-labelled white cells	Infection, abscess imaging	40	2.8 days	i.v.	Spleen	5.5	0.59
Iodine-123	Sodium iodide capsules and solution	Diagnosis of thyroid function; thyroid imaging	20	13.2 h	p.o.	Thyroid	0.9	0.15
Iodine-125	Human serum albumin	Plasma volume determination	0.2	60 days	i.v.	Heart	0.69	0.34
Iodine-131	Sodium iodide capsules and solution	Diagnosis of thyroid function	0.2	8.1 days	p.o.	Thyroid	500 (35% uptake)	15
		Treatment of hyperthyroidism	600		p.o.	Thyroid	790 (55% uptake)	
		Treatment of thyroid carcinoma and metastases	8000		p.o.			24
Iron-59	Ferrous citrate	Ferrokinetic studies of iron metabolism	0.4	44.6 days	i.v.	Heart	32	13
Krypton-81m	Gas	Pulmonary ventilation	3600	13 s	Inhalation	Lungs	0.0002	0.00003
Phosphorus-32	Sodium phosphate	Treatment of polycythaemia vera	300	14.3 days	i.v.	Bone surfaces	11	2.2
Selenium-75	Selenomethyl	Adrenal imaging	8	119.8 days	i.v.	Adrenals	5.1	1.7
Technetium-99m	Sodium pertechnetate	Brain imaging	500	6 h	i.v.	GI tract	0.062	0.013
		Thyroid imaging	80		i.v.			
		Diagnosis of Mechel's diverticulum	400		i.v.			
Technetium-99m	Albumin aggregated (MAA) Albumin microspheres (HAM)	Lung perfusion imaging	100		i.v.	Lungs	0.067	0.012

Technetium-99m	Etefenin (EHIDA) injection	Hepatobiliary imaging	150		i.v.	Gall bladder	0.11	0.024
Technetium-99m	Exametazime	Region cerebral blood flow	500		i.v.	Lacrimal	0.068	0.018
	HM-PAO	Leucocyte labelling	200		i.v.	Spleen	0.157	0.016
Technetium-99m	Glucoheptonate	Brain imaging	500		i.v.	Bladder wall	0.056	0.009
		Kidney imaging	300		i.v.			
Technetium-99m	Medronate (MDP) injection	Bone imaging	600		i.v.	Bone surfaces	0.063	0.008
Technetium-99m	Pentetate (DTPA)	Brain imaging	500		i.v.	Bladder wall (4 h void)	0.08	0.063
		Kidney imaging, renograms	300		i.v.		0.047	0.007
		Lung ventilation imaging	80		Aerosol inhalation			
Technetium-99m	Stannous fluoride	Heart blood pool (Tc-RBC)	800		i.v.	Heart	0.023	0.0085
Technetium-99m	Succimer (DMSA)	Kidney imaging	80		i.v.	Kidneys	0.17	0.016
Thallium-201	Thallous chloride	Myocardial perfusion imaging	80	73.1 h	i.v.	Kidneys	0.54	0.23
Xenon-133	Gas	Pulmonary ventilation imaging, cerebral blood flow	40	5.25 days	Inhalation	Lung	0.0011	0.0008

Table 8.4 Effective dose equivalent (EDE) from some common investigations using (1) radiopharmaceuticals and (2) radiology (data extracted from ARSAC (1998) and Shrimpton et al (1986))

Radiopharmaceutical	Activity (MBq)	EDE (mSv)	Radiological examination	EDE per examination (mSv)
[^{99m}Tc]pertechnetate	500	7	Chest	0.05
[^{99m}Tc]MAA	80	1	Abdomen	1.4
[^{99m}Tc]phosphonate	600	5	Pelvis	1.2
[^{57}Co]vitamin B_{12}	0.04	0.2	Barium meal	3.8
[^{131}I]iodide	0.2	3	Barium enema	7.7
[^{201}Tl]thallous ion	80	25		
[^{67}Ga]gallium citrate	150	15		

- identifying the site of disease in the face of rising tumour markers, e.g. colorectal cancer, germ cell tumours
- establishing the response to therapy by imaging before, during and after therapy
- identifying the primary site of tumour for biopsy or therapeutic purposes, e.g. in paraneoplastic syndromes from an unknown primary tumour.

Sites of primary and secondary tumour in which PET can have a role in patient management include central nervous system tumours, head and neck tumours, lung cancer, Hodgkin's and non-Hodgkin lymphoma, malignant melanoma, breast cancer, cancers of oesophagus, pancreas and large bowel, primary and secondary liver tumours, tumours of adrenal glands, testicular and ovarian cancer.

Radiation dose and critical organs

The localisation of the isotope material even temporarily in some organ or tissue means that the absorbed dose of ionising radiation which a patient receives following the administration of a radioactive material is rarely uniform. In any isotope test it is always necessary to ensure that the whole body and each organ in the body receives an acceptably low dose. Some knowledge of the metabolic processes involved is essential in calculating the doses received by the patient in these procedures. It is possible that, because of retention of the isotope in one particular organ, that organ may receive a dose approaching the reasonable limit for that organ before the limit for the whole body is reached. The organ which is most vulnerable in this sense is called the *critical organ* and calculations of absorbed dose involved must take account of the possible concentration of the isotope in the critical organ.

The definitions for absorbed dose, dose equivalent and effective dose equivalent are given in Chapters 5 and 6. Absorbed dose, measured in grays, is the quantity of energy imparted by ionising radiation to a unit mass of tissue. The dose equivalent, measured in sieverts, is equal to the absorbed dose multiplied by a factor that takes into account the way in which different radiations deposit their energy in tissue. The effective dose equivalent, also measured in sieverts, is the sum of the products of the dose equivalent to various organs and a risk weighting factor for each organ. The effective dose equivalent is very important in nuclear medicine procedures as it allows for a variety of non-uniform distributions of dose equivalents in the body to be expressed as a single number representing the risk to health.

Dosimetry

The radiation dose to a patient resulting from the administration of a radiopharmaceutical depends on the amount of energy deposited by the radiation in the patient. When a radionuclide is absorbed in a local site in the body it disappears from that site roughly exponentially, with an effective half-life determined by the physical decay and the metabolic process which may remove it from the site. The energy of the beta particles which it emits is absorbed almost entirely in the immediate vicinity of the active material. However, the gamma rays emitted by the active material will not be absorbed appreciably in the immediate vicinity. In general, depending upon the energy of the photons, a proportion will be absorbed elsewhere in the body, but most will escape altogether from the body. The photons that are absorbed will produce secondary electrons by the processes, described further in Chapter 4.

Calculation of the dose distribution of a radiopharmaceutical requires a knowledge of the *cumulative activity*, the *equilibrium dose constant*, and the *absorbed fraction*. Organs are divided into *source* organs, in which activity is accumulated and which therefore become a radiation source and irradiate other organs, and *target* organs which are the organs for which the dose is being calculated.

The cumulative activity, A_c, measured in kBq h, in each organ depends upon the percentage uptake in the organ, the effective half-life and the administered activity (i.e. the time integral activity). The equilibrium dose rate, Δ, measured in joules per becquerel per second or kg Gy kBq^{-1} h^{-1}, depends only on the radionuclide used and for gamma rays is analogous to the specific gamma ray constant. It represents the average amount of energy, either beta or gamma, emitted per disintegration. The absorbed fraction, ø, (no units), depends on the organs involved, their sizes and relative distances apart. The absorbed dose, D, is given by

$$D = \frac{\Delta \times ø}{m} \times A_c$$

where m is the mass, in kg, of the organ whose absorbed dose is being measured. The contribution to the absorbed dose from the beta particles and the gamma rays must be calculated separately. If mathematical modelling is used, values for the masses and separating distances of the organs can be assumed and Δ and ø can be used to draw up a table of the dose from one organ to any other organ for unit deposited radioactivity, of a given radionuclide, in unit time. These are known as S values. Tables of Δ, ø, and S can be found in the publications of the Medical Internal Radiation Dose Committee (MIRD), the International Commission on Radiation Units and Measurements (ICRU 1979) and the International Commission on Radiological Protection (Publication 53) (ICRP 1987).

Let us consider the absorbed dose to the thyroid gland from an administered dose of 200 kBq of iodine-131, where the uptake is 35% and the mass of the gland is 20 g. The equilibrium dose rate for the beta particles is 0.110×10^{-6} kg Gy kBq^{-1} h^{-1} and for the penetrating radiations 0.217×10^{-6}. In this example the source and target organ are one and the same so the absorbed fraction for the beta particles will be 1; the absorbed fraction for the penetrating radiations is 0.03.

If we assume that none of the radioiodine leaves the thyroid gland then the effective half-life equals the physical half-life of 8.1 days (194.4 h) and the mean life (p. 25) will be 1.44×194.4 h. The cumulated activity, A_c, will therefore be:

$$200 \times 1.44 \times 194.4 \times 0.35 = 1.964 \times 10^4 \text{ kBq h}$$

From the above equation the absorbed dose can be calculated as follows.

The absorbed dose from the beta particles will be:

$$\frac{0.110 \times 10^{-6} \times 1}{0.02} \times 1.964 \times 10^4 = 0.108 \text{ Gy}$$

the absorbed dose from the gamma rays will be:

$$\frac{0.217 \times 10^{-6} \times 0.03}{0.02} \times 1.964 \times 10^4 = 0.006 \text{ Gy}$$

and hence the total dose to the thyroid gland is 0.114 Gy.

The effective dose equivalent can also be calculated. Once the cumulated activity in the source organ is known, then the dose to other target organs can be calculated by use of the S value tables. Each target organ dose can then be weighted according to the risk factor for that organ. The sum of the weighted doses in the target organs gives us the effective dose equivalent. For the 200 kBq of iodine-131 used in the example above the effective dose equivalent is 3 mSv.

RADIATION PROTECTION IN NUCLEAR MEDICINE

There is a great deal of legislation governing the use of radioactive materials, and the protection of persons against ionising radiations arising from their medical use. In general, in the following pages the United Kingdom regulations have been quoted. However, these are based on the Recommendations of the International Commission on Radiological Protection (ICRP 1977a, 1977b and 1982), the International Atomic Energy Agency Regulations (IAEA 1985, 1986), and the relevant Directives of the Council of the European Communities. (Regulatory documents are listed in Notes for Guidance on the Clinical Administration of Radiopharmaceuticals and Use of Sealed Radioactive Sources 1998 HMSO, London.)

Supply of unsealed sources

The use of radionuclides in liquid form for either therapy or diagnosis involves a number of procedures which are different from those in other hospital departments, and which arise from the radioactivity of the material used. Arrangements must be established for the regular receipt of supplies of radiopharmaceuticals. Radioactive materials with a long physical half-life, such as chromium-51 ($T_{½} = 27.8$ days), may be retained in the hospital radiopharmacy and dispensed as required. For other radioisotopes with a shorter half-life, such as thallium-201 ($T_{½} = 73.1$ h), orders must be placed with a commercial supplier in sufficient time to guarantee delivery when they are required. A third group of radioisotopes consists of those in which the half-life is so short that they are generally only available by production in the hospital from relatively longer-lived generator columns (p. 35) The most common example is technetium-99m ($T_{½} = 6$ h) produced from a molybdenum-99 column ($T_{½} = 67$ h). Weekly purchase of a new generator column is necessary in this case.

Transport

A second consideration regarding supplies of radioactive materials is that they must be transported and stored under conditions such that they are secure and that the leakage radiation from the container presents no hazard either to any worker or to a member of the general public. The transport of a pure beta emitter such as phosphorus-32 is generally an easy matter, but for isotopes with penetrating gamma radiation such as sodium-24 the protection during transit is more difficult and involves large and heavy shielded containers.

The transport of radioactive materials falls into two categories: transport outside the hospital by means of road, sea and air; and transport and movement within the hospital. There are national and international regulations governing the transport of radioactive materials which take care of the leakage of ionising radiation from the intact container and also prescribe packaging methods so that, in the event of an accident, leakage of the contents, and therefore the spread of contamination, are most unlikely. The international regulations are the IAEA Regulations for the Safe Transport of Radioactive Material (IAEA, Vienna 1990, Safety Series No 6, ISBN 92–0–123890–8). These regulations have been enacted as The Radioactive Material (Road Transport) (Great Britain) Regulations 1996.

Packaging

Three types of packaging are defined by the IAEA: *excepted*, *type A* and *type B*. Table 8.5 lists the maximum activities of radionuclides in common hospital use which may be transported with type A packaging. It can be seen that, in general, type A packaging is adequate for hospital users of unsealed radionuclides. All packaging is designed to withstand minor accidents.

Table 8.5 The maximum activities, for various radionuclides, which may be transported with type A packaging

Radionuclide	Max. activity (TBq)
^{198}Au	0.5
^{51}Cr	30
^{57}Ga	6
^{131}I	0.5
^{99}Mo	0.5
^{24}Na	0.2
^{32}P	0.3
^{201}T1	10
^{90}Y	0.2

Labelling

An internationally recognised design of warning label, known as white and yellow labels, specifying a transport category between I and III must be affixed to the package. The label must identify the contents of the package, the activity of the radionuclide and, by use of the category rating and the transport index, give an indication of radiation dose rate on the external surface of the package and at 1 m from it. The *transport index* is defined as this latter quantity measured in mSv h^{-1} multiplied by 100. Table 8.6 lists the surface dose rate for each transport category and the transport index.

A package may contain so little radioactive material or the material may be in such a dilute form that the risk of contamination is negligible. In this case, provided the surface dose rate is less than 5 μSv h^{-1} the package can be excepted from most of the packaging and labelling requirements. For example, 800 MBq of technetium-99m or 50 MBq of iodine-131 per package could be transported as excepted packages. Nevertheless the contents of the package must be described in the accompanying paperwork.

Movement of radioactive sources within the hospital are not subject to the various transport regulations. However, these movements are subject in the UK to the Ionising Radiation Regulations 1999 (HSE, 1999, Reg. 29). The requirements for moving radioactive substances include ensuring that the substance is kept in a suitable receptacle and that it is suitably labelled. General principles for internal movement include:

Table 8.6 The surface dose rate for each transport category

Category	Max. surface dose rate	Max. transport index
I (white)	< 5 μSv h^{-1}	—
II (yellow)	< 500 μSv h^{-1}	1.0
III (yellow)	< 2 mSv h^{-1}	10.0

1. The material must be securely contained in a double container. The outer container should be rigid and capable of leakage containment should the inner container break.

2. Both inner and outer containers must be clearly labelled with the radionuclide, its chemical form and the activity at a specified time.

3. The radioactive material must not be left unattended during transit.

4. Adequate shielding must be provided to protect the person carrying or accompanying the radionuclide.

Custody and storage

On arrival at the hospital a suitable place for the receipt of the containers must be arranged and the sources themselves must be placed when unloaded in a suitable shielded store. Small cupboards with 1–2″ (25–50 mm) of lead wall are convenient for many of these sources. However, to reduce the weight of lead it is often preferred to store individual vials in lead pots, where the thickness of the lead is appropriate for the energy and activity of the particular radionuclide. Any container holding a radionuclide should be marked with the radiation symbol.

Regulations 28 and 29 of the IRR-99 relate to accounting for and keeping of radioactive substances. Accounting procedures are essential to ensure that all radioactive sources are traceable and that losses of significant quantities are identified as quickly as possible. The records to be kept of each substance should include:

- A means of identification of the radionuclide by name and by batch
- The date of receipt
- The activity of the radionuclide at a specified time and date
- Any activity used and date and time of use
- The location of storage
- The date and manner of disposal.

These records must be kept for at least 2 years from the date of disposal. Inevitably some radionuclides will have undergone significant radioactive decay before disposal and this must be allowed for in the accounting procedure.

Design of facilities

The facilities in a nuclear medicine department are designed to minimise the hazard from: (1) external radiation arising from the radioactive materials or from the patient following injection of a radiopharmaceutical; (2) surface contamination; and (3) ingestion, inhalation, or skin absorption of a radioactive material.

Shielding from gamma radiation is in general a problem very similar to that encountered in dealing with small sealed radioactive sources. The gamma ray exposure rates normally met are, however, smaller than when working with sealed sources so that quite simple shielding arrangements, such as small lead bench shields, are adequate.

All surfaces should be smooth and impervious, with the main aim being to prevent retention of surface contamination in the event of a spill. Bench tops and floors are always covered with a continuous non-absorbent surface such as plastic laminate and seam-welded linoleum. Walls and ceilings are covered with good-quality gloss paint which can be cleaned easily. Covings should be used where the walls meet floor and ceiling and at the rear of laboratory benches.

Hand-washing facilities, with elbow- or foot-operated taps, must be provided in rooms where unsealed radioactive sources are handled. Drainage from sinks and wash basins should pass directly to a main sewer in order to avoid accumulation of radioactive waste and to allow rapid dilution by non-active waste.

Some radioactive materials may have to be handled in conditions under which active products may escape into the atmosphere as volatile products from the surface of a solution, as dust from dry preparations or as gaseous products. To prevent ingestion or inhalation from any of these products, work of this type must be conducted in a fume cupboard. To give adequate containment of escaping products the fume cupboard requires an exhaust system which provides an air flow inwards across the whole of the open working window at a rate of at least 0.5 metres per second.

Controlled and supervised areas

Different areas within the nuclear medicine department may be classified as *controlled* or *supervised* (p. 77). The designation is based on an assessment of the potential radiation dose which may be received by those who enter the area, which may take into account the occupancy factor as well as other factors such as dose rate and surface and airborne contamination levels. Entrances to all rooms in which radioactivity is used must display appropriate warning signs bearing the international radiation warning symbol (trefoil, see Plate 1.3) and an indication of the classification of the area and the nature of the hazard, e.g. 'Supervised area. Unsealed Radioactive Sources'.

Examples of controlled areas might be the radiopharmacy or the room of a patient undergoing iodine-131 thyroid ablation therapy. A waiting room may be designated as a controlled area. Gamma camera rooms may be designated as either a supervised or a controlled area depending on the dose rate, contamination levels and occupancy. In general, radioisotope laboratories in which only radioactive samples are analysed will be designated as a supervised area.

Monitoring

Suitable monitoring equipment must be available to sensitively detect all radionuclides in use in the department. The calibration of such monitors should be traceable to national standards.

The IRR-99 requires that levels of ionising radiation are adequately monitored for any area where unsealed radioactive materials are in use or stored. Monitoring is an important means of ascertaining the efficacy of techniques in use and in restricting exposure. Contamination monitors must be checked regularly and must be calibrated annually. Where there is high background count rate caused by the presence of nearby radioactive sources, the contamination of work surfaces may be established by wipe testing.

Hands, clothing and work surfaces should be monitored at the end of each working period and the results recorded. If the monitoring shows levels of contamination greater than those given in Table 8.7 then decontamination procedures should be followed.

Safe administration

The administration of radionuclides for diagnostic or therapeutic purposes requires great care, to ensure that the patient receives the correct isotope and dose, any possible spillage is contained, and that exposure to personnel is kept to a minimum. All staff involved in this type of work must receive appropriate training (under the Ionising Radiation (Medical Exposure) Regulations HSE, 2000).

Staff administering radiopharmaceuticals will be exposed to radiation during the administration and when it is inside the patient. To minimise the risk of ingestion, eating, drinking, smoking and the application of cosmetics or contact lenses are strictly forbidden in the presence of radioactive materials. Similarly, to prevent personal contamination, staff should wear protective clothing such as disposable gloves, a lab coat or overall buttoned up, and possibly a plastic apron, so that any spilt radioactive solution will not contact the skin. The hands should always be washed after handling radioactive materials. Examples of potential ingestion and contamination hazards to staff from diagnostic and therapeutic procedures are found in ventilation lung scanning where radioactive gases or aerosols may leak into the air and subsequently be inhaled, and in the oral administration of liquid iodine-131 where a risk of contamination exists. The availability of therapeutic doses of iodine-131 in capsule form has greatly reduced this latter risk, as well as being a simpler and quicker method of administration.

There are three principal factors which staff can use to help reduce their external radiation exposure. These are distance (inverse square law), shielding and time. Good radionuclide working practice includes the use of long-handled forceps, syringe shields, protective screens and swift yet careful working practices commensurate with the adequate and safe administration of the radionuclide (p. 76).

The majority of radiopharmaceuticals are administered by intravenous injection. Equipment required for this purpose includes a shielded container in which the radiopharmaceutical can be transferred from the dispensary to the injection area, a tray over which any transfer of radioactive solutions can take place, and an impermeable shielded receptacle for discarded materials.

For sources to be dispensed or administered using a syringe, a syringe shield made of a suitable shielding material with a window in the side so that the contents are visible can be fitted over the barrel of the syringe

Table 8.7 Maximum permissible contamination levels

Category	Surface	Level of contamination that should not be exceeded (Bq cm^{-2})		
		Class III	Class IV	Class V
B	Surfaces in controlled areas including any equipment therein	30	300	3000
C	Surfaces of the body	3	30	300
D	Supervised and public areas, clothing, hospital bedding	3	30	300

Classification of radionuclides in common use in hospitals (for surface contamination purposes only): class III, ^{32}P, ^{111}In, ^{59}Fe, ^{90}Y, ^{131}I; class IV, ^{123}I, ^{125}I, ^{99m}Tc, ^{67}Ga, ^{201}Tl; class V, ^{51}Cr

(Fig. 8.17). The use of syringe shields must be considered in order to minimise the exposure to the fingers and hands. These shields, which are designed to absorb the majority of the beta particles, as well as to attenuate the gamma ray photons, are typically made of metals with high atomic number such as tungsten, or thick cylinders of transparent Perspex. There are, however, further considerations in the use of each type. Metallic syringe shields are used for the majority of radionuclides, but they are not ideal for pure beta emitters as bremsstrahlung radiation can contribute significantly to the finger and hand dose. Perspex syringe shields, which can be 7–15 mm in thickness, are used for this purpose.

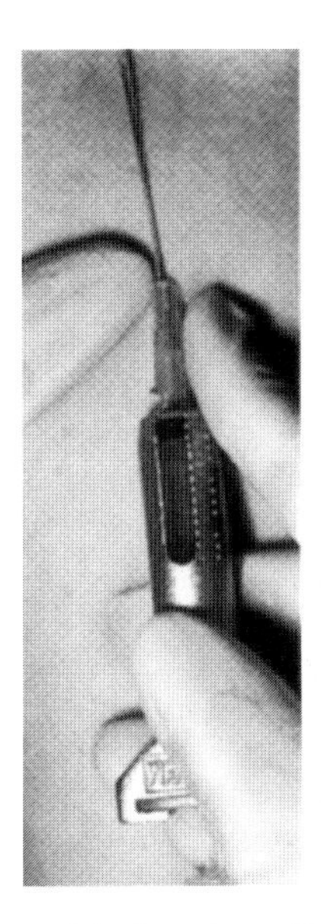

Fig. 8.17 Intravenous injection of a radioactive material using a shielded syringe.

Safety of the patient

The administration of any radioactive material to the patient has an associated risk factor. Any member of staff concerned with carrying out nuclear medicine procedures on patients has a responsibility to ensure that the techniques used are appropriate for their purpose, and that the radiation dose to the patient is no higher than is absolutely necessary to achieve this purpose and that the benefits of carrying out the test outweigh the risks. Effective dose equivalents for some common nuclear medicine procedures, together with average values for some common radiographic procedures, are given in Table 8.4. It is essential that each investigation is justified on clinical grounds and that there is no lower-risk alternative.

SECTION 3

Physics of radiotherapy

SECTION CONTENTS

CHAPTER CONTENTS

9

Kilovoltage beam generators

Keith Bomford

INTRODUCTION

The generators and control circuits described in this chapter are used over the range of X-ray energies from 8–300 kV, covering the ranges commonly known as:

- Very low-energy X- (or Grenz) rays: 0.035–1.0 mm Al HVL, 8–50 kV
- Low-energy (or superficial) X-rays: 1.0–8.0 mm Al HVL, 50–160 kV
- Medium-energy (or orthovoltage) X-rays: 0.5–4.0 mm Cu HVL, 160–300 kV.

The need for X-ray energies greater than this has been recognised for many years, but other techniques have to be used to generate megavoltage radiations and are the subject of the next chapter. X-ray energies between 500 and 1000 kV are of no value in radiotherapy for reasons to be explained in Chapter 12, and 300–500 kV are rare.

X-RAY TUBE INSERT

We have seen that X-rays are produced whenever an electron stream travelling at high speed is brought to rest in a solid target. To produce an X-ray beam it is necessary to have an evacuated tube in which the electron stream can be produced and accelerated on to a suitable target by a voltage generator. Thus the basic components of an X-ray set are :

- an evacuated tube
- an electron stream
- a target, and
- a voltage generator.

The X-ray tube insert is a highly evacuated envelope containing two electrodes and, as such, its electrical behaviour is the same as that of a diode valve (p. 6). In construction, however, there are important differences.

The accelerating voltage used to generate X-rays may be up to 500 kV and, therefore, great care has to be taken to electrically insulate the anode from the cathode. The two electrodes may be sealed into a re-entrant glass envelope—re-entrant to maximize the insulation path—enclosed in a bath of insulating oil. In the metal–ceramic insert, the electrodes are supported within the metal housing using ceramic insulators and the insulating oil bath may be replaced by epoxy resin—oil is still used as a coolant. In both the glass and metal–ceramic inserts, the electrodes are rounded and highly polished to avoid sharp corners because the intense electrostatic field created at any rough edges would give rise to internal sparking and electrical breakdown.

The electron stream is produced by thermionic emission from a heated tungsten filament (the cathode). The filament is a helix of tungsten wire at the centre of a semi-cylindrical focusing cup (Fig. 9.1). This cup is maintained at the lower potential of the filament and so focuses the electrons on to the X-ray target (anode). As in the case of the thermionic diode under saturation conditions, the number of electrons emitted is determined by, and therefore controlled by, the temperature of the filament and increases rapidly with that temperature. The filament of an X-ray tube is heated using a highly stabilised circuit, and the X-ray tube current is controlled by varying the current through the filament (Fig. 9.2).

So far the word *target* and the word *anode* have been used interchangeably, but it is important now to differentiate between the two. The anode is the positive electrode in the X-ray tube and usually made of copper. The target is the piece of tungsten bonded into the surface of the anode (Fig. 9.1). The electrons bombard the tungsten to produce the X-rays. Tungsten is commonly chosen as the target material for its high atomic number ($Z = 74$), which leads to a relatively efficient conversion of electron energy to X-ray energy, and for its high melting point (3387°C), which reduces the chance of melting the target under the intense heat generated. Furthermore, the target material should not evaporate readily when heated in a vacuum since, if it does, it is deposited on the walls causing a breakdown in the electrical insulation of the tube. In the hooded anode, this deposition is on the hood and rendered harmless.

Target angle and heel effect

It has been seen in Chapter 2 that kilovoltage X-rays are produced in a *reflection* target and the useful beam is considered to be at right angles to the electron stream. In this context the word *reflection* is used to describe the fact that the useful X-rays are emitted from the surface bombarded by the electrons; the laws of optics do not apply. The target angle is the angle between the axis of the X-ray beam and the face of the target (Fig. 9.3). The effect of this angle is threefold. The thin target theory suggests that although the (lower-energy) X-rays are produced predominantly in the direction at right angles to the electron beam (Fig. 2.9), closer examination shows that the X-ray intensity is somewhat greater at angles of less than 90° than at angles of greater than 90° to the direction of the electrons. In order therefore to achieve a greater degree of symmetry to the X-ray beam, it is necessary to attenuate the radiation on the anode side of the beam axis to a greater extent than that on the cathode side. Figure 9.3 shows the effective source of X-rays at a point O below the surface of the target and the two X-rays OA and OB. From this simple construction, it can be seen that OB is attenuated by a greater thickness of target material than OA. Since the relative lengths of OA′

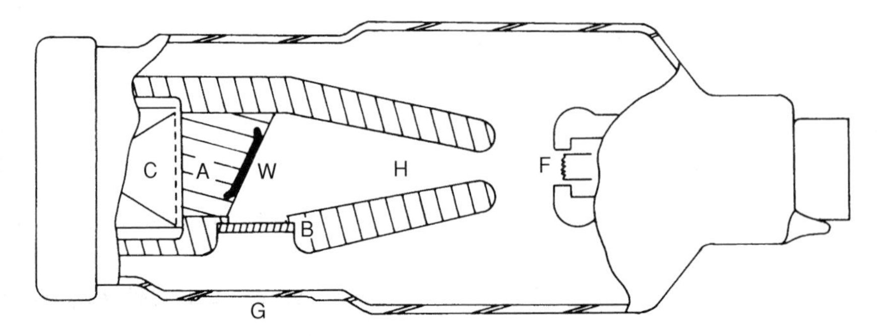

Fig. 9.1 A 250 kV X-ray tube showing the copper anode A, the tungsten target W, the cooling oil spray C, together with the copper anode hood H and the beryllium window B. The filament F and the thin window in the glass G are also shown. (Adapted from a diagram supplied by Elekta Ltd.)

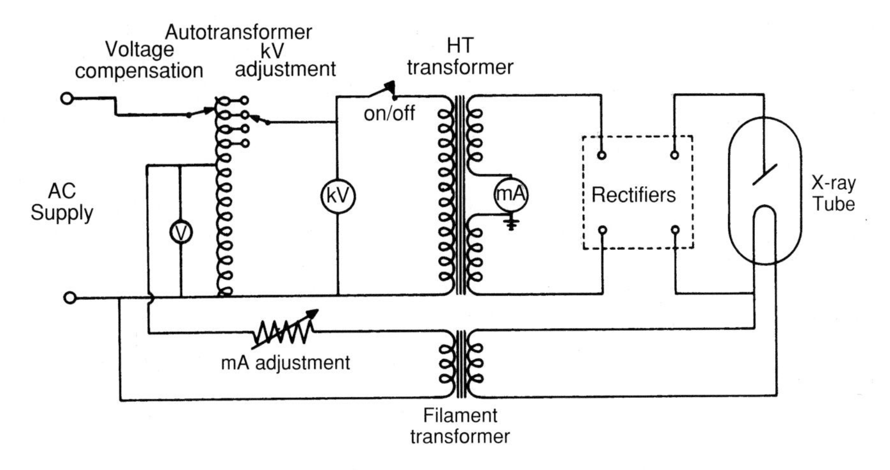

Fig. 9.2 A simplified (single-phase) X-ray generator circuit.

and OB′ are dependent on the target angle, the angle can be chosen to produce a symmetrical beam of radiation by attenuating the more intense beam OB by a suitably greater thickness OB′.

Attenuation is, however, dependent on photon energy as well as atomic number. It follows, therefore, that a particular target angle will only produce a symmetrical beam of radiation for one photon energy, the *design energy*, and to operate the X-ray tube at lower energies will result in an asymmetric beam. The effect of small changes in accelerating voltage may not be clinically significant. At voltages between 200 and 300 kV, the target angle is usually about 30°.

The second important parameter that is dependent on target angle is the overall field size or maximum beam divergence. It can be seen from Figure 9.3 that as the beam divergence increases, the thickness OC′ increases rapidly and the intensity at C falls, producing a beam edge. It follows that the half angle of beam divergence cannot exceed the target angle and, in practice, the useful beam is limited to a few degrees less than the target angle.

Thirdly, the geometry of the target is such that the area of the tungsten bombarded by the electrons is larger than either the cross-sectional area of the electron beam or the area from which the X-rays are seen to emanate (Fig. 9.4). The latter is known as the *effective focal spot size* and decreases with target angle. In diagnostic X-ray tubes, where the effective focal spot size is of greater importance, small target angles are used—15° is common and some are as low as 7°. In therapy, however, large symmetrical beams are of greater importance than the size of the focal spot. In either discipline, the larger the area of target bombarded by electrons the larger the area for the dissipation of heat.

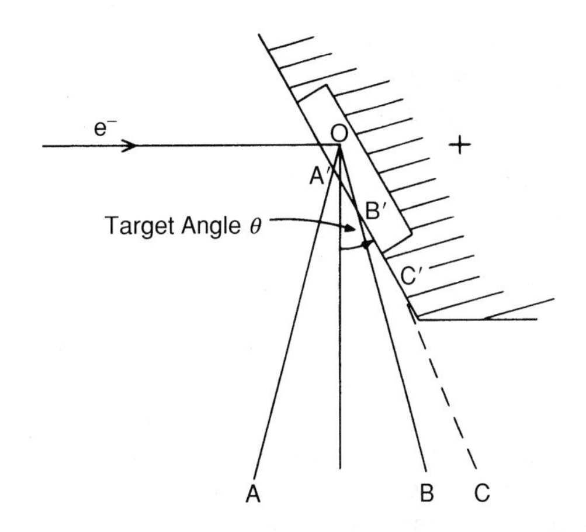

Fig. 9.3 The definition of target angle and the heel effect.

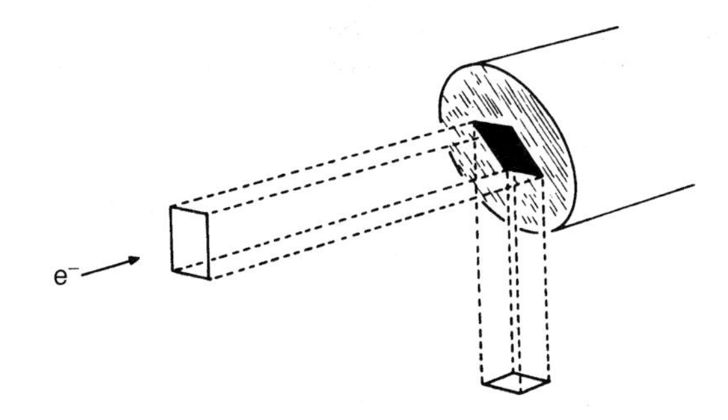

Fig. 9.4 The effective focal spot size.

Cooling the X-ray target

The generation of heat in the target bombarded by high-energy electrons leads to real problems of cooling in kilovoltage X-ray tubes. Only about 1% of the energy dissipated in the target is converted into X-rays and 99% into heat. The method of cooling depends on the design of the target and the voltage at which it operates (Fig. 9.5). X-ray tubes with only one HT cable have a target at earth potential and can be cooled directly by a flow of cold water through the anode behind the target (Fig. 9.5B). Where the target is not at earth potential, as in bipolar tubes, it must be cooled by the forced convection of cool insulating (transformer) oil. The cool oil is sprayed onto the back of the target (Fig. 9.5A) and the oil, now warmed, will flow over the outside of the insert as a part of the electrical insulation around the envelope before passing out of the tube housing to a heat exchanger where the heat is dissipated either into water or into the atmosphere and so to waste. The heat exchanger will be a separate unit, preferably located in an adjacent room, connected to the X-ray tube housing using two flexible oil pipes.

Warming the X-ray target

The need to cool the target is readily understood when the heat dissipation in the target is rated at several kilowatts but there is another adverse effect to be taken into account. If this quantity of heat is dissipated into a cold anode, it can cause mechanical damage. Owing to their different coefficients of expansion, the heated target will expand more than the cold copper anode causing the target to buckle and crack. A severe example of this is shown in Figure 9.6 where the target is seen to be cracked and partially detached from the anode. (This radiograph was taken using an 8 MV linear accelerator and also shows the cooling spray behind the anode and the section through the anode hood.)

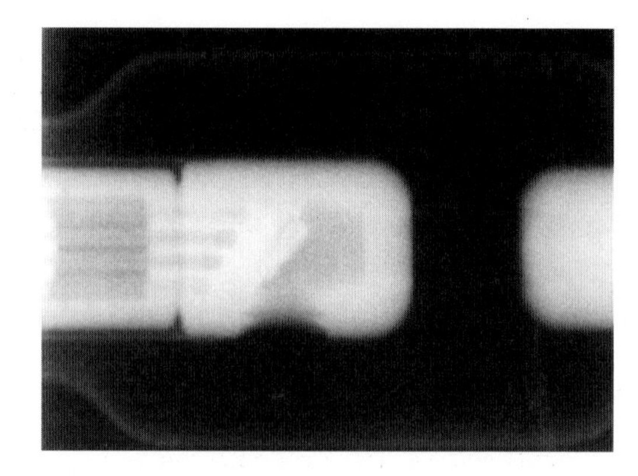

Fig. 9.6 An 8 MV radiograph of a 250 kV tube insert showing the damaged target; the cooling spray on the back of the target and the anode hood are clearly shown.

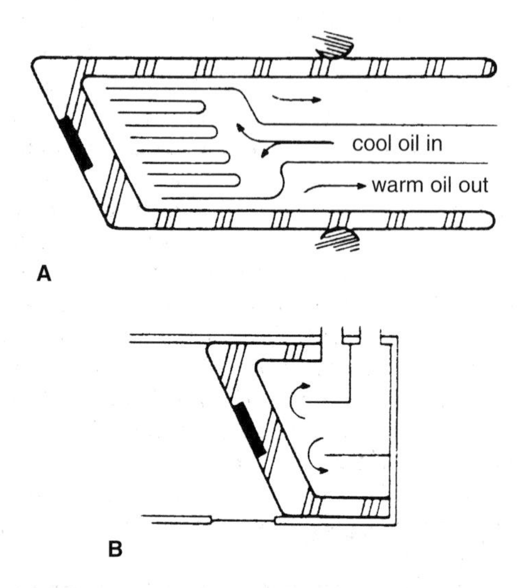

Fig. 9.5 The cooling of X-ray targets using forced convection: **A** with oil and **B** with water.

To overcome this problem of differential heating, it is important to slowly increase the heating of a cold tube insert. This *warm-up* process must be carried out first thing each morning and repeated during the day if the workload is insufficient to keep the tube warm. The manufacturer's guidance should be followed, but in general the warm-up period will be between 10 and 20 min. Microprocessor-controlled generators are protected by a sensor which demands that their automatic warm-up program is followed through whenever the tube is below its operating temperature.

X-RAY TUBE HOUSING

The X-ray tube itself is often referred to as the *insert* and is the principal component contained in the *X-ray head*. The X-ray head is a metal tank in which the insert is rigidly mounted and connected to the high-tension (HT) supply cables. The head contains the insulating transformer oil and two temperature-sensitive devices (thermal cut-outs) which will prevent the use of the tube when its temperature rises above a predetermined level or when the temperature is too low.

Other essential features of the X-ray head include:

- The X-ray window and primary collimator through which the useful X-ray beam emerges

Table 9.1 Permitted leakage radiation from kilovoltage X-ray therapy tube housings

Maximum operating potential	At 1 m from the target	At 5 cm from the housing surface
50–500 kV	10 mGy h^{-1}	300 mGy h^{-1}
Less than 50 kV	—	1 mGy h^{-1}

- Lead protection around the head to reduce the leakage radiation (i.e. unwanted radiation) to a safe level (Table 9.1)
- An assembly on the primary collimator to house and electrically interlock the added filtration (p. 154)
- An ionisation chamber or diode to monitor the output beam dose rate (p. 151)
- An assembly to mount the secondary collimation in the form of an adjustable diaphragm or interchangeable applicators (p. 151)
- At medium energies, means of fixing a back pointer (p. 174).

Tubestand

The X-ray head will be mounted on a gantry or tubestand to enable the beam to be positioned and directed in a way appropriate to the treatment in hand. The gantry may be:

- ceiling mounted to suspend the tube housing from an adjustable column
- wall or floor mounted with the tube housing on the end of a cantilever arm, the latter being raised or lowered on a fixed vertical column, or
- mounted on an isocentric gantry like the linear accelerator (p. 174).

Whatever the type of gantry, the tube housing will need to be adjustable in three orthogonal directions and about two or three axes of rotation, each with a reliable (fail-safe) braking system (i.e. the brakes should be applied when the electrical supply is off). This fail-safe facility is of particular importance where the weight of the tube housing is counterbalanced by a weight or a spring connected by cables.

X-RAY GENERATOR CIRCUITS

A simple X-ray generator circuit is shown in Figure 9.2, and for simplicity, this circuit assumes a single-phase power supply, whereas, in practice, most generators are three-phase (as in Fig. 7.12). The input voltage is fed to the autotransformer via a *voltage compensation* circuit, which may be manually controlled at the control desk or automatically controlled by a servo-system. Compensation is essential because the supply voltages can vary by typically ±6% and the local demand (e.g. by hospital lifts) can also influence the supply to the X-ray unit. In the manual system illustrated in Figure 9.2, the voltmeter V monitors the voltage appearing across a fixed number of turns on the autotransformer coil, and the voltage compensator control is adjusted so that the incoming *volts per turn* on the autotransformer remains constant.

The *autotransformer* is a transformer with only one winding, acting as both primary and secondary, and its function is to provide a secondary voltage only slightly above or below the primary. Having ensured that the volts per turn is correct on the primary, by selecting the correct number of turns from the secondary winding, it is now possible to obtain the required input voltage to the HT transformer. Because the HT transformer has a large but fixed turns ratio, the selector may be calibrated in kilovolts although only a few hundred volts exist at that point in the circuit. The primary circuit carries a high current at the supply voltage to be transformed into a high-voltage, low-current supply for the X-ray tube. If the supply is at the normal frequency (50 Hz in the UK) then a massive soft iron core is required to maximise the flux linkage between the primary and secondary windings, making the transformer more efficient but very heavy.

The safety interlocks built into the X-ray control are in the secondary circuit of the autotransformer and the primary circuit of the HT transformer. They will include the door interlocks, filter interlocks, the treatment timer, over- and under-temperature interlocks, etc. and the X-ray beam on/off switches. Switching an inductive circuit at high power can cause considerable sparking and damage to the contacts. Here the heavy-duty contactor will be immersed in insulating oil and will only energise when the kV is set low, the kV being increased to the required value during the first few seconds of the X-ray exposure (see Timer-error, p. 56). In this case, a kV meter must be connected to the HT primary circuit to ensure the correct value is reached after switch-on.

The filament transformer is situated in the same housing as the HT transformer but for two very different reasons. The tube filament is at the full kilovoltage below earth potential wherever the target is at earth potential or at half the full kilovoltage below for bipolar tubes. Although this step-down transformer is only reducing the supply voltage to a few volts to heat the tube filament (typically 60 watts), the potential difference between the primary and the secondary is considerable requiring complete electrical isolation. Secondly, because the X-ray tube operates under saturation conditions, the tube current is determined by the temperature of the filament, and thermionic emission varies rapidly with small changes in temperature and filament voltage. The filament transformer, therefore, must guarantee a very stable voltage supply to the filament once its primary voltage has been set by the 'mA adjust' control. The filament transformer is therefore more accurately described as a *stabilised isolation transformer*.

HT cables

The HT generator and the X-ray head are separate assemblies connected by *shockproof HT cables*. The cathode cable requires two inner conductors to carry the filament supply and the negative HT connection. Although the anode cable only requires one inner conductor, it is cost-efficient to use a cathode cable with two inner conductors connected in parallel. (An earthed anode tube does not require an anode HT cable.) The inner conductors are individually insulated and surrounded by flexible solid rubber insulation covered by an earthed metal sheath (offering less than 1 ohm m^{-1} resistance) connected to both the tube housing and the transformer tank. Electrical or mechanical failure of the rubber insulation can result in an electrical breakdown between the inner HT conductors and the earthed sheath. Such a breakdown will often be accompanied by the smell of burning and the sound of sparking!

Because of the high voltages involved, all the principal components of an X-ray generator will be bonded to a common electrical *earth reference terminal* by a thick continuous copper wire (in a green/yellow sheath) or a thick bare copper tape to minimise the risk of electric shock to staff or patient. (The sheath of the HT cables must not be relied upon for this purpose.) These earth connections must be clearly labelled and not tampered with under any circumstances.

Greinacher circuit

Although the X-ray tube itself behaves as a rectifier, a circuit without additional rectifiers is of little practical value for two reasons: (1) the X-ray tube has to be made to withstand the full reverse voltage; and (2) the heated anode can become a source of electrons—by thermionic emission—which will bombard and damage the filament during the negative half-cycle of the applied voltage. The HT circuit will therefore usually incorporate a rectifier–capacitor network to produce a nearly constant potential and a constant tube current. Half- and full-wave rectified circuits have been used but the Greinacher circuit is more common.

The Greinacher circuit is illustrated in Figure 9.7. Two series-connected rectifiers, R_1 and R_2, and two series-connected capacitors, C_1 and C_2, are in parallel with the tube. The HT transformer secondary is connected to the midpoints of the two capacitors and of the two rectifiers. During the half cycle, in which end A of the transformer winding is positive, the capacitor C_1 is charged through the rectifier R_1 to the peak voltage of the transformer, while rectifier R_2 is not conducting. During the next half cycle, C_2 is charged to the same potential through R_2. Now C_1 and C_2 are series connected and their potentials are additive, thus, a voltage equal to twice that of the transformer is seen across the X-ray tube. It is sometimes known as a *voltage doubling circuit*. When the secondary voltage on the HT transformer falls, the capacitors discharge through the tube (not through the rectifiers), and providing their capacitance is large and the tube current small, the fall in the voltage applied to the tube will be small. So there will be a *ripple* on the tube voltage (of, say, 5%) but the tube current will remain steady, as the tube continues to operate under saturation conditions.

Cockcroft–Walton circuit

Increasingly, X-ray generators are being fitted with *high-frequency generators*. The frequency of the supply voltage is increased from 50 Hz to typically 15 kHz, thereby reducing the need for the massive soft iron core. The high-frequency Cockcroft–Walton generators are therefore comparatively smaller and lighter in

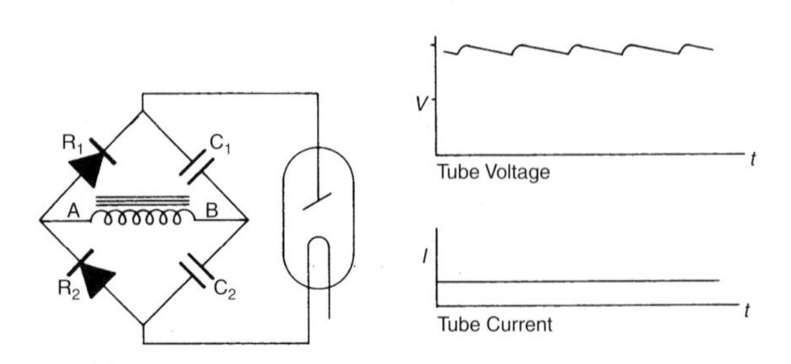

Fig. 9.7 The Greinacher voltage-doubling circuit, the voltage applied to the X-ray tube is twice that of the HT transformer.

weight than the conventional generator (Fig. 9.8A). The HT transformer in the conventional circuit (Fig. 9.2) is replaced by one fed by a 15 kHz power inverter to step the voltage up to about 10 kV (Fig. 9.9A). The transformer output is then fed into a modified Cockcroft–Walton circuit—a stack of rectifiers and capacitors—which multiplies up the voltage and rectifies it to produce a DC voltage with less than 0.2% ripple (Fig. 9.9B). A high degree of stability in output dose rate, of less than 0.1%, is achieved by a servo-system in both the kV and mA control circuits. The multiplication factor is fixed and a variable kilovoltage output is achieved by varying the input to the HT transformer as before. A single unit can cover the low-energy X-ray range. For medium-energy X-ray generators, two identical units may be used back-to-back, i.e. one supplying the negative supply to the filament and one, the positive supply to the anode.

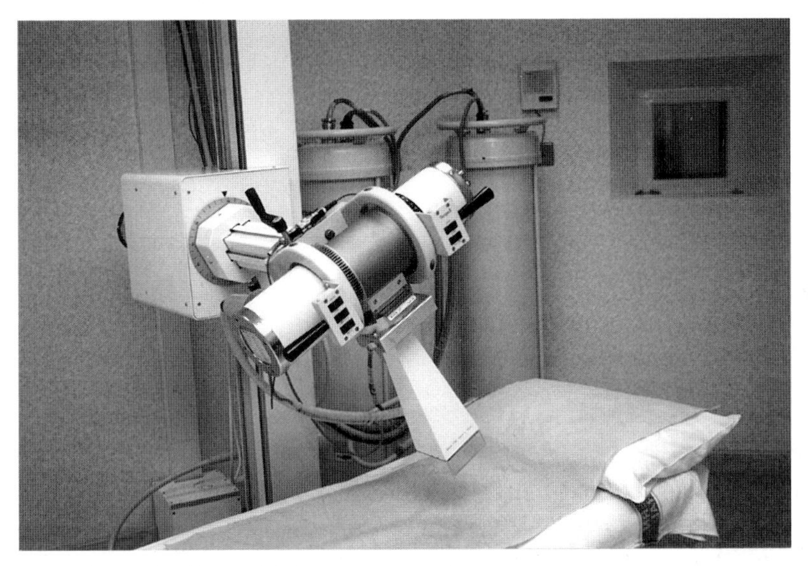

Fig. 9.8A A 300 kV therapy Cockcroft–Walton high-frequency generator.

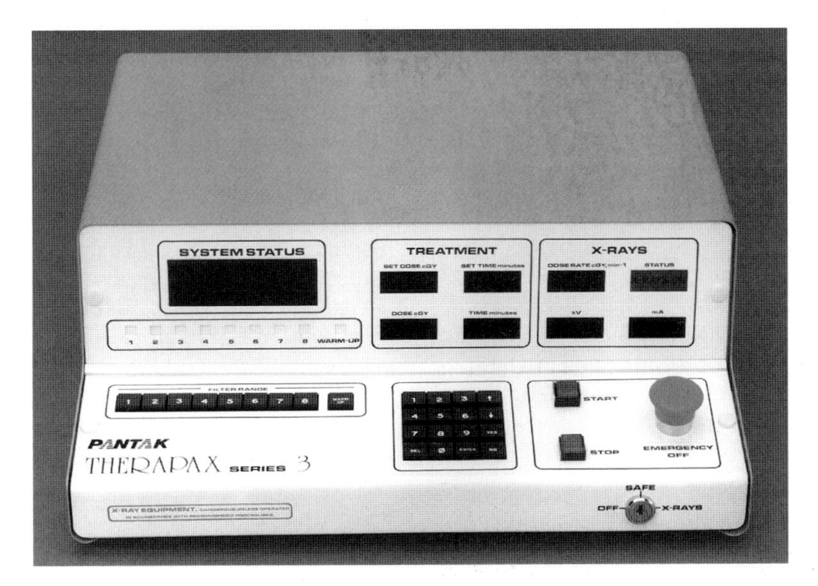

Fig. 9.8B The control desk of the Pantak Therapax. (Courtesy of Pantak Ltd.)

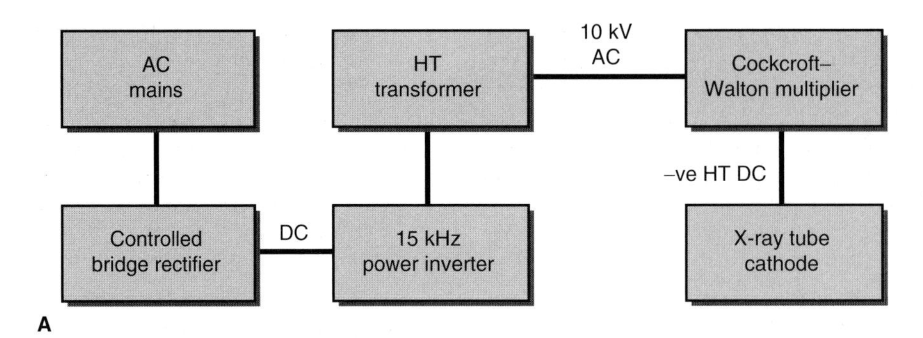

Fig. 9.9A A block diagram of a Cockcroft–Walton generator for an earth anode X-ray tube. (Adapted from a diagram supplied by Pantak Ltd.)

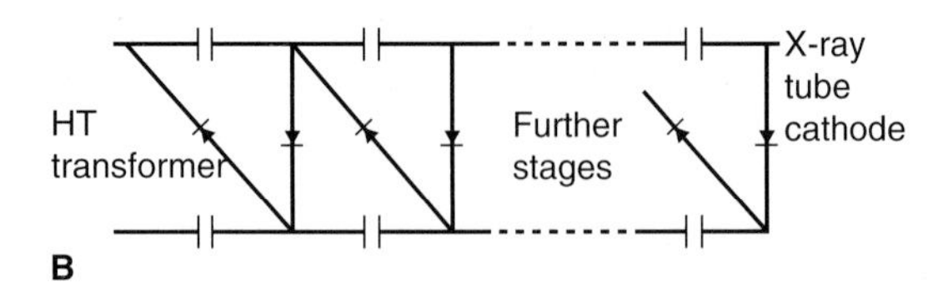

Fig. 9.9B The Cockcroft–Walton multiplier circuit. (Adapted from a diagram supplied by Pantak Ltd.)

The control desk

The control desk may use the traditional moving-coil meters, switches and indicators, a dedicated processor (Fig. 9.8B) or a microprocessor, video display and keyboard. In either case it will feature the following.

Mains voltage compensation

Most units will have an automatically controlled mains voltage compensator, while older units may require manual control to a datum line on a meter.

Kilovoltage control and kV meter

Both the kV control and kV meter will be in the primary circuit of the HT transformer. The operating kV and mA will be interlocked with, and selected by, the added filtration, and on switch-on; the kV will be automatically ramped up to the operating potential during the initial stages of the exposure. The kV, mA and added filter must all be clearly indicated at the control desk throughout the exposure.

Tube current control and mA meter

The operating mA will be automatically selected, again by the added filtration. The mA control is in the primary circuit of the filament transformer. The mA meter will be connected at that point in the HT circuit which is at earth potential—at the positive terminal for an earthed anode circuit or at the midpoint of the secondary winding for a bipolar tube. Where the generator is to be used at more than one beam quality, it is advisable to adjust all the normal operating tube currents to produce approximately the same dose rate at each quality, particularly where treatment exposure is determined from a dose rate–time chart. Rapid fluctuations in the value of mA are the first signs of an HT breakdown either in the tube insert or the HT cable.

X-ray on/off switch

While there may be many means by which the beam can be switched off (e.g. by opening the treatment room door) there must be only one beam-on control switch and that must be located on the control desk. The useful beam is switched by switching the supply to the HT transformer, the filament is usually heated continuously while the generator is connected to an electrical supply.

Treatment timers

Switching on the X-ray beam starts two independent exposure timers; the purpose of the primary timer is to switch off the X-rays automatically after a pre-set exposure time, measured in minutes and *decimal minutes*. Both timers must count up from zero to the time prescribed—continuing beyond that pre-set time if, for any reason, the beam is not switched off. The second, back-up, timer is independent and designed to terminate the exposure at an agreed interval above the pre-set time. It should only terminate the exposure in the event of a failure of the primary timer, but its ability to do so is checked in the timer reset procedure. Where the exposure is controlled by the use of timers alone, the output dose rate should be continuously monitored or checked daily using an appropriate instrument. Because the kV is ramped up to the operating voltage after the beam has been switched on—and the timers started—the correction for timer error (p. 56) must be added to each exposure, unless it has been shown by measurement to be insignificant.

Dose meters

The output dose rate is predetermined by:

- the treatment distance
- voltage waveform
- target material, and
- inherent filtration

and controlled by the choice of:

- added filtration
- kilovoltage, and
- tube current.

Since the output is proportional to $(\mathrm{mA}) \times (\mathrm{kV})^2$, these two parameters need to be continuously monitored, electronically or by observation. Wherever possible, an ionisation chamber or solid-state detector is fitted in the beam (on the patient side of any additional filtration) to continuously monitor the intensity of the emerging X-ray beam (Bomford 1976).

The preferred technique is to have two independent ionisation chambers feeding into two independent integrating dose meters (as required for linear accelerators, p. 166) each calibrated to display the dose delivered to the patient. At kilovoltages, however, this is complicated by the energy dependence of the detector (ion chamber), the wide variations in dose rate with field size and the range of beam qualities to be accommodated.

Indicator lamps and interlocks

There are several safety devices which can protect an X-ray unit against overheating, overvoltage, overcurrent, etc., all of which may be indicated on the control desk/panel. The essential indicators are those to indicate the status of the door interlock and the selected kV, mA and added filtration. It is essential the filter, kilovoltage and the tube current are interlocked together so as to prevent a wrong combination from being used—the only exception to this is where only one combination is used, in which case the filter should be fixed in place with a tool. 'Beam-on' warning lights should be duplicated on the control desk, outside the treatment room door and also inside the treatment room. They should be energised on completion of all the interlocks but before the beam-on switch is operated, for they are intended to indicate that the unit is 'in a state of readiness to emit' radiation as well as staying lit for the duration of the exposure.

Safety fuses or circuit breakers safeguard the equipment from electrical failure. Any failure of this sort must be identified and corrected by a competent engineer.

BEAM COLLIMATION

In general terms *beam collimation* means the limiting of the spread of the *useful beam* of radiation to a predetermined direction and size. In practical radiotherapy, it is necessary to be able to vary the size of the field to suit the needs of each patient's treatment. The collimating system can be divided into primary collimation and secondary collimation.

Primary collimation

The maximum divergence of an X-ray beam is limited by the target angle (p. 145). The *primary beam collimator* is a conical aperture in the kilovoltage tube housing. It defines the maximum divergence of the beam and, therefore, the maximum field diameter at a specified distance from the source. The axis of that aperture defines the beam axis and should pass through the centre of the focal spot when the insert is correctly aligned.

Interchangeable applicators

The *secondary collimation* provides a means of varying the field size to suit the particular requirements and the means of rotating square and rectangular fields about the beam axis. Secondary collimation at kilovoltage energies will usually be achieved using interchangeable applicators. *Interchangeable applicators* (Fig. 9.10) are preferred wherever the SSD is short, as they provide an accurate means of setting up the source–skin distance, thereby reducing errors due to the inverse square law. To provide an adequate choice of size and shape of field up to 20 applicators may be required for each machine.

Each type of applicator has a base which serves as a means of attaching the applicator to the tube housing and incorporates a diaphragm which limits the beam to the size required. The diaphragm reduces the transmitted intensity outside the useful beam to less than 2% of that of the useful primary beam. The distal end of the applicator wall may be transparent to enable the coverage of the beam to be checked visually when the

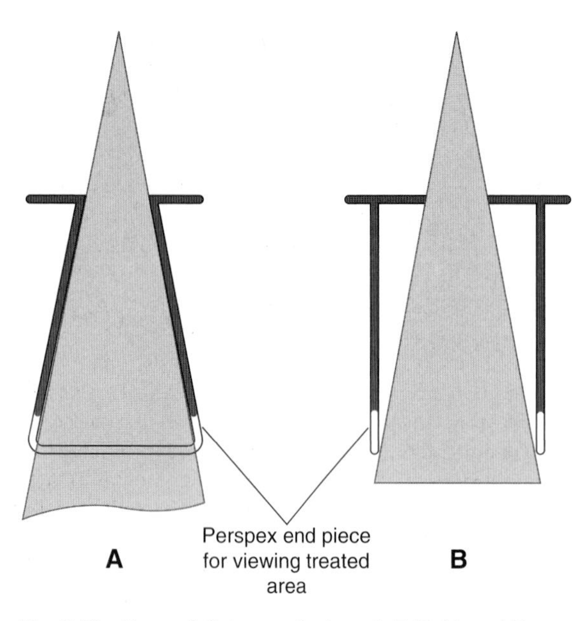

Fig. 9.10 Beam-defining applicators: **A** Fulfield; and **B** parallel-sided.

applicator is in contact with the patient. The final collimation is achieved at a point within approximately 5 cm of the skin surface. The face in contact with the skin indicates the actual area irradiated by the beam. The 'Fulfield' applicator (Fig. 9.10A) has lead-lined walls parallel to the rays at the edge of the field and the Perspex end (typically 3 mm thick) is taken across the face of the applicator to absorb secondary (recoil) electrons from the lead. The Perspex face is inscribed with the principal axes, which of course intersect on the beam axis, thereby simplifying the setting-up of a patient and the use of 'bolus'. In the design shown in Figure 9.10B the walls are not irradiated and can be made of steel; however, the straight sides make larger applicators particularly bulky and difficult to handle.

Non-standard field sizes and tailored shapes can be made by attaching lead cut-outs of adequate thickness over the end of a slightly over-large applicator—Table 9.2 shows the lead thickness required to attenuate the incident beam to less than 2%. The surface dose rate will be reduced due to the reduced back-scatter and the increased SSD, and an appropriate increase will be required to the treatment time (p. 197). (Wherever lead is handled, the bare surfaces should be covered with wax, paint or plastic film to minimise the lead contamination of the skin of both the patient and the staff.)

Table 9.2 The lead equivalence required to reduce the transmitted primary beam to less than 2%

Therapy beam	mm lead equivalence (approx.)
50 kV 1 mm Al HVL	0.25
100 kV 2 mm Al HVL	0.5
150 kV 4 mm Al HVL	1.0
250 kV 2 mm Cu HVL	2.0

Applicator checks

Applicators from time to time should be checked for accurate alignment. The check is twofold. First, set up a reference pointer to mark the beam axis on the surface of the applicator, then on rotating the applicator in its mounting, the pointer should remain at the same point on the applicator surface or describe a circle less than 2 mm diameter (Fig. 9.11A). Second, a film should be set up, with markers indicating the corners of the applicator and with minimal back-scattering material, and exposed to a density of about 1.5—the processed film should show coincidence of the markers with the corners of the blackened area. The blackened area should also be checked carefully for any 'pincushion' effect, as 'Fulfield' applicators tend to be handled in such a way that the lead lining is deformed inwards and separated from the applicator wall material. This effect is shown exaggerated in Figure 9.11B.

If these checks suggest that the alignment on rotation is satisfactory, but the coincidence of the blackened area and markers is poor, then the focal spot may not be correctly aligned to the axis of rotation of the applicators. To check this requires a special device called a *pin-hole camera* (Fig. 9.11C). This device is

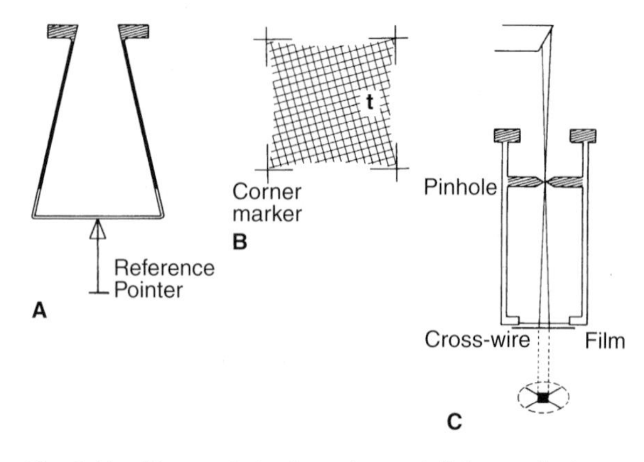

Fig. 9.11 Alignment checks on beam-defining applicators: **A** the reference pointer to check mechanical alignment; **B** the mechanical/photon alignment is checked using corner markers and film; and **C** the pin-hole camera to check alignment of the tube insert and applicator mounting.

mounted in place of the applicator and checked for rotational accuracy. A film is then exposed and the focal spot is imaged on the film together with the shadow of the cross-wires, the intersection of which should be in the centre of the image of the focal spot. (A regular focal spot film can give useful information on the condition of the focal spot (Bomford 1976).)

Beam direction

At low and very low energies, the beam penetration is minimal and the treatment restricted to superficial disease. Beam direction is usually restricted to positioning the applicator symmetrically over the visible disease at normal incidence and in skin apposition. At medium energies, deeper tissues may be treated and beam direction will be achieved using a back pointer in conjunction with the beam axis defined by the applicator. For quality assurance checks on a back pointer, see page 174.

BEAM QUALITY

An X-ray beam is of practical use only after it has emerged from the target and passed through the wall of the tube insert, the tube shield, and any other material placed in its path. Since the attenuation of photons increases with decrease in photon energy, the spectral distribution of the X-ray beam changes in passing through any material between the target and the point of use. Figure 9.12 illustrates the effect by plotting the spectral distribution of a beam generated at 140 kV and the same tube current from a tungsten target with (curve A) and without (curve B) some additional filtration. It will be noted that the total intensity, as represented by the area under the curve, is reduced by the addition of the filter, but at the lower energies the relative reduction in intensity is much greater than at the

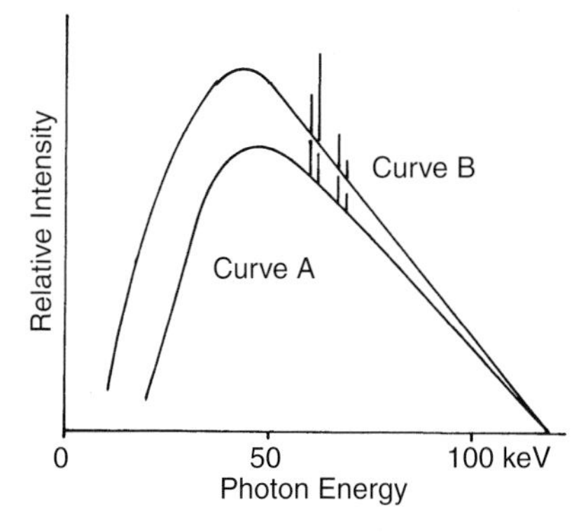

Fig. 9.12 X-ray spectra showing the effect of filtration.

higher energies. This process is known as *beam hardening*. The *added filtration* is a vital parameter of any kilovoltage X-ray beam as it affects the ability of the beam to penetrate the tissues.

The penetrating ability of the primary radiation as it emerges from the X-ray head is often referred to as the *beam quality*. It has been seen in previous chapters that the X-ray beam is a continuous spectrum of photon energies and the extent to which any of the photons interact with matter depends on their energy and on the atomic number of the attenuating medium. If the photons are not absorbed they will be transmitted. Therefore, to know fully the penetrating ability of an X-ray beam requires a knowledge of the number of photons of each energy and the method by which each is absorbed and attenuated. Fortunately, for radiotherapeutic purposes, such a detailed knowledge is not required and some approximation is adequate.

The quality of a kilovoltage X-ray beam is stated in terms of the first half value layer, HVL_1, *and* either the generating voltage (kVp) or the homogeneity coefficient. The first *half value layer* is defined as the thickness of a specified absorber which reduces the air kerma rate in a narrow beam to one-half its original value (IPEMB 1996b). The homogeneity coefficient is the ratio of the HVL_1 divided by the thickness of the same material required to further reduce the intensity of the beam from 50% to 25%, i.e. the second half value layer, HVL_2. For a homogeneous (monochromatic) beam (e.g. caesium–137) the first and second HVL will be the same and the homogeneity coefficient will be equal to 1; for X-ray therapy beams, it is generally between about 0.5 and 0.7.

The X-ray beam quality depends on various factors:

- The accelerating voltage
- The voltage waveform
- The target material
- The inherent filtration
- The added filtration.

Taking these briefly in turn, the accelerating voltage (kVp) determines the minimum wavelength in the spectrum. If the generator provides a constant potential then this minimum wavelength will be present throughout the exposure, whereas if a half- or full-wave rectified circuit is used, it is only present instantaneously giving the spectrum proportionately more lower-energy photons. The target material will superimpose on the continuous spectrum its own characteristic line spectrum (Ch. 2). The *inherent filtration* includes the target material, the glass envelope, the X-ray window, etc., over which there is no operator control. Added filters will be used to remove more of the low-energy photons and their effect will now be discussed in detail with particular reference to the HVL.

Filtration

The mass attenuation curves of Figure 4.12B show that, in the photoelectric region, an absorber will attenuate low-energy photons more readily than the higher-energy photons. This property is exploited in the use of *beam-hardening filters* applied to kilovoltage X-ray beams. In the range from about 1–10 MV, the absorption graph for lead is relatively flat and there is little preferential absorption of lower-energy photons; filters, therefore, have no hardening effect. Above 10 MV, in the pair-production dominated region, the higher-energy photons are absorbed in preference to those of lower energy. Beam-hardening filters are, therefore, not used at megavoltages. (They must not be confused with beam-flattening filters (p. 166) and beam-modifying filters (p. 205).)

In Figure 9.13, the two horizontal axes cover the same photon energy range. The upper graphs show the linear attenuation coefficients for aluminium, copper and tin. The lower curves show a 250 kVp X-ray

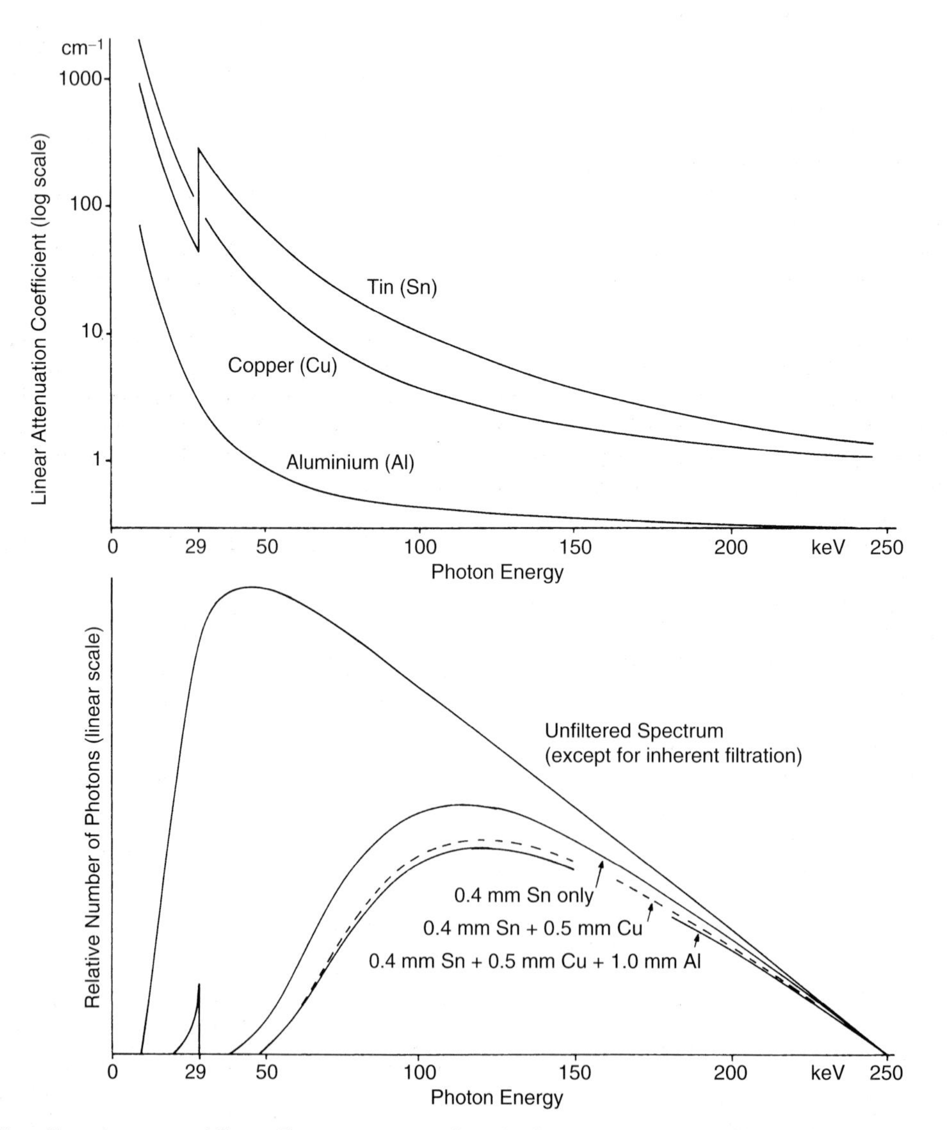

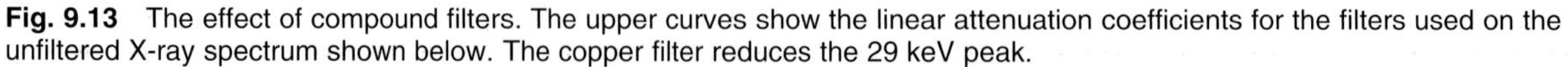
Fig. 9.13 The effect of compound filters. The upper curves show the linear attenuation coefficients for the filters used on the unfiltered X-ray spectrum shown below. The copper filter reduces the 29 keV peak.

spectrum under different degrees of filtration. Under only inherent filtration, the (unfiltered) spectrum shows that the majority of the photons are of such low energy that they will be absorbed in the superficial tissues. In order to preserve the high-energy photons while removing the unwanted low-energy photons, a filter material which is highly attenuating below 40 keV and offering little attenuation to the photons in the 200 keV region is required. Aluminium (Z = 13) is of little value in this situation, but may be used as a primary filter for X-rays generated at energies up to approximately 120 kVp. Copper (Z = 29) may be used up to 250 kVp, but tin (Z = 50) is preferred for energies above 200 kVp. However, copper and tin are never used in isolation. In Figure 9.13, when a beam-hardening filter of 0.5 mm tin is added to the unfiltered beam, the spectral peak is moved from 45 keV to about 115 keV, but there is a lesser peak at 29 keV owing to the K-absorption edge of tin. To attenuate this 29 keV peak, a copper filter is added to the tin. Copper, however, adds its K-absorption edge at 9 keV which has to be filtered out by adding the aluminium–the K-edge of aluminium is less than 2 keV and is negligible. It needs to be remembered that tin and copper not only have a low attenuation coefficient at 20 keV and 9 keV respectively, but that they become sources of their own characteristic radiations with photon energies just below these edges. These are not shown in the diagram, but constitute an addition to the spectrum. It is important therefore that, when using such a *compound filter*, the metals must be fitted in the correct order—highest Z closest to the target, lowest Z to the patient.

The tin–copper–aluminium filter is often referred to as a *Thoraeus filter* after the Swedish physicist who found the most efficient filter for his 200 kVp X-ray beam was 0.4 mm Sn + 0.25 mm Cu + 1.0 mm Al. By 'efficiency' in this connection he meant getting the desired hardening effect with the minimum loss of beam intensity, i.e. the maximum output dose rate. At that time, dose rates were 20 cGy min^{-1} at best!

Beam-hardening filters can, therefore, improve the relative penetration of the beam and raise the value of the homogeneity coefficient. The actual measurement of these parameters will now be considered.

Measurement of HVL

The method of measuring HVL is the same over the whole range of energies found in the radiotherapy department providing the characteristics of the radiation are observed, namely that the ionisation chamber wall is air equivalent over the range of photon energies being measured—the same chamber could not be used for both 10 kV and 10 MV—and its energy response does not vary by more than, say, 5%. It should also be remembered that the penetrating ability of the beams will vary considerably and the choice of absorbing material is important—those normally used are shown in Table 9.3.

The apparatus required is shown schematically in Figure 9.14. The HVL_1 is determined by measuring the intensity of the beam transmitted through various thicknesses of the chosen metal (aluminium or copper) and interpolating to find the thickness that would transmit 50% of the intensity measured with zero thickness of material added (Fig. 9.15).

To measure the HVL, the basic requirement is a means of collimating the beam, C, to a small size but large enough to cover the ionisation chamber, D, which will be referred to as the detector. (The error resulting from the use of a large beam size will be explained later.) If repeat exposures cannot be given very accurately, a second monitor chamber, M, will be required on the tube side of the collimator to detect the variation in the

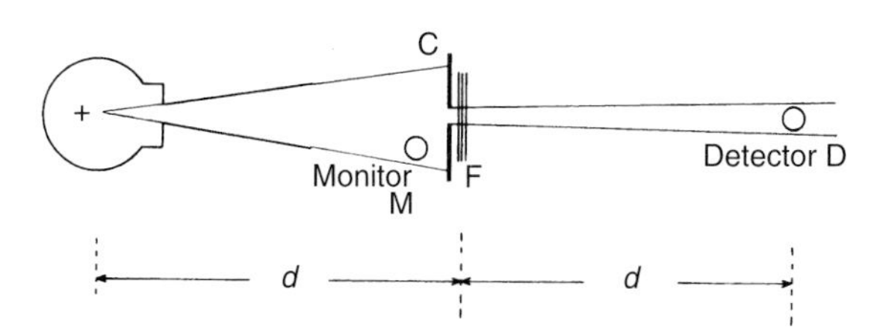

Fig. 9.14 The layout for the measurement of half value layer.

Table 9.3 Typical values of added filtration and beam quality

Energy	kVp	Added filter (mm)	HVL	Effective photon energy	Equivalent wavelength
Very low	10	Nil	0.02 mm Al	6 keV	0.207 nm
Low	80	1 Al	2.5 mm Al	30 keV	0.041 nm
Medium	250	1 Cu + 1 Al	2.1 mm Cu	108 keV	0.011 nm
Medium	300	0.8 Sn + 0.25 Cu + 1.0 Al	3.8 mm Cu	155 keV	0.008 nm

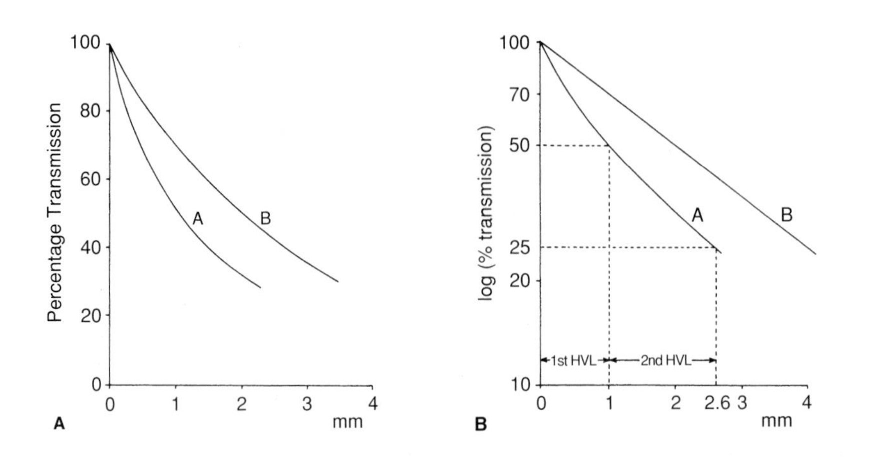

Fig. 9.15 The attenuation of a radiation beam by the addition of filters plotted **A** on a linear scale and **B** on a logarithmic scale. Curve A is for an inhomogeneous X-ray beam and curve B for a homogeneous beam.

exposure incident on the filters, F, as they are added during the experiment; the reading obtained on this monitor chamber must not influence or be influenced by the other variables. The exposure time chosen should be typical of the exposures in clinical use, as it can influence the outcome because each measurement will be affected by the timer error and the shape of the voltage ramp (Heales et al 1998). The focus-to-filter distance should be approximately equal to the filter-to-detector distance and greater than the range of the electrons emitted from the filter material; the focus-to-detector distance should be more than 50 cm and preferably between 80 and 100 cm (Klevenhagen & Thwaites 1993).

With the apparatus carefully and rigidly aligned and a table in which to record the results (Table 9.4), the measurements can begin. (If the monitor, M, is not used then it is assumed that the readings that would have been obtained would all be equal, namely $M_0 = M_1 = M_2$ etc. in Table 9.4 and columns 4 and 5 would not be required.) The maximum thickness of the filters to be added will depend on the radiation and material being used and the exact purpose of the experiment but the transmission should be reduced to less than 20%. The calculation of percentage transmission for the final column of the table is:

$$\%\ \text{transmission} = \frac{D_n \times M_0 \times 100}{D_0 \times M_n}$$

where D_n and M_n are the readings taken on inserting a thickness t_n making the total filtration equal to t. On completion of the readings and calculations, a graph of the percentage transmission through the chosen filter material is plotted as in Figure 9.15A. If possible, the logarithm of the percentage transmission should be plotted as in Figure 9.15B. In this example, it can be seen that 1.0 mm is required to reduce the intensity to 50% and a further 1.6 mm to reduce it to 25%. The HVL_1 is, therefore, 1 mm and the homogeneity coefficient is (1.0/1.6) or 0.67.

The graphs in Figure 9.15 reveal a good deal more. First, it has been said that a homogeneous beam of radiation would obey the law of exponential absorption and would have a homogeneity coefficient of unity. The law of exponential absorption states, using the same nomenclature:

Table 9.4 The measurement of half value layer

Added filter	Total filtration	Detector reading, D	Monitor reading, M	Ratio D/M	Percentage transmission
Nil	Nil	D_0	M_0	D_0/M_0	100.0
t_1	t_1	D_1	M_1	D_1/M_1	$\frac{1/\ \ 1}{0/\ \ 0} \times 100$
t_2 etc.	t_1+t_2	D_2	M_2	D_2/M_2	$\frac{2/\ \ 2}{0/\ \ 0} \times 100$

$$D_n = D_0 \, e^{-\mu t} \text{ or } \ln (D_n / D_0) = -\mu t$$

The straight-line graph (curve B) in Figure 9.15B may be the graph of this equation and its gradient is $-\mu$. The gradient of curve A is also $-\mu$, but the magnitude of μ decreases with increasing filtration. Now consideration of the photoelectric region shows that the linear attenuation coefficient (or rather μ/ρ, but ρ is constant) decreases with increasing photon energy (Fig. 9.13). This, therefore, is another way of explaining that the peak of the spectrum is moved to a higher photon energy by the preferential absorption of the low-energy photons by the addition of filters.

Effective photon energy and equivalent wavelength

From the above equation, $D_n/D_0 = ½$ when $t = \text{HVL}_1$, by definition, and the equation simplifies to:

$$\text{HVL}_1 = 0.693/\mu \text{ or } \mu = 0.693/\text{HVL}_1$$

since $-\ln(½) = 0.693$. From the attenuation data appropriate to the filter material, μ can be used to derive the energy of a homogeneous beam of photons having the same HVL_1 as the X-ray beam under examination. This energy (in keV) is known as the *effective photon energy* of the X-ray beam. This is particularly useful when attempting to compare X- and gamma ray beams. A third alternative specification of the quality of the beam is to calculate the *equivalent wavelength*, λ, using Duane–Hunt's law (p. 17). Some typical values of effective photon energy and equivalent wavelength are given in Table 9.3.

Broad beam attenuation

It was stated earlier that a narrow beam should be used for the measurement of HVL. This is necessary to minimise the radiation scattered by the added filters by an excessively large beam of radiation. Such scattered radiation would increase the reading D_n which when plotted on the transmission graph would give an overestimate of the HVL_1. Such *broad beam* data have their usefulness in radiation protection (Ch. 6) but for radiotherapy treatment, *narrow beam attenuation* is required.

CALIBRATION OF OUTPUT DOSE RATE

A *definitive calibration* of the output dose rate must be carried out as a part of the commissioning procedure or following any major repair (e.g. a new tube insert) or modification which might affect the output beam (IPSM 1992). It must be derived from two independent sets of measurements based on two different instruments carried out by two physicists experienced in radiotherapy physics. (The two instruments may be calibrated against the same secondary standard.) For each generator, the output dose rate is measured under the operating conditions used clinically. If more than one combination of kV, mA and filter are used, then the output must be measured for each combination. There is a mandatory requirement (HSE 1998a) that regular calibrations of the reference field size are made on all kilovoltage generators at least once every 4 weeks, and continuous monitoring of dose rate is preferred (Bomford 1976) to a daily check.

It is normal practice to measure the output dose rate for each treatment applicator available using the appropriate technique, always ensuring that the chamber is adequately covered, particularly by the smaller applicators. Where a phantom is used, it must extend at least 5 cm outside the nominal field size and the measurement at depth should be corrected using the appropriate depth dose data. The output dose rate for each applicator is tabulated for use at the control desk.

Medium-energy X-rays (160–300 kV)

The field chamber will be centred 2 cm deep in a water (equivalent) phantom of no less than $20 \times 20 \times 12$ cm^3, with the stem parallel to the larger face. The surface of the phantom will be at the normal treating distance (i.e. in contact with the treatment applicator) and at right angles to the beam axis of a 10×10 cm^2 field (the set-up is similar to that shown in Fig. 10.17). Several instrument readings should be taken and corrected to the standard temperature and pressure and the mean corrected reading, M, calculated. (Ideally the phantom and chamber should be kept at room temperature.) The dose-to-water at 2 cm deep, D, in the set (exposure) time, t, will be:

$$D = M \, (N_K \, k_{ch})_f \, [\mu_{en}/\rho]_{water/air}$$

The quantity, $[\mu_{en}/\rho]_{water/air}$ varies with both beam quality and field size. For the derivation of $(N_K \, k_{ch})_f$, see page 60. Where the exposure has been controlled by monitor units, then the measured dose D divided by the percentage depth dose at 2 cm for the 10×10 cm^2 field size in use should be within 1% of the set monitor units. The output dose rate is calculated by dividing the integrated dose, D, by the percentage depth dose at 2 cm deep for the 10×10 cm^2 field size in use and by the exposure time, $(t - \Delta t)$, where Δt is the timer error (p. 56).

Low-energy X-ray beams (50–160 kV)

The field chamber will be in air, centred on and at right angles to the beam axis of the selected treatment applicator and at a small, but known, distance from the applicator surface—e.g. if the stem of the chamber is in contact with the edge of the applicator and at right angles to the beam axis, that distance will be the radius of the stem (Fig. 9.16). Several instrument readings should be taken and corrected to the standard temperature and pressure and the mean corrected reading, M, calculated. The dose-to-water at the centre of the chamber, D_c, in air and in the set time, t, will be:

$$D_c = M\, N_{K,f}\, [\mu_{en}/\rho]_{water/air}$$

The quantity, $[\mu_{en}/\rho]_{water/air}$, varies with both beam quality and field size. For the derivation of $N_{K,f}$, see page 60. The output dose-to-water, D, needs to be known at the surface of the applicator and therefore the dose, D_c, at the centre of the chamber needs to be increased by the inverse square law to correct for the stand-off and corrected for the fact that the surface dose will be further increased by the radiation scattered back from the tissues irradiated. The back-scatter factor, B, is dependent on the beam quality and the size and shape of the beam. The surface dose, D, delivered in the set time, t, will be:

$$D = M\, N_{K,f}\, [\mu_{en}/\rho]_{water/air}\, B\, \{(S + x)/S\}^2$$

where S is the source–skin distance for the applicator and x the stand-off distance to the chamber centre. (The validity of the inverse square law in this context should be checked as radiation scattered from the applicator may affect it.) The output dose rate is calculated by dividing the integrated dose, D, by the exposure time, $(t - \Delta t)$, where Δt is the timer error (p. 56).

Very low-energy X-ray beams (8–50 kV)

The field chamber should be of the parallel-plate design and mounted at the surface of a water (equivalent) phantom of more than 5 cm thick to provide full back-scatter. The chamber should be exposed within a beam large enough to give at least a 2 cm margin around the chamber. The front surface of the phantom should be at the normal treating distance, i.e. in contact with the treatment applicator. Several instrument readings should be taken and corrected to the standard temperature and pressure and the mean corrected reading, M, calculated. (The phantom and chamber should be kept at room temperature.) The dose-to-water at the surface of the phantom, D, in the set time, t, will be:

$$D = M\, (NK\, k_{ch})_f\, [\mu_{en}/\rho]_{water/air}$$

The quantity, $[\mu_{en}/\rho]_{water/air}$, varies with both beam quality and field size. For the derivation of $(NK\, k_{ch})_f$, see page 60. The output dose rate is calculated by dividing the integrated dose, D, by the exposure time, $(t - \Delta t)$, where Δt is the timer error (p. 56).

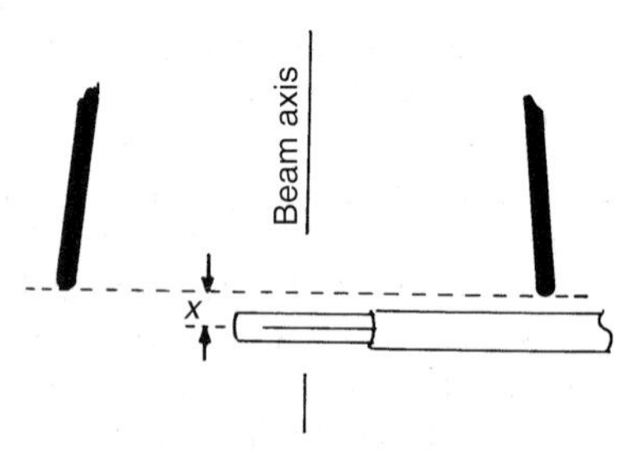

Fig. 9.16 The calibration of output dose rate in air for low-energy X-rays; the stand-off, x, must be carefully measured.

COMMISSIONING NEW EQUIPMENT

Acceptance tests

New radiotherapy equipment should only be ordered after close scrutiny of the manufacturer's technical specification and discussion about the customer's particular requirements. Compliance with local, national or international requirements should not be assumed. After the equipment has been ordered and delivered, it will be installed by the manufacturers or their agents, but before it is accepted the customer's Medical Physicist should ensure the installation complies with the agreed specification. The acceptance tests will be designed to demonstrate that the details of the agreed specification have been satisfied—in five main areas:

- The radiotherapy beams—each beam energy and beam modality—are of the specified quality and intensity and can be controlled and monitored in the specified manner and to the specified accuracy. The range of applicator sizes and their alignment must be checked. The kV, mA and filter combinations must be interlocked.
- All the movements of the tubestand cover the specified ranges and that the brakes operate effectively throughout the range and fail-safe. Where motorised movements are involved, the speed and control must be checked.
- All the electrical aspects of the equipment must be checked for safety—the connections to earth (the ERT must be clearly labelled), the operation of limit switches, interlocks, built-in safety circuits, particularly where the equipment could malfunction and

where maintenance staff may be put at risk. The consequences of a mains supply failure must be included.

- The radiation safety requirements must be met—leakage radiation levels from the tube housing, applicator transmission, beam dosimetry and control, etc. The installer will have had the adequacy of the structural shielding checked at an early stage, but checks should be made on other aspects such as door interlocks and warning signs (unless the manufacturer has supplied and fitted these, he will not accept sole responsibility).
- The inventory of the accessories, spare parts, instruction and maintenance manuals, circuit diagrams and safety manuals, etc., all in English.

A careful record of all these checks and operating parameters must be kept for future reference as they will form a basis for quality control.

Equipment peripheral to the radiotherapy generator, e.g. the closed-circuit television viewing system, intercom, etc. may or may not be the responsibility of the supplier of the therapy equipment. The structural work on the treatment and control rooms may be the subject of a separate contract.

Commissioning tests

Once new equipment has been accepted then the customer will repeat most of the checks listed above with a view to making detailed measurements to ensure the equipment can be used safely to treat patients. This commissioning of the equipment will be the responsibility of a competent Medical Physicist and take about a week; more for complex equipment. Commissioning will include:

- Full radiation protection survey of the treatment room and adjacent areas—not forgetting above and below—to ensure the requirements of the safety legislation are satisfied within the accepted use of the equipment. Any failure in structural protection may be difficult to correct at this stage and may impose limitations on the use of the equipment or the occupancy of the adjacent areas. This survey will include interlocks and warning signs and the systems for audiovisual contact with the patient during treatment in compliance with the Regulations.
- Full radiation protection survey of the equipment itself—leakage radiation levels when the beam is on—for compliance with the permitted maxima.
- Confirmation of the accuracy of all the beam-direction devices in all their modes of use.
- The measurement of depth dose, beam profiles and isodose chart data for all beam modalities in sufficient detail for the treatment planning of patients. The measurement of the output dose rates for all the applicators and the correct correlation between monitor units and the delivered absorbed dose in grays.
- The output dose calibration over the full range of the dose (rate) meter (if fitted) to check linearity over the range of available dose rates and to check saturation. To check all the facets of the double dosimetry / timer system, including timer error.

It is important that all the staff involved with the new equipment are given time to become familiar with it before it is handed over for the treatment of patients. Radiographers need time to practice the controls both inside and outside the room. Maintenance staff need time to study drawings and circuits and to locate principal components within the equipment—the simplest repair can take many hours if the technician does not know where to find the faulty component!

Quality assurance

Throughout the life of the equipment, 15 years, say, it is essential to ensure that the data collected during commissioning is fully documented and continues to be relevant by monitoring the performance of the equipment through a programme of regular checks. These checks will take a variety of forms and be repeated at different intervals.

A separate *fault book* must be maintained by the radiographer (and others) in which all the faults which develop on each equipment are logged—however trivial they may appear. This is important for two reasons. Where radiographers work in shifts on one piece of equipment or whose duties rotate through several pieces of equipment, no one person will be able to remember all the quirks of that equipment. The written log will reveal the frequency at which faults occur, the dates on which major repairs have been undertaken and, over a period of time, trends will be detectable which may assist in the preventive maintenance programme. The fault book records the random and intermittent events that inevitably occur. The quality control technician and the maintenance technician should examine the fault book regularly.

A planned quality assurance programme does not wait for faults to happen, but looks for consistency in general and thereby finds discrepancies before they manifest themselves as faults. The programme will usually consist of daily, weekly, monthly checks and, maybe, 6-monthly or 12-monthly checks. The actual frequency of a particular check will be determined for each particular item of equipment. For example, the output dose rate of kilovoltage X-ray generators should be calibrated at least once every 4 weeks if an output dose rate monitor is fitted, but checked daily if there is no monitor fitted. If a prescribed attenuator is then placed in the primary beam, a second measurement can confirm the quality or penetration of the beam—this type of measurement may not be a precise measurement of HVL, but over a period of months the consistency of the result builds confidence in the equipment. Other beam parameters which should be included in the QA programme will include beam symmetry, applicator alignment and the ability of the dual timer/dosimeter system to terminate the exposure.

All the devices used for setting-up a patient's treatment should be included in the programme. These will include the mechanical pointers, scales, movements and their brakes, etc. and other accessories. It should not be necessary to check indicator lamps, because any failures should have been reported previously in the fault book. The operation of interlocks and limit switches should be included, particularly if they are rarely used in clinical practice. Quality assurance is a shared responsibility between radiographers and medical physics staff and close cooperation is essential.

The preventive maintenance inspection is a vital part of the overall quality assurance programme carried out by the maintenance technician. The details need not concern the radiographer but will include checking water flows and air filters, tightness of electrical connections as well as the more intimate operation of the equipment itself.

The quality assurance programme is vital to any radiotherapy equipment and takes time to implement, just how long depends on the complexity of the equipment. Half a day per month plus 2 full days per year is typical for kilovoltage therapy equipment. This investment in time does not preclude the possibility of breakdown but can minimise the unexpected interruptions to the treatment schedule.

In the event of an equipment malfunction, be it in the generator or in the dosimetry, causing an error of more than +20% of the intended dose fraction (+10% of the total course dose), the incident must be reported to the Health and Safety Executive once an investigation has confirmed beyond reasonable doubt that an overexposure has occurred—guidance on the content of the investigation/report is given in a Health and Safety Executive publication (HSE 1998a). In the event of an underexposure of similar size, the employer should instigate an investigation but the incident is not notifiable to the HSE.

DESIGN OF KILOVOLTAGE THERAPY ROOMS

Protective barriers

Adequate protection in a beam therapy room begins with the generator itself and the protective requirements of kilovoltage equipment have been detailed (Table 9.1). For X-ray generators with a maximum operating potential of less than 50 kVp, it is permissible, but undesirable, to have the operator and control desk in the same room as the X-ray tube; for all generators capable of operating at more than 50 kVp, the control desk must be outside the protected treatment room.

The versatility of the kilovoltage tubestand is such that the primary beam can be directed at any part of the ceiling, floor and walls and it is unwise to make any distinction, other than giving the instruction that the primary beam must not be directed at the door or window. (This restriction should be borne in mind when making the decision about the position of the tubestand within the room.) Ideally, the entrance door and observation window will offer the same degree of protection as the wall(s) in which they are located and the protection must be maintained by suitably lapping lead through the frames and over the joints (Fig. 9.17). There should be no other (entrance/exit) doors or windows in the protected room.

The calculation of the protective material required follows the same pattern as outlined for the primary barriers in a megavoltage room (p. 179)—and gives a similar result, namely approximately 6 TVLs. For a new medium-energy treatment room, concrete is the preferred protective material, but where an existing room is being modified then lead panelling may be added to the existing walls. For low- and very low-energy treatment rooms, lead panelling may be the preferred material. On a practical note, lead panelling

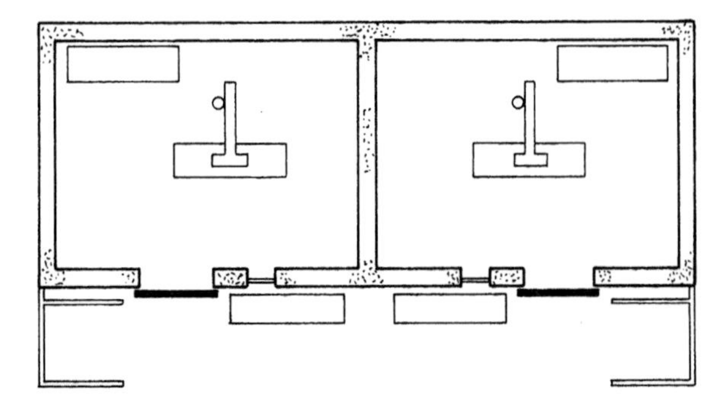

Fig. 9.17 The layout of two typical orthovoltage treatment rooms showing the transformer cabinets, the protected sliding doors and control desks with lead glass observation windows.

is heavy and needs to be well supported and secured and itself protected from perforation by water pipes, electrical conduits, etc.

Entrance doors

The entrance door will be lead lined and heavy, both to hang and to use—the operation of sliding doors is more reliable than hinged doors. The door must operate an interlock to inhibit or terminate any exposure when the door is open. The interlock must be a fail-safe device and only reset by the positive action of the operator at the control desk—when all but the patient have left the room. 'Positive action' usually means operating a second switch within a pre-set time.

All X-ray therapy rooms (including those very low-energy X-ray rooms where the operator is inside) will be *radiation controlled areas* (p. 77) whenever the generator is energised, and warning signs, preferably electrically operated, must be displayed to that effect at the entrance. An additional warning sign should display 'DO NOT ENTER' or otherwise advise of the hazard (Plate 1.2) from the moment the generator is *in a state of readiness to emit* (HSE 1988b) radiation until the termination of the exposure. Visible and audible warnings are required in the treatment room to indicate that radiation is imminent or present, together with a mains supply isolation switch for use in an emergency.

Observation of the patient

Therapy rooms are controlled areas when the beam is emitted and everyone, except the patient, must be outside the protected area. However, in the interests of safety, the patient must be kept under observation. At kilovoltage energies, lead glass windows are commonly used—with lead as an added ingredient, glass can be made with an increased density ($\rho \sim 4000$ kg m^{-3}) and increased atomic number for use in protective barriers but it must be handled with care as the lead makes the glass very soft and easily damaged. Glass of up to 2 mm Pb equivalence is readily available and widely used, although more than one thickness may be required. The window must be large enough to provide a clear view of the room and of the patient for more than one operator. Closed circuit television, with a pan and tilt camera fitted with a zoom lens, is an ideal alternative to lead glass—to improve the privacy for the patient, the TV monitor can be blanked out when the treatment room door is open. The CCTV system does not offer the patient a view of the operator and this is often cited in favour of the window.

Communication with the patient

A hands-off intercom should be available so the patient can speak to the operator during the treatment without having to move. Again, if this is linked through the door interlock circuit, it can be muted while the operator is in the room.

CHAPTER CONTENTS

10

Megavoltage beam generators

Keith Bomford

INTRODUCTION

The need for X-ray energies greater than the kilovoltage range has been recognised for many years, but basic transformer technology is not suited to voltages for radiotherapy above about 500 kV. Other techniques have to be used. X-ray energies between 500 and 1000 kV are of no value in radiotherapy (Ch. 12). There has been a variety of suggestions as to the optimum megavoltage X-ray energy for radiotherapy. The earliest recommendation was 8–10 MV but, because of large 'exit' doses, this was discarded in favour of 4 MV. 4 MV was subsequently discarded because the penetration was inadequate for the 'larger' patient, albeit ideal for many head and neck treatments. 6 MV is the currently popular choice. Dual energy accelerators will often have one beam energy of 6–8 MV and a second of 10–15 MV, for the 'larger' patient, although energies above 10 MV present difficulties in radiation protection.

THE LINEAR ACCELERATOR

The linear accelerator now dominates the market; the *betatron* was widely used in some countries but it proved more suited to electron beam than X-ray beam generation.

The dual modality accelerators today offer both one or two X-ray energies and a range of electron beam energies. The electron beam energy is usually variable from 6 MeV up to an energy somewhat higher than the maximum photon energy. A range from 6–20 MeV electrons permits the treatment of the superficial tissues up to 20–60 mm deep.

We have seen that X-rays are produced whenever an electron stream travelling at high speed is brought to rest in a target. To produce a megavoltage X-ray beam it is necessary to have an evacuated tube (the waveguide) in which the electron stream can be accelerated on to a suitable transmission target using the energy of a radiofrequency wave.

The electron gun

The source of electrons may be a directly heated filament or an indirectly heated oxide-coated cathode which will release electrons by thermionic emission. The cathode is mounted in an *electron gun* at the input end of the corrugated waveguide. The cathode will sit within a focusing cup held at a slightly lower potential to 'push' the electrons in the direction of the waveguide while the negative potential (of a few kV) on the gun itself will cause the electrons to accelerate towards the input end of the corrugated waveguide, which is held at earth potential. The electron gun may be demountable to facilitate the replacement of the filament.

The radiofrequency generator

As the name linear accelerator implies, the electrons are accelerated in a straight line and this is achieved using radiofrequency (rf) waves of approximately 10 cm wavelength. These radio waves are generated either in a specially designed vacuum diode valve called a *magnetron* or in an rf oscillator called a *klystron*. In either case, the radio waves pass down a smooth rectangular waveguide containing gas under pressure, through a rf window and into an evacuated waveguide.

The magnetron is a vacuum tube containing a cylindrical indirectly heated oxide-coated cathode coaxially mounted within a cylindrical anode and supported between the poles of a permanent magnet whose field is parallel to the common axes of the electrodes. The magnetic field causes the electrons to follow spirally curving paths as they travel from cathode to anode, which in turn cause a resonance with keyhole-shaped cavities in the anode. The frequency is predetermined by the geometry of the cavities but may be varied slightly by adjusting a plunger built into the anode; the plunger is servo-controlled to maintain a stable output. The magnetron is water-cooled. It is mounted directly on to the end of the rectangular waveguide and the radiofrequency wave is released from an 'aerial' within the magnetron.

The klystron is essentially a power amplifier, taking a low-powered oscillator of the required frequency and amplifying it through resonant cavities. A steady stream of electrons pass a gap in the primary cavity (of the low-powered oscillator), the oscillator causes the electrons to bunch together so that when a bunch of electrons passes the gap in the second resonant cavity, that cavity will be excited more powerfully albeit with the same frequency. The stream of electrons is emitted by a heated cathode and ultimately the bunches of electrons are absorbed in an 'electron catcher' where their energy is dissipated into cooling water. As with the magnetron, some adjustment of frequency is possible, by adjusting the frequency of the primary oscillator. The output radiofrequency wave is taken from the second cavity. Because the klystron requires a high electron current and an accelerating potential of 100 kV, it must be operated within a protective metal case; both electrical and radiation safety measures must be followed when servicing the klystron or working in its vicinity.

The corrugated waveguide

When a radiofrequency wave passes through a smooth waveguide of conducting material and circular cross-section with a diameter comparable to (but slightly greater than) the wavelength, an electric field is established as in Figure 10.1A. If a free electron is placed on the axis of the tube at point A, for instance, it will be accelerated to the right by the electric field but it will only

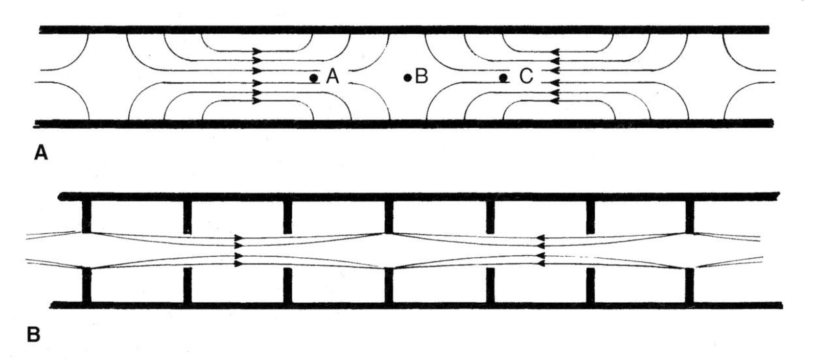

Fig. 10.1 The electric field pattern created by an rf wave passing down **A** a smooth tube and **B** a corrugated waveguide.

continue in that direction if the electric field moves with it. (At B, it would not move whereas at C it would move to the left.) Now, radiofrequency waves in free space travel at the velocity of light, 3×10^8 m s^{-1}, and cannot be accelerated. They can, however, be made to move more slowly by the introduction of iris diaphragms into the waveguide, which is then referred to as a *corrugated waveguide*. The hole diameter and the spacing of the iris diaphragms control the wave velocity (Fig. 10.1B) by controlling the electrical capacitance of the waveguide. The closer the irises, the slower the wave velocity. Two modes of operation will be described below.

The dimensions of the corrugated waveguide are critical, not only requiring very accurate machining during manufacture, but also temperature stabilisation during operation. The whole of the radiofrequency circuit, the magnetron or klystron, corrugated waveguide and rf load, together with the target is temperature controlled to better than ± 1°C. This is achieved by pumping distilled or de-ionised water through a simple network of cooling pipes and a heat exchanger where the surplus heat is transferred to the atmosphere. A linear accelerator dissipates tens of kilowatts of heat when the beam is energised, although the X-ray efficiency is much higher than for kilovoltage X-rays, typically being about 40%.

The travelling wave accelerator

In the travelling wave accelerator (Fig. 10.2), the (negative) voltage pulse applied to the magnetron is also applied to the gun so that the electrons enter the corrugated waveguide with the rf wave. The wave velocity is reduced in the *bunching section*, where the iris diaphragms are closer together, to about 0.4*c*, but as the wave travels down the guide, the wider spacing of the diaphragms allows it to accelerate carrying the electrons with it. (This phenomenon is familiar to those who enjoy surf-boarding!) At the end of the guide the rf wave will be diverted and absorbed (i.e. the wave energy is converted into heat) in the rf load, while the electrons enter a field-free region prior to striking the target.

In Figure 10.3, the electrons to the left of A will experience a stronger field and therefore a greater acceleration, while electrons to the right experience a lesser acceleration, thereby adding to the bunching effect. But the mean acceleration will depend on where the bunch is centred on the wave, or to put it more technically, the acceleration of the electrons depends on the phase relationship between the wave and the electron pulse. The final energy achieved by the electrons will be determined by the length of the corrugated waveguide, typically 4 MV per metre, and the frequency of the rf wave.

The standing wave accelerator

If the corrugated waveguide is closed at both ends, the rf wave will be reflected back at each end and, at the resonant frequency, a standing wave will be established; in such a system the radiofrequency power

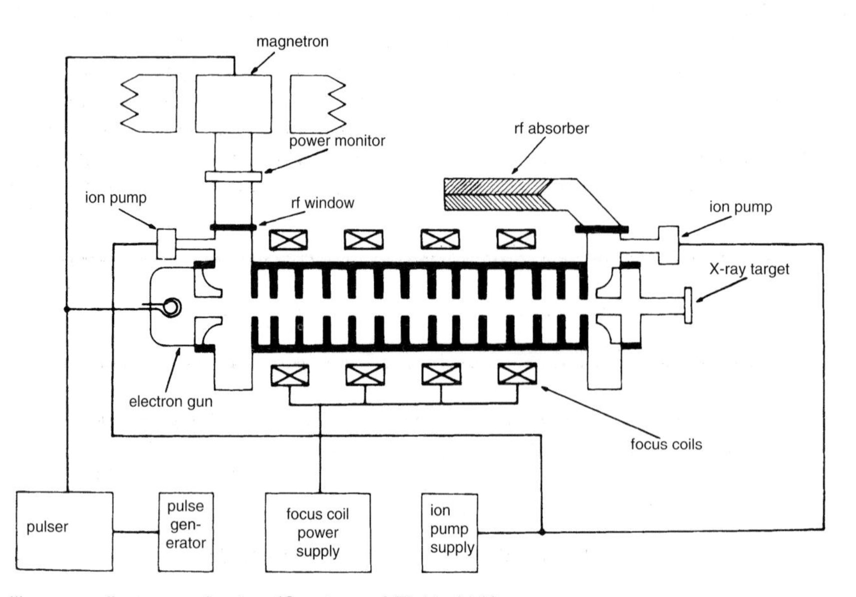

Fig. 10.2 A travelling wave linear accelerator. (Courtesy of Elekta Ltd.)

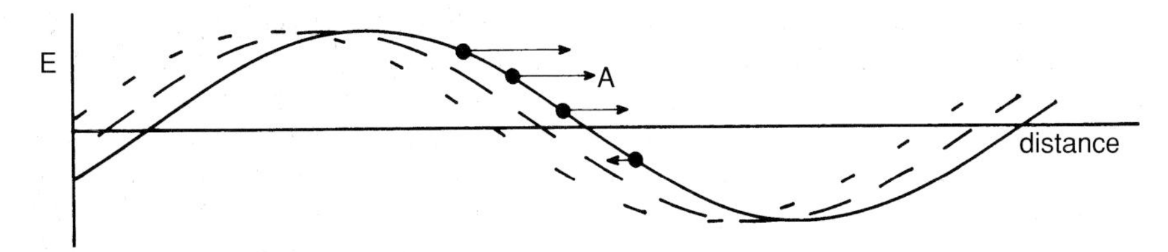

Fig. 10.3 The travelling wave—on the leading positive edge the electrons bunch together as they are accelerated in proportion to the electric vector.

may be input at any point along the guide. In the standing wave accelerator, the irises are equally spaced and the wave pattern is established as shown in Figure 10.4. In alternate cavities, at the nodes of the standing wave, the electric field is always zero, while in the intermediate antinode cavities, the direction of the field changes direction with time. Now, if the induced field changes direction each time the electron traverses a 'node' cavity, then the electron will be accelerated through each 'antinode' cavity in succession thereby gaining energy. The length of each cavity is designed to conform to the acceleration of the electrons. In the so-called *side-coupled waveguide*, the 'node' cavities are taken out of line and attached to the side of the guide, thereby shortening the overall length of the guide (Plate 1.7).

The two ends of the guide have to be closed to reflect the radiofrequency wave, but in practice a small hole is left through which the electrons are injected from the electron gun and ultimately leave the waveguide and strike the transmission target.

For low-energy accelerators, the side-coupled guide is short enough to enable a transmission target to be attached directly to the end of the corrugated waveguide, thereby producing the X-ray beam in the same direction as the electron acceleration (for example a 6 MV guide is only 300 mm long). In operation, the beam energy is more stable than with the travelling wave accelerator because the corrugated waveguide is less tolerant of small changes in the radiofrequency.

The energy of the standing wave accelerator can, however, be varied by using separate guides in tandem and varying the phase difference between them; for example, it is possible to accelerate to a middle energy in the first guide and then, by changing the phase, either to accelerate further in the second to a higher energy or to decelerate to a lower energy, thereby providing two very different energies.

The X-ray head

Within any corrugated waveguide there is a radial component to the electric field which would cause the electrons to disperse unless its effect was opposed by the magnetic field produced by externally mounted focusing coils. These coils seek to restrict the final focal spot on the X-ray target to only a few millimetres in diameter.

Where the waveguide is short enough to be in line with the X-ray beam axis, the transmission X-ray target will be mounted directly on to the end of the guide. Where longer waveguides are required, they will be mounted within the cantilever arm of the isocentric gantry and the electron beam will emerge from the accelerating guide and enter into a field-free *flight tube* and pass through one or several magnetic fields to

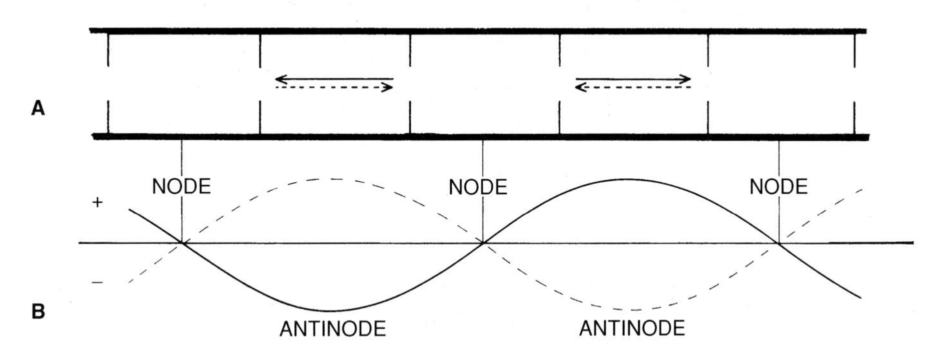

Fig. 10.4 The standing wave accelerator: **A** the waveguide and **B** the wave.

steer the electrons through an angle of up to 270° before reaching the X-ray target (Fig. 10.5 and Plate 1.8). The current required by these electromagnets may be used to monitor the energy of the electrons—the higher their energy the larger the required current.

The X-ray target

The spatial distribution of the X-rays produced (Fig. 2.9), suggests megavoltage X-rays are emitted predominantly in the same direction as the bombarding electrons. To maximise the X-ray beam intensity, the transmission target will be thick enough to stop all the electrons bombarding it but thin enough to minimise the self absorption. Usually the target is at earth potential, a few millimetres thick of, say, tungsten, gold or platinum and cooled by a flow of water as described above.

The flattening filter

Although the thick target will cause some modification of the spatial distribution, the theory has two consequences particularly relevant to photon energies above 4 MV. Firstly, the photon energy sets a maximum practicable field size, in that the higher the energy the smaller the divergence of the X-rays produced. Secondly, the intensity along the central axis of the beam is greater than at the edges; that is, the dose distribution across the beam is not uniform.

Beam uniformity is achieved by the introduction of a *beam flattening filter* close to the target (Fig. 10.6). This is a metal filter, preferably of low atomic number and

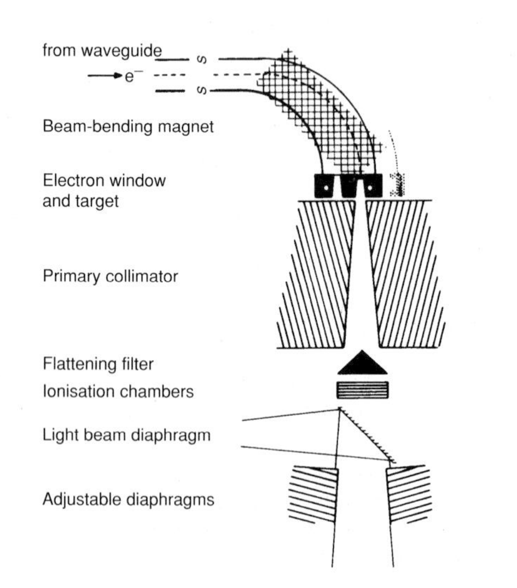

Fig. 10.5 The X-ray head assembly of a linear accelerator.

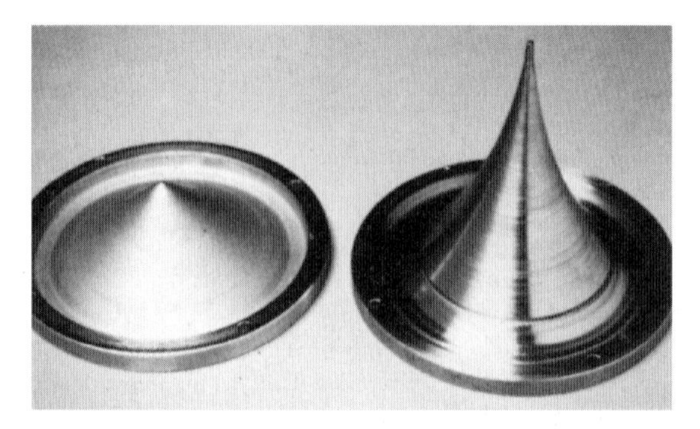

Fig. 10.6 Typical flattening filters. (Courtesy of Varian Medical Systems UK Ltd.)

conical in section, being thick at the centre to reduce the intensity of the central axis beam and tapering to zero at the edges so as not to reduce the intensity of the peripheral beam. A different flattening filter is required for each photon beam energy. The distribution across the flattened beam should be such that within the central 80% of the width of the beam, the intensity does not vary by more than ±3% at d_{max}. The flatness, being dependent on the distribution of the scattered radiation, does vary with depth and any definition of flatness must specify a depth. At depths greater than that specified, the beam will be under-flattened, i.e. the central axis dose will be greater than the off-axis dose, whereas at lesser depths the reverse is true.

The dual dosimeter

Immediately beyond the flattening filter, i.e. nearer the patient, there will be an ionisation chamber whose primary function is to provide a measure of the integrated dose at the isocentre. In practice the chamber is quite complex. It may be sealed so that its response does not vary with the ambient conditions (p. 54) or it will be unsealed and temperature and pressure transducers will be used to correct the signal electronically. For dual modality accelerators, the electrodes will be sufficiently thin to minimise the energy loss and attenuation of the electron beam. The regulations on *dual dosimetry* system require two independent chambers feeding signals to two independent integrating dosimeters—each capable of terminating the exposure at the selected preset level, or of continuing to count up should the exposure termination circuit fail. They are to be independent in the sense that any failure of either circuit must not affect the operation of the other. In addition, the chamber will give a measure of dose rate. Where very short exposures are given, for example where field weighting factors are used or hyperfractionation is practised, both the linearity of the dosimetry system and the initial stability of the beam must be checked thoroughly—the latter can be checked using the technique used to measure timer error (p. 56).

Other segmented sections of the chamber will provide signals to monitor parameters such as beam symmetry and, via a servo-system, correct the beam operating parameters.

Although the X-radiation from a linear accelerator is pulsed at between 100 and 500 pulses per second (the prf or *pulse repetition frequency*), the average dose rate of the flattened beam may be several gray per minute at 1 metre from the target. Each pulse lasts about 2 microseconds. The final output dose rate is determined by the gun filament temperature and the pulse rate and tuning to the optimum radiofrequency.

Nearer the patient again will be the light beam diaphragm system (p. 170), the adjustable collimators (p. 168), provision for the insertion of wedge filters (p. 205), tissue compensators (p. 203) and local shielding blocks (p. 172) and facilities for attaching beam-direction devices (p. 174).

Leakage radiation

The unwanted radiation, i.e. that emitted in directions other than the useful beam, will be reduced by the addition of lead or some other heavy metal around the X-ray head and as close to the target as possible. (Where the protective material used to reduce this leakage radiation is depleted uranium, this will require registration under The Radioactive Substances Act of 1993 (RSA 1993).) The permitted radiation leakage through the housing of the linear accelerator is quoted as a percentage of the useful beam dose rate at 1 metre from the target, and is divided into several components. At a distance of 1 metre from any point along the flight of the electrons—from gun to target—the leakage dose rate shall not exceed 0.5%. Over a 2-metre radius, measured from the normal treating distance and at right angles to the beam axis, the leakage dose rate shall not exceed 0.2% except within the central area defined by the primary beam collimator. Again at the normal treating distance and at right angles to the beam axis, the area within the primary beam collimator but outside the useful beam, the transmission of the primary beam through the secondary (adjustable) collimators shall not exceed the values in Table 10.1.

At energies above 10 MV, where neutron activation may occur, the permissible leakage of neutron radiation at 1 metre from the electron beam and over the 2-metre radius beyond the limits of the primary collimator, is limited to 0.05%. Maintenance staff working on these machines are advised to have a radiation monitor available to check for hazards which may result from residual neutron activation of the X-ray target and collimators after the exposure has been terminated. Any such activation is likely to fall within the provisions of The Radioactive Substances (Testing Instruments) Exemption Order 1985 (RSEO 1985).

Conversion to the electron beam modality

The dual modality linear accelerator is designed for both photon and electron therapy. The conversion from the photon mode to the electron mode requires changes in the operation of the accelerator. The X-ray target is replaced by a thin window. A scattering foil, to disperse the finely focused electron beam, replaces the flattening filter. The electron gun temperature is reduced to lower the beam current and this in turn may require adjustments to the steering and focusing magnetic fields along the waveguide. Most of these adjustments will be made automatically when the modality switch is changed, but each of these mechanical and electrical changes will be selected and independently confirmed before the beam can be energised. The adjustable X-ray diaphragms will need to be opened wide unless they are required at particular settings for use in conjunction with the interchangeable electron beam collimators (p. 169). Any material, particularly metals, in the electron beam will generate X-rays. The X-ray contamination of an electron beam should not contribute more than 1% per 5 MeV of beam energy of the total electron dose delivered (p. 221).

The control panel

The control panel of the linear accelerator may be of the traditional type with a range of indicators, switches

Table 10.1 Maximum permitted leakage radiation through beam-limiting diaphragms

Maximum field size (cm)	20 × 20	30 × 30	40 × 40	50 × 50
Permitted transmission	2.0%	1.1%	0.6%	0.4%

and meters or a video display and keyboard backed by a microprocessor. Whichever type is used, the control panel must clearly show the beam modality, photons or electrons, and their energy. There must be a means of presetting the dose to be delivered and the expected treatment time. In conjunction with these there will be two independent displays of the dose given and the elapsed treatment time—any one of these three displays being capable of terminating the exposure on reaching its preset value, or on developing a fault in its circuitry. Any changeable (wedge) filters or scattering foils will be interlocked and identified on the control panel. Beam on/off controls will be clearly identified. In addition to these basic requirements the control panel may display any number of parameters relating to the running conditions of the accelerator, the beam direction and couch position relating to the patient on treatment, and may identify the patient as well.

Select and confirm systems

Select and confirm systems should be incorporated in the design of the equipment so that any selection made on the controls is independently confirmed before the beam can be energised—for example, a change in photon energy will require a change of flattening filter; the selection will cause the change, the confirmation signal will not be given unless that change has been implemented and the new filter is correctly located.

Likewise, where a microprocessor is used to confirm the treatment set-up, the patient's ID will automatically select a range of treatment parameters. The system will compare or display any serious discrepancies between the parameters on file and those set on the patient, for example the orientation of a rectangular field, to draw the radiographer's attention to the error. In some situations, the system will prevent treatment being given until the discrepancy is put right or reduced to an acceptable level. Only selected senior staff should be authorised to override such a discrepancy. The patient identification may be a punched card, bar code or magnetic strip, perhaps on the wrist band of the inpatient.

QUALITY INDEX OF THE X-RAY BEAM

The dose at a point within the patient depends on many factors:

- The ability of the primary radiation to penetrate the tissues
- The contribution made by the radiation scattered by the surrounding tissues
- The dose delivered to the surface (or just below the surface) of the tissues.

Table 10.2 Typical values of quality index

Energy	SSD	Quality index
Cobalt-60	80	0.57
4 MV	100	0.58
6 MV	100	0.65
8 MV	100	0.68
10 MV	100	0.75

The penetrating ability of the primary radiation is referred to as the beam quality. The beam quality of an X-ray beam generated at less than one million volts is stated in terms of the HVL and either the generating voltage (kVp) or the homogeneity coefficient (p. 153). Above one million volts, the statement of the X-ray beam energy in MV used to be considered adequate, but there is an increasing interest in a specification in terms of a *quality index* defined in a $10 \times 10\ cm^2$ field at 100 cm source–chamber distance where:

$$\text{Quality index} = \frac{\text{Ionisation measured at a depth of 20 cm } (J_{20})}{\text{Ionisation measured at a depth of 10 cm } (J_{10}) \text{ at the same source–chamber distance}}$$

The measurements are most easily made in a horizontal beam by mounting the ionisation chamber at 10 cm deep in the water phantom and adding/removing 10 cm of solid water material to/from the entry wall of the phantom, or in a vertical beam and adding/removing 10 cm depth of water. Typical values of quality index are given in Table 10.2. In the case of gamma ray beams the isotope and its mass number are normally adequate although the quality index may be specified for comparison purposes.

BEAM COLLIMATION

In general terms, beam collimation means the limiting of the spread of the radiation to a predetermined direction and solid angle. In practical radiotherapy it is necessary to be able to vary the size of the beam to suit the needs of each patient. This is referred to as field size or beam size. The collimation system can be divided into primary collimation and secondary collimation.

Primary collimation

Primary collimation is achieved by a conical hole in a suitably thick metal block close to the source of radiation.

The axis of the hole defines the beam axis and should pass through the centre of the X-ray target and the isocentre. It also defines the maximum divergence of the beam and, therefore, the maximum field size at the specified treatment distance. If this primary collimator is circular then the larger square fields defined by the secondary collimators, which may be 40 × 40 cm or 50 × 50 cm, will usually have rounded corners.

Secondary collimation

Having defined the overall maximum field size and the beam direction, the secondary collimation provides a means of adjusting the field size to suit the particular requirements and the means of rotating square and rectangular fields about the beam axis.

Interchangeable applicators

A selection of, say, six open-ended applicators are invariably used in electron therapy. Their design may be similar to that in Figure 9.10A, namely a remote diaphragm limits the electron beam to a size only marginally larger than the aperture in contact with the patient. The size of the margin is critical to the uniformity of the beam profile. Electrons striking the inner surface of the applicator wall will be scattered back into the beam and ideally boost the dose delivered to the edge of the field to the level on the beam axis; too many or too few contributing to a non-uniformity at the edge. Alternatively, the electron beam will be collimated through a series of apertures mounted on an otherwise open frame (Fig. 10.7). The final beam is shaped by a cut-out cast into low-melting-point alloy inserted into the end of the applicator.

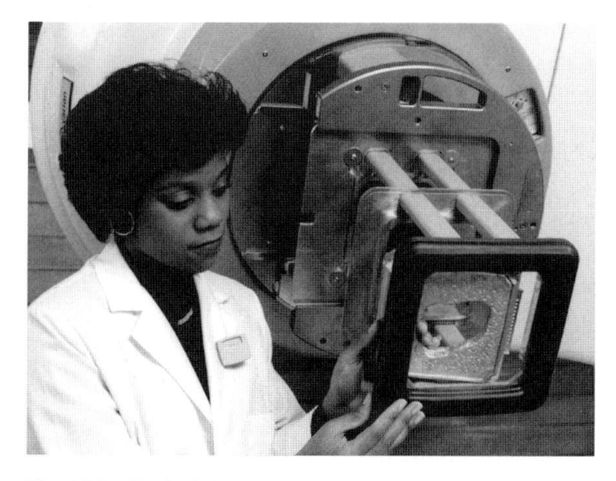

Fig. 10.7 Typical electron beam applicator. (Courtesy of Varian Medical Systems UK Ltd.)

Adjustable diaphragms

Adjustable diaphragms are used for megavoltage units as the penetrating photon radiation requires a large thickness of a heavy metal to reduce the transmitted intensity to less than the permitted maximum (Table 10.1). In addition, the high-energy radiation produces in the diaphragms secondary electrons which have a considerable range in air and so, if the diaphragms were close to the skin, these electrons would contribute to the skin dose, negating one principal advantage of megavoltage radiation—the skin-sparing or build-up effect (p. 197). The optimum diaphragm–skin distance is based on the consideration of skin dose and penumbra width and should not be less than 20 cm, but the precise value depends on the beam energy and the design of the unit. In practice, the diaphragms are approximately half way between the source of radiation and the patient and may have a transparent electron filter over the aperture.

The adjustable diaphragms in common use limit the choice of field shape to squares and rectangles within the overall circle defined by the primary collimator and consist of two pairs of parallel collimating blades, one pair closer to the target, the other closer to the patient (Fig. 10.8A). In general, each pair of blades are symmetrically placed about the beam axis and should be parallel to an accuracy of ±1°, and at right angles to the second pair, again to an accuracy of ±1°. This double plane system has the clear disadvantage in that the collimated length of the two pairs of blades—which may be 10–12 cm thick—is very different, giving rise to different geometric penumbra widths on the two principal axes of the beam.

To minimise the size of the penumbra (p. 171), the collimating faces of the thick diaphragm blades are made to move in such a way that they always lie along the direction of propagation of the radiation from the target, i.e. along a radius from the source, and the collimated length—the distance from the source to the distal part of the diaphragm blade—is made as large as possible. A compromise has to be reached between the collimated length and the range of the secondary electrons from the diaphragm blades. The field or beam size is simply defined by its two dimensions (p. 200) and there may be a locally agreed convention about the orientation of rectangular fields, e.g. the cephalocaudal dimension is always quoted first and underlined—$\underline{H} \times W$.

In asymmetric mode, each of the four blades may be moved independently of the other three, creating

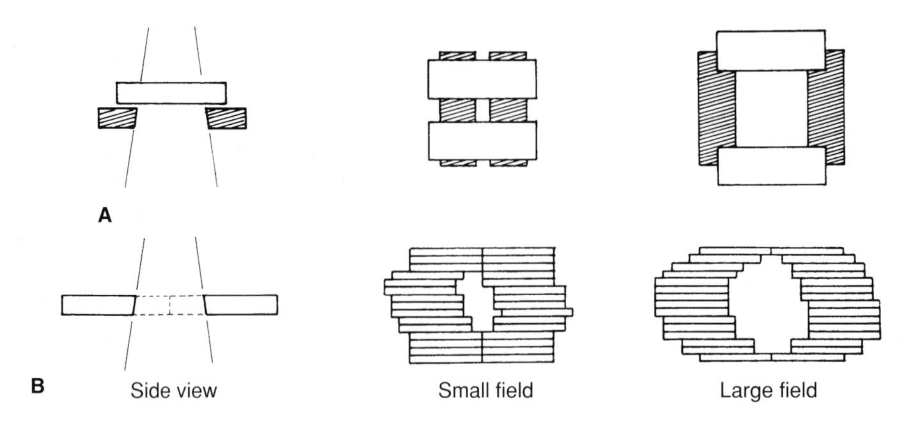

Fig. 10.8 Adjustable diaphragm systems modified: **A** double plane; **B** multileaf.

asymmetric fields which may or may not contain the mechanical beam axis. The design and accuracy of the blades is the same as for the symmetric mode, but the size of the field must now be defined by four parameters, each defining the distance of the edge of the beam from the mechanical beam axis and using a negative sign where the blade crosses over that beam axis. For many treatment techniques, asymmetric control is only needed on one pair of collimator blades but to have the facility on only one pair may prove restrictive where the wedge orientation is restricted to one pair of collimators.

Multileaf collimators

Multileaf collimators may replace the adjustable diaphragms or may be an accessory used in conjunction with the adjustable diaphragms. A multileaf collimator system consists of two coplanar sets of blades, each blade capable of moving parallel to, but independently of, the other set. Each set may consist of, say, 26 or more blades, each blade presenting a 1 cm shadow at the normal treating distance. Larger systems (80 or 120 blades) are also available where several blade widths are incorporated so that small fields may be more accurately defined by narrower (½ cm) blades than those used to define outer edges of larger fields. Multileaf systems can offer square or rectangular fields, while almost any other shape of field can be approximated within the limitations of the blade width, thereby reducing the dose to the healthy tissues otherwise exposed in the corners of a circumscribed square or rectangular field (Fig. 10.8B). The system is microprocessor controlled and the preset position of each blade, based on the planned treatment volume (PTV) as defined by the treatment planning computer, may be logged into the patient's record and called up and set each day of treatment. The size and shape of the field is displayed on a monitor on the control desk and ideally confirmed by portal imaging (p. 109).

To enable each blade to move independently of its two neighbours, there will inevitably be a small gap between them and a potential path for radiation to 'leak' through, particularly where that gap is close to the principal axis of the field and therefore 'radial' from the source. With wear and tear, this leakage may increase with time and must be subjected to quality assurance checks. Where the multileaf collimator can be used in conjunction with the adjustable diaphragms, closing the latter to the smallest circumscribed rectangle will restrict any gap leakage to within that rectangle.

Light beam diaphragm

Since the collimating system is some distance from the patient, a light beam is incorporated into the unit to indicate the area covered by the radiation. The light beam (Fig. 10.9) is provided by a small filament lamp or fibreoptic positioned in such a way that its virtual image is coincident with the source of X-rays. In this way, the visible light is seen to emanate from the same source as the radiation beam and, therefore, illuminates the area irradiated as defined by the diaphragm system. A thin surface-silvered mirror does not appreciably affect the photon beam. A specially constructed mirror is, however, required if it is to be used in conjunction with an electron beam. A suitable cross-hair 'object' is incorporated to produce an 'image' on the patient identifying the principal axes of the beam and their intersection on the beam axis. A simple optical pointer may project an illuminated scale on which the

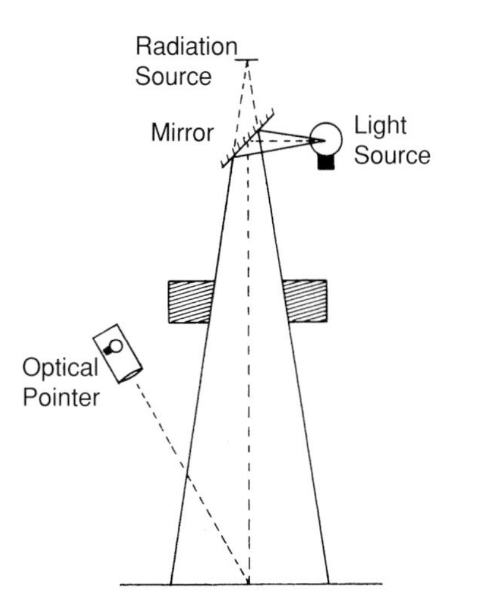

Fig. 10.9 The principle of the light beam diaphragm and optical front pointer—for simplicity, the projected SSD scale is not shown.

SSD may be read at the point indicated by the beam axis.

Periodic checks are carried out to confirm the accuracy of the light beam and the adjustable diaphragm system. First, a reference mark—a cross on a piece of paper—is attached firmly to the couch at the isocentre. The cross is aligned to the beam axis as delineated by the light beam. Rotating the diaphragm should not cause any deviation of greater than 2 mm. Second, check with a ruler that the light beam delineated correlates correctly with the set field size at the normal SSD. Then, using film or radiation-sensitive paper and radio-opaque corner markers check the optical/photon alignment by making an appropriate exposure with a minimum of back-scattering material. The setting-up is simplified if the corner markers are incorporated into one surface of a piece of Perspex, say, 12 mm thick. The markers are then in close contact with the film and the Perspex provides the necessary build-up. This test should be repeated over a range of field sizes. Close examination of the films should confirm the coincidence of all four corner markers, the orthogonality of adjacent and the parallelism of opposing diaphragms. The light beam gives a sharp image of the beam edge and can be misleading as the photon beam will have a penumbra edge of finite size—the corner markers will be seen within this penumbra edge.

Penumbra

If the source of radiation in the therapy unit were a point source, the precise direction of the radiation would be known and the size of the beam would be uniquely defined. In practice it is not a point source. The X-rays may emanate from a small area on the target, typically 3–5 mm on a linear accelerator. Gamma rays, on the other hand, emanate from all points within a finite cylindrical source of, say, 17 mm diameter and 25 mm long. This presents a problem. In Figure 10.10A the point marked A is in the beam of radiation and point B is outside the beam. In Figure 10.10B this is also true, but point C is neither inside nor outside the beam, it is said to lie in the *geometric penumbra*. It is in a region where it can receive radiation from some parts of the source but not from the whole source. In the case of a point source, the dose gradient between points A and B is sheer, while in the case of a finite source, the dose gradient is gradual and depends principally on the size of the source. Applying the principle of similar triangles to Figure 10.10B, the geometric penumbra, p, is defined by:

$$p = s\,(f - c)/c$$

where s is the diameter of the source, f the source–skin distance and c the collimated length. The geometric penumbra is independent of field size. It is easy to see from the equation above that to reduce the size of the geometric penumbra, the source diameter must be reduced ($s = 0$ for a point source) or the collimated length, c, must be increased and made more nearly

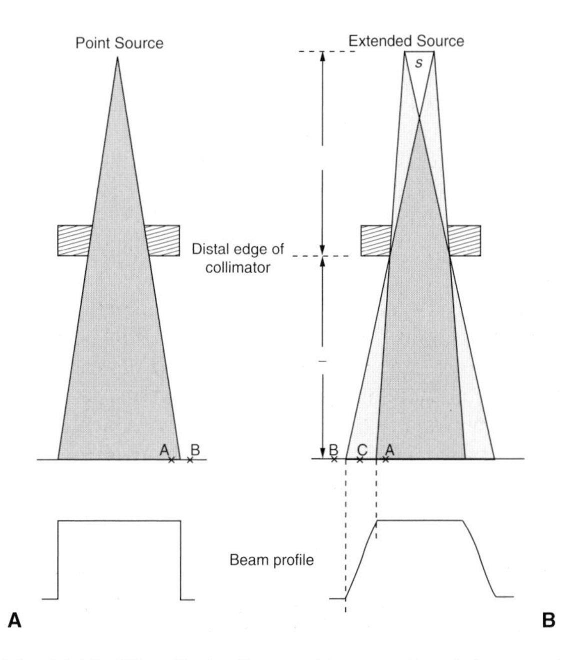

Fig. 10.10 The effects of geometric penumbra: **A** from a point source and **B** from a finite source.

equal to the source–skin distance, f. It should be noted that the geometric penumbra rapidly increases with the source–skin distance, being proportional to $(f - c)$. The collimated length, c, is measured to the distal edge of the diaphragm blade from the source.

By changing the angle of the collimator face as the field size is changed, the face can be maintained parallel to the rays from a point source, thereby presenting the full thickness of the blade to the rays to be absorbed. Because the source will be of finite size, there will always be some rays that will traverse less than the full thickness of the collimator blade and will give rise to a further blurring of the edge of the beam which is referred to as *transmission penumbra*. The combined geometric and transmission penumbra width can be estimated by reducing the collimated length, c, in the above formula to $(c - t)$, where t is the thickness of the diaphragm or by redefining the collimated length to the proximal edge of the collimator.

Beam shaping and local shielding blocks

Unless a multileaf diaphragm system is available, any modification to the shape of the otherwise square or rectangular field must be achieved by the addition of heavy metal blocks (of lead, tungsten or one of the low-melting-point alloys). Areas in the centre of the field may be protected in a similar manner. The thickness of the blocks will be determined by the degree of protection required, but will be at least 6 cm lead equivalent or 4 HVLs. The dose in the shadow of the block will be increased by the scatter from the adjacent irradiated tissues, with the result that to reduce that dose to much less than 10% is difficult (Fig. 10.11).

These blocks may be suspended from the front of the unit or mounted above or below a *shadow tray* similarly suspended. Alternatively, they can be supported on a table over the patient but the blocks will be larger and heavier. The weight of these blocks is of serious concern to the safety of both staff and patient and some mechanical lifting device should be employed. The shadow tray or table may be a sheet of Perspex or a perforated aluminium plate. The actual means of suspension adopted must be decided from a consideration of the penumbra width and the electron contamination. Minimal penumbra and therefore accurate shielding requires the blocks to be close to the patient. On the other hand, electron contamination requires the blocks to be distant from the patient. The electron contamination can be reduced by fitting each block with a material which will absorb these secondary electrons and which will not itself produce additional contaminating electrons. Brass is often used both as a filter and a means of protecting lead blocks from physical damage—lead is soft and easily distorted if accidentally dropped. Brass has the further advantage that it can be tapped to accept fixing screws through a perforated shadow tray so that the blocks can be fixed in position for use when the beam axis is not vertical. Blocks of complex shape, e.g. for mantle treatments (p. 216), may themselves be attached to a Perspex plate which can carry marks to aid its alignment in the light beam.

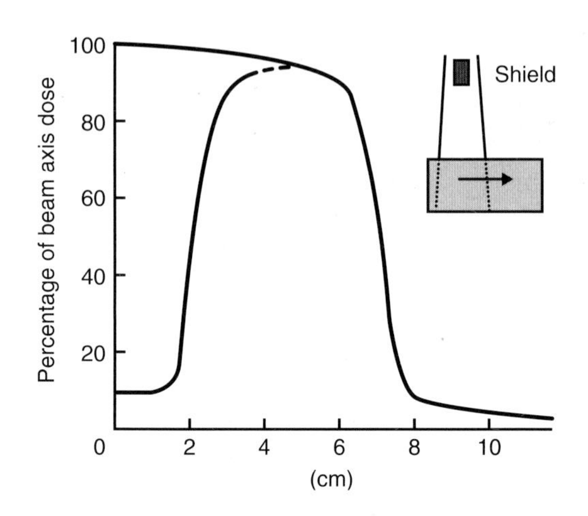

Fig. 10.11 The dose profile under a local shielding block.

Lead shielding blocks intended for general use are often rectangular in section with the (collimating) faces parallel to the beam axis and not to the radiation they are intended to absorb. These give rise to the maximum transmission penumbra and, therefore, a poor X-ray shadow. Wherever possible the blocks should be tapered to minimise the transmission penumbra effect (Fig. 10.12).

Low-melting-point alloys of lead, bismuth and cadmium are readily available and enable shielding blocks to be tailor-made to the patients' individual requirements and later melted down and recycled. The density and atomic number of the alloy, about 9.7 g cm^{-3} and 75 respectively, are less than those of lead, 11.4 g cm^{-3} and 82, and therefore, the blocks need to be proportionately thicker, 8 or 10 cm. The simplicity of manufacture and the accurate shaping (in all three planes) far outweigh the problem of thickness.

To tailor-make shielding blocks

One method used to tailor shielding blocks is as follows:

- A radiograph is taken using the simulator so that the SSD and field size match those to be used during treatment.

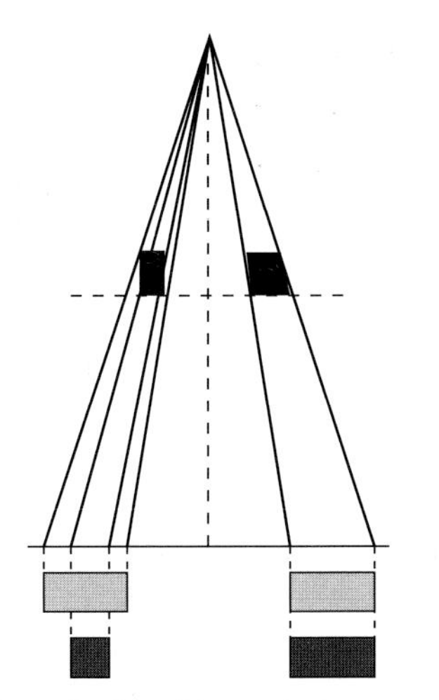

Fig. 10.12 The reduction of transmission penumbra by the use of tapered (tailor-made) shielding blocks.

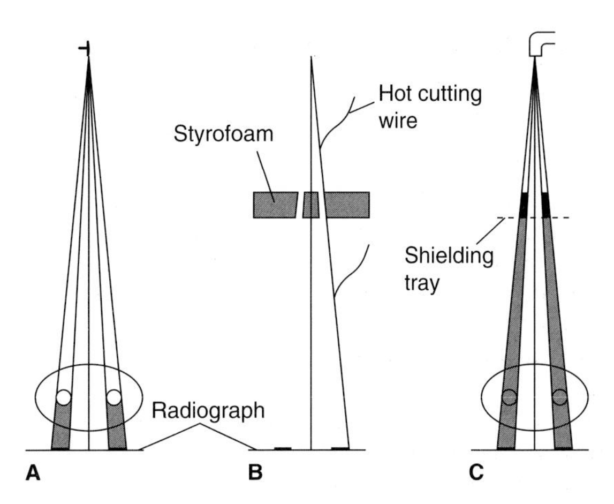

Fig. 10.13 The making of tailor-made shielding blocks. **A** Patient radiographed on simulator under treatment geometry. **B** The cast cut to shape using the hot wire and marked-up radiograph. **C** Patient treated using the cast shielding blocks.

- The area to be shielded and the beam axis are marked carefully on the film (Figs 10.13A and 10.14). The pattern on the film is then used in conjunction with the hot wire to cut a hole in the styrofoam (Fig. 10.13B) using the focal–film distance from the simulator and the source-shielding tray distance from the treatment unit.
- The styrofoam is then used directly as a cast for the low-melting-point alloy. The cooling rate of the alloy needs to be carefully controlled to minimise the risk of cavitation—the formation of cavities as the apparently solid material shrinks. The blocks then produce the precise shadows to protect the areas originally marked on the film (Figs 10.13C and 10.14).

Low-melting-point alloy can be recycled many times, but eventually its melting point rises as the balance of metals in the alloy is disturbed. The alloy can, however, be replenished by adding the lost component to the molten alloy. Providing the alloy is never overheated and is handled according to the manufacturer's instructions, it is not considered a health hazard, although protective gloves are often advised. New alloy should be checked for radioactivity as the bismuth may contain isotopes from the radium decay scheme (p. 30).

BEAM DIRECTION DEVICES

All the radiation treatment planning and the immobilisation of the patient is of little value unless the day-to-day treatment beams can be set up accurately on the patient. This requires that the treatment unit and

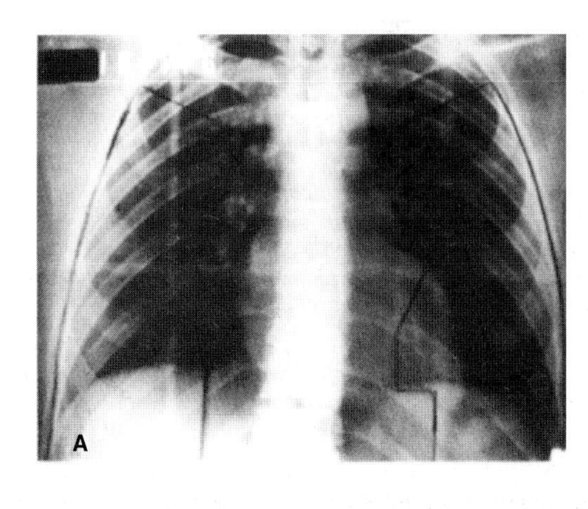

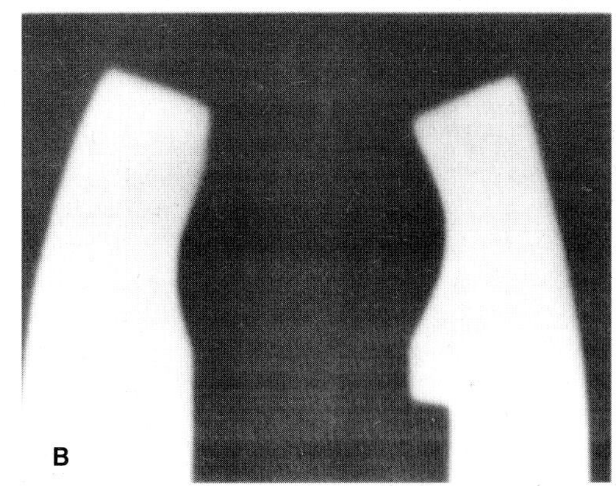

Fig. 10.14 Planning film: **A** from the simulator used in the preparation of tailored shielding blocks and the check film and **B** on the linear accelerator confirms their accuracy.

the patient are correctly aligned for each radiation field. In simple terms, beam direction devices are those which:

- define the beam direction
- centre the beam axis
- set the source–skin distance

and thereby enable the radiation treatment plan parameters to be reproduced on the treatment unit. The simplest and most widely used devices are the front and back pointers.

Front and back pointers

Mechanical front and back pointers are mounted on the unit in such a way that they lie and move along the beam axis (Fig. 10.15), the front pointer being calibrated to show the distance between its tip and the source of radiation, the SSD; the back pointer may be scaled to show the distance of its tip from the isocentre.

In use, the front pointer is set to the normal treating distance and the patient positioned so that the entry point (of the beam axis) on the patient coincides with the tip of the pointer. The gantry angle and the couch rotation are then adjusted until the back pointer coincides with the exit point. If the entry point is not at the isocentre, some further adjustments to the couch will be necessary. The entry and exit points must be clearly marked on the patient's skin or immobilisation device. The pointers must be removed before the beam is switched on.

The mechanical front pointer may be replaced by a light pointer system. Similarly back pointers have been replaced by other devices, too numerous to mention, but which fulfil the same purpose, namely to define the direction of the beam in relation to the entry point on the patient. A *laser back pointer* is a bit of a misnomer. It is mounted in the counterbalance of the gantry and projects a sheet of laser light, which contains both the axis of rotation of the gantry and the axis of rotation of the diaphragm system. In practice therefore, it projects onto the patient a line which, somewhere along its length, intersects with the beam axis. The beam direction is therefore correct when that line passes through the beam exit mark on the patient (assuming the front pointer is correctly centred).

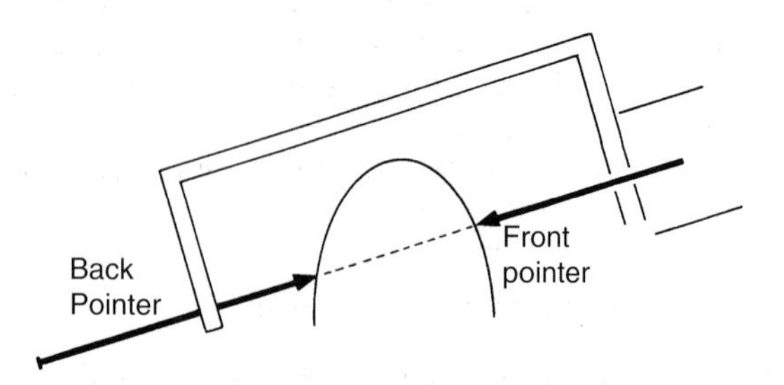

Fig. 10.15 The principle of the front and back pointer.

Quality assurance checks

The accuracy of any pointer system needs to be checked periodically. In this case, this is done by rigidly mounting a reference marker, say on the couch, such that it coincides with the tip of the pointer to be checked. On rotating the beam diaphragm system about the beam axis, the tip of the pointer should not deviate from the reference marker by more than 1 millimetre. This check should be repeated with the pointer set at several positions along its length and at several gantry angles. The same tests should be applied to the back pointer bearing in mind it will be used over a wider range of distances from the isocentre. The back pointer mounting is susceptible to mechanical misalignment and needs to be checked carefully.

Isocentric gantry

Reference has already been made to the isocentric gantry but its description is included here for it is essentially a beam-direction facility. The *isocentric gantry* has three principal axes of rotation:

- the beam axis or axis of rotation of the diaphragm system
- the horizontal axis of rotation of the gantry
- the vertical axis of rotation of the couch.

These three axes of rotation intersect at a point called the *isocentre* (Fig. 10.16). The position of this point in space may also be identified by two or three lasers mounted on the side walls of the treatment room and high on the wall opposite the gantry. The two side lasers each project two intersecting sheets of light to define a horizontal line across the room at right angles to the gantry axis, each passing through the isocentre and the lens of the opposing laser. The third, sagittal laser, projects a single sheet of light vertically through the isocentre and containing the gantry and couch rotation axes. The sagittal laser therefore identifies the position of the isocentre along the horizontal line defined by the two side lasers. Furthermore, the sagittal laser greatly assists in getting the patient straight on the couch and, if appropriate, centring the patient's midline on the isocentre.

The value of the isocentric gantry lies in the fact that in setting up the patient a rotation about any of these

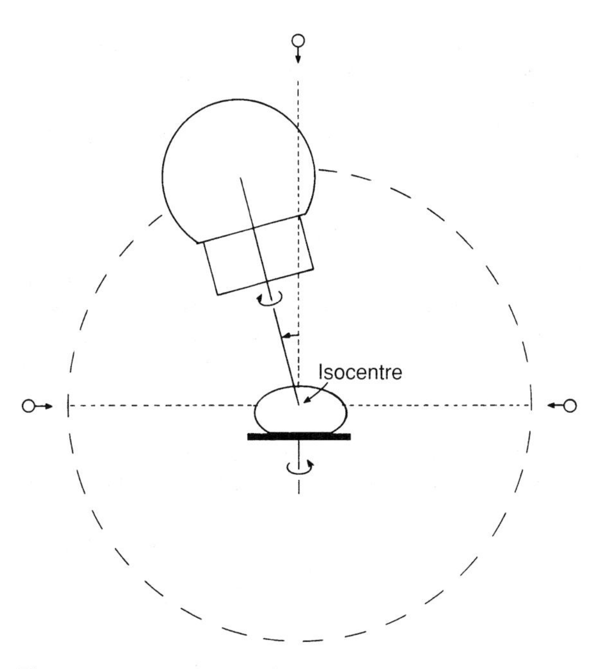

Fig. 10.16 The principle of the isocentric gantry.

three axes can be carried out knowing that the position of the isocentre is not altered. In practice, this is a considerable help whether the patient is being treated with the isocentre on the skin or inside the lesion.

To set up to a skin mark

Using the optical or mechanical front pointer the skin mark is positioned at the isocentre using the linear movements of the couch, i.e. couch height, lateral and longitudinal movements. This fixes the source–skin distance. The beam direction is then set using the rotational movements, i.e. gantry and couch rotations to the specified angles or until the back pointer locates the beam exit mark. The diaphragm rotation completes the set-up. Do not use the linear movements after the entry mark has been set up. It is easy to remember: linear movements set the entry point, rotation movements set the exit point.

To set up to a point inside the patient

At the planning stage the intersection of the beam axes is located as being at a depth, d cm, vertically below an appropriate skin mark. The front pointer is set at the source–axis distance less the value of d. With the beam axis vertical, the pointer and the skin mark are brought together using the linear movements as before, so positioning the planned intersection of the beam axes at the isocentre. The patient couch is now rotated to align lateral skin marks with the side lasers or to define the plane containing the planned beam axes. The gantry and diaphragm rotations can now be set for each field in turn. Once the patient has been positioned, there is no need to move the patient or the couch between the treatment of different fields.

Quality assurance checks

The isocentre is defined as a point, whereas, because of mechanical tolerances and the effects of gravity, it is usually a small sphere or ellipsoid having a maximum diameter of less than 2 mm. Its accuracy is most readily checked by setting up reference pointers to check each of the three rotations in turn as follows. Fix a mechanical front pointer to the X-ray head with its tip at the isocentre and a reference pointer horizontally and overhanging the end of the couch, again with its tip at the isocentre. With the beam axis vertical, rotate the couch between its two extremes of movement, measuring the deviation from the front pointer; then repeat the procedure fixing the couch and rotating the gantry. Once that has been completed, repeat the procedure again, but this time measuring the deviation of the front pointer from the couch pointer on rotation of the diaphragms at selected gantry angles. This is a purely mechanical check because the isocentre is mechanically defined; the check on the couch rotation is more realistic if the couch is loaded with a distributed weight of 135 kg.

Finally, a word of warning. The rotational movements referred to above are those about the principal axes which define the isocentre. The unit may have other rotational facilities, one being the rotation of the couch about an eccentric support. To avoid confusion, this rotation should be positively locked into its central position whenever it is not being used.

CALIBRATION OF OUTPUT DOSE RATE

For each generator and for each beam quality, a *definitive* calibration must be carried out as a part of the commissioning procedure or following any major repair or modification which might affect the output beam (IPSM 1992). A definitive calibration must be derived from two independent sets of measurements based on two different instruments carried out by two physicists experienced in radiotherapy physics. (The two instruments may be calibrated against the same secondary standard (p. 59).)

Megavoltage photon beams

A water phantom of adequate size, at least $20 \times 20 \times 12$ cm^3 is used such that the *field* ionisation chamber is positioned with its centre at the prescribed depth (Table 5.2) below one of the larger faces and with at least 5 cm to the exit surface. The face of the phantom is centred at the normal treating distance with the ionisation chamber on the central axis (Fig. 10.17) in a 10×10^2 cm field. The chamber is in its close-fitting Perspex sheath. The chamber is then exposed for a typical treatment time or for a known number of monitor units on the integrating dosimetry system, say 2–3 Gy. As before, several readings are taken and the average reading, M_f, corrected using the air mass correction factor based on the atmospheric pressure and the temperature of the phantom—if that is likely to be different from the ambient temperature of the room (p. 54). The percentage depth dose (PDD) factor corrects the measured value to d_{max} without the need for inverse square or back scatter factors. The dose, D, to a point at d_{max} on the central axis will then be given by:

$$D = N_{Df}\, M_f\, 100/\text{PDD}$$

and should be within ±1% of the monitor units set for the reference field size. For the derivation of N_{Df}, see page 59. If the calibration is based on time, the dose, D, divided by the time (corrected for any timer error, will give the dose rate. This calibration should be repeated at least once a week and ideally every day. Unless the calibration is repeated daily, then a daily consistency check should be instituted using a protocol which includes tolerance levels outside which specified action should be taken.

Output factors

The routine output dose rate measurements are made using a reference field size (usually 10×10 cm^2). At the initial calibration of the unit, and at regular intervals

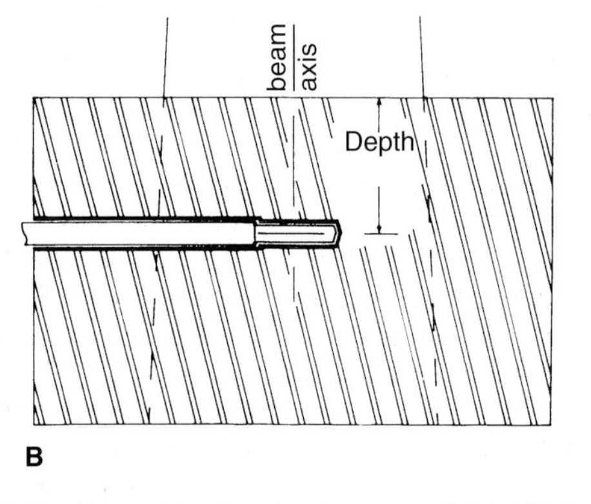

Fig. 10.17 The calibration phantom—see Table 5.2 for the value of d.

thereafter, the output dose rate will be measured for all field sizes which will be encountered in the clinical use of the unit and output factors tabulated for the (equivalent) square fields. This variation in output dose rate is principally due to the increase in scattered radiation with field size. The output factor is unity for the reference field size and, for other field sizes, the output factor is defined as:

$$OF_S = \frac{\text{Output dose rate for field size, } S}{\text{Output dose rate for the reference field size}}$$

The measurements should be made in a water phantom at least 10 cm larger than the maximum nominal field size being measured. Output factors may be used alongside a table of equivalent squares (or diameters) (Table 12.4) to determine the monitor units required to deliver the prescribed dose to any other field size available on the generator.

Electron beams

The electron beams used clinically should be calibrated every day or at least twice a week using the calibrated parallel-plate chamber set at d_{max} in a water phantom of adequate size—the thickness should be sufficient to stop all the electrons within the phantom. It is common practice to take a further measurement at depth, at say $d_{50\%}$, to confirm the energy of the electron beam. If a solid water-equivalent phantom is used, it should be made up of loose sheets to minimise the risk of electric charge building up and invalidating the measurements. As explained in Chapter 5, the reader is referred to the definitive protocol (IPEMB 1996a) as the conversion from $N_{D,air,c}$ to dose-to-water, D, is too dependent on the choice of chamber to elaborate here.

COMMISSIONING NEW EQUIPMENT

Acceptance tests

New radiotherapy equipment should only be ordered after close scrutiny of the manufacturer's technical specification and discussion about the customer's particular requirements. Compliance with local, national or international requirements should not be assumed (e.g. the international convention on the movement scales is not universally accepted). After the equipment has been ordered and delivered, it will be installed by the manufacturers or their agents, but before it is accepted the customer's Medical Physicist should ensure the installation complies with the previously agreed specification. The acceptance tests may take a week, more for very complex equipment.

The acceptance tests will therefore be designed to demonstrate that the details of the agreed specification have been satisfied—in five main areas:

- The radiotherapy beams—each beam energy and beam modality—are of the specified quality, intensity and range of sizes and can be controlled and monitored in the specified manner. Wedges, filters, applicators, etc. must be interlocked.
- All the movements of the gantry, collimators and couch cover the specified range and that the brakes operate effectively throughout the range of movement. Where motorised movements are involved, the speed and control must be checked. The accuracy of the isocentre must be checked.
- All the electrical aspects of the equipment must be checked for safety—the connections to earth, the operation of limit switches, interlocks, built-in safety circuits, particularly where the equipment could malfunction and where maintenance staff may be put at risk. The consequences of a mains supply failure must be demonstrated.
- The radiation safety requirements must be met—leakage radiation levels from the tube/source housing, collimator transmission, beam dosimetry and control etc. The installer will have had the adequacy of the structural shielding checked at an early stage, but checks should be made on other aspects such as door interlocks and warning signs (unless the manufacturer has supplied and fitted these, he will not accept sole responsibility).
- The inventory of the accessories, spare parts, instruction and maintenance manuals, circuit diagrams and safety manuals, etc.

A careful record of all these checks and operating parameters must be kept for future reference.

Equipment peripheral to the radiotherapy equipment, e.g. the closed-circuit television viewing system, intercom, lasers etc., may or may not be the responsibility of the supplier of the therapy equipment. The structural work on the treatment and control rooms will be the subject of a separate contract.

Commissioning tests

Once new equipment has been accepted then the customer will repeat most of the checks listed above with a view to making detailed measurements to ensure the equipment can be used safely to treat patients. This commissioning of the equipment could take several weeks and will be the responsibility of a competent and experienced Medical Physicist. It will include:

- Full radiation protection survey of the treatment room and adjacent areas—not forgetting above and below—to ensure the requirements of the safety legislation are satisfied within the accepted use of the equipment. Any failure in structural protection may be difficult to correct at this stage and may impose limitations on the use of the equipment or the occupancy of the adjacent areas. This survey will include interlocks and warning signs and the systems for audiovisual contact with the patient during treatment.
- Full radiation protection survey of the equipment itself checking for leakage radiation levels when the beam is on. Further assessments will be necessary in the 'beam-off' mode of gamma ray beam units.
- Where an accelerator generates X-rays at greater than 10 MV, checks must be made of residual radiation from the short-lived isotopes produced by neutron activation both within the generator and within the structure of the treatment room.
- Confirmation of the accuracy of all the beam- direction devices, the collimators and the coincidence of the photon/electron beams with the mechanical/optical delineators, including the isocentre and sagittal projection lasers, if fitted.
- The measurement of depth dose, beam profiles and isodose chart data for all beam modalities in sufficient detail for the treatment planning of patients. The measurement of output factors, wedge and shadow tray correction factors, etc. to enable the correct correlation between monitor units and the delivered absorbed dose in grays.
- The output dose calibration over the full range of the dose monitor to check linearity and over the range of available dose rates to check saturation. To check all the facets of the double dosimetry system.

In addition to the commissioning work of the Medical Physicist, the Radiographers and the Mould Room staff will need to familiarise themselves with the equipment and with the accessories supplied—e.g. couch head rests—to assist with the setting-up of patients.

It is important that all the staff involved with the equipment are given time to become familiar with it before it is handed over for the treatment of patients. Radiographers need time to practice using the controls both inside and outside the room. Maintenance staff need time to study drawings and circuits and to locate principal components within the equipment—the simplest repair can take many hours if the technician does not know where to find the faulty component.

Quality assurance

Throughout the life of the equipment, probably 12–15 years, it is essential to ensure that the data collected during commissioning continue to be relevant, by monitoring the performance of the equipment through a programme of regular checks. These checks will take a variety of forms and be repeated at different intervals.

A separate fault book must be maintained by the radiographer (and other users) of all the faults which develop on each equipment—however trivial they may appear. This is important for two reasons. Where radiographers work in shifts on one piece of equipment or have duties that rotate through several pieces of equipment, no one person will remember all the quirks of that equipment. The written log will reveal the frequency at which faults occur, the dates on which major repairs have been undertaken and, over a period of time, trends will be detectable which may assist in the maintenance programme. The fault book records the random and intermittent events that inevitably occur. The quality control technician and the maintenance technician should examine the fault book regularly.

A planned quality assurance programme does not wait for faults to happen, but looks for consistency in general and thereby finds discrepancies before they manifest themselves as faults. The programme will usually consist of daily, weekly, monthly checks and 6-monthly or 12-monthly checks. The actual frequency of a particular check will be determined for each particular equipment. For example, it is mandatory that the calibration of the output dose (rate) of an accelerator is repeated at least weekly for photons and at least twice weekly for electrons. The procedure may be extended to placing a prescribed attenuator in the primary beam and taking a second measurement to confirm the beam quality—this may not be a precise measurement of quality index, but over a period of months the consistency of the result builds confidence in the equipment. Other beam parameters which should be included in the QA programme will include beam flatness and symmetry, wedge correction factors, photon/optical beam alignment and beam size indication—particularly where there are no mechanical indicators.

All the devices used for setting up a patient's treatment should be included in the programme. These will include the alignment of the lasers, optical and mechanical pointers, scales, rotations about the isocentre, the security and alignment of headrests, shadow trays, etc., the security of shielding blocks, wedges and other accessories.

It should not be necessary to check indicator lamps, because any failures should have been reported previously in the fault book and replaced. The operation of interlocks and limit switches should be included, particularly if they are rarely used in clinical practice. Quality assurance is a shared responsibility between radiographers, medical physicists and maintenance staff and close cooperation is essential.

The preventive maintenance inspection is a vital part of the overall quality assurance programme carried out by the maintenance technicians. The details need not concern the radiographer but will include checking water flows and air filters, tightness of electrical connections, cleanliness of insulators as well as the more intimate operation of the equipment itself.

The quality assurance programme is vital to any radiotherapy equipment and takes time to implement. How long depends on the complexity of the equipment. 15–20% of the machine time is typical for megavoltage therapy equipment. This investment in time does not preclude the possibility of breakdown but can minimise the unexpected interruptions to the treatment schedule.

In the event of an equipment malfunction, be it in the generator or in the dosimetry, causing an error of more than +20% of the intended dose fraction (or +10% of the total course dose), the incident must be reported to the Health and Safety Executive once an investigation has confirmed beyond reasonable doubt that an overexposure has occurred—guidance on the content of the investigation/report is given by the Health and Safety Executive (HSE 1998a). In the event of an underexposure of similar size, the employer should instigate an investigation but the incident is not notifiable to the HSE.

DESIGN OF MEGAVOLTAGE X-RAY BEAM THERAPY ROOMS

Adequate protection in a beam therapy room begins with the generator itself and the protective requirements of the equipment have been detailed elsewhere in this chapter.

Primary and secondary barriers

The walls of a megavoltage therapy room are frequently identified as primary barriers or secondary (or scatter) barriers (Stedeford et al 1997). The *primary* barrier is that part of the wall (and ceiling and floor) which may be irradiated by the primary beam, while those parts unlikely to be so irradiated are termed *secondary* or *scatter* barriers. The secondary (leakage) radiation from the X-ray head is limited to approximately 0.5% of the primary beam dose rate (p. 167), but of the peak photon energy. The scattered radiation comes from the patient and other material in the beam and will be lower in energy, depending on the angle of scatter, and of an intensity dependent on the angle, the area irradiated and, to a lesser extent, on the scattering material. For all megavoltage radiations, the 90° scatter has an energy of about 0.5 MeV and therefore the broad beam absorption data for 1 MV radiation may be used in calculations. Table 10.3 shows the energy of the scattered radiation for a range of primary photon energies and scattering angles calculated using the formula for Compton shift (p. 43). The primary barriers are typically about 6 or 7 TVLs thick, and the secondary barriers about 3 or 3½ TVLs, to bring the time-averaged dose rate outside the room down to a level consistent with the dose limit applicable to those not occupationally exposed.

For example, consider a 4 MV linear accelerator producing a primary beam dose rate of 1.6 Gy min^{-1} at 1 m SSD (Fig. 10.18). If a point 6.4 m from the focus is to be protected to reduce the dose rate to 0.3 mSv per year (0.3 mGy per year) when the beam-on time is expected to be no more than 2 hours per day, 5 days per week, then the barrier thickness may be calculated as follows:

Primary beam dose rate at 1 m

$$= 1.6 \times 2 \times 60 \times 5 \times 52 \text{ Gy/year}$$

Primary beam dose rate at 6.4 m

$$= \frac{1.6 \times 2 \times 60 \times 5 \times 52}{6.4 \times 6.4} \text{ Gy/year}$$

Primary beam dose rate at 6.4 m

$$= 1220 \text{ Gy/year}$$

Wall attenuation required

$$= 0.3 \text{ mGy}/1220 \text{ Gy} = 0.25 \times 10^{-6} = (1/2)^2 \times 10^{-6}$$

or = 6 TVL + 2 HVL

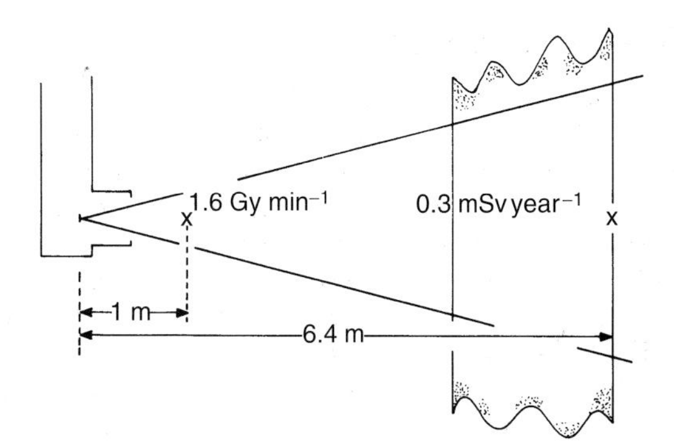

Fig. 10.18 The calculation of primary barrier thickness.

The data from Table 6.4 give 1 TVL = 275 mm and 1 HVL = 85 mm concrete, making this primary barrier 1.82 m thick. Under these conditions, the average dose rate at the point will be $1.6 \times 0.25 \times 10^{-6}/6.4^2$ Gy min^{-1} or 0.6 mGy h^{-1}.

Entrance maze

At megavoltage energies, protected doors are too heavy and are replaced by maze entrances, through which the scattered radiation is attenuated by multiple scattering and distance (Fig. 10.19). At the outer end of the maze—which should be in full view of the operator at the control desk—there must be an interlocked door or gate or a light beam sensor to terminate any exposure in progress should the barrier be broken. This door interlock should be a fail-safe device which can only be reset by the positive action of the operator at the control desk—when all but the patient have left the room.

All megavoltage X-ray therapy rooms will be controlled areas (p. 77) whenever the generator is

Table 10.3 The energy of scattered radiation

		Energy of primary photon (MeV), $h\nu$						
		0.26	0.51	1.02	2.56	5.11	10.22	25.55
$\alpha = h\nu/0.511 =$		0.5	1.0	2.0	5.0	10.0	20.0	50.0
Angle of scatter		Energy of scattered photon (MeV)						
ϕ	$1 - \cos\phi$	$h\nu/(1 + \alpha(1 - \cos\phi))$						
30	0.13	0.24	0.45	0.81	1.55	2.22	2.84	3.41
60	0.50	0.20	0.34	0.51	0.73	0.85	0.93	0.98
90	1.00	0.17	0.26	0.34	0.43	0.46	0.49	0.50
120	1.50	0.15	0.20	0.26	0.30	0.32	0.33	0.34
150	1.87	0.13	0.18	0.22	0.25	0.26	0.27	0.27
180	2.00	0.13	0.17	0.20	0.23	0.24	0.25	0.25

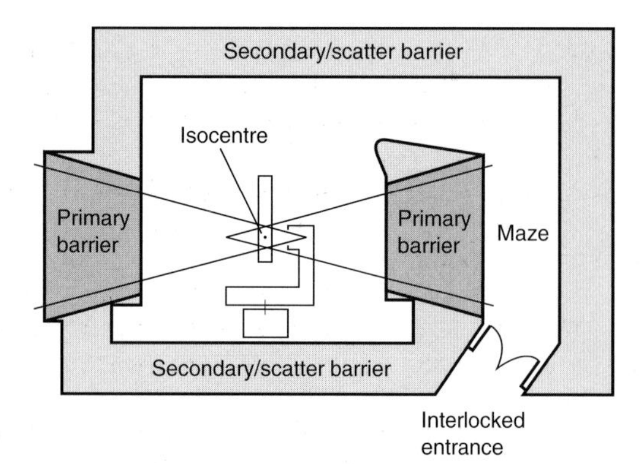

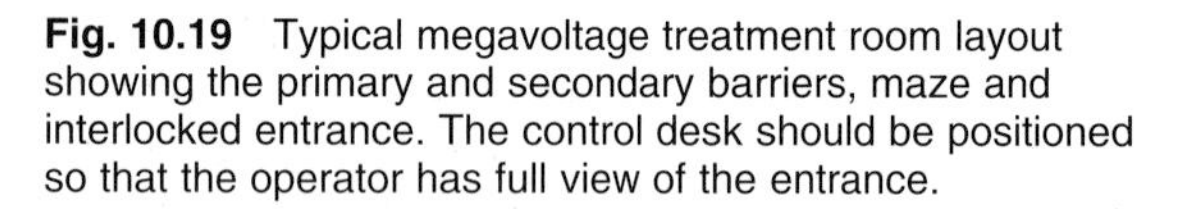

Fig. 10.19 Typical megavoltage treatment room layout showing the primary and secondary barriers, maze and interlocked entrance. The control desk should be positioned so that the operator has full view of the entrance.

energised, and warning signs, preferably electrically operated, must be displayed to that effect at the entrance(s). From the moment the generator is *in a state of readiness to emit* radiation until the termination of the exposure, an additional warning sign should display 'DO NOT ENTER' or otherwise advise of the hazard (Plate 1.2).

Visible and audible warnings are required inside all treatment rooms to indicate that radiation is imminent or present, together with emergency mains isolator switches for the safety of anyone accidentally shut in the room.

Observation of the patient

For megavoltage therapy rooms, lead glass has been used but closed-circuit television—in black and white or in colour—has proved more convenient and somewhat cheaper. Closed-circuit television, with a pan and tilt camera fitted with a zoom lens, is ideal in that the patient can be viewed either in close-up or from a distance. Two systems enable the operator to have two angles on the patient and provide some insurance against the failure of one system. The vantage points commonly used are (i) close to the sagittal laser, looking along the gantry axis, and (ii) at about 45° to the first, to give a more lateral view without being obscured by the rotation of the gantry head. Providing the vantage points are carefully chosen, they can both pan to observe a patient having total body irradiation against the side wall (p. 217). If the video signal is interrupted by a second door interlock circuit, then the monitor screens can be blanked out while the radiographer is in the room attending the patient, thereby increasing their privacy. The CCTV system does not offer the patient a view of the operator and this is often cited in favour of the window.

Communication with the patient

A hands-off intercom must be available so the patient can speak to the operator during the treatment without having to move. Again, if this is linked through the second door interlock circuit, it can be muted while the operator is in the room.

GAMMA RAY BEAM GENERATORS

Much of what has been said above relating to the megavoltage beam from a linear accelerator applies equally to the gamma ray beam from a teleisotope unit and therefore only the principal differences will be highlighted in what follows.

The isotope source

Gamma-rays are in nature identical to X-rays except that they are spontaneously emitted from certain radioactive isotopes. A gamma ray beam is produced by suitably housing an isotope source in a substantial shield to attenuate the unwanted radiation while permitting its useful gamma radiation to emerge through an appropriate aperture in that shield.

To produce a useful gamma ray beam for radiotherapy, a high specific activity source emitting megavoltage gamma radiation is required to provide an adequate dose rate at the chosen treating distance. Caesium-137, with its long half-life has been used but now its main application is in brachytherapy (Ch. 14). Cobalt-60 is the isotope most widely used in teletherapy. Cobalt-60 is produced by neutron bombardment of cobalt-59 in a reactor and decays to nickel-60 by emitting a beta particle and two gamma rays of 1.17 and 1.33 MeV. Its half-life of 5.26 years requires a new source to be fitted every 3½ years, by which time the treatment times will have increased by about a half. Cobalt-60 is available to a high specific activity which, combined with an air kerma rate of 0.3 $Gy\,h^{-1}\,TBq^{-1}$ at 1 m, produces a source with a high useful beam dose rate (1 TBq = 10^{12} Bq; T = tera). Cobalt-60 at 100 cm SSD produces a beam with depth doses equivalent to an X-ray beam of approximately 3 MV. Under the Radioactive Substances Act (1993), the premises must be licensed to hold a source of this specification.

The source design

To guard against the leakage of radioactive particles and to simplify the handling of the source, the radioactive cobalt is doubly encapsulated in stainless steel (Fig. 10.20). The cobalt metal is in the form of discs approximately 2 mm thick and, typically, 17 mm diameter. These discs, probably 10–15 of them, depending on the required air kerma rate, are inserted into the inner capsule of stainless steel and any remaining space is taken up by similarly sized inactive discs. The inner capsule is then closed with a screw cap which is sealed in place by brazing. The sealed inner capsule is then mounted in an outer case which is again closed with a screw cap and brazed. (It should be noted that although a unit may be designed to accept sources of a certain activity, say 200 TBq, the source is often specified in terms of the air kerma rate at a metre to overcome any misunderstandings over the effects of self absorption within the source.)

The source change procedure

The manufacturer of the cobalt unit provides the supplying isotope laboratory with a *source pencil* which will accept a doubly encapsulated source of standard design. The laboratory will load the source into the pencil and the pencil into the manufacturer's transit container. To facilitate the changing of a source on site, an empty container is linked to the cobalt unit and the pencil containing the spent source is transferred from the treatment head to the transit container. A second container with the new source pencil is then linked to the unit and the procedure reversed. The whole procedure may take a whole day, although the actual source transfers will only take a second or two.

The alternative procedure is to dismantle the source housing from the gantry and send it to an isotope laboratory to have the new source fitted using their hot cell facility. This results in a considerably longer 'down time'.

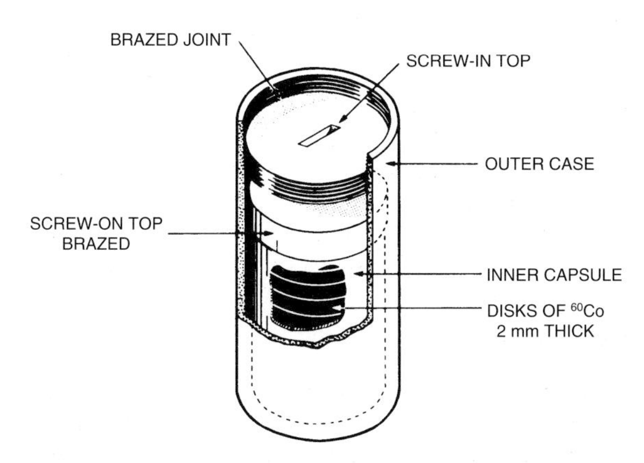

Fig. 10.20 A double encapsulated teletherapy cobalt-60 source. (Reproduced from Meredith and Massey, Fundamental Physics of Radiology, Wright, Bristol, 1977.)

Despite all the precautions, it is good practice to take a wipe test soon after a new source is fitted and periodically (e.g. annually) after that. To do this, all readily accessible surfaces—especially the collimating system—are wiped with a damp swab. Providing the free activity collected on the swab is less than 200 Bq the source is considered leak free.

Two definitive output dose rate measurements must be made before the new source is used to treat patients and the results must be compared with the supplier's certificate of calibration and the previous source data and any differences reconciled. (The supplier's test report on the source will relate to specific laboratory conditions and not to the clinical application, but a comparison with test reports on previous sources should confirm the result of the output dose rate measurement.) A full QA procedure should also be carried out before returning the unit for clinical use.

The beam control

One fundamental difference between an X-ray unit and a gamma ray beam unit is that the gamma radiation cannot be switched off. If the mains supply fails or is interrupted by a switch the X-ray beam is automatically safe. The gamma ray beam is not—unless it is designed to be so—but safety mechanisms can fail.

The *moving source* unit (Fig. 10.21A) has a mechanism whereby the source can be moved from the centre of the protective shield to the apex of the beam collimating system—i.e. the point from which the useful beam emanates. The mechanism moves the source between the 'beam off' and the 'beam on' positions. In the *fixed source* unit (Fig. 10.21B), however, the source is fixed at the apex of the collimating system and a shutter absorbs the useful beam or allows it to pass out of the head—the open shutter may form part of the collimating system. Whichever mechanism is employed, it is mandatory to provide a spring return mechanism and a manual return system to make the unit safe in the event of a power supply failure in addition to the design control mechanism. The failure of the electrical supply, or of the spring, must not leave the source stranded in the 'beam on' position. The manual return system needs to be understood by everyone who may be required to operate the unit and a written protocol must be kept readily available and rehearsed by selected members of staff. Mechanical indicators are incorporated in the design of the unit to show when the shutter (or source) is in the safe 'beam off' position. Indicator lamps show the position of the source as 'source safe', 'in transit' or 'beam on'. Supplementary electrical and mechanical indicators may also be fitted.

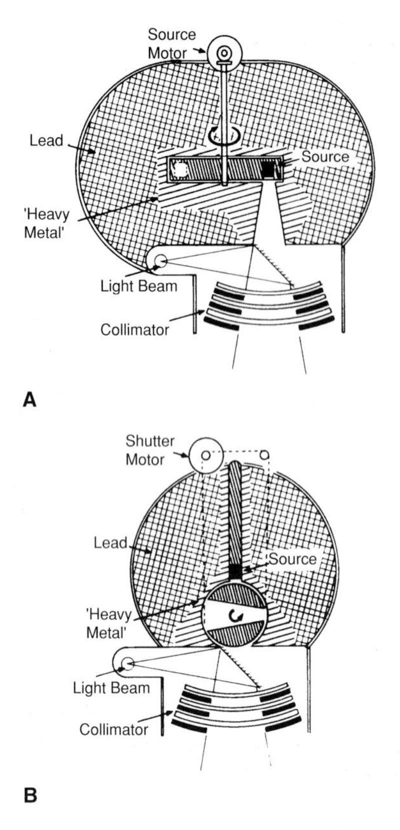

Fig. 10.21 Typical cobalt-60 teletherapy units of **A** the moving source type and **B** the fixed source type.

It must be possible to mechanically lock the mechanism in the 'Beam Off' position whenever the unit is left unattended.

Since the radiation is emitted spontaneously, the only controls required are those to operate the beam on/off mechanism. The control desk is, therefore, very simple. A double treatment timer is used to terminate the exposure after a preset time. The primary timer should measure the length of the exposure to the patient while the secondary back-up timer should measure the time the source/shutter is out of the 'beam off' position—the difference between the two timers on completion of the exposure is therefore the overall 'transit time'. Any change in this overall transit time may give advanced indication of a mechanism malfunction and should be reported. As for kilovoltage X-ray generators, the timers should count up to the preset value and continue beyond that value if the exposure fails to terminate; each timer should be capable of terminating the exposure and operate independently. The significance of any timer error (p. 56) should be assessed.

To correct for the decay of the source, treatment times will need to be increased by approximately 1.1% each month (in the case of cobalt-60)—but the output dose rate should be also confirmed by regular measurement as well.

Leakage radiation

The source housing will usually be a steel, lead-filled, casting with a central core of either steel or a heavy metal alloy (where this heavy metal is depleted uranium, see the note on p. 167). The head of a 200 TBq cobalt unit will weigh more than 1000 kg. The function of this protection is primarily twofold. First, when the beam is on, to reduce the level of radiation reaching those parts of the patient other than the treated area and to reduce the level of radiation reaching the walls of the treatment room, thereby reducing the wall thickness required. Second, there is the need to make the unit safe in the 'beam off' condition to enable the radiographers to attend to the patient, and other staff (e.g. cleaners) to carry out their duties in the treatment room in safety. The source housing must reduce the gamma ray air kerma rates at (5 cm from) the surface and at 1 metre from the source to below the accepted safety limits (Table 10.4). This protective material will surround the source in all directions except one—the direction of the useful beam.

In any new installation or following any modifications which may affect the protection surrounding the head, a complete check is required to ensure the intensity of the leakage radiation is below the accepted limits and to ensure there are no weaknesses, such as cracks or pinholes, in the material used. The former is measured using a large-volume (e.g. 500 ml) ionisation chamber and the latter by wrapping X-ray film around the surface of the housing. (Students should not confuse the leakage of active material from the source detected by the wipe test (p. 181) and the leakage of unwanted radiation through the limited attenuation afforded by the source housing.)

Beam collimation

The primary collimation will be a square or circular divergent hole, of which the shutter may be a part, through the source housing. It will define the beam axis and will limit the overall maximum field size available. Secondary collimation and beam direction devices will be of similar design to the linear accelerator and subjected to the same quality assurance programme.

Table 10.4 Leakage air kerma rates permitted from gamma ray beam units

	At 1 m from source		At 5 cm from the surface
	Maximum	Average	
Beam OFF	0.1 mGy/h	0.02 mGy/h	2.0 mGy/h
Beam ON	0.1%*	—	—

* Of the useful beam kerma rate at 1 m

Penumbra trimmers

The diameter of the gamma ray source gives rise to a large geometric penumbra and, where the treatment technique permits, it is possible to increase the effective collimated length by the use of *penumbra trimmers*. These are heavy metal bars mounted between the diaphragm system and the patient (Fig. 10.22) and positioned in such a way that the inner surfaces lie in the same plane as the faces of the diaphragm blades themselves.

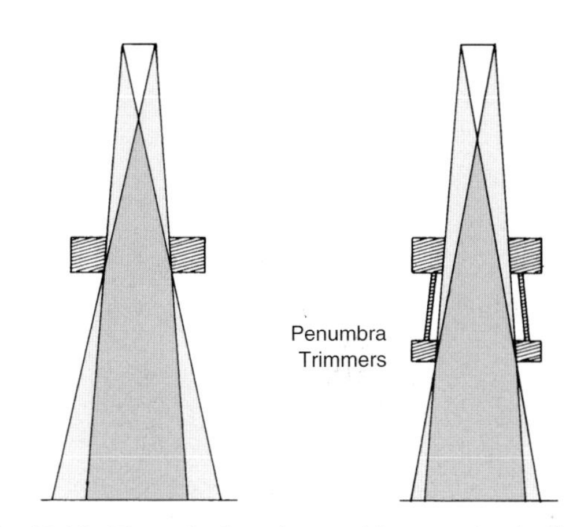

Fig. 10.22 The reduction of geometric penumbra by the use of penumbra trimmers.

Design of gamma beam therapy rooms

The gamma beam therapy room will be of the same basic design and have the same facilities as the linear accelerator room. All the walls, ceiling and floor should be considered as primary barriers as the versatility of the gantry is such that the gamma beam can be directed at any point of the room. At an early stage of planning, consideration must be given to the access route for the replacement source procedures every few years and for access to the source housing, relative to the primary beam, should the manual source procedure have to be implemented. A gamma alarm must be installed in the room, powered from an independent electrical supply with battery back-up, to indicate, visibly and audibly, whenever the beam is 'not safe'. As a further precaution, staff entering the room should carry pocket radiation alarms (p. 84). The gamma beam therapy room will be a radiation 'controlled area' 24 hours a day, and a permanent warning sign (Plate 1.3) to that effect will be required together with an electrically operated 'DO NOT ENTER' or similar warning sign.

CHAPTER CONTENTS

11

Radiation treatment planning: immobilisation and contouring

Keith Bomford

INTRODUCTION

The phrase *radiation treatment planning* (RTP) as applied to external beam therapy is used to describe the work involved in displaying graphically a dose distribution which results when one or more radiation beams converge on the target volume. This chapter deals with the provision of immobilisation and patient contouring devices, two vital precursors to any practical treatment planning.

For treatments in the abdomen and thorax reliance is usually placed on the radiographer's ability to position the patient in the same way each day of treatment by paying particular attention to the position of the limbs and the extremities.

Immobilisation devices may be advantageous in selected cases. Whenever the treatment site may be subject to movement during the few minutes of treatment, e.g. in a young child or a very nervous patient, then some form of immobilisation must be considered. The obese patient will have a contour which is not reproducible from day to day making the use of skin marks unreliable, while very slim patients will find the hard couch top so uncomfortable that they will find it difficult to lie still for the duration of the treatment. In either case an *immobilisation device* becomes important.

For treatments of the head and neck, some immobilisation device (e.g. patient mould or shell) becomes essential as a means to ensuring the same position is reproduced each day and to avoid a geographical miss when the treatment fields are small. Various techniques are available.

Knowledge of the external patient contour—in two or three dimensions—is required before any treatment planning for megavoltage radiation therapy and while these data are readily available from CT scans other options are available. It is most important that the contour data are taken from the patient in the treatment position while using the prescribed immobilisation devices.

PATIENT IMMOBILISATION

Patient shells

A patient shell, which accurately fits and immobilises the patient, enables the planning and treatment to be carried out with greater accuracy. It will be worn by the patient at every stage of localisation, simulation, verification and treatment and must maintain its shape for several weeks. The good shell locates on the bony protuberances of the patient and:

- enables the localisation of the lesion to be accurately determined from surface markers attached to the shell
- enables an accurate position of the patient to be reproduced each day
- guarantees an accurate and constant patient contour
- can be labelled and marked clearly and avoids the need to draw marks on the patient
- offers accurate beam entry and exit points
- provides a base for the addition of build-up material and/or local shielding.

Space does not permit a detailed description of all the procedures involved in making a shell but the traditional method of making a vacuum-formed clear plastic shell using a plaster bandage impression is outlined. The transparency of the plastic enables the accuracy of the fit to be checked, minor adjustments may be made by applying local heat. There is no place for a badly fitting shell. There is no place for a good shell, badly fitted.

If the proposed treatment demands the skin-sparing effect to be maximised, the entry ports for the treatment beams may be pared away from the shell, leaving only a narrow strap across the centre on which to uniquely define the central axis of the treatment field—the need for this should be borne in mind from the beginning as any cut-outs will tend to weaken the shell making it less effective as an immobilisation device.

The making of a clear plastic shell using a plaster bandage impression

1. Preparation of the patient. When the impression is taken, the patient should assume the position to be adopted in the treatment room (Fig. 11.1A); the clinician should be consulted if there is any doubt. The impression of a patient's head will be more accurate if any long hair is cut short or shaved if the hair is likely to be lost during treatment. Hair should be covered with a tight swimming cap and the face well coated with a separating medium. The patient should be warned that the plaster may feel cold at first, but will become quite warm as it hardens.

2. If a full head shell is to be made, the impression of the back half should be made first. The edge of the plaster bandage should be neatly finished to define the coronal plane through the centre of the ears. Once the impression has hardened, a separating medium should be put on the outside extending about 3 cm from the edge.

3. Before commencing the front half, it must be decided how far the impression should extend—upwards and downwards—bearing in mind that the finished shell needs bony protuberances on which to locate, e.g. the nose, the eyebrows, the chin, the shoulders. Secondly, how is the patient going to breathe during treatment? The patient may breathe normally through the nose in which case the impression will be made with the mouth closed, and the position of the chin will be determined by the teeth. (If any dental work is anticipated before the end of treatment, it should be completed before the impression is made; it must also be decided whether treatment will be given with or without dentures). Alternatively, the patient may breathe through the mouth in which case a mouth insert with a short breathing tube should be made to fix the position of the chin and to depress the tongue. This mouth insert should preferably be made of a tissue-equivalent material.

4. The front impression can now be commenced. The plaster bandage should be shaped carefully round the bony points and round the prepared edge of the back half of the impression, if present (Fig. 11.1B)—the two halves must fit uniquely together once they have been removed from the patient. The impression will usually require about six thicknesses of plaster bandage suitably overlapped to give rigidity to the finished impression. Weaknesses can be strengthened after the impression has been removed from the patient but distortions cannot be corrected. Once the impression has hardened, it should be eased carefully off the patient.

5. The two halves should now be fixed together by adding a further three layers of plaster bandage over the joint. If only a front half has been made then the open side should be closed using plaster bandage, taking care not to distort the impression. The mouth or nose aperture should also be closed. After rinsing with a separating medium, fill the impression with a fairly thin mix of plaster of Paris (adequate support round the impression must be provided so that it is not distorted under the weight of plaster) and allow it to set without applying additional heat, e.g. overnight.

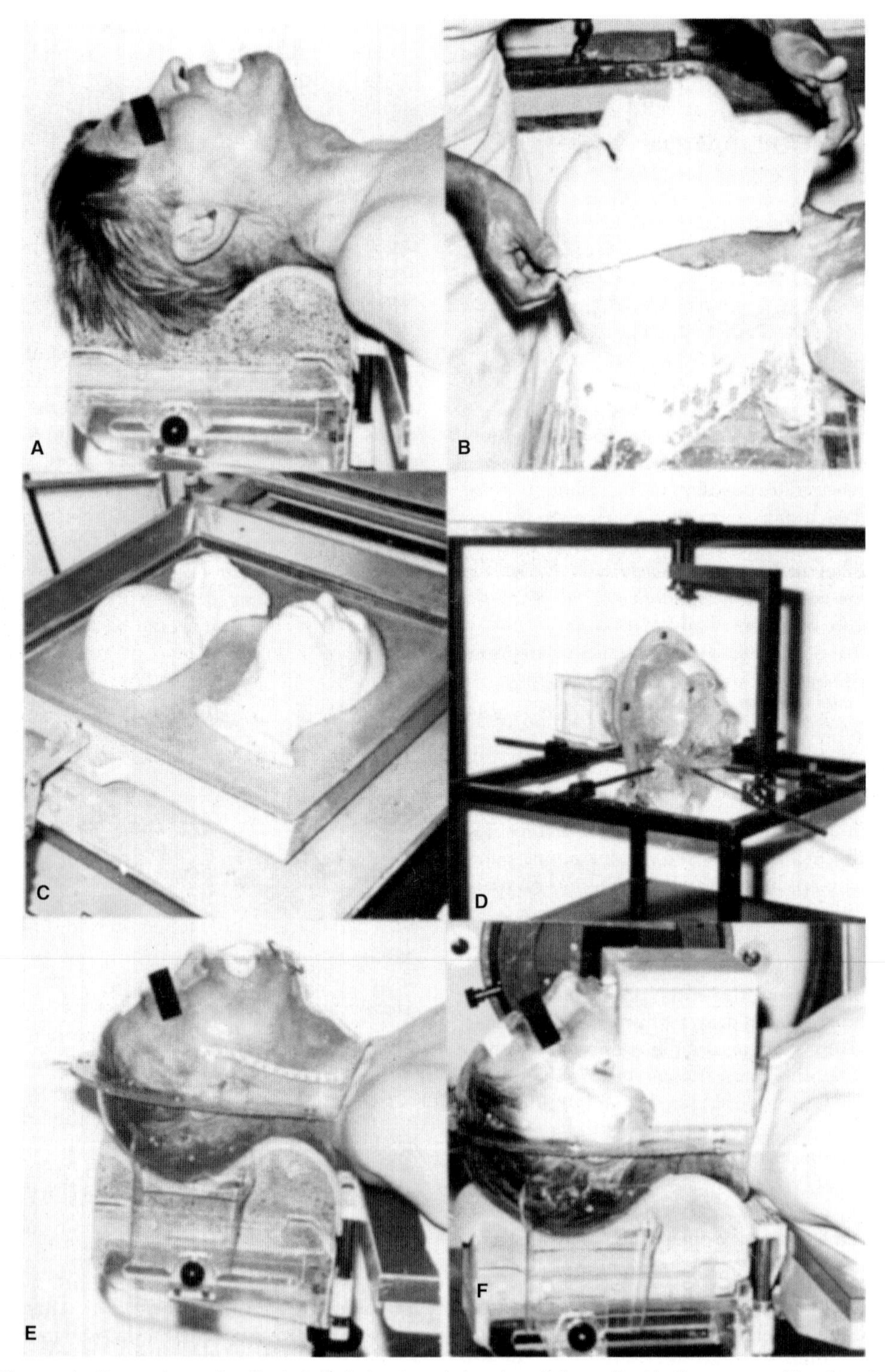

Fig. 11.1 The production and use of patient shells in treatment planning: **A** the patient in the proposed treatment position with a breathing tube; **B** the removal of the front half on completion of a whole-head impression: **C** the two halves of the case in position for vacuum forming; **D** the complete shell in the contouring jig; **E** the patient in the shell in position for the localisation films on the simulator; **F** the shell complete with tissue-equivalent wax block in use on the accelerator.

6. The impression can now be peeled off the solid cast, leaving an exact replica of the patient. Small pimples on the cast, resulting from air pockets in the impression, can be pared away with a knife. The cast of a full head should be sawn into two halves along a diameter chosen to avoid the proposed treatment beam ports.

7. The casts are now ready for vacuum forming (Fig. 11.1C). The flat surface of each half cast is placed on the platform of the vacuum forming machine. The plastic sheet is clamped around its edges and heated until it is pliable. Compressed air is used to pre-stretch the plastic into a bubble and the cast is raised into that bubble before the vacuum is applied to form the plastic tightly round the cast.

8. The plastic is trimmed off the casts leaving a flange approximately 3 cm wide all round to accept press-studs to hold the two halves of the full shell together (Fig. 11.1D). If only a half shell is being made the excess plastic may be cut away completely. The breathing aperture can be cut away using a dental saw. The patient shell is completed by polishing all the edges.

9. Supports will be moulded (by hand) and securely attached to the shell to allow it to be fitted to a head rest or the couch of the treatment unit so that the patient is uniquely positioned (Fig. 11.1E).

10. Treatment accessories, e.g. TE wax, local shielding, etc., can be attached to the shell after the target localisation and treatment planning has been completed (Fig. 11.1F).

Alternative impression materials

Although plaster bandage has been used almost exclusively as an impression material, other materials are available and can be used to advantage in certain cases. They may be used in conjunction with plaster bandage. Certain materials (e.g. dental impression compounds) are used dry, relying on heat to soften them during the impression stage and hardening as they cool. Other water-based materials (e.g. alginates) are mixed and applied to the patient where they set into a gel. Once set, they can be peeled off. Used carefully they can reproduce the very texture of the skin. These materials are particularly valuable if impressions are required from moist open wounds.

Another alternative is to use perforated thermoplastic. This material may be softened in a hot water bath or warm oven and shaped directly onto the patient and onto the headrest or couch, before it cools and hardens (Fig. 11.2). It is available in different sizes and may be pre-cut for selected purposes to reduce the wastage which inevitably results during the moulding procedure. At 55°C, the material becomes mouldable and transparent. The perforations are small and remove some 10–20% of the material and permit the final fit of the shell to be assessed either visually or by measuring the stand-off through the perforations; reheating allows minor adjustments to be made for changes in body contour during treatment.

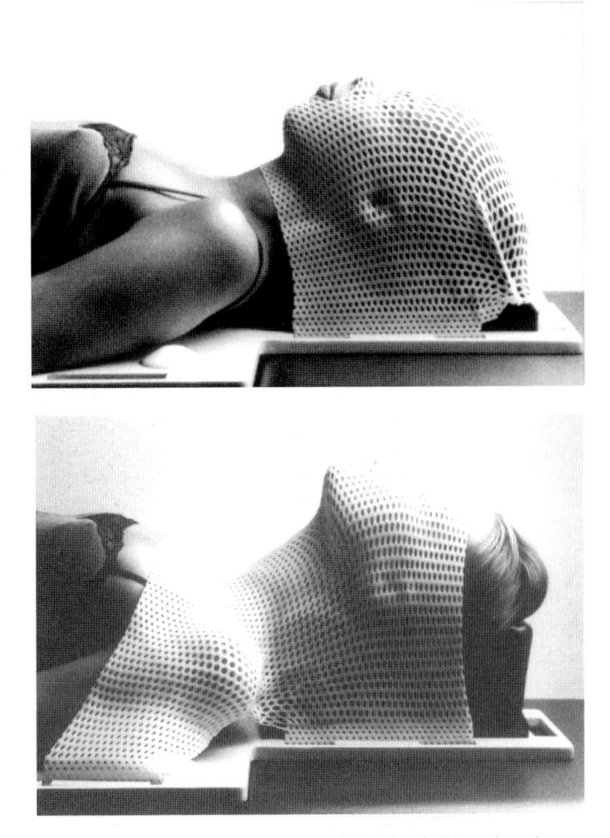

Fig. 11.2 Thermoplastic shells: **A** for the full head and **B** for the neck. (Courtesy of Nuclear Associates.)

Apertures may be cut in the shell around the eyes and for breathing through the mouth or nose while taking care not to weaken the shell. Once finished, the shell must be kept away from radiators and any source of heat. As with the clear plastic, re-use is not recommended although uncut areas may be salvaged and reshaped for immobilisation devices

Immobilisation techniques

Patient shells are essentially dual purpose in that they both immobilise the patient and provide a facility for beam direction devices and other aids to the treatment.

Where immobilisation is the sole requirement, other techniques and materials may be adopted.

Effervescent materials

Self-hardening effervescent materials can be used to immobilise a patient. A rough frame of, say, expanded polystyrene is formed round the part to be immobilised. A large empty polythene bag is then flattened in the frame and the patient positioned on top of the bag. The materials are mixed and introduced into the polythene bag; the mixture rapidly expands to fill the gaps between the frame and the patient and hardens, forming an accurate impression of the patient's position. Being aerated like the expanded polystyrene, the immobilisation device produces negligible attenuation of the treatment beam and, providing adequate access to setting-up marks has been left (the foam is opaque), it can be used on the treatment set without modification (Fig. 11.3). Two words of caution: the chemicals are toxic and toxic fumes may be produced and therefore the polythene bag must not be perforated; and heat is generated during the hardening process which some sensitive skins may find unacceptable. The setting up procedure is simplified if the polystyrene frame is designed to fit uniquely to the treatment couch. The frame may be re-usable, the foam bag will not.

Vacuum bags

An alternative to the foam bag is to use a sealed plastic bag loosely filled with small expanded polystyrene spheres. The same crude frame may be used and the patient again positioned on top of the bag. The bag is manually formed round the patient whilst the air pressure in the bag is gradually reduced using a vacuum pump. At approximately half atmospheric pressure, the bag becomes rigid and 'fits' firmly round the patient, preventing any significant movement. The rigidity can be maintained throughout a course of treatment and until the vacuum is released, when the bag and contents may be re-used for another patient. A variety of shapes and sizes of bag are available to immobilise any part of the anatomy or the whole of the patient, for total body irradiation (TBI), for example. As with the foam, the attenuation in the polystyrene is minimal, but being opaque, consideration must be given to the beam entry ports during the initial evacuation. Radiation damage to the plastic will eventually cause vacuum failure and necessitate the replacement of the bag.

Bite blocks

The head may be immobilised using a bite block (Fig. 11.4). This is a dental impression suspended from a rigid gantry attached to the couch. The patient lies supine on the couch in the treatment position with the bite block in the mouth. The bite-block gantry is then adjusted to fix the position of the bite block with respect to the couch. Providing its adjustment and the patient's grip on the bite block are both maintained, then the position of the patient's head will be accurately held secure. To assist the patient maintain the grip on the bite block, a vacuum may be applied between the block and the upper dentition.

Breast jigs

One of the most difficult treatment set-ups is that for the treatment of the breast (Ch. 26), often requiring the use of up to four fields, two coplanar to the breast and two coplanar to the supraclavicular tissues. All

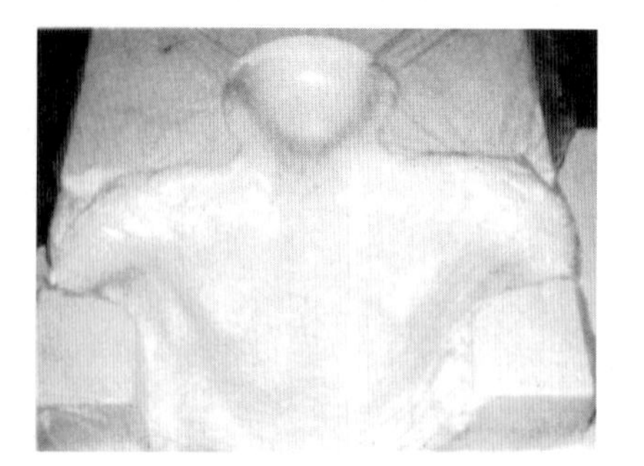

Fig. 11.3 Self-hardening effervescent foam impression.

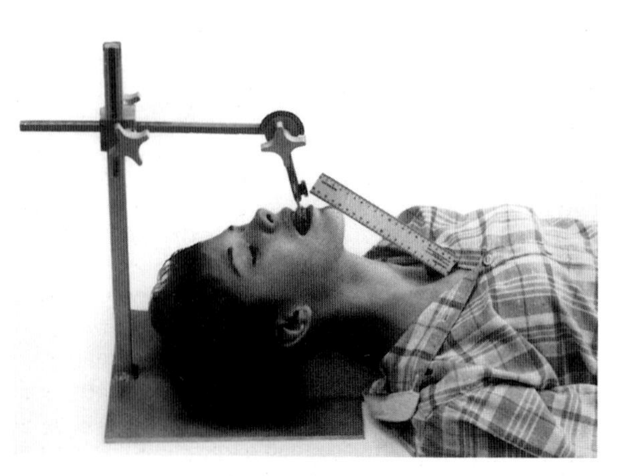

Fig. 11.4 The bite block. (Courtesy of Nuclear Associates.)

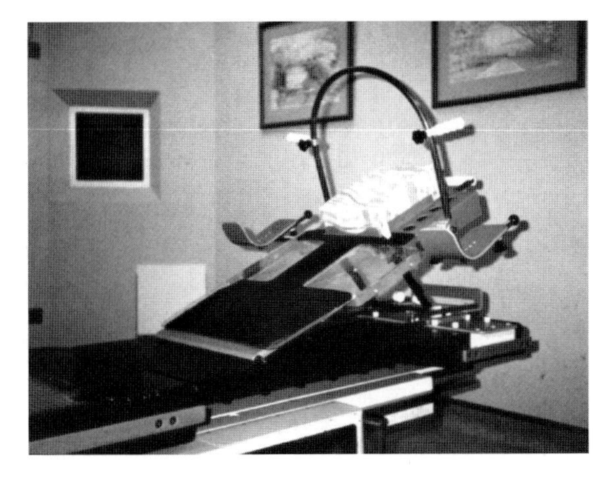

Fig. 11.5 The Sheffield breast jig.

four fields will often make use of the 'beam-blocking' technique or the asymmetric collimators to bring one edge of each field to the mechanical axis, thereby removing the effect of beam divergence from that one edge. This does not remove the penumbra, and the alignment of the superior edges of the breast fields with the inferior edges of the supraclavicular fields is critical. To achieve accuracy in this set-up requires careful positioning of the patient so that all four fields can be treated without moving the patient. The use of a specially designed breast jig (Fig. 11.5) is preferred. The jig may consist of a support which raises the patient's shoulders and provides an elbow support and/or a hand-grip for the patient to grasp while holding her arm above her head; all these positions can be varied to meet the individual requirements of the patient's treatment and locked into position, the positions are scaled so that they can be reproduced to each patient's requirements each day.

PATIENT CONTOURING DEVICES

The value of radiation treatment planning depends on the reproducibility of the shape of the patient on a day-to-day basis throughout the course of treatment. The couch where the patient contour will be taken therefore should be identical in every respect to the couch on which that patient will be treated. It is imperative that the patient is correctly positioned before the contour is taken for planning purposes. A variety of devices are available for taking patient contours. The very simple lead strip (say, $10 \times 3 \times 600$ mm^3) may be used. Such a strip can be easily bent round the patient and skin marks transferred to the lead using a piece of

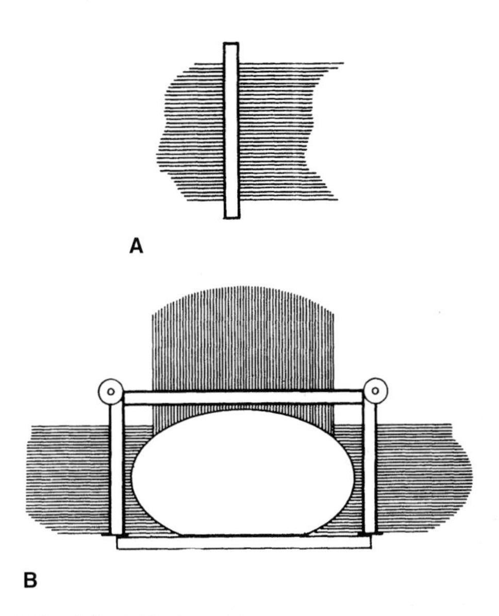

Fig. 11.6 Adjustable templates.

chalk or marker pen. The strip is then carefully transferred to a drawing board and the contour marked onto paper. As with other devices, it is advisable to check the principal dimensions of the contour by an independent means, e.g. callipers or a height bridge. The strip should be varnished to avoid direct contact with the (toxic) lead.

Other optical–video and electromechanical devices based on the pantograph have been developed in various centres, but the most widely adopted devices are described below.

Adjustable template

Adjustable templates are invaluable for taking complex contours (e.g. round the head and neck). They are made up of a large number of parallel rods or pins which can be adjusted lengthways to fit any shaped contour and then clamped in position (Fig. 11.6), the finer the rods the more detailed the contour; rods of 3 mm diameter are usually adequate. The template is then transferred to a drawing board and the contour traced onto paper round the ends of the rods. Three such templates can be mounted on a frame and used to take complete contours (except where the patient is in contact with the couch).

Rotating jig

A simple jig is shown in Figure 11.1D for taking the contour from the outside of a patient's shell. (Wherever the contour is taken from the shell in the absence of the patient, as here, it is imperative that the shell is not deformed.) The shell is supported on four pins which define the plane of the contour. A fifth pin rotates about an axis at right-angles to the plane and scaled in degrees of rotation about the axis and in centimetres radius from the axis. By measuring these two parameters for a variety of points round the surface of the shell, the contour can be readily plotted on polar graph paper. Providing the range finder on the simulator is sufficiently accurate, it may be used in conjunction with the gantry angle in a similar manner.

A simple device of similar design can reproduce the contour from the inside of the shell to represent the patient contour. If the treatment beam passes through the shell then the outer contour is required, whereas if the shell material will ultimately be cut away, to maximise the skin sparing, the inner contour is required.

CT scanner

External and internal patient contours can be obtained from CT scan data, thereby enabling the anatomy to be accurately mapped within the external patient contour in multiple planes throughout the irradiated volume (e.g. Fig. 12.13). Providing the CT slices are close together (e.g. 3 mm spacing), the treatment planning computer can reconstruct the contour and the internal anatomy in a plane oblique to the normal CT scan by interpolating the data from the closely spaced scans. (Never tilt the CT gantry!) Such reconstructions can be particularly useful in sites, such as the middle ear, where the complex anatomy presents particular problems. The contours produced from CT data are, however, often too detailed for planning purposes and some manual smoothing of the contour may be required. Care has to be taken to ensure the CT couch is as flat and as hard as the treatment couch and, where necessary, the patient is restrained or constrained (e.g. using a shell or immobilisation device) in the planned treatment position. The CT scanner is perhaps the ideal contouring device giving, as it does, both the external contour and internal anatomy with optimum registration, but its use can never be justified solely as a contouring device, and care must be taken if contours are taken from diagnostic scans unless the patient's position at the time of the scan can be guaranteed.

The principal dimensions of any external contour should be checked manually and any electronic display checked for distortion of the image as part of the routine QA.

CHAPTER CONTENTS

12

Principles of radiation treatment planning

Keith Bomford

INTRODUCTION

The phrase *radiation treatment planning*, as applied to external beam therapy, is used to describe the work involved in displaying the dose distribution which results when one or more radiation beams converge on the target volume. To achieve this involves bringing together both the patient data and the therapy beam data. The patient data comes from clinical examination (palpation, endoscopy, etc.) and the results of one or more imaging technologies, such as X-ray (Ch. 7), nuclear medicine (Ch. 8), ultrasound and magnetic resonance. The therapy beam data are the main subject of this chapter. (Radiation treatment planning in brachytherapy is dealt with in Ch. 14.)

At megavoltage photon energies, the differential absorption in the tissues is minimal and an understanding of the dose distribution in a homogeneous medium is generally considered sufficient except where the beam traverses healthy lung (p. 202)—as imaging techniques improve other tissue inhomogeneities will be taken into account. At kilovoltage photon energies, where differential absorption is more significant and where the beam penetration is such that the treatment is of superficial disease with a single field, the treatment planning is minimal. Where multiple kilovoltage beams are used, the treatment planning is usually limited to the manual calculation of the dose at selected points (p. 221). Megavoltage electron therapy is largely confined to single-field treatments although a few centres will attempt multiple electron field treatments or a mixture of electron and X-ray fields (p. 219). (It should be noted that the terms *beam* and *field* in this context tend to be used interchangeably to describe the radiation passing into the patient.)

DISTRIBUTION OF DOSE IN A UNIFORM PHANTOM

In earlier chapters, the quality of a beam was discussed in terms of its ability to penetrate through attenuating materials (i.e. half value layer, p. 155, or quality index, p. 168). It is now necessary to investigate the penetration and the distribution of the beam within the body tissues. Owing to the complex structure of the body and the problems of measuring the radiation within the body itself, most measurements are made using a uniform phantom which is carefully chosen to be *(soft) tissue equivalent*, that is, to attenuate, absorb and scatter the radiation to the same extent as soft tissue. (What is soft tissue equivalent will be different from bone or fat tissue equivalent for X-rays, and different again from those deemed to be tissue equivalent in other situations, e.g. in magnetic resonance imaging.)

Tissue-equivalent materials

If the photon interactions in a material are the same as those that would take place in soft tissue then that material is said to be soft tissue equivalent and sometimes referred to as a tissue substitute. From an analysis of the absorption processes (Ch. 4), it is clear that such a material for photon therapy must have:

- an effective atomic number close to that of the tissue it simulates because of the dependence of photo-electric absorption and pair production processes on the atomic number, Z
- an electron density close to that of the tissue it simulates because of the dependence of the Compton scattering process on the number of electrons per gram, and
- the density (in g ml^{-1}) should be as close as possible to that of the tissue it simulates because spatial measurements will be made in the phantom material.

Table 12.1 lists some properties of soft tissue and of some tissue-equivalent materials. Water is the most commonly used and distilled or de-ionised water is preferred. In many ways, water is the ideal material in that it is homogeneous and yet permits ionisation chambers (or other radiation detectors) to be moved freely within it. Its major disadvantage is that ionisation chambers need to be kept very dry! A waterproof sheath is essential. There is no simple chemical compound that matches the atomic composition of body tissue and a variety of mixtures have been developed which satisfy the requirements of one or more radiation interactions. Lincolnshire bolus is a mixture of sugar and magnesium carbonate made up into small spheres. While the density of this material is greater than that of soft tissue, the packing density of its spheres produces good tissue equivalence. (It is important, therefore, to check from time to time the condition of the bolus and remove fragmented or powdered spheres from it.) A variety of tissue-equivalent materials are

Table 12.1 Properties of tissue and tissue-equivalent materials

Material	Atomic number Z	Elemental composition (% by weight)*				Density g ml^{-1}	Electron density e/g × 10^{23}	Physical form
		H	C	N	O			
Average soft tissue	7.35	10.1	11.1	2.6	76.2	0.98–1.00	3.36	
Muscle (skeletal)		10.2	14.3	3.4	71.0	1.05	3.31	
Water	7.4	11.2	—	—	88.8	1.00	3.34	(Pure) clear liquid
'Solid water' (WT1)		8.1	67.2	2.4	19.9	1.02	3.25	Cold-cured red-brown resin
Mix D	7.5	13.4	77.8	—	3.5	0.99	3.40	White brittle solid
Temex®	7.1	9.6	87.5	0.1	0.5	1.01	3.28	Black flexible solid rubber
Lincolnshire bolus	7.3	5.9	37.9	—	52.7	1.05	3.18	Regular granules
A150		10.1	77.7	3.5	5.2	1.12	3.30	Black conducting plastic
Acrylic	6.5	8.0	60.0	—	32.0	1.17	3.25	Clear rigid thermoplastic
Paraffin wax		15.0	85.0	—	—	0.93	3.45	Brittle, malleable when warm
Polystyrene		7.7	92.3	—	—	1.05	3.24	Clear rigid thermoplastic

* Where the percentages do not total 100, small quantities of other elements are present

available commercially in solid sheet form of various thicknesses from 2–50 mm, the thicker sheets may be machined to accept ionisation chambers. Phantom materials for other body tissues are also available but not in common use.

The calculation of dose within a patient is invariably based on the dose distribution in a uniform soft-tissue-equivalent phantom and the rest of this and the next chapter will be devoted to this. For the measurement of basic beam data, the phantom will be a semi-infinite cuboid phantom and the beam axis will enter at right angles. A phantom is said to be *semi-infinite* if the measurements being undertaken are not affected by any further increase in its size; in practice this means the radiation detector should never be used within ~ 50 mm of the sides or exit surface to ensure the scatter component is complete. To measure a $50 \times 50\ cm^2$ field requires a phantom of at least $600 \times 600 \times 600\ mm^3$.

Percentage depth dose

The term *percentage depth dose* expresses the dose at any point within the phantom as a percentage of the maximum dose on the central axis of the beam, it is not confined to points within the geometric beam. The formal definition is:

> The percentage depth dose (PDD) is the ratio, expressed as a percentage, of the absorbed dose at any given point to the absorbed dose on the beam axis at the depth of maximum dose.

For some purposes, it is advantageous to separate out the primary radiation dose from the scattered radiation dose and, to this end, the *zero area percentage depth dose* is formally defined as:

> PDD (zero area) in a water phantom irradiated by a photon beam is the ratio of the absorbed dose at the given point to that at the maximum dose, both being due to primary photons only.

The *central axis depth dose curves* are often plotted against depth as a means of comparing one radiation beam with another (Fig. 12.1 and Table 12.2), while a map of the dose distribution will be shown as an *isodose chart* where each isodose curve (line) is the locus of points of equal dose; in many respects they are analogous to height contours on a geographer's map. Typical isodose charts are shown in Figure 12.2, where the charts represent the distribution of dose in one of the principal planes of the beam, the principal plane is parallel to the edge of the (rectangular) beam and

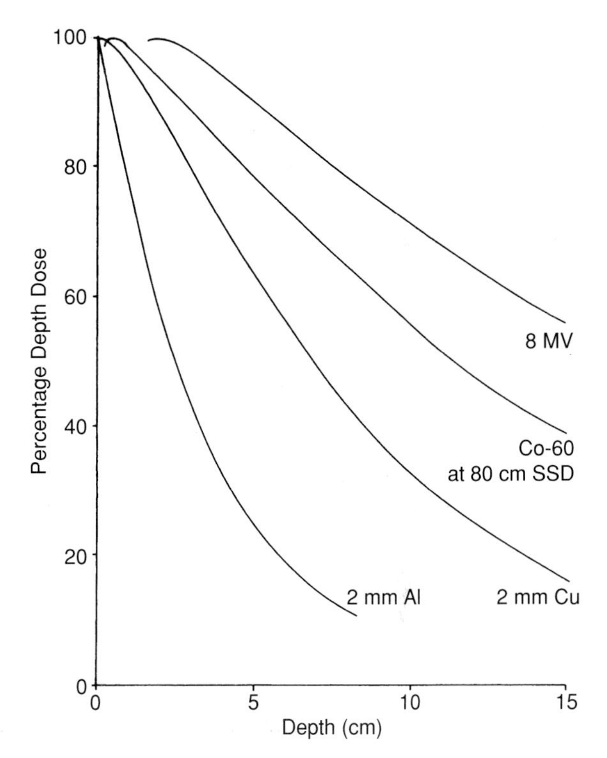

Fig. 12.1 Typical central axis depth dose curves for X- and gamma ray therapy beams.

Table 12.2 Some depth dose data for $10 \times 10\ cm^2$ fields

Energy	SSD	HVL/QI	d_{max}	$d_{80\%}$	$d_{50\%}$	$\%DD_{10\ cm}$
100 kV*	20	2 mm Al	0	0.7	2.2	5.2
250 kV	50	2 mm Cu	0	3.0	6.9	32.3
Cobalt-60	80	0.57	0.5	4.7	11.6	56.4
4 MV	100	0.58	1.0	5.9	13.7	62.7
6 MV	100	0.65	1.5	6.8	15.7	67.7
8 MV	100	0.68	2.0	7.4	17.1	71.0
10 MV	100	0.75	2.5	8.5	19.1	74.5

* 5 cm circle

contains the central axis. (In Fig. 12.2 only half of each chart is shown.)

A graph of the percentage depth dose at 10 cm deep against beam quality (Fig. 12.3.) is an alternative means of comparing one beam with another; the 10 cm depth is chosen as being typical of the clinical applications. At megavoltages, the depth dose does not vary significantly with field size, whereas at kilovoltages, field size is a significant factor. A closer examination of the data presented in Figure 12.3A, shows that the depth dose at 10 cm deep does not increase with half value layer above, say, 4 mm Cu while at 20 cm deep it decreases.

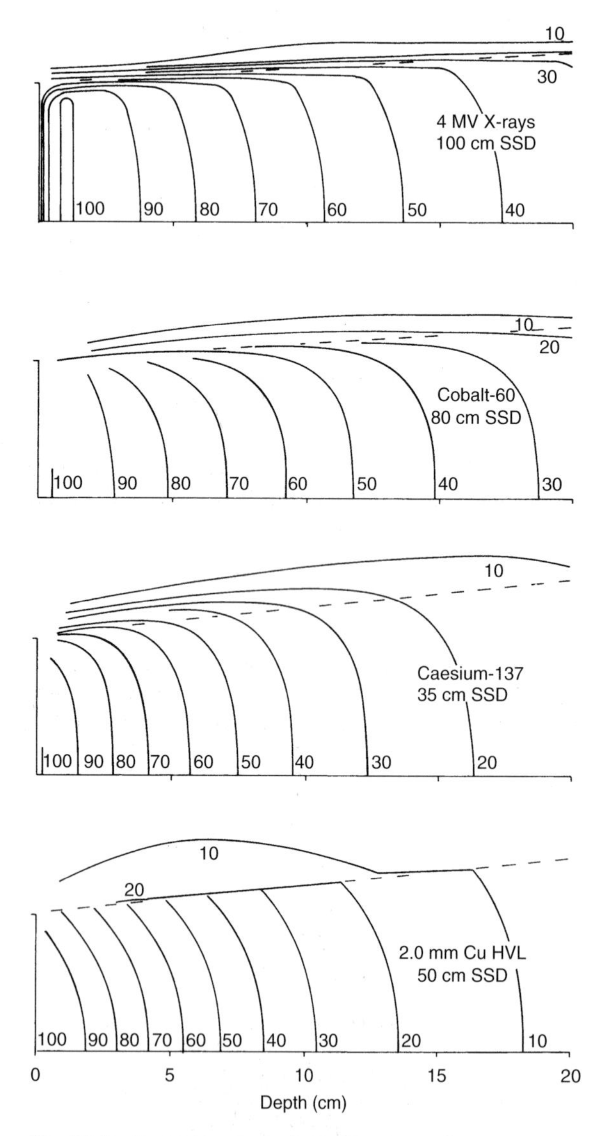

Fig. 12.2 Typical isodose charts for megavoltage, teleisotope and kilovoltage beams.

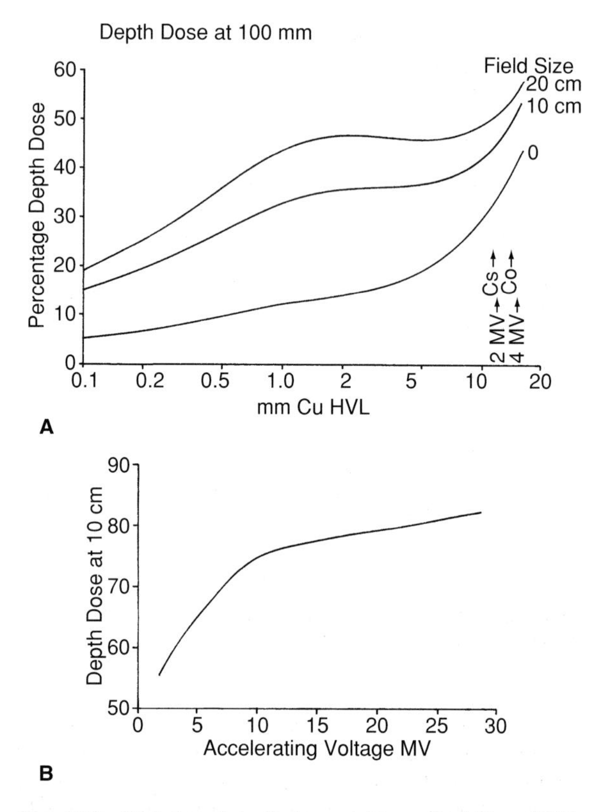

Fig. 12.3 Variation of depth dose at 10 cm: **A** at 50 cm SSD with HVL and **B** at 100 cm SSD with accelerating voltage.

This follows from the Compton scattering process—the generation of scatter is reduced and increasingly in the forward direction as the energy increases and, at photon energies between about 500 kV and 1 MV, the reduction in scatter generation is greater than the increase in primary penetration.

Central axis depth dose

There are many factors which affect the distribution of dose along the central axis of the beam. The dose will fall with increasing depth owing to the absorption and attenuation in the successive layers of tissue and with the increasing distance from the target. (The inverse square law has to be obeyed.) Superimposed on this primary radiation (from the target) will be the scattered radiation which results from the Compton scattering processes taking place within the tissues.

The magnitude of these effects will depend on the quality and the size and shape of the radiation beam and the nature of the tissue itself. Figure 12.4 shows the central axis depth dose curves for a 6 MV and a 250 kV beam with the contribution from scatter plotted sepa-

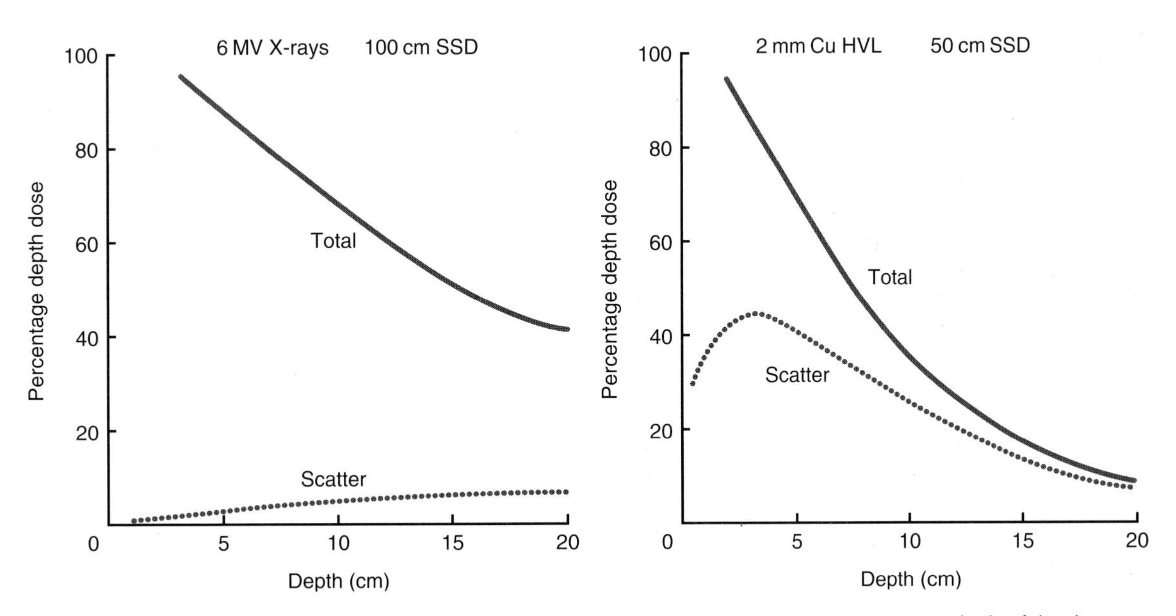

Fig. 12.4 Percentage depth dose curves for 6 MV and 250 kV X-ray beams showing the relative magnitude of the dose contributed by the scattered radiation.

rately. The scatter contribution plays an important role at all depths in kilovoltage therapy, not least at the surface (zero depth) where the dose is significantly increased by the radiation scattered back from the tissues at depth. In contrast, the scatter contribution is minimal, but not negligible, at megavoltage energies.

Effect of changes in source–skin distance

It has already been stated that the central axis depth dose is dependent on the inverse square law and, therefore, on the source–skin distance (SSD). As a general rule, other factors remaining unchanged, the depth dose at a point in the beam increases as the source–skin distance increases. If primary radiation from the source alone is involved, then the simple application of the inverse square law would be all that is necessary to derive depth dose data for different SSDs. However, the field width measured at depth varies with the SSD owing to the changing beam divergence (Fig. 12.5). Therefore, assuming the same field size at the surface, the scatter component at depth will decrease with increasing SSD. Furthermore, at megavoltage energies the 100% reference point is at a depth, d_{max}, below the surface and this must also be taken into account in applying the inverse square factor.

To quantify the basic assumption that the depth dose at depth, d, increases with source–skin distance, f, we define a factor:

$$F = \frac{(f_1 + d) \times (f_2 + d_{max})}{(f_1 + d_{max}) \times (f_2 + d)}$$

in which d_{max} is equated to zero when the 100% is at the surface, i.e. for beam qualities < 4.0 mm Cu HVL. The modified depth dose D is then given by:

$$D(d, f_2, S) = D(d, f_1, S/F) \times \frac{\text{PSF}(S/F)}{\text{PSF}(S)} \times F^2$$

where PSF(S) is the *peak scatter factor* for the *equivalent square* field of side S. This simple formula is only approximate, giving results accurate to about 2%.

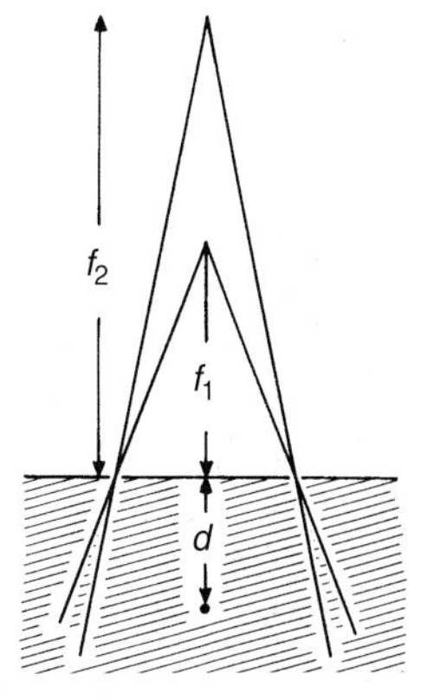

Fig. 12.5 The effect of changing from one SSD to another.

Since F is a function of d, the use of this formula without a computer is usually limited to evaluating a few points in any clinical situation, e.g. the midpoint and exit dose for a parallel-opposed pair. Any radiation treatment planning software will handle changes in SSD as a matter of course.

One of the principal reasons for using extended SSDs is to achieve a field size larger than the collimator will allow at the normal treating distance, e.g. when treating the CNS (Ch. 30). An alternative approach to this problem is to abut one beam to the edge of another; this is less satisfactory insofar as it is impossible to align two divergent beam edges and expect a uniform dose throughout the combined penumbra as the dose profile through the penumbra is non-linear. Furthermore, although careful alignment of the two 50% isodose lines at a selected depth may produce a reasonably uniform dose on the planning computer display, it is almost impossible to reproduce with sufficient accuracy in setting-up the patient. At the more shallow depths there will be a serious underdosage and a corresponding overdosage at greater depths owing to the divergence of the beams. However, the overall uniformity may be improved by *feathering*, a technique whereby the alignment of the beams to each other is maintained from day to day, but the position of the abutment relative to the patient is deliberately changed by, say, 2 cm.

Back scatter

At kilovoltage energies below 400 kV, the dose at the surface of the irradiated phantom is substantially greater than the dose at the same point if no phantom were present. The phantom material is scattering back to the surface a fraction of the primary radiation and this contribution is known as *back scatter* (Fig. 12.6). The contribution due to back scatter at the point where the beam axis enters the phantom is expressed as a percentage of the contribution due to primary radiation and called *percentage back scatter*. It increases with the area of the field irradiated and with the thickness of the underlying tissues. This is to be expected,

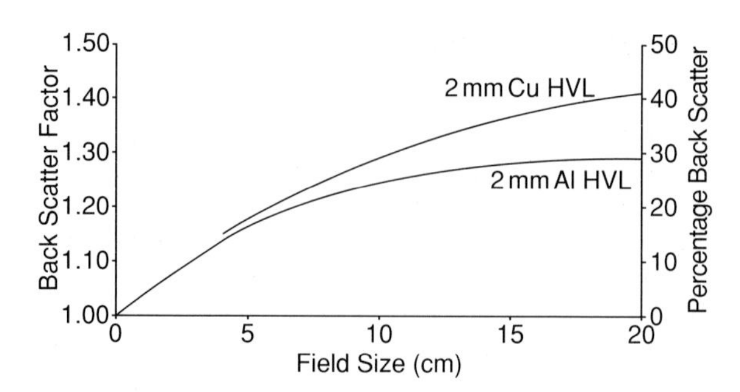

Fig. 12.6 The back scatter factor increases with the equivalent square of the field size.

although with very large fields and very thick tissues the extremities of the irradiated tissue are a long way from the centre of the incident field and contribute very little. The back scatter, therefore, approaches a maximum. For the same reason, the back scatter from a square or circular field will be greater than that for an elongated field of the same area.

The percentage back scatter at the surface of an irradiated phantom varies in a complex manner with radiation quality. It is largest for a beam quality of ~ 0.8 mm Cu HVL—in the medium X-ray energy therapy region—and falls as the quality increases, i.e. as the Compton scatter produced decreases in magnitude and becomes increasingly in the forward direction. It also falls with lower-quality beams where Compton interactions are swamped by photoelectric interactions by which most of the radiation is absorbed. At its maximum the percentage back scatter can reach 50% and is, therefore, very important.

At megavoltage energies, where the maximum dose is at some depth, d_{max}, below the surface, and for energies above 400 kV, the term *peak scatter factor* (PSF) is defined and used in much the same way as the back scatter factor, although its magnitude and its degree of variation with field size and phantom thickness are much smaller than for kilovoltage energies. The peak scatter factors may be normalised to a reference field size, usually 10×10 cm^2 (Table 12.3).

Table 12.3 Some normalised peak scatter factors (NPSF) (BJR 1983)

	Field size (cm^2)					
	5 × 5	7 × 7	10 × 10	15 × 15	20 × 20	30 × 30
Cobalt-60	0.984	0.990	1.000	1.014	1.023	1.034
4 MV	0.984	0.990	1.000	1.013	1.025	1.038
6 MV	0.983	0.990	1.000	1.014	1.023	1.035
10 MV	0.961	0.982	1.000	1.027	1.041	1.048
21 MV	1.000	1.000	1.000	1.000	1.000	1.000

Equivalent square

It has been seen above that percentage back scatter (and percentage peak scatter) cannot be simply related to the area of the field. Elongated fields produce less back scatter, as measured on the central axis, than square fields of the same area. Nevertheless, the elongated rectangular field will give rise to back scatter of the same magnitude as a square (or circular) field of smaller area (Fig. 12.7, Table 12.4). It is therefore possible to define for each rectangular field an *equivalent square field* (or an *equivalent diameter field*) which produces the same percentage scatter. This concept is of particular value when using non-standard field sizes for it is not only the back scatter that is the same, but the forward scatter is also the same and this gives rise to the same central axis depth dose. The same logic may be applied to any irregular-shaped field but there is no simple means of determining the equivalence. The primary contribution is the same for all beam sizes (of the same quality and SSD), the scatter contribution is the only variable.

Tables are available (BJR 1996) which give the size of the equivalent square for all rectangular fields commonly encountered; an abridged table is given in Table 12.4. The relevant tables are often made available at the control desk on kilovoltage generators where a lead cut-out (p. 152) may be used in conjunction with a standard beam applicator. The charted dose rate for the applicator must be *reduced* by the ratio of the two back scatter factors (for the equivalent square of the cut-out and the equivalent square of the applicator), thereby increasing the treatment time (or set monitor units) required to deliver the prescribed dose using the cut-out.

Build-up

At megavoltage energies, the scattered radiation is more in the forward direction and gives rise to less scattered radiation outside the edges of the beam. This is clear as soon as you compare the isodose charts for kilovoltage and megavoltage beams (Fig. 12.2). Analysis of the Compton scattering process also shows that the recoil electron is ejected in the more forward direction and with increasing kinetic energy. The range of the recoil electron at 200 kV is extremely small (and measured in microns) but at megavoltages it is considerable (and measured in millimetres, Table 4.3) and an electron dose build-up to d_{max} manifests itself below the surface of the irradiated tissue.

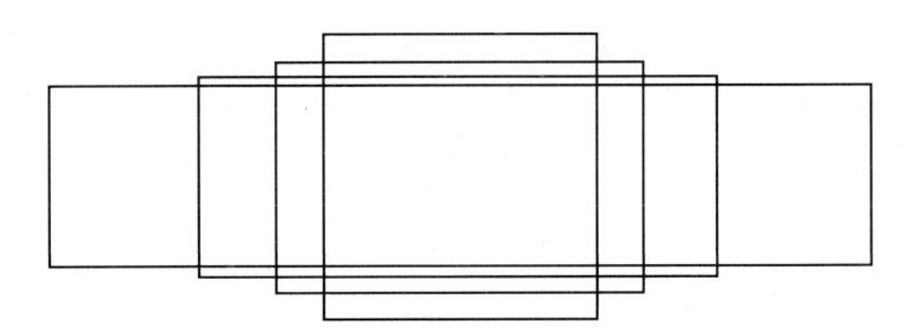

Fig. 12.7 Rectangular fields of different size and elongation having the same equivalent square.

Dose build-up may be explained in simple terms as follows. Each successive thin layer of tissue produces its quota of recoil electrons which in turn deposit their kinetic energy through several successive layers of tissue beyond their point of origin. Although the kinetic energy released in each layer (the kerma) may be constant, the energy deposited in each layer (the absorbed dose) will be determined by the total number of electrons passing through the layer, and that number increases as each layer adds its quota of recoil electrons to the electron flux from the preceding layers. This number only continues to increase until the new electrons released only replace those which have come to the end of their range. The electron dose build-up thus reaches a maximum at a depth determined by the range of the electrons and therefore by the energy of the photon beam. In practice, the kerma is not quite constant but falls, as the primary radiation undergoes absorption and attenuation, with the result that the depth of the dose maximum is less than the maximum

Table 12.4 Abridged table of equivalent of squares of rectangular fields (BJR 1996)

Long axis (cm)	Short axis (cm)							
	2	4	6	8	10	15	20	30
2	2.0							
4	2.7	4.0						
6	3.1	4.8	6.0					
8	3.4	5.4	6.9	8.0				
10	3.6	5.8	7.5	8.9	10.0			
15	3.9	6.4	8.5	10.3	11.9	15.0		
20	4.0	6.7	9.0	11.1	13.0	17.0	20.0	
30	4.1	6.9	9.4	11.7	13.9	18.9	23.3	30.0

range of the secondary electrons; d_{max} is further reduced because the recoil electrons do not all travel in the direction of the primary radiation. In summary, the kerma falls from the surface; the absorbed dose builds up to a peak before beginning to fall with increasing depth (Fig. 12.8).

As a rule of thumb, the depth of the peak, d_{max}, in centimetres equates to approximately one-quarter of the X-ray energy in megavolts (2 cm at 8 MV, etc.) while cobalt-60, being approximately equivalent to 2–3 MV X-rays, has a peak at approximately 5 mm.

The almost exponential shape of the dose build-up curve is primarily determined by the recoil electrons from within the tissues being set into motion in the (mainly) forward direction, and therefore it will not be affected by the curvature of the skin or the obliquity of the incident beam. In general, the depth of d_{max} should be measured in the direction of the radiation from the source irrespective of the skin curvature. This thinking has only to be modified when the angle of incidence is less than, say, 20° (i.e. when the beam is almost tangential to the surface). Although the recoil electrons are predominantly in the forward direction, they do not travel in straight lines, but deviate and distribute their energy over a small volume. There is still some build-up of dose below the tangential surface, but the skin dose is higher than that at normal (90°) incidence and builds up to a maximum over a depth considerably less than the normal value suggests.

This analysis of build-up implies that the dose at any surface is zero. The surface dose in practice is not zero because of the recoil electrons ejected from other materials in the beam—diaphragms, beam-shaping blocks, etc.—and the intervening air itself. The value of the surface/skin dose and the shape of the build-up curve will therefore vary from one machine to another of the same photon energy and with both photon energy and field size (Fig. 12.8). In practice, the surface dose will be in the range of 20–50% for most megavoltage photon beams, and lower values can be expected as the photon energy increases. This problem is then one of *electron contamination* of the photon beam (and not to be confused with photon contamination of the electron beam; p. 221) and may be reduced by the use of an electron filter; brass or copper filters are ideal, but Perspex or lead glass is usually preferred because these do not interrupt the light beam.

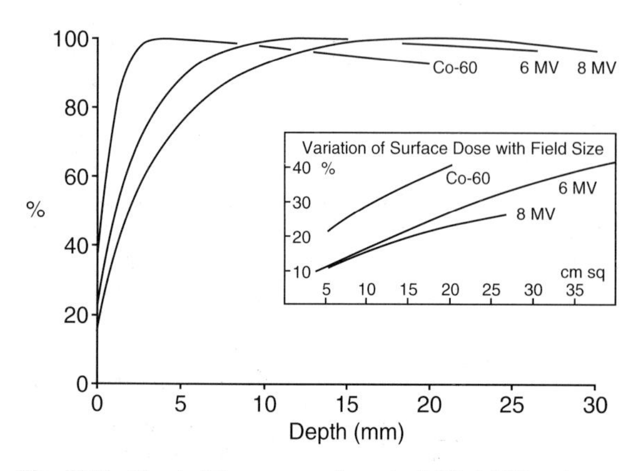

Fig. 12.8 The build-up curves for cobalt-60, 6 MV and 8 MV. The inset shows the variation in skin dose with field size for the same three beams.

ISODOSE CHARTS

Measurement of isodose charts

An *isodose chart* is a family of isodose lines. Owing to the complexities of the isodose distribution within the radiation beam, approximation methods may be used, (i) to minimise the number of measurements required before the isodose chart can be uniquely specified and stored in the treatment planning computer, and (ii) to calculate the dose at any point by interpolation of that stored data. Some of these models are entirely empirical. Any one treatment planning computer system will require a unique set of measurements and this in itself may cause considerable delay in commissioning a replacement planning system.

Water phantom measurements

The basic requirement is a water tank, probably 600 × 600 × 600 mm^3 in which a small detector can be moved in all three orthogonal directions by remote control (Fig. 12.9). A tank of this size weighs more than 216 kg and should be mounted on its own trolley as it is likely to exceed the cantilever weight specification of the treatment couch. The radiation beam may enter the tank vertically, so enabling the measurements to be made at the water surface, or horizontally, through the wall of the tank which may be thinned to permit measurements close to the surface. The detector will be a small ionisation chamber or solid state detector (Fig. 12.10) or, in certain circumstances, an array of detectors (Fig. 12.9). A second (reference) monitor will be rigidly mounted in the beam to monitor any fluctuations in the output of the X-ray generator but out of the plane of movement of the detector. After normalising the detector/monitor ratio and selecting the relative doses required, the detector may be constrained to move in a single plane and to follow each isodose in turn. The controlling computer

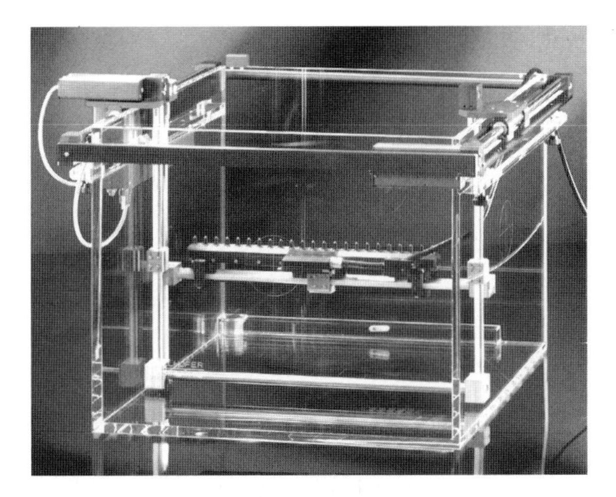

Fig. 12.9 A water phantom for measuring isodose data. Note the linear array of 24 ion chambers for measuring isodose data for conformation therapy beams. (Courtesy of Wellhofer Dosimetrie GmbH.)

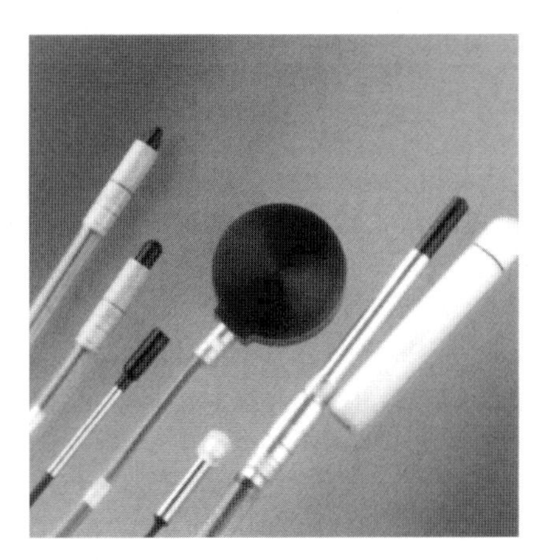

Fig. 12.10 A selection of diode and ion chamber detectors, including the scan diode and the parallel plate electron chamber (3rd and 4th from the left respectively) for use in a water phantom. (Courtesy of Wellhofer Dosimetrie GmbH.)

will automatically record the relative signal and the coordinates of the detector at many thousands of points while scanning through the plane of measurement either for immediate display in a compatible form or for later analysis on a treatment planning computer system (TPS). One complete isodose chart may take an hour to produce by this method.

Where the TPS requires a unique set of dose point measurements then the plotting system may be programmed accordingly, e.g. to measure the central axis depth dose curve and several profiles at selected depths.

Film measurements

Where a water tank is not available, useful information regarding the dose distribution in a megavoltage beam can be determined using film. If a slow radiographic film is sandwiched firmly between sheets of tissue-equivalent material of adequate size and exposed in such a way that the film contains the beam axis, then, after processing, isodensity lines may be plotted using a *densitometer*. The calibration of these isodensity lines must be based on measurements of dose along the central axis in the same phantom material. This technique is equally applicable to electron beams. It may also be used to investigate the dose distribution in a non-uniform and/or non-rectangular phantom irradiated by one or more fields.

The technique may be improved by darkening the room so that unwrapped film may be used to ensure good contact with the phantom material and by inclining the beam axis at a few degrees to the plane of the film (Fig. 12.11) to ensure the primary radiation traverses the phantom and not only the film.

At kilovoltage energies, the energy response of the film in the changing X-ray spectrum with depth in the phantom make the interpretation of the film too difficult to be of any practical value.

Some isodose curve characteristics

Before leaving the subject of isodose charts it is worth summarising some of the characteristics of the different photon energies encountered in the radiotherapy department. Any isodose chart (Fig. 12.2) may be identified by examination of the following three aspects:

- Central axis depth dose distribution, particularly the depth of the maximum dose and, say, the 50% depth
- Beam profile or the dose distribution across the beam
- Penumbra region (p. 171).

The kilovoltage X-ray beam has a central axis dose which falls fairly rapidly from 100% at the surface to 50% at less than 6 cm, the profile is quite curved due to scatter and the penumbra is sharply defined and clearly diverges from the source. The scattered radiation generated within the beam by Compton interactions is

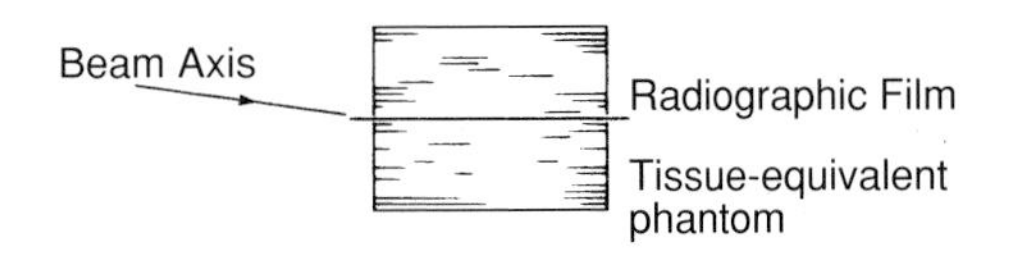

Fig. 12.11 The use of film for the measurement of megavoltage isodose charts.

released in all directions, some of which will pass from within the irradiated beam to beyond the geometric edge. In the medium-energy range, this scatter will result in a dose of 10–25% being given to the healthy tissues immediately outside the penumbra. These low decrement isodose lines may appear to be discontinuous with those of the same value within the beam, but only because the penumbra is so narrow the lines are difficult to show.

A cobalt-60 beam is readily identified by the 5 mm depth of maximum, a well-defined beam edge but fairly wide penumbra, and a profile that is less rounded than for the kilovoltage beam, except close to the beam edge; the 50% depth lies between 7 and 12 cm depending on field size and SSD.

Megavoltage X-ray beams are characterised by their narrow penumbra, flat profile and a depth of peak dose greater than 10 mm; the 50% depth will be between 10 and 20 cm depending on energy and SSD but largely independent of field size.

Definition of field size

One characteristic of isodose charts is the width of the penumbra and here we are referring to the penumbra as measured in the water phantom and, therefore, includes the effects of both geometric and transmission penumbra (p. 171) and the scattered radiation. Because of this diffuse edge, we need to clearly define what we mean by *field size*. The preferred definition is 'the width of the 50% isodose line at the depth of maximum dose and at the normal treating distance'. This definition is used whenever data are published for general use and it is increasingly being adopted in clinical practice, replacing a multitude of similar but different definitions. It has a practical advantage where one field abuts the edge of another because it 'fits well' with the edge of the light beam diaphragm as projected on the patient. At the same time, that gives cause for concern insofar as seeing the edge of the light beam as a sharp line, it is easy to forget there is a penumbra. In multicentre trials and where the results of treatment are published, any different definition should be quoted alongside any statement of field size.

Asymmetric beams

Traditionally, each radiation beam has been symmetrical about the axis of rotation of the diaphragm system. This is no longer the case. Asymmetric control is widely available on one or both pairs of diaphragm blades (Fig. 10.8) and in any beam specification, the distance of each of the four blades from the central axis has to be clearly stated, as X_1, X_2, Y_1 and Y_2, and whether that measurement is positive or negative—a negative value is used where the blade has crossed the midline.

The initial demand for asymmetric diaphragm systems—and probably one of their main applications—is in the treatment of the breast (Ch. 26) where the junction between the edges of two tangential fields to the breast need to be aligned with the edges of the supraclavicular fields. Previously, the alignment was technically not possible because each of the beams was a divergent beam. By moving one collimator blade to coincide with the axis of rotation of the diaphragm system, it is possible to generate a beam of radiation which is asymmetric and, in particular, where one geometric edge does not diverge but follows the axis of rotation of the diaphragm system, while the other edge diverges in the normal way. (A similar beam shape can be produced by aligning a local shielding block (p. 172) with the axis—a technique sometimes known as *beam blocking*.) Now, in the case of the breast treatment, when three or four asymmetric or blocked beams are used, then the superior borders of the two tangential fields to the breast can be made to coincide with each other and with the inferior borders of the supraclavicular fields, all the beams being set up to a common isocentre. This opens up the possibility of abutting the fields to deliver a more uniform dose, although abutting fields can present dose uniformity problems as we have seen above. The edges of the asymmetric or beam-blocked beam will still exhibit a penumbra affect (p. 171) and, as before, this must be taken into account when interpreting the area delineated by the light beam diaphragm.

This is but one example of the use of asymmetric collimation. With two pairs of asymmetric diaphragm blades, a square or rectangular field can be defined anywhere within the confines of the primary collimator and may or may not contain the axis of collimator rotation. Where the asymmetric blades cross over this axis, both edges diverge from the axis in the same direction—offering unique possibilities in rotation therapy.

Experience in the use of asymmetric systems is limited and there is no accepted definition on which to base the dosimetry—the previously accepted reference point at d_{max} on the axis being no longer meaningful—but several methods have been developed and are discussed by Tsalafoutas et al (2000). To refer the relative dose to a point at d_{max} in the centre of the beam may be a logical approach. For absolute dosimetry, or dosimetry relative to the normal reference point (at d_{max} on the axis of rotation), an off-axis correction factor will need to be defined. All these data will need to be measured locally and carefully evaluated. The isodose chart for an asymmetric beam will appear to be wedged because of the natural curvature of the symmetric beam profile. The addition of wedges to the asymmetric beam will further complicate the dosimetry.

Multileaf collimation

Multileaf collimators enable the shape of the beam to be varied from the normal rectangular format, although all the many 'corners' will remain right angles (Fig. 10.8). The 'serrated' appearance to the edge of the field will give rise to an effectively broader penumbra, while the isodose distribution and the absolute dosimetry will have to be defined in terms similar to those outlined above for asymmetric fields. New protocols are urgently awaited. The size and shape of the multileaf field will be recorded and referenced within the controlling computer, not by recording manually the position of each of the, say, 52 collimating blades. The computer takes the collimator positions directly from the field shape drawn on the treatment plan or planning film. Portal imaging (p. 109) is an essential complement of any multileaf collimator system for it is through the portal-imaging system that the day-to-day field size, shape and position is checked against the original specification (Fig. 12.12).

EFFECTS OF INHOMOGENEITIES

The fundamental measurements on the relative distribution of dose and the absolute magnitude of the dose in a single beam of radiation have all assumed that the patient is accurately represented by the homogeneous water tank. This is far from true! Yet in most of our treatment planning little cognisance is given to the inhomogeneities within the patient, largely because of the complexities which arise as soon as any inhomogeneity is introduced. Until CT became widely available, the geometric data were imponderable. Lung was the one exception, but now CT gives the internal anatomy at least in multiple planes if not in three dimensions.

The effect of an inhomogeneity can be described in qualitative terms and first we concentrate on the effects of lung and bone inhomogeneities within soft tissue, but improvements in imaging techniques are on-going and other tissue inhomogeneities will be taken into consideration in the future by using the CT data to determine the relative absorption.

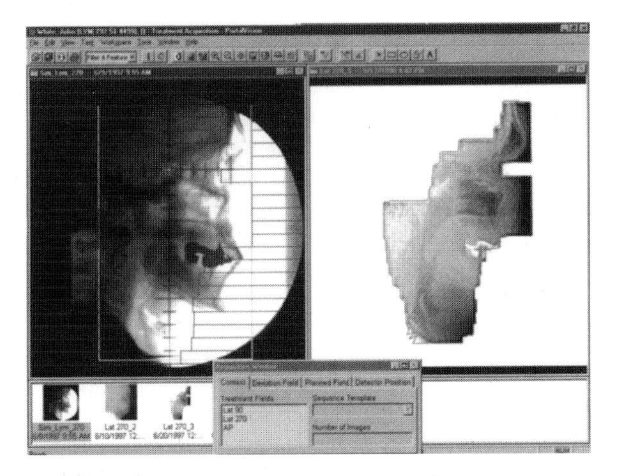

Fig. 12.12 The portal image (right) confirms the accuracy of beam size and shape relative to the simulator image (left). (Courtesy of Varian Medical Systems UK Ltd.)

Lung

Healthy lung tissue has the same atomic number but only one-third the density of soft tissue (the emphasis on *healthy lung* is necessary because diseased lung tissue will have a density closer to that of soft tissue). The radiation will therefore suffer less attenuation in passing through healthy lung than it would in soft tissue with the result that the tissues beyond healthy lung, and within its geometric shadow, will receive a greater dose than that predicted from the standard isodose charts. The effect of correcting for the lung inhomogeneities is illustrated in Figure 12.13 where in A the tissues are assumed to be homogeneous soft tissue, whereas in B the application of a lung density correction results in an increase of more than 15% in the tissue dose while all the other parameters remain unchanged.

Effective depth

Where treatment planning is carried out using manual techniques, the sheer complexity of the inhomogeneity problem makes anything more than a crude adjustment of the dose distribution for the presence of inhomogeneities prohibitive. It is possible, however, to crudely predict the lung density correction factor on the assumption that, on passing through lung, the dose is increased by, say, 2.5% per cm of lung. Alternatively, the dose beyond an inhomogeneity can be calculated using the effective depth method, where:

$$d_{\text{eff}} = d_t + d_i\rho$$

where d_t and d_i are the thicknesses of soft tissue (of density 1) and the inhomogeneity (of density ρ) respectively, and then applying an inverse square factor, $(\text{SSD} + d_{\text{eff}})^2 / (\text{SSD} + d_t + d_i)^2$, to reduce the dose at d_{eff} for the actual depth, $d_t + d_i$.

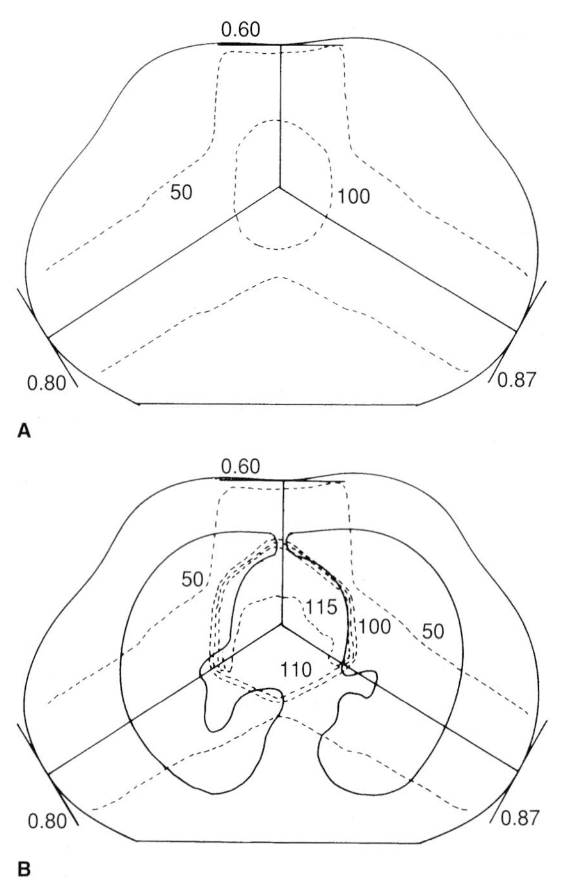

Fig. 12.13 The effect of lung correction factors: in **A** the contour is assumed to be homogeneous, whereas in **B** allowance is made for the lower density in the lungs—no other beam parameter is changed.

To make any serious attempt to take inhomogeneities into account it is necessary to use a treatment planning computer and bring in the internal mapping of the patient's anatomy from the CT or MR scanner so that the full three-dimensional size and shape of the inhomogeneity within the patient contour can be accurately assessed. (The CT image is derived from the photoelectric absorption while the treatment beam is absorbed by Compton scattering and therefore dependent on electron density. The so-called *CT numbers* can, however, be calibrated using a phantom containing known electron density elements to facilitate inhomogeneity correction, away from the tissue interfaces. The MR image may aid the visual differentiation of the tissues but cannot provide other useful data on inhomogeneities; the cross-registration of the CT and MR images is complex.)

Bone

Bone has a greater atomic number and a greater density and will absorb more radiation than soft tissue at the kilovoltage energies (Fig. 5.1) with the result that the tissues beyond the bone will receive less dose. At megavoltages, bone may absorb less dose, gram for gram, than soft tissue because of its lower electron density. But bone is nearly twice as dense as soft tissue and therefore concentrates twice the mass into the same volume. This increased absorbed energy per unit volume explains why bone still appears whiter than soft tissue on megavoltage images (Fig. 7.1).

Scatter

This relatively simple analysis is further complicated by the fact that the radiation scattered by bone and lung is different and so is the electron flux. At kilovoltage energies, the dose to soft tissue beyond lung is higher due to increased transmission through the lung and lower due to the reduced scatter produced by healthy lung, while beyond a bone inhomogeneity the dose is reduced by the high absorption in bone and increased by the increased scatter from the bone. One clinical consequence of this differential absorption is that, while underlying bone is at a greater depth than the more superficial tissues and therefore overtly receiving a lesser dose, because of the bone's greater absorption coefficient in a low-energy X-ray beam, the absorbed dose in the bone may be significantly higher than that in the overlying soft tissue. Where this may seriously affect the clinical outcome, electron therapy is preferred.

Tissue interfaces

At megavoltage energies, the secondary electron flux is greater in a higher-density medium and, since the electrons have a range of several millimetres, the electrons generated in bone close to a bone–tissue interface will increase the dose to the immediately adjacent tissue and to a depth where electronic equilibrium is restored. Those soft tissue elements and the bone marrow actually living within trabecular bone always receive a higher dose than they would if the bone were replaced by soft tissue. Similarly, healthy lung will receive a higher dose the closer it lies to the tissue–lung interface and the soft tissue close to a lung–tissue interface will receive a lower dose. So, although there may be clearly defined interfaces between the soft muscle tissues and the inhomogeneities, the dose distribution across the interfaces is far from easy to calculate! Computer planning systems make no attempt to calculate the dose distribution in these build-up or *roll-off* regions at interfaces other than at the first air–tissue interface as the beam enters the patient. It should, however, be remembered that where diseased tissue infiltrates an internal air–tissue interface, e.g. the larynx, the mucosa may receive a lower than predicted dose as illustrated in Figure 12.14.

Prostheses

Before leaving the question of inhomogeneities, mention must be made of those artificially introduced in the form of *prostheses*. Prosthetic surgery is on the increase and therefore more patients with prostheses in situ are being referred for radiotherapy and they cannot be ignored. While the general rule is not to irradiate any prosthesis, it cannot always be avoided. Electronic devices, such as pacemakers, must be kept out of the primary beam and if there is any doubt as to the radiation effects on the device, then careful checks must be introduced.

Metallic prostheses, such as replacement hip joints, will cause a greater shadowing effect on the tissues beyond because of their higher density and atomic number, but of greater concern is the effect of the radiation on the adhesives used to secure the prosthesis. As with bone, the dose immediately adjacent to the metallic prosthesis will be enhanced by the electron flux generated within the metal both penetrating the adhesive and the bone itself. As a general rule, adhesives lose their adhesion under radiation. New materials are continually being developed and the effects of radiation on each one will have to be evaluated (Erianson et al 1991).

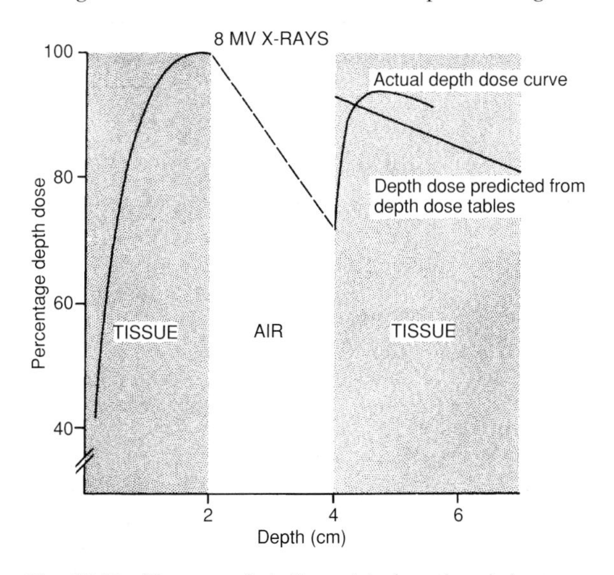

Fig. 12.14 The second air–tissue interface dose is lower than predicted from the depth dose data owing to recovery of the 'skin-sparing' effect as the beam passes through an air inhomogeneity.

OBLIQUE INCIDENCE

Owing to the curvature of the skin, most radiation beams applied to the patient will enter a curved surface at an angle other than the normal 90° incidence. Such oblique incidence may be quite deliberate or simply due to the fact that the patient's skin is curved rather than flat; in either case the dose distribution in the patient will not be that shown on the appropriate isodose chart. There are two alternative ways of dealing with this, either to correct the dose distribution or to correct the skin curvature.

Isodose shift technique

If the skin-sparing properties of a megavoltage beam are to be maximised, then the isodose distribution may be corrected from that of normal incidence to that for oblique incidence. The computer will use a mathematical approach to the problem based on the inverse square law (and the varying SSD) or the changes in exponential attenuation through the tissue excess or tissue deficiency. These techniques would be too complex to contemplate for routine manual treatment planning techniques but a 'rule-of-thumb' correction may be applied.

A rule of thumb is an approximation to the truth which is sufficiently accurate for the purpose providing it is used within its limitations. The rule here is to move the charted isodose curves through a distance equal to a fraction of the thickness of the tissue excess or tissue deficiency as measured along the ray from the source of radiation to the point of interest (Fig. 12.15). The distance moved depends on the beam energy and the depth of the isodose line. The recommended fractions are 0.67 (or two-thirds) for cobalt-60 and 0.60 for X-rays of 5–15 MV. This correction is not applied in the build-up region where the build-up continues to follow the expected pattern with the result that the isodose lines follow the curvature of the skin surface. See the discussion on build-up above for the effect of steep angles of incidence.

Tissue compensators

The charted isodose curve may be used while maintaining the skin-sparing properties of the megavoltage

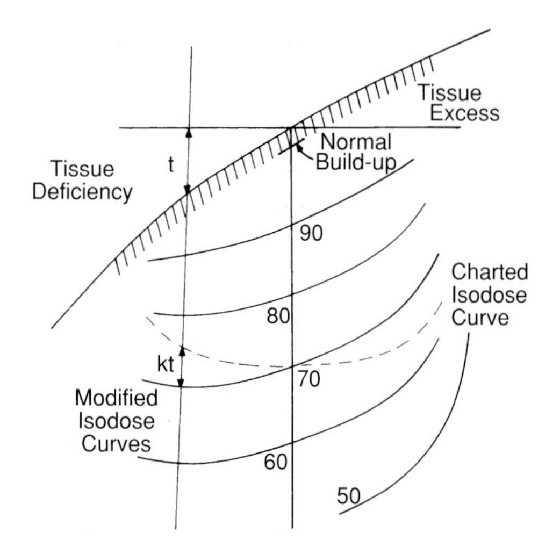

Fig. 12.15 The correction for oblique incidence using the shift technique.

beam by the use of *tissue compensators*. Here the lack of attenuation in the region of tissue deficiency is made good by using an attenuator in the primary beam sufficiently removed from the skin that the build-up region is unaffected by secondary electrons from the attenuator (Fig. 12.16). This technique is particularly valuable in regions where the skin curvature is complex, e.g. in the region of the neck. Tissue compensators are often used for treating small body sections, one compensator for each treatment field. A compensator correction factor will need to be applied to the set monitor units based on the attenuation through the baseplate and the changed SSD.

Where the curvature is sufficiently great to justify a tissue compensator, the accuracy of alignment of the compensator and patient during the treatment demands the use of an immobilisation shell (p. 185). The shell will extend over the treated region and therefore all the data required to make the compensator may be obtained from the shell, providing the shell does not distort in the absence of the patient.

Having determined accurately the position and direction of the beam axis, the stand-off or thickness of tissue deficiency may be measured at regular (say, 1 centimetre) intervals over the whole of the field area, and preferably beyond, and using 'bricks', each equivalent, say, to a cubic centimetre of tissue (Fig. 12.17), to build the compensator. These 'bricks' will be less than 1×1 cm^2 in area owing to the fact that the compensator will be mounted about half way between the source and the skin and 1 g cm^{-2} thick in whatever material is chosen, e.g. 3 mm of aluminium. The bricks will be glued to a baseplate which can be uniquely

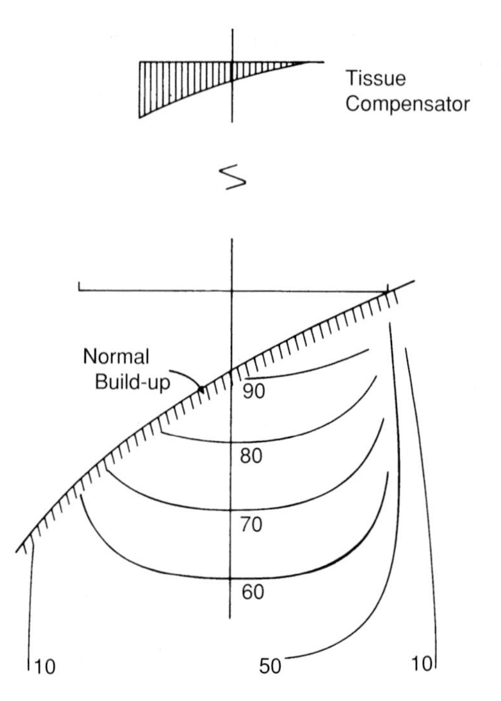

Fig. 12.16 Using a remote tissue compensator, the skin-sparing effect and the charted dose distribution are both maintained, providing the SSD is increased by the compensated thickness.

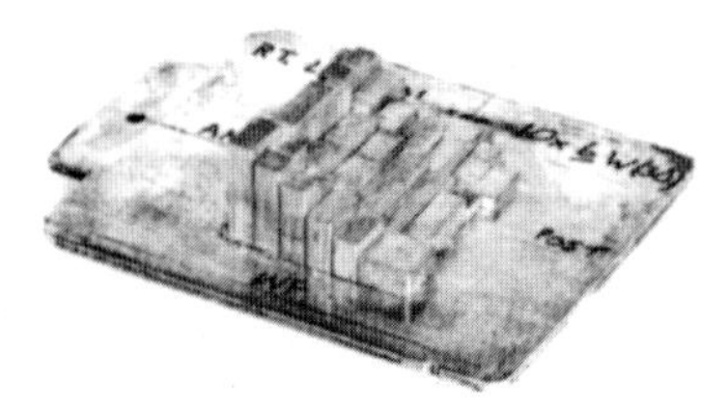

Fig. 12.17 A tissue compensator.

positioned in the beam to guarantee the correct alignment. Layers of thin lead sheet (approx. 1 mm per cm of tissue deficiency) may be cut and used in a similar manner (Jani & Pennington 1990).

An alternative technique is to carve a hollow in styrafoam and to use that as a cast for a low-melting-point alloy compensator. The carving may use profile data taken from the shell or digitised data taken from the treatment planning computer. In either case, the data are processed through a computer directly to the cutting device. The relative thickness of the compensator (to that of water) will be governed by the choice of material—tissue-equivalent wax ($\rho = 1$ g cm^{-3}), low-melting-point alloy (ρ 9 g cm^{-3}), or a stainless-steel granulate ($\rho = 4.5$ g cm^{-3}) have been used and can be recycled (Partridge et al 1999). It has been suggested that the multileaf collimator can be used in place of a tissue compensator in much the same way as the asymmetric collimator can be used in place of the discrete wedge.

Where the curvature is mainly in one direction, then tissue compensation may be achieved by using a small angle wedge (p. 214). What is more exciting is the possibility of not compensating for skin curvature but actually modifying the beam profile to deliver the desired dose profile at the target site by correcting for the combined effects of oblique incidence, skin curvature and tissue inhomogeneities in the incident beam (Thomas 1985).

Although scattered radiation plays a less significant role in megavoltage therapy, the loss of scatter generation in the tissue deficiency does result in a reduction in the dose to the first few centimetres relative to the dose to tissues at greater depth where the scatter contribution is not affected. A small correction may be required for this.

The tissue compensators used in total body irradiation techniques are more crude than those described above, insofar as they seek to compensate only for large changes in the separation of the parallel-opposed beams due to the varying body diameters, particularly in the head and neck region, caudally from the lower third of the thighs and to correct for the lack of absorption in the lungs (p. 217).

The use of bolus

At the kilovoltage energies, where there is no skin-sparing effect, the normal practice is to correct the oblique skin contour back to the flat surface of the beam-defining applicator by filling the gap with 'bolus' or tissue-equivalent material, thus making good the tissue deficiency. The 'bolus' then provides both the attenuation of the primary radiation and the scattered radiation so vital to the dose distribution. Where a kilovoltage beam is so oblique that 'shine past' is possible, then the added bolus should extend laterally to envelop the whole beam to maximise the generation of scattered radiation. This approach may be used at megavoltage energies where skin sparing is not required (Fig. 12.18 and Fig. 11.1F). In either case, normal incidence is effectively restored and the appropriate isodose chart can be used without correction.

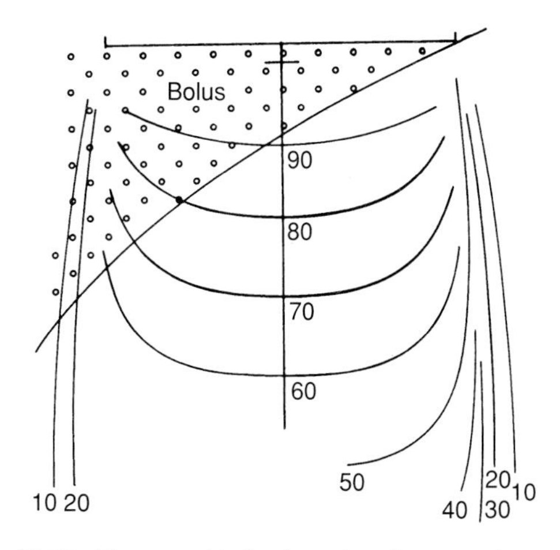

Fig. 12.18 The use of bolus to restore the normal incidence and so maintain the charted dose distribution, but note the loss of skin sparing.

WEDGES

Where the clinical target volume (p. 208) is close to the surface of the patient but too thick to be adequately treated by a single field, it is often convenient to use two photon beams with wedges. A *wedged pair* can be used to treat regions such as the antrum (p. 213), the larynx and the middle ear. A wedge attenuates the radiation at one edge of the field preferentially to that at the other, thereby tilting the isodoses away from their normally symmetrical position (Fig. 12.19). The wedge may also seek to straighten out the inherent curvature of the isodose lines.

A wedge is identified by its wedge angle. The *wedge angle* is defined as the angle through which the 50% isodose line is turned (Fig. 12.19). The *wedge factor* defines the increase in set monitor units required to deliver the same dose at d_{max} with the wedge as without the wedge present for the same field size. Each wedge will be designed for use up to a maximum field size, which may be significantly less than the maximum available without the wedge, to avoid having an unnecessarily large wedge factor. The clinical use of wedges is such that wedge angles below 45° are required in fields up to about 20 cm wide and above 45° in fields up to about 15 cm wide. The wedge interlocks should inhibit the setting of fields larger than their design maxima. The wedge will usually cover the whole range of field sizes perpendicular to the wedged direction.

There are three different methods of producing the wedging effect required. Traditionally, *discrete wedges* have been used to produce a limited range of wedge angles, typically 15°, 30°, 45° and 60°. These are wedge-shaped pieces of metal—aluminium, brass or steel—mounted on a baseplate, which in turn would be mounted and interlocked in the space behind the mirror of the light beam diaphragm system (LBD, Fig. 10.9) or mounted externally on the exit port of the X-ray head. The latter have the advantage that their presence and orientation are clearly visible, but

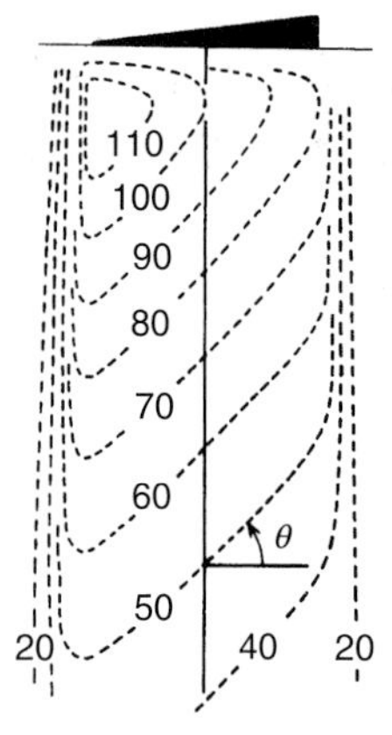

Fig. 12.19 An 8 MV isodose chart for a wedge of angle θ.

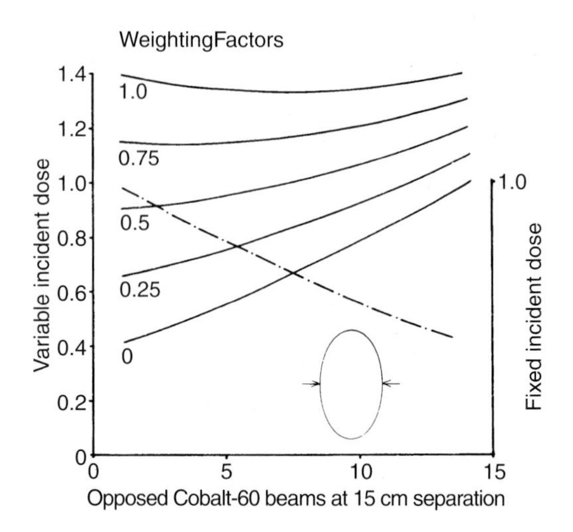

Fig. 12.20 The effect of weighting factors on the dose gradient of a parallel-opposed pair.

the disadvantages of being heavier, increasing the out-of-field scatter and blotting out the light beam.

With computer controlled linear accelerators, it is possible to produce a wider variety of wedge angles by other means. With the so-called *flying wedge* or *dynamic wedge*, located behind the LBD mirror, a wedged isodose for any angle, up to 60°, can be produced by delivering a fraction of the set monitor units with the discrete 60° wedge in the beam and the remaining fraction without it—the larger the fraction with the wedge, the greater the effective wedge angle. Having set the controls, the beam is interrupted while the wedge is electrically driven out of the beam at the appropriate point during the exposure. The advantages of the dynamic wedge are that there is no handling of the wedge, the wedge angle is infinitely variable up to the maximum and the out-of-field scatter is reduced.

Thirdly, the wedging effect may be produced simply by using the asymmetric diaphragm facility. One beam edge is fixed throughout the exposure. The opposing collimator blade is positioned to irradiate a narrow slit beam initially, but moves, in a controlled manner throughout the exposure, opening to the prescribed field size on completion of the exposure. This technique has several advantages in that there are no wedges to handle, no interruption of the light beam and no beam-hardening effect by the filter material. The principal disadvantage lies in the complexity of measuring the isodose data both initially and routinely for QA purposes; rather than using a single detector, a linear detector array is required (Fig. 12.9) so that the signal can be integrated throughout the movement of the collimator blade. Insofar as the profile of the movement against monitor units is computer controlled and infinitely variable, it will be possible to prescribe the profile as a means of optimising the treatment plan.

WEIGHTING FACTORS

In many situations, each field in a cross-firing technique is given the same exposure to d_{max}. Some distributions, however, may be improved by reducing the dose given to one or more fields in the multifield treatment plan. These fields are said to be weighted against the others. *Weighting factors* of 50% (half dose) or 75% (three-quarter dose) may be used when using manual planning techniques but any factor can be readily applied using computer techniques. Their effect is to alter the *dose gradient* and thereby improve the uniformity of dose. To illustrate the effect, consider the dose distribution along the common axis of two equal parallel-opposed beams (Fig. 12.20). The dose gradient is zero at the midpoint because the dose gradient of one beam is exactly balanced by the gradient of the other, whereas away from the midpoint, the dose gradient of one beam dominates over the lesser gradient of the other. Reducing the incident dose to the dominant beam will reduce the resulting dose gradient at the point in question. The effect of weighting factors on a four-field box technique may be seen by comparing Figures 13.2C and 13.6.

Weighting factors are so simple to apply when using computer-based planning systems that they may be trimmed by 1 or 2% simply to improve the 'appearance' of the final plan while making little difference to the dose distribution.

CHAPTER CONTENTS

13

Practice of radiation treatment planning

Keith Bomford

INTRODUCTION

The phrase *radiation treatment planning* (RTP) as applied to external beam therapy is used to describe the work involved in displaying graphically a dose distribution which results when one or more radiation beams converge on the target volume. Chapter 11 stressed the need to be able to reproduce the position of the patient correctly throughout the planning and treatment procedures and discussed some of the immobilisation devices in common use. The previous chapter outlined some of the principles of radiation treatment planning and should be studied before starting this chapter. This chapter does not include any assessment of the dose fractionation or of dose rate effects, which are dealt with in Chapter 18.

In Part 2, examples will be given for different treatment sites, whilst in this chapter we concentrate on the effects of different field combinations. It should be borne in mind that the relative distribution is not altered appreciably by changes in the size of the patient section or the size of the radiation beams used, e.g. four small oblique fields to the head treating the pituitary produce the same relative distribution as four large oblique fields to the abdomen treating the bladder. Here we concentrate on how to produce that distribution and how to implement the clinician's prescription.

BASIC CONCEPTS IN RADIATION TREATMENT PLANNING

During the whole treatment planning process, it is recommended that six volumes of tissue are identified for record purposes; each volume, except for one, is larger than the preceding one (ICRU 1993, ICRU 1999).

Before the treatment planning process is started:

- The *gross tumour volume* (GTV) is the palpable or visible extent of the malignant tumour.
- The *clinical target volume* (CTV) is the GTV together with that margin added to include the local subclinical spread of the disease. If the GTV has been surgically removed, the CTV will only include the subclinical disease.

During the actual treatment planning process:

- The *planning target volume* (PTV) is that volume defined by the radiation beams required to envelope the CTV after taking into account variations in size, shape and position due to patient movement, breathing, and, for example, bladder volume. Ideally, the PTV will be the same as the CTV; in practice it will usually be larger.
- The *organs at risk* are those normal tissues whose radiosensitivity may significantly influence the position of the fields and/or the prescribed dose, e.g. lens of the eye, spinal cord, etc.

After the completion of treatment:

- The *treated volume* (TV) is that volume enclosed by the isodose surface defined by the treatment plan and deemed to have received the dose prescribed by the clinician.
- The *irradiated volume* is that volume deemed to have received a radiation dose considered to be significant in relation to the normal tissue tolerance.

For many years the PTV has been estimated to be, say, 10 mm beyond the boundary of the GTV but as treatment planning has become more sophisticated such an arbitrary figure has been disputed; the ICRU (1999) suggests an internal margin to take into account patient movement and variations in size, shape and position of the CTV while a set-up margin accommodates the variations in patient position and dosimetric uncertainties. For some further discussion on this see McKenzie (2001). A conformity index may be defined as the quotient of the TV and the PTV when the former encloses the latter.

The treatment planning process may be a simple calculation using central axis depth dose data and take only a few minutes to perform but it may be so complex as to take several hours even with the aid of one of the powerful computer planning systems in use today. There are three levels of dose evaluation (ICRU 1993) which approximate to 1D, 2D and 3D treatment planning. These may be thought of as the dose-to-a-point, the dose-in-a-(mid)plane and the dose-throughout-a-volume respectively.

However detailed the radiation treatment planning may be, it is a matter of judgement as to whether the result of that planning is acceptable to the clinician, and the only constraint on the clinician is that the prescription of dose must be within what is considered to be accepted practice (HSE 2000). The following list of criteria gives a guide as to what is generally accepted, although some centres may beg to differ on the detail:

1. The dose throughout the CTV should be uniform to within ±5%.
2. The PTV should as near as possible be the same as the CTV in position, size and shape.
3. The dose to the PTV should exceed that to any other volume by at least 20%.
4. The dose to the organs at risk (e.g. eyes, spinal cord, etc.) should, where practicable, be kept below their tolerance dose.
5. The integral dose should be kept to a minimum.

These criteria also provide guidelines on how the treatment planning of any site should be approached. Criterion (3) suggests that unless the PTV includes the skin surface, then two or more fields should be used to converge on the PTV. Criteria (2) and (5) suggest that the radiation beam size should be kept to a minimum and the beams should enter the patient as close to the PTV as possible providing criterion (4) is not broken.

While it is widely accepted that the dose should be uniform, it is also recognised that there will be variations of dose within the PTV. It is therefore necessary to decide whether the dose prescribed should be the *maximum* or the *minimum* dose to the PTV. On the other hand, if the PTV is considered to be divided into a regular matrix and the dose at each matrix point tabulated, then the dose prescribed could be applied to the *modal dose* point (the most frequently occurring dose value in the matrix), the *average dose* point (the arithmetic mean of all the matrix dose points) or the *mean dose* point (the central value when sorted by magnitude). In any one centre, there may be a general policy on dose prescription, or it may be determined by the clinician in respect of each patient, provided it is clearly documented. However, when it comes to interdepartmental trials, this flexibility is not acceptable and ICRU (1993) recommends that the dose to the ICRU *reference point* is reported together with the maximum dose and the minimum dose to the PTV. This reference point will be in the PTV. It should be a clearly defined point, a point where the dose can be quoted with some accuracy (e.g. in a region of low dose gradient) and a point where the dose is clinically relevant. In simple beam configurations, this point is mostly likely to be the intersection of the beam axes and close to the centre of the PTV. Any point outside the PTV receiving a dose greater than that prescribed is referred to as a *hot spot*.

TREATMENT PLANNING BY HAND

Most of the examples given in Part 2 will be from a computer treatment planning system (TPS). However, simple treatment planning with coplanar beams can be developed without a computer by manually using the data on the basic isodose charts (Fig. 13.1). Corrections for inhomogeneities are rarely attempted without the use of a computer, but corrections for oblique incidence (p. 203) and simple field weighting (p. 206) can be accommodated. The resulting isodose lines are normalised to the applied (given) dose to each (unweighted) field, as in Figure 13.2.

Planning by hand is simplified if a *planning table* is available, i.e. a light box set into a desk top and inclined at an angle of, say, 10° to the horizontal. Each isodose chart should be available on a separate acetate sheet, so it can be adjusted to the desired position and angle under a sheet of tracing paper on which the patient contour is drawn. The resulting distribution is then drawn on the tracing paper. (If a single beam isodose chart needs modifying, e.g. to allow for oblique incidence (p. 203) or for weighting factors (p. 206), this should be completed before attempting the following procedure.) If a three-field plan is to be drawn, the third field will be added to the summation of the first two; a four-field plan is the addition of the summation of adjacent fields one and two to the summation of adjacent fields three and four.

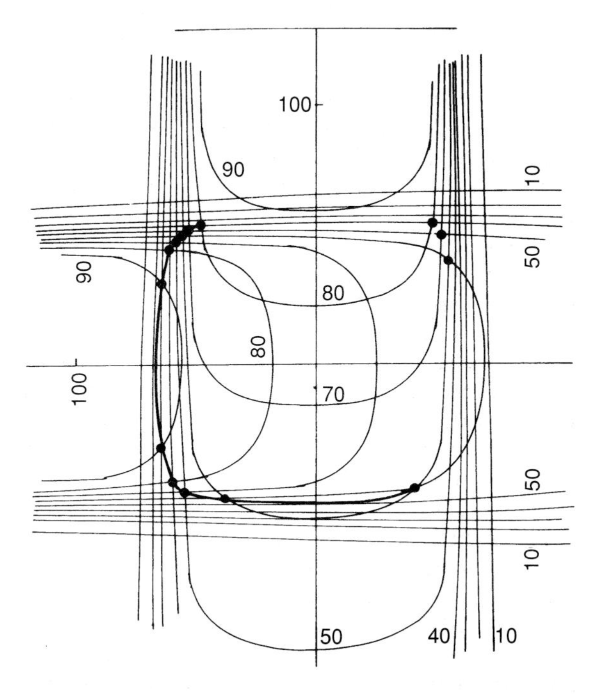

Fig. 13.1 The manual addition of isodose curves assuming the two beams enter at normal incidence with a hinge angle of 90°.

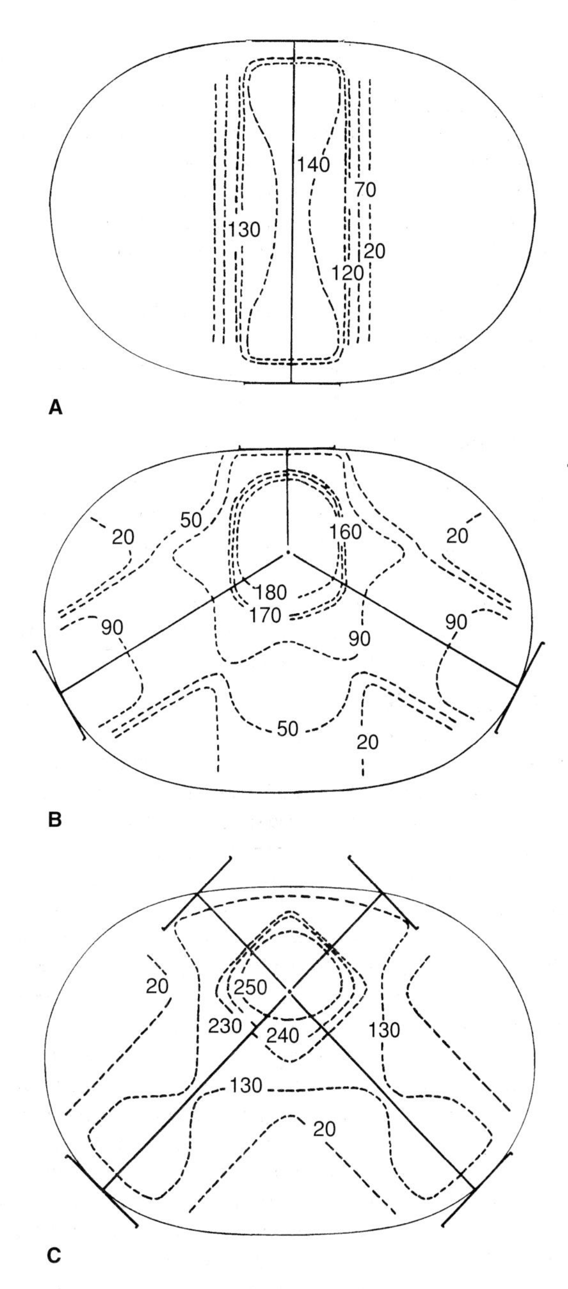

Fig. 13.2 **A** The parallel-opposed pair distribution; **B** the three-field distribution; **C** the four-field box distribution.

• In Figure 13.1, two isodose charts are shown each normalised to 100% at d_{max} with the isodose lines at 10% intervals. In practice it is easier to add the distributions of two intersecting beams, as shown, than of two parallel opposed beams. It is important to draw every isodose line in the resulting distribution, again at 10% intervals. Thus, to draw the 120% isodose line the planner will look for and mark the intersections of the individual isodose lines which add up to 120%, as shown, i.e. 100 + 20, 90 + 30, 80 + 40, 70 + 50, 60 + 60, 50 + 70, 40 + 80, 30 + 90, 20 + 100.

• Having marked all the points, notice that the consecutive points are at the diagonally opposed corners of each quadrilateral. Now join up all the points in order as smoothly as possible and without crossing any isodose line except at the intersection of two. Occasionally two adjacent points are the addition of the same two isodose lines, which may appear inseparable—the resultant isodose line lies between the two! Occasionally, too, there may be too few points of intersection to know where the resultant isodose line should be drawn; to solve this, the planner must interpolate the individual isodose charts to find points of the required value, in this example, 75 + 45, 63 + 57, etc. Remember isodose lines in the resultant distribution will never intersect and will always be continuous within the patient contour—isodose curves of low value may be discontinuous (only) at the patient contour.

TREATMENT PLANNING BY COMPUTER

Treatment planning by hand is largely a thing of the past as a range of computer planning software is now widely available from simple PC systems to complex three-dimensional (3D) planning systems with data links to the CT scanner, treatment simulator and the therapy beam generator itself. With the complexities involved in radiation treatment planning, it is not surprising that this saw the first application of computer technology in medicine and within about 10 years a computer optimisation program was available which recommended the optimum field parameters for a three-field plan (Hope et al 1967)—the software took about 48 hours to run a single plan! Since then complete computer optimisation has given way to *user optimisation* whereby the software allows the user to modify the beam parameters with an almost instant response to demonstrate the effect.

The radiation beam data in the early systems were often stored as a matrix because the basic isodose data for any beam were difficult to reduce to a mathematical formula. This matrix proved cumbersome to store and slow in calculation, and empirical formulae were developed to try to overcome this limitation (Haywood et al 1979). Today, for basic PC systems and 2D planning with regular fields, several beam profiles are stored which, together with the central axis depth dose curve, enable off-axis doses to be readily calculated although allowances for shielding blocks and/or multileaf collimation are limited. Further development of the computer model now enables the scatter contribution from the whole irradiated volume to be included with the primary 'ray' data and thereby details a full 3D dose distribution whatever the shape of the field (Conway 1998). Whichever system is used, the final isodose curves are interpolated from a dose matrix of about 3 mm interval.

In practice, most treatment plans currently comprise a 2D dose distribution through the midplane of the target tissues and containing the axes of all the (square or rectangular) fields; occasionally planes parallel to that midplane may be computed (Plate 1.9). Full 3D plans are becoming more widely used and the dose distributions in all three orthogonal planes can be displayed (Plate 1.10).

3D plans are far more time-consuming and require greater operator skill and fast graphics workstations to handle the contouring of external and internal anatomy in orthogonal or oblique planes from CT images, tissue inhomogeneity corrections, multileaf collimators and/or shielding blocks, etc. (The CT images will usually be produced with slices of less than 3 mm thick and 3 mm spacing and once the GTV and CTV contours have been marked on the principal plane, they may be copied on to adjacent planes and emended as necessary on each plane.) All these parameters may be handled through the keyboard and displayed in tabular form or through the 'mouse', but full colour display is essential to identify the information superimposed on the patient section. The graphics display may be in the standard midplane, but equally it could be the sagittal or coronal section or an oblique plane based on the appropriate computer reconstruction of the anatomy. A split-screen facility enables several of these images to be displayed at the same time (Plate 1.5).

The so-called *beam's eye view* (BEV, Plate 1.11) facility is ideal for determining the size and shape of the field as it enables the actual coverage of the beam and therefore the exclusion of the critical tissues to be checked (but, as on the simulator, the beam edge displayed does not include any representation of the beam penumbra) and the *digitally reconstructed radiograph* (DRR) is produced for comparison with the simulator film or the therapy portal image (Fig. 13.3). Some TPS

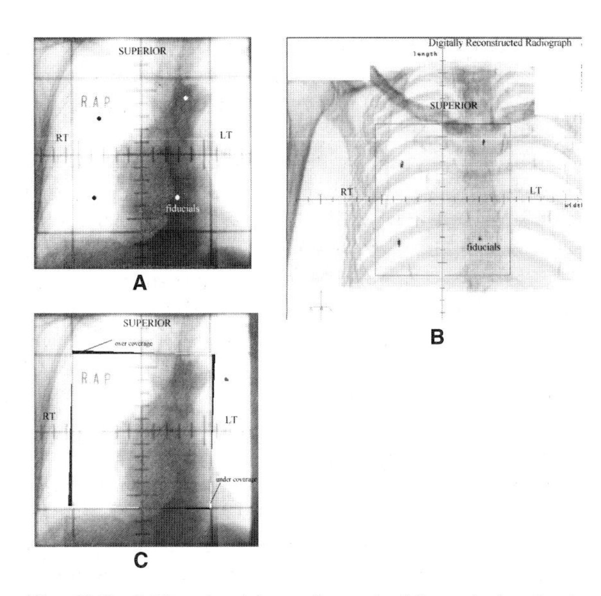

Fig. 13.3 **A** The simulator radiograph of the anterior chest; **B** a digitally reconstructed radiograph (DRR) from the virtual simulator; and **C** overlaying the two shows the slight rotation of the patient between the two procedures.

packages include facilities for scoring the plan in terms of the dose uniformity or for compiling a cumulative *dose–volume histogram* (DVH) of the target tissues (p. 222) to show how much of the PTV is above/below the nominal prescribed dose; the DVH for each critical organ may also be displayed (Fig. 13.4, Table 13.1). This scoring facility is particularly valuable in assessing which of several alternative plans is the best.

The TPS is therefore a complex mix of hardware and software and quality assurance is vital if errors are going to be avoided. The hardware QA must include the performance of all the input/output devices while the software QA must check not only the routine calculations but also the accuracy of the fundamental data sets and the boundaries of calculation, etc. (Whilde et al 1993, IPEMB 1996c).

SIMPLE DISTRIBUTIONS

Atlases of dose distributions

Atlases of dose distributions are no longer used as an aid to treatment planning because of the limitations inherent in such distributions. They are, however, a valuable teaching aid for students and an aide-memoire for those involved in treatment planning when faced with an unfamiliar case. Each chart in the *atlas* provides the dose distribution resulting from fields of a stated size, relative angle, separation and beam quality.

Parallel pair

The radical treatment plan demands the distribution to be tailored to the individual patient and will often involve two, three or four fields. Two directly opposing fields are known as a *parallel-opposed-pair* and the distribution is typified in Figure 13.2A. In general,

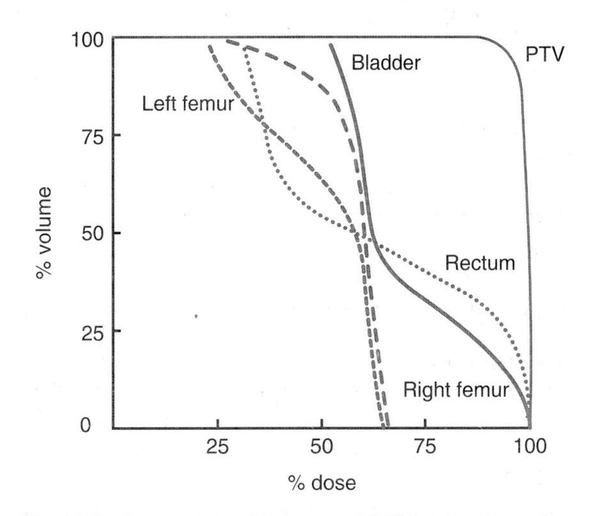

Fig. 13.4 Dose–volume histograms (DVH) for the planned tumour volume (PTV) and several critical tissues—in this case neither femur exceeds two-thirds of the PTV dose while small parts of both bladder and rectum receive the full PTV dose.

Table 13.1 Computed data relating to the DVHs shown in Figure 13.4; the prescribed PTV dose is 55 Gy

	Bladder	Right femur	Left femur	Rectum	PTV
Volume (cm^3)	172	43	43	86	180
Minimum dose (Gy)	28.0	14.1	11.4	16.4	47.9
Maximum dose (Gy)	55.4	36.2	35.8	55.6	55.8
Modal dose (Gy)	32.5	34.4	34.1	55.0	55.0
Standard deviation (%)	16.5	8.1	13.9	26.7	1.6

the distribution is symmetrical about the beam axes where both beams enter at normal incidence. In particular, the midpoint receives the minimum dose along the central axes (except within the build-up region) and the maximum dose at right angles to the central axes. The actual variation of dose along these axes of symmetry depends on the quality of radiation and on the separation of the fields (Fig. 13.5). The variation in dose is reduced by reducing the separation and by increasing the energy of the radiation. Within these limits, the enclosed tissues receive a fairly uniform dose.

It should be remembered (Fig. 12.2) that the dose to the edges of the beam, while being lower than on the central axis when the beams enter a flat surface at normal incidence, may be increased where there is excessive curvature of the entry surfaces, e.g. frontal and occipital fields to the head. The edge of the beam will always define the edge of the PTV; a uniform dose distribution cannot be achieved through the penumbra of a beam (p. 171).

This two-field technique is valuable where large volumes of tissue are to be irradiated and/or where the treatment is palliative. The use of very large fields, as for total body and mantle irradiations, will be discussed later in this chapter (p. 216).

Box technique

If the parallel pair gives a relatively uniform irradiation to the enclosed tissues, then two intersecting parallel pairs will produce a uniform distribution over the centrally placed volume enclosed by all four fields. This is true regardless of the angle between the axes of the two pairs, i.e. the 'box' is not necessarily rectangular. For example, two pairs at right angles produce a 'square-shaped' distribution (Fig. 13.2C), while two pairs at, say 120°, will produce a 'diamond-shaped' distribution. The advantage of the *box technique* is the steep dose gradient on the four sides of the PTV, while the disadvantage is that some of the irradiated tissue outside receives half the dose to that inside—an effect exacerbated when small fields are used at large separations. There is no reason against using three parallel pairs, but the improvement is rarely justified.

The four-field box technique is ideal for treating tissues centrally placed within the patient contour. Where the box technique is used to treat a volume which is off-centre (as in Fig. 13.2C), then the distribution may be improved by weighting those fields closer to the treated volume so that they can contribute the same dose to the centre of the volume as the more distant fields (Fig. 13.6).

Three-field technique

By arranging three fields so that they overlap only in the target volume (Fig. 13.2B), it may be possible to bring more of the tissue outside the PTV to less than half the target dose while the *irradiated volume* may be larger than in the box technique, i.e. to spread the *unwanted dose* more thinly over a larger volume of tissue. Be aware that if this technique is applied to a large patient section with too low a photon energy beam, then significant dose may be given to the tissues around the d_{max} of the more distant fields, as in the two oblique fields shown in Figure 13.2C. It will be also noticed that the dose gradient at the edge of the PTV is less steep than that in the box technique, while the PTV will approximate to a circle within the six field edges approximating a hexagon. These three- and four-field techniques are widely used in radical treatments using quite small fields—providing the beam direction can be guaranteed and the target is close to the centre of the patient section. Off-centre CTVs are better treated using wedged beams.

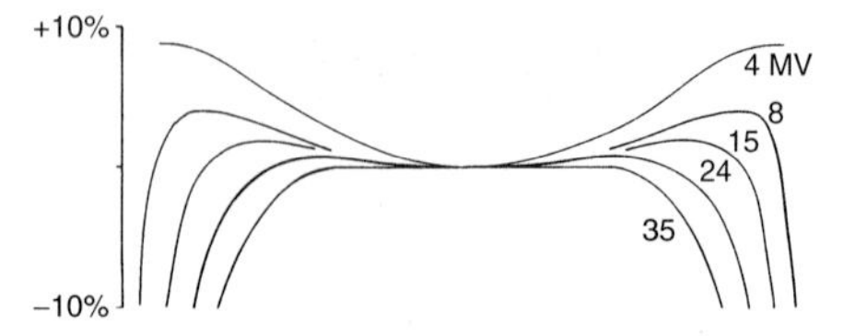

Fig. 13.5 The variation of dose uniformity along the common axes of a parallel-opposed pair with photon energy.

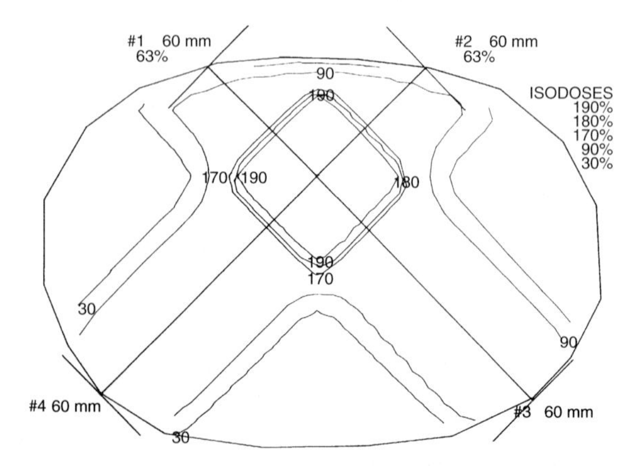

Fig. 13.6 The four-field box distribution of Figure 13.2C improved by the use of weighting two fields by 63%.

Wedged pair dose distribution

The wedged pair technique is ideal for the treatment of tissues which extend deep into the patient contour from a point close to the surface (e.g. the antrum)—tissue-equivalent material may be added to the skin surface to bring the PTV even closer to the skin itself, if that is required. A single wedged beam is characterised by its *wedge angle* (p. 205), and the ideal dose distribution is obtained when each of two beams of the same wedge angle, θ, enter at normal incidence (Figs 13.7 and 13.8A) with a *hinge angle* of (180 - 2θ) degrees. The hinge angle, *H*, is the angle between the beam axes at their point of intersection (angle *qps* in Fig. 13.7). In cases such as the middle ear, the CTV is almost triangular, and aligning the two beam edges with two sides of that triangle, effectively defines the hinge angle and, by implication, the wedge angle (Fig. 13.8B). The additional *wedging effect* produced under conditions of oblique incidence effectively reduces the wedge angle and increases the optimum hinge angle. This suggests, in practice, one should start the planning process with a wedge angle steeper than might be expected.

The student should note that wherever wedges are used, they are used in pairs with the 'thick edges together' irrespective of the hinge angle. Rarely will two wedges of different wedge angle be used together as the difference in their dose gradients will need to be compensated by introducing weighting factors, which in turn modifies the wedge angle.

The three-field wedged pair

If the disease is confined more to the superficial tissues, then the addition of a third unwedged field between the two wedged fields may be preferred. In this context, the concept of hinge angle is not appropriate. The aim is to use a large hinge angle and large wedge angle to create a reversed dose gradient and then to use the intermediate unwedged beam to counter that dose gradient to give the required uniformity. Figure 13.9 shows two examples of this technique, both giving the desired uniformity of dose to the same CTV (not shown). Their difference lies in the choice of wedge angle and weighting factors. (The comparison of two dose distributions is simplified when they are normalised to the target dose, as here; all three fields will carry a weighting factor, they may be equally weighted as in Fig. 13.9A or differently weighted as in Fig. 13.9B.)

Any application of external beam therapy means there will be some irradiation of the healthy tissues outside the PTV, but this technique offers some choice as to which tissues get the *unwanted dose*. Note, for example, the 50% and 20% isodose lines. In Figure 13.9A, the greater weighting of the unwedged field increases the dose to the deep-seated tissues, whereas

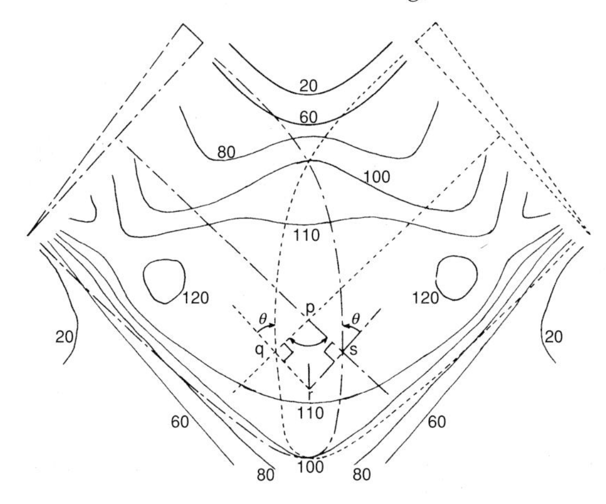

Fig. 13.7 The optimum hinge angle for a wedged pair assuming the two beams enter at normal incidence with a hinge angle of 180–2θ.

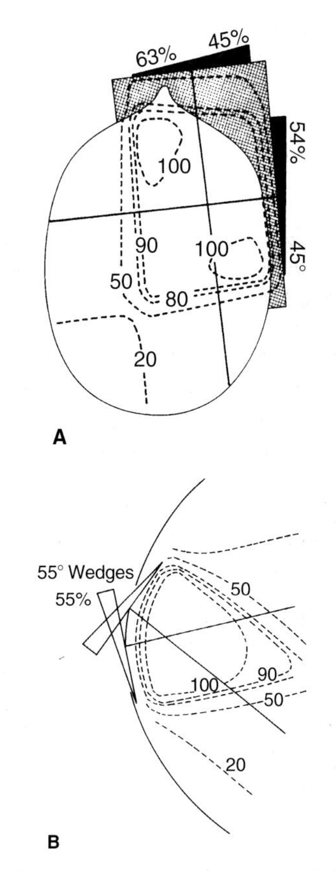

Fig. 13.8 **A** A wedged pair to the antrum with full TE build-up, and **B** a wedged pair to the middle ear without build-up.

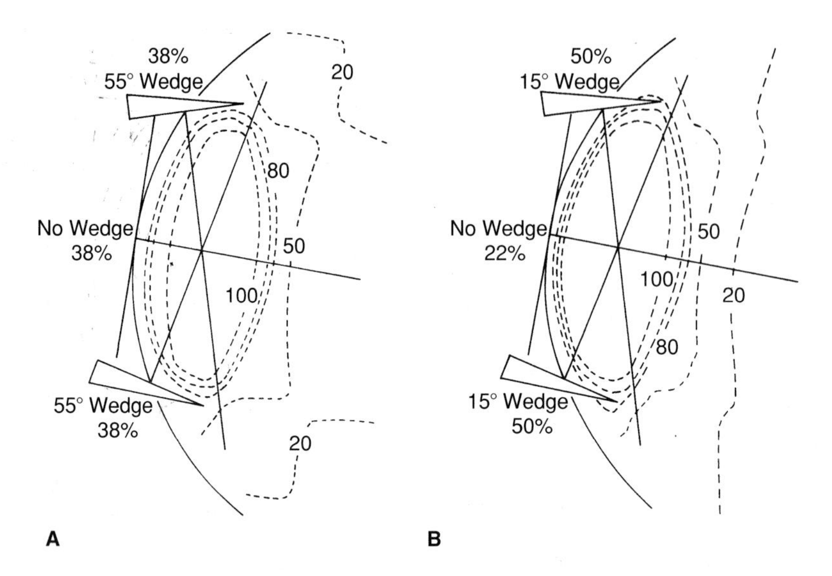

Fig. 13.9 The use of a wedged pair and an intermediate third plane field and illustrating how the dose to tissues outside the PTV can be modified by changing the weighting factors and wedge angle—the lower weighting on the plain field reduces the dose at depth at the expense of increasing the dose to the exit tissues of the wedged beams.

in Figure 13.9B, the wedged beams carry the greater weighting factor and deliver a larger dose to the superficial tissues beyond the CTV but less dose to the deep-seated tissues.

This technique can be applied to superficial targets, as shown, but is equally applicable to deep-seated targets, e.g. treating the nasopharynx, the bladder or the cervix with an anterior plain field and two opposed lateral wedged fields.

Wedges as tissue compensators

The wedging effect of oblique incidence can sometimes be compensated by the use of wedges of shallow wedge angle, say 15°. For example, when treating a larynx with a parallel-opposed pair, it may improve the final dose distribution if wedges are used such that their thick edges are (together) to the anterior. This technique is of limited value but can, with care, be used to advantage wherever the skin curvature is predominantly in one plane. The use of the dynamic collimator blade system of wedges (p. 205) would enable the beam profile to be tailored more accurately to the requirements.

ROTATION THERAPY

A logical extension of multiple fixed field techniques is to have an infinite number of fields all aimed at one centre. This is achieved by moving the source of radiation in an arc whilst irradiating the patient. In *arc therapy,* the source of radiation moves through a prescribed angle, while in *rotation therapy* the source moves through a full 360°. Rotation therapy was developed in the 1920s as a means of maximising the dose at depth without exceeding the tolerance dose to the skin using 200 kV radiation. Although skin dose should no longer be a problem, thanks to the skin-sparing effect of megavoltage radiation, arc therapy is still used in some centres, particularly where cobalt-60 provides the only megavoltage radiation. The dose distribution resulting from a full rotation of the source of radiation is essentially circular or elliptical—the major axis of the ellipse being at right angles to that of the patient contour (Fig. 13.10). There are no steep dose gradients at the edges of the PTV because the beam edges are blurred by the rotation. In arc therapy as the arc is reduced from a full 360°, the volume of uniform dose moves away from the centre of rotation in the direction of the centre of the arc. As the angle of arc falls to zero, the distribution reduces to a single beam isodose as one would expect.

Not all arc therapy uses a single centre of rotation; multiple centres have been used to good effect. Kidney-shaped (re-entrant) dose distributions can be achieved using arc therapy in conjunction with asymmetric collimators, offering yet one more variable to an already complex treatment regime.

The dosimetry is complicated by the fact that the source–skin distance (SSD) varies while the source–axis

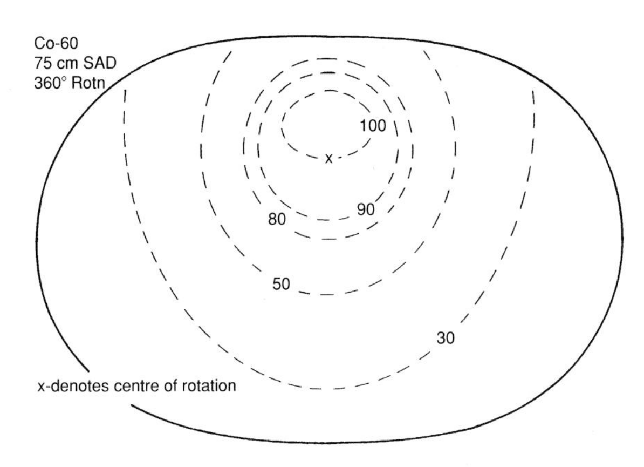

Fig. 13.10 A dose distribution resulting from rotation therapy.

distance (SAD) remains constant. The dose rate at the centre of rotation can be estimated using tissue–air ratios (TAR) or tissue–phantom ratios (TPR).

Tissue–air ratio

The *tissue–air ratio* (TAR) is the ratio of the dose rate at a point in the patient to that at the same point (at the centre of a minimal mass) in air when there is no patient present.

$$\text{TAR} = \frac{\text{Axis dose rate in tissue}}{\text{Axis dose rate in air}}$$

(The phrase 'minimal mass in air' is open to interpretation and dependent on the photon energy). The dose rate at a point is dependent on the distance from the source (inverse square law), the thickness of the overlying tissues (attenuation) and the scatter contribution appropriate to the field size. Since the TAR is the ratio of dose rates at the same point in space, the ratio is independent of distance from the source. For a given field size (and, therefore, scatter contribution), it is possible to tabulate the TAR against the thickness of the overlying tissue (Table 13.2).

By definition, the dose rate at the isocentre point in the patient is the dose rate in air at that same point in space (the isocentre) multiplied by the TAR. The mean value of the TAR, for no less than 20 radii of the patient contour, may be used to determine a mean dose rate on the axis of a full rotation.

Tissue–phantom ratio

The TAR is equal to the PSF (p. 196) multiplied by the TMR, the tissue-maximum ratio. The TMR is the special case of TPR where the reference point is at d_{max} on the central axis. These are defined as:

Table 13.2 Tissue–air ratios for cobalt-60 (BJR 1983)

Depth (cm)	Field size			
	5 × 5	10 × 10	15 × 15	20 × 20
5	0.849	0.905	0.936	0.957
7	0.763	0.830	0.870	0.893
10	0.642	0.718	0.765	0.795
12	0.570	0.646	0.696	0.730
15	0.474	0.547	0.600	0.638
20	0.348	0.411	0.462	0.500

$$\text{TMR} = \frac{\text{Axis dose rate at depth } d \text{ in a phantom}}{\text{Axis dose rate at depth } d_{max} \text{ in same phantom}}$$

$$\text{TPR} = \frac{\text{Axis dose rate at depth } d \text{ in a phantom}}{\text{Axis dose rate at reference depth in same phantom}}$$

The tissue–phantom ratio (TPR) may be used instead of the tissue–air ratio above to determine the mean dose rate at the axis of rotation providing the reference dose rate is known at the reference point in the phantom. The use of TPR is a little more straightforward in practice than that of TAR because the reference dose rate can be measured directly under standardised conditions.

CONFORMATION THERAPY

Field shape

For nearly a century, the radiotherapy of deep-seated tissues has used co-planar, regularly shaped symmetrical fields, with the result that the treated volume has approximated to a simple geometric volume enclosing the target tissues while trying to minimise the volume of adjacent healthy tissue irradiated. The only real exceptions to this have been when lead cut-outs (p. 152) or local shielding (p. 172) have been used to protect tissues at risk; these techniques today might be rightly referred to as *conformation therapy* for their aim has been to conform the PTV to the CTV in position, size and shape (p. 208). Many uses of local shielding blocks have now been replaced by the use of multileaf collimators (p. 170) to shape the beams to the contours of the CTV.

An early attempt to minimise the irradiation of healthy tissue involved reducing the field size as the tumour regressed but, of course, not all tumours regressed during the fractionated course of treatment and the technique carried the risk of underdosing the subclinical spread of the disease.

Another early attempt at conformation therapy was to computer-control the field size, gantry angle and couch position using a specially adapted cobalt-60 gamma beam unit (Davy et al 1975). The technique was not widely adopted, but with the greater sophistication of computer control available on linear accelerators today variations on this technique are being adopted, particularly in the control of field size and shape.

Multileaf collimators are now widely available and provide opportunities to shape the field to conform more closely to the shape of the target tissues. To maximise their usefulness multileaf collimators must be used in conjunction with:

- a CT scanner/virtual simulator facility (p. 108) to provide the patient data in three dimensions
- a three-dimensional treatment planning system using pencil-beam data to calculate the dose distributions from the irregular-shaped fields, and
- a portal imaging system (p. 109) to verify the accuracy of the collimation and patient set-up on a daily basis throughout the course of treatment.

Beam profile

Conforming the fields to the shape of the diseased tissues is one thing but this is likely to make it more difficult to obtain the dose uniformity required for an acceptable plan because the scatter component at depth is dependent on the size and shape of the beam and the more irregular the shape the more irregular the scatter component of the dose.

The use of 'bolus' in kilovoltage therapy (p. 205) sought to correct the dose distribution in the patient to that shown on the isodose chart and thereby simplify treatment planning. Tissue compensators (p. 204) in megavoltage therapy sought to correct the beam profile for irregularities in the skin surface while maintaining the skin-sparing effect. The so-called *difference compensators* sought to present the optimum beam profile to the target tissues in addition to correcting for the surface irregularities (Thomas 1985).

We have already seen in the last chapter that the independent control of one collimating blade may be used as an alternative to a discrete wedge-shaped attenuator (p. 206) to produce a wedged beam profile. Developing this technology one step further suggests the collimator blade can be moved during the beam exposure, not to produce a smooth wedge profile but to produce the optimum beam profile prescribed by the TPS for the treatment plan and after applying inhomogeneity corrections to the overlying tissues. Applying this principle to the multileaf collimator introduces the concept of *intensity modulated radiotherapy* (IMRT) and optimising both the beam shape and beam profile to the target tissues (Nutting et al 2000).

Cohen (1966) and Bomford (1969) both foresaw the day when treatment planning would become analytical rather than syntactical; working backwards from the needs of the CTV to obtain the optimum beam parameters for the treatment plan—maybe varying the energy of the beam as well as the beam size, shape and profile for each patient.

MANTLE TREATMENTS

The treatment plans considered so far have involved radiation fields of dimensions smaller than the patient so that, with some modification, the isodose data measured in the semi-infinite phantom can be regarded as adequate. There are situations, however, where the field dimensions are larger than the patient—in the treatment of the whole thorax using mantle fields and in total body irradiation, for example.

The radiation treatment planning of mantle fields is complicated because it always involves substantial lung shielding (Fig. 10.14) and the considerable variation in the separation of the parallel-opposed AP–PA pair over the length and breadth of the fields. The minimum separation is in the upper half of the field where the local shielding is also minimal; both factors increase the dose to the midplane tissues. The aim of treatment planning is to deliver a uniform dose to this midplane while minimising the dose to the lungs.

The lung dose is unlikely to be much below 10% in that the major component to the dose in the shadow of the shielding block (p. 172) will be scattered radiation from within the adjacent irradiated tissues. The presence of the shielding, in turn, reduces the scatter component to the irradiated tissues, and the equivalent square concept cannot be simply applied. The scatter component near the centre of the T-shaped field will be greater than along its three arms. At the higher photon energies, the scatter component is small and therefore variations in scatter will have a smaller effect on the dose uniformity.

The effect of the variation in beam separation may be minimised by the use of higher photon energies (Fig. 13.5) and extended SSDs as both these factors reduce the dose gradient and therefore reduce the variation of midpoint dose with field separation. Modern collimators will cover these large fields at the normal treating distance, but this benefit of using extended SSDs should not be ignored.

The third area of concern in this technique is the lateral aspect of the chest wall which may be included in the field outside the lung shield. The lung shields should be tailor-made and tapered to minimise the effects of transmission penumbra. The scatter component of the chest wall dose will be negligible—there will be no scatter generated by the photons lateral to the chest wall (they will shine past) and there will be no significant scatter generated from within the shielded lung. The primary radiation component, however, will be increased because the beam separation is small. Together, these factors leave some uncertainty in any estimate of the delivered dose to these tangential tissues.

While manual planning techniques can be applied, the full 3D TPS will produce a more accurate dose distribution in the central areas, but its accuracy in the peripheral tissues will need to be assessed as it may be jeopardised by the computer modelling.

TOTAL BODY IRRADIATION

The use of *total body irradiation* (TBI) with megavoltage (6 MV) photons is an established preliminary to *bone marrow transplantation*. This poses organisational problems as well as problems in radiation treatment planning. The treatment is usually given in six or eight fractions over 3 or 4 days (Ch. 29). Whether the patient adopts the fetal position or lies down, the treatment beams will be horizontal and parallel opposed. The very large field sizes required usually mean that the patient is treated close to the treatment room wall which, together with the over-large fields, means the dose to the patient may be increased by the radiation scattered back off the walls. A few centres will add AP and PA fields, but only where the necessary patient position can be maintained and reproduced with sufficient accuracy—e.g. using vertical rather than horizontal beams.

The aim of the radiation treatment planning is to deliver a uniform dose to the midline at the different levels within the patient despite the variations in (lateral) beam separations from typically 10 cm at the neck to 40 cm at the shoulders. These major variations in beam separation can be accommodated using tissue compensation to the head and neck and caudally from the lower third of the thighs (Fig. 13.11). Lateral beams to the thorax will, however, traverse considerable thicknesses of lung, where the attenuation is less than in normal tissue and because the dose to the lung is critical, careful lung compensation is essential. The lung compensators are best designed using the 3D data from a full CT investigation of the thorax, careful treatment planning and attention to the position of the upper arm through which the beam may or may not pass. The patient is treated through a transparent

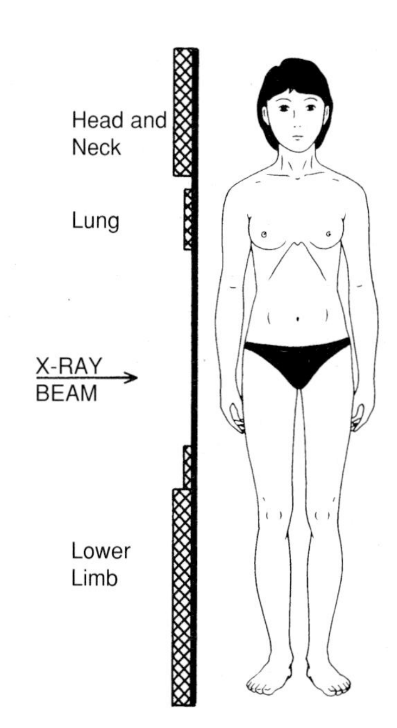

Fig. 13.11 Tissue compensation for lateral fields in total body irradiation.

screen, positioned close to the patient to bring the peak dose closer to the skin (skin sparing is not required), and the compensators are most conveniently attached to that screen. The screen will be of a thickness approximately equal to the d_{max} of the radiation, say, 15 mm acrylic. The head and neck, lung and lower limb compensation is readily achieved using aluminium, brass and sheets of acrylic respectively—the shape of the lung compensator will need to be tailored to the individual patient.

It is customary to monitor the dose given to the patient using TLDs or silicon diodes attached to the patient at selected and critical points. This survey of dose may be carried out as either a preliminary to the treatment using a low-dose trial irradiation or at each fraction throughout the treatment. Logically, the probes will be placed on the anterior and posterior midlines at various locations, but more useful information is gained from probes in the coronal midplane measuring the entrance and exit doses than from probes in 'shine past' locations. As with all patient dose measurements, the results must be interpreted carefully in the light of conditions prevailing at the time of irradiation (p. 67). Where three or four fields are used, the weighting of each field will be determined from the separate dose survey of each field.

Trials have been started where the patient stands, with appropriate support, in which case AP and PA fields may be used with suitable tissue compensation. This simplifies the setting-up in that a simple turntable may be used to turn the patient between fields (Jones et al 2000).

RADIOSURGERY

In contrast to TBI, radiosurgery is the use of very small fields—less than 25 mm diameter—to treat brain disease (Leksell 1968). Its principal use is in the treatment of artereovenous malformations which are often too deep within the brain for conventional surgical techniques to be used, but are readily accessible to accurately collimated and defined radiation beams.

The technique has been established using a large number of cobalt-60 sources arrayed over a spherical sector and individually collimated to focus their radiation on to the target tissues. The unit in Sheffield (Fig. 13.12 and Plate 1.12) uses 201 1-mm diameter cobalt sources to irradiate a volume of tissue at the focus within a 50% isodose surface as small as 4 mm diameter or as large as 18 mm. The interchangeable helmets provide the final collimation. Larger targets can be accommodated by treating multiple foci.

Figure 13.13 shows the two orthogonal views of the distributions using the 4 mm and the 18 mm collimators. The very nature of the technique precludes the measurement of the isodose distribution using an ionisation chamber in a water tank and it is measured in a tissue-equivalent head phantom using a solid-state detector probe, within which the position of the crystal sensor is accurately known, and moving through a matrix of points (Walton et al 1987).

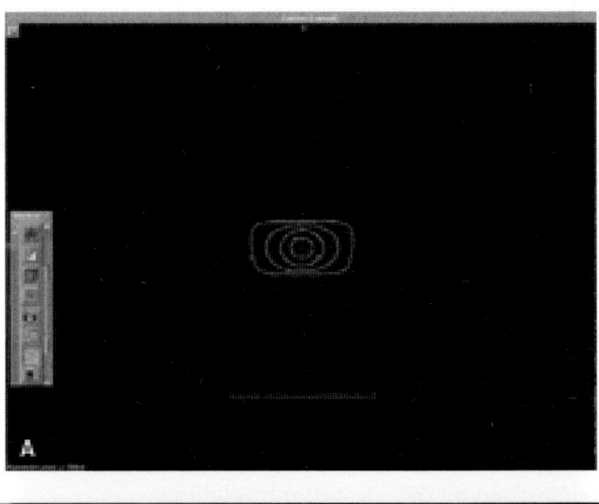

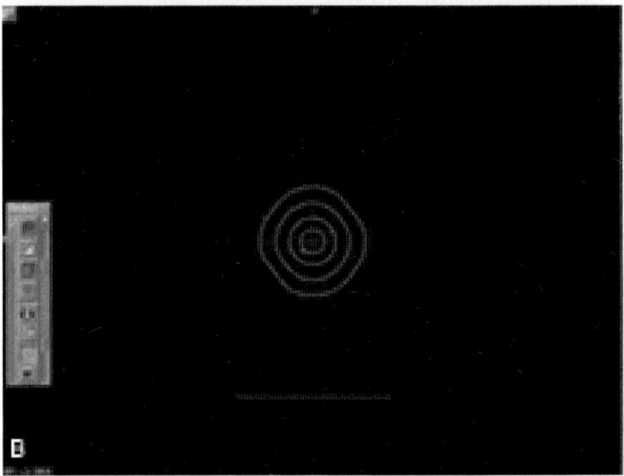

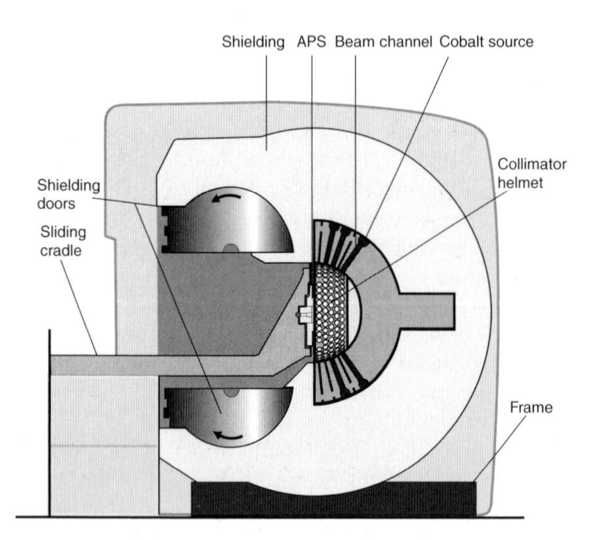

Fig. 13.12 The Sheffield stereotactic radiosurgery unit—schematic diagram showing the helmet in the treatment position. (Leksell GammaPlan®, courtesy of Elekta Instrument AB, Stockholm.)

To achieve this level of accuracy in the clinical situation demands that the localisation, the treatment planning and the treatment are completed in a single session during which the patient 'wears' a reference frame (Plate 1.12B). The frame is attached rigidly to the outer table of the skull under local anaesthetic and defines the coordinate system to be used for both the localisation of the CTV and the positioning of the patient for treatment. The localisation of the target will be carried out by subtraction angiography, CT or MR imaging. The whole procedure takes some 4–6 hours to complete and the patient is usually allowed to leave hospital the following day.

Radiosurgery is now being practised in some centres using a linear accelerator as the source of radiation, but a special collimator has to be fitted to give the necessary field size at the isocentre. Four or more arcs of gantry rotation, each at a different setting of couch rotation, are used to achieve the high concentration of dose

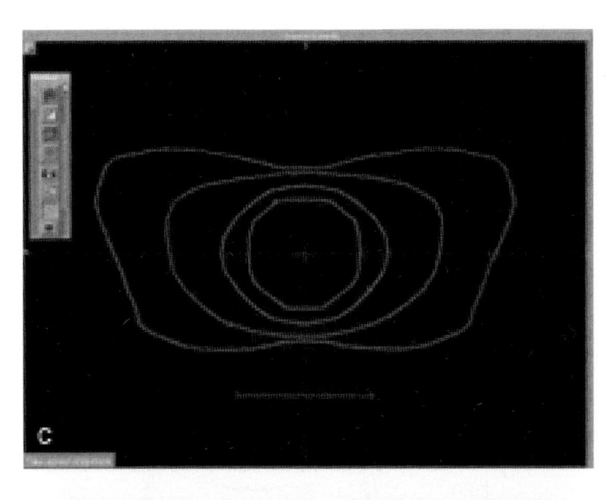

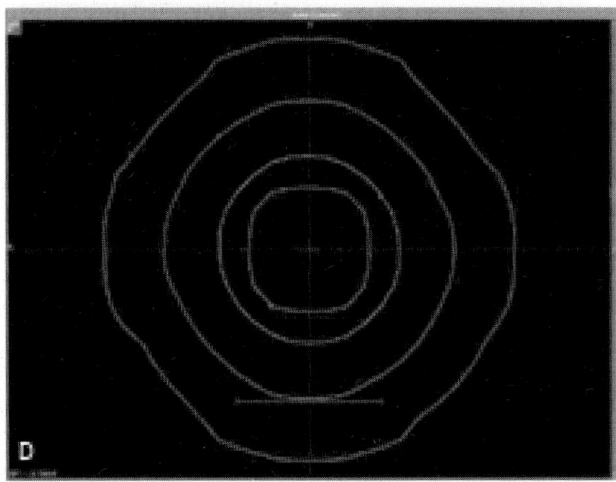

Fig. 13.13 **A** The coronal and **B** the axial isodose distribution for the 4 mm collimator; **C** and **D** for the 18 mm collimator, respectively—the straight line is 20 mm in length.

required. As may be expected, the dose gradient at the edge of the irradiated volume is less steep than on the cobalt unit and the smallest PTV is about 15 mm.

TREATMENT OF SUPERFICIAL LESIONS

So far in this chapter we have dealt with the treatment of deep-seated lesions using multiple fields. If the lesion is superficial and only involves the skin or underlying tissues to a depth of a few centimetres, then a single treatment field may be all that is required.

Depth dose is a function of photon energy and the source–skin distance and it may be reduced by reducing either or both. Traditionally, low-energy X-rays of between 50 kV and 160 kV have been used at source–skin distances of 15–30 cm. Owing to the dominance of photoelectric absorption in tissues at these photon energies, the irradiation of surface lesions has lead to greater doses being absorbed in the underlying bone than in the overlying soft tissues. The higher photon energy of cobalt-60 beams at 5–20 cm SSD and of *radium surface applicators* have been used to advantage in these critical situations, but both these techniques have now been replaced by the use of electron beams below about 10 MeV. *Beta plaques* are valuable in selected circumstances (Ch. 14).

Typical isodose curves for some of these radiation beams are shown in Figure 13.14 and their relative merits will be dealt with briefly.

Low-energy X-ray beams

Low-energy X-rays still treat over 90% of the superficial lesions in the radiotherapy department, particularly sunburn-related cancers. The advantages are:

- the simplicity of the X-ray unit both in design and operation
- a wide range of field-defining applicators (usually circular), and
- the ease of collimation and field-shaping to individual requirements (with only 1 or 2 mm lead).

The disadvantages are the high bone absorption and the minimal penetration. Over the range of energies and field sizes in common use, the 80% depth, d_{80}, varies from only 6 mm to 16 mm (Fig. 12.1 and Table 12.2). Medium-energy X-rays (say, 2 mm Cu HVL) may be used at the normal 50 cm SSD for the treatment of some thicker superficial lesions.

Electron beams

High-energy beams for clinical use may be produced by dual modality linear accelerators over a range of energies from about 3 MeV up to about 25 MeV. For clinical purposes, the nominal energy of the electron beam has been defined in terms of its *half-value depth*, HVD, i.e.

$$\text{Energy (MeV)} = 2.5 \times HVD\ (\text{cm})$$

$$\text{or} \quad d_{50}\ (\text{mm}) = 4 \times E\ (\text{MeV})$$

where the HVD or d_{50} is the depth of the 50% isodose line on the central axis. A more useful parameter by which to define the electron beam is the depth of the 80 percentile, d_{80}. The build-up curve for the electron beam is less marked than for photons and usually gives a skin dose of greater than 80%. The d_{80} value, beyond d_{max}, may therefore be used to define the treatable depth and the approximation that

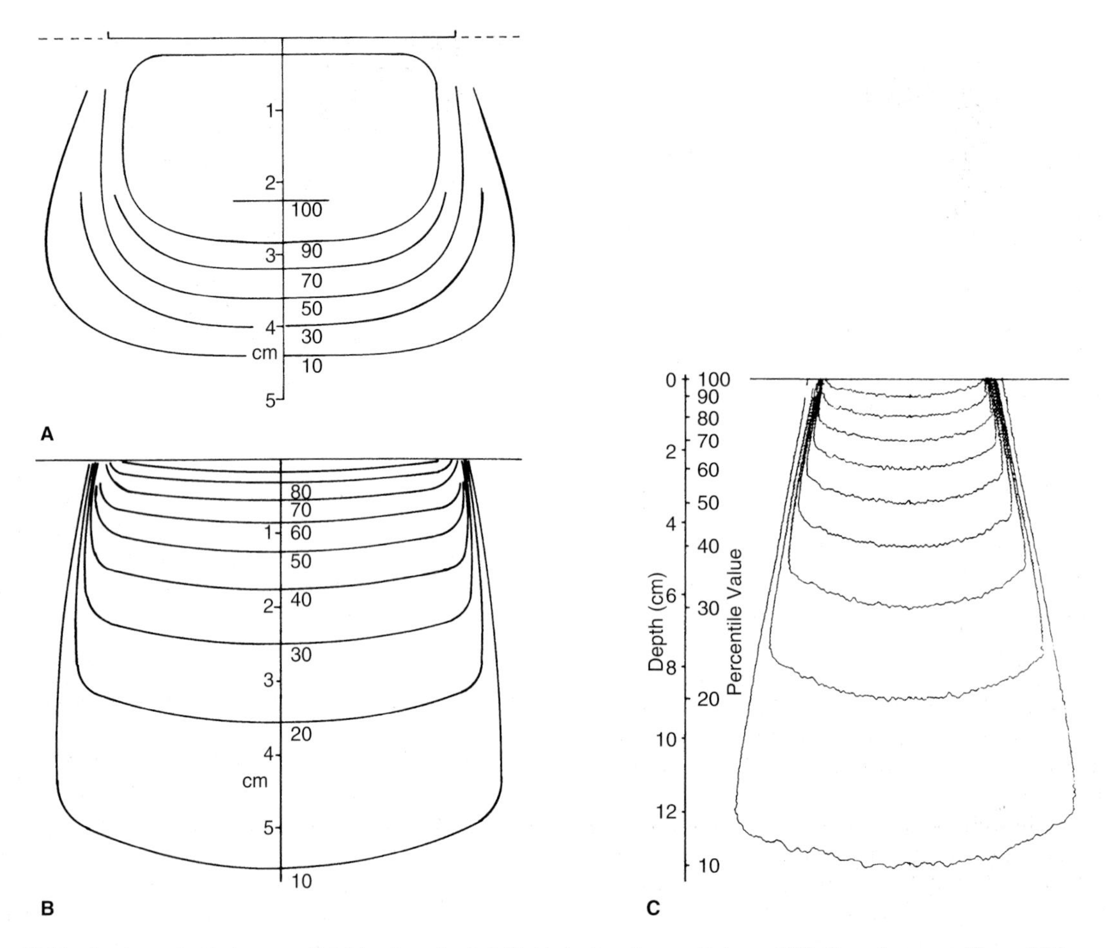

Fig. 13.14 Isodose charts for superficial treatments: **A** 9 MeV electron beam; **B** 1 mm HVL X-ray beam at 15 cm SSD; **C** cobalt-60 beam at 10 cm SSD.

$$d_{80}\ (\text{mm}) = 3 \times E\ (\text{MeV})$$

is a useful aide-memoire, but it can vary with different methods of electron beam generation (the maximum dose gradient is steeper and the d_{80} is greater with a *scanned* electron beam than with a *scattered* electron beam).

The depth dose curve (Fig. 13.15) for electrons is characterised by its flat peak and the steep dose gradient which flattens into the X-ray contamination 'tail'. The maximum gradient of the depth dose curve is less steep for the higher energies since these electrons undergo many more interactions (ionisations and excitations within the tissues) and their paths are correspondingly more tortuous.

The advantages of electron beams (up to 10 MeV) for the treatments of superficial lesions are clear. The dose is satisfactorily uniform to a depth determined by the energy of the electrons and the sharp fall-off of dose leads to the sparing of tissues at greater depths. The temptation to add shielding to further protect underlying tissues, e.g. the gums and/or teeth when treating around the mouth, is to be avoided because the electrons scattered back off the shield can increase the local dose to the proximal tissues by some 50% of the local dose. Collimation is relatively simple over a wide range of field sizes, local beam shaping requires a few millimetres of lead (or, say, 9 mm of LMP alloy) (p. 172) depending on electron energy. Arc therapy with electrons offers a useful means of irradiating the post-mastectomy chest wall, with minimal irradiation of the lungs, although posing complex problems in terms of dosimetry.

The higher electron energy beams (10–25 MeV) may be used in single or multi-fixed field treatments or in combination with photon beams. However,

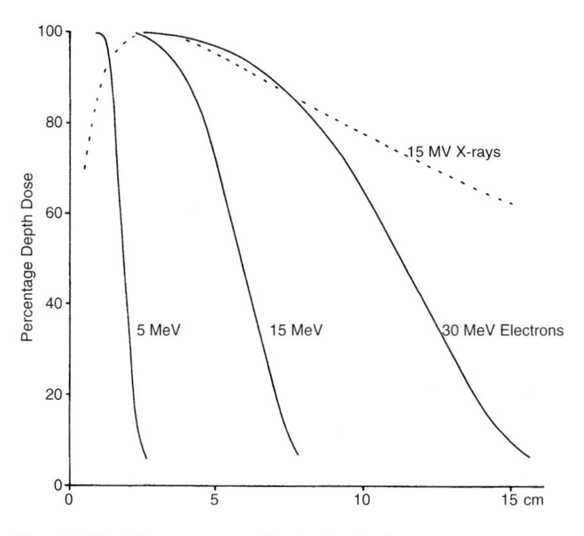

Fig. 13.15 Electron central axis depth dose curves—note the maximum gradient is less at the higher energies.

accommodating the steep dose gradients associated with electron beams and the penumbra edges of photon beams in the treatment planning computer is one thing; the accurate reproduction of the patient set-up on a daily basis is quite another, if over- and under-dosage are to be avoided at the abutment of the beams.

Every electron beam suffers from *X-ray contamination*. The X-rays are generated at the same peak energy when the electrons are stopped in the electron window, the ionisation chamber, the collimators, the air and in the tissues. The contribution made by this high-energy X-ray contamination to the total dose is measured at twice the depth of the maximum range of the electrons and quoted as a percentage of the peak dose; it should be kept to a minimum, typically less than 2% and never greater than 5%.

The toxic ozone produced by the high electron dose rates encountered in research work and in some clinical applications at large SSDs can reach unacceptable levels and high rates of air exchange in the treatment room are required for the safety of staff.

CALCULATION OF DOSE

No treatment plan is complete without a specification of the dose to be given to the tumour. The dose prescription will be the responsibility of the Oncologist and will be quoted in terms of the target dose to a specified percentile value within an overall treatment time and total number of fractions (Ch. 18). The actual number of fractions per week of treatment will be an important factor, but does not come into the calculations.

- The prescription will be a target dose, D, to some prescribed percentile value, $\%TD$, within the PTV, in F fractions. In the simplest case of a single field treatment, this means the total peak (applied) dose, P, may be obtained by rearranging the definition of percentage depth dose, viz.:

$$P = D \times 100 / \%TD$$

and the peak (applied) dose per fraction, P/F. If the peak dose rate, say on the cobalt-60 unit or linear accelerator, is P', then the exposure time per fraction will be:

$$t = \frac{(P/F)}{P'} + \Delta t$$

where Δt is the timer error (p. 56). The quoted peak dose rate, P', may be specified only for a reference field size, say 10×10 cm^2, in which case it must be adjusted by multiplying by the appropriate output factor before calculating the exposure time. The output factor is defined as:

$$\text{OFs} = \frac{\text{Peak dose rate for the equivalent square}}{\text{Peak dose rate, } P'\text{, for the reference field}}$$

and will vary from a few per cent below to a few per cent above unity depending on field size (p. 176).

- Similarly, on a kilovoltage X-ray unit, the dose rate quoted for the applicator should be reduced when a lead cut-out modifies the field size, by multiplying by the ratio of the back scatter factors for the cut-out and applicator respectively, i.e. $\text{BSF}_{\text{cut-out}}/\text{BSF}_{\text{applicator}}$ If there is a small stand-off between the applicator surface and the skin surface, then the treatment time should be further increased by the inverse square factor $[(f+x)^2/f^2]$ where f is the normal SSD and x is the stand-off. At megavoltagae energies, the factor would be $[(f+x)^2/(f+d_{max})^2]$. If the stand-off is so significant as to produce a change in both field size and in SSD, then the change in the depth dose distribution may also have to be taken into account (p. 195).
- In all the above examples, it has been assumed that the exposure to the patient will be controlled by time alone. Where a dual dosimetry system is being used on a linear accelerator or medium-energy kilovoltage generator, the exposure will be determined solely by the *monitor units* (mu) set on the primary channel of the dual dosimetry system—the secondary dose channel and the treatment timer being for back-up purposes only. The monitor units will usually be calibrated in grays or centigrays for a reference field size (10×10 cm^2) at the normal treating distance (say, 100 cm). As before, the peak (applied)

dose per fraction, P/F, will be calculated, and for a field size other than the reference, the monitor units required will be

$$\text{mu} = (P/F)/\text{output factor}$$

The monitor units to be set will be further increased by multiplying by any wedge factor, shadow tray correction factor, etc. as appropriate to the treatment in hand.

- Providing a dose distribution involving two or more fields is based on the premise that the peak dose to each of the fields is 100%, e.g. as in Figure 13.2, then the calculations are as described above. However, if the distribution assumes that the peak dose to any one of the fields is not 100%—either because weighting factors have been used or the distribution has been normalised to the target dose, $\%TD = 100$, e.g. as in Figure 13.9, then the total peak (applied) dose, P, must be calculated separately for each field using the formula:

$$P_i = D \times 100 \times W_i/\%TD$$

where W_i is the weighting factor for field i. This new value, P_i, may then be used to replace P in the equations above.

By way of example, in Table 13.3, the dose distributions illustrated in Figures 13.2C and 13.9B are used in conjunction with a typical dose prescription to derive the exposure time or monitor units required for each fraction of treatment.

Dose histograms

In the above analysis, the dose, D, was prescribed to a particular value of the percentage tumour dose ($\%TD$) without reference as to how that $\%TD$ was chosen. As we have seen, the choice may be the maximum, minimum, mean, average or modal dose to the PTV. While the first two are uniquely defined, the other three will lie somewhere between the two. An alternative analysis is to base the prescription on the *cumulative dose–volume histogram*, i.e. the percentage of the target volume receiving a dose greater than $\%TD$.

- These five different quantities, the maximum, minimum, mean, average and modal dose, are most easily understood by the following example. Let us assume the dose to each of 1000 matrix points of the PTV has been rounded to the nearest 1%, and they are distributed as in the dose histogram shown in Figure 13.16 and Table 13.4.
- Using the definitions given above (p. 208), the modal dose is the peak of the histogram at 98%, the mean dose is $\frac{1}{2}$(min. + max.), i.e. $\frac{1}{2}(89 + 105)$ or 97%, while the average dose is $\Sigma(TD \times N)/\Sigma N = 97464/1000$ or 97.5%. Where the target tissues have been treated before, the oncologist may decide to prescribe to the maximum (105%), but if the tissue is known to be particularly radioresistant then prescribing to the minimum (89%) may be more appropriate. The modal dose is probably the most commonly used prescription.
- From the third line of Table 13.4, we can see, for example, that 0.8% of the target tissues will exceed a dose of 103 and only 5% will receive a dose below 93 or, alternatively, 94.2% of the PTV will receive a dose within 98 ± 5. These data are plotted as the cumulative dose–volume histogram in Figure 13.16.

Table 13.3 Calculation of treatment time and monitor unit settings for typical treatment plans

Treatment plan shown in Figure	13.2C	13.9B	
Prescribed target dose, D, say	50 Gy	60 Gy	
Prescribed % target dose, $\%TD$	240%	100%	
		Wedged	Non-wedged
Weighting factor, W_i	100%	50%	22%
Total applied dose, P_i (Gy)	20.8	30.0	13.2
No. of fractions, F	20	25	25
Applied dose per fraction, P_i/F (Gy)	1.04	1.20	0.53
Output factors, say	0.98	0.96	1.00
Wedge factors, say		1.12	
Set monitor units, mu*	1.06	1.40	0.53
Treatment time, t (min)*	0.68	0.90	0.34

* Assuming the dose rate at d_{max} for the reference field size is 1.56 Gy per minute, the timer error is negligible and the integrating dose meter (mu) is calibrated in grays

Table 13.4 The data used for the dose histogram in Figure 13.16

Dose value,	*TD*	88	89	90	91	92	93	94	95	96	97
No of points,	*N*	0	2	3	12	33	70	84	93	98	105
Vol. > *TD*,	%	100.0	100.0	99.8	99.5	98.3	95.0	88.0	79.6	70.3	60.5
Dose value,	*TD*		98	99	100	101	102	103	104	105	106
No of points,	*N*		106	104	93	79	73	37	6	2	0
Vol. > *TD*,	%		50.0	30.4	29.0	19.7	11.8	4.5	0.8	0.2	0

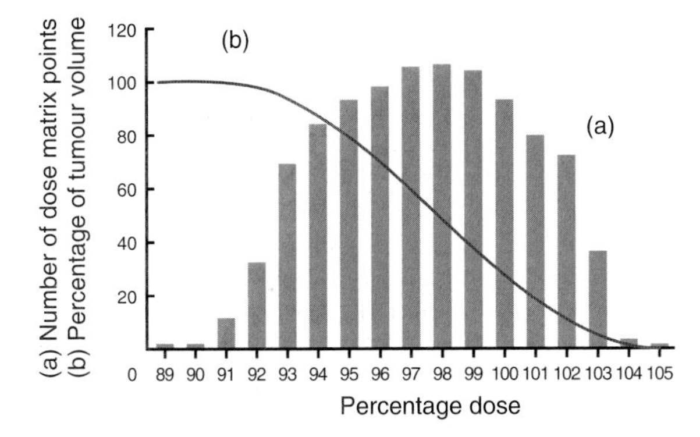

Fig. 13.16 **A** The dose histogram based on the data in Table 13.4 where the ordinate is the number of matrix points at each dose interval. **B** Superimposed is the DVH for the same dose matrix.

Integral dose

Dose has been defined as the energy absorbed per unit mass of tissue in a small element of tissue, i.e. $D = \delta E/\delta m$. The integral dose is the summation of the dose to all elements of the irradiated tissue and represents the total absorbed energy, viz. $E = \Sigma D\delta m$. The unit of integral dose is the joule (in diagnostic X-ray, the phrase *the total energy imparted* is used and quoted in mJ). The detailed evaluation of the integral dose is complex, but it is readily appreciated that the integral dose will increase with the incident dose, it will also increase with both the field size(s) and thickness of the patient treated. It is less easy to appreciate that in a particular treatment situation the integral dose decreases with increasing photon energy and varies only slowly with the number of fields used.

Integral dose in this context is confined to the tissues deliberately irradiated during a course of radiotherapy. In addition, there is a whole-body component of integral dose arising from radiation scattered from the exposed tissues and leaking through the source/tube housing. It is in recognition of this whole-body irradiation that the acceptable levels of leakage radiation are set (Chs 9 and 10).

Patient dosimetry

It is generally accepted that the dose delivered to the clinical target volume should be accurate to better than ±5% with ±3% being the aim. There is a belief that the final proof that all the treatment planning and dose calculation has been completed correctly lies in the measurement of the dose delivered to the patient on treatment, but it is not so simple. In Chapter 5, it was suggested the small size and tissue equivalence of thermoluminescent dosimeters and solid-state detectors made these techniques ideal for such measurements. The solid-state detector has the advantage that the results are immediately available and discrepancies can be investigated while the patient remains on the couch. The results of TLD measurements will not be available for several hours.

The measurements cannot be made in vivo at the point of interest, the detectors have to be placed as close as practicable, usually on the entrance or exit skin surface. The results of such measurements therefore need to be carefully interpreted as they cannot be compared directly with the doses expected. The reasons lie in the detector encapsulation, if any, and in the depth of maximum ionisation associated with megavoltage radiations.

The sensitive element in solid state detectors is very small and usually encapsulated in sufficient material to establish electronic equilibrium and therefore should only be used at the design photon energy specified. This encapsulation makes the probes useless for assessing skin dose or lens of eye dose, the latter being one of the critical tissues of concern in radiotherapy. On the other hand, thermoluminescent materials are invariably encapsulated in insufficient material to establish electronic equilibrium and therefore may be used for skin dose measurements if the encapsulation is thin enough, or for lens of eye dose if the encapsulation is matched to the depth of the lens. It must be remembered that the dose in the build-up region initially increases very rapidly with depth (Fig. 12.8). There may be uncertainty too, insofar as lens of eye dose is usually measured because of its proximity to the edge of the beam and the detector is likely to be within the steep dose gradient of the beam penumbra; the small day-to-day variations in beam set-up and/or the placing of the detector will be critical to the consistency of the results of measurement.

The second factor is a geometric one due to the inevitable spatial separation of the detector and the point of interest. If a solid-state detector probe is placed on the entrance surface of a patient and irradiated at normal incidence, the centre of the probe is at a point d_{max} (plus the radius of the probe) closer to the X-ray target than the point at which the dose is prescribed and, by the inverse square law, the dose measured will be some 3–4% higher (at 6 MV and 100 cm SSD). Add to this the effects of oblique incidence and differences in scatter component at the points of interest and of measurement and there will be considerable uncertainty in the results of measurement.

The solid state detectors should always be irradiated from a direction at right angles to their axis; not along their axis. They may also show a temperature sensitivity requiring a correction factor of some 2% for a change from room to body temperature and a radiation sensitivity change as the total accumulated dose to the detector increases; regular recalibration is essential. Correction factors can be derived and selectively applied to match the clinical application and thereby convert the initial reading into a true assessment of the delivered dose. Solid state detectors should not be used at kilovoltage energies.

CHAPTER CONTENTS

14

Brachytherapy

Keith Bomford

INTRODUCTION

Choice of isotope

Radioactive materials are widely used in medical practice. Chapter 8 dealt with the use of unsealed radioactive materials, i.e. liquids, gases, etc. in radiodiagnosis. Chapter 10 dealt with their use in the production of gamma ray beams for radiotherapy. Chapter 15 will highlight those radionuclides used in therapy. The present chapter describes the physical aspects of their use in the form of discrete sealed sources, i.e. where the radioactive material is contained in a metal capsule. The use of radium-226 ($T_{1/2}$= 1640 years) to produce gamma radiation effects in limited volumes of tissue is one of the oldest established practices of radiotherapy. Radium-226 is an alpha emitter but within its decay scheme (Fig. 3.7) are radium B (lead-214) and radium C (bismuth-214) emitting gamma rays with energies in the range from 0.2–2.4 MeV; the higher energy photons in the spectrum make radiation protection difficult and the inert gas, radon-222, is a constant additional hazard (p. 72).

Caesium-137 ($T_{1/2}$ = 30 years) largely replaced radium as the nuclide of choice in the 1960s. It is a by-product of nuclear fuel reprocessing and has a lower photon energy of 662 keV. It is an alkaline metal but, as a compound of chloride or sulphate, it is chemically stable. These salts are soluble and therefore, for clinical sources, the caesium is incorporated into glass for high-activity sources or into zirconium phosphate for needles and tubes. Caesium sources are doubly encapsulated and carry a recommended working life of 10 years, during which their activity falls by approximately 20%.

All sources have a *recommended working life* beyond which the manufacturer will not guarantee the integrity of the source.

Iridium-192 ($T_{½} = 74$ days) is now being used more widely, taking advantage of its high specific activity and the properties of a flexible wire (p. 232). Other nuclides, e.g. gold-198 grains ($T_{½} = 2.7$ days), have been used in selected applications, but are no longer widely available. Each of these has the disadvantage of a shorter half-life requiring some correction to be made for radioactive decay either before or during the treatment.

Cobalt-60 has been used in brachytherapy but only to a limited degree. Essential data on some of these alternatives to radium are summarised in Table 14.1. Iodine-125 is described later (p. 238) but it cannot be described as a radium substitute because of its very low energy emission.

This use of discrete gamma ray sources to irradiate the tissues is usually referred to as *brachytherapy* and it falls into three distinct applications. *Interstitial therapy* is where the sources are implanted directly into the diseased tissues (Ch. 22). *Intracavitary therapy* is where the sources are arranged in a suitable applicator to irradiate the walls of a body cavity from inside (Ch. 27). The use of *surface applicators* is where an external surface of the patient is treated by locally applied sources arranged on an appropriately shaped applicator. While the use of gamma-emitting surface applicators has been largely replaced by the use of electron beams and will not be covered in this chapter, limited use is made of *beta plaques* and these will be briefly described (p. 238).

The point source

Before considering complex arrays of sources, consider the simplest source of all—an isolated point source. Gamma rays are emitted isotropically. It follows, therefore, that the intensity of radiation will decrease with the inverse square of the distance from the source (p. 40) and the intensity will be uniform over a spherical surface centred on the point source. The dose rate will be proportional both to the activity of the source, A (the number of photons emitted per unit time), and to the inverse square of the distance, d, from the source. Figure 14.1 represents a line of five equally spaced point sources, each emitting gamma rays in all directions and producing a complex pattern of isodose lines, but each line representing the cumulative effect of the inverse square law applied to each source. From this one figure several important conclusions may be drawn.

1. Despite the complex nature of the isodose lines shown, each one will be circular in cross-section, i.e. when viewed from one end of the line of sources.
2. At points close to any one source, the isodose surface will be essentially spherical, the influence of the neighbouring sources being negligible.
3. The dose distribution along a line close to and parallel to the line of sources will be very uneven, being high close to each source and lower between adjacent sources.
4. Each low point could be raised by inserting a further source half way between each existing source, making the distribution more uniform.

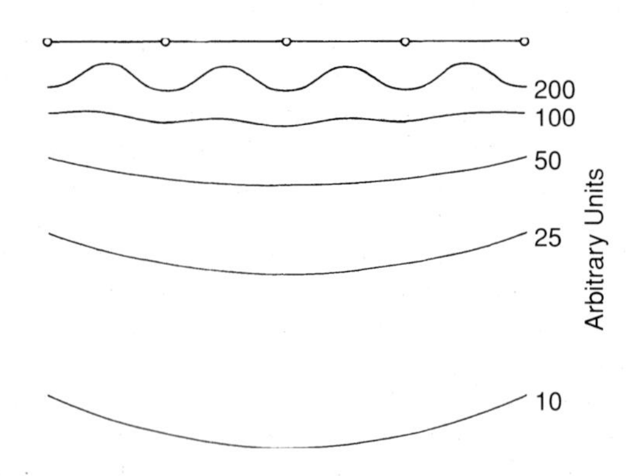

Fig. 14.1 The complex isodose distribution from a line of five point sources.

Table 14.1 Isotopes used in brachytherapy

Isotope	Half-life	Photon energy MeV	Air kerma rate per GBq at 1 m	Sources available
Caesium-137	30 years	0.662	0.078 mGy h^{-1}	Needles and tubes. Beads for afterloading
Cobalt-60	5.26 years	1.17, 1.33	0.307 mGy h^{-1}	Needles and tubes. Beads and pellets for high-dose-rate afterloading
Iridium-192	74 days	0.3–0.6	0.113 mGy h^{-1}	Wire and pins for manual afterloading Pellets for remote afterloading
Iodine-125	60 days	0.027–0.036	0.034 mGy h^{-1}	Seeds for permanent implantation or surface applicators
Radium-226	1600 years	0.2–2.4	0.195 mGy h^{-1}	Needles and tubes

5. The dose uniformity improves as the distance between the line of interest and the line of sources is increased.

6. The dose uniformity improves as the distance between the sources is reduced.

The student will appreciate that the extension of (4) is to make a continuous line source and the extension of (5) and (6) is that the five sources become effectively a single point source. The corollary of (1) is that the distribution shown is essentially that of a section through five parallel line sources viewed end-on. The three valuable consequences drawn from this analysis are:

- The uniformity of dose achieved is dependent on both the distance from the sources and the spacing of those sources.
- A line source may be thought of as a line of closely spaced point sources and vice versa.
- The uniformity of dose is further improved by increasing the activity of the sources at the end of the line.

Localisation of sources

One consequence of the inverse square law, when considering the dose distribution surrounding implanted sources, is that, at the short distances of interest, the accuracy of the dose calculation is critically dependent on the accuracy of localisation. The accurate geometry of the treatment simulator (p. 101), together with its remote control facility makes it the ideal means of localising implanted sources or 'dummy' sources if the final activity is to be afterloaded. The sources are metallic or enclosed in a metallic sheath and will show up clearly on a radiograph or image intensifier.

Orthogonal films are taken and the relative positions of the sources within the adjacent anatomy can be determined using the same procedures as outlined earlier (p. 104). If the dose calculation is to be done on a computer then the program may accept data from two non-orthogonal films providing some other correlation of the films is available. The program may also have a facility for matching the two sets of end coordinates of line sources automatically. The implant will be checked immediately on completion in theatre using the C-arm X-ray/image intensifier equipment so that any deviations from the planned insertion can be corrected without delay, but the C-arm does not have the geometric accuracy required on which to base dosimetry calculations.

Dose–volume histograms

In brachytherapy, there is no clearly defined clinical target volume (CTV) and the maximum target dose is undefined. Furthermore the computed dose distribution generally relates only to the relative position of the implanted sources rather than to the anatomy of the patient although, with CT becoming increasingly accessible, scanning the patient with dummy markers (in place of the radioactive sources) in situ is now a more practical proposition. This is particularly advantageous for patients whose brachytherapy is to be supplemented with external beam therapy, e.g. in the treatment of the cervix, as a means of correlating the two dose calculations. A patient with brachytherapy sources in situ must not be taken to other departments for routine procedures.

The concept of dose–volume histograms (DVH) was introduced in the context of external beam treatment planning (p. 211) and the DVH is equally valid in brachytherapy. The tissue dose immediately adjacent to an implanted source is inevitably very high and providing the sources are not too widely spaced, the dose to the tissues between the sources will be significant. The dose–volume histogram will demonstrate the volume enclosed by successive percentile isodose surfaces and aid the correlation with the known gross target volume (GTV).

Recommendations from the International Commission on Radiation Units and Measurements (ICRU 1985) suggest that in any brachytherapy treatment, the *total reference air kerma* is recorded; that is, the summation of the air kerma rate at 1 metre multiplied by the insertion time for each individual source used.

TREATMENT OF THE CERVIX

Perhaps the most common use of sealed sources is in the treatment of cancer of the cervix (Ch. 27) and for many decades the technique has involved inserting preloaded sources into the uterine canal and vagina in the operating theatre. More recently remote afterloading techniques have been widely adopted—these will be discussed in the next section. Radium tubes, and subsequently caesium tubes, were loaded into applicators designed to fit the uterine canal and the lateral fornices of the vagina. Three lengths of uterine applicator were used incorporating one, two or three tubes in tandem, the uppermost source being of higher activity. Two vaginal applicators were used and again in three sizes with one tube in each. The Manchester vaginal *ovoids* were designed so that the dose rate was uniform over the whole surface—the ovoid was therefore circular with the tube at the centre and approximately elliptical in the orthogonal plane. The vagina was slightly distended by placing a 'spacer' or 'washer' between the ovoids and the vagina packed to push the ovoids away from the rectum and to hold them in situ (Fig. 14.2A). The Sheffield kidney-shaped vaginal applicator contained two caesium tubes but, being firmly supported from a perineal bar, the vagina did not require packing and the rectal dose was reduced by the two built-in tungsten shields (Fig. 14.2B).

Despite the possible variations, the basic shape of the dose distribution remains essentially pear-shaped (Fig. 14.2A) and the duration of the insertion is based on the dose rate to two defined points, namely point A and point B. These are not anatomical landmarks. Point A is simply a reference point defined as 2 cm lateral to the uterine canal and at a level 2 cm above its external os or above the level of the lateral vaginal fornices. Being so close to the sources, the dose gradient at point A approaches 10% per mm. Point B is taken at the same level but on the pelvic wall—taken to be 5 cm lateral to the midline. The dose gradient at point B is much lower. (If the uterus is not midline then the distance between points A and B will not be 3 cm.) However, the dose rates at these two points may be tabulated for a range of standard insertions and used as an alternative to calculating each individual case. Where individual calculations of dose rate are required, then it is necessary to determine the dose rate each tube contributes to each point. In most cases the inverse square law approximation may be applied for point B as its distance from each individual tube is large with respect to the active length. For point A, however, it is necessary to total the dose rate contributions from each source from a knowledge of its relative position and using isodose charts or a mathematical approach such as the Sievert integral (Sievert 1932) or Young and Batho tables (Young & Batho 1964). For a more complete and accurate estimation of the dose distribution, the calculation is most conveniently done on a computer using the accurate localisation films from the treatment simulator to provide the patient input data.

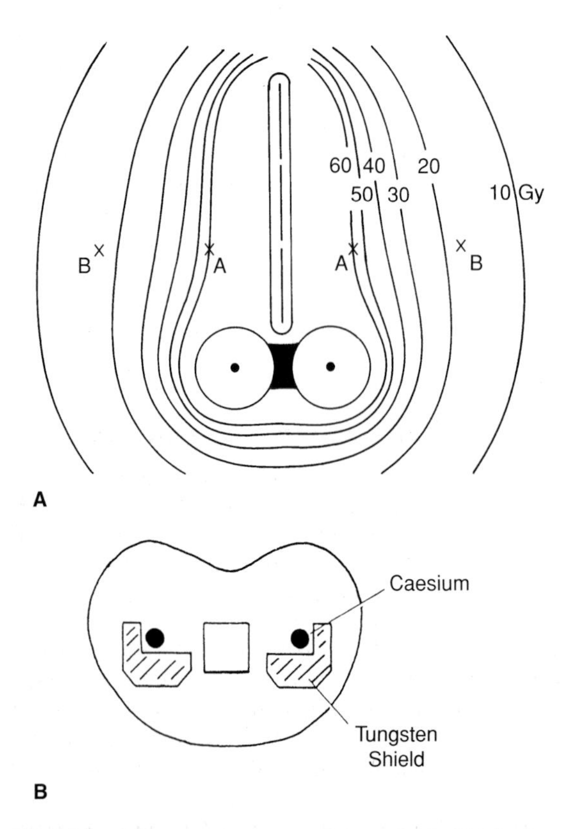

Fig. 14.2 **A** The source array and dose distribution for the treatment of the cervix using a uterine tube and two vaginal ovoids separated by a spacer. **B** The Sheffield vaginal applicator showing the rectal shielding.

Although the quotation of the dose at points A and B has sufficed for several decades, other dose points have been regularly calculated to estimate the dose to other organs at risk. These have included the bladder and the rectum in particular and the sigmoid colon and ureters. The estimations have often been based on direct measurements using special *rectal probe* dosimeters, but clearly the results of such measurements are very dependent on the position of the probe and the relative anatomy at the time of measurement; in the steep dose gradients surrounding intracavitary sources these errors may be gross. Specific recommendations have been laid down on how these points should be defined on lateral and AP radiographs (ICRU 1985) so that the computer can calculate the dose to each organ at risk.

In addition to the quotation of the dose at each of those organs, it is recommended that the treatment specification should also include the total reference air kerma. Typically this will be in the range from 40–60 mGy. And finally the length of the three principal axes of the pear-shaped 60 Gy isodose surface is to be recorded, the principal axes being along the intrauterine source and those orthogonal to it at the widest point of that surface. In calculating the 60 Gy isodose the subsequent external beam therapy (if any) should be taken into account. This precise specification is not intended to replace the locally determined treatment schedules, but primarily to justify multicentre intercomparisons.

REMOTE AFTERLOADING SYSTEMS

The manual insertion of preloaded sources into the cervix was the one medical application which gave rise to the highest radiation exposure to staff—in the operating theatre, in the transfer to the ward and to all those attending the patient in the ward—during the subsequent treatment time of some 48 hours. While non-essential procedures (e.g. mopping the floor) could be deferred until the sources had been removed and the essential procedures were performed from behind 25 mm lead bedside shields (Plate 1.13), the exposure to staff is now considered unacceptable and contrary to the ALARA principle (Ch. 6). The preferred alternative is to use a *remote afterloading system*. Such a system provides safe storage for the sources (leakage air kerma rate < 10 mGy h^{-1} at 1 m) and facilitates for transferring the required sources from the safe through connected transfer tubes to the catheters in the patient by remote control.

Remote afterloading systems have four essential advantages over the manual insertion of preloaded sources:

- the elimination of exposure in transporting the patient and minimising the exposure to theatre and ward staff
- maximising the time available to improve the geometrical arrangement of the source catheters
- the opportunity to increase the activity used and thereby reduce the treatment time
- the overall treatment time is preset and terminated by the remote afterloader.

There are three recognised dose rate regimes (Table 14.2), each one somewhat higher than the traditional dose rate of ~ 0.6 Gy h^{-1} to point A obtained with manual loading of 'live' sources, and requiring some adjustment to the prescribed dose to accommodate the change in *dose rate effect* (Ch. 18).

The basic technique in each is essentially the same, namely to insert catheters into the patient under anaesthetic (in this context the word catheter will be taken to include any rigid or flexible tube into which a source may be introduced; it is important to avoid any sharp bends in any catheter). The catheters are then secured in place. If appropriate at this stage, very low activity sources may be temporarily inserted to allow a pro rata measurement of the rectal dose rate to be made. The precise position of the catheters, as identified by the insertion of a train of dummy sources or markers, will be checked using a mobile or C-arm X-ray unit in theatre. Accurate localisation films of known magnification will provide the geometric data from which to compute the overall treatment time required to satisfy the dose prescription.

Two methods of source transfer are in common use. A source train can be made up from an array of discrete (e.g. caesium) sources interspersed with inactive spacers which can then be transferred to and from the patient under pneumatic control. In the case of the cervix treatment, three such trains will usually be required and each will be irradiated simultaneously. The alternative is to use a single (e.g. iridium) source pellet fixed to the end of a *drive wire* which is capable of causing the source to oscillate over a prescribed length of the catheter or of positioning the source at preselected points within the catheter for different intervals of time, the so-called *dwell time*. The one source is then repeatedly cycled through its programme of positions and times in each of the catheters until the prescribed dose has been delivered; the cycling of this *stepping source* may be continuous for low-dose-rate (LDR) or high-dose-rate (HDR) or discontinuous for pulsed-dose-rate (PDR) techniques. In units using a drive wire, a second wire, with a 'dummy' source, is driven in and out of each catheter to check for blockages or unacceptable bends in the catheter before the source wire leaves the safe position.

Table 14.2 Dose rates in brachytherapy

Low dose rate	0.4–2.0 Gy h^{-1}	2 fractions
Medium dose rate	2.0–12 Gy h^{-1}	2 fractions
High dose rate	12–60 Gy h^{-1}	> 6 fractions

NB: On the experience gained at low dose rates, the total prescribed dose may need to be modified once the dose rate exceeds about 1 Gy h^{-1}. The number of fractions refers to the brachytherapy component only of the treatment of the cervix.

Low/medium-dose-rate techniques

The low-dose-rate regime seeks to reproduce the dose rates established over several decades with radium and caesium preloaded sources for the treatment of the cervix. With the preloaded source technique, the range of available sources was very limited and offered a dose rate of ~ 0.6 Gy h^{-1} to point A. The sources for LDR/MDR remote afterloading systems are usually caesium-137 and the activity per source may be chosen, within the overall design maximum for the afterloader, to offer either low or medium dose rates. The freedom to tailor the source trains to the requirements of the patient is an added bonus. The treatment planning program will take these requirements into account and specify the distribution of activity in each source train and overall treatment time for each catheter.

The patient from theatre is returned to the specially equipped single-bedded side ward where the catheters are connected through flexible *transfer tubes* to the remote afterloading machine (Fig. 14.3). Each source train will be composed in accordance with the treatment plan and its overall treatment time programmed into the remote afterloader. Only after all the staff have left the protected room will the prepared source trains be transferred from the machine to the patient and the treatment started (or resumed after an interruption) using the remote control. As with external beam therapy, the treatment may be interrupted at any time—i.e. the sources may be remotely transferred from the patient to the safe within the machine—whenever the patient needs the nursing staff or visitors to enter the room. The treatment is automatically terminated on completion of the preset time. Interruptions to treatment for nursing care and/or visitors should add no more than 10% to the overall treatment time.

Although designed around the treatment of the cervix, LDR equipment has also been used in the treatment of the nasopharynx and the oesophagus.

High-dose-rate techniques

The high-dose-rate systems reduce the actual irradiation time to less than 1 hour with dose rates often in the region of 150 Gy h^{-1}. This enables the treatment to be given on a day-case basis in an area not dissimilar from a gamma ray beam therapy room (p. 183), in or adjacent to the operating theatre. However, the preparation of the patient and the dose calculation times will not be reduced and the number of treatment fractions will generally be increased as part of the dose rate correction.

HDR treatment of the cervix may be given using equipment based on the design of the LDR equipment described above but upgraded to accommodate higher-activity sources of cobalt-60 rather than caesium. However, stepping source equipment is more widely available.

The single stepping source pellet (of, say, 400 GBq iridium-192 of 10 mm length), incorporated in the end of a drive wire (of, say, 1.5 m long), will be programmed to 'dwell' at different points in turn along a prescribed length of each catheter. By adjusting the dwell time at predetermined dwell positions, almost any conceivable linear dose distribution can be achieved, with the more uniform distributions being achieved when the dwell positional interval is equal to, or slightly larger than, the source length. The dwell times should be kept short and the programmed cycle repeated several times to average out the rate at which the dose is delivered to the adjacent tissues.

These systems are not confined to the treatment of the cervix. They have been used to treat the nasopharynx, prostate, oesophagus, bronchus, etc. (Plate 1.14) and, where extra-fine sources and catheters are available, they can be used for interstitial therapy (Fig. 14.6),

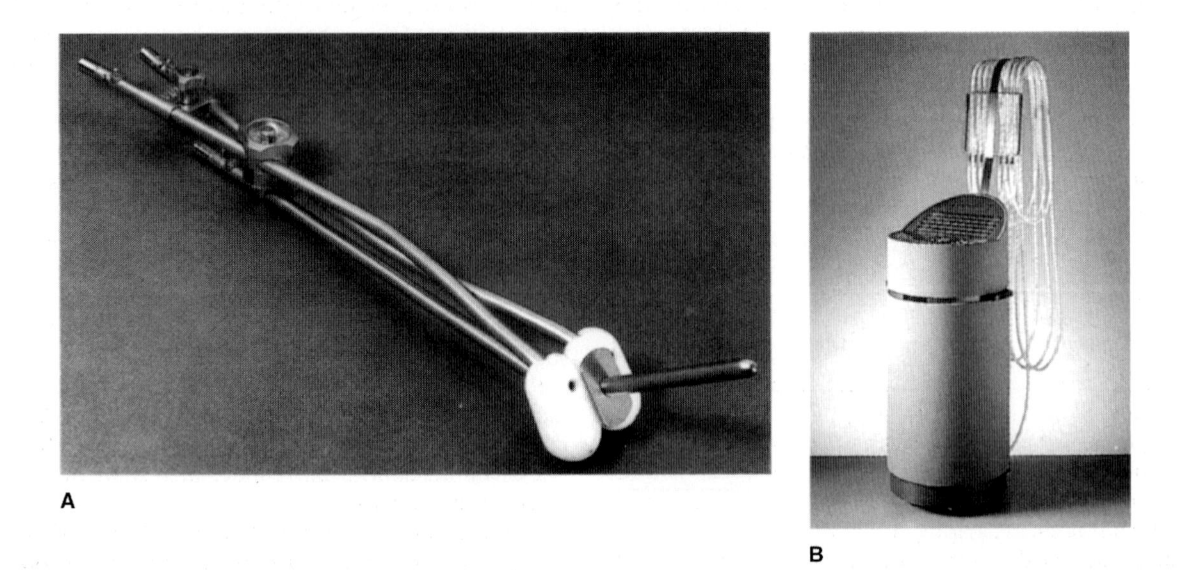

Fig. 14.3 **A** The vaginal and uterine catheters used with the remote afterloading equipment shown in **B**. (Courtesy of Nucletron Trading Co., Chester.)

e.g. in breast conservation therapy. Furthermore, HDR equipment is often sufficiently mobile to enable it to be taken into a protected operating theatre for intraoperative radiotherapy (IORT) to be practised—for colorectal cancer, retroperitoneal sarcomas, advanced gynaecological and thoracic tumours and various neoplasms.

Pulsed-dose-rate techniques

The pulsed-dose-rate (PDR) technique uses high-dose-rate equipment to simulate a low-dose-rate regime by repeating the programmed cycle but with a prescribed time interval of, say, 1 hour between cycles. There is no recognised definition of dose rate but an irradiation of 10 minutes every hour giving a mean dose rate of ~ 0.5 Gy h^{-1} while that during the pulse is ~ 3 Gy h^{-1} is typical. The source may be of smaller dimensions and of lower activity than in the HDR application.

Quality assurance

Remote afterloading equipment is regarded as a gamma ray beam unit for radiation protection purposes, and requires all the associated facilities: independent gamma alarm, regular 'wipe' tests, door interlocks and warning lights, patient intercom and viewing systems, etc. (pp. 180 and 183). An infrared CCTV may be preferred where treatments continue through the night. The unit itself will contain a large single source or a number of radioactive sources and will therefore incorporate a secure protected safe with leakage radiation levels below the relevant limits. Under normal operation, remote afterloading equipment minimises the exposure of staff to radiation. However, staff should be subjected to personnel monitoring, rehearse emergency procedures and have ready access to a radiation monitor and a protected container of a size capable of accepting the catheters should they, and their sources, need to be removed from the patient in an emergency.

A strict QA protocol must be set in place, practised and documented at every stage. The daily QA checks should seek to confirm the routine operation of all aspects of the equipment: the operation of door warning and control indicator lights/CCTV/intercom, the radiation monitor, the interrupt/emergency/door interlocks, the date/time/activity of the source data and an adequate supply of printer paper. A visual inspection of the catheters and transfer tubes should be used to check for signs of damage. Monthly checks should be made on the accuracy and linearity of the timer and back-up timer and an autoradiograph on the sources.

Dosimetry

A strict QA protocol must be followed whenever the sources are replaced to ensure the integrity of each source and its activity. Iridium-192 sources will need to be replaced every 3 months while caesium sources may last the lifetime of the equipment, but both will need careful assay to guarantee the dosimetry. Re-entrant ion chambers or 'well' counters may be used for the intercomparison of two or more sources of identical geometry, but may not be suitable for absolute measurements. Farmer type (thimble) chambers, with calibrations traceable to national standardising laboratories, may be used for in-air measurements providing the source–chamber separation is large enough to make both the source and the chamber dimensions negligible, but this often means the dose rate is too low to be measured accurately. The alternative is to place the chamber closer to the source and to apply detector (geometry) response correction factors and inverse square deviation factors to the readings obtained—to have the chamber centred between three or more straight catheters is better (e.g. Vollans & Wilkinson 2000). Such measurements should be made annually for caesium sources and monthly for iridium sources.

Facilities will also be required—and kept readily available—for measuring and checking the make-up of source trains or stepping cycle before the commencement of treatment. Techniques will vary but will usually involve autoradiography, preferably in a scatter-free environment, using a jig to superimpose a calibrated scale on the image.

The accuracy of the patient dosimetry is also dependent on the accuracy of the localisation of the sources and on any movement of the catheters (relative to the target tissues) throughout the duration of the treatment. Both these should be monitored regularly and, as always, care should be taken to ensure that the localisation films are taken while the patient adopts a position that can be maintained throughout the treatment.

Regular checks should be made on the computer hardware and software to ensure that the source data are correct for the date and time of treatment and that the algorithm used is handling that data correctly and within its limitations.

The final checks should include monitoring of the patient and the empty catheters for radioactive contamination on completion of treatment and a careful review of the print-out to ensure the prescription has been fully implemented; the print-out should be filed with the patient's records.

In the event of an equipment malfunction, be it in the generator or the dosimetry chain, causing an error of more than +20% of the intended dose fraction (or +10% of the total course dose), the incident must be reported to the Health and Safety Executive once an investigation has confirmed beyond reasonable doubt an overexposure has occurred—guidance on the content of the investigation/report is given in a Health and Safety Executive publication (HSE 1998a). In the event of a similar but underexposure, the employer should instigate an investigation but the incident is not notifiable to the HSE.

MANUAL AFTERLOADING SYSTEMS

Where remote afterloading equipment is not available manual afterloading may be used. The same theatre procedures are followed as for remote afterloading but laboratory-prepared source trains (Fig. 14.4) are loaded manually—using appropriate forceps, etc.—either into guides before leaving theatre (iridium pins) or into catheters on arrival in the ward (iridium wire or gynaecological caesium source trains). It is not practical, however, to unload and reload the source trains for each interruption for essential nursing and therefore the same ward procedures have to be followed as for preloaded source treatments (p. 239). The improved geometry and reduced exposure to theatre staff make manual afterloading preferable to the use of preloaded sources.

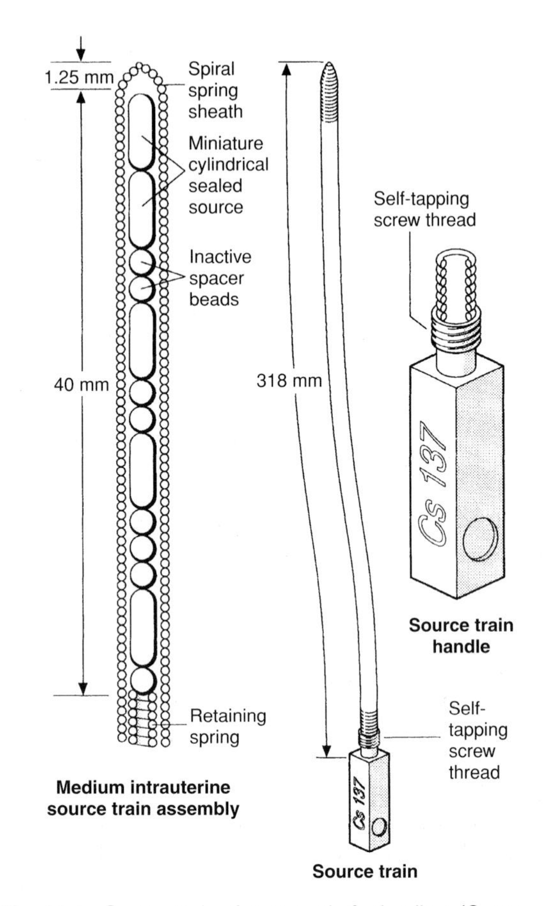

Fig. 14.4 Source trains for manual afterloading. (Courtesy of Amersham International plc.)

Iridium wire

Iridium-192 ($T_{1/2}$ = 74 days) is activated in a reactor by the neutron bombardment of a platinum and iridium-191 alloy wire and decays to platinum-192. The gamma ray spectrum is complex, covering a range from 0.3–0.6 MeV while the beta emission is absorbed by a 0.1 mm Pt coating. It is available as a thin flexible wire (0.3 mm diameter × 500 mm maximum) or as a double (hair) pin (0.6 mm diameter × 60 mm maximum). In clinical practice, both may be cut to length at the time of the implant and, therefore, iridium cannot be technically regarded as a sealed source. Special precautions have to be taken (p. 248) as radioactive contamination can occur, e.g. small fragments of active metal may be left behind on the cutting device. The iridium is usually purchased with the activity per unit length required for the application in hand while the radioactive decay during the few days of treatment may be ignored. Both the off-cuts and the used material will need to be stored (for 2 or more years) prior to arranging for their disposal (p. 243).

The use of thin wire involves the implantation of nylon tubes into the superficial tissues, often during the surgical removal of the bulk disease, the tubes being secured at both ends with nylon balls. The position of these tubes can then be checked radiographically by inserting inactive wire into the tubes. The active iridium wire is cut to length and inserted into a second nylon tube of a smaller diameter than the first in the sealed source laboratory. This tube is then taken to the ward and threaded into the implanted tubes (preferably leaving at least 5 mm between the end of the wire and the skin to avoid long-term skin damage) and secured by crimping lead discs outside each nylon ball as shown in Figure 14.5. After the required treatment time, one lead disc is cut off each source assembly and the other is used to withdraw it.

An alternative technique is to insert rigid *steel guide needles* into the tissues through a template—and, if possible, through a second template where the guides exit from the tissues. This rigid framework not only

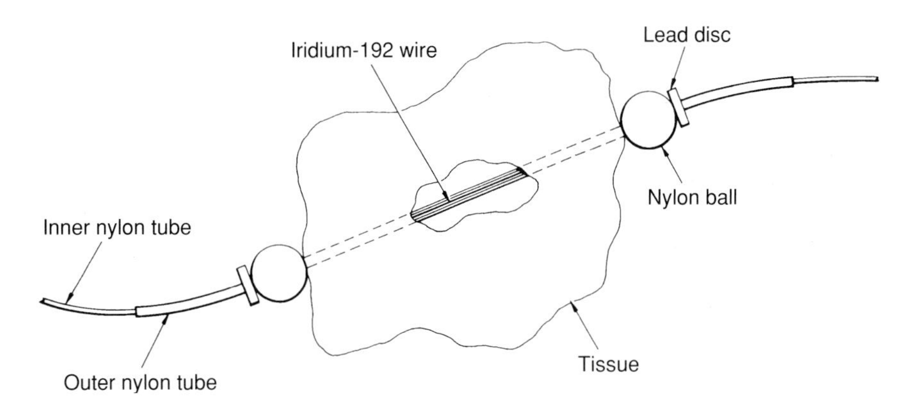

Fig. 14.5 A typical assembly of the Pierquin/Paine manual afterloading technique for iridium wire. (Courtesy of Amersham International plc.)

provides a predictable geometry, but maintains the configuration throughout the duration of the treatment. This technique is often used in the treatment of the breast by remote (Fig. 14.6) or manual afterloading.

Where the implant is not superficial, rigid slotted steel guide needles may be inserted under anaesthetic, and their position checked, using the C-arm in theatre, prior to inserting iridium (double) pins. Once the pins are in position, the guide needles can be removed by allowing the bridge of each pin to slide down the slots in the guide, leaving the pins in situ. Figure 14.7 shows two iridium pins inserted in the vulva, together with the computed dose distribution. The pins are readily removed on completion of the

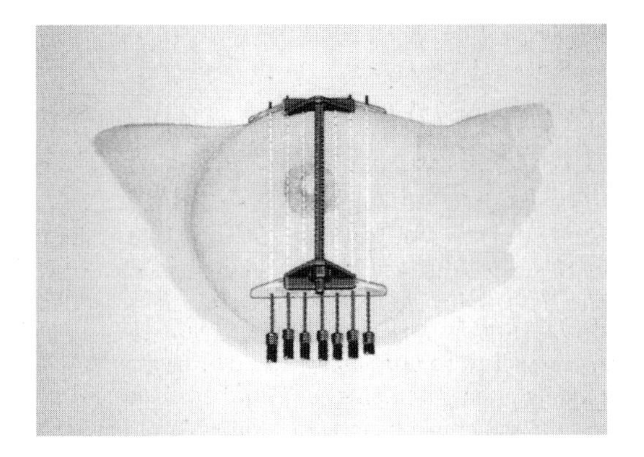

Fig. 14.6 Interstitial therapy of the breast using a remote afterloading technique. (Courtesy of Nucletron Trading Co., Chester.)

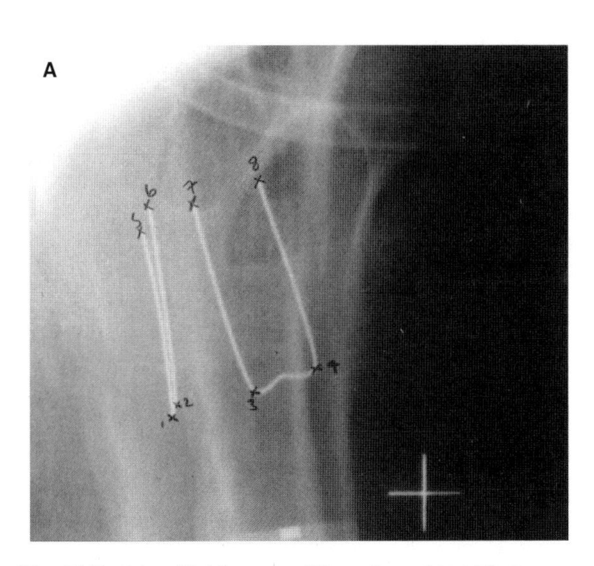

Fig. 14.7 Interstitial therapy of the vulva using iridium hairpins: **A** lateral

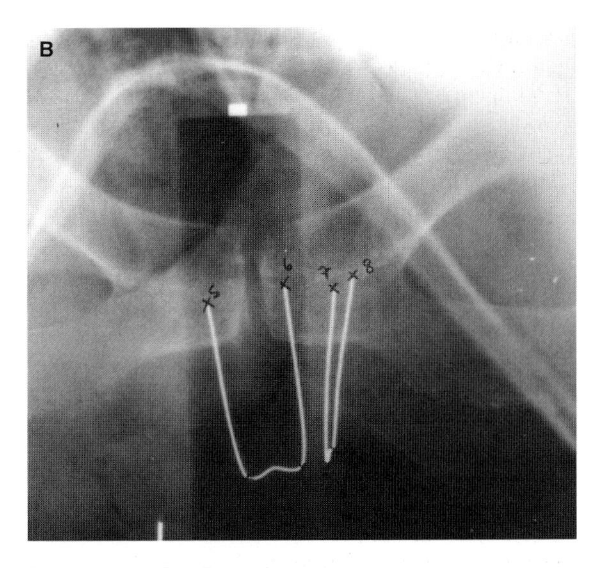

Fig. 14.7B AP radiographs

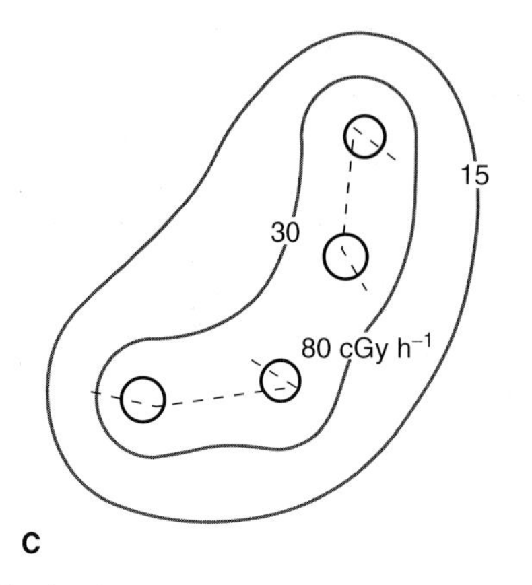

Fig. 14.7C the dose distribution.

treatment, using forceps to hold the bridge and draw them out of the tissues.

Paris system

The Paris system of dosimetry accommodates equally spaced straight sources distributed over one or two planes—each source will be of the same activity per unit length, but of a length primarily determined by the target size (Pierquin et al 1987). The volume treated to the prescribed dose is some 30% less than the length of the sources while the thickness depends on the separation of the sources—approximately 60% of the source separation for a single plane and 120% of the plane separation for a two-plane implant. The basic dose data for wire may be tabulated or presented in graphical format (Fig. 14.8). The data for pins will be slightly different from those for wire because of their greater diameter and self filtration.

The space between any two adjacent sources is referred to as a *corridor*, and the *basal dose rate* is calculated as the mean of the dose rates at the centre of each corridor. These are determined by measuring or calculating the distance from each source, summing the dose rates given in the tables/graphs at these distances and correcting for the activity per unit length. The treatment is prescribed to the *reference dose rate* (85% of the basal dose rate) or at a prescribed point.

Where the wires are not straight, the computer software will usually accept their subdivision into several shorter (approximately straight) lengths.

Calculation of an iridium implant

- For example: A prescription may read 'A wire implant is required to cover an area of 3×4.5 cm and to deliver 60 Gy at 85% of the basal dose rate in 5 days'.
- Dividing the area into two corridors of 15 mm width uses three wires of length 60 mm. The basal dose rate could be calculated as in Table 14.3 where the three wires are identified as ABC and the centre of each corridor as X and Y; the dose rate figures are taken from Figure 14.8. The mean basal dose rate calculated in the table is 0.837 Gy h^{-1} and 85% of this is 0.711 Gy h^{-1} (when using sources of 8.8 MBq mm^{-1}).
- The prescription requires a dose rate of 60 Gy in 5 days, or 0.50 Gy h^{-1}. The source activity required is therefore only $8.80 \times 0.50 / 0.711 = 6.19$ MBq mm^{-1}. Incidentally, the calculated dose rate at point Z (5 mm from point Y in a direction perpendicular to the implanted plane) is 0.695 Gy h^{-1} and confirms that the 85% prescription encloses 5 mm tissue either side of the plane.
- Using three 60 mm wires of 6.19 MBq mm^{-1} means the total implanted activity is $3 \times 60 \times 6.19 = 1114$ MBq. Given that the air kerma rate at 1 m for iridium is 0.113 mGy h^{-1} per GBq and the treatment is 120 h, the total reference air kerma is 15 mGy.
- Figure 14.9 shows the dose distribution around four 60 mm iridium wires implanted at the corners of a 2 cm square. The basal dose rate is calculated at the centre of the square by summing the dose rates from each of the wires. In this example all the wires are the same length and equidistant from the centre, i.e. at 1.4 cm distance. Figure 14.8 gives the dose rate at 1.4 cm from the centre of a 60 mm source as 0.2 Gy h^{-1}. The basal dose rate is therefore $4 \times 0.2 =$ 0.8 Gy h^{-1} when the activity is 8.8 MBq mm^{-1}. Pres-

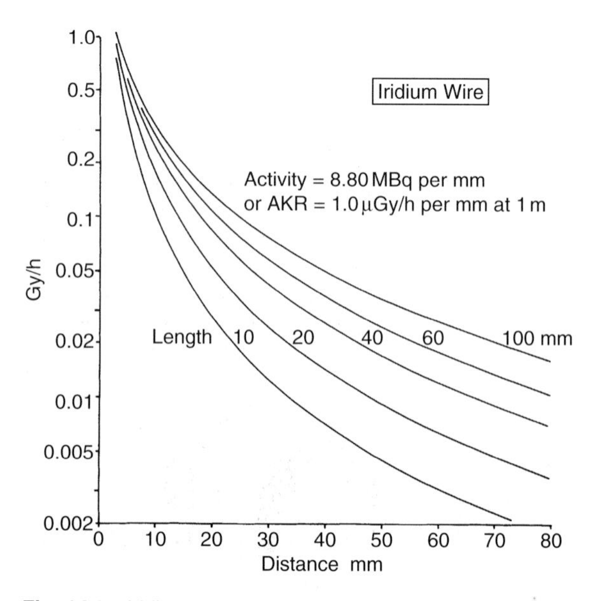

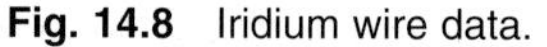

Fig. 14.8 Iridium wire data.

Table 14.3 Calculation of iridium wire planar implant

	Point X		Point Y		Point Z	
	d (cm)	Gy h^{-1}	*d* (cm)	Gy h^{-1}	*d* (cm)	Gy h^{-1}
Source A	0.75	0.373	2.25	0.091	2.30	0.087
Source B	0.75	0.373	0.75	0.373	0.90	0.304
Source C	2.25	0.091	0.75	0.373	0.90	0.304
Total dose rates		0.837		0.837		0.695

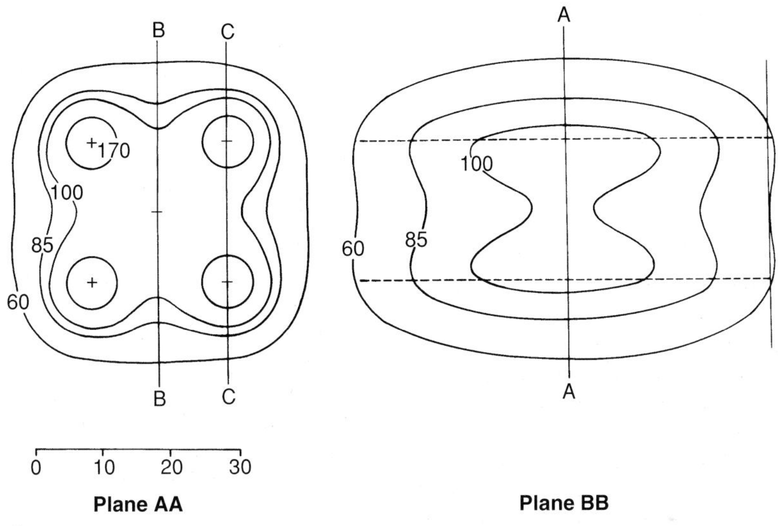

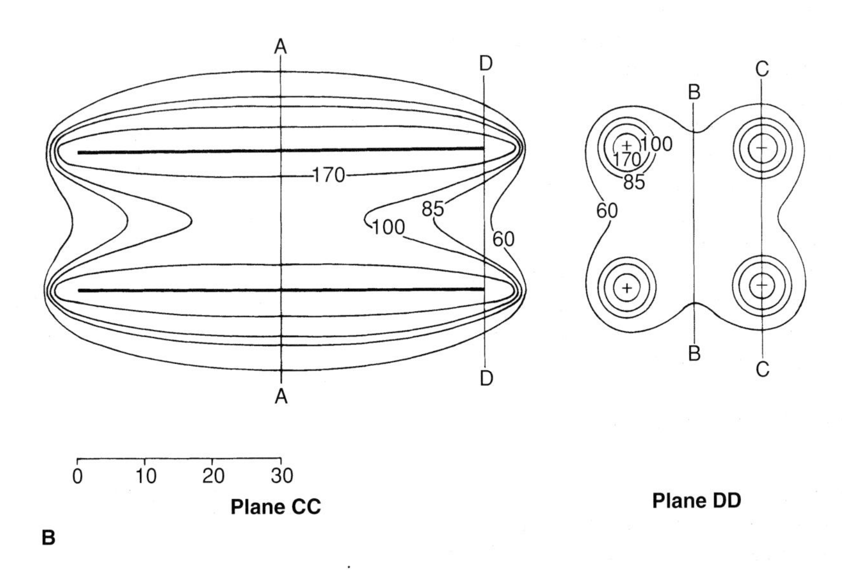

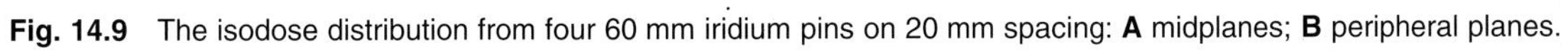
Fig. 14.9 The isodose distribution from four 60 mm iridium pins on 20 mm spacing: **A** midplanes; **B** peripheral planes.

cribing to the 85% isodose gives a dose rate of 0.68 Gy $^{-1}$. Thus a typical prescription of 10 Gy per 24 h (0.417 Gy^{-1}), requires a linear activity of the sources of $8.8 \times 0.417/0.68 = 5.4$ MBq mm^{-1}. In the figure, the 170% isodose curves are shown enclosing each source and indicate the volume of tissue irradiated to twice the prescribed dose.

MANUAL SYSTEMS

Needles and tubes

The manual implantation of preloaded sources has now largely been replaced by other techniques for reasons of radiation safety, but where the workload is small and access to other techniques is denied, the use of preloaded sources may be the only practical solution. Figure 14.10 shows the isodose distribution surrounding an interstitial *caesium-137 needle* and its construction. The activity is distributed uniformly down the length of the needle by packing it into several individual cells, to minimise the spillage of active content should the needle become damaged. It is important to distinguish the *overall length* (as visualised on the radiograph) from the *active length* (as required for dosimetry purposes)—the two 'inactive ends' are of equal length.

Each source will have an identification number or code engraved on it. This is necessary for record keeping, especially for the *leakage test* (p. 242) and any repairs, as detailed records must be kept of every individual radioactive source with a half-life of more than a few days. In practice, a system of coloured threads helps to identify the source type and its ultimate removal from the patient.

Paterson–Parker system

The *Paterson–Parker* system (sometimes called the *Manchester system*; Meredith 1967) of dosimetry was originally developed for use with radium needles and tubes. It sets out rules relating to the distribution of sources in various regular geometric configurations to deliver a uniform dose to the prescribed plane or volume. Here we shall only consider the rules for the rectangular planar implant (using needles) and the line source (using tubes).

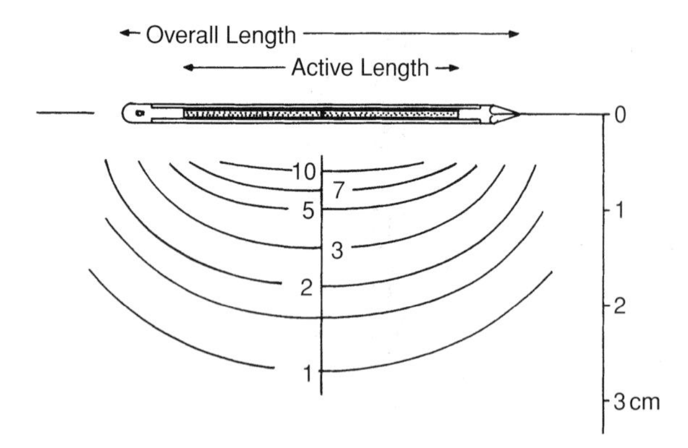

Fig. 14.10 The construction and isodose distribution for an interstitial needle.

Planar implants

The single plane interstitial implant is designed to treat a volume of tissue of the same area to a thickness, h, of 5 mm on either side. For the rectangular implant, the activity is distributed uniformly around the periphery and the area divided into strips of less than 2 h wide, parallel to the longer sides. If one extra line is required, a half-strength needle is used, for more than one extra line then two-thirds-strength needles are required. Where the rectangle has sides in the ratio of 2, 3 or 4, the overall activity implanted should be increased by 5%, 9% and 12% respectively.

The Paterson–Parker system of rules assumes the use of radium, but the data may be used for other nuclides providing their photon energy is similar and their activity is converted to *milligrams-radium-equivalent* by multiplying by the ratio of the air kerma rates. Once this has been calculated and provided the decay during the proposed treatment is negligible, radium data may be used. (All radium sources are assumed to be filtered by 0.5 mm Pt, unless otherwise stated.) A fundamental concept of the system is the *milligram-hour*, the product of the total activity and the treatment time. Paterson and Parker produced tables and graphs which give the milligram-hours (mgh) of radium required to deliver 1 Gy to a particular geometry (Fig. 14.11). The calculation may need to be repeated three times, based (i) on the theory of the intended implant, (ii) on the practical sources available and (iii) on the actual geometry of the implanted sources.

- For example: A prescription may read 'A needle implant is required to cover an area of 3×4.5 cm and deliver 60 Gy to a plane at $h = 0.5$ cm distance in 5 days'.
- Stage 1: To calculate the required activity for the prescribed treatment:

Area of implant = 3×4.5 cm^2 = 13.5 cm^2
To deliver 1 Gy at 0.5 cm distance requires 30 mgh (Fig. 14.11)
To deliver 60 Gy at 0.5 cm distance requires 30×60 mgh
To deliver 60 cGy in 5 days ($\times$ 24 hours) requires $(30 \times 60)/(5 \times 24) = 15$ mg.

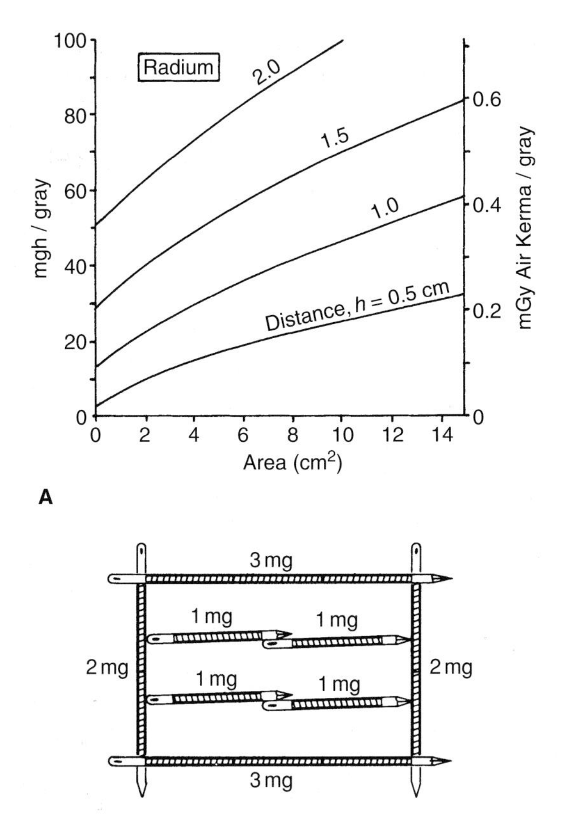

Fig. 14.11 **A** Paterson–Parker data and **B** a typical needle planar implant.

- Stage 2: To satisfy the 'rules', we must use the layout of needles illustrated in Figure 14.11B, and calculate the actual treatment time.

Periphery 2×3 mg + 2×2 mg = 10 mg plus
Two extra lines of 2×1 mg = 4 mg
Total activity used = 14 mg

- The dose of 60 Gy at 0.5 cm distance requires 30×60 mgh and therefore the revised treatment time = $30 \times 60/14 = 128.5$ h. The total reference air kerma is 13 mGy.
- Because of the inherent non-uniformity of dose in the implant situation, a relaxation of the above rules is permitted, namely to implant a fraction of the total activity round the periphery and to distribute the remainder as evenly as possible over the enclosed area. The peripheral fraction for areas less than 25 cm^2 is two-thirds of the total, one-half for areas between 25 cm^2 and 100 cm^2 and one-third for areas greater than 100 cm^2. Using this approximation in the above calculation would have lead to the same 10 mg round the periphery and 5 mg over the enclosed area and precisely the treatment time of 120 h prescribed.
- Stage 3: Postoperative radiography of the implanted sources will demonstrate how closely the implanted sources have followed the plan envisaged at Stage 2. A recalculation of the implanted area may required a revision of the treatment time based on the actual implanted area and the implanted activity.

Linear sources

For intracavitary therapy, a line source, e.g. to treat the uterine canal, may be made up of several collinear tubes mounted in an applicator. The cylindrical

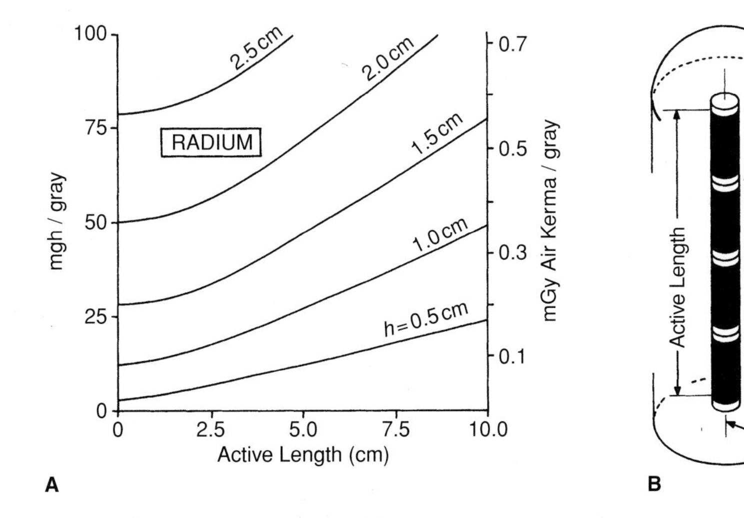

Fig. 14.12 **A** Paterson–Parker data and **B** a typical line source applicator.

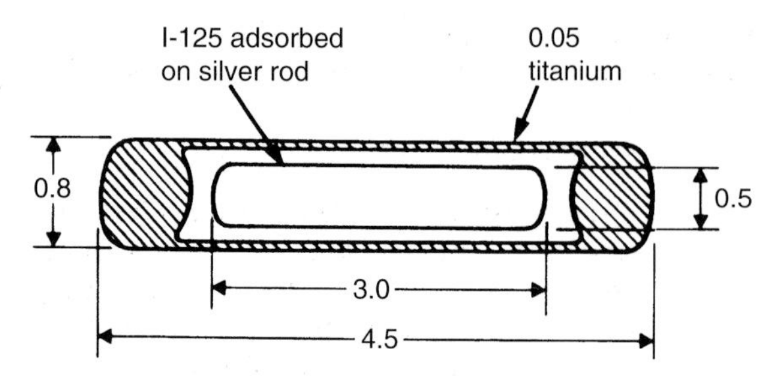

Fig. 14.13 Iodine-125 seeds. (Courtesy of Amersham International plc.)

surface treated is that defined by its radius, *h*, and the active length of the source. Only two rules apply. First, the active length is defined as the distance between the two active ends of the composite source. Secondly, the inactive space between the active ends of adjoining sources should not exceed the source–surface distance, *h*.

The dose calculation follows the same pattern as in the previous example using the line source data in Figure 14.12, the dose uniformity over the surface will be ± 10%.

IODINE SEEDS

Iodine-125 seeds have been used both for permanent implant in the pituitary and for surface applicators to treat the cornea. Iodine-125 is the daughter product of xenon-125 ($T_{½}$ = 18 h) which is produced by neutron bombardment of xenon-124 and decays by electron capture to tellurium-125 ($T_{½}$ = 60 days). The iodine-125 is adsorbed on a silver rod to form a seed with an overall length of 4.5 mm when encapsulated in 0.05 mm titanium (Fig. 14.13). The silver rod acts as an X-ray marker to locate the seed in radiography. Iodine-125 emits two primary photons of 27 and 35 keV, both of considerably lower energy than from any other brachytherapy source. These photons are absorbed in soft tissue by photoelectric absorption, make the assay of the seeds difficult and the emission anisotropic.

OPHTHALMIC APPLICATORS

Ophthalmic applicators should be handled using rubber-tipped forceps to protect the very thin active 'window' from physical damage. Theatre procedures for inserting these applicators should be rehearsed using non-active applicators and, where possible, the sutures should be positioned using the non-active applicator to minimise the handling of the active applicator. In addition to iodine-125, several other isotopes have been used in combating eye disease.

Strontium-90

The strontium-90 ($T_{½}$ = 28 years) compound is incorporated in a rolled silver foil bonded into the silver applicator and formed so that it presents an active concave surface of 15 mm radius to the cornea, with a surface filtration of 0.1 mm silver. Strontium-90 is only useful when in (secular radioactive) equilibrium with its daughter product, yttrium-90 ($T_{½}$ = 2.7 days). The 0.1 mm Ag filter is designed to absorb the low-energy beta particles from the strontium decay (0.54 MeV max., range in water 1.2 mm) while transmitting the higher-energy beta particles from the yttrium-90 (2.27 MeV max., range in water ~ 11 mm). The back of the applicator is finished with a much thicker (0.9 mm) layer of silver to reduce the transmitted dose rate to a relatively safe level. A variety of plaques are available, each designed to give a useful dose rate of approximately 1 Gy min^{-1} at the surface reducing to 50% at ~ 2 mm (Fig. 14.14).

The measurement of the beta dose rate is complex and involves the comparison of the dose rate of the ophthalmic applicator and that of a plane strontium-90 plaque which has been measured using a special ionisation chamber known as an extrapolation chamber. Such a chamber enables the dose rate at a surface to be extrapolated from a series of readings at different distances from the surface.

Ruthenium-106

Ruthenium-106 ($T_{½}$ = 369 days) is a fission product of uranium and decays with a low-energy beta emission

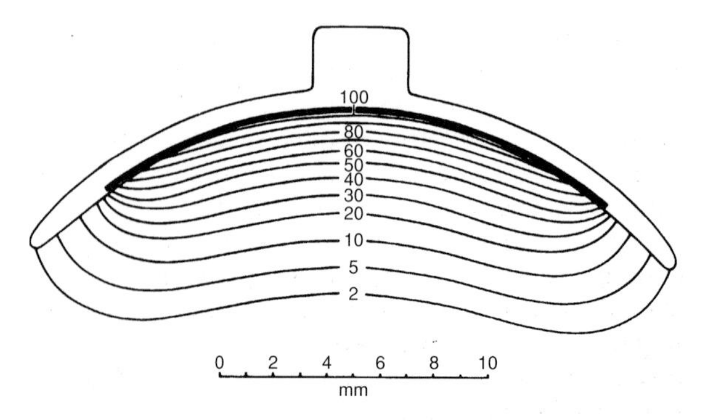

Fig. 14.14 The isodose distribution for an 18 mm diameter strontium-90 ophthalmic applicator. (Courtesy of Amersham International plc.)

to rhodium-106 ($T_{½}$ = 30 s) which has a higher-energy beta emission, namely 3.54 MeV max. The ruthenium applicator is made of silver with a window thickness of 0.1 mm Ag and a thicker protective layer of 0.9 mm Ag on the back. The spherical radius of the window is 12 mm. The applicator is designed for suturing to the sclera for 7–10 days (Plate 1.15). The useful dose rate is typically 0.1 Gy min^{-1} at the surface reducing to 50% at ~ 2.7 mm. A 15 mm acrylic visor is recommended to protect the eyes of the operator when using the ruthenium applicators.

Cobalt-60

Treatments of retinoblastoma have been effected using cobalt-60 ophthalmic applicators of similar construction to the ruthenium applicator. Their longer half-life was an advantage, but the high-energy gamma radiation gave high doses to other vital structures, e.g. the lens, macula and optic nerve, than with the ruthenium beta particle radiations. The cobalt-60 applicators had a useful dose rate of typically 0.06 Gy min^{-1} at the surface, reducing to 50% at ~ 2 mm.

PROTECTION IN BRACHYTHERAPY

Brachytherapy is one of the most hazardous radiation procedures in health care and is further complicated by the fact that we have to consider not only the safety of the staff involved and that of other patients, but also the safety and security of the sources themselves. For a fuller explanation, reference should be made to the current regulations (HSE 1999) and their supporting documents.

Safety of staff

Handling

The principal hazard of small sealed sources is that of their high energy, and therefore penetrating beta and/or gamma radiations, unless the sealed source is damaged. Unsealed sources present both the hazards of external radiation and of radioactive contamination. (Iridium is technically an unsealed source in that fragments of active material may be left contaminating the cutting jig, drapes, etc.) **Under no circumstances should a sealed source be handled—contact with the fingers or the skin must be avoided.** The use of finger dosimeters (p. 82), in addition to whole-body dosimeters, must be considered.

In general, there are three methods of reducing the external radiation hazard:

- reducing the time spent in manipulation
- increasing the distance between the source and the operator, and
- using protective barriers or screens.

These three measures will often work against each other in practice; for example, the time spent manipulating the source may be increased by either increasing the distance or by the use of protective screens. Invariably a compromise has to be reached.

A simple *lead bench* (Fig. 14.15) made from two pieces of lead approximately 35 × 35 cm^2 × 5 cm thick can rest on a laboratory bench so that the operator can sit or stand behind it with only the head and arms exposed to the sources on the horizontal section. The alternative is to use a specially constructed bench where the protective material is built up all round and incorporates a protected observation window of lead glass. All the surfaces should be impervious and continuous for ease of handling the sources.

Special care must be taken to avoid excessive irradiation to the fingers. Under no circumstances should the operator pick up a radioactive source with the fingers. A selection of long-handled forceps must always be available. In some larger departments, *slave manipulators* (Fig. 14.16) may be available. Wherever the manipulation requires skill, the procedure should be practised using inactive 'dummy' sources and specially designed tools, e.g. the threading of needles can be simplified by the use of a needle threader and a lead block to hold the needles securely with only the 'eye' exposed.

Nursing on the wards

Single-bedded ward accommodation is essential and the door should carry a radiation trefoil warning sign with the words 'Controlled Area—Gamma Rays' (Plate 1.3). A protected container, capable of accepting all the sources in use, must be available on the ward at

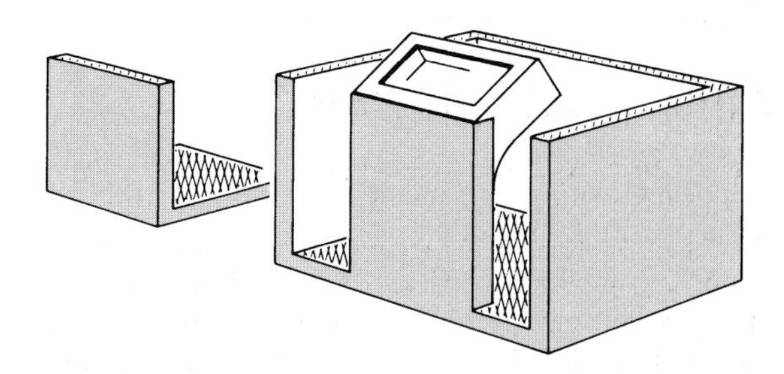

Fig. 14.15 Protected lead benches for the small sealed-source laboratory.

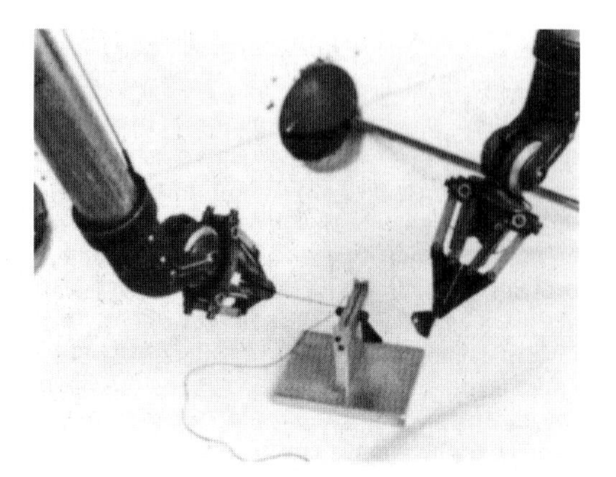

Fig. 14.16 Slave manipulators may be used to thread interstitial needles—note the use of a needle threader in the fingers on the right.

all times for use should the sources have to be removed in an emergency.

Nursing staff who undertake responsibilities for the removal of sources to terminate the brachytherapy treatment or for interrupting the treatment by remote afterloading will come under the Ionising Radiations (Medical Exposure) Regulations 2000 (HSE 2000) which demand they undergo special training in radiation protection.

Where remote afterloading equipment is being used, the sources may be temporarily withdrawn from the patient to allow essential nursing and other procedures to be carried out in a radiation-free environment. Emergency procedures must be available should the source transfer mechanism fail. Where remote afterloading equipment is not available and the treatment requires the sealed sources to be in situ for several days, mobile *lead bed shields* (Plate 1.13) should be placed by the bed so that the staff are protected whilst carrying out the essential nursing procedures. Non-essential procedures should be postponed until after the removal of the sources. The Radiation Protection Supervisor (RPS) will assess the hazard presented by each patient and restrict the time spent by the staff nursing the patient. Routine procedures should be shared by using a rota system in order to minimise the exposure to individual members of staff. The RPS will also restrict the patient's visitors, and children and pregnant women should not be allowed to visit patients with brachytherapy sources in situ.

A procedure must be clearly documented for the artificial resuscitation of a patient to minimise the risks to staff from radiation sources still in situ.

Nursing in theatre

The basic principles of speed and distance and the use of protective barriers must be followed during the actual insertion of the 'live' sources in theatre and during their removal. The use of non-active applicators during the preparation of the patient is to be recommended as a means of reducing staff exposure. The use of protective barriers in the recovery area should not be overlooked. Where (C-arm) X-ray equipment is used in theatre, then all staff must stand clear when instructed to do so by the radiographer making the exposures.

The discharge of the patient

A patient undergoing treatment with long-lived sealed sources must not be discharged until all the sources have been removed. In the interests of safety—of the public and of the sources—a patient determined on self-discharge must be detained long enough to recover the sources.

Where the isotope is not removable, then the patient must be detained so long as the total activity exceeds the limits laid down (Table 15.2). The limit for discharge of the patient is dependent on the isotope, its form, the mode of transport and the duration of the journey. The decision to discharge such a patient should also take into account the home circumstances to which the patient is returning, particularly if there are young children or pregnant women at home. The patient must be given written instructions about any necessary restrictions to be observed, e.g. about nursing young children, returning to work, etc. and the date from which the restrictions can be relaxed (Fig. 15.1)

The death of the patient

It is unlikely that the radiation sources will have contributed to the death of the patient and all sealed sources must be removed immediately. If, for any reason, this is not possible, then the Radiation Protection Adviser must be called upon to advise on the precautions to be taken at post-mortem and in the recovery of the sources before the disposal of the body. If non-removable sources are involved, the RPA must be consulted also about the funeral arrangements.

Safety of sources

Supply and registration

The hospital site must be licensed to hold radioactive sources (RSA 1993) and the practitioners must hold valid

ARSAC certificates before administering sources to patients (or to research volunteers) (ARSAC 1988). It is normal practice to appoint a *custodian* or *curator* to take the overall responsibility for the safety of (un)sealed sources held by the hospital and to ensure that the requirements of the site licence are met. Each new source must be assayed using a calibrated ionisation chamber and the result of the measurement justified against the supplier's certification (Poynter 2000). It will be the responsibility of the curator/custodian to ensure that adequate records are kept. These should include:

- A register of stock of all sealed sources, having a half-life greater than a few days, will contain the detailed specification of each individual source, its supplier, its identification marks, its serial number, both the certificated and the locally measured activity and the reports of leakage tests and repairs. In addition the record will contain the date and mode of disposal of the source and to whom; such records shall be kept for at least 2 years after the disposal of the source.
- A record of all sealed sources issued from and returned to the main store, together with date and time, and the signature of the responsible person making the transfer. This record may be accompanied by some visual display system to indicate what is in the store and available for issue. It is vital to be able to readily identify the location of every source in the event of an emergency.
- A record of the administration of radioactive sources to patients and of the removal of temporary implants.
- An annual audit of the total stock must be made by an independent observer.

Storage

Normally all laboratory procedures will be carried out in specially designed accommodation designated as a 'Controlled Area—Gamma Rays'. This *sealed source laboratory* should not be used for any other purpose. The main safe for the storage of sources will be designed so that sources may be distributed into individually protected drawers, each drawer being fitted to accommodate a specific type and number of sources in an orderly fashion (Fig. 14.17). It should be possible to check the number and type of source in each drawer at a glance. The storage safe should be ventilated to the open air by a fan operated both before and during the transfer of sources to and from the safe.

Every transfer must be accompanied by an entry in the record book and the signature of a responsible individual. The safe should be kept locked whenever it is not being used. Both the room and the safe should be marked with the black and yellow warning trefoil (Plate 1.3).

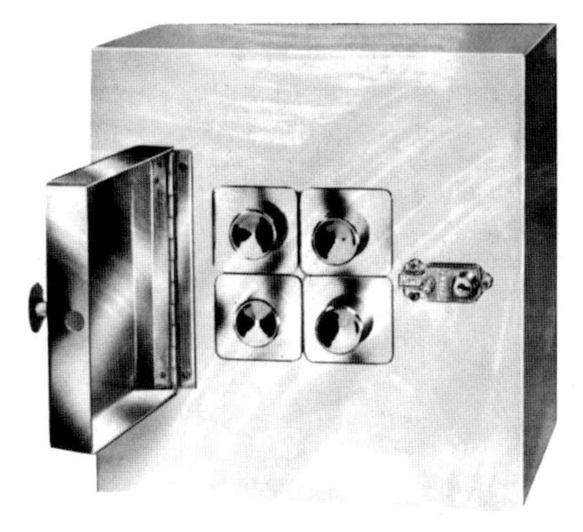

Fig. 14.17 The multi-drawer protected storage safe for sealed sources. (Courtesy of Nuclear Associates.)

Sterilisation

Sterilisation should be carried out in the protected environment of the sealed source laboratory. Sources should be examined for any defects before any sterilising procedure is undertaken and any source thought to be defective should be taken out of use until it has been thoroughly examined and tested. Sterilisation of sealed sources may be achieved by a variety of means—ethylene oxide gas sterilisation, immersion in cold sterilising liquid, boiling in water, etc.—and care must be taken to reduce the risk of damage to the source or corrosion of the surface. Where heat is used (as in boiling) care must be taken to ensure that in the event of failure (e.g. boiling dry) the temperature cannot rise above 180°C. Sources used for remote afterloading do not require sterilising because they do not come into contact with the patient—the catheters used can be sterilised in the usual way taking care to keep fluids out of the catheters.

Cleaning

Cleaning of used sources can contribute significantly to the exposure of the technician's fingers unless some automatic devices are used and a rigid procedure followed. For example, the immersion of the sources in hydrogen peroxide solution or normal saline solution immediately after their removal from the patient will ensure that any tissue deposits adhering to the sources do not harden and become caked to the surface. The use of a low-power ultrasonic cleaning bath—suitably surrounded with lead or behind the lead bench—reduces the handling of the sources to a minimum. The replacement of acrylic applicators before they become roughened or cracked will reduce the time required to clean them. Abrasive substances should never be used for cleaning.

Movement

Movements outside the hospital complex are governed by the Radioactive Material (Road Transport) (Great Britain) Regulations (HMSO 1996) outlined in Chapter 8 and must be strictly followed. Movement of sources within the hospital premises must be fully documented so that, in the event of fire or the suspected loss of a source, the exact location of each source can be readily identified. Regular movements within the hospital should follow specified and documented routes which should be the easiest if not the shortest. The design of new departments should be drawn up with this requirement in mind. Movements of the sources should be in long-handled containers (pots or trolleys) specially designed for the purpose, i.e. providing adequate protection and security, appropriate labelling and minimising the risk of loss or damage.

Patients with sealed sources in situ should not be allowed to leave their ward without permission and that should only be granted if there is good reason and the radiation safety of others can be guaranteed.

The use of permanently installed gamma alarms at strategic points along the corridors, in sluice rooms and at doorways to detect the unauthorised passage of any source is to be recommended. Such installations need to be checked regularly.

Leakage (wipe) tests

All sealed sources should be checked for free activity, i.e. radioactive content that has leaked out of the encapsulation, at least annually and whenever there is any suspicion of damage to the source. Any source is capable of being damaged, but needles are the most vulnerable as they may be bent by mishandling, by being dropped or by being pushed against a bone during implantation. They may be easily checked for straightness by rolling them on a hard flat surface—a piece of plate glass is ideal. No attempt should be made in-house to straighten a bent needle—it should be immediately sealed in a glass container.

Three *leakage* tests are recognised: The *wipe test* is readily carried out by passing the source—using forceps—through a foam pad moistened with ethanol. The activity on the pad should then be measured in a calibrated *well counter*. A *bubble test* may be performed by immersing the source in water and reducing the pressure to 100 mm mercury—no bubble must be observed. A third alternative is the *immersion test*, immersing the source in warm (50°C) water for 4 h and then measuring the activity of the water. Higher-activity sources may be tested by the immersion test or by wiping/testing the catheters through which the source has passed several times. Any catheter used in association with afterloading equipment should be tested for free activity before repair or disposal.

If any leakage test suggests a free activity greater than 200 Bq, the source must be regarded as leaking and steps taken to get the source examined and repaired accordingly. Any source suspected to be leaking must be sealed in an airtight (preferably glass) container pending its repair or disposal by a competent authority.

Suspected loss

Every effort must be taken to prevent the loss of a sealed source but despite each movement of sources being recorded, it is still possible for sources to get mislaid in transit or lost from a patient. In the event of a source being suspected lost, the documented procedure must be invoked. Notices outlining the procedure should be posted in all areas where sources are routinely used. (If the lost source could put the public at risk, the police and the Health and Safety Executive must be alerted.) The local procedure should be along the lines shown below.

The (suspected) loss of a source

1. All avenues by which the source may have been removed from its last known location must be closed immediately. There should be no flushing of toilets or sluices, no removal of dirty dressings, laundry or rubbish of any sort, no sweeping of floors, no movement of patients, staff or visitors away from the area. No further material should be placed in the hospital incinerator or removed from the site.
2. The persons responsible for the radiation safety in the department or ward and the RPA must be notified as soon as possible.
3. A search for the source must be initiated immediately, bearing in mind that other sources known to be in the vicinity will also be detected by the monitor used in the search. If at any stage the search suggests the lost source is damaged, then the further precau-

tionary measures relating to unsealed sources (p. 248) should be observed.

4. If the initial search is unsuccessful, consideration must be given to calling in specialist assistance from outside the hospital.

Disposal of sources

Long-lived isotopes (e.g. caesium) with half-lives of several years must be sent to an approved organisation for disposal. If the sources are being replaced, the supplier may be willing to accept the spent sources for disposal. The alternative is to employ the services of a specialist disposal company. Under no circumstances must the sources be allowed into inexperienced hands, either deliberately or accidentally, or put away and forgotten. Long-term storage of sources awaiting disposal is to be deprecated. Where the isotopes have half-lives of less than a few months (e.g. iridium), the spent sources may be stored in lead pots either until they can be disposed of as inactive waste or until sufficient have been accumulated to justify their disposal as outlined above. Full details of each source sent for disposal must be recorded together with the date, activity and method of disposal. These records must be kept for the number of years specified in the legislation. Disposal of radioactive material can be expensive and should be budgeted for in advance.

DESIGN OF BRACHYTHERAPY FACILITIES

Sealed source laboratory

Brachytherapy sources will be stored in a secure protected safe and handled in a specially prepared room equipped with a protected bench (p. 239) and remote handling facilities (p. 240). The cleaning and sterilising facilities are most conveniently situated in the same room. In many respects, the laboratory requires the same facilities as those described in Chapter 8 for unsealed sources and in Chapter 10 for gamma beam therapy equipment, including the radiation trefoil and controlled area sign. There is no 'useful beam' or primary beam of radiation and it must be assumed that the ceiling, floor and walls will be irradiated isotropically. The thickness of the protected walls etc. will be determined from the maximum possible activity of sources and an assessment of the maximum exposure time in any one day. In determining the protection on the safe itself no such time allowance is relevant. The design of protected benches for use within the laboratory was discussed above.

Brachytherapy ward/theatre

When patients have 'live' sources implanted, then both the operating theatre and the single-bedded protected room on the ward will be designated a temporary controlled area (p. 77) from the moment the sources arrive until the sources are finally removed.

The structural protection will be calculated in much the same way as for the laboratory, ignoring the attenuation within the patient and paying particular attention to patients in adjacent wards who again will be exposed 24 h per day and subject to dose limits. To minimise the risk of loss and radioactive contamination, the floors should be impervious and continuous with coved skirtings. The need for personal monitoring will need to be assessed for the ward / theatre staff.

Remote afterloading suite

The afterloading suite, whether it is for low- or high-dose-rate treatments, will require a maze entrance with an interlocked barrier, a means of observing the patient, an intercom and an independently powered gamma alarm as for a gamma ray beam unit (pp. 81 and 183). As with the gamma beam unit, the single-bedded room will be without windows although by careful design, daylight can be admitted through the protected barriers. If the remote afterloading equipment, which contains the stock of sources when not in use, is not in the single-bedded ward then the warning signs may be removed and the designation as a controlled area is only temporary. The room housing the equipment will be permanently so designated.

- The calculation of the protective barriers is based on the air kerma rate for the isotope in question (Table 14.1). For example, a low-dose-rate remote afterloading unit has the capacity for 48 caesium sources, each of 1.6 GBq activity. Assuming the sources will be at the centre of a 3×3 m room, typical of a single-bedded room, and the nearest point in an occupied area outside the room is 2 m from the sources, then:

$$\text{Air kerma rate at 2 m distance} = 48 \times 1.6 \times 0.078/4 \cong 1.5 \text{ mGy h}^{-1}$$

- If the occupancy is unlikely to exceed 40 hours per week then, potentially, the annual total air kerma in that occupied area will be:

$$1.5 \times 40 \times 52 \cong 3000 \text{ mGy}$$

- If the dose limit applicable to the adjacent area is 0.3 mSv per year (0.3 mGy per year) then the attenuation required in the wall will be:

$$0.3 \text{ mGy}/3000 \text{ mGy} = 10^{-4} \text{ or } 4 \text{ TVL}$$

- Table 6.4 gives the TVL for caesium as 160 mm and 4 $\times$ 160 = 640 mm concrete.

The low-dose-rate afterloading suite will need to be situated close to 24 h nursing cover and therefore close to a full-time ward, whereas high-dose-rate equipment may be accommodated close to the theatre suite or the radiotherapy department and under the control of the therapy radiographers.

CHAPTER CONTENTS

15

Therapy with unsealed radionuclides

Keith Bomford

INTRODUCTION

Chapter 8 has dealt with the diagnostic imaging techniques using unsealed radiopharmaceuticals. This chapter discusses their use in therapy and concludes with aspects of radiation protection matters relevant to both but particularly to therapy. Therapeutic applications involve the administration of a radiopharmaceutical with the intent of selectively destroying diseased tissue. There is a growing interest in targeted radiotherapy where specific tissues and organs are targeted using specially prepared radiopharmaceuticals (Fleming & Perkins 2001). The biological effects of the emitted ionising radiations are maximised to produce local therapeutic results in the tissues in which the radionuclide is deposited.

If a suitable radioactive compound can be concentrated in one particular organ, it seems feasible that a therapeutic radiation dose could be given to that organ. Unfortunately this possibility is only feasible if the ratio of the concentration in the tumour to that in other healthy tissues is very high. For example, a *concentration ratio* of 1000 to 1 is required if a therapeutic dose of 50 Gy is to be delivered to a particular organ while keeping the general whole-body dose to 0.05 Gy. Unfortunately, the concentration ratio normally observed is at most 100 to 1 and while this may be suitable for diagnostic purposes, it is not for therapy. However, a limited number of radionuclides are suitable for therapeutic administration (Table 15.1), having the following properties:

- The radionuclide emits a large proportion of its energy in the form of beta particles. Beta particle radiation is completely absorbed by the tissue in which the isotope is lodged and delivers a localised radiation dose. Radionuclides which decay by beta particle emission and have a high gamma ray yield may be used if their chemical and biological properties outweigh other undesirable physical properties.

- A physical half-life of about 10 days is desirable because radionuclides of shorter half-life require the administration of higher levels of activity to achieve the required dose, posing a greater hazard to staff, while nuclides of longer half-life pose a greater radiation hazard to the patient.
- The effective rate at which the radioactivity disappears from a particular site is important. The effective half-life has been shown to be a combination of the physical and biological half-lives (p. 117). Occasionally, the administration of isotopes of long physical half-life may be justified if, in the chemical form used, the biological half-life and therefore the effective half-life is very short.
- The specific activity, i.e. the ratio per unit mass of radioactive to non-radioactive atoms in the element, should be as high as possible. This will allow very small quantities of the agent to be used and will ensure that the radio-label does not significantly alter the chemical or biological properties of the pharmaceutical.

PHOSPHORUS-32

Phosphorus-32 ($T_{½}$ = 14.3 days) comes close to being the ideal unsealed therapeutic radionuclide. It is a pure beta particle emitter with an average energy of the beta particles of 695 keV, resulting in a maximum range in tissue of about 8 mm (Fig. 3.5B). It is normally administered intravenously as sterile sodium phosphate, and may be used in the treatment of polycythaemia vera and related blood disorders. Treatment regimens vary and are a matter for clinical judgement with typical activities administered in the range 150–350 MBq. Following intravenous injection, approximately 50% of the phosphorus-32 accumulates in the blood-forming bone marrow. The absorbed dose to the bone surface and to the red bone marrow is 11 mGy/MBq and the effective dose equivalent is 2.2 mSv/MBq. In order to control the disease, treatment may be repeated at intervals of 6–12 months. (Note: The effective dose equivalent (p. 74) is very important in nuclear medicine procedures as it allows for a variety of non-uniform distributions of dose equivalents in the body to be expressed as a single number representing the risk to health.)

STRONTIUM-89

The average energy of the beta particles from strontium-89 ($T_{½}$ = 50.5 days) is 500 keV and the maximum range in tissue is about 7 mm. It may be used for the palliation of pain from bone metastases secondary to prostatic and breast carcinoma. Administered activity is typically 150 MBq given intravenously as sterile strontium chloride. The absorbed dose can be expected to be of the order of 300 mGy/MBq, dependent upon the degree of concentration of the strontium within the metastases. The effective dose equivalent is 2.9 mSv/MBq.

YTTRIUM-90

The average energy of the beta particles from yttrium-90 ($T_{½}$ = 2.7 days) is 923 keV and the maximum range in tissue is about 11 mm. Although yttrium-90 is a pure beta emitter the high energy of the beta particles can give rise to bremsstrahlung radiation. An injection of a sterile suspension of colloidal yttrium silicate in aqueous solution is given for a variety of disease states. The activity administered will vary. For example 120–240 MBq is injected into joints for the intra-articular treatment of arthritis, while 1–4 GBq is injected intrapleurally or intraperitoneally for the intracavitary treatment of malignant effusions. The absorbed radiation dose to the patient will depend upon the nature of the disease state.

IODINE-131

Iodine-131 ($T_{½}$ = 8.1 days) is the most important and most extensively used unsealed therapeutic radionuclide as it allows a high radiation dose to be delivered to the thyroid and a low dose to the rest of the body (Ch. 24). It decays by beta particle emission and a complex gamma spectrum; the principal gamma ray energy is 364 keV (in 80% of disintegrations). The average energy of the beta particles is 246 keV and

Table 15.1 Some properties of the radionuclides used in therapy

	Radionuclide			
	^{32}P	^{89}Sr	^{90}Y	^{131}I
Half-life (days)	14.3	50.5	2.7	8.1
Average energy of beta emission (keV)	695	500	923	246
Max. range in tissue (mm)	8	7	11	3

their maximum range in tissue is about 3 mm. Iodine is chemically very reactive and is readily concentrated in the thyroid gland. It may also be trapped in the salivary glands and the gastric mucosa. As a precursor to therapy, it is important to know the percentage uptake of iodine in the thyroid (p. 121) before calculating the therapeutic dose to be administered.

It should be noted that other thyroid function studies may use technetium-99m because it gives a lower absorbed dose to the gland while the pertechnetate ion (TcO_4) behaves in a similar way to the iodine ion in the thyroid. Figure 8.9 shows a static image of the thyroid gland acquired approximately 30 minutes after an intravenous injection of 40–80 MBq of [^{99m}Tc]pertechnetate. Such a study provides an assessment of the size of the gland in hyperthyroidism and the localisation of metastatic thyroid cancer.

Thyrotoxicosis

Two distinct disease states may be treated by iodine-131 therapy. The first is the non-malignant condition of *thyrotoxicosis*, where the thyroid gland is overproducing thyroid hormones. The administered activity will depend upon the size of the gland and the degree of hyperactivity, but is usually in the range 150–500 MBq. With a normal-sized gland, typical figures will be a percentage uptake of 55%, an absorbed dose to the gland of 790 mGy/MBq and an effective dose equivalent of 24 mSv/MBq. About 90% of the absorbed dose will be due to the beta particles and 10% to the gamma rays (p. 135). This form of treatment is contraindicated in persons under the age of 40 and in pregnant or lactating women (p. 250).

Thyroid tumours

The second condition is the well-differentiated thyroid tumours and their metastases. The administered activity is very high, being of the order of 2–8 GBq, as the aim of treatment is to ablate all the thyroid-like tissue. The treatment may be repeated at 6-monthly intervals until no residual thyroid tissue remains. The radioactive iodine is supplied and administered as a solution of sodium iodide, preferably in capsule form, though in the body it is the radioactive iodide ion whose behaviour is of importance.

Because of the high activity involved, this treatment must be carried out in the specially equipped single-bedded suite. The safety measures will remain in place for at least 48 hours after the administration and until the residual activity in the patient has fallen below the levels laid down in the regulations for return of the patient to the main ward or to his or her home circumstances.

RADIATION PROTECTION

Insofar as the external radiation hazard is concerned, the accommodation of the patient and the precautions will be similar to those relating to low-dose-rate afterloading brachytherapy and much of what has been said in the previous chapter in connection with sealed sources is equally applicable to unsealed source therapy. In addition, special precautions against radioactive contamination must be observed in the care and management of patients undergoing unsealed radionuclide therapy. The principles outlined in Chapters 6 and 8 are relevant, bearing in mind that the activities in therapeutic applications are much greater than in diagnostic procedures—there is always the potential for radioactive contamination:

- of the accommodation
- of the equipment
- of the patient and of anything or anyone that is likely to come into contact with the patient.

All the staff attending the patient must wear protective clothing when handling the patient or any articles which may be contaminated. Any goods or clothing found to be contaminated must be kept separate and stored for assay and approved disposal by the medical physics staff. Staff must be familiar with and practised in the use of a (de)contamination monitor and regularly record the results of monitoring. These matters are discussed in more detail below. In addition to film/TLD badge monitoring, there may be a requirement for periodic monitoring of the staff for inhaled or ingested contamination, e.g. of the thyroid when nursing iodine therapy patients.

Accommodation

The following facilities are required:

- The patient must be confined to a single-bedded room with impervious wall finishes and flooring with coved skirtings to ease decontamination. The door will carry a trefoil sign and the area be designated as a controlled area.
- The patient must have exclusive use of an en suite toilet and shower facility connected directly to a main drain. Manhole covers to the drain need to be labelled appropriately.
- Bed linen, towels and clothing must be monitored for contamination before being sent to the laundry (see maximum permissible contamination limits in Table 8.7).

- Visiting by adults should be discouraged for the first 24 hours and restricted thereafter; visiting by children and pregnant women is forbidden.
- An emergency decontamination kit and radiation monitor should be readily accessible.

Control of contamination

- All the patient's body fluids, including perspiration and saliva, may be contaminated with radioactivity; staff must wear at least gowns and gloves to protect their own skin and clothing. Overshoes should be worn if there is any chance of the floor being contaminated.
- Wherever possible, utensils such as cutlery and crockery should be disposable and must be collected together and retained in the room together with other contaminated material, such as disposable handkerchiefs, until dealt with by authorised personnel.
- All nursing procedures should be carried out in the minimum time compatible with good nursing care. In particular, a procedure must be clearly documented for the artificial resuscitation of a patient which minimises the risks to staff from both the external radiation hazard and from radioactive contamination.

Discharge of patient

Patients who have received radionuclide therapy will present a radiation hazard to anyone with whom they come into contact and must not be discharged until their residual level of activity has fallen below the prescribed limit. Table 15.2 lists the activity levels at which the patient may be discharged and any restrictions on the mode of transport used. Self-discharge must be deprecated on the grounds of the hazards to others.

All patients who exceed the 50 MBq MeV activity level at the time of discharge should be given written instructions about precautions to be taken on leaving hospital. This may take the form of a card, as shown in Figure 15.1. Following discharge, the room may not be re-used until it has been monitored and declared free from contamination.

In the case of the death of a patient following the administration of a therapeutic dose of radioactivity, due regard must be given to the safety of the relatives, pathologists and undertakers, etc. A local policy should be written for each application practised in that centre.

Spillage

The remainder of this chapter is relevant to both diagnostic and therapeutic applications of unsealed radionuclides, but the hazards are that much greater in therapy because of the higher activities involved.

In spite of every care and attention to technique, accidental spillage of radioactive materials does occur and a clinical unit which handles unsealed radioactive sources should have fully documented procedures and equipment for dealing with emergency spills. Staff should also be trained to deal with spills. In the clinical situation there are various ways in which the spill of a radionuclide can occur. These include accidental spillage in dispensing or administration, and contamination resulting from urinary incontinence or the patient vomiting following the oral administration of a radioactive material. For diagnostic procedures radioactive urine presents the main contamination hazard. This is particularly so in patients having bone scans, where a high proportion of the injected radiopharmaceutical is excreted in the urine and patients are required to empty their bladder before imaging commences.

Decontamination

Two principal criteria pertain when implementing decontamination procedures. Firstly, the safety of the individual is paramount. Secondly, it is essential to contain the spill and avoid spread. In the event of a major spill,

Table 15.2 Maximum activity levels of unsealed therapeutic radionuclides for discharging patients from hospital

Radionuclide	< 10 MBq MeV No restrictions	< 50 MBq MeV No transport restrictions*	< 150 MBq MeV Travel by public transport †	< 300 MBq MeV Travel by private transport
^{131}I	30 MBq	150 MBq	400 MBq	800 MBq
^{32}P	300 MBq	1.5 GBq	4.5 GBq	9 GBq
^{90}Y	100 MBq	500 MBq	1.5 GBq	3 GBq
^{198}Au	30 MBq	150 MBq	400 MBq	800 MBq

* Continue to avoid close contact with children and pregnant women.
† Includes ambulances and hospital cars.

RADIONUCLIDE INSTRUCTION CARD		
Name: Address: Hospital No: Department: Address: Consultant:	It is important that you carry this card with you at all times and observe the following instructions until .... a) Avoid journeys on public transport until .... b) Avoid going to places of entertainment until .... c) Do not return to work until .... d) Avoid prolonged personal contact at home until .... and observe the verbal instructions given to you before leaving hospital. e) other .... Signed .... On	Radionuclide administered:............. Activity:............. On:............. If an accident occurs or you have any difficulty, Please telephone: .... and ask for ....

Fig. 15.1 Radionuclide instruction card for patients leaving hospital with significant residual activity. (The card should be of a distinctive colour, preferably yellow.)

e.g. 30 MBq of iodine-131, the following actions should be taken:

1. Take immediate action to contain the contamination; all persons not contaminated and not involved in the incident should leave the area.
2. Notify the radiation protection supervisor and obtain appropriate assistance (from outside the hospital, if necessary).
3. Give priority to the treatment of injuries, but decontaminate personnel (see below) as soon as possible.
4. Decontaminate the room (see below).
5. Remove all contaminated materials for appropriate storage or disposal.
6. Prepare an incident report and report to the radiation protection adviser.

An emergency decontamination kit and radiation monitor (a 'spill kit') containing appropriate tools and equipment to deal with a radioactive spill should be available at all times. This kit might include overshoes and protective clothing, plastic bags, radioactive warning tape, pens, appropriate decontamination materials, tools for handling contaminated articles, and portable monitoring equipment.

Personal decontamination

Any person, who is contaminated with radioactive material, must be decontaminated as quickly as possible to prevent absorption through the skin, ingestion, and spread of the contamination. The following steps should be carried out:

1. Use the (de)contamination monitor to assess the extent of contamination.
2. Remove all contaminated clothing.
3. Wash the contaminated area with soap and water (avoid the use of abrasives); a designated commercial decontaminant such as 2% Decon-90 may be used where soap and water have failed. Take special care to avoid spreading contamination to the eyes or mouth. If the eyes or open wounds are contaminated irrigate with copious amounts of water.
4. If the skin contamination is extensive and a shower is required then this should be taken after dealing with any localised high-activity contamination.
5. Decontamination procedures should be continued until the activity is below the levels listed in Table 8.7.

Room decontamination

To decontaminate the ward/laboratory area, the following steps should be carried out:

1. Persons not involved in the decontamination procedure should leave the area.
2. Wear the appropriate protective clothing, e.g. gloves, lab coat, overshoes.

3. Use the (de)contamination monitor to assess the extent and mark the edges of the area of contamination.

4. Mop up the spill with an absorbent material such as paper towels working from the outer edge of the area towards the centre; scrub the surface with soap and water, a detergent or a decontaminant.

5. Monitor the area to check activity has been reduced to an acceptable level (Table 8.7); if contamination above these levels persists, cover the area, display a warning sign and allow time for the activity to decay.

Waste disposal

Radioactive waste arises from decontamination following spills; the excreta of patients undergoing diagnostic and therapeutic nuclear medicine procedures; the syringes, swabs, paper tissues, etc. used in the preparation and administration of the radiopharmaceutical and from expired stock solutions. Waste products therefore will be either liquid or solid, although gaseous waste may be encountered from fume cupboards and lung ventilation scanning. The disposal of radioactive waste from a hospital must be organised, carefully controlled and documented in compliance with the UK regulations, not only to avoid hazard to staff and patients in the hospital, but also to avoid any hazard to the general public. Her Majesty's Inspectorate of Pollution, Department of the Environment, will have set limits of activity for both liquid and solid waste for each site and ensure compliance with the relevant legislation.

Liquid waste

In most cases, the disposal of radioactive excreta from patients is best dealt with by discharging to the sewage system. In this way, the hazard to staff involved in collection and disposal is avoided. This is permitted where there is an adequate inactive effluent flow from the hospital to dilute the waste to a low concentration level, and when the toilets reserved for radioactive waste are connected directly to the main drainage system. Similar conditions must also be applied to the disposal of radioactive liquid waste from the laboratories. The waste pipes between the ward/laboratory and the main sewer should be labelled as potentially radioactive.

Some storage facilities are, however, always required for samples, sometimes excreta, needed for assay or for highly concentrated residues of radioactive stock solutions. Such storage facilities must be adequately shielded, designed to prevent risk of escape of material and labelled.

Solid waste

Solid waste from the nuclear medicine department, such as used swabs and syringes, is usually of low activity and may be collected separately in a special container. If the contaminating radionuclide is one with a short half-life, such as technetium-99m, this material can be stored for a few days until the isotope activity has decayed away. Dustbin disposal level waste is limited to 400 kBq in 0.1 m^3 of waste material with no single item containing more than 40 kBq of isotope activity. Larger concentrations of activity in solid waste or long-lived radionuclides will require special arrangements for disposal through authorised routes, but once again strict activity limits are imposed.

Detailed records must be kept of all disposals of radioactive materials irrespective of which route has been used. These records should include the type of radionuclide, its activity at disposal, the route of disposal and the date of disposal.

ARSAC requirements

It is a legal requirement that all administrations of radiopharmaceuticals are carried out under the direction of a medical practitioner who holds an appropriate certificate from the Administration of Radioactive Substances Advisory Committee (ARSAC 1998). The authorisation certificate details the radionuclide; its chemical form; the purpose for which authorisation is allowed; the route of administration; the maximum isotope activity; and the institution where the procedure can be undertaken.

Special conditions

Pregnancy

The greatest care must be exercised when carrying out diagnostic procedures on women of child-bearing age as there is increased risk to the unborn child of mental retardation and carcinogenesis. If the woman is or may be pregnant, then the clinician requesting the investigation must balance the risks against the benefits, and the minimum activity possible must be administered, commensurate with obtaining a diagnostic result. Pregnancy testing should precede therapeutic procedures. Notices must be displayed inviting patients who may be or are pregnant to inform a member of staff.

Lactating mothers

For an appropriate time period following any administration of a radionuclide non-essential close contact with infants should be discouraged. This is generally no longer than 24 hours for a diagnostic procedure. If a radionuclide is administered to a lactating mother then radioactivity may be secreted in the mother's milk and the breast-fed infant will receive a radiation dose from ingested radioactivity. In addition a child may be exposed to external radiation from retained activity within the mother. The magnitude of this problem depends upon the radiopharmaceutical administered, but may require an interruption to, or even cessation of, breast-feeding.

Children

There is an increased risk of carcinogenesis in children and the amounts of radioactivity administered should always be reduced compared to the normal adult dosage. The administered dose is normally reduced in proportion to the child's body weight or body surface area relative to that of the average adult.

PART 2

Radiotherapy and oncology

PART CONTENTS

CHAPTER CONTENTS

16

Cancer: epidemiology, prevention, early diagnosis and education

Ian Kunkler

THE CANCER PROBLEM

Globally, cancer is a growing problem. From 2000–2025 a significant rise in the number of cases is anticipated worldwide. At present, from a world population of 6 billion about 10 million cases are diagnosed annually with 6 million deaths. However, 50% will occur in developing countries, which have 5% of the resources to treat it. This figure will rise to 20 million by 2020 from a world population of 12 billion, with 12 million deaths. Of these 20 million cases, 70% will occur in developing countries.

Cancer is a major cause of death in industrialised societies where life expectancy encompasses the maximum incidence of cancer in middle and old age.

Cancer in the USA

Cancer, after heart disease, is the second leading cause of death. It is projected that at current rates two men and one woman in three will develop cancer during their lifetime. Two out of every three families are affected. New diagnoses were projected to be over 1.2 million in 2000 with over 555 000 deaths. More than half of the new cancers and deaths in the USA are accounted for by cancers of the lung, breast, colon and rectum. Cancer is likely to be a major health care burden among older people. By 2000 more than 60% of new cancers and 70% of new cancer deaths are anticipated to occur after the age of 65.

Cancer in Europe

With closer ties in the provision of health care within the European Community (EC) and with Eastern Europe, a European perspective is needed on the size of the cancer problem. The planning of the provision of cancer prevention and treatment within Europe will need to take account of the different current and future trends in cancer mortality. Within the combined population of 322 million in the EC, there are about three-quarters of a million deaths from cancer each year. The incidence of malignancy within the EC is rising. It is estimated for example in Sweden that the prevalence of a wide range of malignancies is likely to increase in number by 2010, particularly breast, rectal and prostate cancer.

In Northern and Western Europe the commonest malignancies in males in rank order are lung, colorectal, prostate, bladder and oral, and in females breast, colorectal, stomach, endometrium and cervix. These top five malignancies represent 60% of cancers for each sex.

Variations in cancer mortality in Europe

Within Europe there are striking differences in cancer mortality. These differences have been highlighted by the EUROCARE studies drawn from 47 cancer registries from 17 European countries. For the EUROCARE2 study, survival data for the period 1978–1989 was accumulated from about 1 300 000 patients diagnosed for 45 cancer sites or aggregations of cancer sites. For example, the mortality from oesophageal cancer is much higher in Northern and Western France than across the border in Belgium. The reasons for this are not clear. Differences in the consumption of alcohol and tobacco are probably important. Less explicable is the higher incidence of oesophageal cancer in Irish and Scottish women or of stomach cancer in Bavaria compared with neighbouring parts of Germany. For the commoner cancers (lung, breast, bowel, colorectal and prostate) the UK has poorer survival figures than many of the countries in continental Europe (Fig. 16.1) and closer to Poland, Estonia and Slovakia, which are much less prosperous. Much higher survival is achieved in France, Germany and Sweden. The reasons for these differences are not clear and are probably multifactorial. For some cancers such as breast cancer the reason may be more advanced stage at diagnosis. In addition there may be shortcomings in the infrastructure and coordination of cancer services, resulting in patients not receiving an optimal standard of care. A national cancer plan has been developed in England, and equivalents are under development in the other home countries to improve the cancer survival by 2010 to match the best in Europe. It is calculated that if Britain could reach the standard of the best survival rates in Europe, over 25 000 lives could be saved per year and, if it reached the European average, approximately 10 000 lives could be saved.

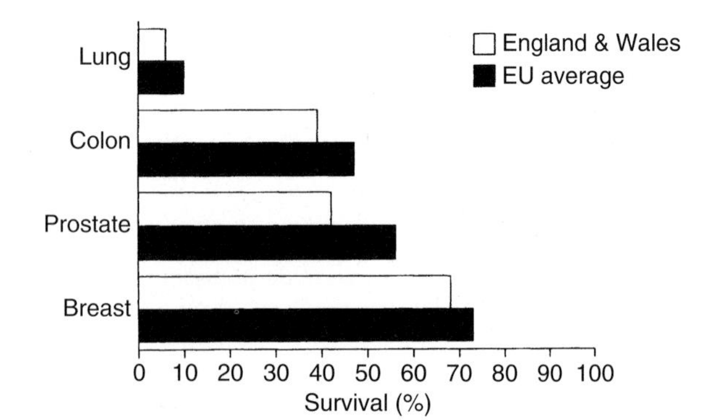

Fig. 16.1 Cancer survival in the early 1990s: England and Wales compared to European average. Data may not be precisely comparable because cancer registration is variable across Europe and relative survival is not age standardised, i.e. does not take account of non-cancer-related but age-related causes of mortality. Percentage surviving 5 years after diagnosis: England and Wales data for cases diagnosed 1986–1990; EU average for 1985–1989. (Source: Cancer Survival Trends, Office for National Statistics, 1999. Reproduced with permission from the Department of Health.)

Future trends in cancer mortality in Europe

When rise in population, increasing age and projected changes in risk are taken into account, increases in common cancers such as lung, large bowel, prostate and breast cancer are predicted in Northern Europe (including Great Britain). Stomach cancer is one of the few cancers likely to fall in incidence.

Cancer in the UK

In the UK 1 in 5 deaths is due to cancer and, after heart disease, it is the commonest cause of death. In England and Wales it accounts for 25% of all deaths. Each year in England 200 000 people are diagnosed with cancer and about 120 000 people will die from the disease. The incidence and mortality of common cancers in men and women in England and Wales are shown in Figure 16.2. Lung and skin cancer are the most common. However, whereas skin cancer carries very little mortality, the opposite is true of lung cancer, which accounts for nearly 40% of male deaths from cancer.

In Scotland similar rises in cancer incidence are anticipated as in the rest of the UK. In 1960 there were 13 600 new cases of cancer diagnosed in Scotland. By 1989 this had nearly doubled to 25 808. This increase was in part due to the aging of the population. In the three decades from 1960 the number of citizens aged 75 years or older had increased

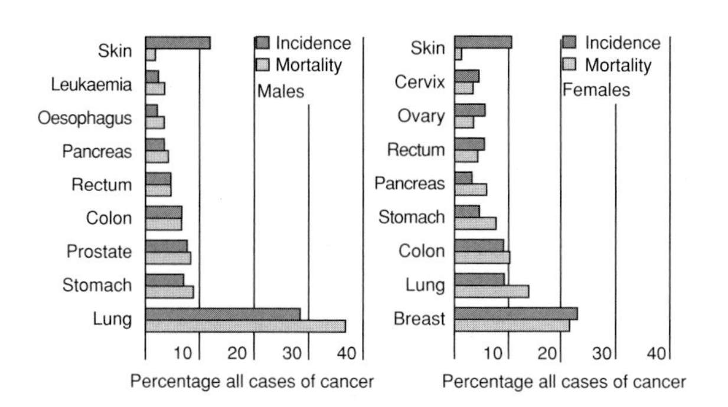

Fig. 16.2 Incidence and mortality of common cancers in England and Wales. (Reproduced with permission from Souhami R L & Moxham J 1990 Textbook of Medicine, Churchill Livingstone, Edinburgh.)

by 71%. The incidence of lung cancer rose from 1960 to 1979 and then declined. Over the same period there was a fourfold rise in female lung cancer. For female breast cancer, incidence rose by about 50%. However, as in the rest of the UK, the death rate from breast cancer has fallen by 30% since 1990. A similar decline in the USA has also been seen and a similar trend is emerging in other European countries. Rates of prostate cancer have nearly doubled, with the highest proportion in older men, among whom there was a threefold rise in the annual number of newly diagnosed cases.

Impact of cancer burden on medical workload

In the UK a consultant in clinical oncology in 1991 would be referred on average 560 patients per year. That represents 12 new patients per week. These are much higher figures than in many other European countries in Europe where, for example, each consultant in Norway would see 75 patients per year, 100 in Belgium and 200 in France, Spain and Portugal. On average there is one clinical oncologist per 224 000 population. Each UK consultant, if one includes patients on follow-up, will have about 2000 patients under his or her care at any one time. It is estimated that 40% of all patients with cancer will require some form of radiotherapy at some stage of the management of their disease. Approximately 110 000 new patients will need radiotherapy every year in England and Wales. To implement the Calman/Hine report on cancer services in the UK, eight non-surgical oncologists (clinical and medical oncologists) will be needed per 1 000 000 population, taking account of an anticipated 4% per annum increase in workload. Even so this is less than half of the number of cancer specialists in other comparable European countries.

EPIDEMIOLOGY OF CANCER

Terminology

Epidemiology is the study of the occurrence and distribution of disease. It can be divided into three main groups: descriptive, analytical and experimental:

- *Descriptive epidemiology* is concerned with the retrospective analysis of the relationship between a disease and suspected aetiological factors.
- *Analytical epidemiology* is the study of the relationship between different risk factors (e.g. age, sex, occupation) and the development of disease.
- *Experimental epidemiology* involves observing the effects of controlling relevant suspected factors (e.g. stopping cigarette smoking).

The *incidence rate* of any disease is the total number of new cases occurring over a given period of time (usually a year) among a given number of people (usually 100 000 for cancer). This is different from the *prevalence rate*, which is the number of cases of a particular disease existing at a given point in time.

The *mortality rate* is the incidence rate for the end-point of death. The *crude death rate* is the number of deaths during a given period of time (normally a year) per thousand population. Crude death rates are of limited value since they do not take account of the differing proportions of people in particular age groups between populations. The crude death rate in a particular population may exceed that of another country simply because it contains a higher proportion of elderly people. The *age-specific death rate* takes account of the effect of age distribution on death rates. It is defined as:

$$\frac{\text{Number of deaths in a specific age group}}{\text{Mean population of that age group}} \times 100$$

It provides a useful means of comparing mortality in different populations.

The *standardised mortality ratio* (SMR) is an overall measure of mortality which compares the observed number of deaths from a disease in a particular population with the expected number of deaths that would have been anticipated in a standard population if the age-specific death rates were the same.

$$\text{SMR} = \frac{\text{Observed numbers of deaths in given region}}{\text{Expected number of deaths in given region}} \times 100$$

SMRs are useful in comparing deaths from cancer in particular socioeconomic groups and occupations.

PROGNOSIS IN CANCER

We know what we mean by 'cure' of a simple fracture. We mean the uniting of the fracture and freedom from further trouble. But what do we mean by 'cure' of diabetes mellitus? We mean control of the underlying disease process but not its eradication. So in cancer we may talk of the 'cure' of, for example, a small basal cell carcinoma by surgery or radiotherapy where recurrence or persistent disease is uncommon. In other cancers such as breast cancer it is more appropriate to use the term 'control' since the tumour may recur locally or at distant sites after many years of freedom from the disease.

Indices of success

Survival rates

In measuring the success of treatment for cancer, a conventional yardstick is the proportion of patients who survive for a certain number of years—usually five. *Five-year survival* is sometimes interpreted as 'cure'. While this is true of many squamous carcinomas of the head and neck, it is not true of breast cancer, as seen above. For breast cancer, 10-, 20- or even 30-year survival figures (Fig. 26.24) are more appropriate end-points because of the long-term pattern of relapse and death from the disease.

Survival may be with or without evidence of cancer. For this reason the terms *disease-free survival* or *recurrence-free survival* are commonly used to define the outcome of treatment. These results require an elaborate system of clinic follow-up. Yet it is only from painstaking analysis of this kind that we can derive a sound knowledge of both the natural history of cancer and the effects of treatment. Survival data are commonly presented plotted graphically as curves (Fig. 26.24) which allow the comparison of different treatments for different stages of disease over time.

Crude survival. In studies of patients treated for cancer, a variety of ways are used for analysing their survival. *Crude survival rate* refers to the number of patients alive a given number of years (n) after treatment. This is not valid unless all the patients included have been followed up for at least n years.

Actuarial survival. If a proportion of patients have been followed up for a shorter time than n years, the *actuarial method* (also known as log rank) is commonly used. The actuarial method assumes that all patients are subject to the same probability of dying from a particular cancer whether or not they have been withdrawn or lost from a study. It also assumes that for patients entering a study over a given period of time the probability of survival is constant. This method is used for calculating survival rates for deaths from cancer alone. Patients who die from causes other than cancer (i.e. from intercurrent disease) are considered to have been withdrawn from the study during the interval in which their death has occurred.

Age-corrected survival. Crude or actuarial survival rates do not take account of the mortality from natural causes of the patients studied. As a result the efficacy of treatment can be substantially underestimated. The crude survival rate can be corrected for age (*age-corrected survival rate*). The age-corrected n-year survival rate is:

$$\frac{\text{Crude } n\text{-year survival rate}}{\text{Expected } n\text{-year survival rate in a normal population of the same sex and age composition}}$$

The age-corrected survival rate enables direct comparisons between cohorts of patients of different ages and sex. It is the mortality specific to that particular disease. If a group treated for the same cancer has the same death rate from all causes as that of the normal population of the same sex and age, that group of patients can be considered cured. When the survival of the normal and treated groups are plotted semilogarithmically, the point at which the two curves begin to run in parallel is the time at which the survivors can be considered cured. In breast cancer the mortality of the disease continues to exceed that of the normal population even up to 30 years after treatment (Fig. 26.24). The curves never cross and patients can rarely be considered cured because of the long-term risk of relapse.

Outcome of palliative care

Survival figures are essential for estimating the success of treatment aimed at cure but are of limited value in assessing the effects of palliative treatment. The main aim of palliative treatment is the relief of distressing symptoms (p. 313). Palliative radiotherapy or chemotherapy may sometimes restrain tumour growth sufficiently to prolong the patient's life for a few months or sometimes years. However, as a goal, survival is subordinate to symptomatic relief.

EPIDEMIOLOGY AND THE PREVENTION OF CANCER

The principal role of epidemiological studies in oncology has been in the prevention of cancer. Such studies have played a major role in establishing occupational hazards in several industries (e.g. bladder cancer in aniline dye workers) and the link between lung cancer and smoking.

Epidemiology can assist in the prevention of cancer in a number of ways. First, it can show differences in the incidence of cancer in different populations and correlate them with differences in the prevalence of a potential causal factor. Secondly, it can test a hypothesis about the relationship between the occurrence of the disease to an aspect of the affected individual's constitution or exposure to some environmental factor. Thirdly, it can test the validity of a causal relationship by seeing whether the disease can be prevented or its incidence reduced by changing the prevalence of the suspected agent. A good example of the latter is the reduction in lung cancer observed among doctors since they gave up smoking cigarettes.

This analytical approach in the field of cancer has a long history. Percival Pott in 1775 was the first to describe an occupational cancer. He established the relationship between cancer of the scrotum and exposure to soot in chimney sweeps. Of wider significance has been the link established between cigarette smoking and lung cancer by Doll and Hill in 1964 in a survey of over 40 000 British doctors. Research of this type is important since it has opened the way to the prevention of certain malignant disease by encouraging the population to avoid carcinogenic risk factors such as smoking and alcohol.

Latent period

One of the factors that make the establishment of causal relationships between risk factors and particular cancers difficult is the long 'latent period' between exposure to the carcinogenic agent and the clinical appearance of the disease. For example, following the explosion of atomic bombs on Hiroshima and Nagasaki in 1945, solid tumours were not apparent until 15–20 years later in survivors. In most cases it is chronic rather than acute exposure to carcinogens that gives rise to cancer.

The latent period before cancer is clinically apparent will vary with the type of carcinogen, intensity and duration of exposure and age at the onset of exposure. Exposure to relatively small quantities of blue asbestos on a very limited number of occasions may induce pleural cancer several decades later. The risk of developing lung cancer is three times higher at the age of 60 for those who begin smoking cigarettes at about the age of 15 compared with those who start smoking 10 years later. It has been estimated that for lung cancer and skin cancer the risk of developing cancer roughly varies in proportion to the fourth power of the duration of exposure. For example, the carcinogenic effect after 40 years of exposure is 10–20 times that after 20 years of exposure. It may be that this biological principle holds true for many other tumours.

Sex, age and race in the distribution of cancer

Each tumour tends to have a typical sex distribution and age range. In some tumours these characteristics hold good anywhere in the world, e.g. for retinoblastoma. The sex distribution of retinoblastoma is roughly evenly balanced, with a peak incidence between 1 and 2 years of age.

In other tumours the age and sex distributions may vary. Bladder cancer in the UK is three times commoner in men than women and occurs in the sixth and seventh decades, with a peak incidence at the age of 65. However, the disease may occur earlier in men in their forties and fifties if they have been occupationally exposed to aniline dyes in the rubber industry. There is wide racial variation in incidence: bladder cancer is twice as common in Caucasians as it is in Blacks. In other tumours the age range is more rigid, irrespective of country and race. Cancer is mainly a disease of the middle-aged and elderly. Skin, lung, colorectal and bladder cancer are typical examples. The rate of increase in incidence with age is non-linear and accelerates at and beyond middle age. Occasionally the disease may have more than one peak. Hodgkin's disease has two age peaks. The first is at about 25 years and the second in the sixth decade (Fig. 16.3). These different age peaks suggest that different aetiological factors

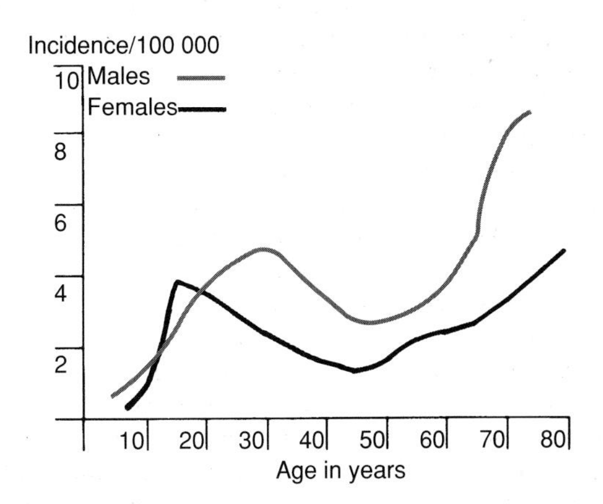

Fig. 16.3 Age-specific incidence of Hodgkin's disease (England, 1984). (Reproduced with permission from Souhami R L & Moxham J 1990 Textbook of Medicine, Churchill Livingstone, Edinburgh.)

may be at work, with different latent periods between exposure and tumour development.

Changing incidence and mortality over time

Both the incidence and mortality of the disease may vary between males and females and change over time.

The male : female ratio for lung cancer increased from 2.0 : 1 after the First World War to 6.7 : 1 in 1959. By 1983 it had fallen to 2.8 : 1. Pipe smoking, virtually a male preserve, was a principal factor in the explanation of the increase in males from 1900 to 1925. In addition, lung cancer was commoner in non-smoking males. Recently there has been a small decrease in the male mortality from lung cancer but in females it continues to rise. The latter is thought to reflect the rise in the number of women who began smoking in the Second World War. The fall in male mortality has no obvious explanation since the number of cigarettes smoked over this period has remained relatively stable.

Sex ratios for some tumours may vary markedly between countries and also influence outcome of treatment. For example the male to female ratio of carcinoma of the oesophagus may vary from nearly 1 : 1 to 20 : 1. The prognosis is slightly more favourable in females.

Variation between populations

Differences in incidence of the same tumour between different countries certainly occur, although some may be explained by variation in case registration and medical practice. The incidence and death rates from breast cancer in the Far East are a tenth of those in the West.

Influence of migration

There is good evidence that the incidence of cancer among migrants often differs from the population that they left. Black migrants from Africa to the USA have rates of cancer more similar to white Americans than to the black population in Africa. Similarly, Japanese migrants to Hawaii have rates of colorectal cancer more comparable with those of Caucasian Hawaiians than of the Japanese in Japan. This suggests that environmental factors in the country to which these groups have migrated play a part in the development of malignant disease.

Variation in incidence of cancer over time

While differences in incidence over time may reflect variation in standards of diagnosis, true changes have occurred. The incidence of cancer of the tongue has substantially declined in the UK. The reasons for this are unclear. It probably relates in part to improved oral hygiene. Gastric cancer has also declined in Western Europe in the six decades from 1930 to 1990 and continues to decline.

Table 16.1 Proportion of cancer deaths attributable to different environmental factors (reproduced with permission from Doll R, Peto R 1987 in Weatherall et al, Oxford Textbook of Medicine, 2nd edn, Oxford University Press)

Factor or class of factors	Best estimate of proportion (%)
Ionising radiation	
Background	1
Medical procedures	0.5
Industry	< 0.1
Ultraviolet radiation	0.5
Occupation	4
Industrial products	< 1
Pollution	
Atmospheric	1
Water	< 1
Medical drugs	< 1
Diet	30
Food additives	< 1
Tobacco	30
Alcohol	3
Reproductive and sexual behaviour	7
Infection	(10)
Others and unknown	?

REDUCING THE RISKS OF DEVELOPING CANCER

Based largely on our current knowledge of the aetiology of cancer, it has been estimated that 80% of malignancies are preventable. To put the environmental causes of cancer in perspective their relative proportions have been summarised in Table 16.1. The striking feature is the high proportion due to dietary factors and to smoking (30% each). Smoking is discussed in more detail in Chapter 25. Changing dietary habits could potentially reduce the risk of cancer, possibly by a third. The main cancers involved are those of the stomach, colon and rectum, and breast.

European code on the prevention of cancer

The EC has produced a 10-point code (Fig. 16.4) for the general public, summarising the ways in which certain common cancers can be prevented.

Reducing tobacco smoking

The UK Government has made health warnings mandatory on commercial tobacco products and on advertisements for tobacco. To achieve substantial reductions in tobacco consumption, additional measures would be required. These could include banning advertising of tobacco, its consumption in public places and working environments, increasing taxation on tobacco, reducing tar content in cigarettes and setting up clinics for smokers to help them break the habit.

Alcohol

After smoking, alcohol is the second most important cause of cancer. It may be responsible in some countries for up to 10% of deaths from cancer. Cancers of the mouth, larynx, pharynx, oesophagus and liver are certainly caused in part by alcohol. It probably has a role in the aetiology of some breast and rectal cancers. For several tumours the risk rises with the quantity consumed to more than tenfold for lifelong non-drinkers.

Alcohol and tobacco smoking act as synergistic carcinogens (i.e. the combined effect is greater than that of either alone). This combination accounts for the very high incidence of these tumours in France, where they are often multifocal. Alcohol probably acts as a co-carcinogen rather than a carcinogen (i.e. it promotes rather than initiates carcinogenesis). Spirits may have a slightly stronger carcinogenic effect than other alcoholic beverages.

Any policy on moderating the consumption of alcohol has to take account of a number of facts. First, many people find it pleasurable. Secondly, moderate amounts (2–3 units per day) protect against coronary thrombosis, though heavy drinking has other undesirable social consequences (e.g. violent behaviour and road accidents). Thirdly, its carcinogenic effects are largely in conjunction with smoking tobacco. Thus the risk of cancer induction by alcohol in non-smokers is relatively small.

Ultraviolet light

Exposure to ultraviolet light has been increasing with the reduction of the ozone layer, caused by chemical pollution. An increase in the incidence of all forms of skin cancer can be expected. The principal culprits are the *chlorofluorohydrocarbons* (CFCs). These are components in, for example, aerosol sprays, refrigerants, and solvents for cleaning electronic equipment. However, to put the contribution of commercial sources of CFCs into context, one volcano in Antarctica emits 100 tons (100×10^3 kg) of chlorine every month, substantially more than the combined output of CFCs from deodorants over the same period. Nitrogen oxides from vehicle exhaust fumes also deplete the ozone layer. International agreements have been reached, aimed at eliminating the use of CFCs.

Occupational exposure

A wide variety of occupations are known to carry the risk of exposure to carcinogens. However, they only represent a relatively small number of cases of cancer deaths (4% in the USA). In 1987, 246 agents were classified by the International Agency for Research on Cancer as definitely (50), probably (37) or possibly (159) carcinogenic to humans. These included industrial processes, industrial chemicals, pesticides, laboratory chemicals, drugs, food ingredients, tobacco smoking and related stimulants. Drugs and industrial chemicals represent the largest risks. There are many other occupations where an agent is thought to be carcinogenic to workers but a causal link has not been established. Some of the known occupational hazards are listed in Table 16.2. Of these, exposure to asbestos dust, aromatic amines and the products of burning fossil fuels are the commonest.

Measures to prevent occupational exposure include labelling of products as carcinogenic, and prohibiting the marketing and use of certain substances, e.g. the four aromatic amines (naphthylamine, 4-aminobiphenyl, 4-nitrodiphenyl and benzidine) and blue asbestos (crocidolite).

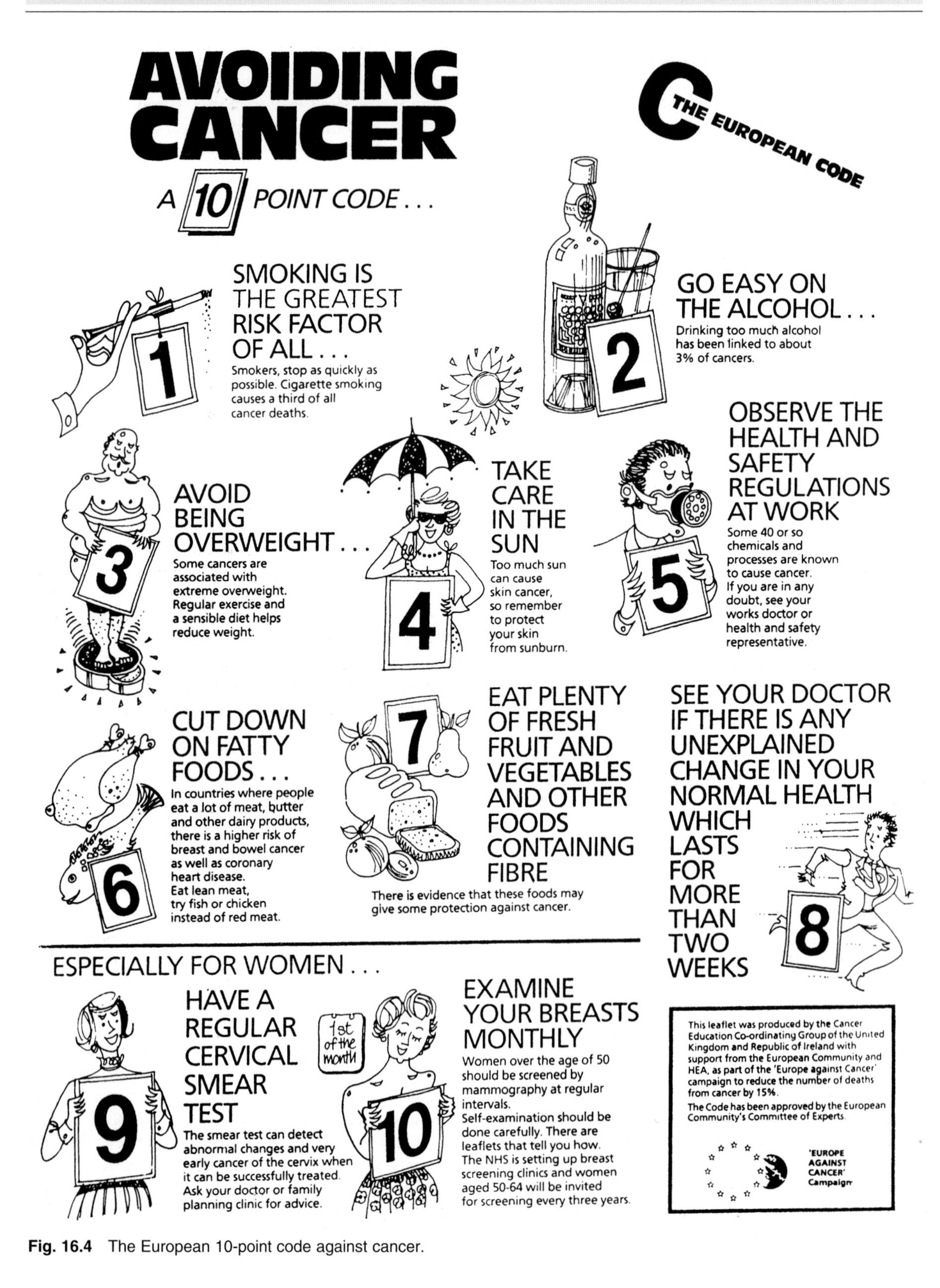

Fig. 16.4 The European 10-point code against cancer.

Table 16.2 Occupational cancers (Modified from Doll R, Peto R 1987 in Weatherall et al, Oxford Textbook of Medicine, 2nd edn, Oxford University Press)

Occupation	Site of tumour	Agent
Dye manufacturers; rubber workers	Bladder	Aromatic amines
Copper and cobalt smelters; pesticide manufacture	Skin, lung	Arsenic
Manufacture of chromates from chrome ore	Lung	Chromium
Asbestos miners; asbestos textile manufacturers; insulation and shipyard workers	Lung, pleura, peritoneum, larynx	Asbestos
Workers with glues and varnishes	Marrow, e.g. erythroleukaemia	Benzene
Uranium and other miners; luminisers; radiologists; radiographers	Lung, bone, bone marrow	Ionising radiation
Nickel refiners	Nasal sinuses, lung	Nickel
Hardwood furniture manufacturers	Nasal sinuses	Agent unknown
Leather workers	Nasal sinuses	Agent unknown
Coal gas manufacturers; asphalters; roofers; aluminium refiners; workers exposed to tars and oils	Skin, scrotum, lung	Polycyclic hydrocarbons (soot, tar and oil)
Seamen; farmers	Skin	Ultraviolet light
PVC manufacturers	Liver (angiosarcoma)	Vinyl chloride

It is thought that preventive methods are likely to have little impact on the mortality from occupational cancers in the near future. The detection of tumours at an early stage by screening is likely to have a greater effect on mortality. Screening of urine by cytology among workers in the dyestuff and rubber industries has long been practised.

Diet

Diet influences carcinogenesis in a variety of ways: carcinogens may be eaten; food substances may be converted to carcinogens once ingested; and dietary components may modify the ways in which the body metabolises and responds to carcinogens.

The only component of food that has been found to be strongly linked to the development of cancer is *aflatoxin*. This is a product of the fungus *Aspergillus fumigatus*, which often contaminates damp cereals in tropical countries. It causes primary liver cancer (see Ch. 25), although the data are unclear since there is a high incidence of hepatitis B, itself associated with liver tumours, in the same group of patients.

Bracken fern containing nitrates is suspected of causing oesophageal cancer, particularly among the Japanese. Salted fish is implicated in the aetiology of nasopharyngeal cancer (p. 362), possibly as a co-carcinogen with the Epstein–Barr virus.

Diet may be indirectly related to carcinogenesis. One example is fibre, which seems to have a protective effect against colorectal cancer (p. 409). A second is obesity, which is associated with an increased incidence of cancer of the endometrium and of the gallbladder in women. Consumption of saturated fat is implicated but not proven as a cause of breast cancer. A third is vitamin A (retinol) and its derivatives, retinoids, which may inhibit the full malignant transformation of cells and prevent tumour formation.

Dietary measures likely to reduce the risk of cancers are:

- High-fibre diet
- Reducing saturated fats
- Plenty of fresh fruit and vegetables (owing to the presence of antioxidants such as vitamin E).

Ionising radiation

The whole spectrum of sources of ionising radiations, both natural and man-made, has been calculated to contribute 1.5% of all fatal cancers. The sources of radiation exposure in the UK are shown in Figure 16.5.

It is estimated that exposure to radon gas from domestic buildings may be responsible for 1% of lung cancer in Europe. Concentrations of radon gas in excess of 400 Bq/m^3 (about 1 in 1000 homes) will expose the occupants to 20 mSv per year. The lifetime risk of fatal cancer from this exposure is about 10%. The carcinogenic risks of ionising radiation have been revised upwards since 1988. Current estimates of risk are two to five times higher. However, it is unclear

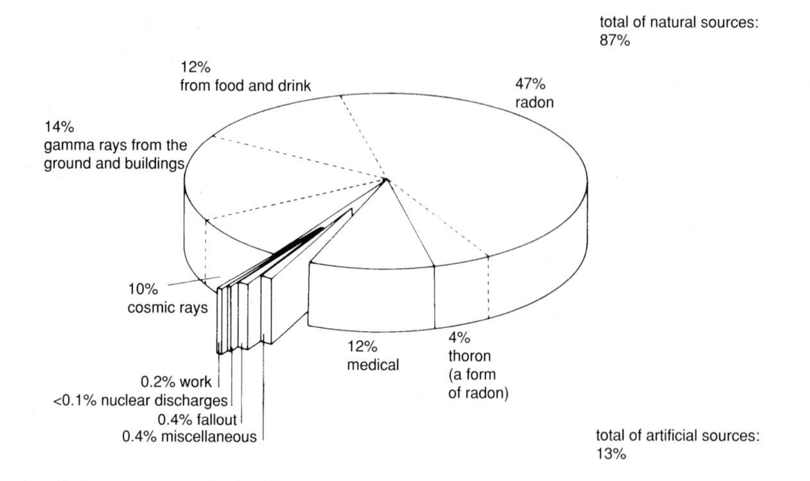

Fig. 16.5 Sources of radiation exposure in the UK population, 1988, based on data supplied by the National Radiological Protection Board. (Reproduced with permission from Reducing the Risks of Cancers, Open University, 1989.)

whether these revised estimates apply to very low levels of exposure to natural background radioactivity.

The role of ionising radiation in the causation of cancer is mainly derived from occupational exposure. Early evidence came from the development of lung cancer amongst miners at Joachimstal in Czechoslovakia and Schneeberg in Germany. Lung disease had been known to occur amongst these workers since the 16th century. It was subsequently appreciated that the disease was lung cancer due to radioactive radon gas in the mines.

The main source of evidence of the effects of ionising radiation in man are the survivors of the atomic bombs dropped on Hiroshima and Nagasaki in 1945. The incidence of acute and chronic leukaemia was significantly raised within a radius of 1.5 km from the epicentre. The highest incidence occurred 6–8 years afterwards. For cancers other than leukaemia the latent period was longer (15–20 years) among victims who received 1 Gy or more; indeed the incidence is still higher 50 years later.

It is assumed that there is no threshold below which cancers cannot be induced by ionising radiation. Indeed children who received only 0.01–0.02 Gy in utero when their mothers were irradiated had an additional 1 in 2000 risk of cancer. At low doses the risk of developing cancer is probably proportional to dose, although much uncertainty remains.

Reducing the levels of radon gas from domestic buildings requires a number of measures. First, systematic surveys are needed to identify buildings which pose a hazard. Levels of radon gas can be reduced by alterations to the floors and installation of extractor fans.

Pollution

Atmospheric. Atmospheric pollution has been suspected to be carcinogenic, ever since the incidence of lung cancer was found to be higher in cities than in the country. The combustion products of coal are known to contain carcinogenic hydrocarbons. However, since the atmosphere is polluted by a wide variety of substances, often in small quantities, the assessment of carcinogenic risk is very difficult. The situation is further complicated by the contribution to atmospheric pollution of tobacco smoking. In the past, pollution probably accounted for about 1% of cancers. Atmospheric pollution in the UK is now falling with stricter rules on the burning of fossil fuels. The evidence suggests that the current burning of fossil fuels, arsenic and asbestos will contribute to much less than 1% of future cancers.

Water. Ingestion of trihalomethanes from chlorinated drinking water may increase the risk of bladder cancer. Reduction of levels of these chemicals in drinking water is desirable.

Chemoprevention

The oral cavity, lung and colon have been the commonest primary sites subject to attempts at chemoprevention. Beta-carotene, synthetic retinoids, calcium and a variety of vitamins reduce the risk of developing oral cancer. A trial of alpha-tocopherol and beta-carotene showed no protective effect against the development of lung cancer.

Among patients in China at high risk of oesophageal or stomach cancer, treatment with vitamin and mineral supplements reduced the incidence and mortality of these tumours. These populations have a 20% incidence of oesophageal dysplasia.

Trials of adjuvant tamoxifen have showed a reduction in the risk of contralateral breast cancer. Trials are ongoing to determine whether tamoxifen can prevent the disease among women at high risk on the basis of their strong family history of the disease.

Antioxidants, e.g. vitamins A and E, are thought to act by reducing DNA damage early in the process of carcinogenesis. It seems most likely that chemoprevention with such agents should occur early in life if they proved to be effective.

The cost-effectiveness of chemoprevention needs to be carefully considered. Preventive treatment may have to be continued for several decades, which may prove very expensive when compared to the numbers of lives saved.

EARLY DETECTION AND CANCER SCREENING

Early diagnosis of some cancers gives the best chance of cure. Sadly, symptoms of many tumours do not develop until the tumours are advanced and the prospect of cure limited (e.g. ovarian and small cell lung cancer). Some patients may conceal advanced tumours, typically of the breast, through fear of confirmation of the diagnosis or through ignorance. Here, however, we are concerned with presymptomatic diagnosis. Although we use the term 'early', it must be remembered that when a cancer is detectable, it is often 'late' in its natural history and may already have seeded distant metastases (e.g. breast cancer). 'Early' is therefore a relative concept applied clinically. An early breast cancer that is only just palpable (or perhaps detected by mammography and not yet palpable) is a very different problem from an advanced tumour invading the chest wall.

Presymptomatic diagnosis

Presymptomatic diagnosis clearly involves a positive search for people who would not otherwise have consulted their doctors or feel the need to submit to any examination or test. *Screening* is the process by which a systematic search is made for particular tumours among individuals who have not sought medical attention because of symptoms. It involves submitting a large population (mass screening) to the same screening test, e.g. in the UK submitting all women between 50 and 69 years to mammography to detect breast cancer.

The evidence for the effectiveness of screening may be interpreted differently in different countries. For example the American Cancer Society recommends screening for prostate cancer by digital rectal examination and serum prostate-specific antigen (PSA) in all men over the age of 50. Its recommendations are accepted by many western countries, but not yet by the UK.

Criteria for screening

A number of criteria must be satisfied to carry out mass screening for a particular tumour:

- Treatment must have a good prospect of reducing the mortality of the disease detected at a early stage.
- The disease must be sufficiently common for a reasonable number of cases to be detected.
- The method of screening must have a high probability of detecting the disease when present (true positive) and a low probability of a positive result when the disease is absent (false positive).
- The screening method must be acceptable to patients, affordable, and practical to apply and interpret in trained hands.

Advantages of screening

1. Reduction in mortality. The main advantage of screening is that it can reduce the mortality from certain cancers (for example in women with breast cancer over the age of 50). Account has to be taken of changing natural histories of some cancers. For example the mortality of breast cancer reached a peak in 1989 and has fallen annually since then. These changes may be independent of the effects of screening. While it has been shown that breast screening does reduce mortality, this has yet to be established for prostate cancer, particularly for men with mild elevations of prostate-specific antigen (PSA).

2. Reduced number of patients requiring radical treatment. The detection of premalignant changes and their eradication by simple measures (e.g. colposcopic laser therapy for severe cervical dysplasia) reduces the need for radical radiotherapy or surgery.

3. Reassurance of patients whose screening test is negative.

Disadvantages of screening

1. Overdiagnosis of non-progressive lesions. Screening may detect different degrees of cellular abnormality (e.g. in cervical smears). These may range from mild dysplasia to carcinoma-in-situ. For some tumours there

may be an orderly progression through these histological changes on the path to invasive malignancy. However, more patients are detected with early changes than would be expected to progress to frank malignancy. Thus not all patients with dysplastic cervical smears will progress to malignancy. Screening is not therefore of benefit to all women with abnormal cervical smears.

2. Psychological and physical morbidity. Anxiety is commonly generated among patients about the technique of screening and its results. This is increased if the patient has to be recalled for further investigations, even if these eventually prove negative. Screening may be uncomfortable. Good mammography requires the breast to be compressed. Similarly laser therapy for a severely dysplastic cervix may be very painful without adequate analgesia.

3. False reassurance. If the screening test is negative, a tumour may still be present. The patient may feel reassured and perhaps ignore the symptoms of the tumour in the belief that she is free of disease. This may occur in early breast cancer where the mammogram is negative or in cervical cancer if the cervical smear has been incorrectly performed.

4. Cost. In general, screening programmes are expensive because very large population have to screened. In countries with limited resources, the priority may be to concentrate on funding the delivery of standard diagnostic and treatment procedures.

Measuring the effectiveness of screening

Before mass screening is introduced, a significant reduction in the mortality from the disease needs to be demonstrated on a large population of patients. This is by far the most important measure of the efficacy of screening. The best design is a randomised prospective trial in which a defined population is assigned randomly to screening or to an unscreened control group. All the deaths due to the particular tumour are recorded among each group over a period of years. Long-term follow-up of such patients is necessary since the transition from premalignant to malignant changes may be in excess of 10 years.

The shorter-term effects of screening can be measured in three ways.

1. The number of cancers detected. In general, the number of cancers detected by screening should exceed the expected annual incidence. This is because screening has detected, and treatment prevented, some cases progressing to invasive cancer. For example, the annual expected incidence of breast cancer in women between 50 and 64 years is 1.6 per 1000. The equivalent figure from the screened population is 5. On subsequent screening the incidence of tumours in the screened population should fall to about the same as the annual expected incidence.

Sensitivity. Ideally the screening test would be 100% sensitive to the presence of a cancer. Unfortunately this is rarely the case. The most reliable way of assessing the sensitivity of a test is measure the number of cancers detected among the screened population between each screening (so called *interval* cancers).

Specificity. The specificity of a screening test is defined as a proportion of negative tests among individuals who do not have cancer. If the test is completely specific, there should be no false negatives or false positives.

2. Earlier stage of disease detected. If screening is effective the proportion of early tumours detected should exceed the expected proportion in an unscreened population. For example, the proportion of early cases of colorectal cancer (Dukes' A) found by screening for faecal occult blood is 50%, compared with 10% in an unscreened population.

3. Comparison of survival of screening detected and unscreened cases—sources of bias. Better survival of patients whose tumours were detected by screening compared with those who were not does not necessarily confirm the benefit of screening. There are two reasons for this. First, the survival of screened cases is measured from the time of diagnosis. This point may be substantially earlier than the time at which symptomatic presentation would have occurred. The time of death may be exactly the same but the survival of the screened cases will be longer. This is known as *'lead-time bias'*.

Secondly, the screened cases are likely to contain a higher proportion of slowly growing tumours. Faster growing tumours are more likely to have presented symptomatically before they are screened. Screened tumours are likely to be slower growing with longer survival.

An additional source of bias is the fact that participation in cancer screening is more likely among the better educated who are more conscious of their health. The difficulty is to obtain the attendance of those from lower socioeconomic groups who have a lesser appreciation of preventive medicine. Women who are prostitutes and at higher risk of cervical cancer frequently default from appointments for screening. Similarly in fee-for-service health care systems there are financial inducements to doctors to include women in screening programmes.

Methods of screening

In addition to simple self-examination, the available methods include:

- Periodic medical examination
- Cytological examination
- Radiological examination
- Highly specialised techniques—radioactive isotopes, biochemical and hormonal estimations, faecal occult blood, endoscopy.

Periodic medical examination

This form of screening has achieved limited popularity, applied either to selected groups such as business executives or offered commercially to those able to afford it. In addition to routine clinical examination, it includes a variety of laboratory blood and urine tests and a chest radiograph. Barium meal or sigmoidoscopy are occasionally carried out. It is unavoidably costly and unsuited to mass screening.

Cytological methods

Cytological methods differ from histological ones. The latter relate to cells organised in tissues, the former to cells isolated singly or in tiny clusters. Growing tumours shed (exfoliate) cells from their surface and these can be fixed and stained on a slide and examined microscopically. The expert can recognise abnormal features of cancer cells, for example of the appearance of the nucleus.

This technique of exfoliative cytology was developed by Papanicolaou in the USA. It is a simpler procedure than surgical biopsy.

Uterine cervix. Premalignant changes or early cancer can be detected by a cervical smear (p. 268). This is the most common application of cytological diagnosis.

Urinary tract (especially bladder). After centrifugation, cells deposited from the urine are examined for evidence of malignancy. This technique is useful for screening workers in dye and rubber industries who are at above average risk for bladder cancer. This method is more acceptable to the public than routine cystoscopy, though less accurate.

Lung. Malignant cells may be detected in the sputum. The need for bronchoscopy in some patients with obvious tumours on chest radiograph may thus be avoided.

Stomach. Gastric washings may yield cancer cells.

It is likely that these traditional manual cytological methods will be replaced by more sophisticated devices which reduce the number of false negative and false positive results. An example is the use of robotic devices which automatically remove blood and inflammatory cells from the cervical cytology sample (see p. 268).

Radiological examination

- Mammography is able to screen for early breast cancer before it is large enough for either the patient or her doctor to feel.
- Chest radiographs have been used to screen for lung cancer.
- Barium meal examination using the double contrast technique, often in conjunction with endoscopy, has been employed to detect gastric cancer in Japan, which has a very high incidence of the disease.

Evaluation of screening programmes

In an ideal world, screening would only be introduced once the costs and benefits had been carefully assessed. Regrettably this is not always the case. Cervical screening, for example, was implemented in the UK before the evidence of benefit was certain. It was instituted because screening was felt by the public and medical profession to be worthwhile but it has never been submitted to a randomised controlled trial.

What can be learned from experience so far? Each cancer will be considered in turn.

Lung

Several mass surveys to detect lung cancer have been carried out by chest radiography and/or sputum cytology. Although there is an increased yield in the first screen, a shift towards the diagnosis of tumours at an earlier stage, and better survival of screen-detected cases, no reduction in overall mortality has been demonstrated. The majority of screened cases were still inoperable. There is no evidence at present that screening for lung cancer is worthwhile. A much greater impact could be made by reducing the smoking of cigarettes.

Cervix

Screening for cervical cancer has been shown from a variety of retrospective studies to reduce the incidence and mortality from invasive cervical cancer. Mass screening was introduced in Europe in the early 1960s in the absence of evidence of effectiveness.

Uncertainty about its benefits was reinforced by the fact that the mortality from the disease was declining in the UK and USA. There was no obvious acceleration in this decline with the introduction of cervical screening. Wide variations in the natural incidence of the disease in Britain, the earlier implementation of effective treatment of symptomatic disease and increasing rates of hysterectomy make the contribution of cervical screening difficult to assess. However, in countries where screening has been quickly and comprehensively introduced the rise in incidence up to the age of 50 is interrupted, showing a fall corresponding to the time when screening was introduced.

The cervical smear is taken using a specially shaped spatula (Fig. 16.6), and the material transferred to a slide. In the UK cervical screening is repeated every 3–5 years in women of 35 years or older.

Although exfoliative cytology remains the cornerstone of current cervical screening, there is a need for more reliable methods, since false-negative rates range from 20 to 40%. About two-thirds of errors leading to false negative tests are due to sampling. One method which could reduce sampling errors is *thin-layer liquid-based cytology*, which is currently under evaluation. In contrast to the Papanicolaou (Pap) smear, the sample is not placed directly on a slide but rinsed from the spatula into a vial containing a preserving transport fluid which keeps nearly all the cellular material in optimal condition for analysis. In making the Pap smear, only about 20% of the cells go onto the slide and the rest remain on the spatula, which is discarded. The cells in the preserving fluid are robotically processed to remove inflammatory cells and blood. The sample is then transferred by machine in a thin layer onto a small circular area of the slide for cytological examination. Blinded randomised trials have shown a significant improvement in slide quality and an 18% increase in cancer detection rate with the thin-layer Pap test compared to the traditional Pap test.

There are computer-assisted automated cytology systems available to try to overcome the variations in quality of manually read cytology. High-resolution images of the smears are acquired using a high-speed video. The images are then digitised. Algorithms are used to identify the morphometric characteristics of individual cells and the slide overall. Automated scanning of smears has been shown to be superior to manually reported cytology by a factor of between 5 and 7.

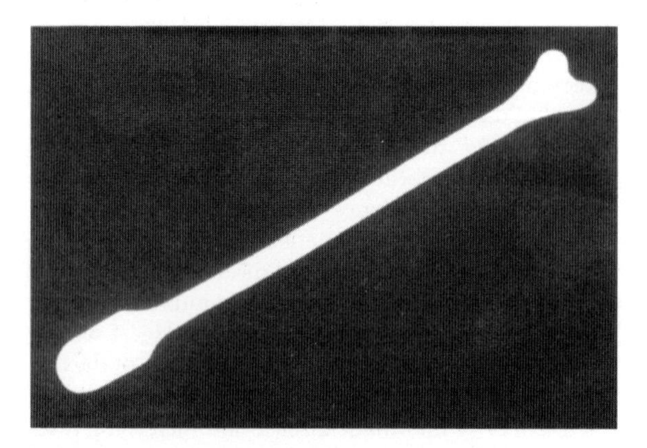

Fig. 16.6 Spatula for taking a cervical smear.

There is an increasing trend towards a rising incidence of the disease in young women. This may be related to sexually transmitted viral infection. Some gynaecologists are recommending changing the criteria for describing a smear as positive to include more women with minimal cellular abnormalities. Such women are being recommended to have colposcopic treatment of even these minimal cellular changes. An assessment of cervical screening using new criteria for reporting cervical smears has yet to be made.

Carcinoma-in-situ has been replaced by the term *cervical intraepithelial neoplasia* (CIN). CIN is divided into three grades, of which CIN III is the most abnormal. All grades of CIN are precancerous. Initially it was thought that CIN I or mild dysplasia was benign. This is now considered to be premalignant and up to 25% of CIN I will progress to CIN III over a 2-year period. Transformation to malignancy has been reported in 18% of CIN III at 10 years and 36% at 20 years.

Patients with CIN should be submitted to colposcopy (illuminated magnification of the cervix). Colposcopic examination allows abnormal areas of the cervix to be biopsied. In many units all patients with CIN are treated. Where the whole abnormal area on the cervix can be seen at colposcopy, it is treated by laser evaporation. If the abnormal area is only partially defined, a cone biopsy (Fig. 27.4) or cylinder excision of the endo- and ectocervix is performed.

Many populations in which cervical cancer is common also harbour some subtypes of the human papilloma virus (HPV). Screening for HPV might identify women at high risk of cervical cancer. For example, signal amplification of samples of cervical cells can be used to identify the five commonest low-risk HPV subtypes. This technique uses hybridisation of low- and high-risk oncogenic HPV RNA probes, the patient's HPV DNA together with an enzyme-linked immunosorbent assay (ELISA). The great and unique advantage of HPV DNA testing is that it can predict the later development of precursors of cervical cancer in women who are HPV positive but have negative cervical cytology. Women with persistent HPV of high-risk type have up to 100 times greater risk of developing cervical cancer within 2–4 years than low-risk HPV types. With double testing by Pap smear and HPV, the negative predictive is nearly 100% for high-grade intraepithelial lesions. Women who are negative on double testing can be given greater reassurance that they do not have the disease. Double testing could also potentially extend the interval between cervical screening. For a women with normal cervical cytology, it normally takes approximately 13 years to develop cervical cancer. It takes 8–12 years for high-grade squamous intraepithelial lesions to progress to stage I cervical cancer. Hence the risk of a woman under the age of 35 developing cervical cancer with negative cytology and negative Pap and HPV tests over intervals of 3–4 years is likely to be very small. Interval high- grade intraepithelial lesions are unlikely to progress to invasive cancer in less than 3 years. Latent HPV infection is uncommon (< 5%) in women aged 35 and older and much higher (20–40%) in younger women. In the majority of these younger women the infection is transient. This argues for the use of HPV screening only in women aged 35 or older. This should avoid unnecessary additional investigations such as colposcopy.

Breast cancer

This is an even more important cancer numerically, with over 13 000 deaths per year in the UK. One in every 12 women will be affected by the disease at some time in her life.

The value of screening for breast cancer has been more intensively studied than at any other tumour site. There is an increased yield of tumours at the first screen, a shift to earlier stage distribution and better survival in the screened population.

Two large randomised studies have shown a 30% reduction in mortality from breast cancer in women aged 50 or over. The reduction persists for up to 18 years, although it falls at that time to 23%. No benefit has been demonstrated in women below the age of 50.

Regular self-examination is the simplest and most obvious means of early detection of a lump in the breast. However, it is not now recommended as a method of screening since it has brought about no reduction in breast cancer mortality. (However, it remains true that at present, self-detection of a lump is the commonest way a breast cancer is detected.) The minimum size that can be detected by this technique is about 1.5 cm.

Mammography is the screening method of choice. Two views are recommended: oblique (Fig. 16.7) and craniocaudal. It is of little value in the small fibrous breast, but very helpful, particularly, in the large breast. It can detect tumours less than 1 cm in diameter.

The classic mammographic features of malignant lesions are: (1) a lesion with a dense centre and an irregular spiculated border (Fig. 16.8); and (2) stippled or punctate calcification (microcalcification), like grains of salt (Fig. 16.9). The presence of microcalcification is virtually pathognomonic of a carcinoma and occurs in about 30% of cases.

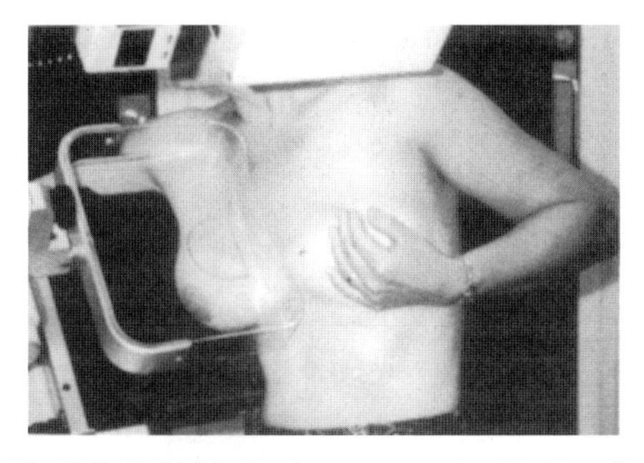

Fig. 16.7 Patient undergoing mammography. (Courtesy of the Rotherham Breast Screening Service.)

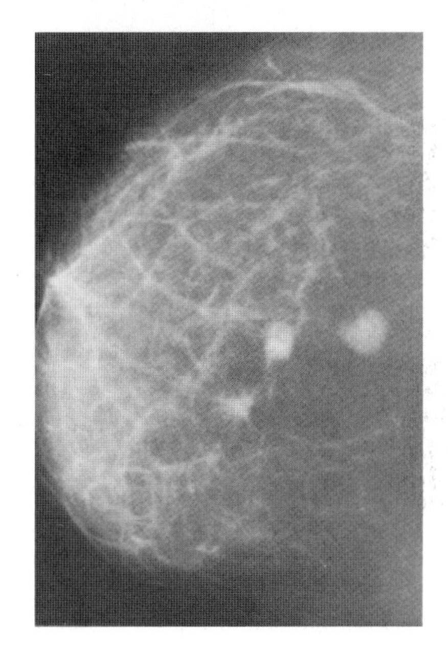

Fig. 16.8 Mammogram showing three spiculated tumours in the breast. (Courtesy of Dr R Peck, Sheffield.)

A national programme of mammographic screening was instituted in the UK in 1988 for women between 50 and 64 years. Two views of the breast (oblique and craniocaudal) improve the sensitivity for the detection of smaller cancers and specificity. Reading of the films by two radiologists (double reading) increases sensitivity by 5–10%. Screening is currently repeated 3-yearly. A UK trial comparing triennial versus annual screening showed a small but insignificant advantage to annual screening. Optimal frequency is therefore probably 2- to

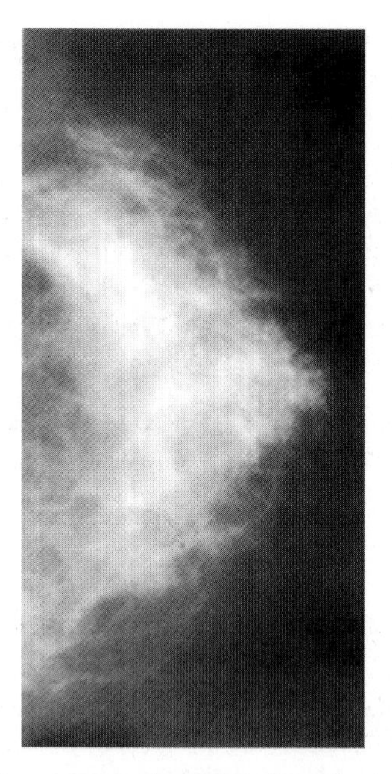

Fig. 16.9 Mammogram showing malignant calcification. (Courtesy of Dr R Peck, Sheffield.)

3-yearly. Patients with abnormal or equivocal mammograms are recalled for clinical examination of the breast and, if necessary, additional mammographic views or ultrasound of the breast. Palpable abnormalities are subjected to fine needle aspiration. Impalpable lesions seen on mammography are localised and needled for cytology under radiological control. Triple assessment by clinical examination, mammography and ultrasound should be carried out by a team of breast surgeon, radiologist, pathologist and radiographer supported by specialist breast care nurse.

Tight quality assurance is applied to the UK breast-screening programme. For women aged 50–52, no fewer than 36 invasive cancers and 4 cases of ductal carcinoma-in-situ cancers (DCIS) should be found among 10 000 women attending breast screening. In excess of 50% should be 15 mm or smaller when measured pathologically.

More women with DCIS (21%) are diagnosed through breast screening compared to symptomatic presentation (3%). In addition more low-grade cancers of special type are detected by screening (27%) compared to symptomatic presentation (12%).

Colorectal cancer

The mortality from colorectal cancer has remained unchanged. It would be of great value if screening could increase the detection of presymptomatic Dukes' A cancers. There is strong evidence that many tumours develop from dysplastic adenomatous polyps. However, the value of screening for colorectal cancer is as yet unproven. A variety of methods have been used, including clinical examination, proctosigmoidoscopy and, if necessary, barium enema. The survival of cases detected by annual proctosigmoidoscopy (64–85%) among over 21 000 men and women was over twice that of symptomatic cases. However, a reduction in overall mortality has yet to be demonstrated in a randomised controlled trial. Approximately 10% of patients with colorectal cancer have a family history of the disease. The value of screening of family members at high risk of the disease is under evaluation.

The most widely used test is that for the presence of faecal occult blood (*haemoccult test*). Disadvantages include the number of false positives, the sensitivity necessary to detect most cancers and polyps and limited acceptability of the technique to the public. It is the most useful test, if positive, for determining the need for proctosigmoidoscopy. There is a need for more specific markers for early colorectal cancer. Alterations in DNA (e.g. mutant *ras*/*p53*) exfoliated from cancers might prove to be more specific markers and are under evaluation. Faecal DNA can be amplified more than a billion-fold by polymerase reaction, so only very small quantities of DNA would have to be collected.

Reliance must still be placed on the immediate investigation of suspicious bowel disturbance or episodes of rectal bleeding, especially at and beyond middle age.

Prostate cancer

The value of screening for prostate cancer has yet to be proven. It meets some but not all the criteria for screening. It is certainly a major health burden with over 85 000 new cases per year in the European Community and 35 000–40 000 deaths, the second commonest cause of death in men. The prevalence of prostate cancer has risen by in excess of 100% in USA and Europe over the last decade. While increased life expectancy accounts for some of the rise, the widespread use of testing for serum prostate-specific antigen (PSA) is a major factor. The difficulty of screening for early prostate cancer is that the optimal treatment is unknown and the available screening methods of serum PSA followed by transrectal ultrasound and biopsy are not sufficiently sensitive or specific. In men aged 50–70, rectal examination and PSA testing will identify clinically suspicious areas in approximately 4%. 10% will have a raised PSA. Further investigation will be needed in 10–15% by transrectal ultrasound and biopsy. The latter causes sepsis in 1–7%, and haematuria in 2–34%. About 2–4% of men with a normal prostate will be found to have prostate cancer, predominantly based on PSA testing. In many cases men with subclinical prostate cancer may die of unrelated causes. It is known for example that over 50% over the age of 70 who have undergone a post-mortem examination will be found to have prostate cancer. It has been estimated that for a 50-year-old man with a life expectancy of 25 years, there is a 42% lifetime risk of harbouring microscopic prostate cancer, 9.5% chance of having clinically evident cancer and 2.9% chance of dying of it. It is likely that a screening programme would identify many men who would not die of prostate cancer. In the USA it has been calculated that among 100 men found to have prostate cancer on screening, on average 16 could have had their life extended by radical prostatectomy. If the estimate is correct, it is unlikely that screening for prostate cancer would result in a fall in the morbidity or mortality of the disease. A large randomised trial is needed to establish the value of screening for prostate cancer.

Hereditary prostate cancer accounts for <5% of cases. Men with first-degree relatives with prostate cancer (especially if diagnosed under the age of 55) or female relatives with breast cancer are at a higher than normal risk. Inheritance is thought to be mendelian dominant or X-linked. However, given the uncertainty of the effectiveness of treatment for early prostate cancer, the value of screening of relatives at risk of prostate cancer is similarly uncertain.

Stomach

No prospective evaluation of screening for stomach cancer has been undertaken. It is not clear what relative contributions the declining incidence and screening have made to the fall in the mortality from the disease. The situation is different in Japan where the incidence is much higher and many early cancers are detected.

Bladder cancer

Screening for bladder cancer by urinary cytology has been used for high-risk groups. While an increased yield at first screening, detection of earlier stage disease and improved survival in screened cases have been demonstrated, no reduction in mortality from bladder cancer has been proved.

CANCER EDUCATION

Understanding about the nature and outcome of cancer treatments tends to vary with educational attainment. The better educated tend to take a greater interest in and are better informed about cancer. They may appreciate that cancer is not a single disease conferring a uniformly poor prognosis. This misconception is sadly still common. For a large proportion of the population, the ugly reputation of cancer persists. They are unaware that about 30% of cancers can be cured or controlled long enough to give patients an expectation of life not far from that of the normal population and that good palliation of symptoms can be achieved in most cases.

Concepts of radical and palliative treatment are not widely understood by the general public or by some members of the medical profession who have little contact with the management of malignant disease.

The need for a coordinated policy

The responsibility for cancer education should be shared between international organisations, national and local governments and the health service professions. A coordinated policy promoting the prevention and detection of early disease is required, to have the maximum impact on the mortality of common disease such as lung, breast and colorectal cancer.

International organisations

Since cancer is a global problem, there is a need for internationally agreed policies. The International Union Against Cancer (UICC) has provided a forum for formulating such policies. It has adopted a number of objectives in relation to tobacco smoking. These include:

- Achieving lower rates of smoking in all age groups.
- Encouraging non-smokers, especially young ones, to remain so.
- Stopping all forms of tobacco promotion.
- Encouraging smokers to reduce, as far as possible, their exposure to harmful components of tobacco smoke.
- Maintaining liaison with other health organisations and authorities to ensure maximum effectiveness and avoid conflicts of interest.

Educating the young about cancer

The behaviour patterns that predispose to some cancers, particularly smoking and cervical cancer, are often established in childhood or adolescence. Peer pressure is often a powerful factor in starting smoking. This pressure is often reinforced by tobacco advertising associating smoking with relaxation, confidence and being adult. Similarly, children whose parents smoke are more likely to do so themselves. However, if their parents smoke but disapprove of their children doing so, children are less likely to become smokers. School policy, teacher and parental example may all contribute to a child's decision whether or not to smoke. Regular smoking is not uncommon among 12- and 13-year-old children. Although smoking rates among boys have fallen, the rates among girls have declined more slowly.

Cervical cancer is known to be associated with starting sexual intercourse in the teens. There is evidence that the age at which the young are starting to have intercourse is declining. Often they have multiple partners. Both boys and girls need to be educated about cervical cancer. Schooling is the only period of a girl's life when her attendance at classes on cancer education is likely. On leaving school, the chances of reaching her with any message on cancer prevention decline sharply.

To prevent lung and cervical cancer it is therefore important to establish programmes of cancer education among children, to encourage behaviour which will avoid cancer and present a realistic picture of the disease in order to avoid unnecessary fear. The latter may reduce the likelihood of attendance for screening.

A child's perspective

A child's perspective of cancer differs from that of an adult. The idea of preventing cancer is difficult for them to comprehend. Children tend not to distinguish cancer from any other illness. The child may regard cancer simply as another type of infectious disease that he or she is likely to catch. Furthermore, talking about a disease which may affect a child several decades later is beyond the comprehension of most children. It seems too far off to have any impact.

Cancer education for children: a different approach

The approach to cancer education among children has to be adapted to take account of the child's different perspective on disease. Teaching about health risks is likely to be non-productive. As one commentator says:

> To children the facts are boring, the distant future is not relevant and some children like to take risks anyway . . . Imagine how many children hold most or even all of the following beliefs: it is part of life to smoke; all my family do; so do my friends and teachers; cigarettes are sold in ordinary shops, so they cannot be that bad; it is attractive to be as thin as possible, if not even thinner; fat people are ugly and laughable; it is good to be calm, cool, confident and sophisticated—cigarettes do this for you, films and advertising tell you so; it is old-fashioned not to have at least one boyfriend or girlfriend and quite unmentionable not to have sexual relations with them; it is beautiful to be tanned; not to eat meat every day is a sign of poverty; it is friendly and sociable to drink alcohol.

After smoking, diet may be responsible for up to one-third of cancer deaths. Collaboration is needed between parents, pupils, schools and the food industry to promote a diet high in fruit, vegetables and cereals and low in fat, salt and sugar. One in five children do not eat any fruit in a week and three in five eat no leafy green vegetables. Children from low-income families are 50% less likely to eat fruit and vegetables than those in high-income families. The UK government as part of its National Cancer Plan is developing a national 'five-a-day' programme to encourage five portions of fruit or vegetables to be consumed by children and adults.

From the quotation above, it is clear that cancer education may conflict with a young person's firmly held beliefs. It is therefore necessary for the health educator to instil healthy behaviour into the lifestyle that the child has chosen.

Cancer education in schools

Successful cancer education within schools is dependent upon teachers having the necessary experience and teaching material. Teachers may have a number of reservations about teaching cancer education. They may feel (1) deficient in their own knowledge about, and fearful of, cancer; (2) that the children are too young to be taught about it; (3) that there is insufficient time within the curriculum.

However, rather than teaching cancer prevention as one subject or focusing a week of teaching on cancer education, teachers may be more amenable to incorporating it into part of their own subject area. For example dietary aspects of cancer prevention could be included in classes on home economics. The carcinogenic properties of certain industrial chemicals could be taught as part of chemistry. Children are more likely to take note of the messages of cancer prevention in this format.

Care needs to be taken that neither children nor adults are given to believe that they are wholly responsible for whether or not they develop cancer. This may induce feelings of guilt and disillusionment if they do contract the disease. It needs to be emphasised that following particular guidelines of behaviour does not always prevent cancer.

Good cancer education packages have been produced for use in schools, e.g. The Cancer Research Campaign Education and Child Studies Research Group package: 'Cells, Cancer and Communities'.

Cancer education within the local community

Each district health authority needs a coherent policy to communicate important information about prevention and early diagnosis of cancer and of services available for the care of patients with cancer and of their families. Such a policy requires coordination of a wide variety of groups, including health professionals, community representatives, schoolteachers and voluntary agencies.

The overall responsibility should lie with the District General Manager. There should be a District Health Promotion Unit which coordinates the publication and dissemination of educational material and organisation of meetings and provides advice to interested parties.

The Director of Education should be involved in developing a programme of cancer education in schools, providing training for teaching staff, encouraging the provision of healthy school meals and adopting non-smoking policies within schools.

The Director of Nursing may incorporate cancer education into basic and post-basic courses. He or she should support non-smoking policies in hospitals.

The role of the general practitioner

Members of the general public have most medical contact with their general practitioner. He or she is in a good position to offer simple advice on the prevention of cancer. Advice on stopping smoking is the most important. Patients may be referred to voluntary classes to help them stop smoking or to use non-carcinogenic nicotine substitutes (e.g. chewing Nicorette gum). The general practitioner can provide screening for cervical cancer and encourage women to accept invitations for breast screening. Young men can be given leaflets on self-examination for testicular cancer. The waiting areas of health centres offer a good site for displaying leaflets on the prevention and early diagnosis of cancer (e.g. the European 10-point code; Fig. 16.4).

Cancer education in the workplace

Cancer education in the workplace can be channelled through environmental health officers, occupational medical and nursing staff, health and safety officers, management and trade unions.

Effective cancer education requires more than simply disseminating information about the causes. More important is the process of persuading people to change their lifestyle to reduce the risk of cancer. Exhorting people to stop smoking is easy. Persuading them sufficiently to stop doing so is much more difficult. One of the most effective methods of educational interventions is directed at small community groups. This may be based on locality, work or social network. Specially trained and influential members of target groups can be very effective in disseminating health education.

Cancer education in the workplace can be very effective if the following criteria are met. It must be part of a general health programme. It needs to be developed in consultation with management and unions. It should use existing networks within the workplace. It should be consonant with workers' own perceived health needs, i.e. what concerns them most. The programme should be popular, e.g. fitness or losing weight, and suited to the company's style.

The essential messages that need to be conveyed are:

1. Many cancers are preventable by changes in behaviour.
2. Some cancers are curable and prognosis for many is improving.
3. The quality of life of many patients with cancer is good.
4. Particular symptoms commonly associated with cancer should be reported promptly to a general practitioner.

CHAPTER CONTENTS

17

Biological and pathological introduction

John Goepel

Radiotherapy is used almost exclusively for the treatment of cancer and related conditions. It is thus very important to have a reasonable understanding of this disease. This chapter contains an outline of the basic characteristics of cancerous cells, and the conditions that can cause cancer. There is consideration of the natural history of untreated cancer, and of the ways that different types of cancer are named and classified.

GROWTH: PROLIFERATION, DIFFERENTIATION AND APOPTOSIS

Growth is the process of increase in size and maturity of tissues from fertilisation through to the adult. When normally controlled, the different parts of the body take on their correct size and specialist functions, and relationship to one another. Furthermore, throughout life these attributes continue despite the need for replacement and repair. This is all a reflection of accurate control of the timing and extent of cellular proliferation, cell-to-cell orientation and organisation, and *differentiation*. Differentiation is the process of a cell taking on a specialised function; this is usually associated with a change in its microscopic appearance. It is also usually a one-way commitment, with relative or complete loss of the ability to continue proliferating. Also important is the ability to delete cells which are no longer needed, by a process called *apoptosis* or programmed cell death. This is used in the development of the fetus, and in maintaining or adjusting the size of a structure in the adult. Apoptosis is also used to delete defective cells.

Growth disorders

Hypertrophy is an increase in the size of an organ due to an increase in the size of its constituent cells. The left ventricle of the heart becomes hypertrophic if it has to work harder because of hypertension.

Hyperplasia is an increase in size because of an increase in the number of cells. The adrenal cortex will become hyperplastic if there is excessive adrenocorticotrophic hormone to stimulate it. However, it will return to normal if the stimulus is reduced again.

Metaplasia is a change from one type of tissue to another. Smoking induces a change of the bronchial lining from the usual respiratory mucosa to a squamous epithelium, with resultant loss of mucus-producing and ciliated cells. It is also potentially reversible.

Neoplasia (literally a new growth), in contrast, is an irreversible process once initiated: it is the main subject of this chapter. It is also called cancer, or a tumour, though the latter is sometimes used to denote any swelling.

NEOPLASIA

A neoplasm can be defined as 'a lesion resulting from the autonomous or relatively autonomous abnormal growth of cells which persists after the initiating stimulus has been removed; i.e. cell growth has escaped from normal regulatory mechanisms'. The abnormality affects all aspects of cell growth and apoptosis to varying degrees. Proliferation continues unabated, irrespective of the requirements of the organ in which the neoplasm is situated. This, combined with loss of control of the normal relationships between cells, often results in the new tumour cells replacing and insinuating themselves between the adjacent normal tissues, a process called *invasion*. Loss of differentiation accompanies, and often correlates with, failure of proliferation control and invasiveness. Failure of apoptosis may also be a major contribution to the survival of abnormal cells.

Benign and malignant neoplasms

Neoplasia is not a single disease, but rather a common pathological process with a multitude of different varieties and clinical outcomes. One fundamental division is between *benign* and *malignant* tumours. Benign tumours will remain localised, with generally relatively little effect on the patient. In contrast, other tumours are locally destructive, may spread to involve other parts of the body, and ultimately result in the death of the patient. Figure 17.1 and Table 17.1 show some of the differences between benign and malignant neoplasms. Further aspects of the classification of tumours are discussed later in this chapter.

The term *cancer* (Latin for 'crab') is very ancient, and there are several explanations for its usage. Some say

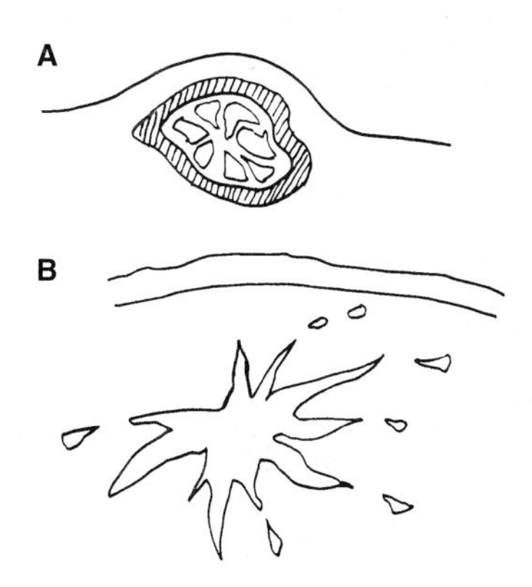

Fig. 17.1 The difference between a benign tumour **A** contained by a definitive capsule and a malignant tumour **B** actively invading the tumour bed.

Table 17.1 Characteristics of neoplasms

Feature	Benign	Malignant
Growth rate	Slow	Variable, may be rapid
Margin	Encapsulated	Invasive
Local effect	Little	Destructive
Differentiation	Good	Variable, may be poor
Metastases	No	Frequently
Usual outcome	Good	Fatal

it reflects the tenacious grip the disease has on its victim, some that it describes the radiating prominent veins that may surround an advanced superficial tumour. Others contend that it describes the irregular infiltrative profile of some tumours, e.g. of breast. Suffice it to say that cancer is a common colloquial term that is generally applied to any malignant neoplasm.

Though the behaviour of tumours, particularly malignant ones, may seem very odd it can generally be explained by the excessive or inappropriate expression of genes that are present in all cells. The tumour continues to be dependent upon an adequate blood supply (though many acquire the capacity to induce new vessels). Also, many of those which arise from hormone-dependent tissues (e.g. breast, prostate) continue to show a degree of dependence on those hormones. This can be exploited to therapeutic advantage by giving antihormone treatment (Ch. 35).

CARCINOGENESIS

The causes of cancer are numerous, and mechanisms of its production are complex, but some of the principles will be presented. There are two avenues of thought to follow: one at the molecular and genetic levels, the other concerned with causative associations. It is not always easy to relate these to each other. Underlying the mechanistic approach is the assumption that cell behaviour is controlled by the genes expressed (which ones, and how strongly), bearing in mind that these can be influenced by chemical messages relayed from outside the cell. Every cell contains the entire genetic code, but only expresses those genes appropriate to its own situation. In cancer this has gone wrong, particularly with respect to proliferation, differentiation or apoptosis. We can generalise to say that multiple abnormalities need to have occurred between normality and cancer, and that this reflects a *multistep* process. Only those cells capable of division are at risk of transforming into a neoplasm. This excludes terminally differentiated cells such as circulating red cells, the uppermost keratinised cells of the skin, and adult voluntary muscle and nerve cells.

Initiation

This describes the first step towards neoplasia. It reflects a change at the molecular level of how a cell can function, escaping in some small way from a control mechanism. Nothing can be seen microscopically at this stage. Substances that can initiate neoplasia are called *initiators* or *carcinogens*.

Promotion

No more will come of the initiated cell unless it continues to divide. Further abnormalities of cell function (i.e. gene expression) arise over a period of time. Substances that enhance this process are called *promoters*.

Progression

Neoplasms are *clonal*, i.e. are derived from a single cell. For this to happen, a cell and its progeny must acquire and sustain a growth advantage over other cells throughout succeeding cell divisions. This eventually results in visible alterations at the microscopic level. Not all the daughter cells will be identical, giving rise to differences between individual cells or subclones; this is called *pleomorphism*.

Clinical cancer

Finally, the neoplasm becomes manifest as a clinically significant tumour. Unless removed, it will continue to progress with a general tendency towards further loss of growth restraint, and acquisition of the capacity to spread to other parts of the body (metastasise).

Oncogenes and tumour suppressor genes

The function of a cell is critically dependent on the expression of its genes. In cancer it has been observed that there may be both inappropriate levels of expression of otherwise normal genes, and abnormalities of genes. Though copying of the genetic code from one cell generation to another is very accurate, it is not perfect. An abnormal copy or *mutation* may give rise to a protein with excessive function or reduced function, or may fail to produce a protein at all, resulting in no function. Alternatively, it may be the control of the gene which is altered, so that there is increased or decreased expression resulting in excess or deficient protein product and hence function. An *oncogene* is an altered gene which contributes to cancer development when its expression is increased. The normally functioning counterparts of these genes are often concerned with control of cell proliferation.

In contrast, *tumour suppressor genes* are those which, when totally absent or non-functioning in a cell, permit the emergence of neoplasia, i.e. their presence prevents neoplasia. Given that all normal cells will have two copies of each gene (one on each chromosome pair), the development of neoplasia by this means requires loss or mutation of both copies.

It must be stressed that clinical cancer does not reflect a solitary abnormality of one of these genes, but rather the final result of a combination of several errors of function. The gradual accumulation of multiple genetic defects is typified by the progression of a benign polyp in the colon to a cancer over about 10 years. How is it that a cell can acquire so many abnormal genes? The explanation in several situations is that there is failure of the screening of the cell's genetic code for abnormalities, or defective repair of incidental genetic damage. The protein p53 is important in assuring the integrity of the genome, and it is frequently defective in cancer cells. Similarly, the failure of DNA repair can result in much more rapid accumulation of mutations – the *mutator phenotype*.

Defective apoptosis has several consequences with regard to cancer. Inappropriately increased expression of *BCL-2*, which inhibits apoptosis, is a major reason for cell accumulation in some tumours, for example follicular lymphoma. Failure of apoptosis may contribute to survival of defective cells and also cell survival in abnormal environments such as occurs during invasion and metastasis. Finally, many cancer treatments rely on induction of apoptosis to kill tumour cells, so these will be less effective if apoptosis is defective.

The development of cancer requires the induction of a new blood supply, *angiogenesis*, and invasion and metastasis: the ability to do this reflects other genetic abnormalities in addition to those mentioned above.

Heredity and cancer

The great majority of common tumours do not seem to have any relationship to hereditary factors. However, some rare tumours do, and have led to an understanding of tumour suppressor genes. The pioneering work of Knudson on families of patients with multiple retinoblastomas (a tumour of the eye) indicated first that there must be two genetic events. In due course it became clear that one defective gene was inherited by the patient, while its corresponding gene on the opposite chromosome became defective, or was lost, in some cells during the growth of the eye. With both retinoblastoma (Rb) genes now defective the cells proceeded to neoplasia.

It is now apparent that a minority of common tumours run in families because of the same sort of mechanism. For example, breast cancer kindreds may be passing on the *BRCA-1* gene; in familial adenomatous polyposis the *FAP* gene results in adenomas and colon cancers, while in familial non-polyposis colon cancer it is a mismatch repair gene that is passed on. This is a rapidly developing field, with many new chromosomal abnormalities reported. An inherited risk of malignancy does not imply a particular cellular mechanism, neither is it certain that a cancer will arise in a particular individual.

Physical agents

Ionising radiation

There is no doubt that ionising radiation can cause cancer. Direct damage to DNA (i.e. the chemical basis of genetic information), and damage mediated via ionisation of water can result in mutation of genes. The damage is randomly scattered throughout the genetic code, but can include sites critical to the development of cancer by the usual sequence of initiation, promotion and so on. Traditionally it has been thought that radiation causes a somatic mutation in a normal cell. The earliest event is probably genomic instability. Subsequently there is a multistep sequence of genetic events. This typically results in an interval of many years between exposure and clinical cancer. The source of radiation does not matter from the point of view of causing cancer, though it will affect the sites at risk.

Ionising radiation can lead to loss of tumour suppressor genes and activation of proto-oncogenes. Oncogenes may also be activated as result of point mutations. Gene amplification can lead to activation and over expression of a proto-oncogene. It had previously been thought that mutagenesis only occurred in normal cells traversed by radiation particles. However, normal cells can undergo change without such damage by virtue of what is termed the 'bystander effect'. The mechanism of this bystander effect is not clear but it could be due to secretion of factors (as yet unidentified) from irradiated cells that influence the survival of adjacent non-irradiated cells.

The dose at which carcinogenesis occurs may be tissue specific. Actively proliferating tissues within or adjacent to the irradiated volume (e.g. in the pelvis), and having a high capacity for proliferation not inhibited by radiation, will carry a risk of radiation-induced malignancy at lower doses than in slowly turning-over tissues such as connective tissue.

Industrial exposure. Early workers with X-rays unknowingly induced tumours, and other radiation damage, in their hands. Today, diagnostic and therapeutic radiation also carry this risk to patients and staff alike, necessitating stringent safety regulations. Some mineworkers are exposed to high levels of radon, which is inhaled and may cause lung cancer (a risk increased by cigarette smoking). Radon- induced lung cancer has been linked to mutations of *p53*, a tumour suppressor gene. This mutation differs from those seen in lung cancer induced by smoking. Another industrial association was with the painters of luminous watch dials. These ladies pointed their brush with their lips, thereby taking in minute quantities of radium. Some of the material remained near the jaw, while some was absorbed and passed to bone marrow, where the alpha emissions resulted in bone necrosis, tumours and marrow failure. In all cases there was the usual long time delay between exposure and clinical cancer.

Atomic bomb survivors have been followed up very carefully. There has been an excessive number of cases of leukaemia, mainly 7–12 years after exposure, and also a larger number of other cancers from about 20 years later onwards.

Ultraviolet light

The shorter wavelengths of solar ultraviolet light, UVB, are capable of damaging the DNA of various skin cells, resulting in mutations and eventually cancers.

Melanin pigment protects against UV penetration to the deeper layers of cells. The common tumours, basal cell and squamous cell carcinomas, seem to result from chronic overexposure; malignant melanoma correlates better with acute and intense exposure.

Chemicals

Coal tars, oils and cigarette smoke

Percival Pott, in 1775, described carcinoma of the scrotal skin in chimney sweeps, and attributed it to the soot. Similarly, mule-spinners in mills developed tumours due to the oil that soaked their clothing, and even today motor mechanics are at risk from lubricating oils. However, the greatest problem at present from this group of chemicals is cigarette smoke. This contains many known *carcinogenic* substances, including benzo[a]pyrene, a potent carcinogen also present in coal tars. Not only do smokers have a very greatly increased incidence of lung cancer, they also have a higher risk of cancer at several other sites, such as the bladder. Chemicals that are able to cause tumours are called *direct carcinogens*, but most require metabolism to the active chemical so are called *procarcinogens*.

Aniline dyes and the rubber industry

Workers in the chemical industry, particularly those involved in making dyes, were found to develop bladder cancer. A similar risk was noted in the rubber-processing industry. The chemical implicated, β-naphthylamine, needs to be metabolised in the kidney, thus releasing the active ingredient into the urine.

Asbestos

Many particulate minerals are now recognised as carcinogenic, including asbestos. The blue asbestos (crocidolite) particles used for insulation are easily inhaled when very small but are then retained within the lung. Over a period of decades they may then cause tumours of the pleura (malignant mesothelioma); they also correlate with bronchial cancer, particularly if associated with smoking.

Hormones

Are endogenous chemicals such as hormones carcinogenic? There is no doubt that hormone levels are important in hormonally responsive organs and their cancers. Whether the hormone is actually carcinogenic, or simply contributes to the process of carcinogenesis by promoting cell proliferation is debatable; the latter is more probable. The relationship between oestrogens and endometrial cancer is discussed in Chapter 27. Breast and prostate cancers are also likely to relate to hormonal influences. As mentioned earlier, hormonal manipulation is an important therapeutic tool in cancer treatment.

Viruses and cancer

As viruses contain genetic material, and gain access to the inside of cells, they have long been suspected of having a role in carcinogenesis. This speculation has been fuelled by finding close similarity between some viral genes and oncogenes. Viruses are clearly responsible for a variety of tumours in several species, such as leukaemias in mice and cats and sarcomas in chickens. In humans, common skin warts are self-limiting benign tumours caused by a virus. Over recent years, these human papilloma (wart) viruses (HPV) have been found to be a large family of related organisms, some of which correlate closely with cancer of the uterine cervix and similar tumours. Similarly, Epstein–Barr virus, which is very widespread and causes infectious mononucleosis, is closely associated with tumours such as Hodgkin's disease, Burkitt's lymphoma (a high-grade non-Hodgkin lymphoma), and nasopharyngeal carcinoma.

Infectivity and cancer. Some patients, or their relatives, worry that cancer may be infectious. It is possible to allay these fears and assure them that this is not the case. The association with viruses mentioned above is a rare sequel to agents widely present in the community; the cancer cannot be passed on.

Immunity and cancer

The immune system exists to detect and eliminate foreign substances, from isolated molecules to whole organisms. This is effected by antibodies and cells, principally lymphocytes. In the development of a tumour, it is quite possible for new or inappropriate substances to be produced. From this one would predict that tumours would sometimes be antigenic, i.e. provoke an immune response. This does seem to be the case. There are several examples of rare and common tumours with evidence of an immune response, generally the presence of numerous lymphocytes within and around the tumour. Tumours of rectum and breast, and seminoma of the testis all vary in the density of tumour-infiltrating lymphocytes. Studies of patients have correlated the density of lymphocytes with survival, often showing an advantage to those with an immune response. However, the effect is not large, and is easily obscured by better treatment to all patients.

With malignant melanoma of skin, there is slightly more evidence to suggest a significant favourable immune response in some patients. Microscopic examination sometimes shows areas of apparent regression within the primary growth. There are also some patients with advanced melanoma who respond to stimulation of their immune system against the tumour (immunotherapy).

Despite these few encouraging observations, it is obvious that the majority of clinical cancer is beyond the capability of the patient's immune system. In some cases there is evidence that tumour cells may simply evade it.

Immune surveillance

The normal immune system actively seeks foreign material, apparently screening everything against its memory bank to distinguish self from non-self. This may allow the detection and elimination of some cancers before they are clinically established. For example, renal transplant patients require drugs to suppress their immune response in order for the new kidney to survive. These patients have many more skin tumours than would otherwise be expected, possibly as a result of loss of immune surveillance. Patients with AIDS suffer from a wide range of tumours, but this does not necessarily imply that loss of immune surveillance is the key event. Many patients with defects of the immune system (either as a result of disease or treatment) have an increase in tumours of lymphocytes, but this is probably a different phenomenon.

Injury and cancer

To be acceptable as a cause of cancer, an injury would need to be severe enough to have caused tissue damage, there must be evidence that the site was previously normal, and that the tumour arose at the site of injury. Finally, the time interval must be long enough to be plausible, generally several years. The mechanism is presumably via a non-specific induction of cell division as part of the repair process, rather than anything actually carcinogenic. There are a few instances that fulfil these criteria, but the usual circumstance is simply that the injury draws attention to a pre-existing tumour.

PRECANCEROUS LESIONS

There are a number of conditions in which there is an increased risk of the subsequent development of cancer. Some are disorders that are not of themselves neoplastic, but carry a risk of cancer. Others are more like a halfway house in which the process of development towards cancer is recognisable as neither normal nor cancer. Some are benign tumours that may change to be malignant. In none is the development of cancer inevitable, though the risk and time scale vary greatly. Some examples are given below.

- *Undescended testis* is an abnormality of development: it carries a high risk of neoplasia (p. 500).
- *Paget's disease of bone*, a condition of middle to late adult life, has a risk of osteosarcoma, a tumour otherwise seen in adolescence (p. 573).
- *Solar keratosis* is a warty skin lesion due to sun exposure; it may progress to cancer.
- *Leucoplakia*, a whitish patch in the mouth (p. 347) or vulva (p. 484), is a descriptive term including several conditions. Some run the risk of cancer later.
- *Dysplasia* may be detected at several sites (e.g. stomach), and indicates a microscopic abnormality of cells with some, but not all, the features of cancer.
- *Carcinoma-in-situ*, may be seen on a surface (e.g. cervix, p. 466) or within the lumen of a duct (intraduct carcinoma of the breast, p. 434). This has all the microscopic features of cancer, but the cells are still confined to their normal anatomical limits, i.e. have not invaded.
- *Adenomatous polyp* of the large intestine is a benign tumour. However, it may develop into a malignant tumour. In the condition familial adenomatous polyposis there are so many polyps (thousands) that malignancy becomes inevitable.

An important consideration is that the detection of some of these conditions allows surgical intervention before cancer becomes established.

Field change

Although an individual tumour arises from a single cell, within the vicinity of that cell there are often other cells part-way through carcinogenesis. Removal of the tumour, or its precursor lesion, may be followed by the local development of further lesions. This is regarded as a field change across the whole area. An example would be the appearance of cancer on the tongue following removal of one from the buccal mucosa.

NATURAL HISTORY AND SPREAD OF CANCER

As stated earlier, *benign* tumours remain localised, often separated from surrounding tissue by a capsule. The tumour has relatively little effect on the adjacent structures, unless it arises in a particularly critical site, and surgical removal is curative. In contrast, *malignant* tumours show a capacity to invade, frequently recur after surgery, spread to other sites and result in the death of the patient. The initial or *primary* site of tumour growth thus gives rise to separate secondary tumours, or *metastases*. Some tumours, such as *basal cell carcinoma* of skin have an intermediate behaviour; they invade locally but do not give rise to metastases.

In summary, spread may occur in several ways (Fig. 17.2):

- by local invasion
- by lymphatic vessels
- by blood vessels
- across cavities.

Local invasion

As the tumour invades, adjacent tissues are displaced and destroyed to be replaced by tumour. The tumour margin is ill-defined and irregular. Surgical removal therefore needs to include a generous extent of normal tissue. Failure to do so results in some tumour being left behind, which proliferates and gives rise to *local recurrence*. Radiotherapy is frequently used after surgery in order to prevent this situation. The invasion often follows anatomical tissue planes; it may be temporarily halted by some dense structure such as bone, until this is also eroded.

Functional effects

The effects a tumour produces will depend upon the site involved; a knowledge of anatomy and physiology allows prediction of many symptoms. Thus a tumour in the head of the pancreas will soon obstruct the bile duct, so that the patient becomes jaundiced. A tumour of the left lung may obstruct its bronchus, with resulting pneumonia from infection of retained secretions. Further local invasion of this mass will compress the recurrent laryngeal nerve; the patient's voice is altered. Further growth may obstruct the superior vena cava passing through the mediastinum, causing swelling of the face and arms.

A tumour just beneath the skin can so stretch it and impair its nutrition that it breaks down to form an ulcer. This is then liable to infection or bleeding. Pain and weakness will occur when peripheral nerves are affected, e.g. Pancoast tumour (p. 421) at the apex of the lung invading upwards to compress nerves to the arm and hand.

The extent of local invasion dictates the extent of surgery necessary to remove it, and indeed may render the tumour inoperable if critical structures are involved. However, the usual reason why a tumour is 'inoperable' is because of metastatic disease. Sometimes it is worth debulking the tumour, but surgery alone is insufficient to cure the patient.

Metastasis

By lymphatic vessels

Invasive tumours readily penetrate the thin wall of lymphatics. Then fragments of tumour are carried downstream to lodge in one or more local lymph nodes. If the tumour cells survive this journey and proliferate in the node they form a *metastasis*, or secondary tumour. Further dissemination may proceed to

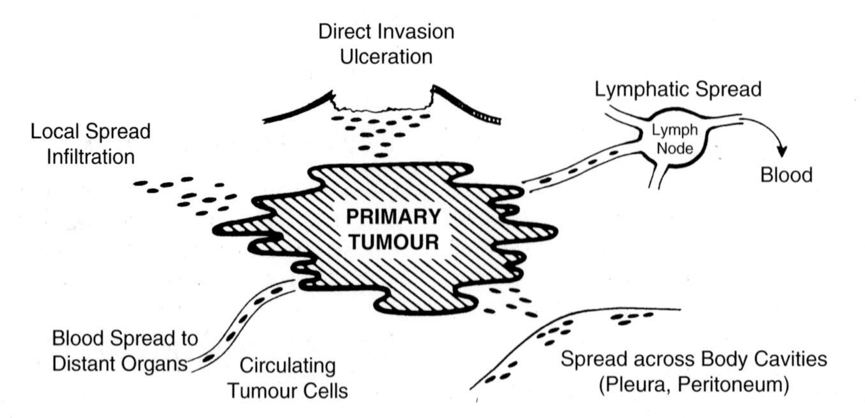

Fig. 17.2 Metastasis or secondary spread. Tumours can spread by a variety of routes including local spread, spread through the lymphatics, via the blood and across cavities. (Reproduced from Calman, Smyth and Tattersall, Basic Principles of Cancer Chemotherapy, Macmillan, 1980 with permission of Palgrave.)

other lymph nodes along the chain, e.g. from pelvic to para-aortic to supraclavicular nodes. Some primary tumours remain tiny, yet have massive nodal deposits. If the node capsule is breached by tumour, the whole mass becomes fixed to surrounding structures.

By blood vessels

Thin-walled blood vessels are similarly at risk of tumour invasion, and again fragments of tumour float passively downstream. (Single tumour cells are generally destroyed by non-specific defence mechanisms in the blood.) These then lodge in the next capillary bed, where they may develop into metastases. Though this can happen in any tissue, the liver, lungs and bone are by far the most frequent sites for secondaries.

Across cavities (transcoelomic)

Access to the *pleura* enables tumour cells to seed themselves around the pleural cavity, forming numerous further deposits or seedlings. These may be associated with secretion of fluid into the cavity, with resultant impairment of respiration. An identical process may occur in the peritoneum; the fluid accumulation is called *ascites*. Malignant cells may settle on the ovaries, or all over the omentum. Related to this, some intracranial tumours, such as medulloblastoma (p. 594) of the cerebellum, may disseminate by the cerebrospinal fluid, seeding over the surface of the brain and down the spinal canal.

Implantation

Occasionally cells may be implanted in the scar by the surgeon's knife while removing a tumour, or through a pleural or abdominal paracentesis drainage site.

Functioning tumours

Many tumour cells continue certain cell functions related to their tissue of origin, but in some this has a profound effect on the patient. Tumours of endocrine glands typically produce an excess of their hormone. The problem is that the tumour is no longer responsive to the usual control of secretion. Thus an adrenal cortex tumour will produce steroids despite switching off its pituitary drive, and Cushing's syndrome will result.

In other circumstances the hormone production is quite inappropriate for the tumour site. Many lung tumours produce substances that mimic the function of parathyroid hormone, antidiuretic hormone, or adrenocorticotrophic hormone (p. 422). Again it is not subject to the normal control of secretion, and the clinical consequences may be severe. Some of the other effects that tumours may have, such as profound weight loss, could be due to secretions as yet unidentified.

Cause of death from cancer

As the word 'malignant' implies, death is the natural consequence of untreated cancer. Sometimes the tumour will have grown locally and spread in a predictable manner. In other cases the primary site remains undetected despite widespread metastatic deposits. Some tumours show relentless progression, and run their course in a few months; others take many years, with long intervals of apparent dormancy.

Many patients with locally advanced or metastatic cancer become bedridden and die from bronchopneumonia, inanition and/or metabolic disturbance. Sometimes there may be liver failure due to numerous liver secondaries. Often the actual cause of death is unclear. It is important to consider carrying out a postmortem examination if there is reasonable doubt about the cause of death. Patients with cancer are still at risk of non-neoplastic conditions such as coronary artery disease. This is particularly likely in patients who smoke. Indeed, smoking may have given rise both to the primary tumour (e.g. in the lung, oral cavity or pharynx) and to ischaemic heart disease.

It is important to make a judgement as to whether the patient died from cancer or from an unrelated condition, since this influences cancer mortality statistics. Where a patient has remained disease free from cancer for more than 5 years, and the cause of death is said to be cancer, this conclusion should be questioned. However, late relapses can occur after 5 years, in breast cancer for example. Alternatively, a new primary may develop, especially in head and neck cancer.

STAGING OF CANCERS

It is of the greatest practical importance in many cases to estimate the extent of the spread of a tumour at the time of initial diagnosis. This process is called *staging*. Staging often influences the choice of treatment, and can provide valuable information on prognosis. Staging may include clinical, pathological, radiological, and biochemical information. This enables similar groups of patients to be compared between different oncology centres nationally and internationally. A number of staging classifications are in use. The simplest and oldest classification is as follows:

Stage 1: Tumour confined to the organ of origin
Stage 2: Local lymph nodes invaded
Stage 3: Distant nodes invaded, or local spread beyond the organ of origin
Stage 4: Blood-borne metastasis present

This is still used with some cancers, though often with slight modification to bring in subcategories, as with the FIGO system for cervix cancer. The UICC (International Union Against Cancer) has worked towards international agreement on the staging of many tumours, coding them on the TNM system.

TNM classification

This includes a description of the primary tumour (T), nodal spread (N), and distant metastases (M). It provides a succinct summary of the extent of malignancy in the patient.

T1–3: Generally based on the size and/or extent of the primary
T4: The most advanced local disease, often with invasion of adjacent structures
N0: No nodes palpable
N1: Mobile nodes on the same side as the primary
N1a: Nodes not considered to contain tumour
N1b: Nodes considered to contain tumour
N2: Mobile nodes on the opposite side (N2a and N2b as above)
N3: Fixed, involved nodes
M0: No evidence of distant metastasis
M1: Distant metastasis present

Thus a very early cancer would be categorised as T1N0M0, and a very advanced one as T4N3M1. The details of how to categorise a tumour vary between sites; the TNM classification for breast cancer is shown in Table 26.3.

The clinical staging may differ from the pathological staging. For example, a tumour in the breast may be measured clinically as 2 cm in diameter and thus be staged as T1. However, when actually measured directly in the mastectomy specimen it might be 3 cm in maximum diameter, and thus be pathologically T2 (abbreviated as pT2). Most staging classifications are based on the clinical extent of spread.

Radiological information may influence staging. For example in carcinoma of the cervix the presence of an obstructed kidney on ultrasound or other investigation (in the absence of a non-neoplastic cause), automatically indicates stage 3b.

The staging of testicular cancer is an example where biochemical information (the presence of serum tumour markers alpha-fetoprotein and human chorionic gonadotrophin) is included. If the tumour is clinically confined to the testis but tumour markers are rising, it is classified as stage 1, marker positive (Mk+).

HISTOLOGICAL GRADING: DIFFERENTIATION

In an effort to predict the future course of a tumour, an estimate is made of how malignant it is for a particular site and type of tumour. Generally speaking, the closer a tumour cell resembles its normal counterpart, i.e. the better it is differentiated, the more orderly and slower its growth. Thus histological examination allows tumour *grading* on the basis of the extent of differentiation. Attention is given to the nucleus (how abnormal it is and how often mitosis is observed), and the cytoplasm (the extent to which normal structures are seen).

For most of the common tumours, the pathologist divides them into descriptive categories: well differentiated, moderately differentiated and poorly differentiated. Undifferentiated tumours lack sufficient features to allow more than a broad classification, as do anaplastic tumours (see below under Classification of neoplasms).

Limitations of grading

Some tumours show a tight correlation between histological grading and behaviour, such that treatment is guided by this information. Cancer of the bladder is one of these. However, the tumour stage is of overriding importance. Some tumours (e.g. pancreatic islet) have a very variable rate of clinical progression, but uniform histology: grading in this circumstance is misleading if attempted. Other tumours vary considerably from one microscopic field to another: in general the outlook will depend upon the worst areas, but these could be missed without adequate sampling. Finally, the organ of origin is important: a well-differentiated cancer of the skin carries an excellent prognosis, whereas in the lung it may not.

GROWTH RATE OF CANCERS

As indicated in the section on carcinogenesis, there is usually a considerable time between initiation of a tumour and its clinical detection. Part of this time is taken by the process of becoming a cancer cell, and part by growing to sufficient size to be found. The latter can be measured as the time taken for it to double in diameter, its *doubling time*. A mass 1 mm in diameter would represent about one million cells: this could result from one cell, and each of its subsequent daughter cells, dividing 20 times. A word of caution is needed before theorising further. Once a tumour exceeds about 2 mm it is essential for it to have its own blood supply: this, together with other supporting structures, is the tumour *stroma*. In some tumours the stroma is very scanty, while in others it constitutes the majority of the mass. (The character of the stroma also influences what the tumour feels like on palpation; most breast cancers are hard because of abundant, dense stroma.) Thus calculations about how many cancer cells there are in a tumour of a certain size will be incorrect if they ignore the stroma.

Another consideration is that the clinical growth of a tumour will be the result of the balance between cell proliferation and loss. It will be influenced too by the growth fraction or proportion of cancer cells actually proliferating. Many cancer cells in a tumour cease to proliferate as they differentiate, or produce non-viable daughter cells. Furthermore, if the vascularity of the stroma is inadequate there will be necrosis.

Though a cancer produces an expanding mass, this is a reflection of loss of control of growth. The actual rate at which individual cancer cells divide is *slower* than comparable normal tissues. If there is a very sudden increase in the size of a tumour, it will probably reflect internal haemorrhage or fluid accumulation. (On the other hand, a slow-growing mass which begins to grow faster may have changed from benign to malignant.)

Observation of established clinical cancers has shown that doubling times vary widely, but average about 2 months. Leaving aside the question of whether this is true for the first 20 doublings to reach 1 mm size, it would require about a further 10 doublings (i.e. 20 months) to reach 1 cm diameter, at which point it might be detectable. Many tumours are 2 cm or more in diameter before they produce symptoms, so a considerable time has elapsed between the first emergence of a clone of cancer cells and the clinical disease. In comparison with that, the remainder of its course, if unchecked, is liable to be over after five or so more doublings. Metastatic deposits may be disseminated during the preclinical period, only to appear after removal of the primary. If the doubling time is considerably more than 2 months the whole process takes on a much longer time scale.

Bearing these matters in mind, there is no fixed length of disease-free interval that equates with a cure. However, for practical purposes 5 years disease free is tantamount to cure for many of the common tumours, with breast cancer as a notable exception. The earlier detection of a cancer at a minute size increases the possibility of removal before metastases develop. However, the tumour has been around for a long time. Prolonged postoperative survival in these patients may simply reflect 'earlier diagnosis' rather than 'longer survival', a phenomenon called *lead-time bias*.

Spontaneous regression of cancer

Occasionally a tumour may regress and disappear without treatment, though the original diagnosis could have been erroneous. Most of the reported cases are renal cell carcinoma, malignant melanoma and gestational choriocarcinoma. In all these instances, immunological mechanisms are thought to be responsible. Some cases of lymphoid tumours fluctuate in size, and may temporarily disappear, only to return later. In some cases of neuroblastoma, a primitive tumour of nerve cells, there is subsequent differentiation and growth ceases.

CLASSIFICATION OF NEOPLASMS

Table 17.2 lists examples of tumour nomenclature. In general, the names are built up from one part to describe the tissue type, and another to indicate its behaviour. All end in 'oma' to denote a lump, a suffix almost restricted to neoplasms, though a few other terms are in use, such as haematoma for an accumulation of blood. Most malignant tumours fall into the following broad categories:

- Carcinoma
- Sarcoma
- Lymphoma.

The majority of tumours arise from epithelium (surface lining cells). Benign ones are called *papilloma* or *adenoma*; malignant ones *carcinoma*, often with a prefix to give the cell type. Carcinoma is Greek for 'crab' but is used in a more restricted sense than cancer and applied only to epithelial malignancy, which makes up 75% of cancer.

Squamous epithelium lines the skin, where it is called epidermis, the upper aerodigestive tract (mouth, pharynx, larynx, oesophagus), anus, vagina and cervix. It is present in the bronchi if there is metaplasia. *Transitional cell epithelium*, (or *urothelium*) lines the renal pelvis, ureters and bladder.

Glandular (secretory) epithelium lines the gut from stomach to rectum, and forms the related secretory glands (salivary, pancreas, biliary tract and liver), endocrine glands (pituitary, thyroid, parathyroids, adrenals), kidneys, ovarian surface, endometrium and breast.

Sometimes the tumour name is combined with a description of shape or function. If a *cyst* is formed it

Table 17.2 Types of neoplasms

Type	Benign	Malignant
Epithelial		*Carcinoma*
Squamous	Papilloma	Squamous carcinoma
Transitional	Papilloma	Transitional cell carcinoma
Basal cell	Papilloma	Basal cell carcinoma
Glandular	Adenoma	Adenocarcinoma
Mesenchymal		*Sarcoma*
Smooth muscle	Leiomyoma	Leiomyosarcoma
Striated muscle	Rhabdomyoma	Rhabdomyosarcoma
Fat	Lipoma	Liposarcoma
Blood vessels	Angioma	Angiosarcoma
Bone	Osteoma	Osteosarcoma
Cartilage	Chondroma	Chondrosarcoma
Lymphoid tissue		*Lymphoma*
		Hodgkin's disease
		Non-Hodgkin lymphoma
Plasma cell		Multiple myeloma
White blood cells		Leukaemia
Intracranial and neural		
Supporting cells		Glioma
Meninges	Meningioma	
Cerebellum		Medulloblastoma
Retina		Retinoblastoma
Sympathetic nerve	Ganglioneuroma	Neuroblastoma
Pigment cells		
Skin or eye	Mole or naevus	Malignant melanoma
Gonad		
Germ cells	Dermoid cyst	Malignant teratoma
		Seminoma
Placenta		
	Hydatidiform mole	Choriocarcinoma

may be cystadenoma or cystadenocarcinoma, both of which are common in the ovary. Mucin-secreting variants would be mucinous cystadenoma.

Sarcoma denotes any tumour of mesenchymal origin (supporting structures). They are much less frequent than carcinoma. Metastasis from sarcomas is generally blood-borne, and few give rise to lymph node secondaries.

Lymphomas are malignant tumours of lymphoid cells; many are classified as Hodgkin's disease, leaving the remainder as non-Hodgkin lymphoma. Some are closely related to leukaemias (tumours of white blood cells).

There are many tumours that do not easily fit the guidelines mentioned: some are in Table 17.2 and others are referred to elsewhere in this book under the relevant organ.

Undifferentiated tumours

Some tumours lack obvious features to allow their identification or classification. An undifferentiated carcinoma or sarcoma cannot be ascribed to any subcategory. An anaplastic tumour could be carcinoma, lymphoma or sarcoma. As these different categories have major therapeutic consequences, it is important to attempt a more detailed diagnosis. Simple microscopy can now be supplemented by special staining procedures, many of which involve detecting cell components with antibodies. The presence of the leucocyte common antigen (CD45), B-cell (CD20) or T-cell (CD3) markers would indicate a lymphoma, whereas finding cytokeratins would suggest a carcinoma. As tumours have deranged genetic function there are sometimes unexpected findings. Electron microscopy sometimes helps. There are other approaches such as cytogenetics, which depends upon finding characteristic abnormalities of the chromosomes. These are most often loss or gain of part or the whole of a chromosome, or translocations in which two chromosomes break and are rejoined with the fragments on the wrong chromosome, for example t(11;22).

Most oncology centres arrange for many of their patients' tumours to be reviewed before treatment. Diagnosis and classification of rare or undifferentiated tumours form a considerable part of such work.

CHAPTER CONTENTS

18

Principles of radiobiology

Trevor J. McMillan

INTRODUCTION

Radiobiology underwent a huge revolution in the 1990s. It has progressed from the description of cellular and tissue response to radiation to the characterisation of genes and proteins that can influence these responses. The key development for the future will be the matching of these two areas, so this chapter aims to describe important features of the cellular response to ionising radiation incorporating some of the recent developments in our understanding of the underlying molecular mechanisms. Further advances will need to introduce this new understanding into clinical radiotherapy. There is every hope that we will be able to use this information to aid individualisation of radiotherapy in terms both of fractionation schedule and the use of effective radiosensitisers. In addition, the combination of radiation and specific gene therapy approaches holds promise for the development of novel treatments that are effective and specific. This is clearly a vast field, so this chapter will concentrate largely on cellular and tumoral response to low LET (linear energy transfer) radiation. Only brief coverage of normal tissue effects and particle irradiation is included.

RADIATION-INDUCED SUBCELLULAR DAMAGE

Ionising radiation transfers energy to the molecules with which it interacts. At the atomic level this can lead to ejection of an electron which can then react with other atoms, causing secondary ionisations. The main product of this process in a cell is an ionised water molecule H_2O^+ which can interact with another water molecule to form OH radicals. These OH radicals have a very high reactivity. Reducing species, $H^{\bullet}$ and e^-_{aq}, are also formed. All these reactive species can go on to damage other molecules, notably DNA, in the so-called *indirect effect*. *Direct damage* is the product of ionisations within the chromatin although the distinction between direct and indirect damage is not always clear, as the close proximity of water to DNA may result in electrons produced in the DNA-associated water directly causing ionisations in the DNA.

Radiation causes a wide range of types of damage in DNA, including strand breaks, base or sugar damage and crosslinks between macromolecules (i.e. DNA–DNA or DNA–protein crosslinks) (Table 18.1). In general it is considered that the DNA double-strand break (DSB) is the most critical for the lethal effects of radiation. The evidence for this is threefold:

- DSB levels vary in parallel with changes in cell killing in most situations.
- One DSB is lethal to yeast.
- Enzymatically produced DSBs (produced by inserting DNA-cutting restriction enzymes into cells) give the same patterns of chromosome damage and lethality as radiation.

However, not all DSB are the same, as the chemical nature of the ends of the DNA fragments and the number of DNA bases that overlap can vary considerably, as can the proximity to other types of lesion. This interaction of lesions has been suggested to be of critical importance to the reparability of the damage and it is relevant because low LET radiation produces ionisations in clusters in a cell so that several lesions may be formed in a stretch of a few nucleotides in the DNA strand (so-called *local multiply damaged sites*, LMDS).

Chromosome and chromatid aberrations

An important product of the DNA damage is observed as *chromosome aberrations* when cells are irradiated in the G_1 phase of the cell cycle or *chromatid aberrations* when cells are irradiated after the DNA replication phase. Frank breaks in chromosomes are commonly induced, and aberrations involving breakage and rejoining of chromosome fragments (e.g. translocations and ring formations) are observed in many irradiated cells. There is a commonly found direct relationship between cell death and chromosome aberration frequency, leading to the conclusion that such damage is an important aspect of the radiation-induced killing of many cells. Chromosome damage also has important usage in environmental radiobiology in that it is a very sensitive indicator of environmental radiation exposure.

Table 18.1 Types and frequency of radiation-induced damage

Type of damage	Number per Gy per cell
DNA double-strand breaks	40
DNA single-strand breaks	1000
DNA–protein crosslinks	150
DNA–DNA crosslinks	30
Base damage	2000
Sugar damage	1500

RADIATION-INDUCED CELL KILLING

At the heart of the biological effects of radiation is the ability to limit the proliferation of cells that would normally divide and produce several daughter cells. In some normal tissues the key targets are the stem cells that form the proliferative driving force of a tissue in that they have an unlimited ability to divide. In tumours there may also be a subset of cells that make the major contribution to tumour growth. The directing of a cell down a differentiation pathway or its existence in a region of low nutrient supply may take cells out of this proliferating compartment (Fig. 18.1).

Clonogenic assays

The evaluation of the loss of reproductive integrity of these cells is best made using so-called clonogenic assays where the surrogate of a stem cell is the clonogenic cell, which is defined as a cell that will produce a colony of 50 cells or more under the defined experimental conditions. This threshold represents an ability to undergo 5–6 cell divisions and is used to eliminate those cells that are undergoing differentiation or that

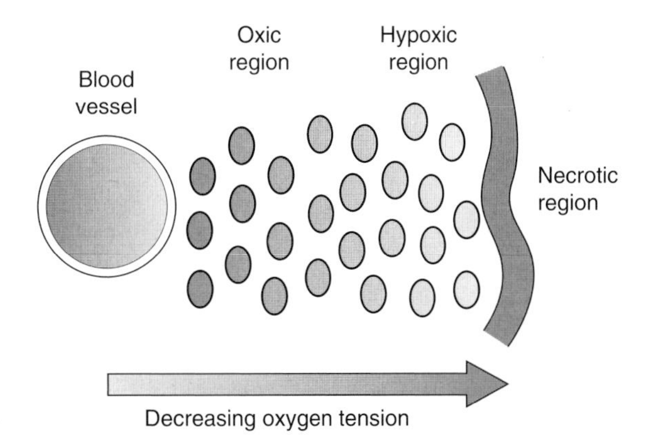

Fig. 18.1 Oxygen gradient away from a vessel. Oxygen generally diffuses a distance of around 200 μm from a blood vessel. Beyond this distance, viable hypoxic cells are first encountered, then hypoxic regions containing dead cells form necrotic regions.

have a limited ability to divide when damaged. The basic experimental procedure is to irradiate the cells, place them in appropriate growth conditions (e.g. in tissue culture nutrient medium in tissue culture flasks or dishes) and allow them to proliferate for several days (7–21 days depending on the proliferation rate of the particular cells) before counting the number of cell colonies that have formed. *The plating efficiency of each group is defined as the ratio of the number of colonies formed and the number of cells seeded.* The efficacy of each radiation dose is then related to the untreated cells by the calculation of the surviving fraction, which is:

$$\text{Surviving fraction (SF)} = \frac{\text{Plating efficiency of treated cells}}{\text{Plating efficiency of untreated cells}}$$

Radiation-induced cell killing is exponential, rather than arithmetic, in nature so the surviving fractions are plotted on semilogarithmic axes to produce so-called *cell survival curves*. Examples of these are shown in Figure 18.2.

The basic shape of these cell survival curves is linear on a semilog plot and for some cell types this does seem to be the true shape. However, for other cell types there is either a *shoulder* on the curve (i.e. a region at low dose where an increment of radiation dose has little or no effect on cell killing) or the curve may be continuously bending. Several mathematical equations exist to describe these curves, including the *multi-target equation*, the *multi-target with single hit equation* and the *linear quadratic equation* (Fig. 18.2). In some cases it has been a matter of personal choice and history that has dictated which equation is used but it is apparent with human tumour cells at least that the initial shoulder is not absolutely flat so that a simple multi-target equation is not appropriate. Fractionation experiments in tumours, normal tissues and tumour cells in culture have produced data that can be accurately described by the linear quadratic equation and hence this is the most commonly used. Many attempts have been made to link these equations to models of radiation action and killing and while these have been useful in proposing hypotheses that have been approached experimentally, in most cases it is more important that the clinical oncologist just recognises the parameters of these equations, has a knowledge of the significance of the range of values of these parameters and can apply them to clinical questions such as those that arise during the derivation of fractionation regimes.

The widest use of the parameters of the linear quadratic equation has been in the description of the dependence of normal tissue response on changes in fraction size. The relationship between *dose per fraction* and *isoeffective total dose* (or *tolerance dose*) is steeper for late-responding tissues than for early-responding normal tissues. In other words, late-responding tissues are more sensitive to changes in dose per fraction. An equation based on the linear quadratic model can be used to describe such relationships and the slope of the curves is determined by the α/β ratio. In general, early-responding tissues have high α/β ratios (around 7–20 Gy) while late-responding tissues have lower α/β ratios of around 0.5–6 Gy. The importance of these values is that they can be used to calculate isoeffect relationships in radiotherapy, and calculations of parameters like the *biologically effective dose* (BED) are important when manipulating fractionation regimes. The BED in effect is the dose required to produce a given biological effect when the radiation is given as an infinitely large number of very small fractions or as a single dose at extremely low dose rate. For a given treatment, the BED can be calculated if the α/β ratio of the dose-limiting tissue and the tolerance dose for a given fractionation regime are known. Using the BED, the relationship between tolerance dose and dose per fraction can be worked out for new fractionation regimes.

The curves in Figure 18.2 are representative of those produced when cells are irradiated over a time of just a few minutes. When irradiation time is lengthened to a period of hours or even days, then the shape of these curves changes and the cells are generally more resistant to treatment (Fig. 18.3). When the treatment is given in vivo then the *dose rate effects* are influenced by the same 'Rs' of radiotherapy as a fractionated regime (see below). In vitro some of these effects are still seen and the trend in Figure 18.3 is usually explained by the cells' ability to repair damage during a protracted treatment and, with irradiation times of several hours, the proliferation of cells during the irradiation. Such effects acquire clinical significance in brachytherapy in which radioactive implants are placed within a tumour. This approach to treatment is largely considered because of the geometry of the dose distribution. The tumour cells close to the source receive a high dose while the more remote normal tissues have a much reduced exposure. In addition, the adjacent cells are treated at high dose rate whereas with increasing distance away from the source the dose rate decreases. Clearly this has advantages for reducing normal tissue effects; however, this combined effect of dose and dose rate can mean that some tumour cells escape effective treatment.

Historically, radiation has been considered to kill cells largely by means of a 'mitotic cell death' in which proliferating cells undergo a general breakdown (necrosis)

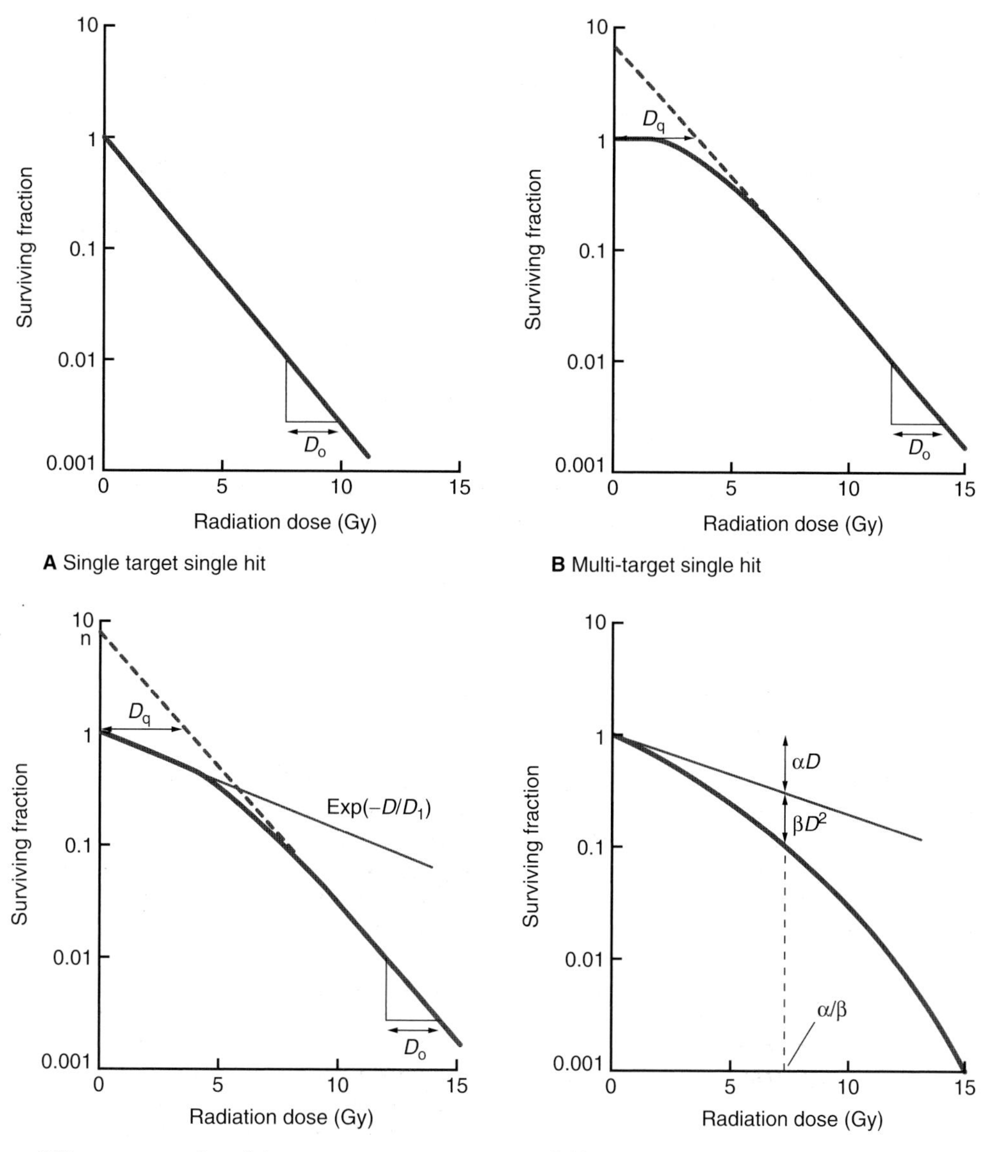

Fig. 18.2 Cell survival curves. The basic nature of a cell survival curve is that it is linear on a semilogarithmic plot **A**; however, variations are commonly observed. The multi-target model assumes a linear portion of the curve preceded by a 'shoulder' in which increases in radiation dose have no effect **B**. The parameters of such a curve are the slope of the curve, D_o (the mean lethal dose, which is the dose to reduce the surviving fraction to 1/e), the extrapolation number, *n*, which is the point at which the extrapolated exponential part of the curve crosses the 0 Gy axis, and the quasithreshold dose, D_q, which is the point at which the extrapolated exponential portion of the curve crosses the 100% survival level. The multi-target with single hit equation **C** has the same parameters as B except that the shoulder has a non-zero slope, D_1. The linear quadratic equation **D** is: Surviving fraction = $\exp(-\alpha D - \beta D^2)$. This is a continuous bending curve, the 'bendiness' of which is dictated by the α/β ratio.

when they attempt to divide with radiation-damaged chromosomes. This holds true for many cells but it is clear that some cells, notably those in some normal tissues, die with apoptotic morphology. *Apoptosis* is a form of 'programmed cell death' that was identified in the early 1970s owing to a characteristic morphology of the

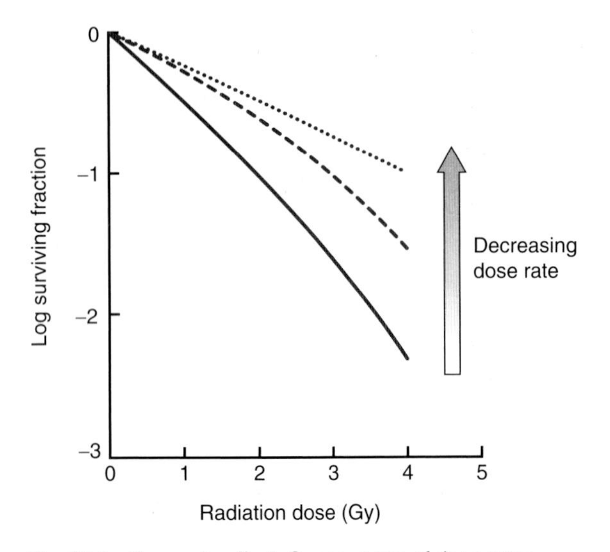

Fig. 18.3 Dose rate effect. Over a range of dose rates (e.g. 0.01–1 Gy per minute) the cellular survival increases as the dose rate is decreased.

chromatin and membranes (Table 18.2). It is now recognised as being the outcome of a sequence of biochemical signals that result in the activation of a series of enzymes (caspases) that degrade cellular proteins and at least one DNA endonuclease that cuts DNA in regularly repeated regions that are not protected by nucleosomal proteins. The latter results in the formation of a ladder pattern when the DNA is separated in an agarose gel. Cells of the haemopoietic system often undergo this classic apoptosis when irradiated, as do cells of the intestine. The significance of this is that apoptosis is under specific genetic control and therefore that susceptibility to radiation-induced apoptosis may be capable of manipulation.

THE OXYGEN EFFECT

Oxygen is important to the effects of irradiation. Cells that are irradiated in the absence of oxygen are much more resistant to radiation than those irradiated in oxygen (Fig. 18.4A). This is due to the oxygen molecules reacting with free radicals to produce chemically unrepairable peroxy radicals ($R^{\bullet} + O_2 \rightarrow RO^{\bullet}_2$). Thus, in effect, oxic cells suffer more DNA damage (Fig. 18.4B). The degree of sensitisation by oxygen in often quoted as an *oxygen enhancement ratio* (OER), which is the ratio of doses needed to produce a given biological effect in the presence or absence of oxygen (Fig. 18.4). For most cells and tissues the OER has a value of around 2.5–3.

The decrease in sensitivity only becomes noticeable at partial pressures of oxygen below around 10 mmHg, which means that most well-vascularised normal tissues (partial pressure of oxygen around 40 mmHg) are not affected by the oxygen effect. However, the vascular supply in tumours usually is not adequate to maintain normal oxygenated conditions for all cells. Oxygen diffusion within a tumour is limited to around 200 μm (Fig. 18.1), so that any tumour with a diameter larger than 400 μm will need to develop a vascular system if the centre of the tumour is to remain oxic. The importance of angiogenesis factors that stimulate and control vascular growth is therefore apparent and the potential usefulness of anti-angiogenesis treatments is explained. Nevertheless, even in a growing tumour, it is not unusual to find a hypoxic fraction of around 10–20% because of the inadequacies of the tumour vascular system. These deficiencies are due to the low production of new vessels leading to chronic hypoxia and physiological defects in the new vessels which mean that they can be closed down for a short time and then open up again. This variation in flow through vessels leads to what has been called *acute hypoxia*. Recent experiments, which have been made possible by the invention of sensitive oxygen probes that can be used in tumours, have shown that the proportion of the tumour that is deficient in oxygen can have an important influence on the success of radiotherapy.

The recognition of the importance of hypoxia in radiotherapy has led to many attempts to circumvent this problem. It has been observed that patients undergoing pelvic irradiation for cervical cancer have a worse prognosis if their pretreatment haemoglobin

Table 18.2 A comparison of some the morphological features of apoptosis and necrosis

Necrosis	Apoptosis
Cells swell	Cells shrink
Mitochondria dilate and other organelles dissolve	Organelles retain definition for a long time
Plasma membranes rupture	Cells dissociate from surrounding cells
Nuclear changes 'unremarkable'	Chromatin condensation and 'regular' DNA degradation

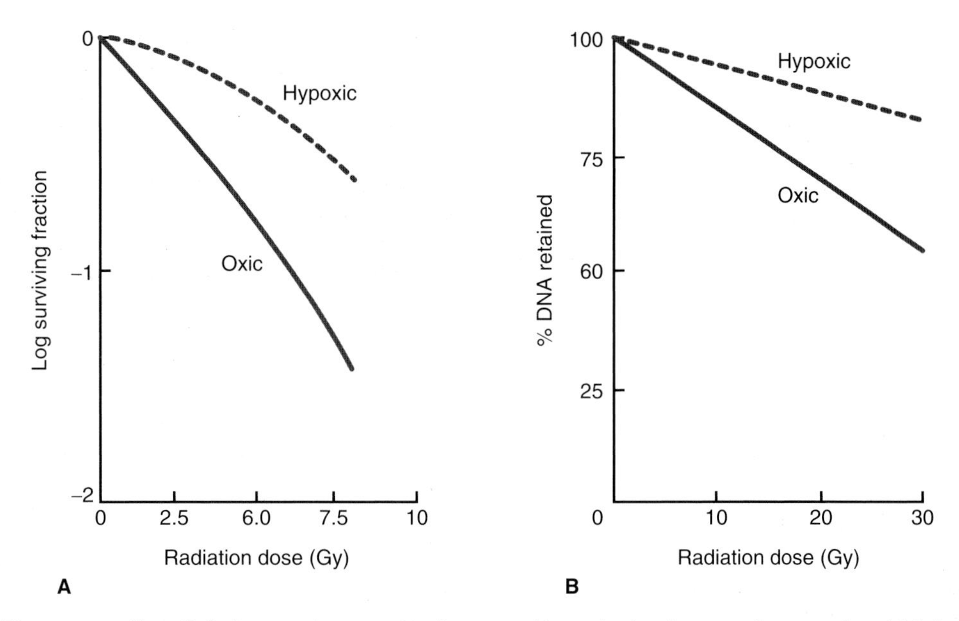

Fig. 18.4 The oxygen effect. Cells have an increased resistance to X-rays in the absence of oxygen **A** and this is largely dictated by a reduction in the amount of damage present immediately after irradiation **B**. **A** shows data from a clonogenic assay. In **B** % DNA retained is inversely related to the amount of DNA strand breakage in gel electrophoresis assays.

level is below 12 g/dl so that it is important to make sure that patients are not anaemic when they start radiotherapy. Some clinical trials have demonstrated a benefit in having the patient breath oxygen at up to three times atmospheric pressure (*hyperbaric oxygen*, HBO) during irradiation. In head and neck cancer, for example, local control and survival have been seen to be 20 percentage points higher at 2 years in the HBO group compared with controls. Such trials demonstrate clearly the importance of hypoxia, though HBO has not been widely adopted, largely for technical reasons.

Major efforts have been directed at developing chemicals that can sensitise hypoxic cells. The largest group of these is the electron-affinic sensitisers which in principle mimic the effect of oxygen and so have no sensitising effect on normal tissues. This general principle of increasing the effect on a tumour without affecting the normal tissue is clearly fundamental to all attempted improvements in radiotherapy and is covered by the concept of a *therapeutic gain*. The most widely studied hypoxic cell sensitiser is misonidazole, a member of the nitroimidazole family. This compound sensitises cells in vitro and was shown to be effective in experimental tumour models, although it was less effective in fractionated regimes than after single-dose treatment. Unfortunately, clinical trials did not prove encouraging, probably because of dose-limiting neurotoxicity, and this raised doubt as to the general validity of this approach. However, improvements have been sought in the toxicity of the sensitising compounds and the ability to identify tumours with significant hypoxic fractions has restored faith in the potential for this approach. One potentially fruitful avenue centres on the recognition that cells can react to hypoxia by switching on specific genes. This will not only allow the identification of hypoxic cells but may allow the specific targeting of hypoxic cells in gene therapy approaches. In addition, the use of drugs that are specifically activated in hypoxic areas is likely to yield beneficial results.

REPAIR OF RADIATION-INDUCED DNA DAMAGE

Many of the important recent advances in our understanding of the cellular response to ionising radiation have come in the field of DNA repair. Several genes and their products involved in the repair of radiation-induced DNA damage have been identified and characterised (Table 18.3). In particular, three of the proteins involved in the rejoining of DNA double-strand breaks have been identified through the characterisation of mutant cells that are sensitive to radiation. The emerging picture of DSB rejoining is that two proteins, Ku70 and Ku80, bind to the ends of the DSB and

Table 18.3 Examples of genes that have a significant influence on the radiosensitivity of mammalian cells

Gene(s)	Proposed function
Ku70, Ku80, DNAPKcs	Attachment of ends of DNA double strand breaks. Non-homologous end rejoining. Initiation of signal pathway?
XRCC2, XRCC3, RAD51	Homologous recombination repair
ATM (ataxia telangiectasia mutated)	Signalling presence of DNA damage?
TP53	Signalling presence of DNA damage?
NBS1 (Nijmegen breakage syndrome 1)	Non-homologous end rejoining? Homologous recombination repair
DNA ligase IV	Non-homologous end rejoining

then recruit a third protein, the catalytic subunit of the DNA-dependent protein kinase (DNAPKcs) to the site of the break (Fig. 18.5). This complex of the three proteins is activated in this way and it is believed that it then initiates signalling pathways that initiate the repair process, though the exact mechanism of this is not known. The importance of this process is demonstrated by the fact that cells deficient in any one of these three components have a reduced ability to rejoin DSB and are extremely sensitive to the killing effects of radiation.

In yeast cells it is clear that DNA repair is most efficient when combined with a slowing down of the cell cycle so that the chromosomes do not attempt to replicate or divide when they are damaged. In mammalian cells this also seems to be the case, with a delay in DNA synthesis acting as a protective mechanism against mutations while a delay in mitosis reduces the persistence of lethal chromosome damage. The cell's ability to make these adjustments comes from the machinery it has in place to regulate the cell cycle and ensure that the DNA synthesis phase and mitotic phase always occur in the right order and at the right time relative to the other cell cycle phases (see Fig. 18.7). The key to this lies in the presence of *cell cycle checkpoints*, which are enzymatic pathways that link particular requirements (e.g. growth factor levels, intact DNA, intact mitotic spindle) to the cell cycle drivers, the cyclins and cyclin-dependent kinases.

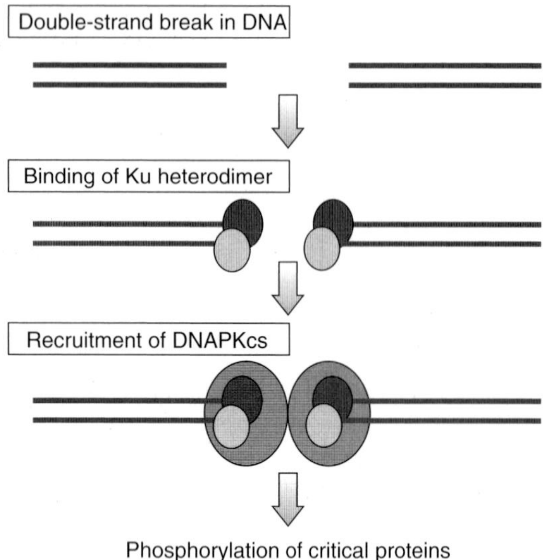

Fig. 18.5 DNA-dependent protein kinase (DNAPK) is a complex of three proteins, Ku70, Ku80 and DNAPKcs. The Ku proteins bind to DNA ends, recruit DNAPKcs and this is believed to initiate a signal pathway and/or recruit repair enzymes to the DNA double-strand break. These are the initial stages of the non-homologous end-rejoining repair pathway.

THE 5 RS OF FRACTIONATED RADIOTHERAPY

The efficacy of fractionated radiotherapy is clearly determined by the physical and technical aspects of radiation delivery and the biological consequences to the tumour and normal tissue. Building on the seminal suggestion of Withers, it is now recognised that there are five factors that are highly influential in dictating the biological response of the tumour. These are the 5 Rs of radiotherapy (Fig. 18.6). Two of these, recovery and repopulation, lead to a decrease in response when treatment is prolonged, while two, reassortment and reoxygenation, are beneficial in a fractionated regime. The fifth, radiosensitivity, is the baseline on which the other modifications work.

Radiosensitivity

It is now well recognised that the inherent sensitivity of tumour cells is not the same in all tumours. Variation exists between tumours of the same type taken from different patients and between tumours of different pathological type. In addition there are some reports of variation in radiosensitivity of the cells

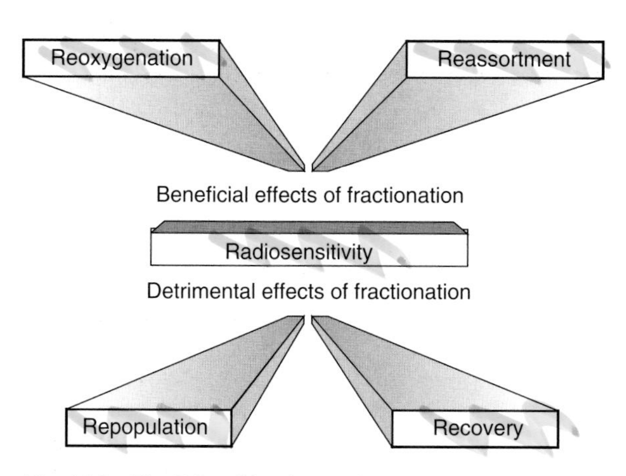

Fig. 18.6 The 5 Rs of fractionated radiotherapy dictate the effect of an extended radiation treatment on a tumour.

within a tumour, although how common this is and its importance are not known. The significance of variation between tumours was first suggested when it was recognised that the clinical responsiveness of different tumour types relates well to the in vitro radiation sensitivity of cells taken from those tumours. Further, there are data to suggest that within a given tumour type the sensitivity of the tumour cells correlates with clinical outcome. It should also be noted that there is variation in the sensitivity of normal cells between individuals. At its extreme this is seen in the rare syndrome ataxia telangiectasia where significant tissue sensitivity to radiation is associated with a sensitivity of the cells from these individuals. In addition, there is now evidence that there is variation within the non-syndromic population.

In tumour cells the theoretical basis of the importance of *intrinsic radiosensitivity* is well demonstrated when one compares the overall effectiveness of a fractionated regime involving multiple 2 Gy fractions. The surviving fraction after a single dose of 2 Gy (SF_2) can vary in the range 0.2–0.6 and if this is maintained for each fraction then a tumour made up of 10^9 tumour cells (around 1 cm^3) would be eliminated after around 13 fractions in the sensitive tumour ($SF_2 = 0.2$) but around 38 fractions if the SF_2 was 0.6. The latter is beyond the total treatment usually given and therefore effectively reflects a lack of curability of a tumour with this degree of cellular radioresistance.

The mechanisms underlying variation in radiosensitivity are diverse. There is evidence to suggest that tumour cells differ in:

1. Their ability to reduce the amount of DNA damage inflicted by radiation
2. Their ability to rejoin DNA double strand breaks, and
3. The fidelity of their repair processes.

Radiation sensitivity has also been associated with differences in apoptotic potential and the ability to regulate cell cycle progression in response to DNA damage (through the activity of cell cycle checkpoints) in some cell systems. The characterisation of these processes has been greatly facilitated by the isolation of genes involved in DNA repair and other genes that can influence the cellular sensitivity to radiation (Table 18.3).

Repopulation

The prolongation of radiotherapy over several weeks means that the cells within a tumour are able to proliferate during treatment. Even if this is at the cell's normal doubling rate, this can lead to an increase in the number of cells that the radiation needs to kill but, in addition, there is evidence that repopulation can actually be accelerated in the treated tumours so that this effect can be significant. A clear decrease in efficacy of radiotherapy with increased overall treatment time as seen in the analysis of Withers et al (1988), is indicative of this consequence of tumour cell proliferation. It has been estimated that every day beyond around 3–4 weeks is equivalent to a loss in radiation dose of about 0.6 Gy. The mechanism underlying accelerated repopulation is not clear but may well be due to the removal of dead cells resulting in an increase in nutrient supply to the surviving cells. If there is a situation where cell loss is reduced, then it is believed that tumour cells may achieve their '*potential doubling time*' (Tpot) which is the extreme situation when cell loss is zero. It is clear that radiation can also affect the production of growth factors and their receptors but the significance of this to repopulation is not known. Accelerated radiotherapy protocols in which the overall treatment time is reduced have been developed to address this proliferation issue and in some cases this is proving effective.

Reoxygenation

As described above, a lack of oxygen can severely limit the cytotoxicity of radiation, and the presence of hypoxic cells in a tumour can therefore be limiting to the success of radiotherapy. One positive aspect of fractionating radiotherapy is that cells that survive one treatment because of a hypoxic environment may become reoxygenated before the next treatment. Again this is a result of the loss of the killed cells leading to a better oxygen supply to the survivors.

Reassortment

Cells alter their sensitivity to radiation as they progress through the cell cycle. Figure 18.7 demonstrates that cells in mitosis, for example, can be twice as sensitive as those at the end of the DNA synthesis phase. A single dose of radiation therefore preferentially kills cells at particular stages of the cell cycle. If there were no cell cycle progression, cells exposed to a second dose would be largely radioresistant. Although cells do not progress normally after treatment because of the activity of cell cycle checkpoints that limit passage through some points in the cell cycle if the cell is damaged, there is usually some progression in between fractions so that cells are reassorted through the various stages of the cycle. This is clearly an advantage of a fractionated course of radiotherapy.

Recovery

The phenomena of *sublethal damage recovery* (SLDR) and *potentially lethal damage recovery* (PLDR) have practical definitions in that they are reflected in the decrease in cell kill when treatment is prolonged (see dose rate effect above) or fractionated (SLDR) or held in a non-proliferative state (PLDR). Both of these are believed to have a basis in DNA repair capacity although there is some evidence that they do not reflect the same repair processes. This is detrimental to a course of radiotherapy treatment.

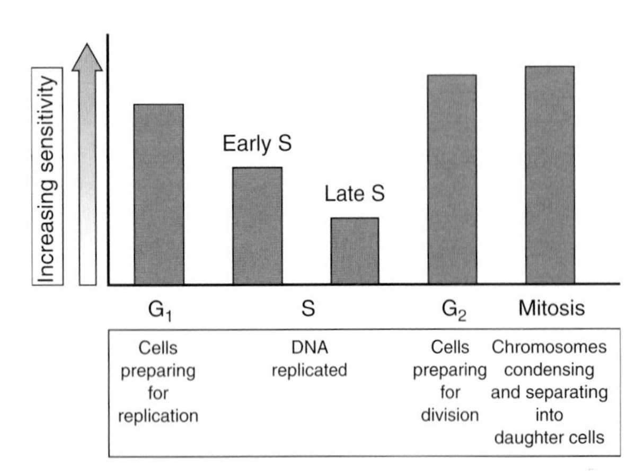

Fig. 18.7 Cell cycle variation in radiosensitivity. The active cell cycle is made up of four primary phases: in G_1 the cells prepare for division, the DNA is synthesised in S, in G_2 the cells prepare for chromosome separation, and in mitosis the chromosomes are separated into daughter cells. Each of these phases has a distinctive radiosensitivity.

INDIVIDUALISATION OF TREATMENT

As we learn to recognise the critical elements of tumour and tissue responses to radiotherapy it is hoped that there will be methods made available that will allow the outcome of radiotherapy to predicted with some precision. The prediction of tumour response could influence whether radiotherapy in any form is indicated for an individual patient. The effect of intrinsic cellular sensitivity has been described above and there are some studies to suggest that a gross measure of cellular sensitivity can predict outcome in some, but not all, tumour types. The search is now on for molecular measures that can substitute for clonogenic assays in this type of analysis in order that the sensitivity information can be available to the clinical oncologist before treatment begins. The expressions of the genes listed in Table 18.3 are obvious candidates for this.

The prediction of tumour factors that can predict other members of the group of 5 Rs should allow patient-specific changes in fractionation schedule and the use of specific sensitisers. The measurement of tumour growth kinetics is an obvious example of this where the speed of growth should, in theory, aid decisions about accelerated fractionation regimes. Early use of measures of proliferation (e.g. the potential doubling time, Tpot) suggested that fast-growing tumour did respond better to accelerated treatment but recent data have been less encouraging. As detailed above there are some indications that the level of hypoxia in a tumour can be predictive of outcome. Even if this is not true for all tumours, tests of hypoxic fraction will be useful in identifying patients that would benefit from hypoxic cell sensitisers.

The approaches outlined above place the emphasis on the tumour but there is currently an increased stress on the normal tissue response. The rationale for this is essentially that radiotherapy regimes are largely dictated by the response of the normal tissues, so by minimising early and, in particular, late effects on these tissues the tumour treatment can be intensified. The difficulty with this approach is that normal tissue reactions are highly complex. The radiosensitivity of normal cells has been found to vary between individuals and this can account for a major part of the overall population variation in normal tissue reactions.

However, the use of a straightforward clonogenic assay on normal cells has had mixed success in its ability to predict clinical outcome. The nature of other aspects of the radiation response, namely expression of growth factors and apoptosis, is now being explored extensively in this context and the discovery of an assay that can predict normal tissue response remains a major goal for radiobiology.

CHAPTER CONTENTS

19

Effects of radiation on normal tissues

Ian Kunkler

The radiobiological events described in Chapter 18, when ionising radiation passes through tissue, result in damage to DNA, mainly through the effects of free radicals. The pathological effects of ionising radiation on cells are due to chemical changes which, although involving only a small part of the DNA molecule, cause major or irreparable damage.

While we understand much about the molecular events following irradiation, it is uncertain how they are converted to changes at a tissue level. Damage to DNA may result in immediate cell death or, at the next mitosis, be fully repaired or result in a permanent change in genotype which is transmitted to future generations of cells. Which of these outcomes is effected will depend on the dose delivered and the radiosensitivity of the cell. Low-dose irradiation is most likely to cause a change in the genotype, since it may be below the threshold for cell death. The abnormal genotype may therefore survive in subsequent cell divisions.

The dose given will influence this outcome, as will the radiosensitivity of the cell. Tissue and organ changes will reflect the overall reactions in the component parts.

Acute cellular effects

The most marked acute effects of radiation on normal cells will be on those with the highest mitotic activity (e.g. gut and bone marrow). The renewal of the cell population from a pool of less-differentiated cells is stopped either permanently or temporarily, while the process of cell loss continues. There is also damage to the vascular lining (endothelium), which results in protein and fluid leakage.

Chronic cellular effects

The pathogenesis of the chronic cellular changes of irradiation is less well understood than the acute ones.

The relative importance of different factors is contested. The lining of collagen is exposed when the vascular endothelium is damaged. Exposed collagen may act as a focus for platelets to gather and thrombosis to be initiated. Vascular endothelial cell loss will result in exposure of the underlying collagen. This will prompt platelet adherence and the formation of thrombus, which is then incorporated into the vessel wall. The intimal lining of vessel wall proliferates. This process is known as *endarteritis obliterans*. Chronic vascular insufficiency may lead to atrophy and fibrosis of the tissues supplied.

Recovery from radiation damage

Recovery from the cellular effects of radical therapeutic irradiation is very limited. The doses given are often close to the tissue tolerance of the particular organ. For this reason radical irradiation is not generally repeated for fear of precipitating tissue breakdown (radionecrosis). It may be possible to repeat palliative courses of radiotherapy (e.g. 30 Gy in 10 daily fractions) as long as the combined dosage remains within tissue tolerance.

Tumour induction

Ionising radiation causes tumours, probably due to mutation in DNA. This is well documented for relatively high doses, but at low dose there is more uncertainty. The risk of malignant transformation and dose is nearly linear. However, as the dose increases, the proportion of cells lethally irradiated also rises. The surviving fraction able to be transformed to malignant cells accordingly decreases. It is tempting but not necessarily justified to extrapolate from the data on tumour induction at high dose to that at low dose. Unfortunately the numbers of tumours induced at low dose are too small to establish a threshold below which neoplastic transformation is unlikely to occur. The role of ionising radiation in carcinogenesis is discussed in Chapter 17.

RADIATION TOLERANCE OF NORMAL TISSUES

The purpose of radiotherapy planning is to confine the X-rays to the tumour and minimise the dose to normal tissues. This is clearly easier for superficial than deep-seated tumours. Inevitably some normal tissue is included in the target volume to cover microscopic spread beyond the visible limits of the tumour. There are definite limits to the amount of radiation that normal tissues will tolerate. This maximum dose of radiation that a tissue will tolerate is referred to as the *tolerance dose*. Exceeding this dose may result in major, and sometimes fatal complications. The tolerance dose will vary with the type and amount of tissue irradiated, the quality of radiation and its fractionation.

Radiosensitivity

The term 'radiosensitivity' means the relative vulnerability of cells to damage by ionising radiation. Radiosensitivity is measurable in cell survival curves (p. 288), using the capacity to reproduce as the end-point. Both normal and malignant tissues have different sensitivities, mainly determined by their different growth rates. This is the basis of the Law of Bergonié and Tribondeau (1904): 'The biological action of Roentgen rays is greater, the higher the reproductive activity of the cell, the longer the period of its mitosis and the less the degree of differentiation.' They studied the testis of the rat and found the radiosensitivity of the rapidly dividing germ cells to be high. It is no surprise that the cells of a malignant tumour of the germ cells of the testis (seminoma) are also very radiosensitive. By contrast, a slow-growing soft tissue sarcoma shares the low sensitivity of its parent tissue. Radiosensitivity is discussed further on page 293.

The various tissues and organs have a wide spectrum of radiosensitivity. The highly sensitive are readily damaged by fairly low doses. The most radioresistant can withstand much higher doses without obvious ill-effects.

High sensitivity

- The epithelium of the skin (epidermis)
- The epithelial lining (inner surface) of the alimentary tract
- The cells in the bone marrow that produce the blood cells, i.e. the haemopoietic tissue
- The reproductive cells of the ovary and testis.

Intermediate sensitivity

- Liver, kidney, lung and many glands (e.g. thyroid).

Low sensitivity

- Muscle, bone, connective and nervous tissue.

RADIATION EFFECTS ON INDIVIDUAL TISSUES

The skin

This is a subject of prime importance since we are bound to irradiate the skin in most treatments, even if it is not the site of the tumour. Before the development of megavoltage irradiation with its skin-sparing property, the tolerance of the skin to orthovoltage irradiation was often a limiting factor in delivering radical radiotherapy to deep-seated tumours. Skin reactions are still of fundamental importance. Inappropriately marked skin reactions should alert the clinician to the possibility of an error in the calculation of the dose to be delivered or in the calibration of the output of the treatment machine.

Microscopic alterations

The changes in the skin reflect its composition from epithelium, connective tissue and blood vessels. Epidermis will suffer the consequence of cessation of mitosis, with desquamation and hair loss. Provided enough stem cells survive, hair will regrow, and any defects in epidermal coverage can be re-epithelialised. The regenerated epidermis will lack rete ridges and adnexa. Damage to keratinocytes and melanocytes results in melanin deposition in the dermis where it is picked up by phagocytic cells; these tend to remain in the skin and result in local hyperpigmentation. Some fibroblasts in the dermis will be killed, while others are at risk of an inability to divide, or to function correctly. As a consequence, the dermis is thinned, and histology shows bizarre, enlarged fibroblast nuclei.

The vessels show various changes depending on their size. Endothelial cell loss or damage is the probable underlying factor; they show vacuolation. Small and thin-walled vessels will leak fluid and protein, and mimic the inflammatory response; in the long term, they can be permanently dilated and tortuous (telangiectatic). Larger vessels develop proliferation of the intima and may permanently impair blood flow.

In summary, the skin is at first reddened with desquamation, and subsequently shows pigmentation. Later it is thinned with telangiectasia; if damage is too severe, it will break down and ulcerate (radionecrosis).

Acute skin reaction

The characteristic acute reaction on skin is erythema (Greek for 'redness'). Before the roentgen and the rad were defined, the 'erythema dose' was actually used as the measure of radiation dosage. In the orthovoltage era, skin reactions were a very useful guide in actual treatment and could give warning signals to the therapist. In a conventionally fractionated course of radical radiotherapy (e.g. over 4 weeks), there is an interval of time (latent period) before erythema appears. This is because the reaction is an inflammatory one following the breakdown of cells in the basal layer, the most actively dividing cells in the epidermis.

Radiodermatitis

Radiodermatitis may be acute or chronic.

Acute. This occurs typically in patients undergoing a radical course of radiotherapy (e.g. postoperative chest wall irradiation for breast cancer).

Chronic. This includes late effects seen in: (1) patients—months or years after treatment; (2) workers exposed to radiation (usually in industry) or patients accumulating small doses over many years without passing through the acute reaction.

Stages of the acute reaction. The acute reaction to conventionally fractionated radiotherapy follows a fairly predictable series of stages. The time at which each occurs will depend on the energy, dose and fractionation. Typically, during a 4–5-week course of chest-wall irradiation following mastectomy for breast cancer, no skin changes are observed during the first fortnight, apart from faint erythema.

At about 14 days, hair loss (epilation) occurs. During the third week the main erythema develops. Initially this is punctuate but then coalesces. The skin is warm, red and oedematous. Dusky pigmentation is common. Itching and discomfort are reported by the patient. During the fourth and fifth weeks of irradiation, dry desquamation occurs, sometimes progressing to moist desquamation. In most desquamation the skin surface is shed, with inflammatory and serous discharge. Regeneration of new skin from the periphery of the irradiated fields or from small areas within the irradiated fields starts about a week after the end of irradiation. Recovery is normally complete by the third week after treatment. Sweat gland function is normally resumed within 2 weeks of the end of treatment. However, the secretion of sebaceous glands usually does not recover, even if most desquamation has not occurred. Hair begins to regrow by about 2 months after treatment. Its colour may be darker in patients with fair or white hair.

The skin reaction increases with both dose and the area irradiated. In practice high skin doses for curative purposes are normally confined to skin cancers where the field diameter is small (2–4 cm). For the cure of skin tumours, the skin is treated to its tolerance. If this is done, radiation-induced skin necrosis will occur in about 5% of cases. It is more likely to occur in treated skin that has been previously damaged and its blood supply compromised, and with increasing field size.

Different parts of the body vary in their skin sensitivity to radiation. The more sensitive areas include those subject to moisture and friction (axilla, groin, vulva, anus) and those with a poor blood supply (back of the hand, back and sole of the foot, midline of back) and areas overlying cartilage (e.g. pinna) and bone (e.g. shin).

Chronic radiation dermatitis. After treatment to high dose, the skin will show some radiation effect for a long time, usually permanently, especially after superficial or orthovoltage irradiation.

All the following changes are now seen far less frequently since the introduction of megavoltage with its skin-sparing effects.

Ischaemia. Many of the late effects of therapeutic doses in the skin or any other organ are due to the destruction and narrowing of local blood vessels with consequent ischaemia, often associated with fibrosis. We shall have occasion to refer to this when discussing particular treatment, e.g. complications of intracavitary caesium therapy in cervical cancer (p. 475) and effects on other tissues, e.g. brain, bone and bowel (see below).

Pigmentation. This may vary from light to very dark brown and will show the size of the irradiated field. It may be distributed in a patchy manner, especially at the edges of a treated area, and may be mingled with whitish patches of depigmented atrophic skin.

Thickening. The skin may heal with considerable fibrosis of the dermis, giving a typical leathery feel with loss of elasticity.

Telangiectasia. Telangiectasia refers to dilatation of thin-walled blood vessels. Destruction or narrowing of the small arteries of the skin may lead to compensatory dilatation of capillaries, which can be very disfiguring.

Late ulceration. An atrophic area is always vulnerable to injuries that would normally be of negligible importance. A scratch or burn, even years later, may lead to a persistent breakdown. This is late necrosis. It is very slow to heal and may require excision and grafting.

Secondary malignancy. This is a complication of chronic radiation exposure. In pioneer X-ray and radium workers, before the dangers were appreciated, skin changes appeared, especially on the fingers. The skin became dry, lost its elasticity and erythema formed around the nails, which became fissured and irregular and might be shed. Later, warts and fissures appeared on the skin and eventually, after some years, malignant change.

Similar changes also happened in some patients subjected to repeated courses of irradiation, especially for non-malignant conditions such as psoriasis and pruritus.

Management of skin reactions

Explanation to patients. Patients should always be given a simple explanation of the probable effects of treatment on the skin and any other organs likely to be affected such as bowel and bladder. It is useful to have a leaflet to hand out at the start, informing them of the likely reactions and of the precautions to take to minimise them. If moist desquamation is expected, they should be warned of the probable breakdown and discharge, crusting and eventual healing after 2 weeks or more. They should be assured that these are normal reactions, not 'burns'.

In milder reactions, little or no special treatment may be necessary, e.g. in dry desquamation, unless the part is exposed to friction, when a simple covering may be useful until the skin has healed. For small areas of moist desquamation (e.g. small basal cell cancer on the face), it is often quite satisfactory to leave it alone, allow it to crust over and leave healing to proceed until the crust drops off the new epidermis. If infection is suspected, the crust may be removed with forceps. If infection is present or threatens during the course of treatment, an antiseptic cream such as chlorhexidine (Hibitane) or cetrimide can be used.

In the first- and second-degree reactions, the chief complaint is usually of simple irritation or itching. An ordinary dusting of talcum powder may be used but, as many of these contain a heavy metal (zinc or bismuth), they should not be put on before treatment has finished, because the metal gives rise to secondary radiation which increases the skin dose and therefore the severity of the reaction. A simple baby powder should be used instead. For the same reason zinc oxide strapping should be avoided and Sellotape or micropore used instead. In areas of friction, lanolin or tulle gras may be applied. When the full course of radiation is over, creams or ointments containing metals may be used freely, e.g. zinc and castor oil. Cold air from a fan also has a soothing effect.

The patient should be cautioned against all forms of irritation to the treated area. The patient was often advised in the past against washing the treated area until the acute reaction had settled. This is usually 2–3 weeks after the end of treatment. Lack of local hygiene over so long a period is unpleasant and inconvenient for the patient. As long as the patient does not rub the treated area vigorously, washing after chest wall irradiation does not significantly worsen the radiation reactions. This is almost certainly true at other sites.

If skin marks have been outlined on the patient for the radiographer's guidance, they must not be washed off. They tend to come off as a result of sweating and friction, especially in hot weather, and then need to be re-marked.

Oropharyngeal mucosa

The mouth and pharynx are lined by mucous membrane covered by non-stratified squamous epithelium. The major and minor salivary glands produce secretions which keep the mucous membranes moist. Below the mucosa lies the lamina propria, containing blood vessels, nerves and minor salivary glands. Since mucous membranes proliferate rapidly, the effects of radiation are expressed at an early stage.

The acute mucosal reaction to conventionally fractionated irradiation is the killing of the stem cells in the basal layer of the epithelium. This has no immediate clinical effects. However, the supply of new cells to replace those lost from the mucosa by wear and tear is cut off. There is therefore a lag phase before the mucosa is denuded. Residual stem cells that have survived irradiation proliferate to try to repopulate the mucosa.

Following the start of irradiation, cells which are dividing in the basal layer degenerate and undergo necrosis. Oedema with neutrophil infiltration develops in the lamina propria and submucosa. This is associated with dilatation of capillaries and swelling of their endothelial lining, accounting for erythema which is observed clinically. When a radical dose (55 Gy) is given in daily fractions over 4–4.5 weeks, a confluent mucosal reaction occurs in which the mucosa is denuded. This starts at the end of the second week. Histologically there is a pseudomembrane consisting of cell debris, fibrin and leucocytes. The mucosal reaction is maximal in the middle of the third week. It has normally settled by the 5th–8th week. If the same dose is given over 5–6.5 weeks, the intensity of the mucosal reaction is reduced.

Where radical irradiation has been given in multiple daily fractions (p. 346) (e.g. 48 Gy over 2 weeks at three fractions of 1.6 Gy 3–4 hours per day, followed by a gap of 3–4 weeks and then further irradiation on the same fractionation schedule to 70 Gy over 6–7 weeks), severe confluent erythema has occurred by day 13 but healed by day 22. Regeneration of mucosal stem cells is thought to be greater during the rest period between a 'split-course' of radiation such as this than between conventional single daily fractions of radical irradiation.

Within a month of a 6–7-week course of radiation, the epithelium has regenerated. Later changes occur as a result of the process of repair, with fibrosis in the lamina propria and the submucosa. Telangiectatic capillaries and thickening of the walls of arterioles are seen. As a result of scarring, the mucosa is subsequently more than normally susceptible to ulceration following minimal trauma.

Salivary glands

Some portions of the major salivary glands (parotid, submandibular and sublingual) are almost invariably included during irradiation of tumours in a variety of sites in the head and neck, especially of the oral cavity. Most of the unpleasant side-effects of head and neck radiation relate directly or indirectly to irradiation of the major salivary glands. Together these glands secrete 60–70% of saliva at rest and following stimulation. The parotid gland is the main source of saliva. Most of the resting saliva is secreted by the submandibular gland.

The minor salivary glands are widely spread in the mucosa of the tongue, cheeks, lips, tonsils and palate. They mainly secrete mucus.

Following irradiation, an acute inflammatory reaction occurs in the major salivary glands. There is rapid loss of secretory acini corresponding to the development of xerostomia (dry mouth). The dose at which xerostomia is permanent varies widely, from 4.5–40.5 Gy. This wide range is probably explained by individual variation in pretreatment salivary flow rates. Permanent inhibition of salivary secretion is probable in 80% of patients after 40–60 Gy, conventionally fractionated. At or beyond 60 Gy total xerostomia occurs in all individuals. If the sublingual and submandibular glands are irradiated and the parotid largely excluded, late sequelae are rare. Patients with the greatest pretreatment taste discrimination tend to experience the quickest loss of taste after irradiation. The relative contribution of direct damage to taste buds by irradiation or as an indirect effect of reduced salivary flow is uncertain. However, saliva is considered important in maintaining the sense of taste.

Intestine

The surface epithelium of the small intestine is renewed every 24–48 hours. A significant dose of irradiation will therefore result in loss of protective and absorptive functions over a similar time scale; diarrhoea and the risk of infection then follow. If a high dose is given to a localised region, the mucosa will regrow, although often with a less specialised cell type, and with the probability of mutations in the remaining cells. The muscle coat will also have been damaged, and there is the risk of granulation tissue causing the formation of a stricture later.

The tolerance dose to limited volumes of the small bowel, as in conventionally fractionated pelvic irradiation for cervical or endometrial cancer, is 45 Gy over 4 weeks.

Clinical effects

In the mouth the membranous reaction is initially white and may be mistaken for thrush. It then becomes yellowish and gradually decreases in size as healing proceeds, as described above.

In the mouth and pharynx these reactions may cause unpleasant dryness, loss of taste, sore throat and dysphagia. In the oesophagus, which is bound to be involved in the treatment of the lung and mediastinum, there may be soreness, painful spasm and dysphagia. Recovery of taste usually occurs 2–4 months after treatment. Xerostomia is permanent if substantial amounts of the parotid glands have been irradiated.

Treatment of mucosal reactions

As a prophylactic measure, dental treatment should be carried out where necessary in cases of head and neck cancer (Ch. 23).

When the mouth and throat are involved, the diet should be light. Drinks of high calorific value (e.g. Build-up or Complan) are helpful. Mouthwashes with aspirin mucilage or a local anaesthetic such as Mucaine before meals are recommended. Hot or spiced food (vinegar or pickles) should not be given. Smoking and alcohol should be discouraged.

Bowel reactions are common and important in the treatment of abdominal and pelvic lesions. Drugs may be required to control vomiting (metoclopramide), spasm (propantheline) or diarrhoea (codeine phosphate or diphenoxylate hydrochloride [Lomotil]). If bowel reactions are marked, treatment may have to be interrupted for a few days or, in extreme cases, stopped entirely.

In the bowel, when abdomen or pelvis is treated, there may be spasm and diarrhoea which can lead to dehydration and also to bleeding. When cancer of the cervix is treated, the rectum (immediately behind the vagina) receives a considerable dose and some degree of proctitis is usual, with irritation, tenesmus, passage of mucus and possibly blood. In the bladder, reactions may cause dysuria with pain and frequency.

Late effects on mucosal surfaces may appear after weeks, months or years. In the mouth, reduction in salivary flow gives rise to dental caries. The fall in pH and in the secretion of antibodies encourages the growth of bacteria responsible for dental decay. These bacteria produce acids from breaking down foodstuffs. The acid in turn dissolves tooth enamel and dentine. There may be malabsorption, adhesions, fibrosis and stenosis, leading to obstruction, fistulae and bleeding. Surgical intervention may be needed for any of these.

Effects on blood-forming tissues

Haemopoietic tissue—mainly bone marrow and lymphoid tissue—is highly radiosensitive. The most marked effects are on the parent (stem) cells of the leucocytes, lymphocytes and platelets. Red cells are much less radiosensitive, as their life cycle is much longer, about 4 months, compared with a day or less for most white cells.

In patients the effect on the blood count is very variable. It depends on a number of factors, particularly the area of bone marrow irradiated and the dose. There is a fall in total white cells (leucopenia) and in platelets (thrombocytopenia) but red cells may hardly be affected at all. If only a very small part of the body is under treatment, the effect on the blood will be negligible, and in superficial therapy, e.g. for skin cancer, there is no need to monitor the blood count. High-dose irradiation of small volumes of the bone marrow will not alter the blood count, but it will result in local loss of haemopoiesis and fibrosis of the marrow cavity. But the larger the field and the more penetrating the radiation, the greater will be the effect on haemopoietic tissue. Whole body irradiation exposure (see below) may result in bone marrow failure. In the absence of a bone marrow transplant this is often fatal.

During most courses of wide-field radical therapy covering substantial amounts of the bone marrow (e.g. mantle or inverted Y for Hodgkin's disease), the blood should be measured twice weekly. More frequent measurements, e.g. daily, are necessary if the blood count is falling rapidly or is close to the threshold for suspending treatment.

There is a risk of inducing leukaemia, as happened in patients who underwent low-dose spinal irradiation for ankylosing spondylitis (p. 597).

Effects on reproductive organs

The gonads (ovary and testis) contain two separate types of tissue:

- Reproductive, for the formation of germ cells (ova and sperm). They are among the most radiosensitive.
- Endocrine, for the production of sex hormones (oestrogens and androgens).

Males

The germ cells of the seminiferous tubules of the testis provide a self-renewing supply of sperm. The Leydig cells of the supporting tissues produce testosterone, the male sex hormone. The germ cells are much more radiosensitive than the Leydig cells. However, there is variation in radiosensitivity between different stages of development into mature sperm. With single doses as low as 2–3 Gy the maturation of spermatocytes is stopped. For spermatids 4–6 Gy causes damage. Doses as low as 0.78 Gy have been reported to cause azoospermia. Owing to this variation in radiosensitivity, depletion of sperm following irradiation is gradual. This may take as long as 22 weeks. Recovery is also dose dependent. The lower the dose the more rapid the recovery. For doses less than 0.1 Gy this occurs in 9–18 months. For doses of 4–6 Gy recovery may take over 5 years. Over 6 Gy no recovery of sperm production occurs. Some dose to the testis is almost invariable from abdominal irradiation (e.g. inverted Y to para-aortic and pelvic nodes for lymphomas or 'dog-leg' irradiation to the para-aortic and ipsilateral pelvic nodes for testicular seminoma). Azoospermia and permanent sterility usually develop after inverted Y irradiation. However, recovery usually occurs 20–40 weeks following 'dog-leg' fractionated irradiation where the dose is less than 0.6 Gy, and 50–90 weeks after doses over 0.6 Gy. In excess of 2 Gy permanent azoospermia is likely.

Total doses of fractionated radiotherapy to the testis should be less than 1 Gy. Sperm storage should be offered to patients with an adequate sperm count prior to treatment. The dose to the testis from scattered irradiation from 'dog-leg' irradiation can be reduced by lead shielding.

At low doses (< 1 Gy), testosterone production from the Leydig cells is maintained, although the levels of the gonadotrophins FSH and LH may rise. Hormone replacement therapy is unlikely to be necessary in the range of doses received by the testis in normal clinical practice.

Females

Sterility can similarly be induced by radiation but depends on physiological age. However, the effects of different doses on the ovary are difficult to assess because it is not possible to measure the absorbed dose to the ovary directly. Hormonal effects are more obvious and of greater clinical significance in the female than in the male. Production of oestrogens can be reduced or abolished with temporary or permanent cessation of menstruation. This effect is used in the induction of an artificial menopause (p. 598). It is not known what the minimum dose is to induce ovarian failure. Amenorrhoea will follow single doses of 6 Gy in prepubertal girls. The dose needed to induce a menopause is probably less with increasing age. This might be due to the reduced number of oocytes in the ovary. Permanent amenorrhoea occurs in only 30% of women aged between 30 and 35 years after 5 Gy but in 80% aged between 35 and 40 years. The dose required to induce the menopause is between 10 and 20 Gy. A dose of 12 Gy in four daily fractions is recommended to induce a radiation menopause for breast cancer.

Genetic effects of radiation

It is well established that ionising radiation does cause gene mutations, i.e. changes in the structure of the genetic material. In man, however, there is little information on which to judge the risks of exposure to particular doses. There was no evidence of an increase in genetic abnormalities among children born to survivors of the atomic bombs dropped on Nagasaki and Hiroshima in 1945 where one or both parents had been exposed to radiation.

The term 'doubling dose' is used to describe the dose of irradiation which doubles the spontaneous mutation rate. The doubling dose in man is estimated to be approximately 1 Gy.

Mutations may occur both in somatic and germ cells. Mutations in somatic cells may be carcinogenic, particularly after exposure to low dosage. Mutations in the germ cells are important since they may have an impact on subsequent generations.

The genetic defects which may be induced are chromosomal abnormalities, changes in autosomal or sex-linked characters, spontaneous abortions and genetic deaths. Genetic death is the term given to the termination of a cell line either due to fetal death early in pregnancy or to reduced fertility. It is thought that most germ cell mutations do not result in offspring that survive. For this reason abnormal children are very rarely fathered by men whose testes have received low-dose scattered irradiation (e.g. from abdominal node irradiation after orchidectomy for testicular seminoma). When it is realised that a single dose of 0.4 Gy to the testis will result in the death of 90% of germ cells, it is understandable that germ cell mutations rarely have the opportunity to be expressed in offspring.

Radiation in pregnancy

Radiation should be avoided in pregnancy. Damage may be done either to the mother's ovaries or to the fetus. Potentially, genetic mutations may occur in the ovaries of mother and fetus, resulting in abnormal later children or future generations. The fetus is particularly vulnerable in view of the relatively enormous growth rate and the extreme immaturity of all its tissues. The first 3 months (first trimester) is the most dangerous period. Even low-dose irradiation (e.g. from diagnostic X-rays) can produce birth defects such as hare lip and cleft palate. More importantly, evidence from women irradiated by the atomic bomb in Japan in 1945 shows that the developing brain may be impaired, causing mental deficiency at low doses (0.04 Gy) and microcephaly at higher doses between 8 and 25 weeks of pregnancy. Larger doses will kill the fetus and lead to abortion.

Fetal irradiation probably increases the risk of childhood leukaemia, although the relationship is not definitely proven. For this reason, diagnostic X-ray departments, before taking films of the pelvis, enquire routinely about the date of the last menstrual period, to avoid exposure in women of reproductive age if there is a possibility of pregnancy.

Kidney

The kidney is an organ of intermediate radiosensitivity. It is mainly a late-responding tissue, although functional and histological changes may be observed within a few weeks of irradiation. The low tolerance of the kidney to irradiation was first appreciated from the study of patients who underwent irradiation for abdominal metastases from testicular cancer. Five clinical syndromes were described:

- *Acute radiation nephritis,* associated with hypertension and proteinuria, occurring 6–13 months after treatment.
- *Chronic radiation nephritis,* associated with urinary protein and casts, nocturia, loss of ability to concentrate the urine, occurring 1.5–4 years after treatment.
- *Benign hypertension,* associated with proteinuria, occurring 1.5–5 years after treatment.
- *Proteinuria,* lasting 5–19 years, as the only evidence of renal damage.
- *Late malignant hypertension,* occurring 1.5–11 years after treatment.

In adults the limit of tolerance if both kidneys are irradiated is 28 Gy in 5 weeks. The risk is less if only part of or the whole of one kidney is irradiated, since the kidney on the opposite side may hypertrophy and compensate for the loss of renal function.

The pathogenesis of renal damage is controversial. It may be due to damage to the endothelial cells lining the glomeruli (parenchymal damage) or to the larger blood vessels (vascular damage). The critical target cell population has not been firmly identified.

Damage to the renal tubules precedes glomerular damage and sclerosis. Radiation nephropathy is slowly progressive and irreversible, in spite of tubular regeneration and epithelial proliferation.

Care should be taken to determine the position of the kidneys when the pelvis, abdomen and spine are treated. The soft tissue shadow of the kidney can often be seen on a plain abdominal film. If there is any uncertainty about their position, an intravenous urogram should be carried out. It should be remembered that pelvic or horseshoe kidneys occur. A pelvic field, which would normally exclude the kidneys in their normal position, may unwittingly include the kidneys in such anomalous positions.

In general, most of one kidney should be excluded from the radiation field or shielded by lead blocks if the other kidney has to be irradiated.

Where part of both kidneys has to be included, for example in abdominal node irradiation for lymphoma (p. 514) and seminoma of the testis (p. 503), the area irradiated should not exceed a third of each kidney.

It is generally safe to irradiate the whole kidney to 20 Gy. Beyond this dose the kidneys should be shielded by lead blocks (e.g. in whole abdominal irradiation for ovarian cancer).

Nervous system and eye

The radiation pathology and tolerance of the central nervous system and the eye are described in Chapter 30.

Bone and cartilage

In growing bone, as in children, irradiation of an epiphysis is likely to retard growth. The tolerance dose for 5% damage at 5 years after irradiation for growing cartilage is 10 Gy. For children under the age of 3 years, the equivalent tolerance dose is lower (8 Gy). The effects on growth are much more marked when the long bones are irradiated than when the vertebral column is irradiated. Both limb shortening and scoliosis may occur in children.

For mature bone, the tolerance dose for 5% damage within 5 years of irradiation is 60 Gy. Both direct damage to osteocytes and indirect damage due to radiation-induced vascular injury may play a part in the pathogenesis of osteoradionecrosis (p. 357). Radionecrosis of the mandible may occur following radical radiotherapy for oral cancer (p. 357 and Fig. 23.12).

The threshold level for osteoradionecrosis may be lowered in patients who have received both radiotherapy and steroid-containing chemotherapy for lymphoma. Radionecrosis of the femoral head is the most important example of this (p. 515).

Cartilage necrosis can occur in the outer ear (pinna and external auditory meatus), nose (ala nasi) and larynx. All these changes are aggravated or precipitated by trauma and infection. Dental caries is an example discussed on page 357.

Lungs

The inflammatory reactions in lung tissue (radiation pneumonitis) may cause serious scarring (fibrosis) which prevents the lung expanding properly. Vital capacity is thus reduced. Care is taken to minimise the amount of lung irradiated in treating the chest wall for breast cancer (Fig. 26.16). Radiation pneumonitis is described in more detail on page 426.

RADIATION SICKNESS

This is a general reaction which is liable to occur during a course of treatment. Its severity depends on the part of the body and the volume of tissue which is irradiated. If a small skin tumour is treated, there will be no general reaction at all. However, if the upper abdomen is irradiated for a deep-seated tumour (e.g. for gastric lymphoma), there may be marked general upset. By contrast, similarly large volumes of a lower limb can be irradiated with minimal systemic upset.

The clinical features of radiation sickness are nausea (sometimes with vomiting), headache, tiredness and weakness. In very sensitive or debilitated patients there may be prostration.

The cause of radiation sickness is unknown. It may be that the products of the breakdown of tissue, particularly rapidly dividing cells of the gastrointestinal tract, contribute largely to the stimulation of the vomiting centre in the brainstem. There is much individual variation between patients in response to the same dose of irradiation to a similar volume. Anxiety about treatment may exacerbate symptoms and can often be relieved by a clear explanation of what is to be expected.

Treatment with sedatives (e.g. Motival) and anti-emetics (prochlorperazine or metoclopramide) may help. More recently the 5-hydroxytryptamine (5-HT) receptor antagonists (ondansetron and granisetron) have proved to be very effective in preventing radiation sickness. An adequate daily fluid intake of 4–5 pints (2–2.5 litres) should be maintained.

WHOLE BODY IRRADIATION

As a therapeutic procedure this is now rarely used except before bone marrow transplantation (e.g. for acute leukaemia). However, chronic exposure is natural and unavoidable (Ch. 16). We are subject to radiation from natural sources and man-made appliances. The current exposure of the population in the UK to these sources is shown in Figure 16.5.

Acute radiation syndrome

The acute radiation syndrome describes the clinical effects of whole body exposure to single doses in excess of 0.5 Gy. The best documented evidence of the effects of such doses is derived from the explosion of atomic bombs at Hiroshima and Nagasaki in Japan in 1945. The radiation doses have been estimated and the survivors followed up and observed. Other episodes have been the unintentional exposure in the Marshall Islands in the Pacific in 1954 in the course of bomb testing, affecting nearly 300 people, and the explosion of the nuclear reactor at Chernobyl in 1986. All these, in addition to observations of experimental animal work, give us a detailed picture of the effects of acute radiation damage.

The time of onset, extent and duration of symptoms are all dose dependent. Three main clinical syndromes are described, reflecting the most radiosensitive organ systems. Their principal features are summarised in Table 19.1.

- The haematological syndrome
- The gastrointestinal syndrome
- The central nervous (CNS) syndrome.

These are preceded by a prodromal syndrome.

Prodromal radiation syndrome

After exposure to whole body doses of 0.5 Gy, radiation sickness begins within 1–2 hours. This is accompanied

Table 19.1 Acute radiation syndromes following whole body irradiation (adapted from Rubin P & Casarett G W 1968 Clinical Radiation Pathology. W B Saunders, Philadelphia)

	Syndromes		
Features	CNS	Gastrointestinal	Haemopoietic
Main organ affected	Brain	Small bowel	Bone marrow
Major pathology	Vasculitis, encephalitis, oedema (CNS)	Depletion of intestinal epithelium, infection	Bone marrow atrophy, pancytopenia, haemorrhage, infection
Threshold dose for onset (Gy)	20	5	1
Threshold dose for death (Gy)	50	10	2
Onset following exposure	0.25–3 hours	3–5 days	2–3 weeks
Typical clinical features	Lethargy, tremor, seizures, ataxia	Malaise, anorexia, nausea, vomiting, diarrhoea, fever, electrolyte imbalance, circulatory collapse	Malaise, fatigue, exertional dyspnoea, leucopenia, thrombocytopenia, purpura
Time of death	Within 2 days	3–14 days	3–8 weeks

by headache, lassitude and sometimes vertigo. At much higher doses of 1 Gy the onset is within minutes.

Haematological syndrome

The threshold total body dose for the development of the haematological syndrome is 1 Gy. At a dose of 2 Gy the syndrome is almost invariably fatal. It comprises two successive phases.

In the first phase the direct target is the bone marrow, where parent cells of the peripheral blood cells are killed or their differentiation inhibited. The immediate result is leucopenia and thrombocytopenia. Of the white cells, the lymphocytes are affected earliest and most profoundly, followed by other white cells and megakaryocytes. The red cell precursors are also sensitive, but since the red cell has a life span of about 4 months, anaemia develops later than leucopenia and thrombocytopenia.

In the second phase a haemorrhagic anaemia develops; this may be a consequence of widespread damage to the vasculature of the viscera and mucous membranes.

The following clinical sequence is seen:

Within hours:	Anorexia, nausea, vomiting, diarrhoea.
24–36 hours:	Symptoms subside; patient feels well
3 weeks:	Malaise, fever, anorexia, fatigue, exertional dyspnoea, alopecia, pharyngitis, swelling and ulceration of tonsils, swelling and bleeding of gums, petechiae and bruising, diarrhoea
5–6 weeks:	Agranulocytosis, anaemia, bacterial infection
8 weeks:	If patient recovers, resolution of symptoms and signs.

Prognosis. The absolute lymphocyte count at 48 hours (without blood transfusion) is a useful guide to outcome:

1200+	Unlikely to be fatal
300–1200	Lethal range
<300	Almost certainly fatal.

Gastrointestinal syndrome

In the gastrointestinal syndrome the main organ affected is the small bowel. The threshold dose is 5 Gy. The time of onset of nausea and vomiting followed by diarrhoea varies from within half an hour of exposure to several hours. These symptoms may persist from the start or subside after 2–3 days, recurring on the fifth day when the gastrointestinal epithelium has been denuded. Diarrhoea becomes bloody. Fluid and electrolyte imbalance develops, eventually leading to circulatory collapse, coma and death.

CNS syndrome

The onset of the CNS syndrome is prompt, with death rapidly supervening. The pathological processes are vasculitis and encephalitis leading to cerebral oedema. Apathy and drowsiness develop, increase in severity and progress to prostration. Seizures ranging from muscle tremor to grand mal type are followed by ataxia if the dose is in excess of 50 Gy.

Effect on unborn children

In those who survived the atomic bomb, a special hazard involved pregnant women. Abortions and stillbirths were brought about. If the child survived in utero, its brain development was liable to be retarded and it might be born with a small head (microcephaly) and mental deficiency.

Late effects of atomic bomb explosions

There are special dangers of radioactive 'fall-out'. This is the radioactive dust containing fission products (p. 70) carried to great heights in the atmosphere with the vaporised material from the bomb. The fine particles are carried in air currents, settling down gradually to earth. These dust clouds can travel great distances, even encircling the earth many times. A bomb exploded in Nevada in the USA produces fall-out detectable in England 5 days later.

A particular hazard of fall-out concerns radioactive strontium, a fission product. This is soluble and is absorbed by plants and grazing animals (e.g. cattle and sheep) and reaches humans in the diet and water. Biochemically it behaves like calcium and is deposited in bone tissue after absorption. It is therefore potentially capable of producing late effects comparable to those in luminous dial painters (p. 277).

CHAPTER CONTENTS

20

Principles of management and dosage

Ian Kunkler

Once a diagnosis of malignancy has been reached, some important management decisions must be made:

1. To select necessary investigations
2. To undertake curative (radical) or palliative therapy
3. To choose appropriate palliative or radical treatment
4. To choose appropriate support services (e.g. nursing and social services) for patient and family.

This chapter concentrates on items (2), (3) and (4). The appropriate staging investigations are covered by tumour site in Chapters 21–32.

Radical or palliative treatment?

This is perhaps the most important decision that the clinical oncologist has to make. The decision will depend on the history, clinical examination and investigations. The oncologist has to weigh the factors outlined below in coming to a decision.

Radical treatment means the attempt to kill or remove all the malignant cells present. Cure or local control is the aim. Some morbidity, and occasionally mortality from treatment has often to be accepted if cure is to be achieved.

Palliative treatment is aimed at relieving the symptoms of cancer (for example pain, dysphagia, dyspnoea) or restraining temporarily the growth of the tumour. Any side-effects should be minor. Palliative and continuing care is considered in detail in Chapter 36.

ASSESSMENT BEFORE TREATMENT

Multidisciplinary management

The increasing complexity of curative cancer management for many tumours, with different combinations of surgery, radiotherapy and chemotherapy for different stages of disease, requires a coordinated multidisciplinary approach. The correct initial choice gives the best prospect for cure or good palliation. Tables 20.1–20.3 summarise the tumours for which surgery, radiotherapy and chemotherapy, respectively, are the treatments of choice. For many early tumours, e.g. of the oral cavity, surgery and radiotherapy give equally good results. The choice between them may depend on local expertise.

In patients with potentially curable disease, inappropriate initial treatment may compromise both the quantity and quality of survival. In curative treatment, it may also increase the risk of complications when surgery or radiotherapy for residual disease has to be added after incorrect primary therapy has failed. Occasionally, for example, a Wertheim's hysterectomy for early cancer of the cervix (p. 469) is not completed because the extent of disease preoperatively has been underestimated. The risk of pelvic morbidity from radical pelvic irradiation following pelvic surgery is much higher than if primary radical radiotherapy had been given alone.

Patients with malignant disease may present before, during or after treatment as a medical or surgical emergency—e.g. with respiratory failure (from large-volume lung metastases from testicular teratoma), with acute upper airway obstruction requiring tracheostomy (laryngeal and thyroid cancer), with spinal cord compression (breast and lung cancer, myeloma) or with pathological fracture (breast cancer)—requiring the attention of the ear, nose and throat, orthopaedic or neurosurgeon.

Table 20.1 Surgery alone—the treatment of choice

Lower oesophagus, stomach, colon, pancreas, kidney
Thyroid
Melanoma
Hepatocellular carcinoma
Keratoacanthoma

Table 20.2 Radiotherapy—the treatment of choice

Oral cavity, lip, tongue, cheek
Nasopharynx
Oropharynx
Hypopharynx
Nasal cavity
Larynx
Skin cancer (except melanoma)
Cervix
Bladder (except T1)
Testis—seminoma
Hodgkin's disease (early)
Non-Hodgkin lymphoma (early)
Medulloblastoma (following surgical debulking)
Astrocytomas (grades 3 and 4)
Retinoblastoma

Table 20.3 Cytotoxic therapy—the treatment of choice

Acute and chronic leukaemias
Hodgkin's disease (advanced)
Non-Hodgkin lymphoma (advanced)
Testicular teratoma
Choriocarcinoma
Small cell lung cancer
Rhabdomyosarcoma
Neuroblastoma

Joint clinics

Where the choice is between surgery, radiotherapy or a combination of both, assessment by an oncologist at a joint clinic with a specialist surgeon, dermatologist, gynaecologist or haematologist is often helpful.

The success of such clinics depends on a collaborative spirit and on each specialist knowing the strengths and limitations of each modality of treatment. In some situations equally good results can be achieved by different treatments, e.g. by surgery and radiotherapy for early cancer of the cervix. The choice may be determined by the relative morbidity of each treatment or by the experience of the specialist or the treatment facilities. For instance, the best results of radical surgery for ovarian cancer are obtained in the hands of a gynaecologist undertaking this form of surgery on a regular basis.

The lines of communication between specialists need to be clear so that the timing of surgery, radiotherapy and chemotherapy are properly synchronised. Each specialist, referring doctor and the patient's general practitioner should be kept informed of the patient's progress. The patient should know which member of the multidisciplinary team to contact for advice.

Advantages. There are a number of potential advantages. Delay incurred by referral to more than one clinic is avoided. The patient may feel reassured that all treatment options have been considered before embarking on the chosen course of treatment. Joint clinics provide a good basis for the audit of treatment and for clinical trials to assess new therapies.

Disadvantages. If the number of medical staff attending the clinic is large, the patient may find attendance intimidating. This can be minimised if, once all the relevant specialists have examined the patient and withdrawn to discuss management, the specialist undertaking the primary management returns alone to explain the planned treatment to the patient and to answer questions.

Information required for a decision on treatment

In every case all the relevant information must be gathered about the patient in general and the tumour and its extent of spread in particular.

Age and general medical condition. The latter includes coincident disease (e.g. diabetes mellitus, chronic respiratory disease, peptic ulceration).

Tumour spread—local, regional nodes, distant metastases. Staging is the term applied to determine the extent of the disease. Staging may include clinical, radiological or laboratory findings. Local, regional or distant spread is assessed by:

1. Clinical examination—especially for accessible cancers, e.g. skin, oral cavity, larynx, cervix and breast. This includes palpation of the regional nodes, e.g. the cervical nodes for the oral cavity, larynx and pharynx, and the axilla and supraclavicular fossae for breast tumours.
2. Instrumental endoscopy—e.g. bronchoscopy for lung, cystoscopy for bladder, sigmoidoscopy for colon and rectum.
3. Radiology—radiographs of the chest for secondary deposits in the lungs, skeletal survey for deposits of myeloma, intravenous urography (IVU) for identification of tumours of the bladder, ureters and kidneys, CT scanning for pelvic, para-aortic and mediastinal nodes.
4. Isotope scans—radioactive tracer studies may detect primary or secondary deposits in thyroid, bone, brain and liver.

Histology. Histological confirmation of the tumour should be obtained, if at all possible. If there is no clinical doubt about the diagnosis (e.g. of a basal cell carcinoma on the face) and the patient's condition is very frail, biopsy may be omitted. Similarly in superior mediastinal obstruction a clinical diagnosis of lung cancer is also often made without pathological confirmation. This is because bronchial biopsy may precipitate serious haemorrhage in the presence of raised venous pressure. Biopsy of brainstem gliomas is often avoided because of the risk of causing a major neurological deficit. Occasionally biopsy of an obvious bronchial tumour is negative. This may happen if the biopsy is taken unwittingly from adjacent inflammatory tissue.

Where the pathological type is likely to influence management, i.e. the patient would be fit for chemotherapy if the histological diagnosis was small cell lung cancer, the biopsy should be repeated. If the patient would only be fit for palliative radiotherapy whatever the histology, further biopsy is often avoided.

Review of histology by specialist tumour pathologist. The histological classification of some tumours, particularly the lymphomas and sarcomas, requires a great deal of experience. In these circumstances, or where the pathologist is uncertain of the diagnosis, the pathological specimens should be reviewed by a specialist histopathologist. The distinction in a neck node between a poorly differentiated carcinoma and a high-grade lymphoma is essential, since the management of each tumour is different. Unless emergency treatment is required (e.g. for stridor from thyroid cancer), a firm pathological diagnosis should be made before starting treatment.

CHOICE OF RADICAL OR PALLIATIVE TREATMENT

When the relevant investigations on these lines have been completed, consideration has to be given as to whether treatment is to be radical or palliative.

The choice between radical and palliative treatment may be straightforward or difficult. A fit young woman with a stage II carcinoma of the cervix should be treated by radical radiotherapy with curative intent. An elderly but otherwise fit patient with localised bone pain from metastatic cancer should be offered a short course or single fraction of palliative radiotherapy. However, often the general condition of the patient is too poor, even if the disease is localised, to sustain the stress of anticancer treatment. Where the decision is borderline, reassessment after correction of anaemia and electrolyte and fluid imbalance is often helpful before a final decision is taken.

The following factors relating to the tumour, the patient and available resources can influence the decision. The importance of each factor will vary from patient to patient.

1. The tumour
   a. Site
   b. Size
   c. Spread (locoregional/metastatic spread)
   d. Operability
   e. Radiosensitivity/chemosensitivity
   f. Histology (including differentiation)
   g. Clearance of surgical resection margins.
2. The patient
   a. Age and general condition (physical and mental)

   b. Morbidity and mortality
   c. Function and cosmesis
   d. Reliability of follow-up after treatment
   e. Preference of patient.
3. Resources: technical expertise, experience and equipment.

1. Features of the tumour

Site. Some tumours are unsuited for primary radiotherapy because of (a) the poor tolerance of the tissues to radical radiation doses, e.g. the skin over the shin, or (b) the proximity of dose-limiting structures (e.g. the spinal cord in head and neck cancer). Other tumours (e.g. nasopharyngeal carcinoma) are unsuitable for surgery because their deep position and proximity to critical structures would require hazardous and mutilating surgery.

Size. In general the larger the tumour, the lower is its radiocurability. This is related to the size of the clonogenic tumour cell population and the increased proportion of radioresistant hypoxic cells. For example, the local control rate of virtually all squamous cancers of the head and neck declines with increasing tumour bulk.

Spread. The pattern of spread of tumour will strongly influence the choice of treatment and will vary with site and histology. Early tumours confined to the primary site, with or without regional nodes, may be suitable for radical surgery or radiotherapy. This applies, for example, to early squamous cell carcinomas of the floor of the mouth. However, carcinomas of the oral cavity which have invaded the mandible are unlikely to be controlled by radical radiotherapy. Radical surgery with reconstruction of the mandible gives a better prospect of cure. Similarly, locoregional spread of Hodgkin's disease to the cervical, axillary and mediastinal nodes can be encompassed by wide field 'mantle' irradiation (p. 512). Chemotherapy also has a role in treating a limited number of chemosensitive tumours with locoregional spread (e.g. pelvic and para-aortic nodes in testicular teratoma).

For metastatic disease, local treatments (with the exception of, for example, the surgical removal of isolated lung metastases in osteosarcoma) are generally inappropriate. For chemosensitive tumours, systemic cytotoxic or hormonal chemotherapy is the main form of treatment. Radical radiotherapy does have a role in the lymphomas in treating residual locoregional disease following clearance of bulky local and metastatic disease by chemotherapy. Palliative radiotherapy may be necessary to relieve local symptoms of metastases (e.g. in bone).

Operability. This depends on two factors.

Fitness for surgery. Patients with a variety of general medical illnesses (e.g. chronic obstructive airways disease or ischaemic heart disease) affecting cardiorespiratory function may represent an unacceptable risk for general anaesthesia. This may, for example, exclude from curative surgery some patients with localised lung cancer. Similarly some patients with endometrial cancer may be too obese for hysterectomy.

Complete removal of the tumour. For radical surgery to be successful the surgeon must be able to remove all the macroscopic disease with a margin of normal tissue. Residual disease at the resection margins is likely to give rise to local recurrence. Early carcinomas of the breast are operable, whereas a more locally advanced breast tumour invading the chest wall is inoperable. Fixity to adjacent structures usually contraindicates radical surgery. This applies, for example, to neck nodes in squamous cancer of the head and neck (p. 356) and to cervical cancer extending to the pelvic side wall.

In the brain, complete tumour removal of high-grade gliomas is impractical because of widespread microscopic dissemination well beyond the macroscopic tumour margins and the need to avoid damage to surrounding normal brain.

Radiosensitivity / chemosensitivity. The sensitivity of tumours to radiotherapy and chemotherapy varies widely (Tables 20.4 and 20.5). Cure may be anticipated in a high proportion of cases of Hodgkin's disease, which is highly sensitive to both chemotherapy and radiotherapy. In contrast, melanoma is relatively resistant to both chemotherapy and radiotherapy, and even palliation is difficult to achieve.

Histology. The degree of differentiation is relevant to management. In general, undifferentiated (anaplastic) tumours are liable to behave more aggressively than well-differentiated tumours. For example, a well-differentiated carcinoma of the thyroid may be curable by subtotal thyroidectomy and radioiodine, whereas anaplastic thyroid cancer is usually unresponsive to any form of local therapy and does not take up radioiodine.

Clearance of resection margins. Curative surgery aims to remove the tumour in its entirety with a margin of normal tissue. If the resection margins are clear of tumour, further therapy is often not required. If there is gross or microscopic disease at the resection margins (e.g. an inadequately excised basal carcinoma of the skin), postoperative radiotherapy is needed to prevent recurrence. Sometimes the pathologist finds that the margin of normal tissue around the resected

Table 20.4 Radiosensitivity of different tumours (reproduced with permission from Souhami R L, Moxham J 1990 Textbook of medicine. Churchill Livingstone, Edinburgh)

Highly sensitive
Lymphoma
Seminoma
Myeloma
Ewing's sarcoma
Wilms' tumour
Moderately sensitive
Small cell lung cancer
Breast cancer
Basal cell carcinoma
Medulloblastoma
Teratoma
Ovarian cancer
Relatively resistant
Squamous cell carcinoma of lung
Hypernephroma
Rectal carcinoma
Bladder carcinoma
Soft tissue sarcoma
Cervical cancer
Highly resistant
Melanoma
Osteosarcoma
Pancreatic carcinoma

Table 20.5 Chemosensitivity of different tumours(reproduced with permission from Souhami R L, Moxham J 1990 Textbook of medicine. Churchill Livingstone, Edinburgh)

Highly sensitive (which may be cured by chemotherapy)
Teratoma of testis
Hodgkin's disease
High-grade non-Hodgkin lymphoma
Wilms' tumour
Embryonal rhabdomyosarcoma
Choriocarcinoma
Acute lymphoblastic leukaemia in children
Ewing's sarcoma
Moderately sensitive (in which chemotherapy may sometimes contribute to cure and often palliates)
Small cell carcinoma of lung
Breast carcinoma
Low-grade non-Hodgkin lymphoma
Acute myeloid leukaemia
Ovarian cancer
Myeloma
Relatively insensitive (in which chemotherapy may sometimes produce palliation)
Gastric carcinoma
Bladder carcinoma
Squamous carcinoma of head and neck
Soft tissue sarcoma
Cervical carcinoma
Resistant tumours
Melanoma
Squamous carcinoma of lung
Large bowel cancer

tumour is very slender, perhaps a few millimetres only. In this circumstance clearance of the tumour may be considered inadequate and postoperative radiotherapy advised or further resection carried out to clear the margins more definitively (e.g. following initial lumpectomy for early breast cancer).

2. The patient

Age and general condition. It is important to assess the patient's fitness for any major procedure, whether it be surgery, radiotherapy or chemotherapy.

Age. Tolerance to both radical radiotherapy and chemotherapy diminishes with age. For example, an elderly person over the age of 70 with inoperable oesophageal cancer may appear medically fit for radical radiotherapy. Such patients often tolerate treatment poorly. Radiotherapy may have to be suspended permanently or the total dose reduced, with consequent compromise of tumour control.

The anticipated rise in the population of elderly in the UK will make this difficult decision a more frequent one. Aggressive treatment of the elderly is likely to result in greater treatment-related morbidity and mortality, without increasing cure rates.

Coincident diseases. A similar argument applies to coincident diseases which compromise fitness to treat. For example, a patient with chronic obstructive airways disease and severely impaired pulmonary function (forced expiratory volume in 1 second (FEV_1) of less than 1 litre) is likely to made more breathless by radical radiotherapy for a lung tumour. Impaired respiratory function may also contraindicate a pneumonectomy. Patients with arteriosclerosis are subject to poorer tissue perfusion. This compromises the ability of normal tissue to recover from radiation injury.

Performance status. An objective assessment of the performance status of the patient (Ch. 37) is a useful guide to fitness to treat. It has been shown, for example, in small cell lung cancer that performance status is a very important prognostic factor in the response to chemotherapy. Poor performance status at presentation tends to be associated with shorter life expectancy. Anaemia and dehydration often accompany malignant disease and impair performance status. They should be corrected before a decision on eligibility for radical treatment is taken, since the patient's general medical state may sometimes be improved sufficiently to undergo radical treatment.

Morbidity and mortality. Surgery may involve unacceptable risks of morbidity and mortality. Examples are:

- *Brainstem tumours,* where cranial nerve nuclei and sensory or motor tracts may be damaged, resulting in serious and permanent neurological deficit.
- *Oesophageal cancer.* Surgery of carcinomas of the middle third of the oesophagus carries an operative mortality as high as 30%.
- *Paediatric cancer,* where the role of radiotherapy has declined with the appreciation of its long-term adverse effects on growth and development. At many sites higher cure rates have been achieved with chemotherapy alone, with fewer long-term complications.
- *Cervical cancer.* In young women with cervical cancer, Wertheim's hysterectomy (p. 469) should enable a functional vagina to be preserved. Radical pelvic irradiation, however, results in progressive narrowing of the vagina owing to fibrosis, limiting sexual intercourse.

Function and cosmesis. Radical surgery, particularly in the head and neck region, can be mutilating, although advances in plastic reconstruction of tissue defects with skin flaps and bone grafts from other sites have improved cosmetic and functional results. Radical surgery of carcinoma of the maxillary antrum involves a maxillectomy. A facial prosthesis is required to fill the tissue defect. Radical radiotherapy of tumours at this site which have not extended into the pterygoid fossa are therefore often treated with radical radiotherapy (p. 368) to avoid facial disfigurement.

Before the advent of cytotoxic chemotherapy, amputation well above the site of the tumour was standard treatment for osteogenic sarcoma of a limb bone. Preoperative and postoperative adjuvant cytotoxic therapy has allowed limb-conserving surgery (Fig. 31.4) to be carried out, with much improved functional results.

In early breast cancer lumpectomy and postoperative radiotherapy can avoid mastectomy in most women with operable tumours 3 cm or less in size (p. 440).

For carcinomas of the lower rectum and anal margin and canal, radical radiotherapy may allow the anal sphincter to be preserved and a colostomy avoided.

Reliability of follow-up. Some patients are less likely to attend follow-up appointments on a regular basis. This may be due to factors such as concurrent physical or mental illness, shift working, unstable home circumstances, lack of transport, distance from the clinic, fear of hospitals or lack of appreciation of the seriousness of their condition or the need for early detection of persistent or recurrent cancer. Early detection of recurrent disease suitable for salvage surgery may thus be compromised. For unreliable attenders, e.g. alcoholics with head and neck cancer, prophylactic neck irradiation carried out at the same time as treatment of a primary tumour may be preferable to treating the neck only when nodes become palpable. Similarly in early breast cancer, a mastectomy, with or without postoperative radiotherapy, may be preferable to lumpectomy and postoperative radiotherapy (breast conservation) where regular clinical and mammographic follow-up of the treated breast for local recurrence is impractical.

The preference of the patient. Some patients prefer surgery or radiotherapy for a variety of reasons. Older patients with operable breast cancer often prefer to have a mastectomy rather than a local excision and radiotherapy because they feel more confident that all the disease has been removed. Young women often prefer a conservation approach because it can preserve breast symmetry and a normal cleavage.

3. Resources

Staff and equipment. Sometimes specialised expertise and treatment may not be available in a patient's district general hospital (e.g. a gynaecologist experienced in carrying out Wertheim's hysterectomy for stage I carcinoma of the cervix in young women). In these circumstances radical radiotherapy by intracavitary, with or without external beam, treatment is preferable. In most cases patients can be referred to hospitals which can provide the necessary technical expertise. In the UK the practice of referring patients with very rare curable tumours, e.g. for retinoblastoma (p. 559) and choriocarcinoma (p. 485), to national treatment facilities is well established. However, in parts of the world where cancer services have a lower health priority, availability of resources may have a greater impact on the choice of anticancer treatment.

Clinical experience. This is one of the most important criteria in choosing treatment. Long personal experience of assessing and treating patients for tumours of different sites and stages is one of the best guides to the probability of cure or effective palliation.

Deciding not to offer anticancer treatment

Occasionally, an oncologist may decide not to recommend anticancer treatment but supportive care only. It is even more difficult to persuade the patient and family that this is the right decision if they anticipate that anticancer treatment will be offered. Some patients have such advanced disease and their general medical condition is so poor that they are unfit for any form of anticancer therapy. Much pressure may be put on the oncologist by the patient, the family or the referring physician or surgeon to offer some form of active anticancer therapy. This must be resisted if the oncologist believes that little benefit will accrue. An open discussion with the patient, the family and referring doctor, emphasising the upset that anticancer therapy would cause, for little benefit, and the positive aspects of symptom control by other means, may persuade all concerned to accept the oncologist's advice.

Clinical assessment in radiotherapy

The radiotherapist and oncologist is both a physician and a technical specialist. Decisions on the management of individual patients depend on balancing clinical and technical factors. If the tumour is a small basal cell carcinoma on the cheek, radiotherapy is a comparatively simple matter. A few brief outpatient attendances suffice. The treatment reaction is predictable and the probability of cure very high. More complex is the choice of target volume, beam directed technique, dose, fractionation and respect for the tolerance of normal tissue and critical organs in the treatment of head and neck cancer.

Inpatient or outpatient treatment?

The majority of patients undergoing radiotherapy can manage to attend as outpatients if they are well enough or within reasonable daily travelling distance of the cancer centre. Relatives may be able to transport them. Failing this, an ambulance can be arranged. Elderly patients often tolerate long journeys poorly and are best admitted. The same applies to patients who are very anxious about their treatment. Hospital admission gives greater opportunity for nursing and medical staff to offer explanation and reassurance about treatment. Many cancer centres have a hostel for patients who are admitted for geographical reasons and who have minimal nursing requirements. Other patients with heavier nursing requirements (e.g. malignant spinal cord compression), undergoing more intensive therapy (e.g. complex chemotherapy regimes) or interstitial or intracavitary therapy (for purposes of radiation protection) will need to be admitted to the main wards.

General medical care

Good medical condition is important in achieving cure, whatever the modality of treatment. Dehydration and poor nutrition are common in advanced malignant disease. Intravenous fluids to correct fluid and electrolyte balance, blood transfusion for anaemia, antibiotics for infection, and calorie and vitamin supplements for malnutrition are often needed.

Review during treatment

A course of radiotherapy, especially to a radical dose, is usually a strenuous undertaking for many patients. One or more of the radiation effects described in Chapter 19 are likely to cause some discomfort and may last for several weeks before healing. Regular weekly review of treatment is necessary to monitor the patient's clinical state and response to treatment. Sometimes the severity of the treatment reaction will require treatment to be suspended, and occasionally stopped definitively. Frequent explanation and reassurance is needed since anxiety often hinders patients' recall of what they have been told initially about diagnosis and treatment.

Palliative radiotherapy

Palliative radiotherapy is aimed at relieving local symptoms of advanced disease. The following criteria should be applied to achieve good palliation:

1. Prompt relief of symptoms
2. Minimal upset from treatment
3. Simple treatment technique
4. Limited number of fractions.

Assessment

Patients with advanced disease may have a life expectancy ranging from a few days to many months. A judgement has to be made as to whether the patient is likely to benefit within his or her expected life span. In most cases benefit from palliative radiotherapy is seen during or within a few days of treatment. Where life expectancy is only a few days, every effort should be made to control the patient's symptoms at home by medical means without recourse to radiotherapy.

Palliative radiotherapy should relieve symptoms with minimal side-effects. The amount of upset varies with site, dose and fractionation.

Site. Sites which tolerate palliative radiotherapy poorly are the upper abdomen (sensitivity of the stomach and duodenum), oral cavity (soreness and dysphagia) and perineum (painful skin and vaginal reaction).

Single fractions of 8 Gy to the lower thoracic and upper lumbar spine are likely to cause vomiting since some of the duodenum will be incorporated in the field. Fractionated treatment is better tolerated.

Palliative radiotherapy is of value at a wide range of tumour sites. Here are a few examples.

- Relief of haemoptysis, cough, dyspnoea and mediastinal obstruction in lung cancer.
- Control of bleeding in advanced bladder, rectal and cervical cancer.
- Relief of pain from bone metastases.
- Relief of symptoms of raised intracranial pressure due to brain metastases.
- Healing of ulcerating breast tumours.

Dose and fractionation

Relatively low doses are adequate to relieve most symptoms. Single fractions of 8 Gy using orthovoltage, cobalt-60 or megavoltage are suitable for ribs, upper thoracic spine, and long bones. Fractionated doses, e.g. 20 Gy in four daily fractions or 30 Gy in 10 fractions are suggested for bony metastases in the cervical, lower thoracic and upper lumbar spine and for malignant spinal cord compression.

Technique

The treatment set-up should be as simple as possible, with single or parallel-opposed fields to limit the duration of each treatment.

Palliative surgery

This may be required for:

1. Obstruction, e.g. transurethral resection in prostate cancer, colostomy in bowel cancer, laser therapy of bronchial and oesophageal cancer.
2. Pain, e.g. pinning of a pathological fracture.
3. Paraplegia—laminectomy for relief of spinal cord compression.
4. Hydrocephalus—ventriculoperitoneal shunting for relief of obstruction of CSF pathways by tumour.
5. Fungation—toilet mastectomy for fungating breast cancer.
6. Ascites—insertion of a LeVeen shunt from the peritoneal cavity into the superior vena cava for recurrent ascites.

Palliative chemotherapy

Palliative cytotoxic chemotherapy is less widely used than radiotherapy because unpleasant side-effects are more common and difficult to justify according to the criteria for good palliation (see above). Palliative hormonal chemotherapy (Ch. 35) is more widely used because of limited toxicity. The use of palliative chemotherapy is considered by site in other chapters.

In general, palliative cytotoxic chemotherapy is best avoided in frail and elderly patients, who are more prone to toxicity. Similarly, poor performance status is associated with poor outcome of treatment. However, poor performance status may be related to the effects of the tumour (e.g. the patient bed-bound due to severe dyspnoea from lung metastases). If symptoms are potentially reversible by chemotherapy, poor performance status is not per se a contraindication to treatment.

1. Hormonal therapy
   a. Antioestrogens, progestogens, steroid inhibitors, androgens in advanced breast cancer
   b. Progestogens in advanced and metastatic endometrial cancer.
2. Cytotoxic chemotherapy
   a. Advanced breast cancer
   b. Lung cancer (except possibly limited stage small cell lung cancer)
   c. Alimentary tract (including liver and pancreas)
   d. Cervix and ovarian cancer
   e. Bladder cancer
   f. Melanoma
   g. Soft tissue sarcomas
   h. Low-grade non-Hodgkin lymphoma.

Technical factors in radiotherapy

In any radiation treatment the clinician has to define the following parameters:

1. Tumour volume
2. Target volume
3. Treatment volume
4. Radiation energy and quality
5. Number of fields
6. Arrangement of fields
7. Use of wedges, tissue compensators or bolus
8. Dose
9. Total number and frequency of fractions
10. Overall treatment time.

(1)–(7) have been covered in Chapter 13. Dose, fractionation and treatment time are considered here.

Dose, fractionation and overall treatment time

It is essential to specify dose, energy, number of fractions and overall treatment time together since each has an effect on the biological response. Stating a dose without specifying its energy, fractionation and overall treatment time is meaningless.

Dose in radical and palliative radiotherapy

Radical. In radical radiotherapy the choice of dose and fractionation regime will depend on the radiosensitivity of the tumour, the size of the treatment volume, the proximity of dose-limiting critical structures and the quality of radiation used.

Relatively radiosensitive tumours such as testicular seminoma can be controlled by total doses of 30 Gy at megavoltage fractionated over 4 weeks. Higher doses of the order of 50–55 Gy are needed to control most squamous carcinomas of the head and neck.

The maximum tolerated dose of radical radiotherapy to different volumes of tissue varies in different parts of the body. For example, field sizes in excess of 60 cm^2 for head and neck cancer rarely tolerate more than 50 Gy in 20 daily fractions over 4 weeks. Similarly, the tolerance of the small bowel limits the dose to the whole pelvis in cervical/endometrial cancer to 45 Gy fractionated over the same period.

The presence of critical structures such as the brainstem and spinal cord may limit the dose that can be delivered to tumours, for example of the head and neck, lung and oesophagus. This problem can be obviated in treating nodal areas overlying the cord in the head and neck by the use of electrons of limited penetration. The appropriate energy can be chosen to ensure that the cord is not overdosed (Figs 23.17 and 23.18).

The relative biological effectiveness (RBE) of the quality of irradiation chosen will influence the choice of dose. Fast neutrons have a higher RBE than photons. The RBE of neutrons varies in different tissues and increases as the dose per fraction falls. The radical doses of neutrons equivalent to photons are therefore much lower.

Homogeneity of dose distribution across the target volume is important to achieve maximum tumour kill. Areas of underdosage may give rise to local recurrence and overdosage to morbidity. For this reason the variation in dose across the target volume should not vary by more than ±5% of the intended dose.

Palliative. Homogeneity of dose distribution is much less important than in radical radiotherapy. Thus simple treatment techniques by single or parallel-opposed fields will suffice for most purposes. Since dose homogeneity is not essential, computerised planning and the use of wedges to improve the dose distribution are not needed. Treatment volumes should be more generous than for radical radiotherapy since the doses delivered should be well below normal tissue tolerance.

Fractionation. Fractionation refers to the division of the total dose into a number of separate fractions, conventionally given on a daily basis, usually 5 days a week (Monday to Friday).

In assessing the value of any fractionation regime, whether for cure or palliation, the effects on both the tumour and the normal tissues have to be considered together. Normal tissue tolerance is dose limiting at many sites in radical radiotherapy (e.g. the spinal cord in head and neck irradiation). At high dose a small increase in cure may be at the expense of substantially greater morbidity. Similarly, high dose per fraction is poorly tolerated with even palliative doses at sensitive sites, as discussed earlier in this chapter.

Hyperfractionation, multiple daily fractions. The terms *hyperfractionated* or *multiple daily fractions* refer to the delivery of more than one fraction per day. It is now appreciated that significant repopulation of some rapidly dividing tumours may occur over the weekend period when traditionally there has been a break in radiotherapy. Tumour repopulation reduces the chance of cure by radical radiotherapy. For this reason hyperfractionated schedules in which the patient is treated every day are under evaluation (continuous hyperfractionated accelerated radiotherapy (CHART). Early experience suggests improved cure rates in non-small cell lung cancer and head and neck cancer (p. 346). The rationale for hyperfractionation is described later in this chapter.

Historical aspects of fractionation. The development of dose and fractionation in the early part of the 20th century was largely empirical. Initially most treatments were given as single large fractions for a wide variety of conditions, both benign and malignant. The energy of the early treatment machines was low and the measurement of their radiation output was clinical and crude (p. 68). Skin reactions were the most frequently used, the so-called *erythema dose*. Later, scientific (as opposed to clinical) methods were introduced to gain a deeper insight into the mode of action of radiation and to find a rational basis for dose, fractionation and overall treatment time, i.e. what factors gave the best probability of tumour cure with acceptable normal tissue morbidity. This is the modern science of *radiobiology*. In Vienna in 1914 a radiologist named Schwarz noted that a mediastinal tumour which had failed to respond to a single large fraction of radiation had regressed several months later when exposed to small fractionated doses. There was still no consensus on the merits of fractionated radiotherapy until, in 1919, Coutard achieved the first cures of tumours of the larynx and tonsil giving one or two small fractions daily over a period of weeks. Coutard's dosage and fractionation were designed to achieve a severe but recoverable acute mucosal reaction. He assumed that the population of cancer cells had the same sensitivity as the normal regenerating epithelial cells. Further confirmation of the therapeutic gain of fractionation was derived from fractionation experiments on the rabbit testis. It was shown that fractionating the same total dose in four fractions caused more damage to the seminiferous epithelium of the testis and less skin reaction than did a single fraction.

In the early 1930s Coutard observed that the acute tolerance of normal tissues treated at high dose per fraction deteriorated with increasing field size. He therefore treated larger volumes with lower daily doses over longer overall times.

In the 1930s Paterson at the Christie Hospital in Manchester combined the low dose rate Paris system of intracavitary radium therapy with the extended treatment times of the Stockholm technique to treat cancer of the cervix. Initially each 48-hour radium insertion was repeated four times over a 4-week period. Subsequently the overall treatment time for intracavitary radium alone was shortened to 2–3 weeks.

In 1935 radical external beam irradiation to small volumes for tumours in the head and neck was initiated in Manchester. Practice at the Christie Hospital was widely adopted in the UK. Daily fractions were given from Monday to Friday over 5–6 weeks to total doses of 5500–6000 R. Reduction in overall treatment time at the Christie Hospital, e.g. 52.5–55 Gy in 15–16 fractions, was brought about because of the pressure on treatment facilities and beds of large numbers of patients. Radical treatments over 3 weeks result in 'hotter' acute reactions. Longer overall treatment times (e.g. 6 weeks) with milder acute reactions have been adopted, particularly in the south of England. Many centres have adopted a middle way (i.e. treating radically over 4 weeks). The cure rates achieved by radical treatments over 3–6 weeks are very similar.

Radiosensitivity. There is a wide spectrum of radiosensitivity among tumours, as illustrated in Table 20.4. Some comment has already been made on radiosensitivity (p. 293).

We know that the sensitivity of a cell, normal or malignant, depends in part on its position in the cell cycle. Those cells in mitosis (M phase) or between G1 and S are more sensitive to killing by radiation than those in S phase. This variation in radiosensitivity during different phases of the cell cycle is less marked with neutrons than with photons and with low-dose-rate brachytherapy (p. 297).

According to the Law of Bergonié and Tribondeau (1904), radiosensitivity increases with the amount of proliferative activity within tissues at the time of radiation. This is now thought not to be the case. The proliferative state of cells at the time of radiation exposure is not critical. However, for radiation to have an acute effect, cells need to be in a proliferative state at or within a short time of exposure. Anaplastic (or poorly differentiated) tumours have a higher proportion of their cell population in mitosis at any given time than do well-differentiated tumours. It follows that anaplastic growths are more likely to be more radiosensitive. This is borne out in clinical practice.

A single dose of 20 Gy may suffice to cure a small basal cell carcinoma of the skin, but if given in five daily fractions (5×4 Gy) it would be insufficient. To achieve a comparable result would require 5×6 Gy (30 Gy). If we took 2 weeks (10 treatment sessions), the dose would be 10×4.5 Gy (45 Gy). As a general rule, the longer the overall treatment time, the higher the total dose required.

Protracted fractionation takes advantage of the better tolerance of the normal tissues and the difference in recuperative ability (see below) between normal and malignant cells. The sequence of events is illustrated in Figure 20.1. Tumour cells suffer progressive damage as the course proceeds and the gap between them and normal cells widens. Eventually, if cure is obtained, all the tumour cells are irreversibly damaged, while normal cells can still recover. If the overall treatment time is too long and the total dose too high (Fig. 20.2A), tumour cure may be obtained but at the expense of permanent injury to normal tissue and inability to heal. If the regime is too short (Fig. 20.2B), the tumour population may remain at a level capable of giving rise to local recurrence.

Fractionation is clearly of great importance in any scheme of therapy, whether radical or palliative. Many patterns of fractionation have been tried, often empirically and without appropriate scientific evaluation of randomised trials.

Influence of time and dose. Both experimental evidence and clinical experience show that variation in the parameters of fractionation influences acute and late normal tissue reactions. The tolerance of normal tissue is affected by the total dose, the dose per fraction, the separation between fractions and the overall duration of treatment.

The severity of the *acute reaction* will depend on the rate of accumulation of dose and the balance between cell killing and regeneration within the irradiated tis-

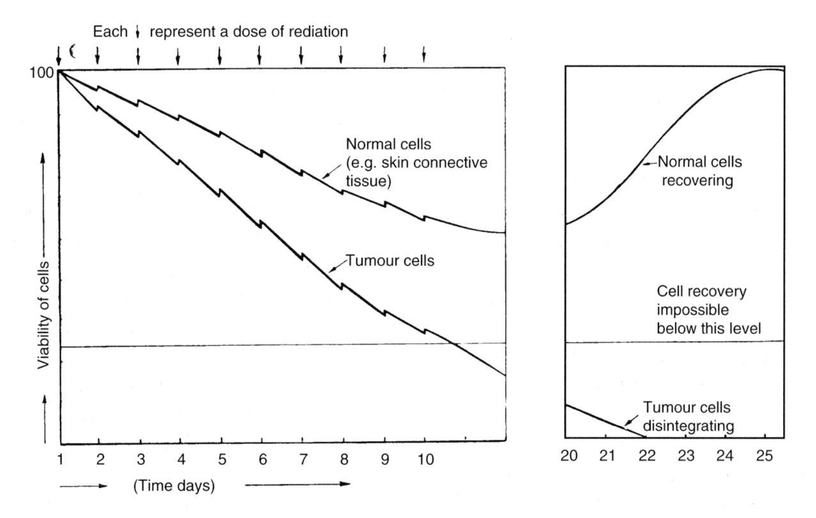

Fig. 20.1 Diagrammatic representation of a successful course of radiation treatment. For explanation see text.

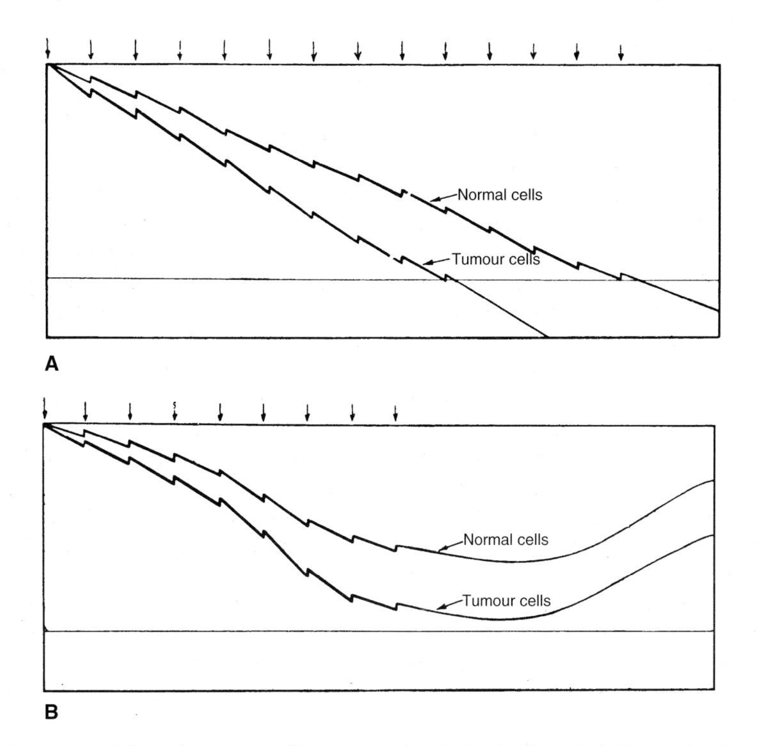

Fig. 20.2 Diagrammatic representation of unsuccessful courses of radiation treatment. **A** Course too long: resultant permanent injury to normal tissues and inability to heal. **B** Course too short: some tumour cells remain active to seed later recurrence.

sues. With shorter overall treatment time (e.g. 3 weeks) acute reactions will be more severe than those given over 6–8 weeks. Healing of the acute reaction requires a minimum number of normal stem cells to survive to allow repopulation of the damaged area. If the rate of accumulation of dose or the total dose is too high, the stem cell population will be eradicated and radionecrosis will occur.

Late reactions typically occur in tissues with a slower cell turnover (e.g. connective tissue). They do not manifest the effects of cell death until after a course of radical radiotherapy has been completed. For this reason the overall treatment time and the rate of accumulation of dose have little influence on late reactions. However, the total dose, size of dose per fraction and the interval between fractions do have a major effect on the severity of late reactions. The rate at which cellular damage is repaired is slower in slow-reacting tissues. For this reason short intervals between fractions may allow inadequate time for repair and result in more severe late reactions. An interval of at least 6 hours is required between fractions for adequate repair in man.

Number of fractions per day

1. *Conventional fractionation.* Daily treatments from Monday to Friday with a gap at weekends remain standard for most radical treatments. However, there is wide variation in the overall treatment time. This varies from 15–16 fractions in 3 weeks in Manchester, with a fraction size of 3.3–3.6 Gy, to 35–40 fractions over 7–8 weeks in the USA, with fraction sizes of 1.8–2.0 Gy.

2. *Hyperfractionation (accelerated fractionation).* Instead of treating once a day, the number of daily fractions can be increased, in practice rarely to more than three. This approach has been explored in tumours where conventionally fractionated radiotherapy has often failed to cure tumours (e.g. cerebral gliomas and advanced lung and head and neck cancer). The rationale for giving more than one fraction per day is based on the 5 Rs of radiobiology (pp. 293–294).

   a. Dose per fraction. There is experimental evidence that as the dose per fraction decreases, so too does the oxygen enhancement ratio (p. 290). Theoretically, with multiple small daily fractions the importance of hypoxia as a cause of radioresistance in tumours should be less marked compared with normal tissues.

   b. Morbidity. In general, accelerated or hyperfractionated treatments are associated with more severe acute reactions. As stated above, acute reactions are determined by the rate of accumulation of dose. Unless small field sizes are used, the mucous membranes of the head and neck will not tolerate fraction sizes of 2 Gy or more given three times a day or more than 55 Gy in 2 weeks.

Late reactions are influenced by fraction size and the interval between fractions. Late reactions are generally worse when the interval between fractions is less than 4.5 hours.

3. *Hypofractionation.* Hypofractionation refers to the practice of giving less than the conventional five daily fractions per week. This approach is illogical for treating most tumour sites since long gaps between fractions may allow tumour repopulation. In a trial comparing three fractions (hypofractionated) versus five fractions (conventional fractionation) per week in laryngeal cancer, there was a tendency for a higher local recurrence rate in the patients treated with three fractions a week.

Hypofractionation is more logical in treating tumours with a higher capacity for repair, e.g. melanomas and soft tissue sarcomas, and in palliative radiotherapy. A limited number of large fractions may take advantage of the higher fractionation sensitivity of such tumours compared with normal tissues.

In palliative radiotherapy single fractions of 4–15 Gy for bone metastases are in general as effective as multiple fractions to total doses of 20–40 Gy. As good and prompt pain relief can be achieved by a single fraction of 8 Gy as by 30 Gy in 10 daily fractions. Two fractions of 8.5 Gy given a week apart are as effective in relieving the symptoms of non-small cell lung cancer as 30 Gy in 10 daily fractions.

Split-course therapy. In split-course treatments, a gap is planned between the first and second halves of the treatment. The duration of the gap may typically be up to a month. The purpose of the gap may be to allow patients, especially the elderly, to recover from the acute reaction of their treatment and to exclude from further morbidity those who have tolerated the first half poorly or whose disease has progressed despite treatment. Split-course therapy is sometimes applied to elderly patients undergoing radical radiotherapy for bladder or prostate cancer. It is commonly used in the radical treatment of lung cancer, since the development of clinically overt metastatic disease during continuous radical radiotherapy over 4–6 weeks is not uncommon. Patients who develop metastases during the month's gap can be spared further toxicity.

Split-course therapy has the disadvantages of the possibility of tumour repopulation during the rest period in rapidly growing tumours and the difficulty of designing split-course regimes biologically equivalent to conventionally fractionated treatments. Furthermore, if both parts of the split course are given, there is no reduction in late morbidity.

Isoeffect formulae. Mathematical formulae, e.g. *nominal standard dose* and *cumulative radiation effect,* have been developed to predict the different dose and fractionation regimes which will achieve the same effect on the tumour (isoeffect). Though these formulae are helpful, their limitations should be appreciated. Observations of the effects of different fractionation regimes in experimental animals, both on tumour cure and morbidity, cannot necessarily be extrapolated to man.

1. Strandquist isoeffect curves. One of the earliest and most influential pieces of work was that of Strandquist. He constructed a series of isoeffect curves to relate total dose to overall treatment time. These included curves for skin necrosis, the cure of squamous skin carcinoma and skin erythema (Fig. 20.3). Each line represents the total dose required to achieve these end-points over a given treatment time. Doses above the middle line resulted in late radiation damage and below the line in tumour persistence or recurrence. In the absence of previous guidelines, Strandquist's isoeffect curves were enthusiastically adopted. However, it was subsequently appreciated that his observations were not applicable to normal clinical practice. It is now accepted that differences in the sensitivity of the skin and squamous skin carcinoma cannot be determined by this method for a variety of reasons. First, the time scale of a third of a day for a single fraction is out of step with normal clinical practice. Secondly, most of his patients had basal and not squamous carcinomas and, thirdly, the number of patients on which his curves were based was small.

2. More recent isoeffect formulae. These include nominal standard dose (NSD), cumulative radiation effect

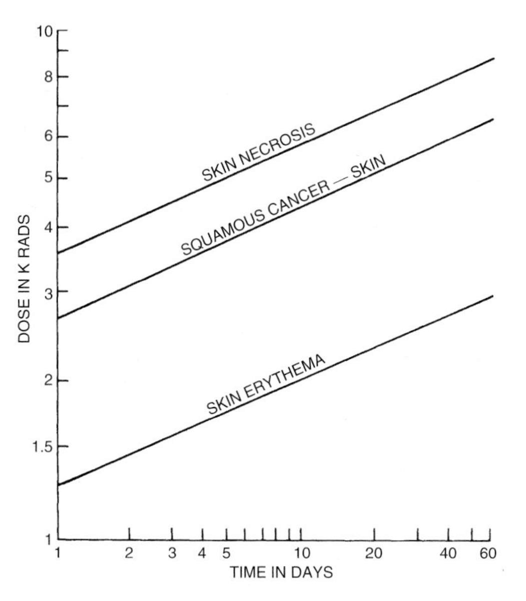

Fig. 20.3 Isoeffect curves relating total dose and overall treatment to skin necrosis, cure of squamous cell carcinoma and erythema. (After Strandquist, 1944. Courtesy of Duncan and Nias, Clinical Radiobiology, Churchill Livingstone, 1977.)

(CRE), time, dose and fractionation (TDF) and, most recently the α/β ratio. The α/β ratio is discussed on page 289. *It should be emphasised that none of these formulae should be relied upon clinically to predict the effects of different fractionation regimes.* All of the predictive formulae have limitations in their applicability to a greater or lesser degree.

Ellis introduced in 1967 an isoeffect formula, the *nominal standard dose.* This proposed that the tolerance of normal tissues (D) could be related to the overall treatment time (T), and the number of fractions (N) by the following formula:

$$D_N = (\mathrm{NSD})\ T^{0.11} \times N^{0.24}$$

The formula was widely adopted, particularly since it enabled less than five fractions a week to be given. This was attractive to centres treating larger numbers of patients. Radical treatments were sometimes reduced to two fractions a week.

Other formulae such as CRE and TDF were derivatives of the Ellis NSD concept.

Cumulative radiation effect (R) was developed to predict the effects of doses below tolerance on normal tissues.

$$R = D_N \times T^{-0.11} \times N^{-0.24}$$

The concept of NSD is only applicable to full normal tissue tolerance doses. It cannot be calculated for two parts of a fractionated course of treatment. The concept of *partial tolerance* is useful for the calculation of the modified treatment regime which has to be given if a continuous course of fractionated radiotherapy is interrupted unintentionally (e.g. by illness or machine breakdown) or intentionally in split-course therapy. The sum of the partial tolerances of the two halves of treatment can be added. Thus if N fractions are needed for a full NSD value of Y rets, then the partial tolerance (PT) from fewer fractions, n, is as follows:

$$\mathrm{PT} = (n/N) \times Y$$

Tables of TDF factors equivalent to the partial tolerance doses have been constructed for fractionation regimes of one, two, three, four or five fractions a week.

Complexity of factors determining biological effects of fractionation. In any fractionated course of radiotherapy, there is a wide range of interacting physical and biological variables operating which determine the biological effect. In addition to the 5 Rs, treatment energy, dose rate, distribution of cells in different phases of the cell cycle, rate of cell loss and of 'scavenging' of dead cells by phagocytosis all play a part. In so complex a situation it is difficult to assess the contribution of any one factor. In the laboratory, where spontaneously occurring animal tumours or human tumours transplanted into animals can be irradiated, the effects of different treatment parameters can be studied. For example. the effect can be observed on normal tissue and tumour of different numbers of fractions of the same total dose while keeping the energy, tissue, field size, dose rate and overall treatment time constant. None the less, great caution should be taken in extrapolating from radiobiological laboratory experiments on animals to man.

Normal tissue tolerance. The tolerance of normal tissue is of great practical importance to the radiotherapist. Exceeding it may result in major morbidity and, sometimes, mortality. Since radical doses often need to be at or close to normal tissue tolerance to achieve cure, some degree of morbidity almost always has to be accepted. For example, a major morbidity rate of up to 5%, mainly due to bowel and bladder damage, has generally to be accepted in treating cervical cancer by radical radiotherapy. The degree of risk accepted will depend on the seriousness of the morbidity. The more serious the complication, the lower the probability of its occurrence is the clinician likely to accept. For example, less than a 1% risk of spinal cord damage would be accepted for 'mantle' radiotherapy (p. 512) for Hodgkin's disease.

Probability of complications. Tolerance doses of ionising radiation are commonly expressed in terms of the doses that give a certain probability of a particular complication. Typically the probabilities cited are 5% ($TD_{5/5}$) and 50% ($TD_{50/5}$). Examples of $TD_{5/5}$ and $TD_{50/5}$ for different tissues are shown in Table 20.6.

There is wide variation (up to 20-fold) in the sensitivity of normal tissues from the most radiosensitive to the most radioresistant. The sensitivity of tumours derived from normal tissues tends to be similar. The testes, ovaries, lymphoid tissue and bone marrow are among the most radiosensitive, as are seminomas of the testis, dysgerminomas of the ovary and lymphomas. Bone, cartilage, nervous tissue and kidney, and correspondingly the tumours derived from them (gliomas, osteosarcomas and renal cancers), are relatively radioresistant.

It is now clear that normal tissue and organ tolerance is relative rather than absolute and can be altered by a variety of factors. These include treatment factors (e.g. dose, volume, fractionation, chemotherapy, radiosensitisers, radioprotectors, biological response modifiers) and patient factors (age, concurrent disease, trauma, direct and indirect effects of tumours). The injury inflicted on normal tissue depends upon the capacity of the stem cell population to supply new cells and the timing of its expression on the cell cycle time for renewal.

Table 20.6 Tolerance doses of normal tissues to conventionally fractionated irradiation (courtesy of Vaeth & Meyer 1989)

Tissue/organ	$TD_{5/5}$–$TD_{50/5}$ (Gy)
Testes	1–2
Ovary	6–10
Eye (lens)	6–12
Lung	20–30
Kidney	20–30
Liver	35–40
Skin	30–40
Thyroid	30–40
Heart	40–50
Lymphoid tissue	40–50
Bone marrow	40–50
Gastrointestinal	40–50
Vasculoconnective tissue	50–60
Peripheral nerve	65–77
Mucosa	65–77
Brain	60–70
Bone and cartilage	> 70
Muscle	> 70

Between 20 and 50 different cell types are represented in normal tissue, although the number of different stem cells is more restricted. This cellular heterogeneity is similar to that observed in tumours. It is therefore hardly surprising that since a fixed dose does not kill all tumour cells, the effect on normal tissues is non-uniform. It also explains why isoeffect formulae (see above) oversimplify normal tissue tolerance and do not reliably predict tolerance in vivo. Each subpopulation of normal cells may vary in its response to different doses, fraction sizes and timing of exposure. The overall response of a given tissue to different dose and fractionation regimes is extremely complex.

Factors influencing radiosensitivity of normal tissues

1. Treatment factors

   a. Quality of radiation and RBE. The quality of radiation and its RBE strongly influence normal tissue tolerance. Megavoltage irradiation with its skin-sparing effects and reduced absorption in bone causes much less skin reaction and risk of bony injury than orthovoltage irradiation. High LET irradiation, such as fast neutrons, with its high absorption in fat can cause substantial damage to tissue with a high fat content (e.g. the bowel). Fast neutrons have a higher RBE (approximately 5.2) for the central nervous system compared with photons, with increased risk of inducing radionecrosis.

b. Dose. The dose that irrevocably damages normal tissue is not absolute but depends on fractionation.

c. Fractionation. The fraction size and the interval between fractions largely influence the severity of acute and late effects. Hyperfractionation and hypofractionation will modify normal tissue tolerance.

d. Volume. Normal tissue tolerance is influenced by the volume of the organ that is irradiated. The tolerance of the whole lung to conventionally fractionated photon irradiation is 20 Gy in 20 daily fractions over 4 weeks. However, limited volumes of lung (e.g. $8 \times 8 \times 8$ cm) will normally tolerate 50 Gy similarly fractionated. The same principle applies to the kidney. If no more than a third of the kidney is treated on each side during prophylactic abdominal node irradiation for seminoma, 30 Gy in 20 daily fractions over 4 weeks are tolerated without serious renal damage. This is because there is adequate functional unirradiated kidney tissue to compensate. The tolerance dose for conventionally fractionated irradiation of the whole kidney is lower (20 Gy).

e. Time. The time interval between exposure of normal tissue to irradiation and the expression of damage is determined by the kinetics of different cell subpopulations.

f. Chemotherapy. Chemotherapy can influence the tolerance of normal tissue. An example is the reduced lung tolerance to radiation following treatment with bleomycin.

g. Other agents. Radiosensitisers such as the hypoxic cell sensitisers (e.g. misonidazole, p. 291) can increase the radiation reaction in some normal tissues (e.g. the skin) and possibly in the CNS, liver and other organs. This may be due to the presence of small numbers of hypoxic cells within normal tissues.

2. Patient factors

a. Age. In utero, in infancy and at puberty, when growth is rapid, normal tissues are particularly sensitive to radiation damage. For example, extended field irradiation before the age of 13 of mediastinal or para-aortic nodes overlying the spine in Hodgkin's disease may impair sitting and standing height by about 5%. Over the age of 13, there is little effect on growth even if it has not been completed.

b. Concurrent disease. A variety of conditions such as anaemia, diabetes mellitus and arteriosclerosis can reduce the supply of oxygen to tissues. This in turn may impair the cellular repair of normal tissue injury and increase both acute and late reactions.

c. Trauma. Irradiated tissue is particularly vulnerable to traumatic damage. For example, if the skin of the nose is irradiated for a basal cell carcinoma, subsequent exposure to very cold temperatures may precipitate skin necrosis. Similarly, radionecrosis of the mandible following radical irradiation for cancer of the floor of the mouth may be precipitated by minor accidental trauma or tooth extraction.

3. Tumour factors

a. Local invasion. The presence of tumour may directly or indirectly affect normal tissue tolerance. Direct invasion of normal structures, e.g. the bowel in extranodal non-Hodgkin lymphoma, may result in perforation of the bowel after abdominal irradiation or chemotherapy. Indirect damage may be caused by mechanical effects, such as ureteric obstruction resulting in hydronephrosis and renal failure.

b. Radiosensitivity. This is another factor of obvious fundamental importance. Tumours, like normal tissues, vary in their vulnerability to radiation and this depends chiefly on their rate of growth.

Table 20.4 lists some of the most important tumours in order of their relative radiosensitivity. It is a useful approximation. There are exceptions: some lymphomas may prove radioresistant, even at high dosage.

The highest proportion of successes is achieved in the epithelial cancers (especially squamous) of moderate sensitivity, such as the skin, mouth and cervix.

The most important factor is the biological nature and behaviour of the particular cell type of an individual tumour. At present there is no reliable method of predicting in advance the responsiveness of an individual patient's tumour to radiation.

FOLLOW-UP

Once patients have completed anticancer treatment, it is customary to assess them on a regular basis as outpatients. In general the longer patients remain well, the less frequently they need to be seen.

Aims

The reasons for following up patients are:

- Confirmation of response to treatment and of resolution of its side-effects
- Detection of persistent or recurrent disease at a stage when curative 'salvage' treatment is possible
- Detection of late complications of treatment
- Reassuring the patient that he or she is free of tumour

- Management of patients with persistent or progressive disease or complications of treatment
- Evaluation of new and existing treatments.

Frequency

The frequency of hospital follow-up will depend on a number of factors. These include:

- The period during which the risk of recurrence is highest
- The development of complications of treatment
- Persistent or progressive disease
- Age and performance status
- Geographical, e.g. distance from the patient's home to the outpatient clinic
- Availability of transport to and from the clinic.

Practice varies widely. For an activity that occupies so large a part of an oncologist's professional time, there is a surprising lack of information on the optimal frequency of follow-up of patients with tumours of different stage and site.

Risk of recurrence

Head and neck cancer. In most cases of head and neck cancer treated with curative intent, recurrence, if it occurs, is most likely to do so within the first 2 years. Thus monthly appointments in the first year after treatment, 2-monthly appointments in the second year and less frequently in subsequent years are generally sufficiently frequent to detect most relapses at a stage when curative salvage treatment can be attempted. A similar intensity of follow-up is applicable to cervical cancer, which has a similar time scale of relapse.

In general, local relapses after 5 years are uncommon in squamous carcinomas. If they do occur they are often due to new primary tumours close to the original site.

Often the distinction between a new primary and relapse of the original tumour is impossible to make. For these reasons such patients probably need at least 10 years of follow-up.

Lymphomas. Relapse more than 5 years after treatment is not uncommon in the non-Hodgkin lymphomas. It is less common in Hodgkin's disease. Lifelong follow-up is recommended.

Breast cancer. The follow-up of patients with breast cancer illustrates a number of principles applicable to other tumours.

Most local relapses tend to occur within 5 years of mastectomy. Surveillance for at least 5 years is therefore desirable.

Although metastatic relapse may occur at any time after treatment, there is no evidence that detection at scheduled as opposed to 'interval' appointments (i.e. arranged between routine appointments) improves survival. Most metastatic relapses are symptomatic. Patients usually present to their general practitioner with symptoms, for example, of dyspnoea from lung metastases or pleural effusion or with pain from bony metastases. The offer of an appointment at the next oncology clinic can avoid unnecessary appointments when the patient is symptom free.

Many clinicians still undertake lifelong follow-up of patients with breast cancer in view of the risk of death persisting for at least 30 years (Fig. 26.24). However, since the tumour is very common, such a policy, particularly in oncology centres serving large populations, can result in very large numbers of women attending the oncology clinic. This pressure can be reduced by surgeon and oncologist seeing patients alternately at an agreed frequency.

SUPPORT SERVICES

Treatment includes not simply the delivery of specific therapy such as surgery or radiotherapy but physical, psychological and social support.

There is a wide range of support services available to meet these needs. Some are specific to patients with particular tumours (e.g. mastectomy or stoma care nurses). Others such as medical social workers have a wide role in assisting patients and their families with their social and financial concerns.

Mastectomy/breast care nurse

Experienced nurses provide counselling to patients who have undergone mastectomy. They are familiar with dealing with the psychological distress of a patient following mastectomy. They can also, in conjunction with the surgeon, offer advice on breast-conserving surgery, the range of prostheses available to compensate for the loss of the breast and the surgical reconstructions of the breast that are possible.

Stoma care nurse

Stoma care nurses provide practical advice on the management of bowel (colostomy, ileostomy) and urinary (urostomy) stomas.

MacMillan nurses

MacMillan nurses are based both in hospitals and in the community. Their role is to provide, in conjunction with the patient's general practitioner, advice on symptom control at home and psychological support for both the patient and the family.

District nurse liaison

District nurses may have a specific responsibility for liaising between the hospital and the community in the care of patients with malignant disease. They may identify nursing needs at home and bring these to the attention of hospital staff. This assists the appropriate provision of support services when the patient is discharged home.

Prosthetic services

The prompt provision of prostheses (to replace, for example an eye, nose or breast) or wigs (following chemotherapy or cranial irradiation causing hair loss) can be extremely important in maintaining a patient's appearance and morale.

Department of social security (DSS) advisory service

Each patient has access to an advisory service within the DSS on sources of financial help. In some areas an adviser may visit a hospital on a regular basis. Financial assistance is of considerable practical importance to patients who are unable to work temporarily or permanently because of disability.

Day care unit

A day care unit can provide patients with support during the period of acute reaction after radiotherapy. The first unit for this purpose was established in Sheffield.

Dietician

Adequate nutrition is important in both radical and palliative therapy of malignant disease. Anorexia and weight loss commonly accompany malignancy and its treatment by chemotherapy and radiotherapy. Maintaining an adequate protein and calorie intake is vital to recovery from radical surgery, radiotherapy and chemotherapy. In incurable disease, dysphagia, vomiting, anorexia and constipation all influence dietary intake.

A hospital dietician should be available to advise inpatients and outpatients with dietary problems related to their malignancy or its treatment. Close liaison is necessary with the hospital catering department and pharmacy to provide for the special dietary needs of patients. This may include selection of foods that are appetising to the patient, oral food supplements (e.g. Complan or Build-up drinks) and nasogastric feeds. Patients being treated with curative intent may sometimes require intravenous feeding (total parenteral nutrition [TPN]). Many hospitals have a team of surgeons, specialist nurses and dieticians who provide such a service.

Medical social work department

Medical social workers are familiar with the social and financial problems faced by patients and their families. They can provide practical advice on grants available, such as mobility and attendance allowances and travel expenses. They liaise with medical and nursing staff and with social services in the community. They may apply on the patient's behalf and with medical support for financial assistance from charitable bodies.

Support and self-help groups

Newly diagnosed patients and their relatives may benefit from attending a support or self-help group. Awareness of how other patients have coped with the emotional and physical side-effects of treatment may enable a patient to cope better with cancer and its treatment.

Bereavement counselling

Some form of bereavement counselling service can help relatives come to terms with the loss of a member of the family.

Spiritual care

Spiritual support of the patient and family can be provided by the church and other religious organisations.

CONFIDENTIALITY

It is important to clarify with the patient, if well enough, what medical information he or she is willing to have disclosed, so that confidentiality is not breached. Often well-intentioned relatives ask to speak to the doctor without the knowledge of the patient. To do so without the patient's permission is a breach of confidentiality. Where the patient is too unwell to grant permission, immediate relatives or, in their absence, close friends may be informed.

CHAPTER CONTENTS

21

Skin and lip

Ian Kunkler

SKIN CANCER

Pathology

Epidemiology

We are seeing an epidemic of skin cancer worldwide. Skin tumours are the commonest of all neoplasms in the UK, as in many other countries with a predominantly white population. Non-melanomatous skin cancer represents 10% of all cancers but only 0.3% of cancer deaths. They are rare in dark-skinned races. They are most common in the seventh and eighth decades of life. There is a male predominance (sex ratio 1.5 : 1). Secondary deposits also occur in the skin.

There are three main varieties: basal cell carcinoma (BCC), squamous cell carcinoma (SCC) and melanoma. Non-melanomatous skin cancer is of considerable importance to the oncologist since it is the most accessible of cancers, tends to present early with localised disease and is eminently radiocurable.

Aetiology

1. *Sunlight.* Ultraviolet light is the most important aetiological factor for skin cancer. It is thought that exposure to sunlight before the age of 20 starts a process of carcinogenesis that results in the clinical development of skin cancer 40–60 years later. The process involves many intermediate steps including activation of oncogenes and deactivation of tumour suppressor genes and other factors. Exposure to the sun also results in changes in DNA in epidermal cells and impairs the capacity of the immune system to eliminate damaged cells. Increased foreign travel to sunny climates and increased life expectancy have also contributed to the rise in the incidence of the disease (238% in the UK over a 14-year period). In addition, outdoor workers (farmers, fishermen) and participants in outdoor sports (golf, tennis, sailing, skiing) are more at risk. Men are at slightly greater risk than women.

Basal and squamous carcinomas arise most frequently on exposed skin, though they can arise elsewhere. For melanoma it is thought that intense exposure to the sun is more important than the total life-time exposure.

2. *Ionising radiation*. Basal and squamous cell carcinomas may occur many years after exposure to therapeutic irradiation for benign conditions in childhood (e.g. for ringworm of the scalp—a practice long abandoned).

3. *Chemical carcinogens*. Prolonged exposure to many oil and tar products may cause squamous carcinomas. Arsenic salts, which used to be prescribed in low dosage for prolonged periods for a variety of common diseases, gave rise to keratoses, typically on the palms of the hands. Some of these underwent malignant change.

4. *Chronic ulcers and granulomas*. Occasionally a long-standing ulcer may develop carcinoma from its margin.

5. *Scar tissue*. Especially after wounds or burns, soft tissue may rarely undergo malignant change.

6. *Immunosuppression*. Squamous cell carcinomas of the skin are commoner following drug-induced immunosuppression (e.g. with steroids) after kidney transplantation.

7. *Genetic factors*. (a) Basal cell naevus syndrome (Gorlin's syndrome) is an autosomal dominant disorder giving rise to multiple basal cell carcinomas developing from childhood onwards. It is associated with odontogenic keratocysts in the mandible, epidermal cysts in the skin, palmar and plantar cysts, other cancers and developmental abnormalities. It is due to a loss of heterozygosity of the 9q chromosome. BCCs may occur on areas of the skin not exposed to the sun. (b) Xeroderma pigmentosum is a rare autosomal recessive disorder in which there is a defect in the capacity to repair DNA. It predisposes to the development of squamous skin cancer after normal light exposure. This seems to illustrate the important normal function of DNA repair enzymes.

Premalignant conditions

There are a number of conditions to consider: some may undergo malignant change.

1. *Hyperkeratosis*. Small warty nodules, may be due to sunlight, actinic or solar keratosis, tar, or X-rays.
2. *Papilloma*. These are generally viral warts.
3. *Bowen's disease*. This is a form of carcinoma-in-situ, and may progress to invasive malignancy.

BASAL CELL CARCINOMA

Pathology and clinical features

This tumour accounts for 80% of skin tumours. It arises from the basal aspect of the epidermis and grows as nests of darkly staining cells, often palisaded peripherally. There are a number of clinical varieties.

1. *Noduloulcerative*. This is the commonest variety (Plate 2.1). It appears as a pearly papule. The epidermis is thinned, and abnormal blood vessels (telangiectasia) can be seen over the surface. As it grows the central part ulcerates. It is associated with haemorrhage.

2. *Superficial*. This variety is a reddish macule with a thin pearly border and atrophy of the epidermis. They are round or oval. Sometimes the border is scalloped or ill defined. The tumour can sometimes be discontinuous or multicentric, so surgical excision sometimes leaves some tumour behind. The multicentricity relates to a tendency to regress, with normal skin between involved areas. However, histologically, even these apparently normal areas of skin are abnormal. Superficial BCCs if greater than 1.5 cm in diameter are commonly associated with a deeply invasive element or have separate tumour islands in the upper and mid dermis.

3. *Infiltrative morphoeic*. This rarer variety appears as a plaque of scar-like tissue (scleroderma) with an ill-defined border making diagnosis difficult and often late. They are flat and detection depends on how much fibrosis they contain. Clinical recognition is assisted by stretching the skin or pressing it with a glass slide. They occur virtually exclusively on the face. Spread is lateral rather than deep. Microscopically, there is a dense stroma with thin strands of basal cells. At the periphery the tumour blends with the surrounding dermis, so there is a great risk of leaving some behind at operation.

4. *Infiltrative non-morphoeic*. This variety differs from the morphoeic form because of the absence of any change in skin colour. Microscopically it is similar to the morphoeic variety with the exception that there is little or no fibrosis. They rarely ulcerate or bleed and may grow to a large size without being clinically detected.

5. *Cystic*. In this form, the tumour is typically raised with a smooth surface and underlying cystic degeneration.

6. *Basi-squamous carcinoma*. Basi-squamous carcinomas have the clinical and histological features of both basal and squamous cell carcinomas. Their growth rate is faster than BCCs and similar to that of SCCs. They have the metastatic potential of an SCC.

General clinical features

The commonest sites are on the face: nose, cheek, temple, eyelid (Fig. 21.1) and scalp. Growth is slow, often over several years, with only a gradual increase in size,

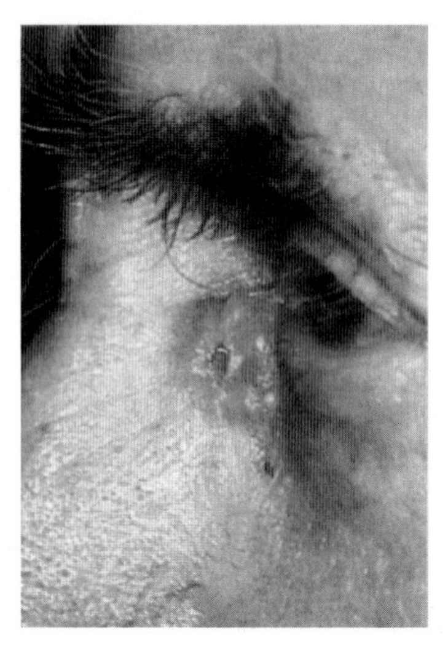

Fig. 21.1 Basal cell carcinoma at the inner canthus.

but superficial ulceration and slight bleeding are common. Infection of the ulcer is common. However, their capacity to grow and destroy tissues locally gives them the common name of 'rodent ulcer'. Typically they are up to 3 cm in diameter at the time of diagnosis. Occasionally, in patients who are mentally impaired or who have neglected themselves or deferred presentation for fear of the diagnosis, the tumour may measure several centimetres in diameter. It may have caused extensive damage by its 'rodent' activity, invading the eye or the skull vault. Very rarely, death in advanced neglected cases may eventually occur from haemorrhage (erosion of a large blood vessel) or meningitis (erosion of the skull). They do not metastasise.

SQUAMOUS CELL CARCINOMA

Pathology

Squamous carcinoma forms about 15% of skin cancer. It tends to grow more rapidly than basal cell carcinomas and may spread to the regional nodes. Microscopically the typical appearance is of a well-differentiated keratinising tumour extending downwards from the epidermis into the dermis. The majority are due to sunlight and are of low-grade malignancy. A small proportion behave fairly aggressively.

Clinical features

Squamous carcinomas may occur anywhere on the body surface but are usually, by reason of occupational exposure, seen on the head and neck, hands, forearms and scrotum. There are two main clinical varieties. The commonest is an ulcer with a raised rolled edge and slough at the base (Plate 2.2). Less common is a slow-growing variety, presenting as a nodular mass. The more advanced form of the latter can be a keratinised horn, for example on the pinna of the ear. Lymph node metastases are commoner with the ulcerated form.

OTHER FORMS OF SKIN CANCER

1. *Malignant melanoma* represents about 5% of skin cancer and is considered later in this chapter.
2. *Miscellaneous*. Sweat gland tumours are uncommon. A variety of cysts and benign tumours also occur.

   a. *Keratoacanthoma* (Fig. 21.2) resembles squamous carcinoma but is distinguished by its well-defined edge and central plug of keratin. It typically develops rapidly over a few weeks. It is a benign lesion and often heals without treatment or after curettage. Biopsy may not distinguish it from a squamous cell carcinoma. If there is any doubt about the histology it should be treated as a squamous cell carcinoma with radical radiotherapy.

   b. *Skin glands*. Sebaceous and sweat glands rarely give rise to tumours, benign (adenomas) or malignant (adenocarcinomas). Tumours of the sebaceous glands occur more frequently on the head and neck. Lymph node spread is rare. Tumours of the sweat glands arise most often in the axilla, scrotum and vulva. Surgery is preferable in these areas since they tolerate irradiation poorly.

   c. *Lymphoma*. Skin lesions (lymphoma cutis) may be an early manifestation of lymphoma. The most serious is mycosis fungoides (p. 524).

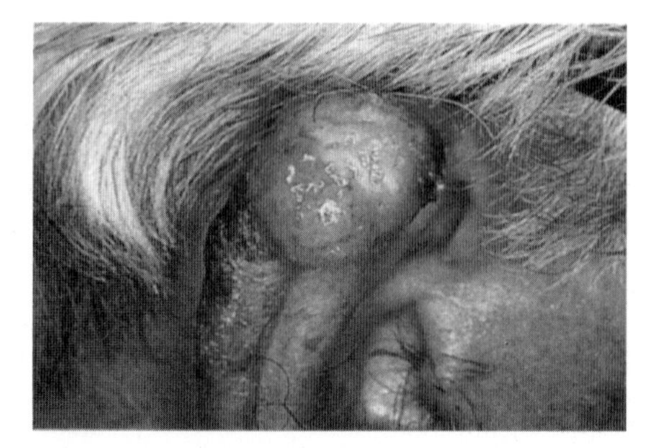

Fig. 21.2 Keratoacanthoma. (Courtesy of Dr D Gawkrodger, Sheffield.)

d. *Secondary carcinoma* often appears as nodules just below the epidermis, especially from a lung or breast primary (of which it may be the first clinical evidence). The diagnosis may be confirmed on fine needle cytology or excision. Local radiotherapy is helpful in relieving pain.

Diagnosis

The diagnosis of basal or squamous carcinoma should be confirmed by biopsy, although the clinical diagnosis is usually clear. Occasionally other tumours such as secondary deposits or primary melanoma are diagnosed. A deep shave biopsy under local anaesthetic (1% buffered lidocaine (lignocaine) with adrenaline (epinephrine) is recommended.

Prevention

The most important element of prevention is the limitation of exposure to the sun, particularly among children but also in adults. Schools should organise outdoor activities early or late in the day. Shade from trees should be available in playgrounds. Long sleeves and hats limit exposure. In addition, reduction in the fat content of the diet (e.g. reducing from 40% to 20% of total calories) can reduce the development of new tumours as can dietary supplements of multivitamins or beta-carotene.

Sunscreens should be used. These are of two types—reflectants (zinc oxide or titanium dioxide) and absorbents (e.g. methoxycinnamates and salicylates). Depending on their content, they protect against ultraviolet A and B. They provide good protection against acute sunburn but must be regularly applied.

Treatment

Basal and squamous cell carcinomas can be cured in over 90% of cases by a variety of techniques, including curettage and cautery, cryosurgery, local excision and radiotherapy. Practice will vary with local expertise and facilities. Curettage and freezing can cure 95% of BCCs of up to 1.5 cm. Similar cure rates (90–95%) are achievable by radiotherapy. The use of liquid nitrogen, although it has high cure rates, means that no histology is obtained and healing may take several weeks.

Close liaison should be established between dermatologist, clinical oncologist and plastic surgeon in determining the best form of treatment, ideally in a multidisciplinary clinic. Lesions in sites which may affect cosmesis, including the eyelids, ear, nose and lips, should be seen by plastic surgeon.

Factors that influence the choice of treatment are the aetiology, site, size, local extent and number of lesions, the cosmetic and functional effect, the age, occupation, general condition and convenience of the patient.

Surgery

Surgery is generally recommended for the following categories:

- Radiation-induced tumours
- Persistent or recurrent disease following radiotherapy
- Scarred or unhealthy skin (e.g. dermatitis or chronic infection)
- Patients under the age of 50 (better cosmesis)
- Sites tolerating radiotherapy poorly (dorsum of the hand, abdominal wall, perineum, shin and sole of the foot)
- Sites adjacent to structures likely to be damaged by radiation (e.g. lateral third of upper eyelid overlying lacrimal gland)
- Very large lesions, e.g. > 5 cm
- Tumours involving cartilage or bone
- Multiple lesions (e.g. Gorlin's syndrome)
- Occupational exposure to extremes of heat and cold.

In general, surgical excision is preferred to radiotherapy in the younger patient because the scar is often less noticeable than the coin-shaped area of pale skin with overlying telangiectasia which characterises the late effects of radiotherapy. However, where loss of tissue is likely to cause cosmetic or functional impairment, e.g. lower eyelid, lip, nose, inner canthus and ear, radiotherapy is generally preferred.

Sites which tolerate radiotherapy poorly (and are more prone to radionecrosis) are the back of the hand, abdominal wall, perineum, shin and the sole of the foot. Surgical excision is preferable at these sites. Similarly, tumours of the upper eyelid are best excised, because of the proximity of the lacrimal gland behind the lateral third. Inhibition of the production of tears from the lacrimal gland will result in a dry eye and the risk of corneal ulceration.

Very large lesions, e.g. over 4–5 cm, are less likely to be controlled by radiotherapy. Surgical excision with skin grafting should be considered.

Tumours invading cartilage or bone, e.g. on the ear or nose, are best treated surgically since radiotherapy may precipitate necrosis of cartilage or bone. Pain is a common symptom of cartilage or bony invasion. This is less of a problem where electrons of suitable energy are available in view of their limited absorption in cartilage or bone.

Multiple lesions, e.g. in basal cell naevus syndrome (Gorlin's syndrome), are best treated by local excision since otherwise many weeks will be occupied by multiple courses of radiotherapy. There may also be difficulty in avoiding overlap with previously irradiated areas.

Elderly patients and those in poor medical condition may not be fit for surgery. However, excision may be possible under local anaesthetic and may be preferable to several visits to hospital for radiotherapy. For the very frail, single fractions of radiotherapy are an alternative.

Patients whose occupations expose them to extremes of heat or cold are best treated by surgery. Such exposure increases the risk of radionecrosis, even many years after treatment.

Small lesions are excised with a margin of normal tissue. This tends to be narrower on the face to achieve a good cosmetic result. Inadequate excision is more likely to occur on the face than in other sites where a more generous margin of normal tissue can be afforded.

Radiotherapy

Target volume

For most basal cell carcinomas the target volume is the tumour with a 0.5 cm margin of surrounding normal skin. Particular care is needed in determining the ill-defined edge of morphoeic lesions. This can often be better appreciated by stretching the lesion between both thumbs. For morphoeic basal cell carcinoma and all squamous cell carcinomas this margin should be larger, i.e. 1 cm.

Technique

Single fields are appropriate for the vast majority of basal and squamous cell carcinomas. Where the contours of the skin may result in considerable fall-off in dose, e.g. over the tip of the nose, a wax block attached to the nose and treatment by opposed lateral fields at orthovoltage makes the dose distribution more even across the target volume. The concavity or convexity of the skin can often be overcome by flattening the tumour and surrounding skin with the treatment applicator.

At some sites (e.g. the inner canthus) it is not possible to bring the applicator to the level of the lesion because the applicator is obstructed by the adjacent nose and cheek or because the lesion is below the surface of the skin (positive 'stand-off') (Fig. 21.3A). In these circumstances, the tumour is treated at a slightly longer SSD (e.g. 20.5 cm instead of the normal 20 cm). Conversely, lesions protruding above the surface of the skin (negative 'stand-off') are treated at a shorter SSD (Fig. 21.3B). The distance from the end of the applicator to the surface of the lesion is measured by passing a thin wooden stick through the middle of the applicator so that it touches the surface of the tumour. The applicator is removed with the stick held in the same position. The distance that the stick protrudes from the end of the applicator is then measured with a ruler.

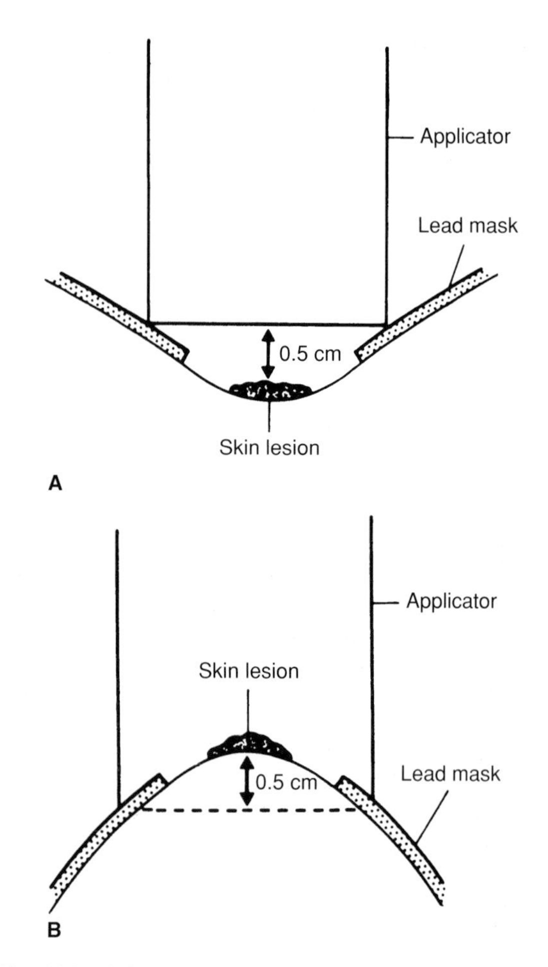

Fig. 21.3 **A** Positive 'stand-off' of 0.5 cm between the lesion and applicator. **B** Negative 'stand-off' of 0.5 cm. (Reproduced from Dobbs J & Barrett A 1985 Practical Radiotherapy Planning, 1st edn, by permission of Edward Arnold, London.)

To avoid a sharply punched out border, which is unsightly, the inner edge of the lead cut-out can be bevelled. This results in a more gradual fall-off in dose at the periphery. The late radiation-induced skin changes are less noticeable since they blend with the surrounding normal skin. Without bevelling, the irradiated area is more clearly demarcated.

Surface radium moulds had a long vogue but are now rarely used as they involve expensive preparation, hospitalisation and unavoidable radiation exposure to hospital staff.

Tumours around the eye. The cornea and the lens of the eye are particularly sensitive to radiation. Every effort should be made to protect the eyes from irradiation where possible.

Eyelid. Lesions on the eyelids are common, usually basal cell carcinomas, e.g. at the medial ends near the bridge of the nose (inner canthus, Fig. 21.1). Tumours of the upper eyelids are generally best treated by surgical excision because a radiation field covering the tumour and 0.5 cm safety margin will almost invariably include the lacrimal gland, which lies behind the lateral third of the eyelid.

Tumours of the lower eyelids can usually be treated by superficial radiation. An internal eye shield is necessary. This is in the form of a contact lens, but made of lead (1 mm thick). It has a smooth surface to avoid scratching the cornea or conjunctiva. Eye shields may be kept in an antiseptic solution (chlorhexidine gluconate) and rinsed before use in sterile water. They should be regularly inspected for damage and cracks. Local anaesthetic (1% tetracaine (amethocaine) hydrochloride) is instilled into the eye, followed by 1–2 drops of sterile paraffin. The patient should be advised that the local anaesthetic will sting briefly before its anaesthetic action takes effect. If the eye shield (Fig. 21.4C) is to be inserted under both lids, the patient is asked to look down and the eye shield is inserted under the upper lid first. The patient then looks up and the shield is placed behind the lower eyelid. For tumours of the lower eyelid, a spatula-like lead shield can be inserted behind the lid margin and taped temporarily to the forehead (Fig. 21.4A).

Tumours of the ala nasi. If the ala nasi is treated, some protection to the inside of the nose can be given by a narrow strip of lead (covered with wax to absorb the secondary electrons from the lead) inserted into the nostril during treatment.

Dose and energy

Choice of energy, dose and fractionation will depend on the site, diameter and thickness of the lesion and the age and general condition of the patient. For superficial and orthovoltage the energy is chosen which delivers 50% of the surface dose to the base of the tumour (the half-value layer). For example, for 100 kV at 15 cm SSD the half-value layer is 1.0 mm of aluminium. The depth doses of different energies are shown in Figure 21.5. Basal cell carcinomas at certain sites, e.g. in the retroauricular sulcus (behind the ear),

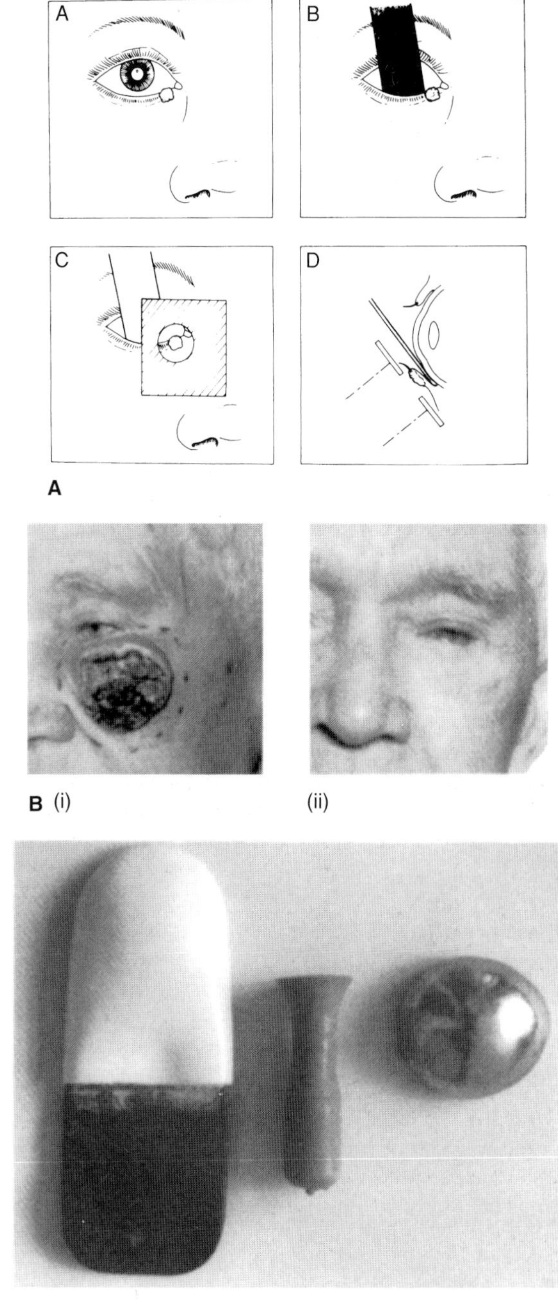

Fig. 21.4 **A** Treatment of skin cancer on lower eyelid (reproduced with permission from Souhami R L & Tobias J S 1986 Cancer and its Management. Blackwell Scientific, Oxford). **B** Squamous carcinoma of the cheek (i) before and (ii) after treatment with 6 MeV electrons (courtesy of Dr A Champion, Sheffield). **C** Protection of the eye during radiotherapy: (left to right) (1) lead shield inserted below lower eyelid, (2) rubber applicator for (3) gold full internal eye shield.

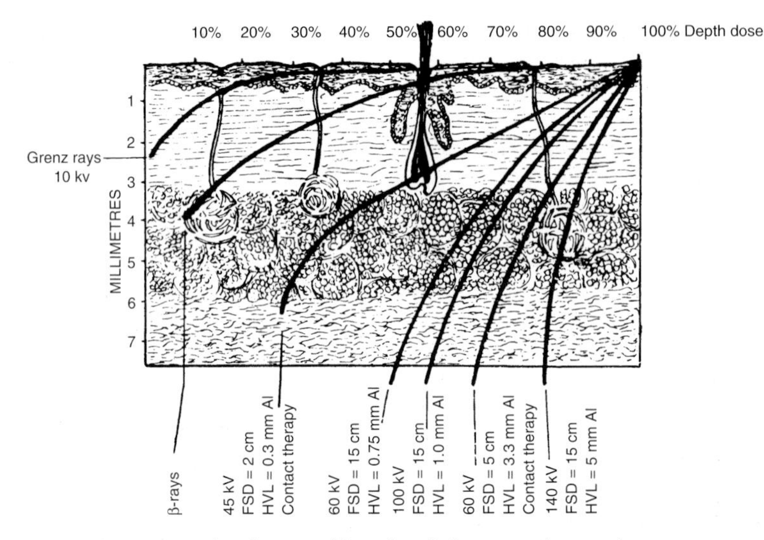

Fig. 21.5 Depth dose absorption curves of various qualities of radiation, superimposed on a cross-section of the skin.

inner canthus and nasolabial fold, are prone to deep extension. This should be suspected if lesions at these sites appear fixed. For deeply penetrating lesions, excision and skin grafting are indicated.

For most basal carcinomas up to 0.5 cm thick, superficial X-rays (90–120 kV) are adequate. For thicker lesions, orthovoltage (250–300 kV), or electrons (6–8 MeV) are required (Fig. 21.4B). Open-ended circular applicators are used (2–4 cm diameter, e.g. on a Pantak machine at 20 cm FSD). A series of lead cut-outs (0.5 mm thick for 90 kV and 2 mm for 140 kV), both circles and ovals, should be available in all standard sizes.

For widespread superficial skin infiltration from mycosis fungoides whole body low energy (3 MeV) electrons or beta irradiation from a strontium-90 source are advised (p. 524).

For lesions up to 3 cm diameter and up to 0.5 cm thick:

45 Gy applied dose in 10 daily fractions over 2 weeks (90–120 kV)

For lesions over 3 cm diameter or > 0.5 cm thick:

50 Gy in 15 daily fractions over 3 weeks (250–300 kV)

or

55 Gy in 20 daily fractions over 4 weeks (megavoltage or 6–8 MeV electrons with bolus to bring the maximum dose to the surface)

Protracted fractionation is particularly important on the cartilaginous areas of the ears and the nose, to minimise the risk of late necrosis.

It is possible to cure small lesions of less than 2.5 cm in diameter with single fractions of 22.5 Gy, and from 2.5 to 4 cm with 18–20 Gy. This is particularly useful for the elderly and frail where a single attendance for treatment is desirable.

Radiation reactions

Acute. When 45 Gy is given in 10 daily fractions, erythema develops in the last few days of the course. The colour deepens for a week and then fades, or goes on to moist desquamation. After moist peeling, a scab usually forms. Healing proceeds underneath the scab. The scab falls off when healing is complete, usually in 4–5 weeks after the end of treatment. Pigmentation may follow, especially in dark-skinned individuals, but usually fades in a few weeks or months.

The acute reaction is more marked in those with fair complexions.

Late reactions. Late skin changes are hypo- or hyperpigmentation, atrophy, alopecia and telangiectasia. These changes become more obvious as the field size increases. Irradiated skin remains at long-term risk of damage. Patients should be advised to avoid excessive exposure of the treated area to sun, cold wind and trauma. The nose and the ear are particularly vulnerable. Cartilage and bone necrosis are now rare with the wider availability of electrons (see above).

Treatment of reactions. If possible, the area should be kept dry and undisturbed, uncovered by any dressing or application. However, for treated lesions which are discharging, some coverage at night to avoid soiling bedlinen is desirable. A simple non-adherent dressing, e.g. tulle gras covered by gauze, suffices in most cases. Thick or infected crusts are best removed to enable the lesion to be cleaned and healing to progress. Greasy applications should be avoided since they prevent natural discharges and encourage infection. Topical antibiotics based on culture and sensitivities of a swab of an infected lesion may occasionally be needed.

Cosmetic creams may help conceal the stigmata of late radiation skin changes.

Patients should be encouraged to apply a high factor sun-blocking cream (e.g. 15) to block UVA and UVB radiation if exposed to the sun.

Other treatments

Oral retinoids can produce tumour shrinkage but are not curative. They have a greater role in chemoprevention in basal cell naevus syndrome and xeroderma pigmentosum or in renal transplant patients with multiple skin tumours. Topical retinoids may reduce the development of solar keratoses and perhaps development of BCCs.

Photodynamic therapy takes advantage of basal cell carcinomas' capacity to take up haematoporphyrin or delta- aminolaevulinic acid in greater concentration than adjacent normal tissue. This renders the tumour sensitive to light of 625–630 nm, 488 nm or 514.5 nm. The tumour is then exposed to laser light which provides selective kill of tumour cells. The efficacy of photodynamic therapy is still under evaluation.

Chemotherapy with cisplatin-based chemotherapy may have a limited role in the palliation of rare cases of metastatic squamous cell carcinoma.

Follow-up

Patients with basal cell carcinomas should be followed up at least until the lesion has healed. This is normally 4–5 weeks after the end of treatment. Longer-term follow-up may be needed if there are other areas of hyperkeratosis or the patient is at particular risk of further skin malignancy (e.g. basal cell naevus (Gorlin's) syndrome, xeroderma pigmentosum) for which lifelong surveillance is warranted.

Closer surveillance is required for squamous carcinomas because of the additional risk of lymph node spread. 3-monthly follow-up in the first 2 years, 4-monthly in the third year and 6-monthly in the fourth and fifth years are suggested. Follow-up can usually be discontinued at 5 years since relapse thereafter is rare. Patients should be encouraged to report back if they notice nodularity or ulceration in an irradiated area which had previously healed.

Recurrences following radiotherapy

Recurrences may occur, especially at the edges, because of a 'geographic miss'. This is more likely in the morphoeic variety of basal carcinoma where the margins are poorly defined. Recurrences are best treated surgically.

Results of treatment

The overall cure rates of surgery and radiotherapy for small basal cell carcinomas of the skin are excellent at about 90–95%. Cosmetic results of surgery are generally better than those of radiotherapy. Cure rates are slightly less good for squamous cell carcinomas owing to their tendency to metastasise.

MALIGNANT MELANOMA

Melanoma is a malignant tumour arising from cells (melanocytes) that produce the black pigment, melanin, and lie in the basal layer of the epidermis. Melanoma of the eye is described in Chapter 30.

Epidemiology

The incidence of melanoma continues to rise. It represents 0.8% of all cancers and 0.6% of cancer deaths. The highest incidence is in Australia and New Zealand (40 per 100 000 population in Queensland). It is lowest in Japan and Hong Kong (0.2 per 100 000). Mortality is falling is some populations, particularly among the young. This may be related to earlier detection of the disease. In the UK the disease is commoner in females (sex ratio 2 : 1). In white races the lower limb and the head are the commonest sites in females, and on the trunk and the head in males. However, melanoma can arise from any part of the skin. Rare sites are the nose, vulva, vagina, anus and penis.

Risk factors

80% or more are thought to be due to exposure to the sun. Intense exposure which causes erythema and inflammation (sunburn) seems to be important in the process of carcinogenesis.

Multiple acquired melanocytic naevi and atypical naevi are risk factors. Benign melanocytic naevi are almost universal. Most people have 10–20 congenital brownish spots or moles. These naevi lie just in the deepest part of the epidermis. The surface may be smooth, warty or hairy. Malignant change is higher in congenital (about 12% for lesions over 2 cm) than acquired melanocytic naevi. The majority of acquired melanocytic naevi do not undergo malignant change. 25–50% of melanomas develop de novo (i.e. in the absence of a pre-existing lesion). Some lesions may develop in areas not exposed to the sun (e.g. sole of the foot).

10% of melanomas are familial. An autosomal dominant gene with incomplete penetrance seems a likely explanation. An oncosuppressor gene, *MTS1*, has been found which corresponds to a known inhibitor of cyclin-dependent kinase that is sited on chromosome 9p21. Some of the mutations were specific to UV-induced DNA damage, supporting the importance of UV irradiation in the pathogenesis of melanoma.

Pathology

Pattern of growth

Situated at the dermal–epidermal junction, proliferating melanocytes may grow either radially (horizontally) or vertically. Most varieties have an initial radial growth phase, with vertical invasive growth later. Nodular melanoma only shows vertical growth. In general the prognosis depends on the thickness of the tumour.

Growth rate is very variable. The clinical course may be very long (10–15 years) or rapidly fatal over a few months. Lymph node and metastatic spread is often rapid. Lymph nodes are often palpable in the absence of satellite nodules around the primary. Spread is then to the regional nodes (to the inguinal nodes from the lower limb, and to the axilla or inguinal nodes from the trunk). Blood-borne metastases are common, particularly to the lungs but also to the brain and liver.

There are four principal clinicopathological varieties:

1. Lentigo maligna
2. Superficial spreading
3. Nodular
4. Acrolentiginous.

Lentigo maligna (Plate 2.3) occurs in an older age group (6th–7th decades) and develops mainly on the face. The superficial spreading variety, which accounts for about 70% of all melanomas, occurs in a younger age group (4th–5th decades), mainly on the legs in women and on the trunk in men. The nodular form (Fig. 21.6) develops in an intermediate age group (5th–6th decades), mainly on the trunk, head and neck in men and on the legs in women. The acrolentiginous form develops on the palms of the hands and on the soles of the feet.

Diagnosis and staging

Early diagnosis is essential for curative treatment. Health professions and the general public need to be

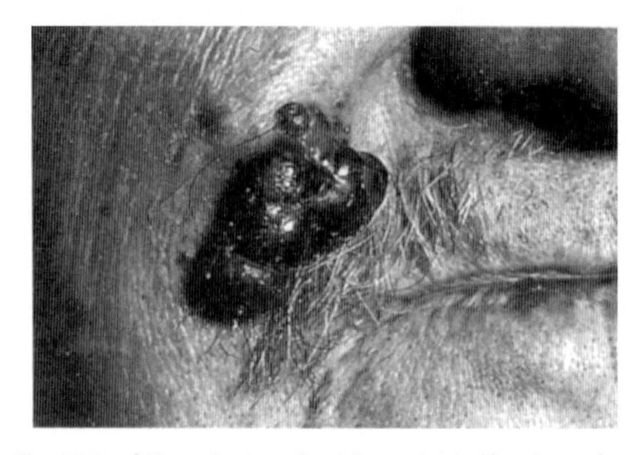

Fig. 21.6 Skin melanoma (nodular variety). (Courtesy of Dr M Kesseler, Rotherham.)

alert to the symptoms and signs of malignant change in any pigmented lesion. There are three major features—changes in shape, colour or size—and four minor features—bleeding or crusting, sensory change, inflammation, or lesion size 7 mm or larger.

Melanoma can be distinguished from an atypical naevus by a number of features. Early melanomas are flat lesions that are often asymmetrical with well-demarcated but scalloped or jagged borders and variegated pigment (browns, black, blue or even pink). An area of depigmentation (regression) is a feature of malignant melanoma. Any pigmented lesion which is changing out of step with its neighbouring lesions needs to be carefully evaluated. A complete examination of the skin including the scalp and soles of the feet is required. Photographs of pigmented lesions with a scale to assess their size assists in documenting any changes in pigmented lesions over time. Ultrasound may also assist in the diagnosis.

The regional nodes are palpated. The clinical diagnosis is confirmed by excisional biopsy and enables the pathologist to assess the depth of invasion. Staging investigations should be influenced by the thickness of the lesion. A baseline chest radiograph is recommended for low-risk melanoma (≤ 1 mm) and for lesions > 1 mm serum LDH. For stage III or IV, CT scan of the brain, chest, abdomen and pelvis is useful. MRI is helpful in the early detection of leptomeningeal disease. Positron-emission tomography with 18-fluorodeoxyglucose may detect subclinical lymph node involvement and visceral metastases. A commonly used staging system for melanoma is shown in Table 21.1. The prognosis of melanoma is principally influenced by the thickness of the primary tumour at the time of diagnosis.

Table 21.1 Staging system for malignant melanoma (American Joint Commission on Cancer and International Union against Cancer)

Stage	Clinical findings
I	Tumour < 1.5 mm in thickness
II	Tumour ≥ 1.5 mm in thickness
III	Regional lymph node involvement
IV	Distant metastases

Prevention

Raising public awareness of the importance of protecting the skin against exposure is important. Avoidance of going out in the sun for the two hours around the solar noon when UV radiation is at its most intense and use of appropriate clothing, hats and of sunscreens is advised.

Treatment

Surgery

For stage I disease, less than 1 mm in thickness, excision with a 1 cm margin of normal tissue can be curative (Clark levels I and II). A skin graft may be necessary. For lesion 1–4 mm, a 2 cm margin is needed. For lesions between 1–2 mm thick, a 1 cm margin is acceptable in a site where a 2 cm margin would require a skin graft or the function of a critical structure (e.g. the eye) would be compromised. For lesions thicker than 4 mm, a wider resection margin of 3 cm is required.

If the regional lymph nodes are not palpable, their removal is probably unnecessary since survival is not altered. Any suspicious lymph node, particularly in the primary drainage area should be investigated by fine needle aspiration cytology or biopsy.

To avoid the need for complete regional node block dissection with its associated morbidity, selective lymphadenectomy using sentinel node biopsy to assess nodal involvement is advised. An intradermal injection of a blue dye is made adjacent to the primary tumour and the first draining lymph node (the sentinel node) is excised. If the sentinel node is histologically involved, a decision can be made to proceed to full block dissection. The sentinel biopsy technique is very sensitive with a false-negative rate of less than 4%.

Radiotherapy

Malignant melanoma is a relatively radioresistant tumour. Radiotherapy (with the exception of ocular melanoma, p. 559), has no primary role in the treatment of the disease, if the patient is fit for surgery. Occasionally radical radiotherapy may be attempted in those unfit for or refusing surgery. The main but limited role for radiotherapy is in palliation of advanced disease. The indications are:

1. Primary or nodes
   a. Painful infiltration
   b. Bleeding
   c. Ulceration
2. Metastases
   a. Bone
   b. Brain.

Technique

For the primary a single field usually suffices, and for the regional nodes (axilla, groin or neck) a parallel-opposed pair. Bone metastases are treated using single fields or a parallel-opposed pair. A parallel-opposed pair of fields is used for brain metastases (Fig. 30.5A).

Dose and energy

For small solitary nodules (< 1 cm) single fractions of 30 Gy using superficial X-rays (90 kV), or 6–8 Gy weekly for larger fields, is recommended. For bone metastases 20 Gy in four daily fractions at orthovoltage or megavoltage is suggested, and for brain metastases 30 Gy in 10 daily fractions over 2 weeks.

Chemotherapy can be given on a regional basis (isolated limb) or systemically. Systemic therapy may be given as an adjuvant to deal with micrometastatic disease or for overt metastases. In none of these situations has a curative role been established.

Regional chemotherapy (isolated limb perfusion)

This involves isolating the limb using a tourniquet under general anaesthesia and injecting cytotoxic agents into the isolated arterial supply. Its use should be restricted to specialist centres with surgical oncologists familiar with the technique. The chemotherapeutic agent of choice is DTIC. The main indication is local recurrence not amenable to surgery. Good palliation can be achieved. Disease-free interval can be extended but overall survival is not improved. Local toxicity is minimal. Bone marrow toxicity is dose dependent. In advanced disease it may delay or avoid amputation for pain and ulceration uncontrolled by other means.

Adjuvant cytotoxic therapy

There is no good evidence that adjuvant cytotoxic therapy given postoperatively following the removal of the primary improves disease-free or overall survival.

Chemotherapy for palliation

Modest palliation is achievable with chemotherapy for advanced disease. Single-agent therapy is as good as and less toxic than combination therapy. Vindesine and DTIC are the preferred agents, with response rates of 20–30%. Suggested doses are shown in Table 21.2. DTIC causes severe nausea and vomiting in most patients and myelosuppression in 15%. For vindesine, bone marrow toxicity is normally the limiting factor. Alopecia occurs in 80–90% of patients. Neurotoxicity is common and cumulative (as with other vinca alkaloids).

Immunotherapy

Immunotherapy may have a role to play in the treatment of melanoma if the body's own immune response is important in influencing the growth of melanoma. Biological response modifiers (interferon, interleukin-2, monoclonal antibodies directed against melanoma cell surface gangliosides) have modest activity. BCG (bacille Calmette–Guérin) can be injected into small areas of local recurrence and skin deposits. Responses can be obtained in over 75% of patients. These indications are very limited, since recurrence is usually extensive and skin deposits multiple.

Human interferon shows about a 10% response rate in metastatic melanoma. Its role in adjuvant therapy is being evaluated in prospective studies but it cannot be recommended for routine use.

Biological response modifiers such as interleukin-2 (IL-2), which stimulate the production of T lymphocytes and may help control the immune response to melanoma, are also under evaluation as an adjuvant and for palliation of advanced disease.

Experimental vaccines against melanoma are under evaluation and appear to improve survival compared to historical controls. Gene therapy involving modifying melanoma cells with genes that encode for interferons, growth factors or cytokines and administered as tumour vaccines is being assessed.

Table 21.2 Palliative chemotherapy for melanoma

Agent	Regime
Vindesine	3 mg/m^2 i.v. weekly
DTIC	250 mg/m^2 i.v. for 5 days. Repeated every 21 days

Prognosis

When the tumour is confined to the epidermis, 5-year survival is 95–100%. It falls to 90% when the dermis is infiltrated and to 65% when tumour extends to the papillary–reticular junction. If there is deeper spread to the subcutaneous tissues or reticular dermis, 5-year survival is about 50%.

Skin metastases

Secondary carcinoma often appears as nodules just below the epidermis, especially in lung and breast cancer. It may be the first evidence of disease. Skin metastases may be symptomless, painful or ulcerate. They often respond well to palliative, superficial or orthovoltage radiotherapy (5 Gy in single fraction or 20 Gy in 4 daily fractions).

LIP

Cancer of the lip is the commonest oral cancer, representing 25% of the total cases. It accounts for 0.2% of cancers and 0.04% of cancer deaths. It arises from the vermilion border of the lip. Strictly speaking, tumours arising from the inner aspect of the lip and the commissures are tumours of the buccal mucosa. The lower lip is involved far more frequently than the upper lip (ratio 10 : 1) and in males more than females (sex ratio 10 : 1).

Pathology

Exposure to the sun and pipe-smoking are the main risk factors. Virtually all are squamous carcinomas. Basal carcinomas on the adjacent skin may impinge on to the lip. Tumours of the lower lip tend to be well differentiated and those of the upper lip less so. The central portion of the lower lip drains to the submental nodes and the lateral portions to the submandibular nodes. The upper lip drains to the upper deep cervical nodes.

Clinical features

Presentation is usually with a superficial ulcer or chronic cheilitis with an overlying scab. Minimal trauma may cause bleeding. Less frequently there is a nodule, indurated plaque, fissure or exophytic growth. There may be associated leucoplakia. Local spread may involve the whole of the lip, the skin below or the oral mucosa, and eventually the mandible.

Tumours at the angle of the mouth are particularly likely to invade the buccal mucosa. This makes radiation treatment more difficult because of the changing tissue contours.

Nodal spread is uncommon at presentation in well-differentiated tumours (10%) but increases with tumours sited at the angle of the mouth, large size and anaplasia. Nodal metastases are present in 40% of poorly differentiated tumours.

Diagnosis and staging

The diagnosis is confirmed by biopsy. Staging is according to the TNM system (Table 21.3).

Treatment

The main treatments are radiotherapy and surgery. T1 and T2 tumours can be treated by surgery or radiotherapy. Radiotherapy is preferable in T2 tumours since excisional surgery may leave a substantial tissue defect which is cosmetically and functionally unsatisfactory.

Surgery

For very superficial tumours, a 'lip shave' and advancement of the vermilion can be carried out. Excision with primary closure is possible for small tumours, with good cosmetic and functional results. Surgery is the treatment of choice for lip tumours with adjacent leucoplakia. T3 and T4 tumours are best treated by surgery since the control rates from radiotherapy are only moderate and overt bone invasion increases the risks of radionecrosis.

There is no advantage in prophylactic block dissection of the cervical nodes. If nodes are > 2 cm in diameter and operable, a radical neck dissection is carried out on the affected side.

Radiotherapy

The choice of technique and energy will depend upon the site and size of the tumour. Electron beam and interstitial implantation with iridium-192 (Fig. 22.5B) are now the preferred methods. Interstitial implantation is discussed in Chapter 22. Previously, superficial and orthovoltage therapy were commonly used before the wider availability of electrons. They have the advantages of the energy being chosen to suit the thickness of the lesion and the sharp fall-off in dose beyond the depth of the target volume.

The cosmetic results of superficial and orthovoltage therapy are less satisfactory owing to greater late radiation fibrosis and contracture of the lip. However, they can still be used if electrons are not available.

A double 'sandwich mould technique' was also used in some centres but has been largely abandoned because of the complex planning and the radiation exposure to staff.

Tumours 1 cm or less in thickness. Such tumours can be treated by interstitial implant alone (Fig. 22.5B) using the plastic tube technique (Fig. 22.4A). Three parallel lines in a triangular configuration are often adequate (Fig. 22.5A). More sources may be needed for tumours extending on to the lip.

Tumours more than 1 cm in thickness

Technique and target volume

Electron beam is preferred. A single field with a lead applicator of suitable size is chosen. The target volume should include the tumour and a 1 cm margin of adjacent normal tissue. The treatment volume should be 1 cm wider than the target volume to take account of the penumbra of the electrons. To protect the buccal mucosa, tongue, teeth and mandible, a shaped lead strip is positioned behind the lip. It is lined with wax to absorb the secondary electrons generated by interaction between the incident beam and the lead.

Dose

50 Gy in 20 daily fractions over 4 weeks

Results of treatment

For tumours less than 3 cm in diameter without palpable nodes, the 5-year local control rate is about 90%. Where nodes are palpable or the tumour exceeds 3 cm in diameter, the local control rate falls to 60%.

Table 21.3 TNM staging of lip cancer

T stage	Clinical findings
T1	Tumour confined to the lip, 2 cm or less in greatest dimension
T2	Tumour confined to the lip, more than 2 cm but not larger than 4 cm in greatest dimension
T3	Tumour confined to the lip, more than 4 cm in greatest dimension
T4	Tumour extending beyond the lip to neighbouring structures, e.g. bone, tongue, skin of neck

CHAPTER CONTENTS

22

Interstitial implantation

Ian Kunkler

Interstitial implantation refers to the temporary or permanent insertion within the body's tissues of sealed radioactive sources. Interstitial implantation together with intracavitary therapy (Ch. 27) make up the two forms of brachytherapy (literally treatment at short distances [from the sources]). Implants are normally employed either alone or in conjunction with external beam therapy in the cure of localised tumours. Occasionally they are used for palliation (e.g. of metastatic neck nodes).

Implants may be temporary with caesium-137 needles or iridium-192 wire or permanent with gold-198 or iodine-125 seeds. Permanent implantation with gold seeds is limited by the unevenness of dose distribution resulting from the difficulty of implanting small individual seeds with good geometry. Implantation with iodine seeds is largely limited by the high cost of each seed. Temporary implants are most commonly practised in the UK, with iridium-192 progressively replacing caesium-137 for reasons discussed below.

This chapter concentrates on the clinical aspects of temporary removable implants. The principles of the two main systems of dosimetry used in the UK (Paris and Manchester) are described in Chapter 14. Implantation of the anterior two-thirds of the tongue using iridium hairpins and caesium needles, and of the breast and anus with plastic tubes and hollow rigid needles, illustrate both systems. The specific indications for implants at these and other sites are considered in the other clinical chapters.

Implantation is predominantly carried out in tumours which are readily accessible to the radiotherapist, e.g. floor of mouth, tongue, lip, skin, pinna, nose, breast, vagina and penis. However, even more deeply seated structures, e.g. the nasopharynx, can be implanted, as can selected prostate, bladder and soft tissue tumours. The latter two require the assistance of the surgeon to provide access but the prostate can be approached percutaneously. More recently, endobronchial (Fig. 22.1) and endo-oesophageal (Fig. 22.2) brachytherapy using

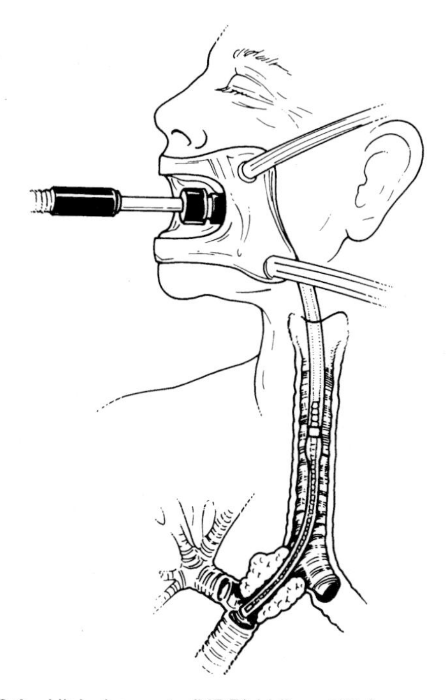

Fig. 22.1 High dose rate (HDR) iridium-192 for endobronchial brachytherapy for palliation of non-small cell lung cancer of right main bronchus using *microSelectron-HDR*. (Source: Nucletron.)

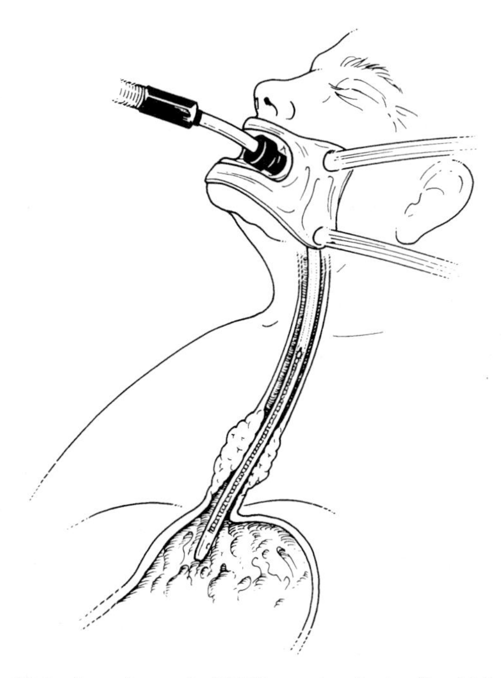

Fig. 22.2 Low dose rate (LDR) remote afterloading iridium-192 oesophageal brachytherapy for palliation of lower third carcinoma using *Selectron-LDR*. (Source: Nucletron.)

high and low dose rate after loading has been applied in the palliation of selected lung and oesophageal tumours.

While the value of implantation has been demonstrated in many personal series of cases by skilled brachytherapists, randomised trials comparing it with other forms of therapy (e.g. surgery or external beam) have rarely been attempted.

HISTORICAL ASPECTS

It was in the 1920s in Paris that the first attempts were made to seal radium salts as a source for brachytherapy. Dosimetry for the early radium tubes and needles was crude. Doses which could eradicate tumours while not exceeding normal tissue tolerance were derived empirically. The Paterson–Parker system (also known as the Manchester system) of radium dosage was described in 1934. This system enjoyed, and in some departments still enjoys, wide usage throughout the world. However, the rigidity of the radium needles (and caesium that replaced radium) meant that the implant was not always best suited to the configuration of the tumour and surrounding normal structures. In addition, radiation exposure to the operator implanting the needles could be substantial.

In the early 1950s the flexible 'afterloaded' plastic tubes containing gold seeds were developed in the USA at the Memorial Hospital in New York. The advantages of afterloading are described on page 470. Afterloaded interstitial iridium-192 has substantially reduced radiation exposure to the operator.

In France in the mid 1950s the techniques of modern afterloading techniques were elaborated. The Paris system of dosimetry for implantation, based on afterloaded iridium-192, was published in 1966. The Paris system of dosimetry and its rules of implantation are described in Chapter 14. In the last 30 years the Paris system has been adopted by increasing numbers of radiotherapy departments in the UK and has largely replaced the Manchester system. However, some departments in other parts of the world where supplies of iridium wire are less reliable have retained stocks of caesium-137 needles because of its long half-life (p. 236). Iridium-192 wire with a much shorter half-life (p. 232) is more difficult to re-use unless a department undertakes implantation very frequently. In some centres permanent implants using iodine-125 are used. Its has a half-life of 59.6 days and emit photons with an average energy of 28.5 keV. As a result of its low energy, fall-off in dose is rapid. This is of particular value at sites where bone or thyroid cartilage are close to the implant. The dose delivered by an iodine implant at the periphery of the tumour is about 120 Gy over 1 year of which half (60 Gy) is over the first half-life of the isotope (60 days).

ADVANTAGES OF INTERSTITIAL IMPLANTATION

Interstitial implantation has the following physical and biological advantages over external beam irradiation.

1. High dose to tumour with reduced dosage to adjacent normal tissues

Because of the inverse square law (p. 226), the dose is inversely proportional to the square of the distance from the source. The dose therefore drops markedly with increasing distance from the source. The implant is normally confined to the tumour-bearing area. This limits the dose, and consequent morbidity, to adjacent normal tissues. By contrast external beam irradiation, e.g. of the head and neck, often includes substantial volumes of normal salivary tissue, resulting in a dry mouth.

The doses around the sources can be very much higher than can be achieved by external beam while still remaining within normal tissue tolerance.

2. Flexible conformation to tumour and normal structures

The flexible nature of iridium-192 wire enables it to follow the changing contours of tumours and adjacent normal structures. For example it can be threaded along the arch of the soft palate. It can be looped around the posterior part of the inner aspect of the cheek where the insertion of rigid needles is hindered by the posterior intermaxillary commissure. Using a mould to keep it in place, it can be inserted into the nasopharynx. The adaptability of iridium wire to local anatomy has permitted the role of interstitial implantation to be greatly extended.

3. Continuous low dose rate

There are a number of radiobiological advantages of low dose rate brachytherapy.

a. Repair of sublethal damage. Repair of sublethal damage increases in importance as the dose rate falls. At low dose rate, accumulated sublethal damage contributes less to cell killing. At very low dose rates (i.e. < 1 Gy/hour), it is direct radiation damage that accounts for most cell death. At low dose rate the tissues with a large 'shoulder' (or low α/β ratio, p. 289), for example late-responding vascular endothelium and connective tissue, are better protected against damage than tissues with a small shoulder (or high ratio), such as basal epidermal cells of the skin. Late-responding tissues thus have a greater capacity to absorb and repair sublethal damage. It also explains why interstitial therapy at lower than conventional dose rates (e.g. 10 Gy per week as opposed to 10 Gy per day) may be tolerated by tissues which have previously received tolerance doses of radical external beam therapy. At higher dose rates (i.e. > 1 Gy/hour) the duration of irradiation is insufficient for sublethal damage to be repaired.

It is uncertain whether any correction to the total dose needs to be made to take account of differences in dose rate. It is thought that at conventional rates of 40–50 cGy/hour (5–$6\frac{1}{4}$) days for a radical dose of 60 Gy) no correction is necessary. For high dose rate some correction would seem appropriate but has yet to be established.

b. Distribution in the cell cycle. It is known that cells in the G_1 phase of the cell cycle (Fig. 18.7) are more radiosensitive than in late S phase. It seems probable that during an implant over 6 days, tumour cells in the more sensitive phase of the cycle have longer periods of radiation exposure than during daily fractionated external beam therapy.

c. Tumour hypoxia. At low dose rates hypoxic tumour cells have a reduced capacity to repair radiation damage compared with normal tissues. This is because repair is an oxygen-dependent process. Better oxygenated normal tissues are preferentially repaired compared with hypoxic tumours cells.

d. Reduced tumour proliferation during irradiation. The short overall treatment times of curative implants, commonly 6–7 days, do not allow increased tumour proliferation to occur during treatment. This is in contrast to external beam irradiation where tumour proliferation may occur in the conventional 24-hour gap between fractions.

CHOICE OF IMPLANTATION TECHNIQUE

In the Manchester system caesium needles are the only sealed sources used, whether it be for the tongue, vagina or anus. In the Paris system, both hairpins (Fig. 22.3), afterloaded plastic tubes (Fig. 22.4) and hollow needles (Figs 22.5, 22.9 and 22.11) are used. Plastic tubes can be used for implanting soft tissue sarcomas where longer target volumes need to be treated than can be encompassed by hairpins. Some radiotherapists also use plastic tubes for breast implants, while others prefer hollow needles. Hollow needles are used with templates to obtain more rigid geometry in the lip (Fig. 22.5A & B), breast (Fig. 22.9), penis (Fig. 22.6) and anus (Figs 22.10 and 22.11).

Anterior two-thirds of tongue

See page 353 for indications.

Iridium

Implantation with iridium hairpins can be carried out under either local or general anaesthesia. Local anaesthesia is less hazardous and has the advantage that the normal tone of the musculature is retained, allowing a similar distribution of the sources during and after the implant. Under general anaesthesia, where muscle relaxants are given, the distal end of the sources tend to bunch together as the normal tone of the tongue's musculature returns postoperatively. None the less, for the comfort of the patient most radiotherapists in the UK prefer to carry out the implant under general anaesthesia.

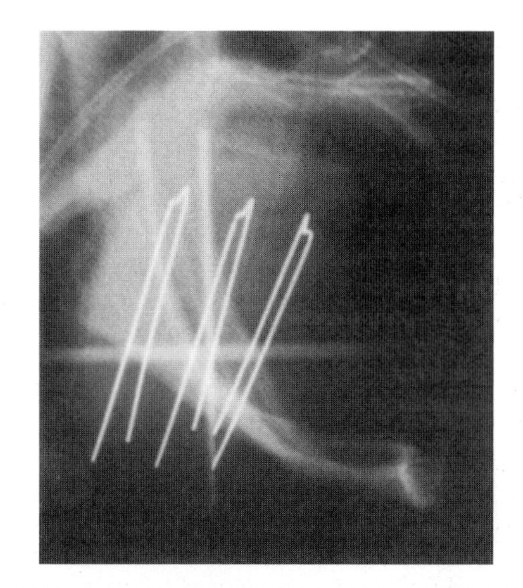

Fig. 22.3 Lateral radiograph showing iridium-192 hairpin implant of squamous carcinoma of the lateral border of the anterior two-thirds of the tongue.

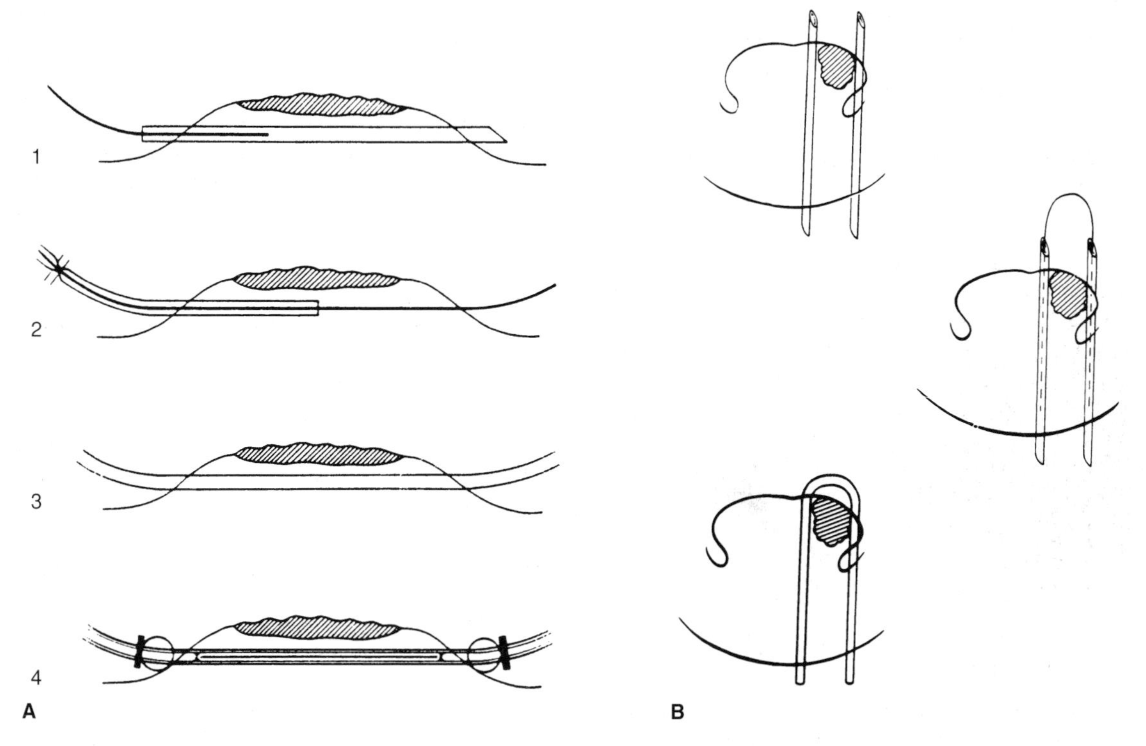

Fig. 22.4 **A** Steps in performing afterloaded plastic tube implant. (1) Stainless-steel guide needle inserted and nylon cord passed down needle. (2) Guide needle removed and outer plastic tubing passed over nylon cord and clamped. (3) Plastic tube in position ready for afterloading. (4) Plastic tube afterloaded with iridium-192 wire encapsulated within inner tubing. Nylon ball and lead discs placed to fix implant in position. (Redrawn from Hope-Stone 1986.) **B** The loop technique for iridium wire implantation. (Reproduced with permission of Arnold from Jane Dobbs, Ann Barrett, Daniel Ash, *Practical Radiotherapy Planning*, 3/e, Arnold, 1999.)

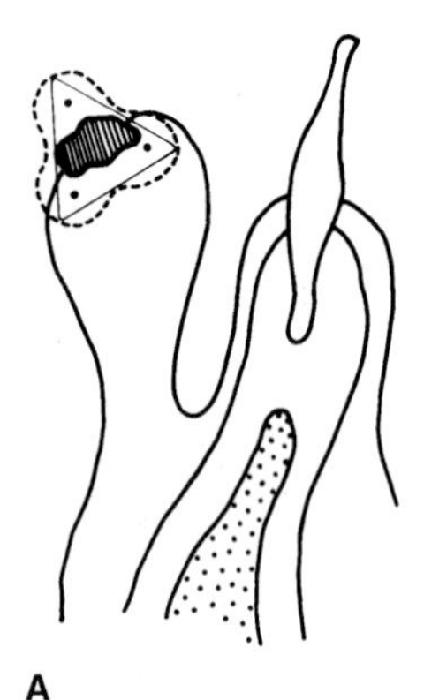

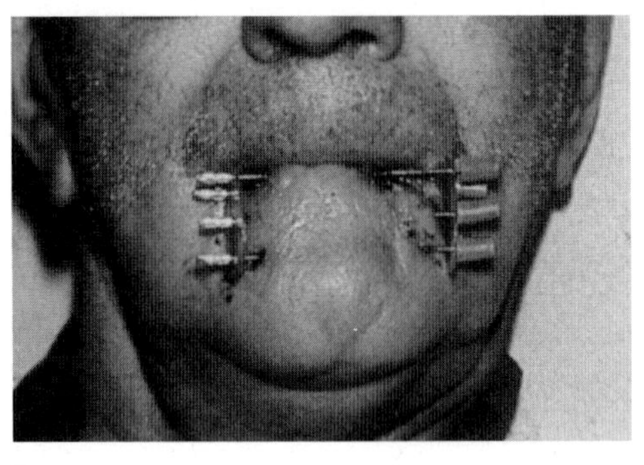

Fig. 22.5 **A** Cross-sectional diagram of a typical triangular implant pattern for a small exophytic lip cancer. References isodose is indicated by the dotted line. (Reproduced with permission from Pierquin et al 1987.) **B** Iridium implant of the lip using a template. (Courtesy of Dr D Ash, Leeds.)

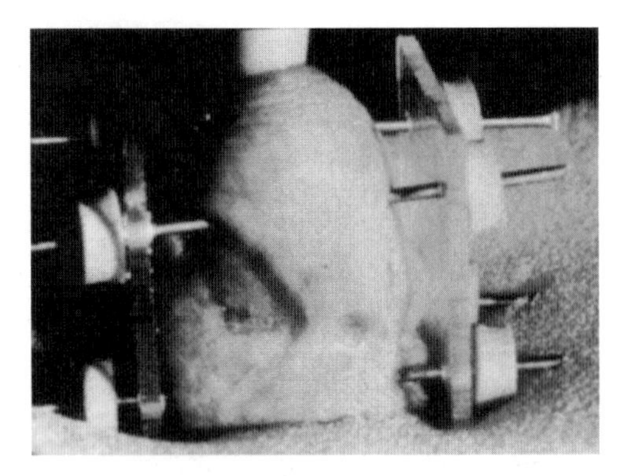

Fig. 22.6 Iridium-192 implant of the penis using hollow needles and template. (Courtesy of Dr D Ash, Leeds.)

A double plane hairpin implant is best suited to most early carcinomas of the anterior two-thirds of the tongue. If the tumour is wider than 12 mm, the standard width of iridium hairpins, additional hairpins or single pins may be required. Alternatively, where the width of the tumour exceeds that of the hairpins, the plastic loop technique may be used, which permits greater widths (up to 20 mm) to be implanted.

A dental impression is made of the floor of the mouth, including that of the tumour. Lead protection is incorporated in the periphery of the mould adjacent to the implant to reduce the dose to the mandible. A similar mould not containing lead (and therefore radiolucent) is used so as not to obscure the position of the pins on the verification radiographs.

For a hairpin implant, the tumour is inspected and palpated to confirm its boundaries. Local anaesthetic is infiltrated around the margins of the tumour.

The most posterior guide gutter is introduced first, with its bridge lying transversely and its limbs at the margin of the target volume. Additional hairpins are implanted anteriorly, keeping an anteroposterior separation of 12–15 mm between each hairpin. The length of the hairpins is chosen according to the depth of extension of the tumour. Ideally, the position of the guide gutters should be verified using a screening facility in theatre. If this is not available, preoperative orthogonal radiographs (Fig. 22.3) are an alternative. Adjustments are made if necessary to the position of the guide gutters to ensure that they are equidistant and parallel. When the geometry is satisfactory, a silk suture is passed under the bridge of the most posterior hairpin and through the substance of the tongue. This is repeated for the hairpins lying anteriorly. The free ends of the threads are clipped to the surgical drapes to the side of the mouth. Each hairpin is gently grasped by one limb and each limb introduced into the guide gutter, starting with the most posterior hairpin. Care should be taken not to bend the hairpins by applying undue pressure when inserting them into the guide gutter. While applying firm but gentle pressure to the centre of the bridge of the hairpin with a specially designed hook, the guide gutter is removed (Fig. 22.7) by forceps held in the other hand. Each hairpin is then sutured to the tongue at the midpoint of its bridge.

For lesions close to the mandible, the dose to the mandible can be reduced by shortening the limbs of the most anterior hairpin by 0.5–1 cm. Rarely are more than three hairpins required. Exceeding this number substantially increases the risk of radionecrosis if the limbs of the hairpin lie close to the mandible.

Dosimetry. This is based on the plane perpendicular to the midpoint of the sources (p. 234). The position of the sources in this plane can be determined from tomograms taken through the central plane or reconstructed from orthogonal radiographs using a computerised

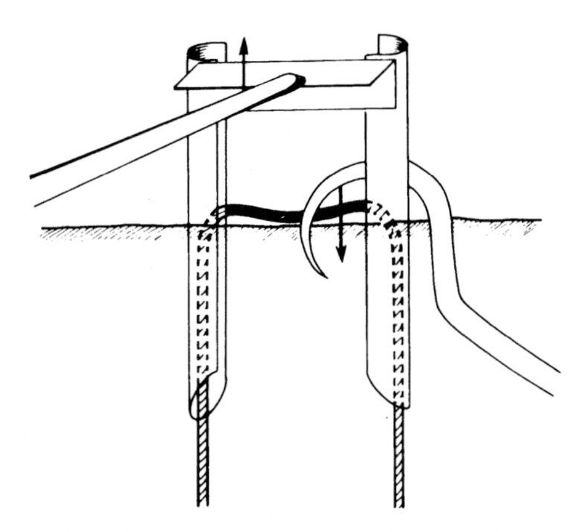

Fig. 22.7 Method of substituting hairpin for guide gutter. The pin is held against the tissue being implanted with a surgical hook while the guide gutter is removed with a needle-holder. (Reproduced from Pierquin et al 1987.)

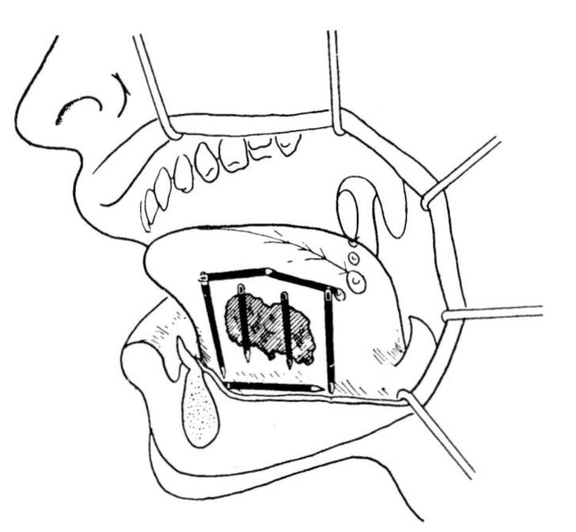

Fig. 22.8 Diagram of radium needles for single-plane implant of the lateral border of the anterior two-thirds of the tongue. The layout is applicable to caesium needles. (Adapted with permission of Arnold from Ralston Paterson, *Treatment of Malignant Disease*, 2/e, Edward Arnold, 1963.)

dose-planning system (p. 235). Ideally both manual and computerised dosimetry should be carried out independently, since errors in one may be exposed by the other.

Caesium needles

While implantation with caesium needles has largely been replaced by iridium-192 in most UK departments, implantation with caesium needles is still practised in departments where resources are limited and access to supplies of iridium difficult to obtain. Caesium implantation is carried out under general anaesthesia in the operating theatre. The therapist can make a preliminary calculation, based on the size of the lesion. In the example shown (Fig. 22.8) a single plane of needles will be adequate, covering a rectangular area. Needles of 1 and 2 mg of caesium are generally of most use in this type of case. Precise details of a typical case using the Paterson and Parker rules are given on page 236. In this case the dose will be worked out at 0.5 cm from the plane of the needles, i.e. it will suffice to dose adequately a 1 cm thickness of tissue, which should include all the malignancy.

Based on these calculations, the operator will have ordered the requisite types and number of needles. It is helpful to pass a suture through the tip of the tongue at the beginning of the procedure. Grasping the threads enables the position of the tongue to be manipulated for the purposes of implantation. The needles are inserted, starting at the posterior margin of the tumour. Needles should be inserted in a posterior oblique direction since they tend to move towards the front of the mouth as the tongue recovers its normal tone after anaesthesia. The distances and separations are carefully measured with a ruler to ensure the correct layout as calculated. A safety margin of 1 cm of normal tissue is included within the area implanted. The needles are held in special grooved long-handled forceps and pushed home with special 'pushers'.

Gold grain implants

Gold grains can be used as a permanent implant, especially in elderly people as they allow free tongue movement and so lessen the risk of postoperative pneumonia. Gold grains are only suitable for small single-plane implants.

Postoperative care (iridium and caesium implants)

The patient is nursed in a protected room. An implant is a painful procedure once the anaesthetic has worn off and adequate analgesia (usually 4-hourly diamorphine) is essential. The position of each hairpin should be checked at least once a day to confirm that the sutures are securely fastened and the position of the hairpin is as intended. A soft diet and fluids are necessary to minimise movement of the tongue.

Iridium hairpins can normally be removed without anaesthetic. A general anaesthetic is usually necessary for the removal of the caesium needles. A soft diet should be continued for a further 3 weeks, by which time the acute reaction has normally settled.

Nasopharynx

Brachytherapy is occasionally applied to nasopharyngeal cancers for patients with recurrent cancer after external beam irradiation or, less frequently, as part of primary treatment. Temporary surface moulds can be used in patients where the whole of the surface of the nasopharynx needs to be treated. An impression is made of the nasopharynx. The applicator is drawn into the nasopharynx and afterloaded through hollow plastic tubes exiting through the nostrils. Radiographic verification of the position of the mould is carried out. Permanent implants via a transoral, transnasal or transpalatal approach are possible using iodine-125. High dose rate (HDR) afterloaded brachytherapy may be an alternative to low dose rate (LDR), although there are no randomised trials comparing the relative effectiveness or toxicity of these different dose rates.

Breast

Interstitial implantation as a boost to the tumour site can be carried out as a peroperative procedure following local excision or, more often, postoperatively following external beam irradiation of the breast. If carried out peroperatively, the radiotherapist has the advantage of knowing the exact site of the tumour. Alternatively, the surgeon can be asked to place radiopaque clips at the poles of the tumour or to draw on the skin, following closure of the wound, the area corresponding to the underlying tumour. If the surgeon makes the incision over the centre of the tumour, the radiotherapist can use the scar as the site to be boosted. In most cases a two-plane implant (Fig. 22.9) is required, where the depth of breast tissue allows. The plastic tubes are loaded with dummy inactive iridium wire. The patient is transferred to the simulator after recovering from the general anaesthetic and anterior and lateral radiographs are obtained for planning. The Paris system of dosimetry is recommended (Ch. 14). To ensure adequate coverage of the tumour-bearing area, the active wire will extend beyond the margins of the target to allow for colder areas occurring between the ends of the wires. Implantation is best done with rigid needles and a template to maintain good geometry.

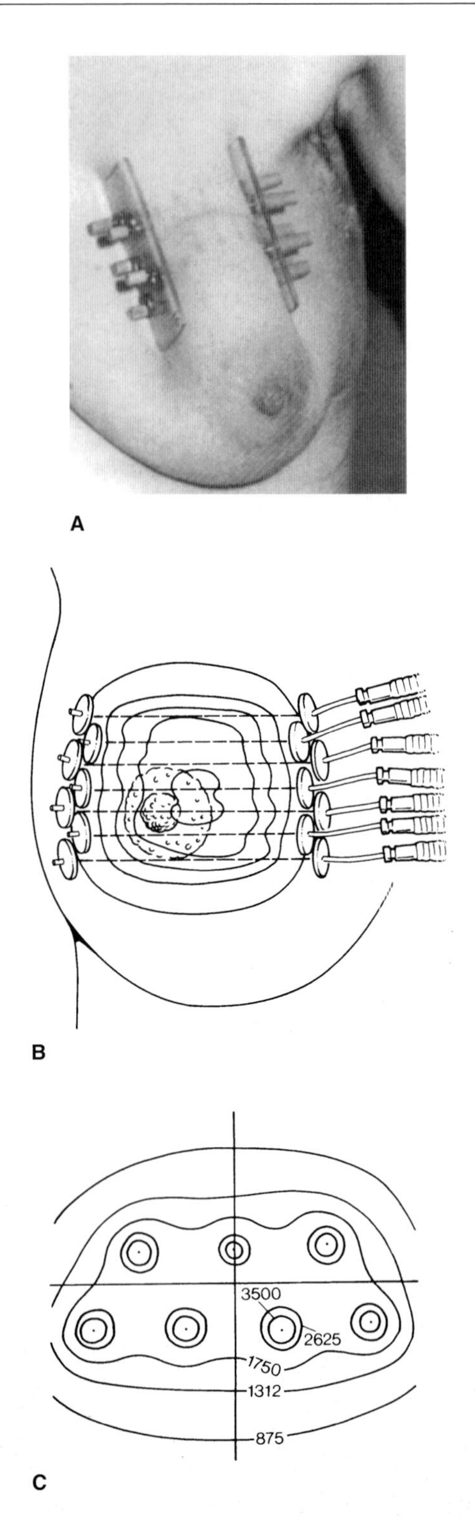

Fig. 22.9 **A** Iridium-192 breast implant with hollow needles and template. (Courtesy of Dr D Ash, Leeds.) Dosimetry of breast implant: **B** in plane of sources and **C** in cross-section.

Anal cancer

Implantation is carried out under general anaesthesia or, for those less fit, under spinal anaesthesia. The patient is placed in the lithotomy position. The circumferential extent, depth and proximal limits are assessed by inspection and palpation. A silver grain is embedded at the proximal and distal limits of the tumour to assist the positioning of the afterloaded sources. To maintain the parallelism of the sources, a crescentic Perspex template, predrilled with holes at regular intervals around its circumference (Fig. 22.10), is sutured against the perineum. Not more than two-thirds of the circumference of the anus is implanted to reduce late anal stenosis. Hollow steel needles of appropriate length are inserted through the holes in the template, through the perineal skin and then under the submucosa of the anus and rectum. Care should be taken not to pierce the rectal lumen. This is difficult to avoid in women in whom it is necessary to place the needles anteriorly in the rectovaginal septum without penetrating either the vagina or the rectum. To verify this it may be helpful to insert the first needle through the rectovaginal septum since, if done later in the implant, the field of vision may be limited. Between five and seven needles are commonly required. The average length is 5–7 cm. Inactive wire is inserted into each steel needle and drawn back under screening until it is correctly positioned in relation to the silver seeds. The appropriate length of iridium wire to be afterloaded can be calculated. Verification lateral and anteroposterior radiographs are taken to confirm the position of the needles and of the inactive wire (Fig. 22.11). It should also be checked that the position of the needles is not significantly altered by extending the patient's legs. The proximal ends of the needles are crimped at their entry points into the template to ensure that the needles are immobilised. Computerised dosimetry is carried out. Sources are afterloaded manually or using an afterloading machine (*microSelectron*).

Care during the implant

One or two enemas to clear the bowel are recommended before implantation. The patient should be nursed prone or on the side in a protected room. Regular 4-hourly opiates are given orally to control the

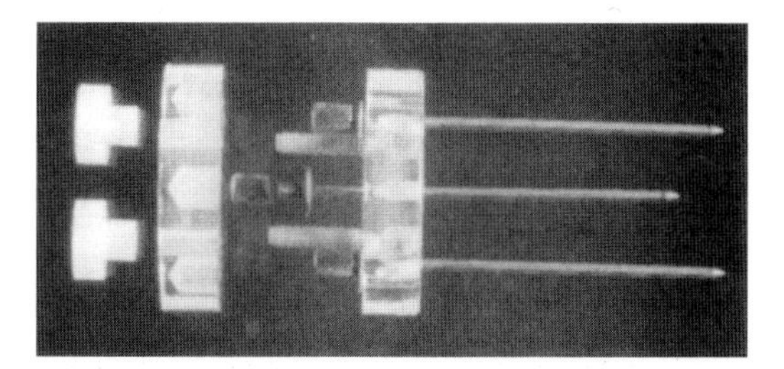

Fig. 22.10 Perineal applicator. (Courtesy of Dr D Ash, Leeds.)

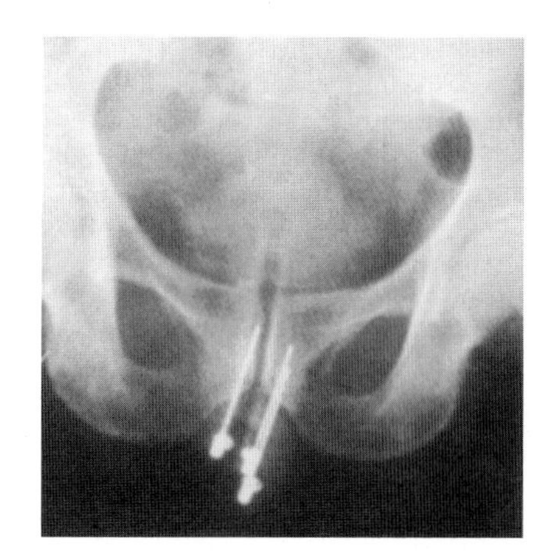

Fig. 22.11 Iridium-192 implant of anal canal using rigid hollow needles and template. (Courtesy of Dr D Ash, Leeds.)

discomfort and to keep the patient constipated during the implant. At the end of the implant, the template and attached needles are removed under a further general anaesthetic.

Prostate

Interstitial implantation

Radium needles were first used to implant the prostate in 1917. There was little enthusiasm for the technique. In the 1960s iodine-125 seeds were implanted at laparotomy. This freehand technique did not produce a precise and regular distribution of radioactive sources. Interest in prostatic brachytherapy has grown with the introduction of transrectal ultrasonography to guide the positioning of seeds. This imaging technique permits direct inspection of the passage of each needle into the prostate. The introduction of a rigid template and computerised dosimetry has improved the homogeneity of dose distribution and allowed intraoperative planning.

Preimplant ultrasound scanning to assess the prostatic volume is a carried out. The borders of the prostate are defined on each transverse 5 mm slice. The coordinates of the sources are defined to give the required distribution. Techniques of positioning the source range from (1) uniform source loading, which risks 'hot spots' at the centre of the volume; (2) peripheral loading, which, if correctly performed, gives a more even distribution; (3) modified uniform loading, which is a compromise between 1 and 2; (4) modified peripheral loading, a modification of the pure peripheral technique, which gives slightly greater activity centrally.

Ultrasound is used to check the position of the tip of the needle particularly around the urethra and near the junction of the bladder and the prostate.

Iodine-125 is the most commonly applied isotope for prostatic brachytherapy but palladium-103 is being increasingly used. The characteristics of the two isotopes are summarised in Table 22.1

Table 22.1 Characteristics of iodine-125 and palladium-103

	Iodine-125	Palladium-103
Half-life (days)	59.4	17
Energy (ke V)	27.4	21.0
Initial dose rate (cGy/h)	10	24
Implant dose (Gy)	144	115

FUTURE DEVELOPMENTS

It is likely that better definition of the target volume will be made possible from computerised tomography, magnetic resonance imaging and ultrasound. Integrating this information with computerised dosimetry from a remote afterloading machine may improve the accuracy of radiation delivery.

The development of high dose rate remote afterloading machines may allow single-fraction peroperative irradiation of tumour sites following surgery.

Newer afterloading machines (e.g. *microSelectron-HDR*) containing iridium-192 for interstitial implantation and cobalt-60 sources for gynaecological applications are able to use a single source which can be switched to different parts of the implant for differing periods of time. The sequence of switching channels will be chosen with the help of computer programmes designed to provide optimal dose distribution over the period of the implant.

CHAPTER CONTENTS

23

Mouth, secondary nodes of neck, tonsil, nasopharynx, paranasal sinuses, ear, salivary glands

Ian Kunkler

PRINCIPLES OF MANAGEMENT OF HEAD AND NECK CANCER

For optimal management, patients should be assessed by a multidisciplinary team of specialised surgeons, oncologists, radiologists, pathologists, nurses, dental hygienists and speech therapists. Support and rehabilitation services are particularly important to this group of patients because they have a high representation of the socially disadvantaged, heavy alcohol consumption with its attendants problems and poor general health.

At present, surgery and radiotherapy (external beam and/or interstitial therapy) remain the only curative treatments for head and neck cancer. Adjuvant chemotherapy has a limited role. Choice of treatment will be influenced by tumour site and locoregional extent, general medical condition and likely cosmetic and functional outcome. Important functional considerations are the ability to breathe, speak, eat and drink. In general, radical radiotherapy is often preferred for early disease because it may offer good prospects for cure while retaining normal anatomy. Surgery is then reserved as salvage therapy for recurrence. For advanced disease, the chances of cure by radiotherapy are lower, and radical surgery, often with postoperative radiotherapy, is often preferred as primary treatment. While there have been considerable advances in head and neck surgery with the use of reconstructive surgery with a free vascular graft or myocutaneous flap (muscle and skin transplant), major functional impairment remains a problem, commonly impairing the patient's quality of life. There still remains uncertainty about the best treatment for many tumour sites, in part because of the absence of randomised trials comparing the benefits of surgery, radiotherapy and chemotherapy. Consideration should be given to recruit eligible patients into prospective randomised trials.

Management by radiotherapy

The anatomy of the head and neck is complex. As a result, target volumes are irregular in shape and close to critical structures such as the eye, brainstem and spinal cord. CT and MRI scanning are essential in identifying the local and regional nodal involvement and can be used in three-dimensional treatment planning. The availability of multileaf collimators in the new generation of linear accelerators allows the tailoring of the radiation beams to the tumour volume while protecting adjacent normal tissues. High standards of verification of treatment fields with verification films or by portal imaging are necessary.

Dose and fractionation schedules

There is good evidence that prolongation of overall treatment time and breaks in treatment (e.g. because of public holidays) compromise local control. A variety of radical radiotherapy schedules are used ranging from 40 Gy in 15 daily fractions to 60 Gy in 30 fractions over 6 weeks. Local control requires about 3 Gy extra per increase in T stage. Radiobiological calculations suggest that about 0.6 Gy per day is needed to compensate for a 1 day increase in overall treatment time.

Hypofractionated schedules (giving fewer fractions, e.g. 2–3 per week) at a higher dose per fraction (3–6 Gy) to a total dose of 60–70 Gy over 6–7 weeks do not improve local control and run a higher risk of late complications and are therefore not recommended.

Hyperfractionated schedules give multiple (e.g. two or three) small 1.1–1.6 Gy fractions per day. An improved therapeutic ratio may be anticipated by delivering a higher total dose over the same overall treatment time as conventional fractionation. Hyperfractionated schedules have been shown to improve local control without increasing late effects.

Accelerated fractionation by giving two or three fractions per day giving the same total dose as conventional radiotherapy but over a shorter time can reduce tumour repopulation between fractions. This is recommended for fast-growing tumours (e.g. of the nasopharynx). One of the disadvantages of accelerated fractionation is an increase in acute side-effects, especially mucositis, and of late effects.

CHART (*continuous hyperfractionated accelerated radiotherapy*) is an approach to fractionation in which the overall treatment time is reduced to about 1.5 weeks with a reduction of the total dose (1.5 Gy given three times daily for 12 consecutive days (including Saturday and Sunday) to a total dose of 54 Gy). In an MRC trial this accelerated schedule was compared to a conventional schedule of 66 Gy, 5 days per week at a dose per fraction of 2 Gy over 45 days. 918 patients were included in the trial for all head and neck cancer sites. Only T1N0 tumours were excluded. There were no differences in locoregional control or overall survival. Acute mucosal reactions are increased but normally heal within 3 months. Late morbidity was less than or similar to that caused by conventional fractionation. In view of the lack of benefit of CHART compared to conventional fractionation, this regime has not been adopted.

An EORTC (European Organization for Research on Treatment of Cancer) trial tested split-course hyperfractionated radiotherapy (SCHAR), a schedule of 72 Gy at 1.6 Gy/fraction three times a day at intervals of not less than 4 hours, 5 days a week over a total of 35 days. In the first part of the schedule 28.8 Gy was given in 18 fractions over 8 days. There was a rest period of 12–14 days and then the rest of the treatment of 43.2 Gy in 27 fractions over 17 days. This was compared with a conventional schedule of 70 Gy in 35 fractions of 2 Gy, 5 days a week over 49 days. 512 patients with squamous cell cancer of the head and neck (except for the hypopharynx or nasopharynx) were randomised. The locoregional control rate at 5 years in the SCHAR schedule was improved (59% versus 46%). Benefits were mainly at the primary site rather than the regional nodes. There was no difference in overall survival. Acute morbidity, particularly mucositis was increased in the accelerated schedule. Late morbidity was, however, greater with grade 3 or 4 toxicity, principally fibrosis, neuropathy, mucosal necrosis or oedema. The actuarial 5-year rate of severe morbidity was 50%. For this reason the SCHAR regime has not been adopted.

Neoadjuvant chemotherapy

Neoadjuvant chemotherapy may be given to reduce the tumour burden before surgery or radiotherapy to improve local control and survival. The commonly used agents are cisplatin and 5-fluorouracil. Although substantial initial tumour responses have been seen, these have not been translated into long-term local control or survival. Accordingly, routine neoadjuvant chemotherapy is not recommended and should only be used in the context of prospective randomised studies.

Concomitant chemoradiation

The aims of concomitant chemotherapy and radiotherapy is to give treatment modalities together to both reduce the tumour burden and take advantage of the radiation-sensitising properties of agents such as cisplatin. A meta-analysis of 23 randomised trials of adjuvant chemotherapy showed that concomitant chemotherapy followed by maintenance improved survival. However, no benefit to induction and maintenance chemotherapy has been shown.

ORAL CAVITY

Anatomy

Cancers of the mouth or oral cavity fall into several anatomical groups with general similarities and some individual differences. They include the lips, the hard palate, the upper and lower alveolus, the buccal cheek, retromolar trigone, and anterior two-thirds of the mobile tongue. A view of the oral cavity is seen in Figure 23.1A.

The anterior limit of the mouth is the vermilion border of the lip. The posterior limits are the circumvallate papillae of the dorsum of the tongue and the anterior margin of the oropharynx (Fig. 23.1B).

The tongue and floor of mouth are the commonest sites.

Pathology

Epidemiology

Cancer of the oral cavity represents less than 1% of all cancer deaths. It is commoner in men, with a male : female ratio of 2 : 1. Its incidence is declining in males and rising in females. Oral cancer is much commoner in India, probably related to chewing the betel nut (with tobacco and caustic lime) and in France due to alcohol and smoking, often in combination.

Aetiology

Environmental irritants predispose—tobacco, chewing betel nut, alcohol, dental sepsis, poorly fitting dentures, syphilis, iron deficiency anaemia and leucoplakia. Improved hygiene, nutrition and dental care, and the decline in incidence of syphilis have lowered the incidence in many countries.

An increased risk has been found among textile workers, particularly if exposed to the dust from the 'carding' of raw cotton or wool.

Histology

Over 90% are squamous carcinomas. The majority are well differentiated. A few are adenocarcinomas or malignant mixed tumours from minor salivary submucosal glands. Soft tissue sarcomas and lymphomas occur rarely.

Spread

Early spread is local, e.g. to the gum, palate, cheek. Bone may be invaded, especially the mandible. There is a rich lymphatic network, predominantly to the submandibular and upper deep cervical nodes (Figs 23.2–23.4). The lymphatics of the oral cavity anastomose in the midline. Contralateral spread may therefore occur.

Blood spread is late and rare. It is mainly to lung, bone and liver.

Clinical features

Most lesions present as ulcers of variable depth and induration. Others are papillary growths or fissured forms. Infection may follow, causing halitosis and excessive salivation. There may be associated leucoplakia. Oral pain may be prominent in the later stages, often radiating to the ear. The tongue may become fixed, with difficulty in eating and speaking.

Diagnosis is usually straightforward on inspection, but a thorough local examination and palpation of the lesion are necessary to reveal the full extent of invasion. The neck is palpated for enlarged nodes. A biopsy should be taken to confirm the diagnosis.

Staging

Tumours of the oral cavity should be staged clinically, using the TNM classification (Table 23.1), by size and local extent. Full blood count and radiographs of the chest and mandible (orthopantomogram) should be arranged. CT and MRI scans are often useful in the assessment of local and regional spread.

Table 23.1 TNM staging of mouth cancer

T stage	Clinical findings
T1	Tumour less than 2 cm
T2	Tumour 2–4 cm
T3	Tumour greater than 4 cm
T4	Invasion of neighbouring structures, e.g. mandible

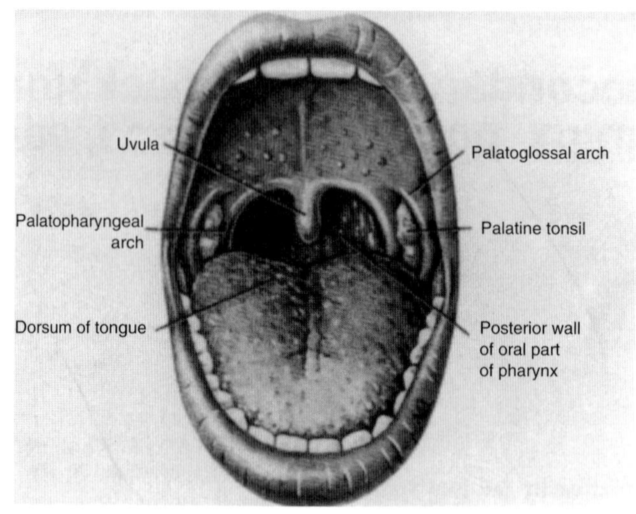

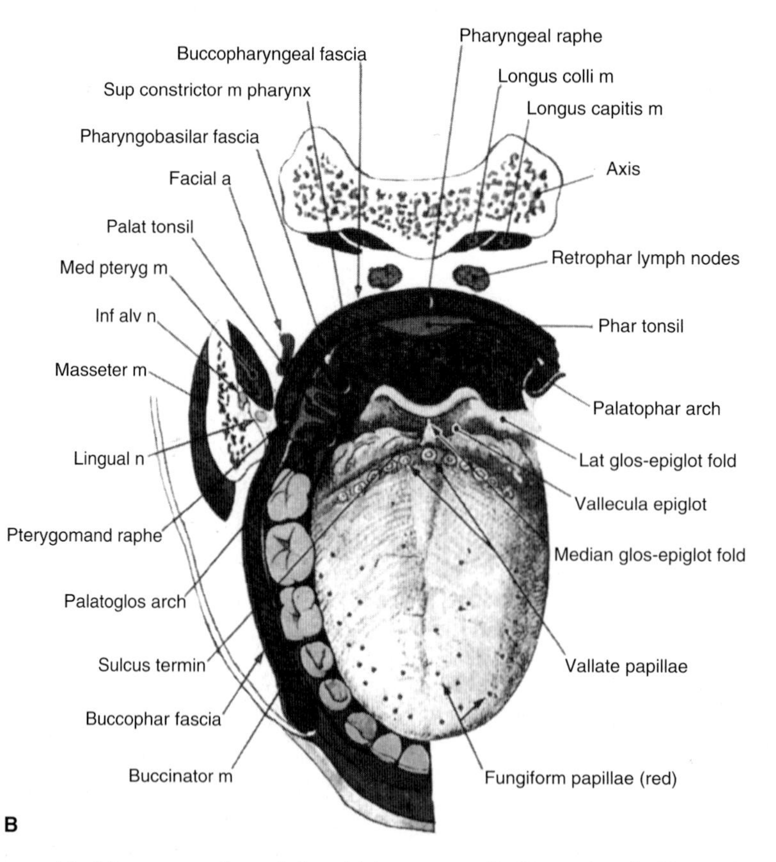

Fig. 23.1 **A** The fauces and its isthmus seen through the widely open mouth. (Reproduced with permission from Romanes G J 1971 Cunningham's Manual of Practical Anatomy, 13th edn, Oxford University Press, Oxford). **B** Horizontal section immediately above the tongue. (Reproduced with permission from Walmsley R & Murphy T R 1972 Jamieson's Illustrations of Regional Anatomy, 9th edn, Churchill Livingstone, Edinburgh.)

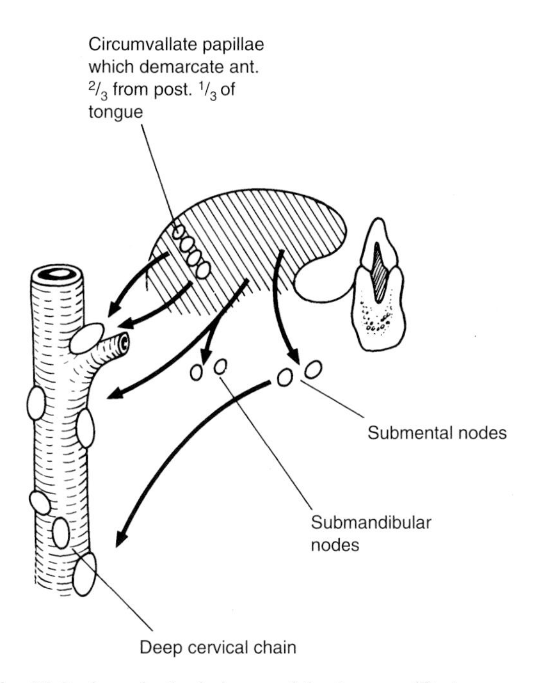

Fig. 23.2 Lymphatic drainage of the tongue. (Redrawn from Ellis H 1975 Clinical Anatomy, 5th edn, Blackwell Scientific, Oxford.)

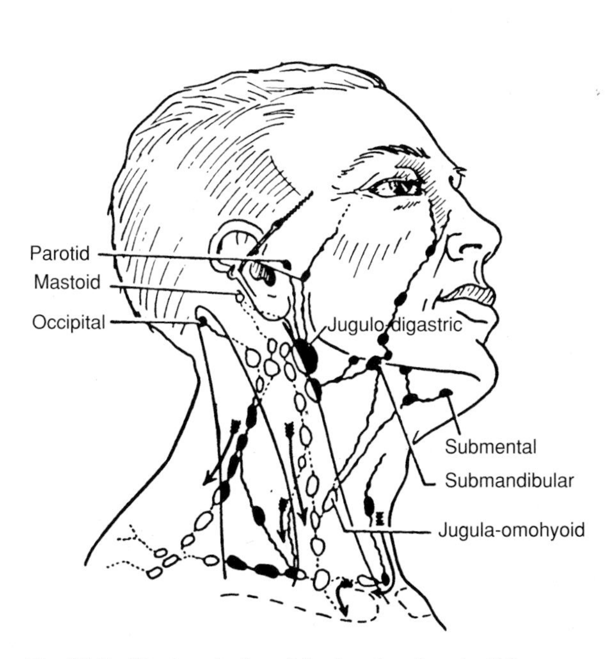

Fig. 23.3 The lymphatics of the head and neck. (After Rouvière; reproduced with permission from Basmajian J V, Grant's Method of Anatomy, 8th edn, ©1971 Williams & Wilkins, Baltimore.)

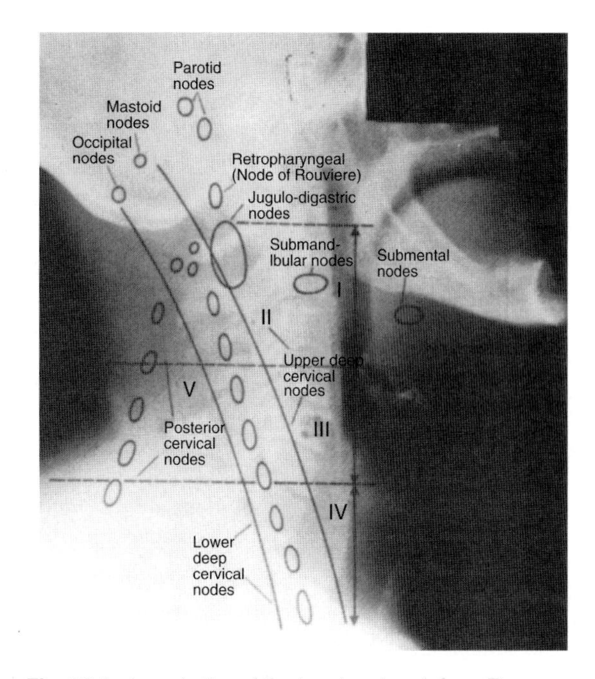

Fig. 23.4 Lymphatics of the head and neck from Figure 23.3, superimposed on lateral radiograph of the neck.

Treatment of tumours of the oral cavity

Ideally the patient should be jointly assessed by a surgeon and a clinical oncologist to decide on the choice of treatment. Surgery and radiotherapy can both be curative. The choice will depend on the aetiology and local extent of the disease, the age and general condition of the patient and the expertise available in radiotherapy and surgery. In general for early disease, radical radiotherapy or surgery may offer comparable local control. For advanced disease, the prospects of cure by local radiotherapy diminish substantially, and radical surgery, if the patient is fit, is generally preferred. Chemotherapy is not curative but useful palliation can sometimes be achieved in advanced disease not controlled by surgery or radiotherapy.

Radical radiotherapy

Radical irradiation of early tumours of the oral cavity should be by small beam-directed megavoltage fields using a full head shell and a mouth bite or by interstitial implantation or a combination of both. Afterloaded implantation using iridium wire is preferable to caesium needles because of the reduced radiation exposure to staff and its greater adaptability to the anatomy of the tumour (Ch. 22). Preparatory dental treatment (see below) should be carried out.

Early disease. Small superficial tumours (T1 and small T2) of the floor of mouth, tongue, lip and cheek in the absence of nodes are curable by implant (Fig. 23.5) alone (65–70 Gy), as long as the tumour can be completely encompassed by the sources in all planes and is not lying immediately adjacent to or invading bone.

More advanced tumours. For more advanced tumours which do not invade bone (larger T2 and T3), radical surgery and radiotherapy each have their proponents. For T4 tumours invading bone, radical surgery is preferred.

Dental treatment. The teeth may be damaged as a direct result of radiation ischaemia or, more importantly, as an indirect effect of a dry mouth (xerostomia) caused by inhibition of salivary secretion.

There is a reduction in the amount of saliva secreted and an increase in its viscosity. Both these factors predispose to bacterial growth and dental decay. In addition, the reduction in the pH of the saliva assists bacterial enzymatic activity, with the production of acids which destroy tooth enamel. Even teeth not in the primary beam are subject to caries. Unless preventive measures are taken, all teeth may be destroyed within 1–2 years of treatment. If later extractions become necessary, osteomyelitis may follow, especially in the mandible, and even bone necrosis.

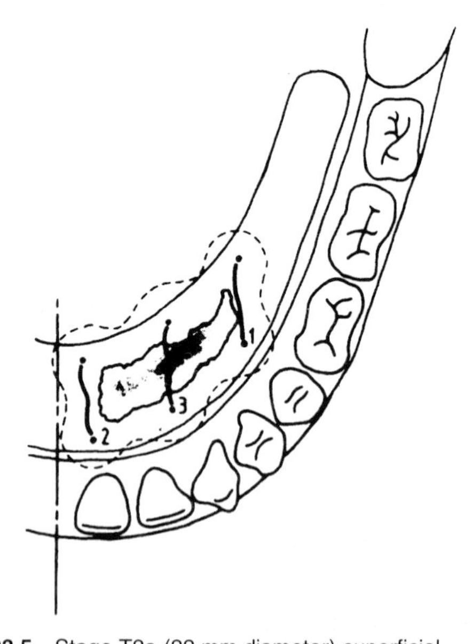

Fig. 23.5 Stage T2a (22 mm diameter) superficial squamous carcinoma, anterior floor of mouth. Implantation with hairpins (2.5 cm long, leg separation = 12 mm). Numbers indicate order in which guides were implanted. Reference isodose indicated by broken line around sources. (Reproduced from Pierquin et al 1987.)

Before irradiation, the patient should be seen by an oral surgeon familiar with the management of patients undergoing irradiation for head and neck cancer. The current trend is towards trying to conserve the teeth since the risk of bone necrosis is reduced if extraction can be avoided. At the least, scaling and cleaning should be done. Any teeth which are nonviable or would require root filling or extensive restoration are extracted. The gums are sutured to encourage prompt healing. There is no fixed period necessary to allow healing of the socket. A week will usually suffice. However, if urgent radiotherapy is required, planning should not be delayed following an extraction.

Scrupulous attention to dental hygiene is essential during and after radiotherapy. A number of measures may help in minimising dental caries. They include:

1. Regular brushing of the teeth.
2. Corsodyl mouthwashes for 1 minute after each meal and in the evening before going to bed.
3. Any extractions required following radiotherapy should be carried out with an atraumatic technique under general anaesthesia and antibiotic cover. Multiple extractions should be stages.

Radical radiotherapy: carcinoma of the floor of mouth

1. T1 without nodes (N0)

Iridium hairpin implant alone (65–70 Gy to reference 85% isodose).

2. T2 without nodes (N0)

Target volume

Radical radiotherapy is given to the primary with at least 2 cm margin of normal tissue and to the submental and submandibular nodes (Fig. 23.6).

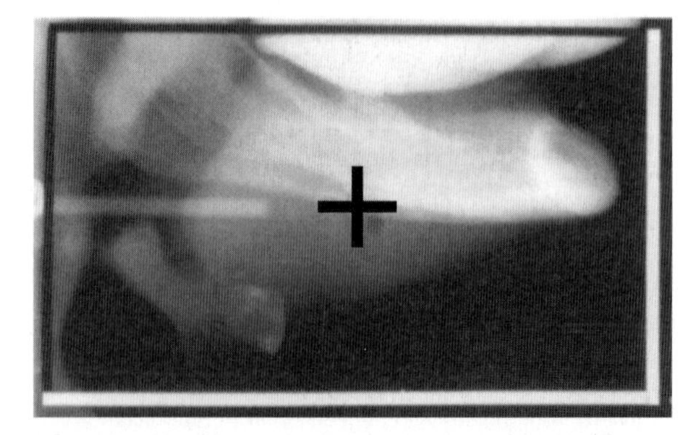

Fig. 23.6 Lateral field margins for early carcinoma of the floor of the mouth. (Courtesy of Dr D Radstone, Sheffield.)

Technique

A right-angled wedged pair of fields (Fig. 23.8) or, for midline lesions of the anterior floor of the mouth, a lateral parallel pair of fields is used.

Dose and energy

48 Gy in 20 daily fractions over 4 weeks (4–6 MV photons), then boost with iridium hairpin implant (20–25 Gy)

If not fit for implant:

60 Gy in 25 daily fractions over 5 weeks (4–6 MV photons)

3. T1 and small T2, mobile nodes (N1)

Target volume

Palpable submental, submandibular or upper deep cervical nodes (level I and II; Table 23.2) can often be encompassed with the primary tumour within the radical irradiation field. If the nodes are mobile and ipsilateral (N1) but cannot be encompassed within a reasonable radical volume (e.g. up to 60 cm^2), a block dissection of the affected side is followed by radical radiotherapy to the primary.

Technique

Parallel-opposed pair of wedged lateral fields.

Dose and energy

60 Gy in 25 fractions over 5 weeks to palpable disease or 50 Gy in 25 daily fractions over 5 weeks postoperatively if necessary

Management of nodes. The principles of management of neck nodes are described on page 355.

The indications for irradiation of neck nodes in cancer of the oral cavity and the levels to be irradiated ipsilaterally or bilaterally are summarised in Table 23.2. In T1N0 tumours treatable by implant alone, no nodal irradiation is necessary.

Surgery

The general indications for surgery in tumours of the oral cavity are:

Table 23.2 Guidelines for cervical nodal* irradiation in squamous cell carcinoma of the head and neck (reproduced with kind permission of Dr M Henk and the CHART steering committee)

Indications	Irradiation
Oral cavity	
T2N0 with well-lateralised primary	Levels I and II on same side
T2N1 with well-lateralised primary	Levels I to V on same side
T2N0 with primary approaching midline, all T3N0 and T4N0	Levels I, II and III bilaterally
All others	Levels I to V bilaterally
Oropharynx	
T2N0 tonsil	Levels I and II on same side
T2N1 tonsil	Levels I to V on same side
T2N0 other sites	Levels I, II and III bilaterally
All others	Levels I to V bilaterally
Nasopharynx	
Squamous carcinoma T1N0	No neck irradiation
Squamous carcinoma T2–4N0	Level II, plus lateral pharyngeal and upper posterior triangle
All undifferentiated carcinoma and squamous carcinoma with node involvement	Levels I to V
Hypopharynx	
All	Levels I to V bilaterally
Paranasal sinuses	
Squamous carcinoma	Lateral pharyngeal nodes only
Squamous carcinoma N+ and undifferentiated carcinoma	Levels I to V bilaterally
Larynx	
T1–2N0 glottic	No nodal irradiation
T3–4N0 glottic	Levels II and III bilaterally
T2N0 supraglottic	Levels II and III bilaterally
All others	Levels I to V bilaterally

* Lymph node levels are defined as follows: level I, submandibular; level II, upper deep cervical; level III, middle deep cervical; level IV, lower deep cervical; level V, posterior triangle

- Tumours attached to or invading the mandible where the risk of radionecrosis is high
- Tumours with widespread associated leucoplakia
- Radioresistant tumours such as melanoma
- Radiation-induced tumours
- Very large tumours unlikely to be cured by radiotherapy because of their bulk (T3 and T4)
- Tumours of the tip of the tongue, which are difficult to immobilise and therefore to irradiate accurately
- Tumours associated with syphilitic glossitis. Syphilis itself may cause ischaemia due to narrowing of small vessels (endarteritis). The addition of irradiation may precipitate necrosis.

Chemotherapy

A curative role has not been established for cytotoxic chemotherapy. It may improve local control in conjunction with surgery or radiotherapy. Tumour shrinkage and symptomatic improvement can occur with one or two courses of cisplatin-containing combination chemotherapy prior to radiotherapy.

Palliative cytotoxic therapy should also be considered in symptomatic patients where surgery and/or radiotherapy have failed. The routine use of cytotoxic chemotherapy in advanced head and neck cancer cannot, however, be recommended. It is essential to ensure that the patient is fit, since agents such as cisplatin and methotrexate, among the most active of drugs, have major toxicities. These are poorly tolerated by the elderly and those in poor general medical condition. Suggested palliative single-agent chemotherapy for up to six courses subject to response and tolerance is:

1. Cisplatin 100 mg/m^2 i.v. infusion in 2 litres 0.9% saline over 6 hours repeated every 3–4 weeks (see Ch. 34 for guidance on management of cisplatin therapy), or
2. Methotrexate 100 mg/m^2 i.v. bolus, with folinic acid 15 mg orally 6-hourly for six doses starting 24 hours AFTER methotrexate injection. Repeated every 2–4 weeks.

CANCER OF THE TONGUE

This is the commonest cancer of the mouth. Approximately 70% occur on the anterior two-thirds, mainly on the lateral or inferior aspects. Locally advanced cancers may infiltrate the musculature of the tongue, the floor of the mouth and base of tongue. Tumours of the posterior third differ. They tend to be more anaplastic and are more likely to metastasise to the regional nodes. Lymphoepithelioma and lymphoma occur more commonly in the posterior third. In addition, tumours of the posterior third tend to present later since they are less accessible to examination by the patient or doctor than more anterior lesions.

Lymphatic spread (Fig. 23.2) from the tip of the tongue is to the submental nodes. The remainder of the tongue drains to the submandibular and deep cervical nodes; 30% of patients with cancer of the oral tongue will have palpable nodes at presentation. Since the lymphatics cross the midline, contralateral nodes may be palpable in patients where the tumour appears clinically confined to one side of the tongue. Bilateral nodes occur in 5%.

Subclinical node metastases occur in about 30% of patients.

For the posterior third of the tongue 75% of patients have palpable nodes. Subclinical nodes are estimated to occur in 40–50% with clinically N0 neck.

Staging

This should include bimanual palpation of the tumour and examination of the neck for lymph nodes. An examination of the tumour and a biopsy should be carried out under general anaesthesia. Staging investigations are as for other oral cavity tumours (see above). A radiograph of the mandible (orthopantomogram) should be requested if there is clinical invasion of the floor of the mouth.

Treatment

Local cure and conservation of function of the tongue are guiding principles. Choice of treatment depends upon the site, stage and pathology and the general condition of the patient.

Tumours of the anterior two-thirds of the tongue are more easily accessible to implantation than those of the posterior third. For early T1 tumours on the lateral border of the tongue similar results are achievable by surgery or radiotherapy. If surgery is used it should only be used where resection of the tumour will not cause functional impairment of the tongue. For T2 and T3 tumours external beam and brachytherapy are advised. T4 tumours are poorly controlled by radiation or radical surgery. Radical surgery followed by postoperative radiotherapy or radical radiotherapy are both reasonable options.

Poorly differentiated and deeply infiltrating squamous carcinomas are more likely to be associated with palpable nodes. Lymphomas, usually of the non-Hodgkin type, occur more commonly in the posterior third of the tongue. They are best treated by external beam alone.

Anterior two-thirds of tongue

Except for small T1 (1 cm or less) tumours, initial surgery is best avoided because the loss of tissue is mutilating and likely to cause functional impairment (speech, swallowing). Surgery is commonly reserved for salvage of tumours not controlled by radiotherapy.

Both surgery and radiotherapy have an equal probability of curing early (T1) well-differentiated squamous cell tumours of the anterior two-thirds of the tongue.

Early disease. Wedge excision gives good functional results in small (1 cm or less) tumours of the tip or lateral border of the tongue.

For T1 and small, not deeply infiltrating T2 tumours on the lateral border of the anterior two-thirds of the tongue, interstitial implantation is recommended (Fig. 23.5 and Fig. 22.3) (see Ch. 22 for details of technique). For larger T2 and T3 tumours of the anterior two-thirds of the tongue which are too extensive for implantation, treatment should be by external beam irradiation initially or surgery.

More advanced tumours (T3–4). A hemiglossectomy is necessary for larger tumours (>4 cm) provided they do not involve the gingival margin or cross the midline. Tumours crossing the midline require more extensive resection. A myocutaneous flap can be used to replace the resected part of the tongue, permitting a reasonable quality of speech and swallowing. For T4 tumours, surgery is preferred to radiotherapy. Radical external beam irradiation to the primary and draining nodes (as for T2 and T3) is the alternative for inoperable T3 and T4 tumours.

External beam irradiation. This is appropriate as primary treatment for patients who are not fit for implantation or for larger T2 and inoperable T3 or T4 tumours. Larger T2 tumours should receive initial external beam followed by a boost with an iridium hairpin implant.

Target volume

This includes the primary tumour with at least a 2 cm margin and the submandibular and upper deep cervical nodes (Fig. 23.7).

Technique

A shell and mouth bite are required. The latter keeps the hard palate out of the field. For lateral tumours an anterior and lateral wedged pair of fields is suitable (Fig. 23.8). If the lesion extends to the midline, a parallel-opposed pair of fields is preferable.

Dose and energy

Implant or external beam alone (T1 and small T2)

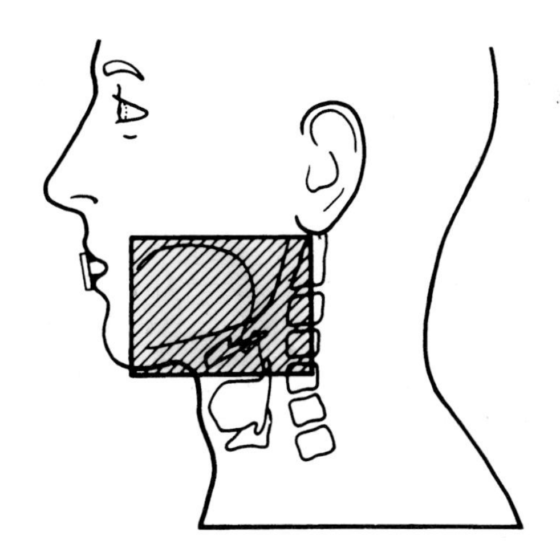

Fig. 23.7 Lateral field margins for localised carcinoma of the tongue. (Reproduced with permission of Arnold from Jane Dobbs, Ann Barrett, Daniel Ash, *Practical Radiotherapy Planning*, 3/e, Arnold, 1999.)

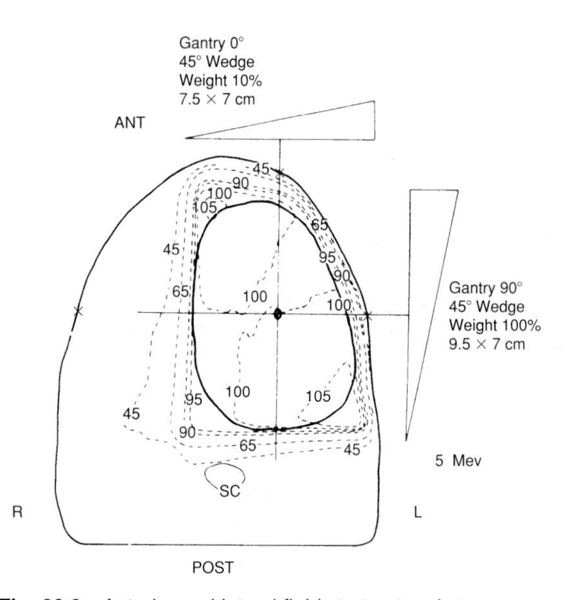

Fig. 23.8 Anterior and lateral fields to treat early tumours of the tongue and floor of the mouth. SC, spinal cord; X, laser reference point. (Reproduced with permission of Arnold from Jane Dobbs, Ann Barrett, Daniel Ash, *Practical Radiotherapy Planning*, 3/e, Arnold, 1999.)

Iridium implant (65–70 Gy to reference 85% isodose)

If unfit for implant:

60 Gy in 25 daily fractions over 5 weeks (4–6 MV photons)

Combined external beam and implant (larger T2)

48 Gy in 20 fractions over 4 weeks (4–6 MV photons) to the primary and neck followed by boost by an implant (20–25 Gy)

External beam alone (inoperable T3 and T4)

60 Gy in 25 daily fractions over 5 weeks (4–6 MV photons)

Posterior third of tongue. For tumours of the posterior third of the tongue, which are usually extensive at presentation, external beam irradiation is recommended since surgery would involve a total glossectomy and major functional impairment. Implantation of the posterior third of the tongue with iridium hairpins is rarely practical because of difficulty of access. An iridium wire boost (30 Gy) can be given using the loop technique (Fig. 22.4B) following external beam (50 Gy in 20 daily fractions over 4 weeks; 4–6 MV photons). Implanting the posterior third of the tongue requires considerable experience.

Target volume

The primary tumour and upper and midcervical nodes are included (Fig. 23.9). In view of the high incidence of nodal involvement, some radiotherapists include all the lymphatics (levels I–V, see Table 23.2) from the base of the skull to the clavicles.

Technique

A parallel-opposed pair of lateral wedged fields cover the primary and upper neck. The lower neck is treated by an open direct field with midline shielding of the spinal cord. A 0.5 cm gap is left at the junction of the upper and lower fields to avoid overlap, unless asymmetric diaphragms are used (Fig. 24.19). If the latter are used, no gap is needed at the junction and the fields are simply matched to avoid any overlap. Wherever a junction between lateral and anterior fields occurs, the junction must lie at least 1 cm below any central disease.

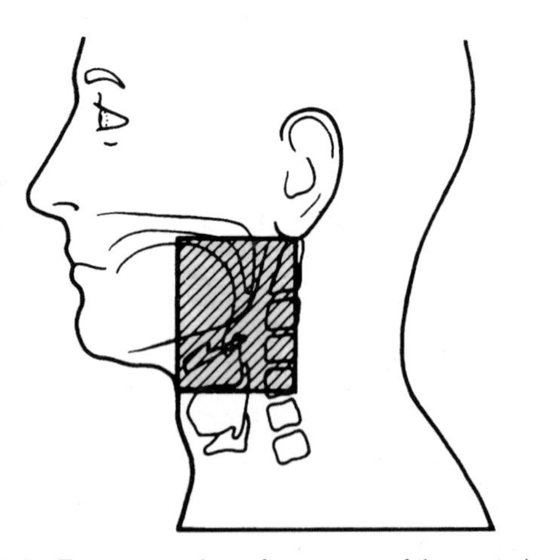

Fig. 23.9 Treatment volume for tumours of the posterior third of the tongue. (Reproduced with permission of Arnold from Jane Dobbs, Ann Barrett, Daniel Ash, *Practical Radiotherapy Planning*, 3/e, Arnold, 1999.)

Dose and energy

If nodal areas not overlying the spinal cord

60 Gy in 25 daily fractions over 5 weeks (4–6 MV photons)

If nodal areas treated overlie the cord. The volume of the upper neck field is reduced at 40 Gy to exclude the spinal cord and the dose to the reduced field continued to 66 Gy in 33 fractions. The anterior lower neck field has midline lead shielding throughout the course of treatment to protect the spinal cord. An additional 26 Gy in 13 daily fractions is given by electron fields to each side of the neck overlying the cord. The energy of electrons needed is chosen using the technique described in Figures 23.17 and 23.18.

66 Gy in 33 fractions over 6.5 weeks (4–6 MV photons or electrons)

Lymphomas. Lymphomas of the posterior third of the tongue are usually of high-grade non-Hodgkin type. External beam irradiation should be the definitive treatment.

ALVEOLUS AND HARD PALATE

Treatment

The management of carcinoma of the alveolus and hard palate is controversial. There are proponents for both radical surgery and radiotherapy. Many of these tumours involve bone, although this may be difficult to demonstrate. If bone is involved, radical surgery is the treatment of choice.

It is essential to exclude a primary tumour arising in the maxillary antrum by tomography or CT scanning. Most lesions are treated by megavoltage irradiation using anterior and lateral wedged fields. However, if the lesion extends to or beyond the midline, parallel-opposed wedged lateral fields are required. Dosage and fractionation are the same as for the floor of the mouth.

BUCCAL CHEEK

Small superficial growths (less than 1 cm) are often best excised in addition to any associated areas of leucoplakia. Otherwise they can be adequately treated by a single-plane iridium implant using the plastic tube technique (65–70 Gy to reference 85% isodose) or by electrons.

Lesions, especially at the back close to the intermaxillary commissure, are difficult to implant and are best treated by external beam or electrons.

For T1 and T2 lesions thicker than 1 cm, implantation alone is inadequate and should be combined with external beam or electrons. Initial electron or megavoltage irradiation to 40 Gy in 20 daily fractions over 4 weeks is followed by an iridium implant (40 Gy to 85% reference isodose).

For patients not fit for surgery or implantation external beam irradiation is an alternative. A direct electron field or anterior and lateral wedged pair at megavoltage can be used. Dosage and fractionation are as for the floor of mouth (p. 351).

For T3 and T4 lesions the probability of local control by radiotherapy is low. Disabling trismus due to severe fibrosis is common. Radical surgery with reconstruction is therefore preferred.

LYMPH NODE METASTASES IN THE NECK

Metastasis to the neck is the most serious aspect of mouth (and throat) cancer, being the commonest cause of death. Prognosis depends more on the presence or absence of secondaries in cervical nodes than on the primary growth.

As a generalisation, it may be said that *operable nodes in a squamous carcinoma are best treated by surgery*, usually radical block dissection, while inoperable nodes must rely on radiation as a poor second best. In a radical neck dissection the submental, submandibular, anterior and posterior cervical nodes are removed in addition to the sternomastoid and omohyoid muscles. The internal jugular vein is divided and tied off above and below.

In squamous carcinoma, four clinical situations have to be discussed:

1. No nodes palpable (N0). At one time 'prophylactic' removal of nodes on the affected side was advised, to remove early microscopic secondaries. The operation of radical neck dissection is a major procedure with significant morbidity and some mortality. However, nine out of ten cases proved to be free of secondaries, and it seemed unjustifiable to penalise the many for the sake of the few. Radical surgery is, of course, unsuitable for patients who are elderly or in poor condition.

'Prophylactic' or 'elective' neck irradiation has a low morbidity compared with radical neck dissection. However, elective neck irradiation, while it does reduce the incidence of the development of subsequent nodal metastases, does not improve survival compared with a 'wait and see' policy. There are three situations where elective neck irradiation is advisable. First, where the likelihood of microscopic nodal metastases is high (e.g. supraglottic tumours); secondly, when the patient is unlikely to be a regular attender at follow-up; and thirdly, where the general condition of the patient would contraindicate a radical neck dissection.

Most therapists prefer a 'wait and see' policy, with regular follow-up at monthly intervals in the first year and every 2 months in the second year. However, elective neck irradiation is becoming increasingly popular. It is within the first 2 years following treatment when lymph node spread is most likely to occur. Indeed, about 50% of block dissections are carried out within 3 months of completion of treatment of the primary. Fine needle aspiration of suspicious nodes can be carried out to obtain histological proof of involvement; the risk of needle track recurrence is very low. Biopsy, however, is contraindicated since it increases the risk of subsequent recurrence. If lymphatic metastases are strongly suspected, the patient should be prepared for a block dissection and the suspicious node examined by frozen section before proceeding to a radical neck dissection.

2. Nodes palpable and operable (N1, N2). Mobile nodes confined to one side of the neck are described as N1 and bilateral mobile nodes as N2.

a. N1 nodes. There are several possibilities, each with its advocates. Some remove the nodes first, then irradiate the primary. Others prefer to irradiate the primary first, then excise the nodes 4–6 weeks later. Others prefer to remove the primary and the nodes in one extensive operation. Alternatively, if the nodes lie close to the primary, they may be included in a volume that is small enough to be treated to a radical dose. A 'wait and see' policy can then be adopted for the neck. If the nodes lie too far from the primary to be included in a radical volume, radical radiotherapy to the primary, followed by neck dissection, is generally the preferred sequence.

If the primary is treated first with irradiation and the nodes are enlarging and/or becoming fixed, a 'holding' single dose of 15 Gy to the involved node can be given. The block dissection can then be carried out as planned.

The local recurrence rate after radical neck dissection is high, of the order of 30%. There are three main risk factors for recurrence, of which extracapsular spread is the strongest predictor of recurrence.

- Invasion through the capsule of the nodes (extracapsular spread)
- The size of the nodes (>3 cm)
- The number of nodes involved by tumour (more than three).

If one or more of these factors are present, postoperative radiotherapy is advisable to the involved side of the neck.

b. N2 nodes. Bilateral nodal metastases are associated with a poor prognosis. Complete radical neck dissection on both sides is not possible since the internal jugular vein has to be preserved on one side. In a bilateral block dissection, the operation on the second side is carried out at a later stage, with preservation of the internal jugular vein. The latter should be followed by postoperative radiotherapy. Because of the poor prognosis and morbidity of bilateral neck dissection, most patients are treated by bilateral radical neck irradiation.

3. Fixed nodes (N3). Fixed nodes are often regarded as inoperable. The interpretation of fixity is often difficult. Indeed nodes which appear fixed to the carotid sheath may sometimes be completely removed. Urgent joint assessment with a head and neck surgeon is essential to determine operability. Occasionally a fixed node may become mobile and operable after a course of radical irradiation. If the nodes are judged inoperable, the situation is almost invariably palliative.

4. Metastatic neck nodes (squamous carcinoma) of unknown primary site. In the upper and midcervical region the most likely primary sites are the nasopharynx, pyriform fossa and the vallecula. If the node is solitary and mobile, a radical neck dissection of the involved side should be considered. If the node is fixed and inoperable and the patient is fit, radical radiotherapy to both sides of the neck shielding the cord is recommended. If the nodes are large and multiple and biopsy shows undifferentiated carcinoma, the pharynx is a likely primary site. Radical radiotherapy should be delivered to the pharynx and nodes.

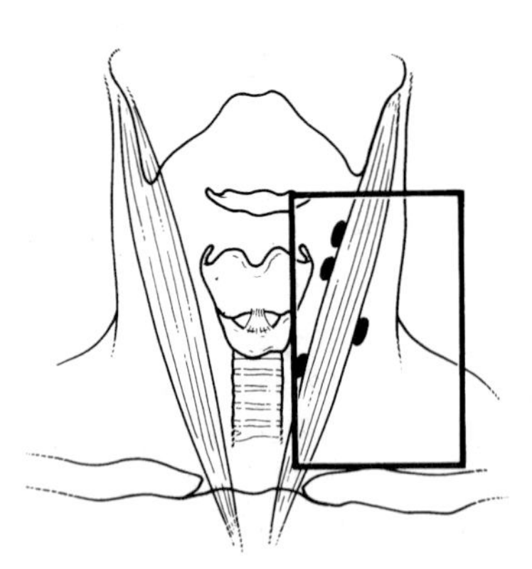

Fig. 23.10 Anterior field for irradiation of secondary neck nodes. A parallel posterior field can be added. The hyoid, thyroid and cricoid and upper tracheal cartilages are shown (from above downwards).

5-year survival for radical radiotherapy of metastatic neck nodes of unknown primary is poor (15%), but long-term survival is occasionally seen and justifies treatment.

Target volume and technique for neck irradiation

For irradiation of one side of the neck, the volume should be treated by a single anterior field extending from the mastoid process to the inferior border of the medial end of the clavicle (Fig. 23.10). The head is extended so that the submandibular and upper deep cervical nodes can be included while limiting dosage to the floor of the mouth. The medial margin of the field lies just lateral to the larynx and spinal cord. The neck nodes may be divided into five levels. The levels which need to irradiated are summarised in Table 23.2.

Avoidance of the spinal cord should be confirmed by simulator or port films. If verification is not available, the anterior field can be angled 10° laterally to ensure avoidance of the cord. The asymmetrical diaphragm technique is also useful. Bolus can be applied to the neck to compensate for the irregular contour of the neck and secure uniform dosage. This does, however, sacrifice the skin-sparing effect of megavoltage irradiation.

For bilateral neck irradiation, a single anterior field is used to encompass the neck, with a 2 cm wide central lead strip protecting the midline structures. Bolus can be applied.

Dose and energy

48 Gy in 20 daily fractions over 4 weeks (4–6 MV photons)

Nodes which were palpable before irradiation are boosted to a further **12 Gy in 5 daily fractions over a week using electrons**. A technique for determining the energy for electrons to treat the nodes adequately without overdosing the spinal cord is shown in Figures 23.17 and 23.18.

Radiation reactions

Smoking and alcohol should be forbidden during the reaction period. About the third week of the course the mucosal reaction will begin (Fig. 23.11) and settle by 3 weeks after treatment. It is always a strain on any patient, with soreness, loss of taste and dysphagia.

Patients need considerable moral support and reassurance from the treatment staff, and must be encouraged to take adequate nourishment and fluid. It is often advisable to admit to hospital during the acute phase, so that the nursing staff can ensure proper

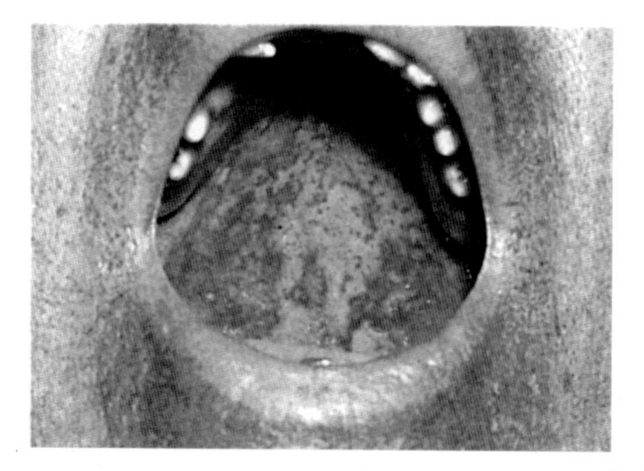

Fig. 23.11 Typical acute reaction on the hard palate during radical radiotherapy.

hygiene and nutrition. Mouthwashes should be frequently used, e.g. Difflam (a local analgesic and anti-inflammatory agent), sodium bicarbonate (a teaspoonful in a pint of warm water), or 0.01% chlorhexidine.

Complications of radiotherapy of cancer of the oral cavity

Late effects. After the acute reaction has passed, late effects follow which may be troublesome. Some degree of dryness of the mouth and throat is unavoidable, owing to inhibition of mucous glands. This will be particularly marked if the major salivary glands, especially the parotids, have been in the high-dose region. It is important to leave at least one parotid gland in the low-dose area if possible, and it is worthwhile adjusting field layouts with this in mind. Loss of taste is another unpleasant side-effect, but one which usually recovers.

Skin changes are generally mild with megavoltage radiation and give no trouble. Submental oedema sometimes occurs, due to lymphatic obstruction, giving a 'dewlap' appearance, but is seldom of sinister importance.

Fibrosis of the submandibular gland, often asymmetrical, may mimic nodal recurrence.

Radionecrosis of soft tissue and bone. Necrosis may occur in the soft tissues of the mouth and in the underlying mandible following both external beam and interstitial implantation. Soft tissue necrosis alone is commoner (15%) after implantation than after megavoltage external beam irradiation but usually heals with conservative measures in a few weeks. Radionecrosis of the mandible (osteoradionecrosis) is more likely to occur if soft tissue necrosis develops on the overlying gingiva. Its incidence is much lower (2%) than soft tissue necrosis. With conventional fractionation, radionecrosis is rarely seen under 60 Gy. The incidence is 1–2% up to 70 Gy and 9% above 70 Gy.

Osteoradionecrosis

Aetiology. Radiation causes damage both directly to bone and indirectly by impairing its vascular supply. The direct effect is considered the more important since the bone damage may occur without obvious vascular damage. Irradiation directly damages some of the bone cells, osteoclasts, which resorb bone and others, osteoblasts, which reconstruct it. These irradiated cells retain their function until some attempt to divide and then undergo mitotic death months or years after irradiation. Gradually the population of bone cells and thus the process of remodelling in the irradiated area diminish. As a result the mandible becomes thinner and loses its structural integrity.

Reduced vascular supply to the periosteum, because of damage to the endothelial cells that line the blood vessels, indirectly contributes to osteoradionecrosis.

Radionecrosis is seen much more frequently in the mandible than in the maxilla. This is because the mandible has denser bone than the maxilla and derives its blood supply only from the periosteum. By contrast the maxilla has a rich blood supply.

Infection may be introduced to the bone by local trauma, tooth extraction or dental infection. Infection stimulates cell division in bone and mitotic death. While tumour involvement may inhibit bone remodelling, it may also precipitate radionecrosis by stimulating the division of osteoblasts to remodel bone following the death of tumour cells. There is a threefold higher incidence of radionecrosis of the mandible in patients who have retained their teeth before radiotherapy compared with the edentulous. Patients with oral cancer are often alcoholic, with poor general medical state and oral hygiene. The latter predisposes to mucosal ulceration and ensuing osteoradionecrosis.

Diagnosis. Presentation is with a flat ulcer with bone visible at its base. It may be painless, even in the presence of a pathological fracture of the mandible. Pain, trismus and general ill health are, however, often present due to associated infection. A radiograph of the mandible (orthopantomogram) typically shows an area of rarefaction, sometimes with evidence of osteomyelitis or pathological fracture (Fig. 23.12).

Management of radionecrosis. Radionecrosis should be managed conservatively since surgical intervention may exacerbate the process of necrosis. Scrupulous attention should be paid to dental hygiene. Mouthwashes with 0.01% chlorhexidine should be carried

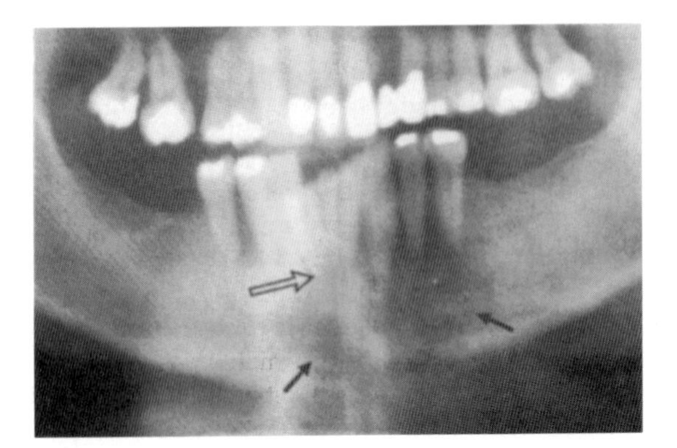

Fig. 23.12 Radiograph of the mandible (orthopantomogram) showing a radiolucent area of radionecrosis (small arrows) and an associated pathological fracture (large arrow). (Courtesy of Mr P McAndrew, Rotherham.)

out after each meal and the patient encouraged to remove food debris.

In most cases small areas of soft tissue necrosis heal within a few weeks with conservative local measures (antibiotics, steroids). If radionecrosis of the mandible occurs, a period of observation, often over months or several years, is worthwhile since spontaneous healing occurs in 50%. The dead bone (sequestrum) may separate spontaneously followed by healing. Once loose, the sequestrum can be carefully removed to avoid abrasion of the adjacent tongue. Surgical resection and reconstruction of the mandible may, however, be necessary to relieve the chronic pain and infection associated with mandibular radionecrosis. All the irradiated bone must be removed. Often both sides of the mandible are involved and require replacement, resulting in substantial deformity.

Results of treatment of oral cancer

Overall about 90% of T1 and 75% of T2 tumours are controlled by radiotherapy. Salvage surgery is successful in approximately half of the failures. For T3 tumours the local control rate falls to 50% and few of the failures are successfully salvaged by surgery.

Anterior two thirds of tongue

For T1 tumours of the tongue, local control varies from 62–100% and 5-year survival from 80–90%. For T2 and T3 tumours, local control is 50–85% and 5-year survival 50–80%. For T4 tumours, local control is 25–45%.

Posterior third of tongue

For T1, local control is 70–95% and 5-year survival 60%. For T2, comparable figures are 50–90% and 50% respectively. For T3 and T4 tumours, local control is 20–50% and 5-year survival about 20%.

OROPHARYNX

Anatomy

The oropharynx (Fig. 23.13) extends from the junction of the hard and soft palate to the level of the vallecula. It contains the posterior third or base of the tongue, the soft palate, tonsils, and the posterior oropharyngeal wall.

The tonsil (Figs 23.1, 23.13 and 23.14) forms part of a protective ring (Waldeyer's ring), a more or less complete circle of lymphoid tissue at the entrance to the pharynx. It includes the two lateral tonsils, the nasopharyngeal tonsil (adenoids) on the roof and posterior wall of the nasopharynx, and lymphoid tissue on the posterior surface of the tongue (lingual tonsil).

The soft palate (Fig. 23.1A) is a mobile muscular flap which extends from the back of the hard palate. It divides the nasopharynx from the oropharynx. From the centre of the posterior border of the soft palate hangs the uvula, which rests on the dorsum of the tongue.

CANCER OF THE TONSIL

Pathology

Tumours in this region are of two main types—squamous carcinoma from the epithelium (75%), and non-Hodgkin lymphoma. Macroscopically they are either an exophytic mass protruding into the throat or infiltrative and ulcerating.

Spread

Local spread is early, beginning with the anterior and posterior pillars and the soft palate. The lower end of the anterior pillar extends to the posterolateral corner of the tongue, which may be invaded. Spread backwards involves the lateral wall of the oropharynx.

Lymphatic drainage of the anterior tonsillar pillar and fossa is to the jugulodigastric (tonsillar) node (Fig. 23.3) lying just behind the angle of the mandible and to the upper deep cervical nodes. If the soft palate is involved, spread may occur to the retropharyngeal nodes, which lie between the pharynx and the pre-

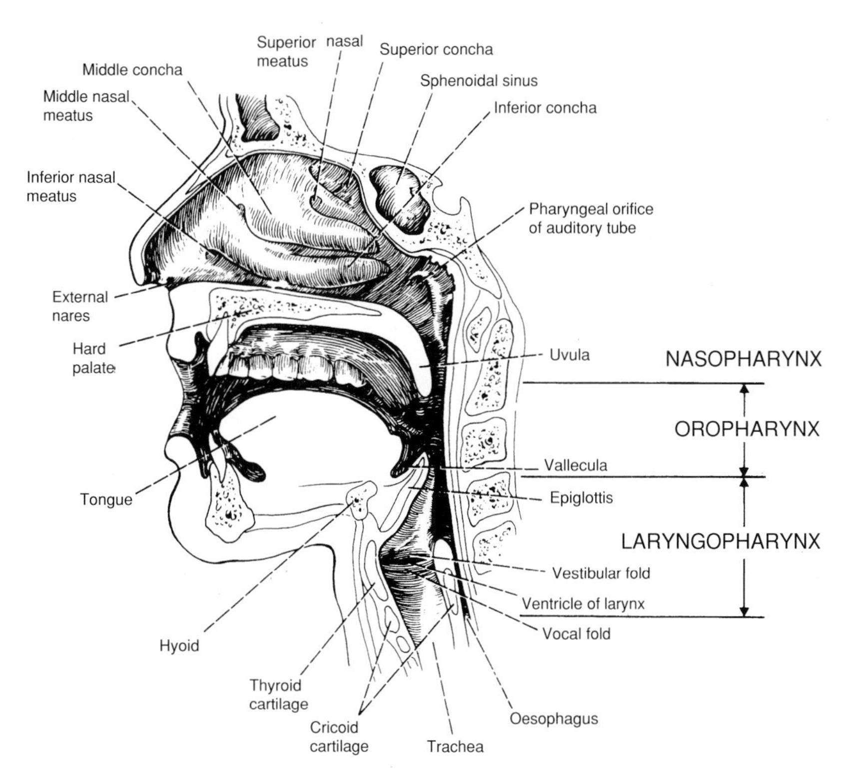

Fig. 23.13 Section of the pharynx, from front to back.

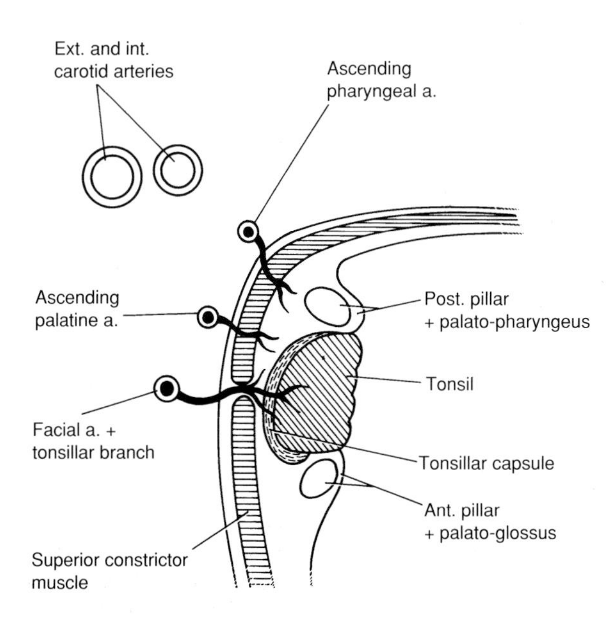

Fig. 23.14 Diagram of the tonsil and its relations in horizontal section. (Reproduced with permission from Ellis, Clinical Anatomy, 5th edn, Blackwells, 1975.)

vertebral fascia on a plane just in front of the mastoid process.

Tumours confined to the posterior pillar are rare. They spread inferiorly to the posterior pharyngeal wall and, unlike tumours of the anterior pillar, may involve the spinal accessory nodes.

Careful local examination by inspection and palpation is essential, since the technique and success of local treatment depend on it.

Clinical features

Symptoms are minimal at the start, with slight sore throat; in later stages, dysphagia and pain may be prominent. Often it is the secondary mass in the neck which brings the patient to the doctor, and the primary is only then discovered.

In general, tumours of the anterior tonsillar pillar are less aggressive and, like tumours of the retromolar trigone and soft palate, present less frequently with palpable neck nodes (40–50%) than do tumours of the tonsillar fossa (75%). Overall 75% of tonsillar tumours are associated with palpable nodes and in 20% they are bilateral.

Treatment

In general, radiotherapy is preferable to surgery since local cure can often be obtained without the functional and cosmetic impairment of radical surgery.

Radical radiotherapy is mainly by external beam since both primary and cervical nodes need to be treated. Some radiotherapists have obtained better local control in early T1 tumours without nodes by boosting the primary with an iridium implant using the 'loop' technique (Fig. 22.4B). Surgery is, however, possible and equally effective for early T1 and T2 tumours. Surgery involves a radical tonsillectomy, partial mandibulectomy and ipsilateral radical neck dissection. Loss of tissue is compensated for by a flap repair.

Radical radiotherapy

Epithelial tumours

Small tumours of the tonsillar fossa or anterior tonsillar pillar without nodes (N0)

Target volume
The primary site and the ipsilateral submandibular and upper deep cervical nodes are irradiated (Fig. 23.15). The superior margin includes the roof of the hard palate. The inferior limit is the lower margin of the hyoid bone. Anteriorly, the field extends through the middle third of the tongue. The posterior border lies just anterior to the spinal cord. The medial limit is the midline.

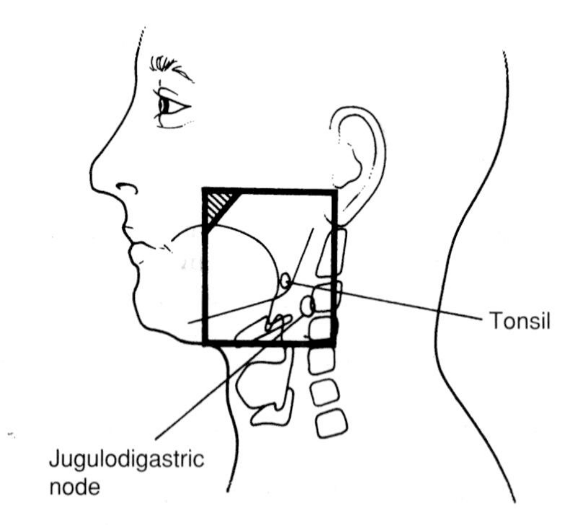

Fig. 23.15 Treatment volume for small tumours of the tonsillar fossa. Lead shielding as indicated for opposing lateral fields. (Redrawn.) (Reproduced with permission of Arnold from Jane Dobbs, Ann Barrett, Daniel Ash, *Practical Radiotherapy Planning*, 1/e, Edward Arnold 1985.)

Technique
An anterior and lateral right-angled wedged pair is used or, for T1 tumours, an oblique lateral wedged pair with CT planning (Fig. 23.16A).

Larger tumours involving the soft palate or base of tongue or crossing the midline

Target volume
These tumours have a higher propensity for bilateral nodal spread. The target volume should therefore

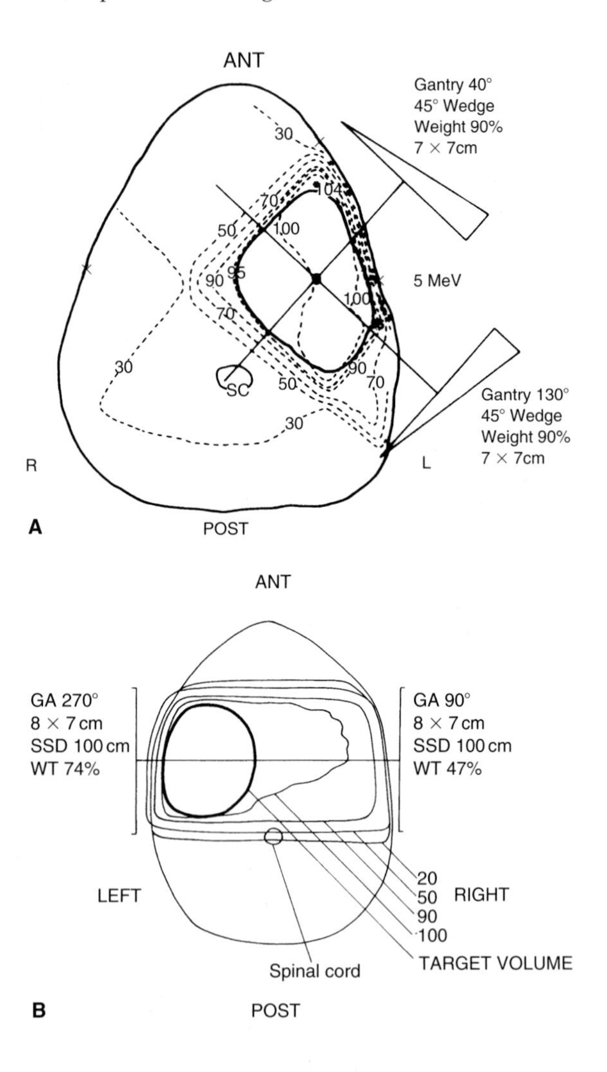

Fig. 23.16 Early carcinoma of the tonsil. **A** Anterior and posterior oblique wedged pair of fields. (Reproduced with permission of Arnold from Jane Dobbs, Ann Barrett, Daniel Ash, *Practical Radiotherapy Planning*, 3/e, Arnold, 1999.) **B** Parallel-opposed fields for treatment of early carcinoma of the left tonsil with 2 : 1 weighting. (Reproduced with permission of Arnold from Jane Dobbs, Ann Barrett, Daniel, Ash, *Practical Radiotherapy Planning*, 1/e, Edward Arnold, 1999.)

include the primary site and the upper deep cervical nodes on both sides of the neck.

Technique

Parallel-opposed megavoltage fields are used with a 2 : 1 weighting on the side of the primary (Fig. 23.16B). The weighting enables a lower but prophylactic dose to the tonsil on the opposite side and the upper deep cervical nodes, while limiting the dose to the contralateral oral mucosa and parotid gland. After 40 Gy, if involved nodes overlie the cord, that part of the volume is treated with electrons of suitable energy (Figs 23.17 and 23.18).

Dose and energy

1. *Nodal disease not overlying spinal cord*

60 Gy in 25 daily fractions over 5 weeks (4–6 MV photons)

2. *Nodal disease overlying spinal cord*

As for tongue (p. 356).

Lymphomas. Lower doses are needed to treat lymphomas compared with squamous carcinomas of the head and neck, since lymphomas are more radiosensitive.

Target volume

Wide field regional radiotherapy is indicated. The volume includes Waldeyer's ring and the lymph nodes on both sides of the neck from the base of the skull to the clavicles.

Technique

There are two chief alternative techniques: (1) lateral opposed fields reaching high enough to include the nasopharynx, and (2) anterior and posterior opposed fields, making allowance for the irregular contour and varying thickness of the neck, either by using bolus on the neck or shielding the laryngeal region with lead for part of the course.

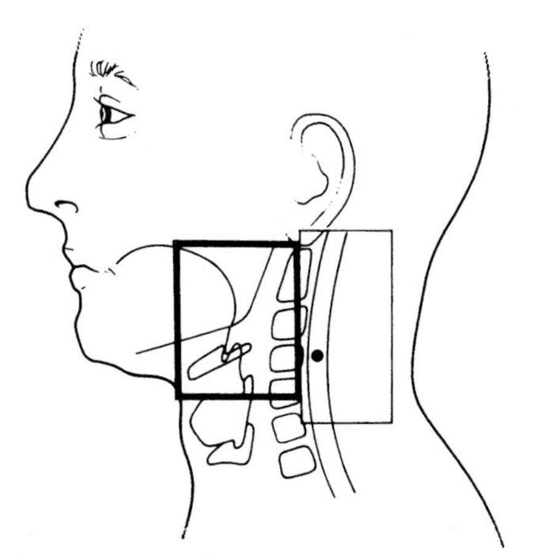

Fig. 23.17 Early tonsillar cancer with nodal involvement. Diagram showing field margins of megavoltage (bold) field to primary tumour and jugulodigastric node and electron beam (light) to posterior cervical nodes. Black dot marks thinnest point of the neck at which depth of spinal cord is measured for choice of electron energy.

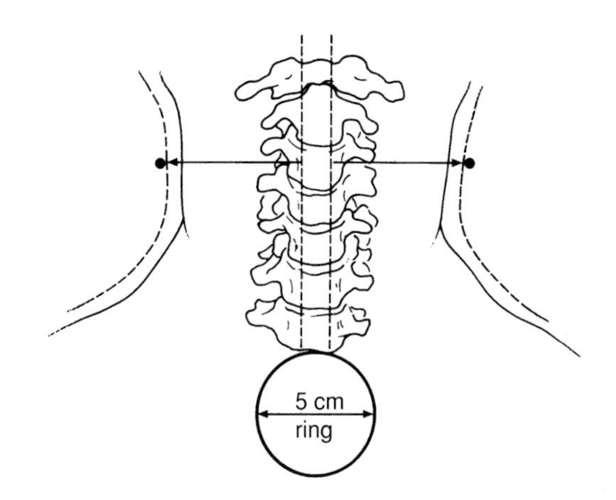

Fig. 23.18 Technique for measuring the minimum depth of the spinal cord in the neck within an electron field. A ball bearing is placed on each side of the shell at the narrowest point of the neck overlying the cord and within the electron field. The surface marking of the spinal cord is a line running inferior to the mastoid process. A simulator film is taken with a magnification ring. The distance from the ball bearing to the lateral border of the spinal cord is measured. Electron energy is chosen to minimise the dose to the spinal cord. (Courtesy of Dr I Manifold, Sheffield.)

Dose and energy

Low-grade non-Hodgkin lymphomas

35 Gy in 20 daily fractions over 4 weeks (4–6 MV photons)

High-grade non-Hodgkin lymphomas

40–45 Gy in 20 daily fractions over 4 weeks (4–6 MV photons)

The primary lesion in the mouth can, if necessary, be raised to higher dosage locally by supplementary small fields after the main course, to give an extra 5–10 Gy. These must avoid the spinal cord and should be checked on the simulator or by portal films. Dosage to the spinal cord should not exceed 40 Gy.

Radiation reactions. Mucositis, especially in radical treatments, is inevitably troublesome, with sore throat, dysphagia, dryness and loss of taste. It is often desirable to admit the patient to hospital towards the end of the course, for nursing care, mouth hygiene and nutrition, especially fluid intake. An aspirin–mucilage mixture before meals helps to make swallowing more comfortable.

Cervical nodes from squamous carcinoma of the oropharynx

The management has been discussed above (p. 355) and most of it is applicable here. The situation is similar to the posterior third of tongue, with a high proportion of anaplastic growths, and involvement of nodes of neck from the start. In such cases treatment should be directed to the primary and the whole of the neck (40 Gy in 20 fractions over 4 weeks) and possible supplementary fields as outlined on page 361.

Results of treatment

The prognosis for growths with no evident secondaries is fairly good, with 5-year survival about 75%, falling to 40% in the presence of secondary nodes. For T1 tumours, local control is 75–95% and 5-year survival 60–80%. For T2 and T3, local control is 60% and 80% respectively and 5-year survival 30–50%. For T4 tumours, local control is 10–35% and 5-year survival 30–50%.

SOFT PALATE

Treatment

For squamous tumours of the soft palate, radiotherapy is the treatment of choice. The target volume is similar to the tonsil, with the exception that the posterior margin should extend back to include the retropharyngeal nodes to which the soft palate drains.

For tumours <3 cm the choice is between external beam (60 Gy in 25 daily fractions over 5 weeks (4–6 MV photons), and implantation (65–70 Gy) using the loop technique (Fig. 19.4B); for tumours >3 cm, external beam to 48 Gy in 20 daily fractions with a boost by implant (20 Gy) to the primary site or external beam alone (60 Gy in 25 daily fractions over 5 weeks).

This is a very difficult site to implant successfully. For superficial lesions a permanent gold grain implant or an iridium wire implant using the loop technique is possible. The latter technique includes excision of the uvula before implantation to avoid underdosage to this outcrop of the soft palate.

Prophylactic neck node irradiation should be considered according to the guidelines in Table 23.2 in view of common and bilateral involvement.

CARCINOMA OF NASOPHARYNX (POSTNASAL SPACE)

Anatomy

The nasopharynx is the nasal part of the pharynx (Fig. 23.13). It is pyramidal in shape. Its roof is the base of the skull, formed by the body of the sphenoid bone and the basiocciput. The roof curves backwards to become continuous with the posterior wall. The latter is formed by the upper cervical vertebrae. Anteriorly, the nasopharynx is continuous with the nasal cavity. On the lateral walls of the nasopharynx are the orifices of the auditory (eustachian) tube which leads to the middle ear. Immediately behind this tubal opening is a deep depression, the pharyngeal recess (Fig. 23.19) (fossa of Rosenmüller). This is a common site of origin for nasopharyngeal cancer (Fig. 23.20). The floor is the upper border of the soft palate. Lymphatic spread is to the node of Rouvière (Fig. 23.4) lying in the retropharyngeal space (Fig. 23.1B) in front of the atlas (first cervical vertebra) and to the posterior, upper and mid-cervical nodes.

Epidemiology

Nasopharyngeal cancer represents 0.1% of all cancers and of cancer deaths. Although rare in Western Europe, nasopharyngeal cancer is very common in parts of the Far East. In areas of Southern China it accounts for the majority of malignant disease. The strongest evidence for a causative agent is the presence of antibodies to a virus (Epstein–Barr) in the blood of patients with nasopharyngeal carcinoma and there is evidence that this virus can persist as a latent infection in nasopharyngeal epithelium. The smoking and curing of fish, common practices in the Far East, have been

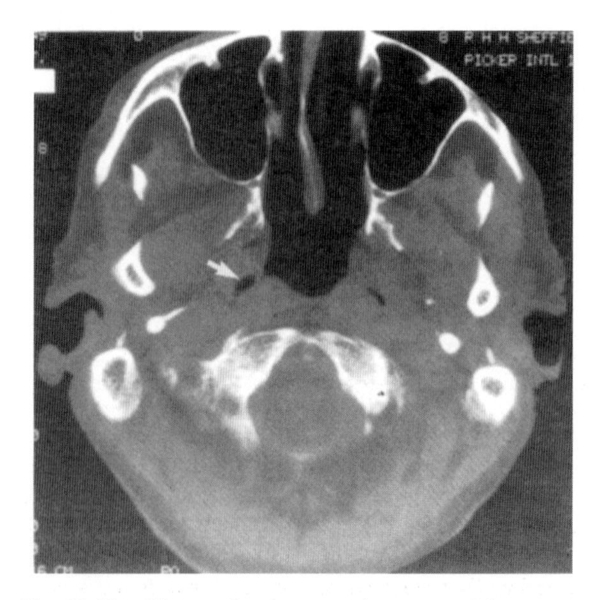

Fig. 23.19 CT scan showing normal anatomy of the nasopharynx. The fossa of Rosenmüller (pharyngeal recess) is arrowed. (Courtesy of Dr R Nakielny, Sheffield.)

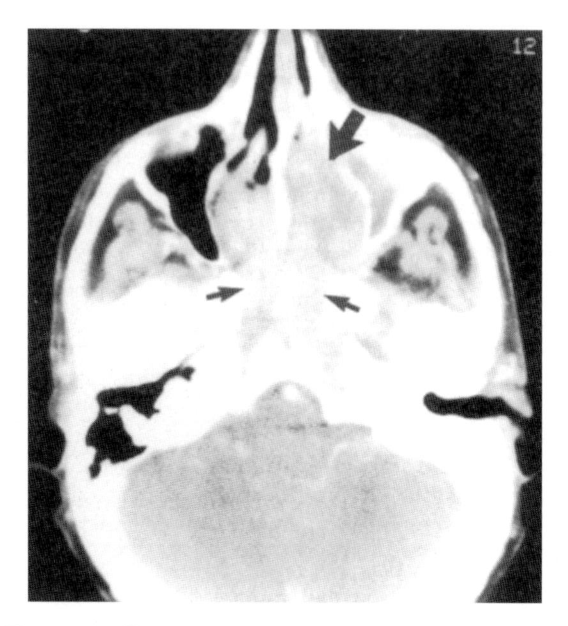

Fig. 23.20 CT scan showing carcinoma of the nasopharynx (small arrows) extending into the nasal cavity (large arrow). (Courtesy of Dr R Nakielny, Sheffield.)

postulated as sources of chemical carcinogens. The disease is commoner in men (sex ratio 3 : 1) and commonest between the ages of 40 and 60.

Pathology

The great majority are squamous carcinomas, often poorly differentiated with a florid lymphocytic infiltrate (lymphoepithelioma); they are difficult to distinguish from lymphoma. Some are lymphomas, almost invariably of the non-Hodgkin type. Adenocarcinomas of salivary type also occur but are rare.

Spread

The mode of spread is important and accounts for the great variety of presenting symptoms—to the posterior part of the nose (nasal obstruction, bleeding), eustachian tube (deafness), upper cervical vertebrae (pain), base of skull (double vision due to involvement of third, fourth and sixth cranial nerves from spread into the cavernous sinus through the foramen lacerum). The ninth, tenth, eleventh and twelfth cranial nerves may also be affected. This can be due to direct extension of tumour into the parapharyngeal space from the lateral wall of the nasopharynx or due to involvement of the node of Rouvière. Invasion of the base of skull is reported in 10–50% of cases. Tumour may be visible in the nose or bulging behind the soft palate in the mouth. Growth is insidious, and the commonest presentation is an enlarged node in the neck just below the lobe of the ear (jugulodigastric) or in the posterior cervical chain. 80–90% of patients present with palpable nodes, of which 50% are bilateral.

Diagnosis and investigation

The nasopharynx should be examined with a mirror or in theatre under anaesthesia and visible tumour biopsied. Even if no tumour is seen, biopsy is still worthwhile since a microscopic tumour may occasionally be revealed. Investigation includes a soft tissue lateral film to show the air cavities and irregularities of the nasopharyngeal wall and special projections to examine the base of the skull for bone erosion. A CT scan of the nasopharynx and neck should be carried out to detail the extent of local spread and nodal involvement. It is also a useful means of assessing the response to treatment.

Treatment

Surgery is quite impractical, and external irradiation is the treatment of choice for both epithelial tumours and lymphomas.

Radical radiotherapy

External beam irradiation is the mainstay of treatment. Brachytherapy is principally considered for disease that has recurred after external beam irradiation.

Epithelial tumours—external beam

Target volume

For squamous cell carcinoma, this should include the primary and the routes of spread, particularly the base of the skull. If the tumour lies less than 2 cm from the midline, the primary site and the upper deep cervical, lateral pharyngeal and upper posterior triangle lymph nodes on both sides of the neck should be included (Fig. 23.21). If the tumour is at least 2 cm from the midline, the primary site and ipsilateral neck alone may be treated.

For all undifferentiated tumours and squamous carcinoma with node involvement, all the nodes on both sides of the neck (levels I–V) should be irradiated (see Table 23.2).

Technique

The patient lies supine with the head extended. A full head shell is required. A large lateral opposed pair of

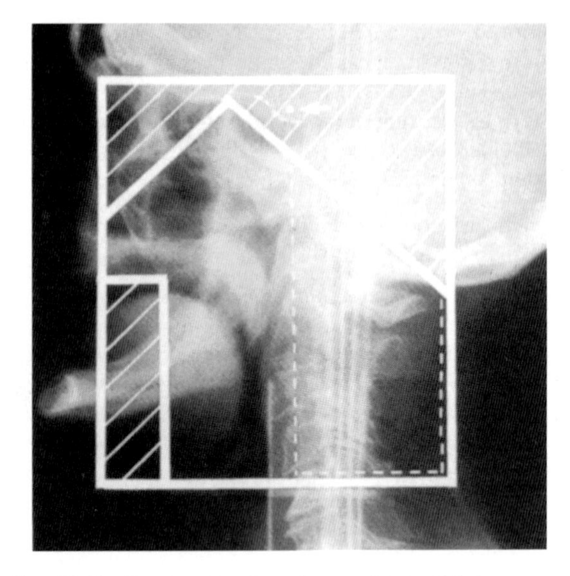

Fig. 23.21 Treatment volume for carcinoma of the nasopharynx (interrupted lines for electrons). Note the shielding of the anterior orbit, optic chiasm (arrowed) and of the brainstem. (Courtesy of Dr I Manifold, Sheffield.)

fields encompass the primary tumour and the nodes of the upper neck. The field includes the nasopharynx, the base of skull, the parapharyngeal space and the posterior half of the orbit (but ensuring full tumour dose is not given to the posterior retina) and any tumour extending into the nasal cavity or the oropharynx. An additional direct anterior field may be required if there is involvement of the nasal cavity. The front half of the orbit, brainstem and optic chiasm are shielded with lead (Fig. 23.21). The doses to the lens are calculated using thermoluminescent dosimetry (p. 66). Once a maximum safe dose to the spinal cord has been reached (40 Gy in 20 daily fractions), the volume is reduced by bringing the posterior margin of the field in front of the spinal cord. Involved nodes overlying and posterior to the spinal cord are boosted with electrons (Figs 23.17 and 23.18).

The lower neck is treated by a direct anterior field with midline shielding of the larynx and spinal cord.

Dose and energy

Primary tumour and palpable nodes

40 Gy in 20 daily fractions over 4 weeks (4–6 MV photons)

Reduced volume (lying in front of cord)

26 Gy in 13 fractions over 2.5 weeks (4–6 MV photons)

Electrons of suitable energy to the same dose to nodes overlying and posterior to the spinal cord.

Total dose: 66 Gy in 33 daily fractions over 6.5 weeks

Prophylactic nodal areas

50 Gy in 25 daily fractions over 5 weeks (4–6 MV photons or photons with electron boost)

The choice of electron energy for treating the nodes is based on the measurement of the depth of the spinal cord from the surface of the neck. A small ball bearing is placed on the shell at the thinnest part of the neck (Fig. 23.18). An anteroposterior radiograph is taken with a 5 cm brass circle to calculate the magnification factor. The distance between the ball bearing and the lateral margin of the cord (approximately 0.5 cm lateral to the midline) is measured and adjusted for magnification.

Boost to primary site

Some centres boost the primary site up a dose of 120–150 Gy with a limited lateral beam using high-energy photons, radiosurgery or intracavitary brachytherapy. This is not widely practised in the UK.

Radiation reaction. Dysphagia due to oropharyngeal mucositis is accompanied by loss of taste. The former usually settles within a few weeks of the end of treatment but the latter may persist for several months.

Complications. The most troublesome long-term symptom is usually dryness of the mouth due to the total inhibition of the secretion of both parotid glands. The risk of dental caries is increased and good dental care is essential.

Secretory otitis media from fibrosis of the eustachian tube is very common. Treatment is by the insertion of grommets.

Damage to spinal cord, brainstem or optic nerves is rare with careful planning. Some dose to the lens may be unavoidable, with resultant cataract. Biochemical evidence of hypopituitarism is not uncommon but clinical hypopituitarism is rare.

Lymphomas. These are managed on the lines laid down for mouth and tonsil (p. 361).

Adjuvant chemotherapy

While some non-randomised studies of adjuvant chemotherapy in squamous cell carcinoma of the nasopharynx have shown improved local control, these have not been confirmed in prospective randomised trials. Routine adjuvant chemotherapy cannot therefore be recommended.

Recurrent disease

In patients with recurrent disease after initial response to external beam, reirradiation with external beam ± brachytherapy boost to the primary site (40–50 Gy with external beam followed by 20 Gy by intracavitary brachytherapy can be considered.

Results of treatment

For squamous cell carcinoma, overall 5-year survival is about 60%. Local control at 5 years is 65–100% for T1 tumours, but drops to 5–40% for T4. 5-year survival following radical radiotherapy ranges from 30–80% and 10-year survival from 20–60%. The lower the anatomical level of nodal involvement in the neck, the worse is the prognosis. In patients with small recurrences after external beam irradiation, 5-year survival of 50% may be obtainable.

Non-Hodgkin lymphomas have a slightly better outlook.

PARANASAL SINUSES

Anatomy

The paranasal sinuses include the maxillary antrum, ethmoid, sphenoid and frontal sinuses.

The maxillary sinus (or antrum) lies in the cavity of the upper jaw (maxilla). It is related (Fig. 23.22) medially to the nasal cavity, inferiorly to the alveolus, superiorly to the orbit and ethmoid sinuses, laterally to the cheek and posteriorly to the pterygoid fossa. The maxillary antrum can be usefully divided into two parts. These are separated by an imaginary line (Ohngren's line) running from the medial canthus to the angle of the mandible. The upper part is known as the *suprastructure* and the lower as the *infrastructure*.

The ethmoid sinuses lie between medial walls of the orbits and upper nasal cavity and superiorly on each side of the cribriform plate below the frontal lobes of the brain.

The sphenoid sinuses lie in the body of the sphenoid bone beneath the pituitary fossa, one on each side of the midline. Each drains into the nasal cavity.

The frontal sinuses are related posteriorly to the frontal lobes. Inferiorly are the ethmoid sinuses, the roof of the nose and the orbits.

Epidemiology

Tumours of the nose and paranasal sinuses are uncommon. They account for 0.2% of all cancers and of cancer deaths. The maxillary antrum is the commonest site, followed by the ethmoids. Causative factors are obscure but exposure to wood dusts in the timber industry and furniture manufacture and leather dust in the shoe industry account for some tumours (adenocarcinoma), presumably due to a carcinogen. The maximum incidence is between the ages of 55 and 75. The male to female ratio is 1.7 : 1.

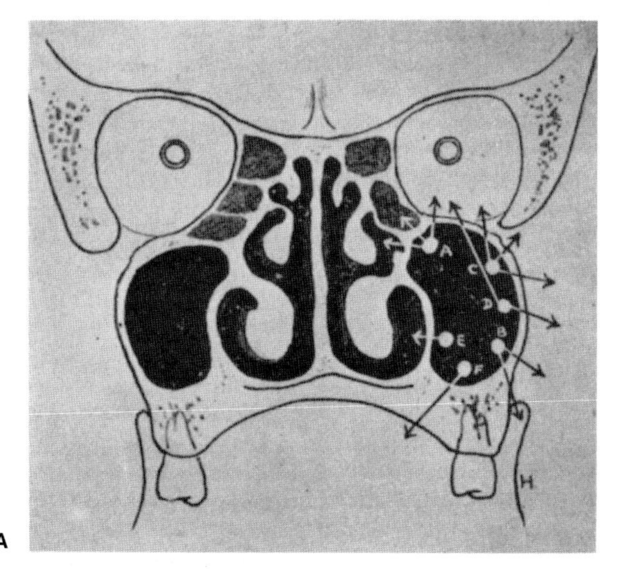

A

Fig. 23.22 **A** Coronal section through the orbit, nose and mouth. The arrows show various possible pathways of tumours arising in different parts of the maxillary antrum. (Reproduced with permission from Rock Carling, Windeyer & Smithers, British Practice in Radiotherapy, Butterworths, 1955.)

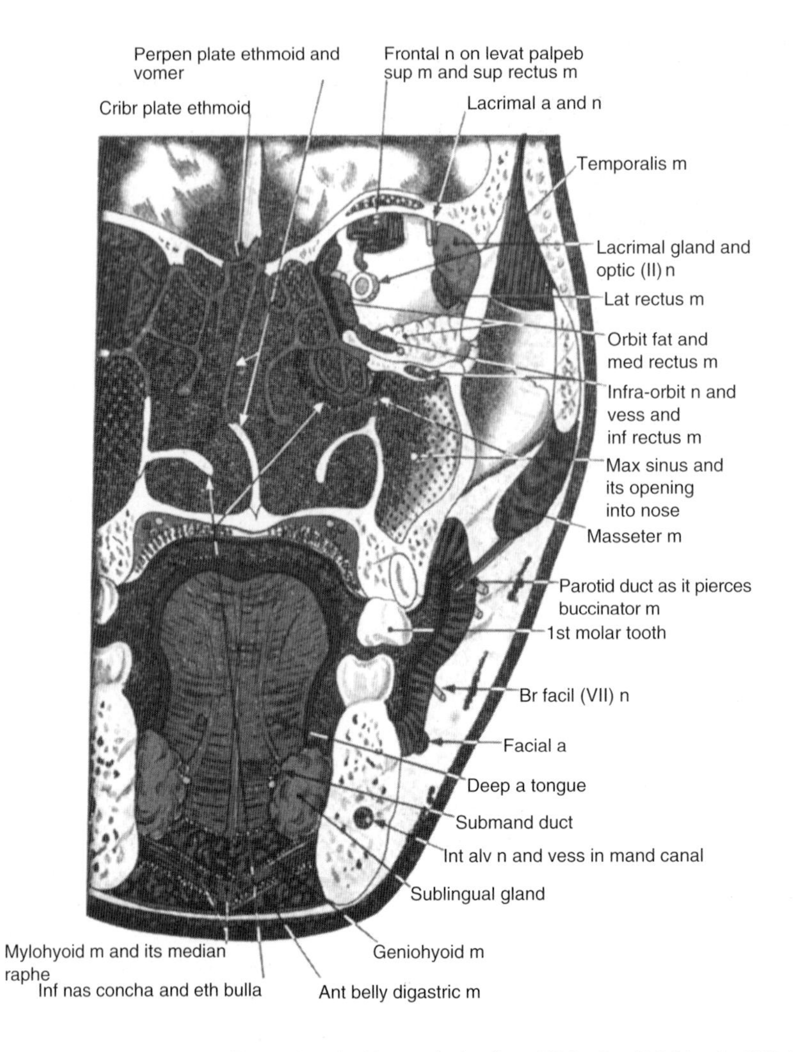

B Coronal section through orbit, nose and mouth. (Reproduced with permission from Walmsley R & Murphy T R 1972 Jamieson's Illustrations of Regional Anatomy, 9th edn, Churchill Livingstone.)

MAXILLARY ANTRUM

Pathology

Squamous carcinoma is the usual type. Adenocarcinoma, lymphoma and various sarcomas (e.g. osteosarcoma, fibrosarcoma) can occur.

Spread

The tumour usually begins in the lining of the membrane of the cavity and can therefore remain silent for a long time. Tumours in the antroethmoidal angle in the ethmoids (A in Fig. 23.22A) may spread to the nose and superficially into the subcutaneous tissues above or below the inner canthus. Tumours of the anterolateral wall (B in Fig. 23.22A), if lying inferiorly, cause swelling of the cheek with depression of the angle of the mouth. Tumours arising in the upper part of the anterolateral wall (C in Fig. 23.22A) may invade the zygoma and cause swelling below the outer canthus. The eye may be displaced upwards if the tumour invades the floor of the orbit. Tumours of the posterolateral wall may invade the orbit from behind, causing protrusion of the eye (proptosis), or the pterygoid region, presenting as a mass in the lower part of the temporal fossa. Tumours at the latter site often cause trismus. Spread to nodes in the neck is late.

Clinical features

Symptoms arise eventually from local spread—nasal blockage, discharge and bleeding, bulging of the

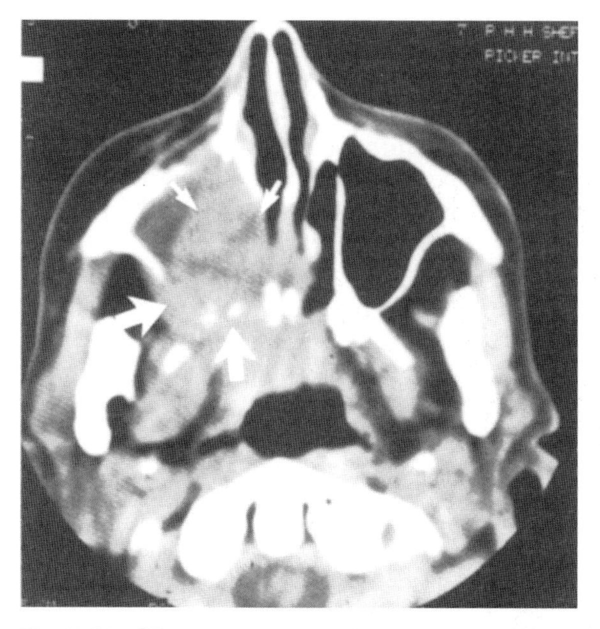

Fig. 23.23 CT scan showing a carcinoma of the maxillary antrum (small arrows) invading the pterygoid fossa (large arrows). (Courtesy of Dr R Nakielny, Sheffield.)

cheek, or ulceration in the mouth. If the orbit is invaded, the eye may be pushed upwards, causing double vision (diplopia), or forwards (proptosis). Palpable nodes are uncommon at presentation (<10%).

Oral pain may at first be thought to be arising from the teeth. Tumour presenting in the mouth may be mistaken for a primary tumour of the gum. It is essential to exclude a tumour originating in the antrum in any patient with malignant disease presenting in the hard palate or upper gums.

Investigation

Plain radiographs or tomograms may show destruction of the antral walls. CT scanning is the most accurate means of assessing local spread (Fig. 23.23) and determining operability.

Treatment

Both surgery and radiotherapy yield poor results since these tumours are usually advanced at presentation.

Surgical excision is suitable for small well-differentiated tumours and may be curative. However, it involves gross mutilation, with the removal of the upper jaw and any invaded structures. A dental prosthesis is necessary to compensate for the palatal defect. If the orbit is involved, removal of the orbital contents including the eye will be necessary. Postoperative radiotherapy is often given, based on the operative findings and histology. Residual disease or moderately or poorly differentiated histology favours the use of radiation.

Radical radiotherapy

Primary radiotherapy is appropriate for patients whose tumours are inoperable or who are unfit for or refuse surgery.

Before radiation begins, it is important to provide adequate drainage of the antral cavity because (1) it is always more or less infected from the start and (2) as radiation proceeds, fragments of growth and dead bone will become foci of further infection, leading to pent-up discharges, necrosis and pain during treatment. Surgical drainage is carried out, preferably by palatal antrostomy, i.e. removal of part of the hard palate and upper alveolus, thus permanently exposing the interior of the antrum. The surgeon removes any loose and decayed teeth, dead bone and necrotic debris and takes a biopsy. The opening has another advantage—the cavity can be inspected later for evidence of recurrence. The gap is closed by an individually made obturator worn like a denture, so the patient can eat and speak normally.

Target volume

The region is awkward for the therapist because of the irregular contours and the proximity of the eyes, both of which must be taken into account in the treatment plan. A full head mould with beam direction is desirable. This is an ideal site for CT planning.

1. If there is no suspicion of invasion of the orbits, the target volume encompasses the tumour, the whole of the maxillary antrum and potential pathways of spread. The lower margin includes the hard palate. The medial limit, the inner canthus of the opposite eye, extends across the midline to cover both ethmoid sinuses and the nasal cavity. The lateral margin is the gingivobuccal sulcus. Anteriorly the limit is the cheek and posteriorly the pterygoid fossa and the lateral pharyngeal node (Figs 23.24 and 23.25).
2. If the overlying skin of the cheek is involved by tumour, wax bolus is used to overcome the skin-sparing effect of megavoltage irradiation. The target volume is otherwise the same as above.
3. If invaded by tumour, the orbit must be included in the treatment volume.

Irradiation of the eye must be fully and carefully explained to the patient, so that he or she understands the vital necessity of irradiating the eye and the likelihood of deterioration of vision in later years.

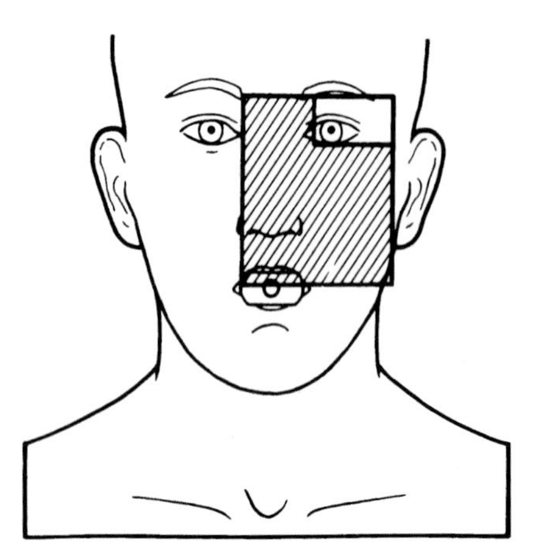

Fig. 23.24 Margins of the anterior field with lead shielding to the cornea, lens and lacrimal gland. (Reproduced with permission of Arnold from Jane Dobbs, Ann Barrett, Daniel Ash, *Practical Radiotherapy Planning*, 3/e, Arnold, 1999.)

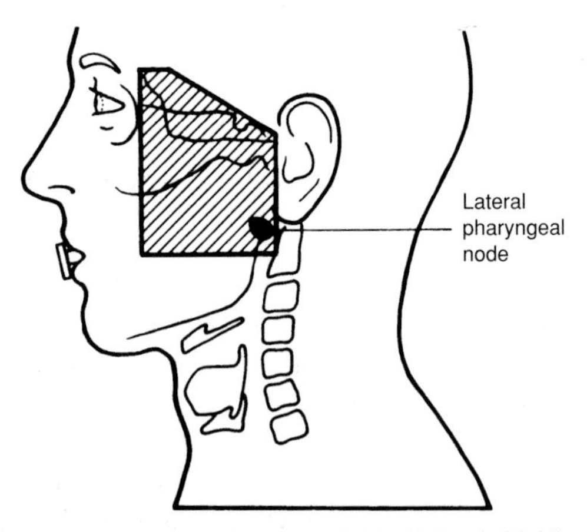

Fig. 23.25 Margins of the lateral field with lead shielding to the optic chiasm and hypothalamus. (Reproduced with permission of Arnold from Jane Dobbs, Ann Barrett, Daniel Ash, *Practical Radiotherapy Planning*, 3/e, Arnold, 1999.)

The fields should extend to the roof of the orbit. The target volume is otherwise as above. No effort is made to spare the eye on the involved side, but every effort is made to avoid the other eye.

Technique
A full head mould with mouth bite is needed. A right-angled wedge pair is the commonest technique. The lateral field is angled about 5–10° posteriorly to avoid the contralateral lens. A third postero-oblique field may be needed from the contralateral side to compensate for the fall-off in dose at the posteromedial part of the target volume (Fig. 23.26).

The brain and optic chiasm are shielded. Whenever the orbit has to be included, the patient should be instructed to keep the eyes open during radiation exposure and look up into the X-ray beam, thus making use of the surface-sparing effect of megavoltages irradiation. If wax bolus is used, cylindrical peep-holes 1.5 cm in diameter should be cut out for this purpose. This minimises damage to the cornea.

Dose and energy
60 Gy in 25 daily fractions over 5 weeks (4–6 MV photons)

The dose to the optic chiasm should be measured and should not exceed 40 Gy.

Palliative radiotherapy

For advanced cases the technique is simpler and it is often adequate to apply a single direct anterior field.
An applied dose of 45 Gy in 15 daily fractions over 3 weeks (4–6 MV photons)

Radiation reactions. Skin and mucosal reactions develop in the usual way and are managed on similar lines.

Irradiation of the eye leads to conjunctivitis, beginning in the latter part of the course. Antibacterial eyedrops (Chloromycetin) should be instilled daily to counteract infection which might damage the cornea.

Late effects on the eye are described in Chapter 30. If full dosage has been given, degenerative changes in the lens (cataract) and retina are virtually certain, commonly about 3 or 4 years later. Vision will be impaired and may be lost entirely. Sometimes a chronically painful eye has to be enucleated. If the eye has been irradiated, follow-up by an ophthalmologist is recommended.

Neck nodes

The management of neck nodes by radiotherapy is summarised in Table 23.2. Unless involved, the cervical nodes need not be treated. If they are palpable, a radical neck dissection may be preferable to irradiation since their inclusion may make the target volume too large for a radical dose.

Results of treatment

The 5-year local control for tumours of the infrastructure is better than for the suprastructure (65% versus less than 50%). For more advanced disease it is about 30%. Failure is usually due to persistent or recurrent disease at the primary site.

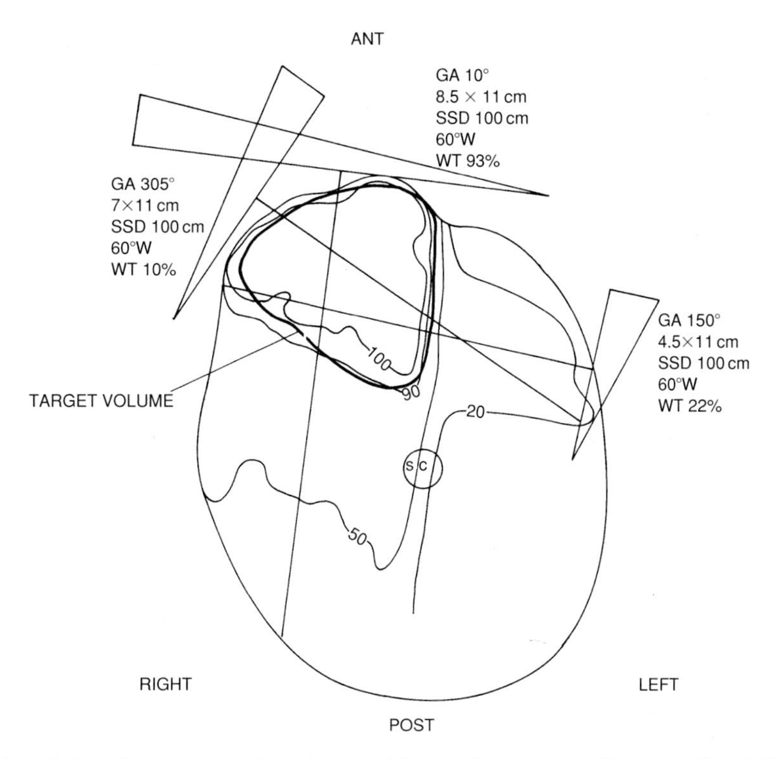

Fig. 23.26 Three-field technique for treatment of carcinoma of the maxillary antrum. (Courtesy of Dr A Champion, Sheffield.)

CANCER OF THE ETHMOID SINUS

Since the ethmoid sinuses lie between the orbits, they are liable to be secondarily involved by tumours of the maxillary antrum and nasal cavity. It is often difficult to say exactly where a growth originated.

Clinical features

It may present at the side of the bridge of the nose, or more often with nasal blockage. The orbit is very liable to invasion and the eye may be pushed laterally.

Investigation and staging

The diagnosis is confirmed by biopsy. A CT scan is essential to assess the extent of bone destruction, especially posteriorly.

Treatment

Surgical treatment is hardly every practicable. Radiation is the usual method and the general principles are similar to those for carcinoma of the maxillary antrum.

Radical radiotherapy

Target volume

The target volume includes the ethmoid sinuses, the maxillary antrum and the nose, but avoiding the eye.

Technique

Figure 23.27 shows a technique for an early tumour, using a heavily weighted anterior field, with supplementary dosage (approximately 10% of the total) from two wedged lateral fields directed behind the lens of each eye, to boost the dosage in the posterior part of the sinus. The front border of the lateral fields lies behind the orbit to avoid the eye. The dose to the optic chiasm must not exceed 40 Gy.

Results of treatment

The 5-year survival for carcinoma of the ethmoid sinus is about 30%.

CANCER OF THE NOSE AND NASAL SINUSES

Tumours of the nose and nasal cavity are rare. Squamous cell carcinoma is the commonest histological

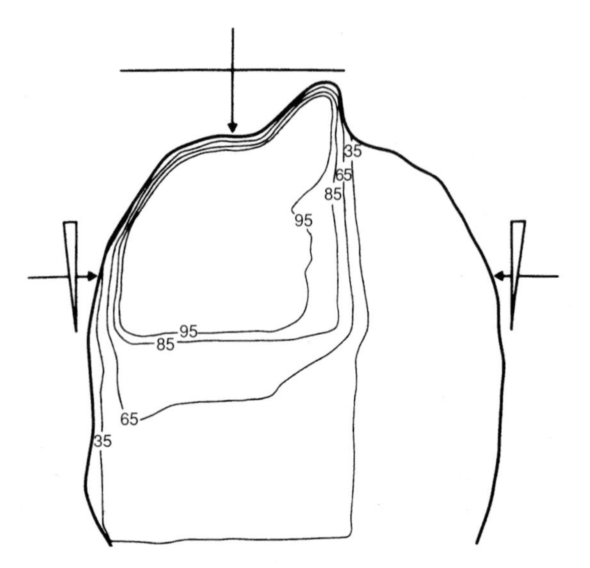

Fig. 23.27 Carcinoma of ethmoid and antrum—three-field technique. (Reproduced with permission from Easson & Pointon, The Radiotherapy of Malignant Disease, 1st edn, Springer-Verlag, 1985.)

type (though its nomenclature has been confusing over the years, and it is often called transitional cell carcinoma). The aetiology of most tumours at these sites is unknown. However, workers in the furniture and timber industries (wood dust) and the leather footwear industry are at increased risk of adenocarcinoma. Adenoid cystic carcinoma, malignant melanoma and olfactory neuroblastoma are rare.

Clinical features

Symptoms are of nasal bleeding, discharge or obstruction. Tumours may be visible on inspection of the nasal cavity. Lymph node involvement is uncommon.

Diagnosis and staging

An examination under anaesthesia of the nasal cavity and a biopsy are required. A CT scan is essential to determine the posterior extent.

Treatment

Radical radiotherapy is the treatment of choice.

Radical radiotherapy

Target volume and technique

For anterior lesions of the nasal cavity a direct anterior field may suffice (Fig. 23.28) to cover the nose. For more posterior lesions an anterior oblique wedged pair is recommended (Fig. 23.29). The eyes should be shielded with lead. The optic chiasm must not be overdosed.

Dose and energy

60 Gy in 25 daily fractions over 5 weeks (4–6 MV photons or 12–16 MeV electrons)

Results of treatment

Overall 5-year local control is 70%.

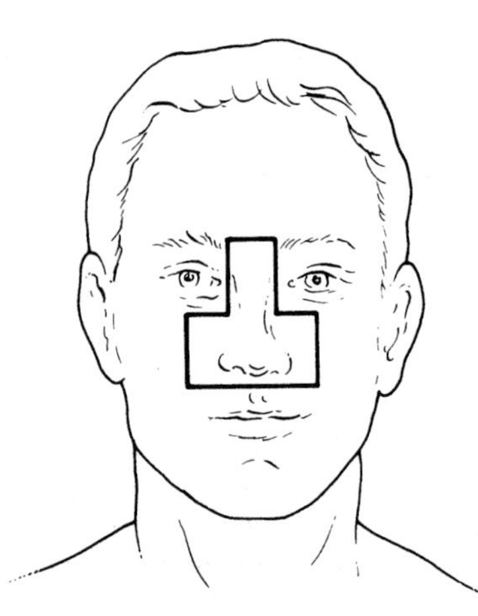

Fig. 23.28 Carcinoma of the nasal cavity—single anterior field. (Redrawn from Easson & Pointon, The Radiotherapy of Malignant Disease, 1st edn, Springer-Verlag, 1985.)

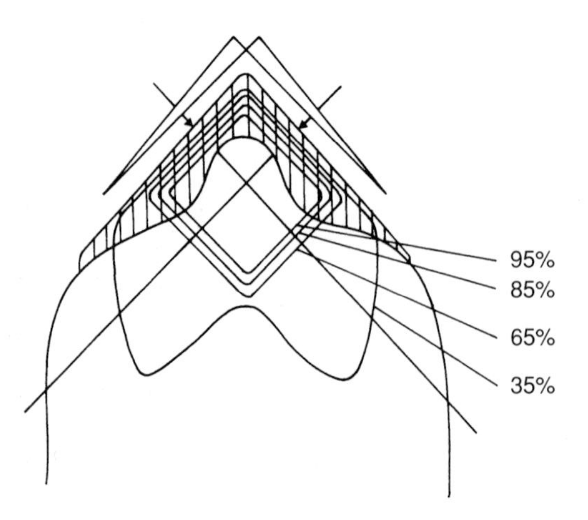

Fig. 23.29 Carcinoma of nasal cavity—wedge pair (5 × 5 cm). (Redrawn from Easson & Pointon, The Radiotherapy of Malignant Disease, 1st edn, Springer-Verlag, 1985.)

THE EAR

CANCER OF THE EXTERNAL AND MIDDLE EAR

Anatomy

The three parts of the ear are the external ear, the middle ear and the inner ear (Fig. 23.30).

The *external ear* consists of the pinna or auricle, the external auditory meatus and the tympanic membrane. The external auditory meatus is the passage leading from the tympanic membrane to the exterior.

It is important to distinguish tumours arising from the anterolateral and posteromedial parts of the ear, particularly if electron beam therapy is not available. In the anteromedial part of the ear the skin is closely adherent to the underlying cartilage. Radionecrosis is likely if superficial or orthovoltage irradiation is employed, owing to the higher absorption in cartilage (see below). In the posteromedial part, the blood supply is richer because of a thin layer of subcutaneous tissue between skin and cartilage. The risk of radionecrosis is less.

The *middle ear* is a narrow cavity in the petrous part of the temporal bone. It contains the auditory ossicles.

The lateral wall of the middle ear is the tympanic membrane. The medial wall separates it from the inner ear. Anteriorly it is connected to the pharynx by the eustachian tube. Posteriorly it communicates with the tympanic antrum and the mastoid air cells. Behind the tympanic antrum lie the sigmoid sinus and cerebellum. Inferiorly lies the jugular vein and superiorly the middle cranial fossa and the temporal lobe of the brain.

The *inner ear* is contained in the petrous part of the temporal bone. It contains the cochlea, the organ of hearing.

The lymphatic drainage of external ear is to the parotid and preauricular nodes anteriorly and to the postauricular and external jugular nodes posteriorly.

CANCER OF THE PINNA

The majority of tumours of the pinna arise from the skin. Basal cell carcinomas are more common than squamous cell carcinomas.

Treatment

These tumours may be treated by both surgery and radiotherapy. Before the advent of electron beam therapy, tumours of the anterolateral part of the ear were treated by excision. This was because of the risk of cartilage radionecrosis resulting from the attenuation of superficial or orthovoltage X-rays in tissues of high atomic number, owing to the photoelectric process (p. 46). With electrons, as with other forms of megavoltage irradiation of high photon energy, attenuation is largely by pair production (p. 46). Absorption in cartilage and bone is therefore much lower than with lower photon energies.

The majority of tumours of the pinna can be treated satisfactorily with electron beam therapy. The energy chosen is suited to the thickness of the lesion. Surgery is recommended for tumours of the external auditory meatus and retroauricular sulcus if they have invaded cartilage or bone.

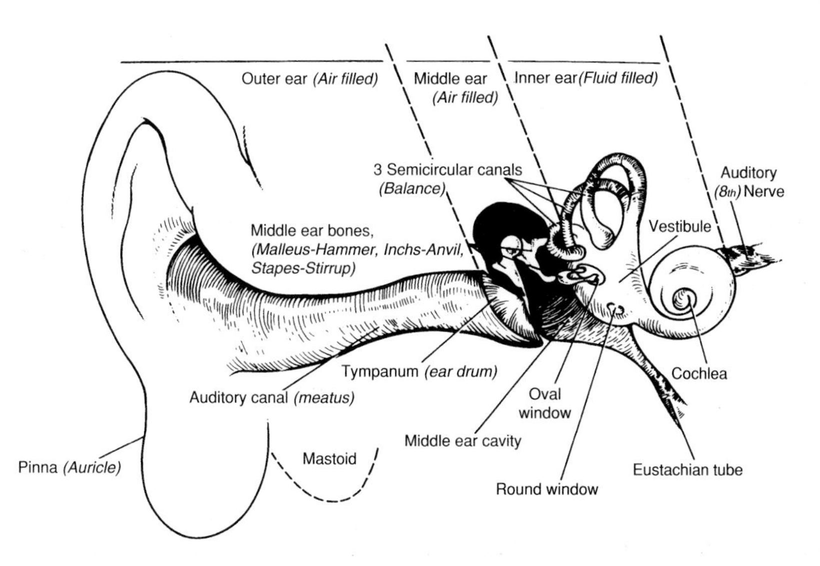

Fig. 23.30 General view of the ear. (Courtesy of Mr P Elliott, Sheffield.)

Radical radiotherapy

Target volume

This should include the tumour with a 0.5 cm margin for basal cell carcinomas and a 1 cm margin for squamous cell carcinomas.

Technique

The ideal treatment is with a direct single field using electrons because of their sharp fall-off in dose at depth and limited absorption in cartilage or bone. In general 6–10 MeV electrons are adequate, depending on the thickness of the lesion. The patient is treated supine with the head turned away from the affected side. A margin of 1 cm of normal tissue around the tumour is included. An impression is taken for a lead cut-out. To compensate for the air gap the ear is filled with wet bolus or a wax cast to the level of the top of the ear. If electrons rather than superficial or orthovoltage are used, the surface of the treated area is bolused to an appropriate thickness to overcome the skin-sparing effect and bring the maximum dose to the surface.

For tumours of the posterior part of the pinna, the skin of the mastoid region can be shielded from the exit dose with a small wedge of wax to absorb the electrons.

Dose and energy

Tumours <3 cm

50 Gy in 10 daily fractions over 2 weeks (6–10 MeV electrons)

Tumours >3 cm

55 Gy in 15 fractions over 3 weeks (6–10 MeV electrons)

Reaction and complications. The skin reaction and its management are as for other sites (see p. 330). However, perichondritis may occur, especially if the cartilage is invaded. The clinical features of perichondritis are pain and exquisite local tenderness, often with evidence of local infection. It is important to start antibiotic therapy early to prevent radionecrosis.

Results of treatment

The results of treatment are excellent, with an overall cure rate of 90%.

CANCER OF THE EXTERNAL AUDITORY CANAL AND MIDDLE EAR

Pathology

These tumours are rare. They occur mainly in middle age. Squamous carcinoma is the usual type. Other tumours include adenoid cystic carcinoma and sarcomas. There is an association with chronic ear infection (otitis media) and a discharging ear in most cases. Because of this, malignant change is insidious and apt to be overlooked.

Spread

Tumours of the cartilaginous part of the canal tend to be expansive while those of the bony part are confined by the bony walls. Spread to the auricle and middle ear is common.

With tumours of the middle ear, local spread with accompanying sepsis occurs early. It may be backward into the mastoid bone, forward towards the nasopharynx, outward to the external auditory meatus, upward to the cranial cavity, downward to the jugular region, inward to the inner ear and petrous part of the temporal bone. The facial nerve is often invaded, causing facial palsy (weakness or paralysis of the muscles of the face). The temporomandibular joint and parotid gland may also be invaded.

Clinical features

The clinical picture is usually of infection, with eventual blood-stained discharge. Examination may show granulation tissue and polypoid fragments. Pain is absent at the start. Later there will be facial palsy and deafness.

Diagnosis and investigation

The ear, parotid and mastoid regions must be examined and the neck palpated for nodes. The integrity of the cranial nerves (especially the seventh) is checked. The nasopharynx should be inspected to exclude anteromedial spread. When suspicion is aroused, examination under anaesthesia is necessary to obtain a biopsy. Most tumours are advanced at the time of diagnosis. Skull X-ray, tomograms, CT (Fig. 23.31) and MRI scanning may help in assessing the degree of bony (base of skull and petrous temporal bone) and soft tissue (mastoid and parotid) spread.

Treatment

The results of both surgery and radiotherapy are equally poor for cancer of the middle ear. Mastoidectomy is appropriate for early tumours. For more advanced tumours (1) biopsy followed by radical radiotherapy or (2) radical surgery followed by postoperative radiotherapy is recommended.

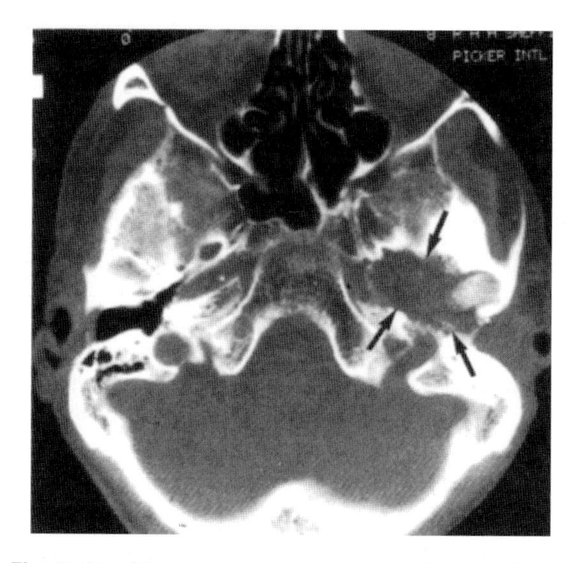

Fig. 23.31 CT scan showing a carcinoma of the middle ear eroding the petrous temporal bone. (Courtesy of Dr R Nakielny, Sheffield.)

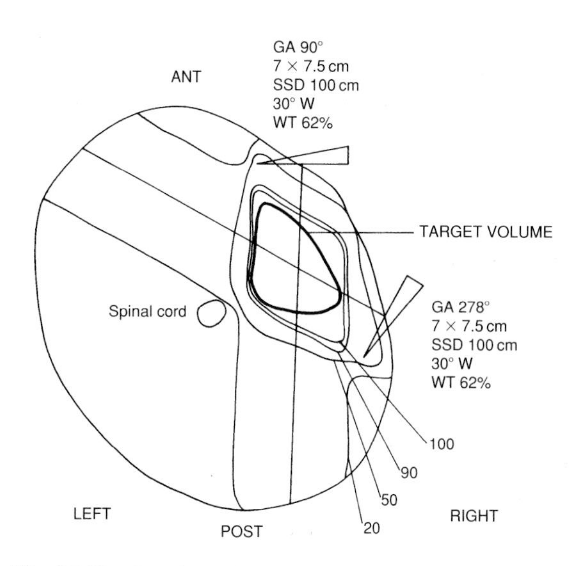

Fig. 23.33 Anterior and posterior wedged pair of fields for carcinoma of the middle ear.

Radical radiotherapy

Target volume

This includes the primary tumour, the mastoid process and the pre- and postauricular nodes (Fig. 23.32). The pre- and postauricular nodes define the anterior and posterior limits respectively. The superior margin lies below the eye. The inferior margin is the tip of the mastoid bone. The wedge-shaped volume with its apex towards the brainstem is illustrated in Figure 23.33.

Technique

A head shell is needed, with the patient lying supine with the head rotated 90′ away from the treated side so that the treated ear faces upwards. The head is extended to avoid irradiation of the eye from the exit beam of the posterior field. Anteroposterior and lateral radiographs are taken and the target volume marked. Anterior and posterior oblique fields are used. Care is taken to ensure the posterior beam exits below the eyes. CT reconstruction of the oblique plane is helpful in confirming this (Plates 2.4 and 2.5). An outline is taken through the centre of the volume, on which the target volume brainstem and lens are drawn. The treated fields can be cut out from the shell if there is no superficial involvement of the ear.

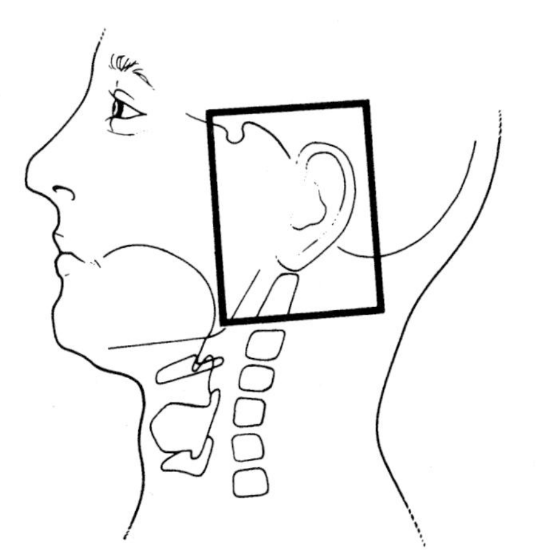

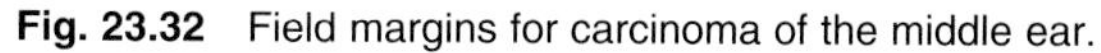

Fig. 23.32 Field margins for carcinoma of the middle ear.

Dose and energy

Primary or postoperative radical radiotherapy:

60 Gy in 25 daily fractions over 5 weeks (4–6 MV photons)

Care should be taken to limit the dose to the brainstem to 40 Gy.

Reaction. The acute reaction is usually not troublesome but hearing may be impaired because of secretory otitis media.

Results of treatment

The outcome of treatment is poor. Radical surgery with postoperative radiotherapy has a better 5-year survival (40%) than primary radiotherapy (15–20%). Bony invasion confers a poor prognosis.

SALIVARY TUMOURS

Tumours of the salivary glands are uncommon and only represent 0.3% of cancers and 0.1% of all cancer deaths. The parotid gland is by far the commonest site (80%). Tumours mainly occur both in the major glands (parotid, submandibular and sublingual) and in the small mucous glands of the mouth and upper air passages, including the nasopharynx, trachea and bronchi.

Anatomy

The *parotid* gland lies in its own fascial compartment in the space between the mandible and the mastoid process. It has both superficial and deep lobes (Fig. 23.34). Its superficial lobe overlies both the masseter muscle anteriorly and the sternomastoid muscle posteriorly. Anteroinferiorly, it is separated from the submandibular gland by a thickening of the parotid fascia, the stylomandibular ligament. Its deep lobe, lying at the level of the transverse process of the second cervical vertebra, is related medially to the styloid process and its muscles, which separate it from the internal carotid artery, internal jugular vein, the lower four cranial nerves and the lateral pharyngeal wall. The superficial part is limited above by the zygomatic arch.

The main anatomical point to note is the relation of the parotid gland to the facial (seventh cranial) nerve, which traverses it. Malignant tumours, unlike benign ones, often cause a facial palsy. The facial nerve may also be damaged when a tumour is surgically removed.

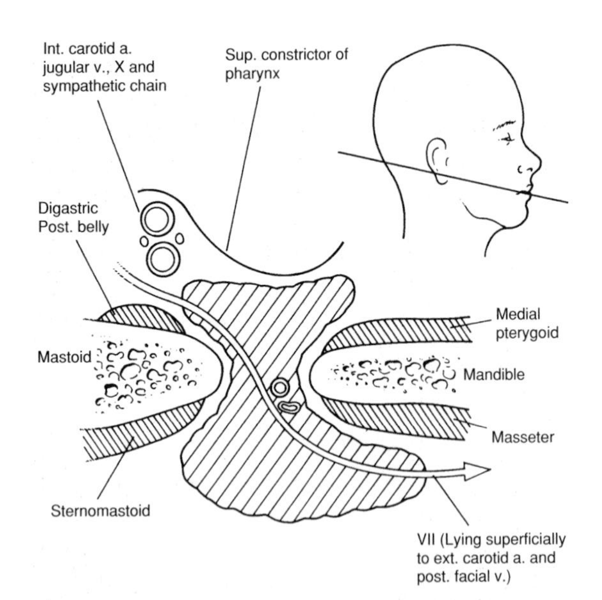

Fig. 23.34 Parotid and its surrounds in a schematic horizontal section—the facial nerve is the most superficial of the structures traversing the gland. (The line of section is shown in the inset head.) (Redrawn from Ellis, Clinical Anatomy, 5th edn, Blackwell Scientific, 1975.)

The parotid drains to the preauricular and deep parotid nodes and thence to the upper deep cervical nodes.

The *submandibular* gland also has superficial and deep lobes. It lies at the angle of the jaw. The superficial lobe is wedged between the mylohyoid muscle and the mandible. The deep lobe is adjacent to the mylohyoid, and posteriorly lies against the hyoglossus muscle. The gland is limited above by the mucous membrane of the tongue and below by the hyoid, to which it has a fascial attachment. The submandibular duct arises from the deep lobe and opens adjacent to the frenulum of the tongue.

The submandibular gland drains to the submandibular nodes and thence to the upper deep cervical nodes.

The *sublingual* gland (Fig. 23.22B) lies just below the mucosa of the floor of the mouth and in front of the submandibular gland. Medially it is related to the submandibular duct and the lingual nerve, which separate it from the base of the tongue.

The gland drains into the floor of the mouth through a number of ducts.

Pathology

About a quarter of parotid tumours and a half of submandibular tumours are malignant. The average age for benign tumours is 40 years and for malignant tumours 55 years. The clinical behaviour of some tumour types is very variable, even among tumours of similar microscopic appearance. Thus attempts at predicting behaviour are in practice of limited use. Table 23.3 shows the pathological classification of salivary tumours.

Benign tumours

The commonest benign tumour is the *pleomorphic salivary adenoma*. It is often called 'mixed parotid tumour'.

Table 23.3 Pathological classification of primary salivary tumours

Benign	Malignant
Pleomorphic adenoma	Pleomorphic adenocarcinoma
Monomorphic adenoma	Adenoid cystic carcinoma
Adenolymphoma	Mucoepidermoid carcinoma
	Adenocarcinoma
	Acinic cell carcinoma
	Non-Hodgkin lymphoma

Though of epithelial origin, it often contains material that stains like cartilage. To the naked eye, the tumour looks well encapsulated. Microscopically, however, there are outgrowths at the periphery of the tumour protruding into the surrounding tissue. Simple enucleation of the tumour is very likely to leave these peripheral remnants of tumour behind and give rise to local recurrence.

Adenolymphoma or *Warthin's tumour* is a rare tumour, almost exclusively occurring in the parotid gland. It probably arises from lymphoid elements. It is the parotid tumour most likely to be bilateral (5–10%).

Pleomorphic salivary adenoma

Clinical features. This tumour presents as a firm swelling, usually near the angle of the jaw. The facial nerve is almost always unaffected.

Treatment. The treatment of choice is a superficial parotidectomy with conservation of the facial nerve. Care should be taken to excise beyond the 'false capsule', otherwise remnants of tumour will be left behind and seed recurrence. If removal is complete, postoperative radiotherapy is not required. If the removal of the tumour is incomplete, postoperative irradiation is advised since there is otherwise a 30–40% risk of local recurrence and further surgery may result in damage to the facial nerve. If recurrence occurs after initial complete excision, further surgical excision should be attempted while preserving the facial nerve. If further excision is inadequate, then postoperative radiotherapy is given.

Technique and dosage are the same as for malignant tumours (see below).

Results of treatment. With adequate excision alone, less than 5% of pleomorphic salivary adenomas will recur. Incomplete excision followed by postoperative radiotherapy yields similar results. The success of further surgery for local recurrence depends upon the number of previous operations and the size and local extent of the recurrence.

Malignant tumours

Pleomorphic adenocarcinomas or *mixed malignant tumours* typically present with a history of a previously slow-growing painless parotid swelling which has suddenly increased in size and become painful. This is an example of malignant transformation within a benign tumour. Sometimes this occurs in a recurrence from previous inadequate excision of a pleomorphic adenoma.

Adenoid cystic carcinomas account for 15% of malignant salivary tumours. They arise in both the major and minor salivary glands (for example in the hard palate). They have a marked tendency to infiltrate along nerves. Primary *squamous cell carcinomas* and *anaplastic carcinomas* of the parotid gland do occur very occasionally and are highly malignant. However, the possibility that they may represent secondary spread from a primary tumour elsewhere in the head and neck should be considered. *Mucoepidermoid carcinomas* contain a spectrum of malignancies ranging from the histologically relatively low grade and benign in behaviour to the high grade and clinically aggressive. *Acinic cell carcinomas* are relatively slow growing. Both Hodgkin's and non-Hodgkin lymphoma may arise in the parotid gland. However, it is often difficult to be certain that the true origin is not in the adjacent parotid nodes.

Clinical features. Malignant tumours are more likely to present with pain and a facial palsy. Lymph node involvement is uncommon. Most malignant tumours do not metastasise to distant sites, with the exception of adenoid cystic carcinoma which may involve the lungs and liver. Lung metastases are often slow growing over many years without giving rise to symptoms.

Diagnosis and investigation. The parotid lump is examined for mobility and the integrity of the facial nerve is tested. The neck is palpated for lymph nodes. Staging investigations should include a chest X-ray and a CT scan (Fig. 23.35) to assess the local extent, particularly medially.

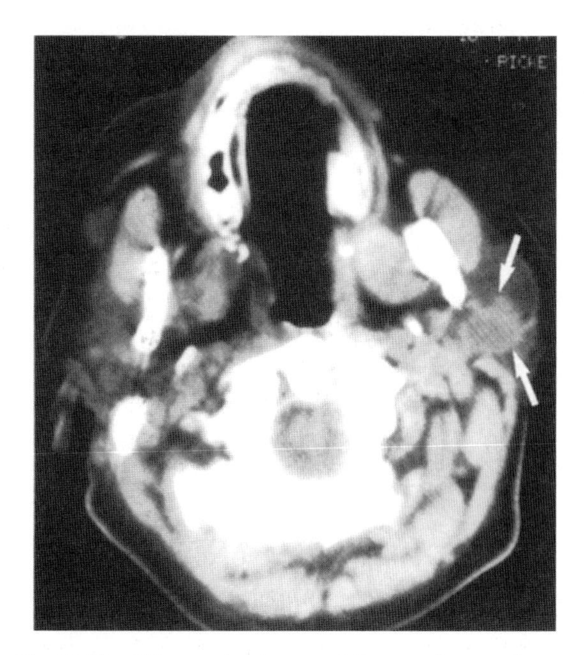

Fig. 23.35 CT scan showing parotid tumour (arrowed). (Courtesy of Dr R Nakielny, Sheffield.)

Treatment. Surgical biopsy and excision followed by radical postoperative radiotherapy is the treatment of choice for most malignant salivary tumours. However, low-grade carcinomas which have been adequately excised do not require further treatment. Lymphomas of the minor salivary glands in the nasopharynx are treated by radical radiotherapy, but surgery or surgery and postoperative radiotherapy are appropriate for minor salivary gland tumours in operable sites.

Indications for radical radiotherapy may be summarised as:

- Inadequate surgical excision
- High-grade malignancy
- Lymphomas,

Palliative radiotherapy is indicated to relieve pain and fungation from advanced disease in patients not fit for radical radiotherapy or in the presence of distant metastases.

PAROTID TUMOURS

Radical radiotherapy

Target volume

This should include the whole of the parotid bed. The upper limit should be the zygomatic arch. The lower border should lie below the inferior pole of the gland and incorporate the upper deep cervical nodes (Fig. 23.36). Anteriorly the field should extend to include the masseter muscle and posteriorly the mastoid process. The medial limit for malignant tumours should cover the whole of the parapharyngeal space. A less generous medial limit is required for pleomorphic adenoma. The lateral margin should cover all the palpable disease and the surgical scar. For squamous or anaplastic tumours, where the risk of lymphatic metastases is high, and in patients with palpable nodes, the ipsilateral neck node groups are treated in addition to the primary.

The target volume is triangular in shape with the apex towards the brainstem. It should allow at least a 1 cm margin of normal tissue around the tumour. This margin may have to be less generous medially to avoid excessive irradiation of the brainstem.

Technique

The choice of technique will depend upon whether the intention is radical or palliative. Uniform irradiation of the parotid region is difficult to achieve because of the changing contour of the neck. The proximity of critical structures such as the brainstem and the eye requires very careful planning and verification.

The best field arrangement is a wedged pair of anterior and posterior oblique fields (Fig. 23.37). A shell is required with the patient supine and the head extended and rotated 90° away from the affected side so that the parotid region faces upward. No mouth bite is necessary. It may be necessary to incline the plane downwards by 10–15° for the posterior beam to exit below the eyes, if the patient is unable to extend the neck adequately or if the target volume needs to include the base of the skull.

The scar and any palpable disease are marked with wire. Anteroposterior and lateral films are taken on the

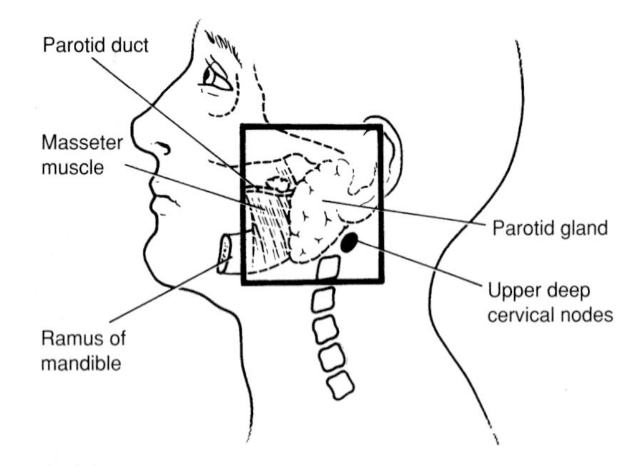

Fig. 23.36 Field margins for treatment of a parotid tumour, in relation to the underlying anatomy. (Reproduced with permission of Arnold from Jane Dobbs, Ann Barrett, Daniel Ash, *Practical Radiotherapy Planning*, 3/e, Arnold, 1999.)

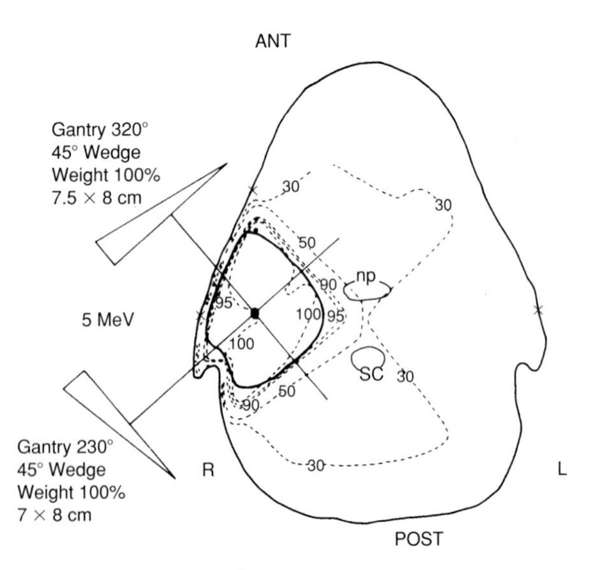

Fig. 23.37 Anterior and posterior oblique wedged fields for treatment of a parotid tumour. (Reproduced with permission of Arnold from Jane Dobbs, Ann Barrett, Daniel Ash, *Practical Radiotherapy Planning*, 3/e, Arnold, 1999.)

simulator. An outline is taken through the centre of the volume. CT planning, with reconstruction, if necessary, of CT images in the inclined plane (Plates 2.4 and 2.5), is helpful in ensuring adequate coverage of the tumour and avoidance of the brainstem and the eyes.

If the lower ipsilateral neck is treated, a direct electron field is used. The energy is chosen according to the depth of the tumour as assessed on CT scan. The target volume should be encompassed within the 90% isodose.

Bolus is applied to overcome the skin-sparing effect of electrons if there is superficial disease or scars.

Dose and energy

60 Gy in 25 daily fractions over 5 weeks at megavoltage (4–6 MV photons or high-energy electrons)

Acute reaction. Skin erythema and mucositis, xerostomia, alopecia and loss of taste occur during treatment. Oral hygiene and dental care are as for other head and neck sites.

Palliative radiotherapy

A simple direct field using orthovoltage, electrons or cobalt is adequate. Bolus is applied for electron or cobalt fields if there is skin infiltration.

Dose

30 Gy in 10 daily fractions or, in fitter patients, 45 Gy in 20 daily fractions

SUBMANDIBULAR TUMOURS

Radical radiotherapy

Target volume

This should include the whole of the submandibular gland and at least a 1 cm margin of normal tissue.

Technique

Small tumours not extending to the midline may be treated by anterior and lateral wedged fields. Larger tumours reaching the midline should be treated by a parallel-opposed pair of fields. Wedges may be required.

Dose is as for malignant parotid tumours.

Palliative radiotherapy

Technique, dose and energy are as for malignant parotid tumours.

Results of treatment of malignant salivary tumours

Prognosis is good for low-grade mucoepidermoid and acinic cell tumours (80–90% 5-year survival), intermediate for adenocarcinoma (50%) and adenoid cystic (60%) and poor for high-grade mucoepidermoid (20%) and squamous cell carcinoma.

CHAPTER CONTENTS

24

Larynx, lower pharynx, postcricoid, thyroid

Ian Kunkler

Anatomy

Lower pharynx

The lower pharynx (hypopharynx or laryngopharynx) extends from the tip of the epiglottis (just above the level of the hyoid bone) to the lower end of the cricoid cartilage, at the junction of the hypopharynx and oesophagus. The anatomy is complicated. Details are given in Figure 24.1.

The larynx

This is best considered as consisting of three sections:

1. The *glottis*—the gap framed by the vocal cords. These are joined at the front and at the back by tendons, the anterior and posterior commissures. Tumours of the anterior commissure have a worse prognosis since at the point of insertion of this tendon there is no perichondrium to act as a barrier to spread. Similarly, tumours of the posterior third of the vocal cords can spread through the posterior commissure into the pyriform fossa. Tumours of the glottis are illustrated in Figures 24.2–24.5.
2. Above the glottis, or *supraglottic*. This includes the epiglottis, the aryepiglottic folds, the arytenoids, the ventricular bands (false cords) and the ventricular cavities. Typical tumours are illustrated in Figures 24.6, 24.9 and 24.10.
3. Below the glottis, or *subglottic*.

It can be seen that the boundaries of the various compartments are not sharply demarcated, and it is often difficult to say where a growth really originated. Overall, 60–70% of laryngeal tumours arise from the vocal cords, 30% from the supraglottic region and less than 5% from the subglottic area. Figure 24.7 shows a typical subglottic tumour.

Lymphatic drainage

The true vocal cords do not have any lymphatic drainage. This explains the absence of nodal metastases in

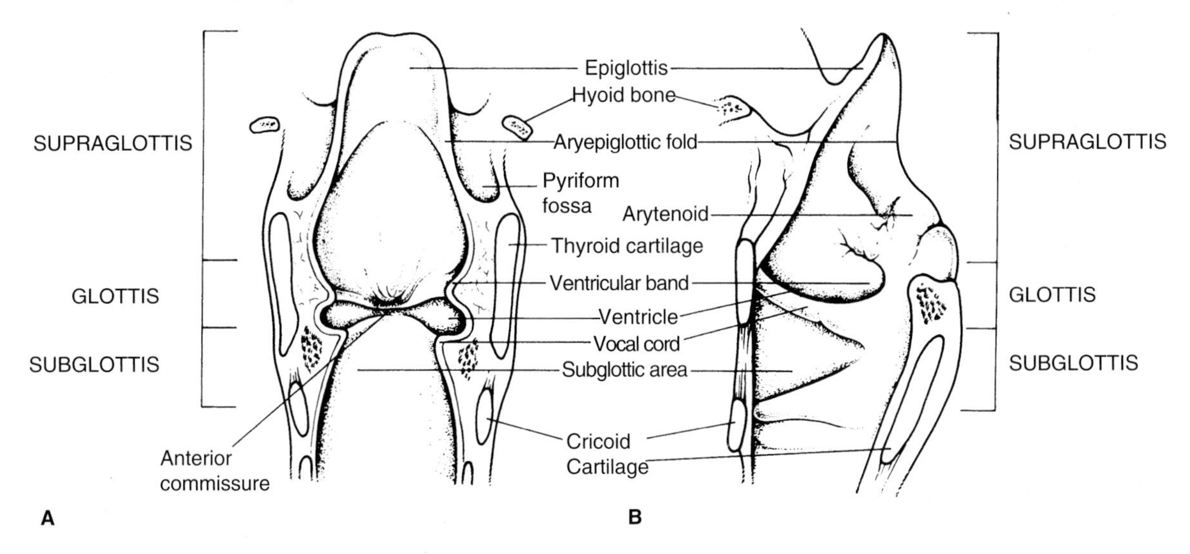

Fig. 24.1 Landmarks of the normal larynx and pharynx from **A** the posterior and **B** the lateral aspect. (Redrawn from Robinson, Surgery, Longmans.)

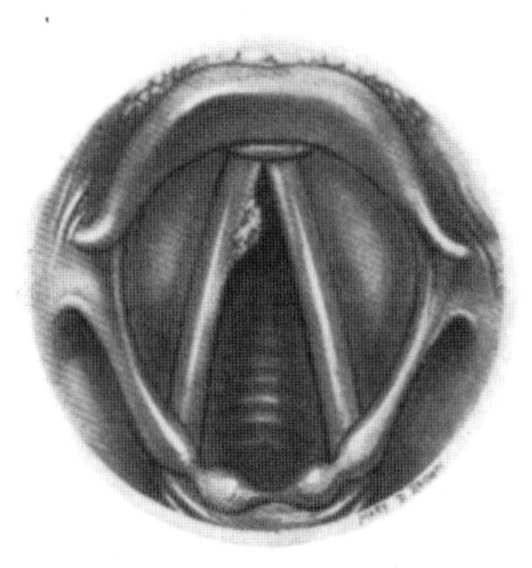

Fig. 24.2 Cordal lesion. Involvement of anterior third of vocal cord. Lymph node metastases rare. (Reproduced from Kunkler and Rains, Treatment of Cancer in Clinical Practice, Livingstone, 1959.)

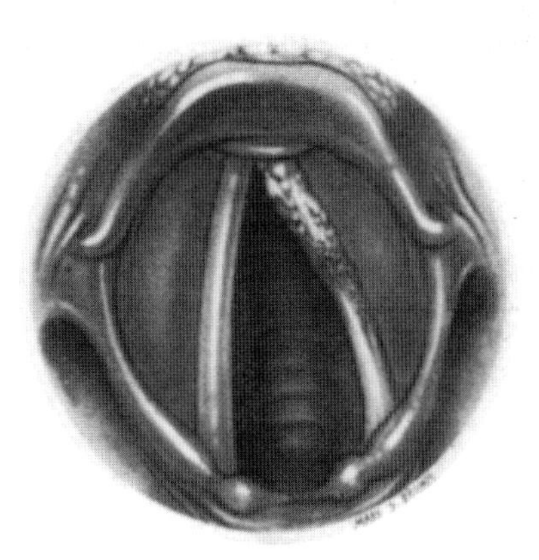

Fig. 24.3 Cordal lesion. Involvement of free edge and upper surface of anterior third of vocal cord. Spread to the anterior commissure. (Reproduced from Kunkler and Rains, Treatment of Cancer in Clinical Practice, Livingstone, 1959.)

tumours confined to cords (T1). For T2 and small T3 tumours arising from the vocal cords the incidence is 2–5%. Tumours of the anterior commissure and anterior subglottis may involve the pretracheal nodes in the midline.

The supraglottic region, by contrast, has a rich lymphatic supply, draining principally to the upper deep cervical nodes. Up to 40% of patients with supraglottic tumours have palpable nodes, and a higher proportion (70%) have microscopic nodal deposits at the time of surgery. The subglottic region drains to the pretracheal, lower cervical and mediastinal nodes. Nodal metastases in subglottic tumours occur late.

Pathology

Laryngeal cancer accounts for 0.9% of all cancers and 0.6% of cancer deaths. The yearly incidence is about 4 per 100 000 in the UK. In Northern Europe it constitutes 20% of tumours of the head and neck. The highest incidence is reported in Brazil and India. Most of these tumours occur in the fifth to seventh decades. The male : female sex ratio is 5 : 1. Smoking is an important aetiological factor. The mortality from laryngeal cancer in smokers is five times that of non-smokers. Some tumours may be related to human papilloma virus infection.

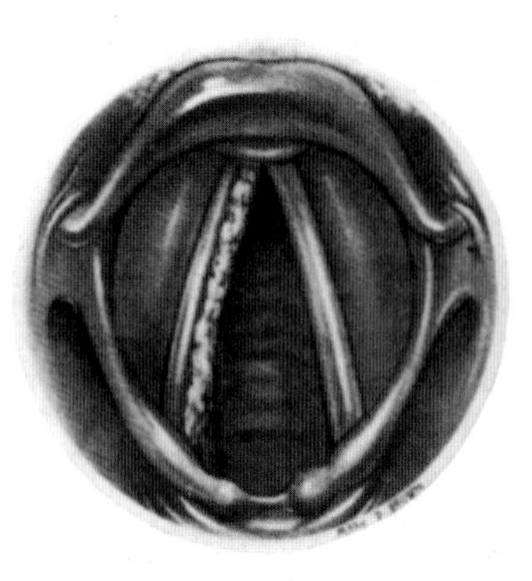

Fig. 24.4 Cordal lesion. Full length of edge of cord involved with slight impairment of mobility. (Reproduced from Kunkler and Rains, Treatment of Cancer in Clinical Practice, Livingstone, 1959.)

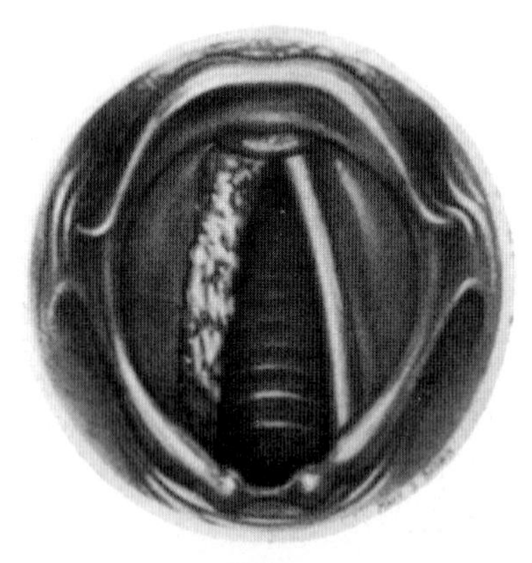

Fig. 24.5 Cordal lesion. Full length of edge and upper surface of cord involved by proliferating and infiltrating growth. Cord fixed. (Reproduced from Kunkler and Rains, Treatment of Cancer in Clinical Practice, Livingstone, 1959.)

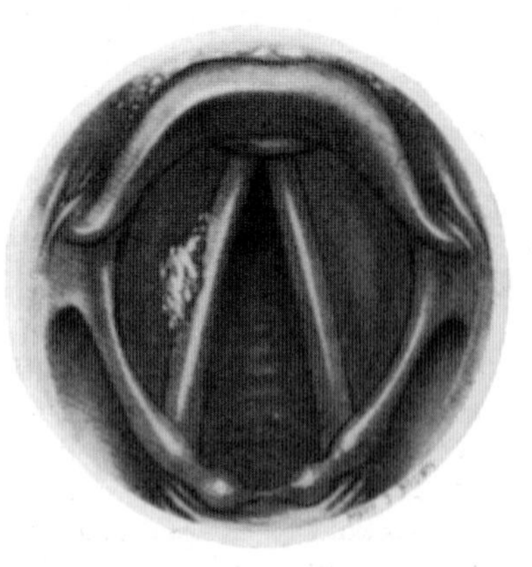

Fig. 24.6 Supraglottic carcinoma. (Reproduced from Kunkler and Rains, Treatment of Cancer in Clinical Practice, Livingstone, 1959.)

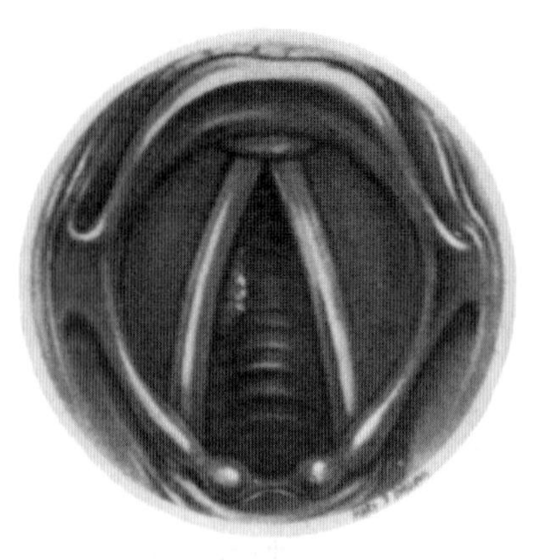

Fig. 24.7 Subglottic carcinoma. (Reproduced from Kunkler and Rains, Treatment of Cancer in Clinical Practice, Livingstone, 1959.)

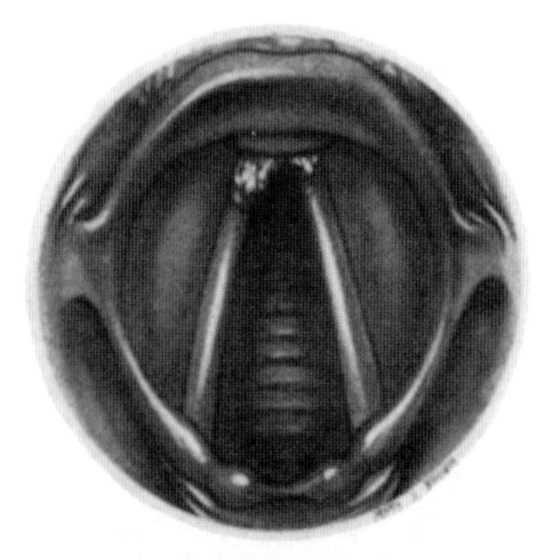

Fig. 24.8 Tumour of the vocal cords. Bilateral or commissural lesion. (Reproduced from Kunkler and Rains, Treatment of Cancer in Clinical Practice, Livingstone, 1959.)

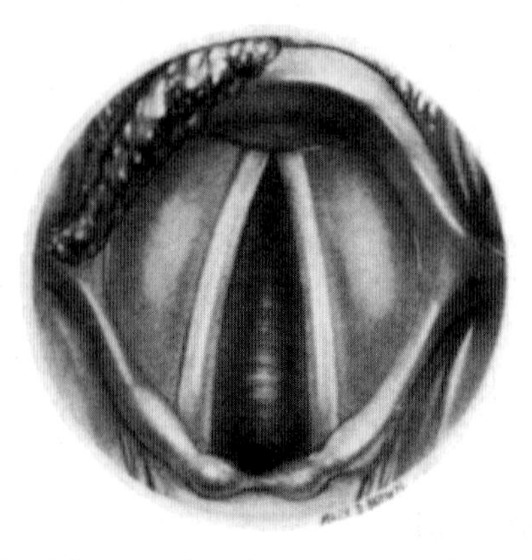

Fig. 24.9 Epilaryngeal carcinoma. Lesion of the epiglottis. (Reproduced from Kunkler and Rains, Treatment of Cancer in Clinical Practice, Livingstone, 1959.)

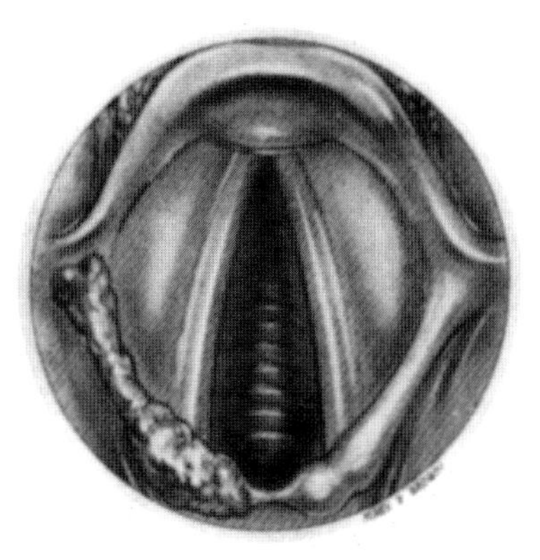

Fig. 24.10 Epilaryngeal carcinoma. Lesion of the aryepiglottic fold. (Reproduced from Kunkler and Rains, Treatment of Cancer in Clinical Practice, Livingstone, 1959.)

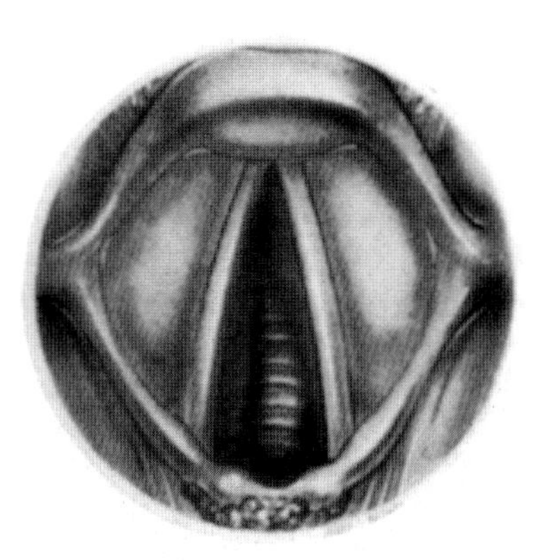

Fig. 24.11 Post-cricoid carcinoma. (Reproduced from Kunkler and Rains, Treatment of Cancer in Clinical Practice, Livingstone, 1959.)

95% of laryngeal tumours are invasive squamous carcinomas, usually well differentiated. Verrucous carcinoma is an uncommon variant of squamous carcinoma, which resembles a viral wart and consequently can be difficult to diagnose microscopically. Another variant is spindle cell carcinoma—a squamous tumour mimicking sarcoma; it usually presents as a rounded nodule. Similar tumours arise elsewhere, particularly in the upper aerodigestive tract. Other varieties of tumour are all rare.

Premalignant lesions may be seen—hyperkeratosis, dysplasia and carcinoma-in-situ. These may follow a prolonged course and be difficult to separate from carcinoma, with repeated biopsies and recurrences.

Local spread

On the vocal cord the lesion commonly begins near the centre and spreads along the cord, later involving the junction of the cords (anterior commissure—Figs 24.3 and 24.8) and then spreading across to the other cord. It is usually slow growing and confined to the cord for a long time. The cords move (apposition and separation) in normal respiration and phonation, and their mobility is maintained until infiltration of the intrinsic muscles of the larynx impairs it and causes some degree of fixation. Late local spread involves the supraglottic region and the laryngeal cartilages; subglottic invasion is less common.

Tumours of the epilarynx (epiglottis, arytenoid and aryepiglottic fold) spread locally to the opposite side, to the pre-epiglottic space and the thyroid cartilage. Supraglottic tumours have a rich lymphatic drainage, which also crosses the midline. 55% of patients with supraglottic tumours will present with palpable nodes of which 16% are bilateral. Subclinical nodal involvement is about 30%. Tumours of the ventricular bands (false cords) spread superiorly to the aryepiglottic folds and arytenoids and anteriorly to the anterior commissure. Tumours arising from the laryngeal ventricle spread to the supraglottis or the contralateral vocal cord and may be transglottic.

Subglottic tumours tend to spread circumferentially and invade the cricothyroid membrane. Posteriorly they may spread to the hypopharynx via the cricoid cartilage. About 10% of subglottic tumours have nodal involvement, mainly in the anterior midline (pretracheal or Delphian nodes) lying low in the neck.

Clinical features

Tumours of the vocal cords tend to present early, with a hoarse voice, since even tiny irregularities of their margins cause enough changes in the vibrating air column to produce hoarseness. Prompt attention to this favours early diagnosis. Advanced growths will narrow the airway 'chink' of the glottis and produce stridor, i.e. audible wheezing on inspiration. Neglect results in increasing dyspnoea, and impending suffocation may have to be relieved by an emergency operation (tracheostomy) whereby an opening is made in the trachea lower down in the neck, and a tube inserted through which the patient can breathe.

Growths in the rest of the larynx or pharynx tend to remain silent for many months. A mass may reach considerable size (3–4 cm) before causing really troublesome symptoms. Lesions in the pyriform fossa are particularly liable to long latency. There may be intermittent vague discomfort or sore throat at first, followed later by interference with speaking (hoarseness, dysphonia), swallowing (dysphagia) or breathing (dyspnoea), depending on the exact site of the growth and the extent of local invasion. By this time—or very often before—there may be secondary cervical nodes, and a lump in the neck is all too commonly the presenting complaint, leading to the discovery of the primary in the throat.

Diagnosis and staging

Preliminary clinical examination is by indirect endoscopy (laryngoscopy) using a long-handled mirror (Fig. 24.12). Except for very early cases, especially on the cords, it is not usually possible to see the whole of the tumour, but only the upper part, or the edge of an ulcer, or an abnormal bulge.

Further detail, to outline the full extent of the mass, is obtainable by radiography. Soft tissue lateral films of the neck are taken and, in addition, tomograms, which will reveal the cords, impairment of their movement and any masses distorting the normal air spaces. Tomograms are helpful in the assessment of local spread (Fig. 24.13), particularly subglottic extension. CT scanning may provide information on the exact size and site of the tumour, but is not usually necessary for planning radiotherapy.

In most cases it is desirable to carry out direct endoscopy, under general anaesthesia, to inspect the whole of the growth and to take a biopsy.

Tumours are staged using the UICC classification (Table 24.1).

Treatment

Preliminary attention is to the patient's general condition, nutrition, and correction of anaemia. Oral hygiene is important, and any dental sepsis should be dealt with at the start.

Glottic carcinoma

The choice of treatment is influenced by the stage of the tumour, likelihood of local control, general medical condition and treatment-related morbidity. As with other head and neck cancers, patients with advanced disease are often in poor general condition and this influences whether treatment is radical or palliative in intent.

The main treatments are surgery and radiotherapy. In general, the best treatment of T1 and T2 tumours is radical radiotherapy, since the cure rates are comparable with surgery (cordectomy or hemilaryngectomy) but there is normally restoration of a good quality voice. Laser therapy has been for very small tumours in the middle of the mobile cord but is reported to result in poorer quality of the voice than with radiotherapy. It is particularly important to avoid gaps in treatment since these may compromise local control.

There is less agreement about the treatment of T3 and T4 tumours. In general, radical radiotherapy is advised as initial treatment for T3 tumours since this will cure about 30% of such patients. Salvage laryngectomy will

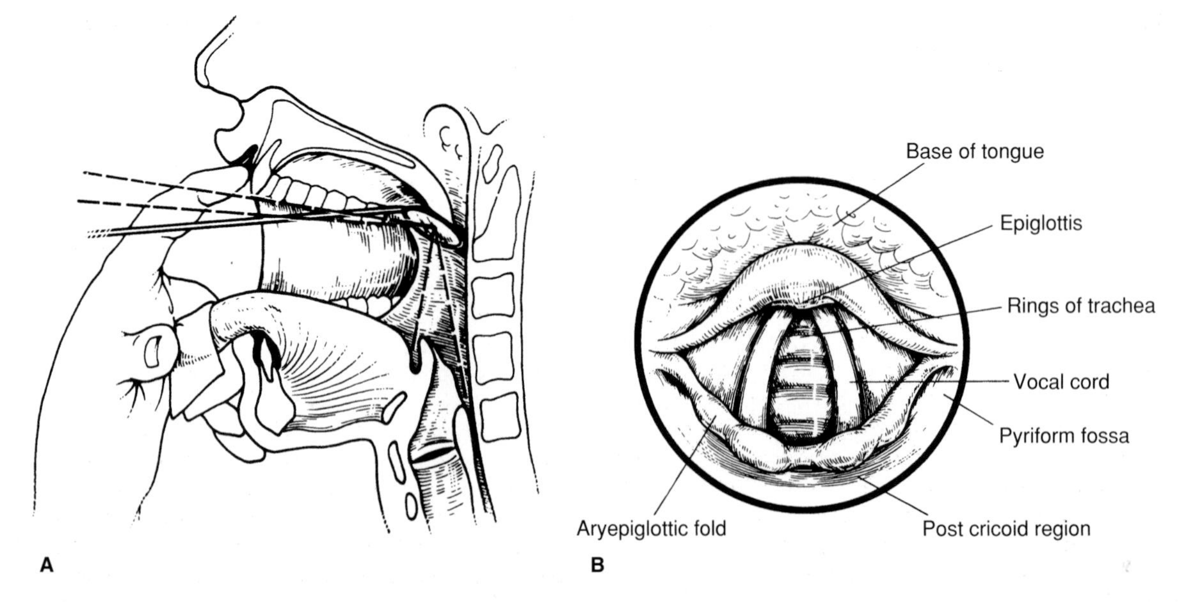

Fig. 24.12 **A** Indirect laryngoscopy and **B** the mirror view of the larynx.

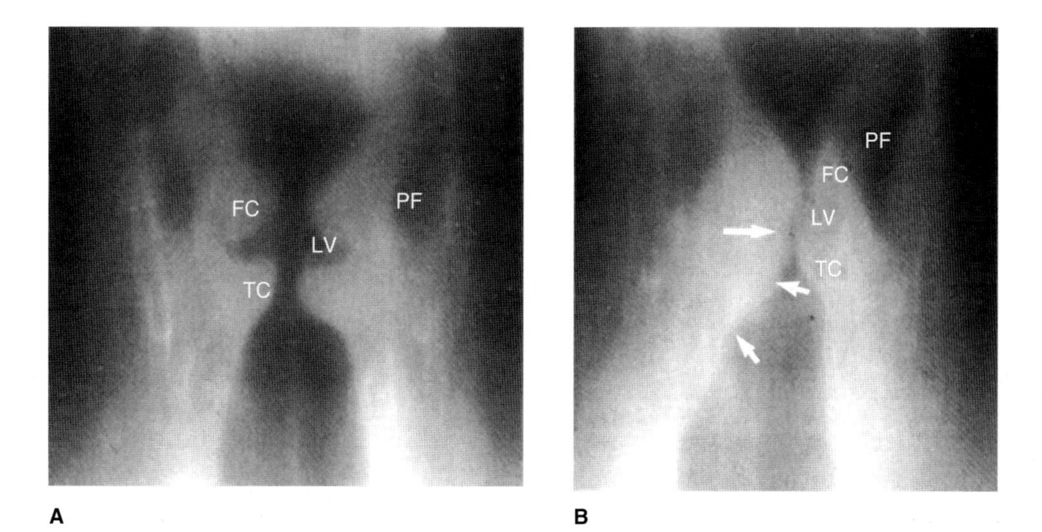

Fig. 24.13 Laryngeal tomograms: **A** normal appearance of vocal cords (TC), laryngeal ventricle (LV), false cords (FC), pyriform fossa (PF); **B** large mass involving the right vocal cord, false cord with obliteration of the ventricle (long arrow) and subglottic extension (short arrows).

Table 24.1 UICC staging of laryngeal cancer

Stage	Clinical findings
Supraglottis	
T1	Tumour confined to the region with normal mobility
T2	Tumour confined to the larynx with extension to adjacent site or sites or to the glottis without fixation
T3	Tumour confined to the larynx with fixation and/or other evidence of deep infiltration
T4	Tumour with direct extension beyond the larynx
Glottis	
T1	Tumour confined to the region with normal mobility
T2	Tumour confined to the larynx with extension to either the supraglottis or the subglottic regions with normal or impaired mobility
T3	Tumour confined to the larynx with fixation of one or both cords
T4	Tumour with direct extension beyond the larynx
Subglottis	
T1	Tumour confined to the region
T2	Tumour confined to the larynx with extension to one or both cords with normal or impaired mobility
T3	Tumour confined to the larynx with fixation of one or both cords
T4	Tumour with destruction of cartilage and/or with direct extension beyond the larynx

cure a further 30% of those with persistent tumour. Radical radiotherapy for failures of primary surgery is rarely successful. For T4 tumours where there is invasion of the cartilage, the risk of radiation-induced necrosis of the cartilage is high after a radical dose and local control rates are poor. Primary surgery is therefore advised for patients with T4 tumours who are in adequate general medical condition.

Secondary nodes of the neck appearing after radical radiotherapy are managed by radical neck dissection if possible.

Radical radiotherapy

Target volume

The target volume for T1 and T2 tumours should be centred on the vocal cords, which lie just below the laryngeal ventricle (Fig. 24.14) and 1 cm below the laryngeal promontory (Adam's apple). Field size should not be less than 20 cm^2 The volume should include the thyroid and cricoid cartilages. If there is supraglottic extension, the upper margin should extend up to cover the hyoid bone and the upper deep cervical nodes (as for supraglottic cancer, Fig. 24.17A).

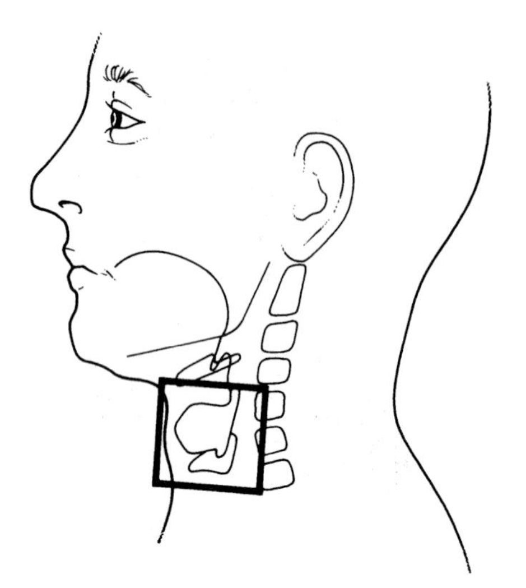

Fig. 24.14 Treatment volume for T1 and T2 glottic carcinoma. (Reproduced with permission of Arnold from Jane Dobbs, Ann Barrett, Daniel Ash, *Practical Radiotherapy Planning*, 3/e, Arnold, 1999.)

A generous margin should be allowed below any subglottic extension.

Technique
A head shell is needed with the mouth closed. A parallel-opposed pair of lateral wedged fields is recommended for most patients. Wax build-up is recommended for tumours involving the anterior commissure to ensure adequate dosage to this region (Fig. 24.15). If the patient has a short neck and lateral fields would pass through the shoulder, a wedged pair of anterior oblique fields as in Figure 24.16 is recommended. The dose to the spinal cord is, however, greater than with lateral-opposed wedged fields.

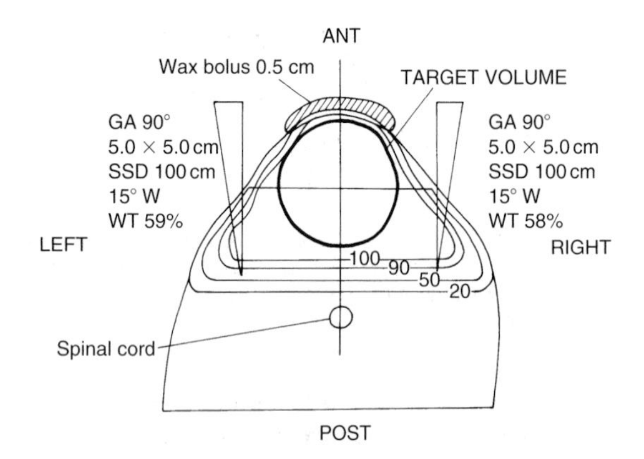

Fig. 24.15 T1 glottic tumour involving the anterior commissure. Isodose distribution for parallel-opposed lateral fields. Note wax build-up to ensure adequate dosage to the anterior commissure.

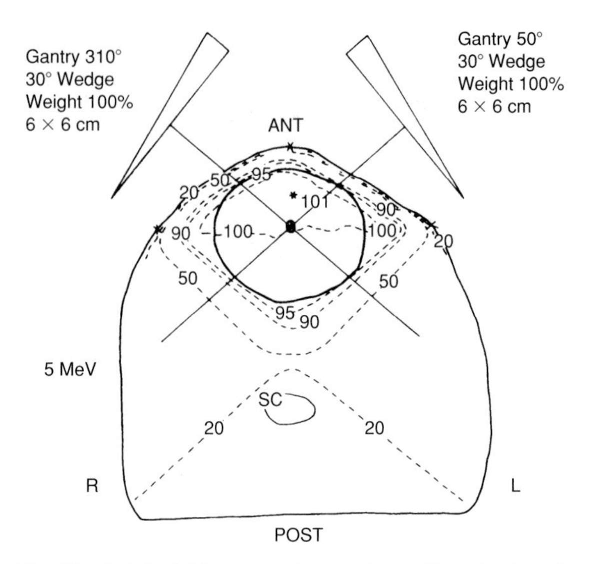

Fig. 24.16 T1 glottic tumour in a patient with a short neck. Isodose distribution for anterior oblique fields. (Reproduced with permission of Arnold from Jane Dobbs, Ann Barrett, Daniel Ash, *Practical Radiotherapy Planning*, 2/e, Arnold, 1992.)

Dose and energy
60 Gy in 25 daily fractions over 5 weeks (4–6 MV photons)

Supraglottic carcinoma

Radical radiotherapy is indicated for supraglottic carcinoma (T1–3) with or without nodes (N0, N1). Laryngopharyngectomy is reserved for recurrence or persistent disease or for T4 tumours.

Target volume
When there is early disease and there are no palpable nodes, the volume (Fig. 24.17) encompasses the primary tumour and the upper deep cervical nodes. The mouth is closed during treatment. The upper margin of the field extends above the hyoid bone and includes the tonsillar region. The posterior border should extend half way across the vertebral bodies.

If the primary tumour is advanced or there are palpable neck nodes, the cervical node chains should be covered on both sides (see Table 23.2).

Technique
A head shell is needed with the mouth closed. In the absence of nodes, a parallel-opposed pair of wedged fields is used. The floor of the mouth is shielded with lead. In the presence of nodes, the lower half of the neck is treated by an anterior 'split neck' field (Fig. 24.18). A lead strip should shield midline structures. The nodes are outlined by lead wire at the time of simulation.

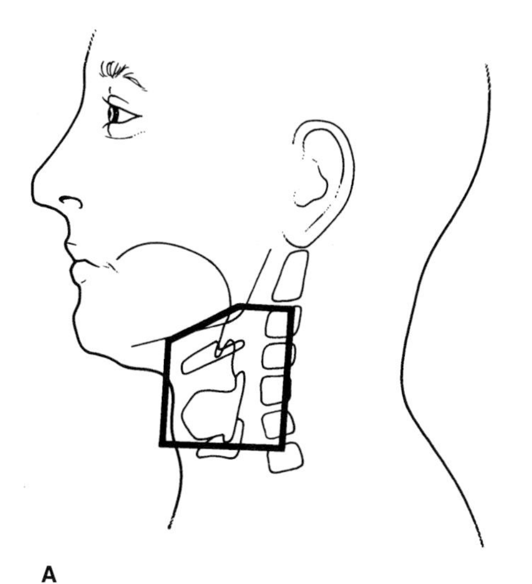

A

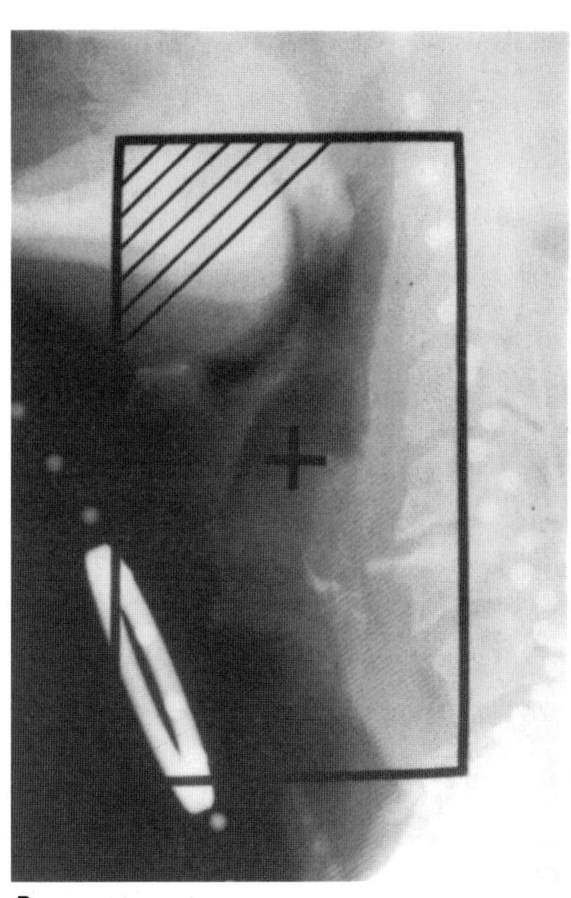

B

Fig. 24.17 Supraglottic carcinoma. **A** Treatment volume for supraglottic carcinoma. (Redrawn from Dobbs & Barrett, Practical Radiotherapy Planning, 1st edn, Edward Arnold, 1985.) **B** Typical lateral simulator film.

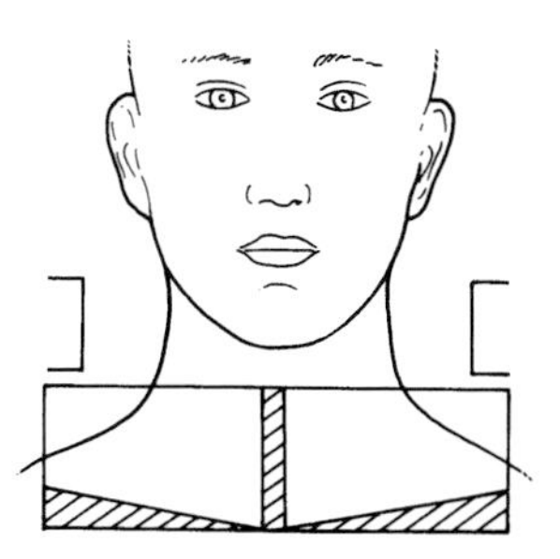

Fig. 24.18 Supraglottic carcinoma. Anterior field to treat lower neck and supraclavicular fossae. (Modified from Dobbs & Barrett, Practical Radiotherapy Planning, 1st edn, Edward Arnold, 1985.)

a.d
a.d
a.d
a.d
a.d
Central Pb

Fig. 24.19 Diagram showing the use of asymmetric diaphragms (a.d) to match adjacent fields at the centre of each beam where there is no divergence. (Courtesy of Dr I Manifold, Sheffield.)

The junction of the upper and lower neck fields should be matched using asymmetric diaphragms (Fig. 24.19). If these are unavailable, a small gap is left between the two fields to avoid overdosage due to overlap. If the nodes overlie the spinal cord, the posterior margin of the upper neck field is moved anterior to the cord after a dose of 40 Gy. The rest of the posterior part of the field is then treated with electrons of appropriate energy. The choice of energy of electrons is based on measurement of the distance between the thinnest part of the neck and the spinal cord (Fig. 23.18).

Dose and energy

T1–T2N0

Primary tumour and, prophylactically, the upper and midcervical nodes in front of the spinal cord

48 Gy in 20 daily fractions over 4 weeks (4–6 MV photons)

Reduced volume to primary and midcervical nodes

12 Gy in 5 daily fractions (4–6 MV photons)

Total dose: 60 Gy in 25 fractions over 5 weeks

More advanced

The volume encompasses the primary and all nodes, including those of the posterior triangle (see Table 23.2).

40 Gy in 20 daily fractions over 4 weeks (4–6 MV photons)

Reduced photon volume to the area in front of the spinal cord. Continue at dose rate of 2 Gy per fraction, 5 days a week, to give:

66 Gy in 33 fractions over 6.5 weeks to primary and palpable nodes

and

50 Gy in 25 fractions over 5 weeks to prophylactic areas

Electrons of suitable energy are used to treat nodal areas overlying and posterior to the spinal cord after 40 Gy, matched to adjacent photon fields.

Subglottic carcinoma

Target volume and technique

The primary tumour and first station draining lymph nodes are treated, using an 'angled down' wedged pair, possibly with wax blocks to compensate for curvature, or the 'twisted wedge' technique is used (Fig. 24.31). The volume is anterior to the spinal cord. Matching posterior electron fields or an inferior field treating the mediastinum anteriorly is difficult and often unsatisfactory. However, lesions at this site with nodal metastases carry a very poor prognosis.

Dose and energy

60 Gy in 25 daily fractions over 5 weeks (4–6 MV photons)

Radiation reactions

Acute. These are managed on the same lines as for the mouth (p. 356). Huskiness may persist for months before improving. Occasionally, especially with large tumours, there may be reactionary oedema very early on, even after the first or second dose, which can be dangerous if the airway is already narrowed. Acute obstruction may be precipitated, calling for emergency tracheostomy to prevent suffocation. If this possibility is anticipated, an elective tracheostomy may be advisable.

If tracheostomy has been carried out, the metal tube must be replaced by a plastic tube before the start of the radiation, otherwise the soft secondary X-rays from the metal will cause excessive reaction in the adjacent skin.

For weeks or months following radical radiotherapy there may be persistent oedema of the laryngeal region and patches of ulceration with infection. It is often difficult to distinguish this from persistent or recurrent growth, and even biopsies may not do so with certainty. Such cases may require laryngectomy to rescue the patient from an intolerable existence, even if there is no residual malignancy.

Late (late cartilage necrosis). Necrosis of laryngeal cartilages is a serious reaction, developing several months after radical radiotherapy. It is rarely seen after megavoltage, but occurred in the orthovoltage era because 200 kV radiation deposits much more energy in calcified cartilage, owing to attenuation by the photoelectric process (p. 442). It is characterised by pain and local tenderness. Infection is likely to follow, with dyspnoea and dysphagia. Tracheostomy may be necessary, or even laryngectomy. The danger of necrosis is a good reason for preferring surgery in cases where cartilage is already invaded by tumour.

Results of treatment

5-year local control is 85–100% for T1 and 75–100% for T2 with 5-year survival of 80–98% for T1 and 60–90% for T2. For T3N0 5-year local control is 30–70% with radiotherapy and 5-year survival 60–74%. Salvage surgery following recurrence for T1 and T2 lesions (about 10–20% of patients) is generally successful. Salvage surgery is feasible in about 60% of T3 lesions with a 5-year survival of 40%. About a third of T3 patients will lose their voice.

The equivalent local control rates by radical radiotherapy for supraglottic cancer are poorer for early disease: about 60–85% for T1 and 40–65% for T2. For T3 and T4 tumours local control is achieved in 30–60% of patients with a 5-year survival of 20–50%. When the nodes are fixed (N3) only 40% are cured.

For early subglottic carcinoma treated by radical radiotherapy results are poor with 5-year survival of 36%.

HYPOPHARYNX

Anatomy

The hypopharynx (Fig. 24.1) lies posterolateral to the larynx and anterior to the fourth and fifth cervical vertebrae. It extends downwards from the aryepiglottic fold at the level of the hyoid bone to the inferior border of the cricoid cartilage. The walls of the hypopharynx are thin. Lateral to it run nerves, blood vessels and muscles in the parapharyngeal space. The distance from the mucous membrane of the hypopharynx to the anterior border of the cervical spine is about 1 cm at the midline. It comprises three areas: the pyriform fossa, the postcricoid region and the posterior pharyngeal wall. Lymphatic drainage of the hypopharynx is to deep cervical chains.

The pyriform fossae are shaped like gutters on either side of the larynx (Fig. 24.1). Behind the larynx lies the postcricoid region, which extends from the arytenoid cartilages to the inferior margin of the cricoid cartilage. The posterior pharyngeal wall runs from the floor of the vallecula to the cricoid cartilage.

PYRIFORM FOSSA

Pathology

Cancer of the pyriform fossa (Fig. 24.20) is the commonest of hypopharyngeal cancers in most parts of the world; 90% of patients are males, principally in the 5th–7th decades. Alcohol and tobacco are thought to be the main aetiological factors. In contrast to postcricoid carcinoma, iron deficiency is not an important aetiological factor. Macroscopically the tumour appears as a fungating mass or deep ulcer. It often extends to other regions of the hypopharynx and to adjacent structures such as the aryepiglottic fold and ventricular bands, so fixing the hemilarynx. Microscopically it is normally a moderately differentiated squamous carcinoma.

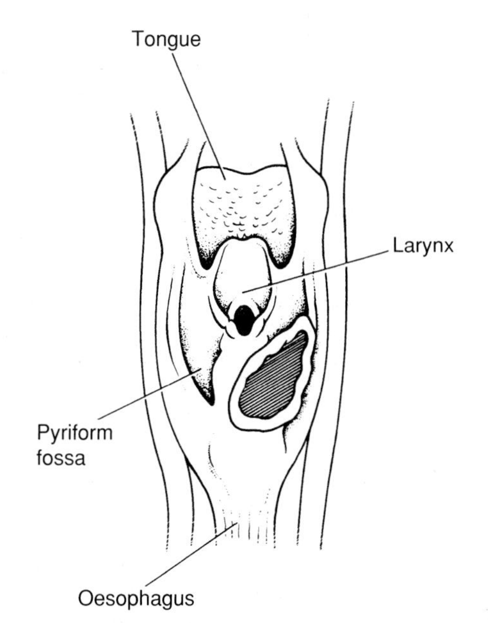

Fig. 24.20 Carcinoma of the hypopharynx (right pyriform fossa). (Reproduced with permission from Macfarlane, Textbook of Surgery, Churchill Livingstone.)

Clinical features

The primary is often symptomless and presentation is normally with a lump in the neck from secondary lymph node spread. Nodes are palpable in 50% of patients at presentation. The primary is normally advanced (T3 or T4). The upper deep cervical nodes may become very large, fungate and become fixed. Symptoms include a sensation of something sticking at the back of the throat, dysphagia, pain and weight loss.

Investigation and diagnosis

Indirect laryngoscopy may show an exophytic tumour associated with pooling of saliva. Direct laryngoscopy and biopsy is required. Tomograms of the larynx may help define the local extent of the tumour and show distortion and obliteration of the affected pyriform fossa. CT scanning is particularly helpful.

Staging

T1 is a tumour limited to one site. T2 extends to an adjacent site or region without fixation of the hemilarynx. T3 is a tumour extending to an adjacent site or region with fixation of the hemilarynx. T4 is a tumour extending to bone, cartilage or soft tissues.

Treatment

Unfortunately the majority of patients are incurable. However, radical radiotherapy is the primary treatment of choice for early tumours and locally advanced tumours with or without ipsilateral lymphadenopathy. When nodes are bilateral the prospect of cure is negligible, and only palliative radiotherapy is worth attempting.

Radical radiotherapy

Target volume

Early tumour (T1–2N0 or small-volume nodes (N1). The target volume should include the primary tumour and upper deep cervical nodes from the angle of the jaw to the inferior border of the cricoid cartilage (Fig. 24.21).

T3 with large nodes (N2). A larger volume includes the primary tumour and the nodes on both sides of the neck extending up to the base of the skull (Fig. 24.22A).

Technique

A head shell is needed in the supine position, the neck straight and the mouth closed.

For early tumours with no or small-volume nodes a parallel-opposed pair of lateral wedged fields is used. For more advanced tumours with bulky ipsilateral cervical nodes on one side, a lateral field on the side of the node and an anterior oblique field on the opposite side are used to limit the dose to the spinal cord (Fig. 24.22). Care is taken to limit the spinal cord dose to 40 Gy. Nodal masses overlying the cord, as for tonsillar cancer, can be boosted by electrons of appropriate energy (Fig. 23.17). If there are bilateral nodes, parallel-opposed fields are needed for palliation.

Dose and energy

Radical

60 Gy in 25 daily fractions over 5 weeks (4–6 MV photons)

More prolonged fractionation with dose modification is needed when including the spinal cord and using electrons (see supraglottic laryngeal cancer, p. 386).

Palliative

30 Gy in 10 daily fractions over 2 weeks (4–6 MV photons)

Radiation reaction. This is as in laryngeal cancer and is managed on the same lines.

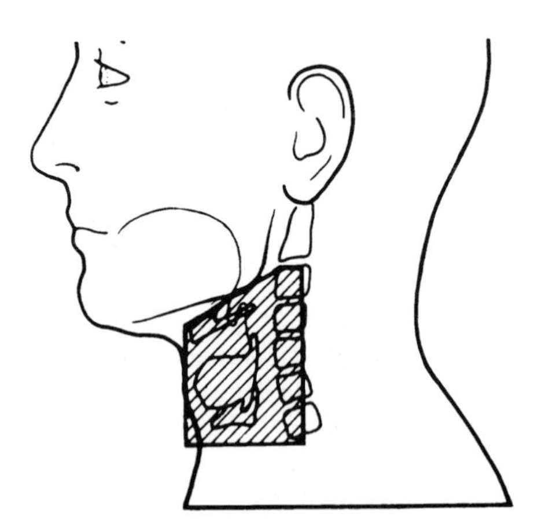

Fig. 24.21 Field margins for early carcinoma of the pyriform fossa. (Reproduced with permission of Arnold from Jane Dobbs, Ann Barrett, Daniel Ash, *Practical Radiotherapy Planning*, 3/e, Arnold, 1999.)

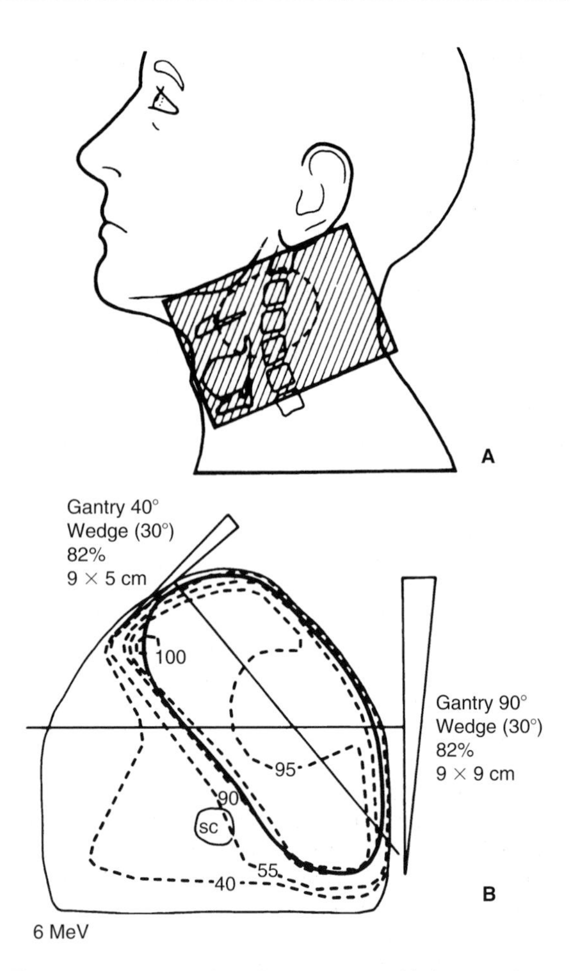

Fig. 24.22 A T3 pyriform fossa tumour with large node mass. **A** Lateral field margins on inclined plane; node mass is indicated by dotted line.(Reproduced with permission of Arnold from Jane Dobbs, Ann Barrett, Daniel Ash, *Practical Radiotherapy Planning*, 3/e, Arnold, 1999.) **B** Isodose distribution. (Reproduced with permission of Arnold from Jane Dobbs, Ann Barrett, Daniel Ash, *Practical Radiotherapy Planning*, 3/e, Arnold, 1999.)

Results of treatment

The results of treatment for cancer of the pyriform fossa are poor. For T1 lesions local control is 85–100% and it is 45–60% for T2–3. Hyperfractionation significantly improves local control. For advanced disease, treatment in predominantly palliative. Overall 5-year survival ranges from 10–40%.

POSTCRICOID AND POSTERIOR PHARYNGEAL WALL

These regions are considered together since they have similar epidemiology, pathology and management. Postcricoid cancer is a special variety of hypopharyngeal growth, just behind the larynx and above the oesophagus (Fig. 24.11).

Pathology

The highest incidence of cancer of the postcricoid and posterior pharyngeal wall cancer is in Egypt and Iraq, affecting principally farm labourers in the fifth decade. Cancer of the posterior pharyngeal wall is commoner in men and postcricoid cancer in women. The precise aetiology in most patients is unknown. However, a small number of cases of hypopharyngeal cancer are radiation induced, occurring after a latency of 20 years following radiation given for thyrotoxicosis. The incidence of postcricoid cancer is falling in the UK as a result of correcting dietary deficiencies. Carcinoma of the postcricoid region is associated, although not invariably, with chronic iron deficiency anaemia and other signs which include a smooth tongue (superficial glossitis) and hollow spoon-shaped nails (koilonychia). This is known, after the workers who described it, as the Plummer–Vinson syndrome in Britain and as the Paterson–Brown–Kelly syndrome in America. About 50% of patients with carcinoma of the postcricoid region have an associated postcricoid web (a small web-like projection of atrophic epithelium projecting in the entrance of the oesophagus). The whole of the epithelium of the upper digestive tract is atrophic, unstable and premalignant, and there may be malignant degeneration in the mouth, pharynx or oesophagus at any time.

Tumours of the postcricoid or posterior pharyngeal wall have usually spread to other areas of the hypopharynx. Macroscopically they appear as a fungating growth or ulcer. This may spread to the pyriform fossa, larynx, oropharynx, cervical oesophagus and thyroid gland. Microscopically it is normally a moderately differentiated squamous cell carcinoma. Spread to lymph nodes (paratracheal, upper and lower deep cervical) occurs in 40% of cases and is late. Nodal involvement is commonly bilateral when the tumour crosses the midline, especially with annular postcricoid tumours.

Clinical features

The cardinal symptom is progressive dysphagia. Indirect laryngoscopy may show only slight oedema or a suspicious pool behind the larynx. The edge of the tumour may be seen in advanced cases (Fig. 24.11).

Diagnosis and investigation

Direct endoscopy should be done, to see the full extent and for biopsy. Soft tissue films of the neck may show widening of the retrolaryngeal and retrotracheal space. A barium swallow shows an irregular filling defect. CT scanning is useful to show invasion of the pre-epiglottic space and the thyroid cartilage.

Treatment

If there is no lymphatic involvement and the primary is resectable, radical surgery gives the best chance of cure. The operation requires the removal of the larynx, hypopharynx and the oesophagus (laryngopharyngectomy). The alimentary tract has to be restored, usually by bringing up the stomach and joining it to the pharynx. Postoperative radiotherapy is not advised in view of the poor radiation tolerance of the stomach, which would lie within the field.

Radical radiotherapy is indicated in patients with an unresectable localised tumour. The prognosis of patients with nodal or mediastinal spread is so poor that radical radiotherapy is not worthwhile.

Radical radiotherapy

Postcricoid

Target volume

This should include the primary tumour and lower cervical nodes (Fig. 24.23). A margin of 2–3 cm should be allowed inferior to the macroscopic limit of the tumour to cater for submucosal spread.

Technique

The patient is treated in a head shell extended below the clavicles, in the supine position with the neck

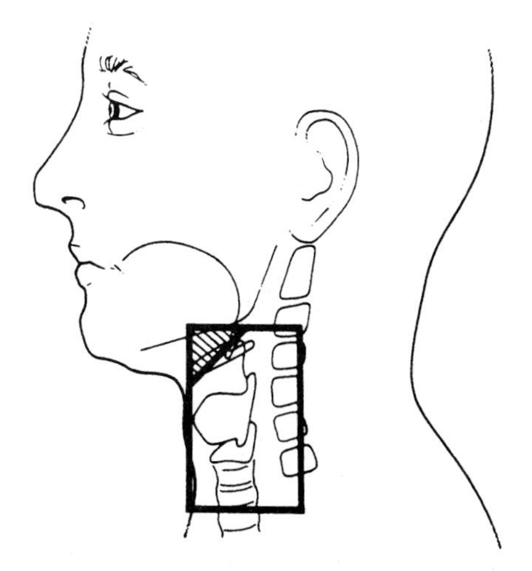

Fig. 24.23 Treatment volume for postcricoid carcinoma. (Redrawn from Dobbs & Barrett, Practical Radiotherapy Planning, 1st edn, Edward Arnold, 1985.)

straight and the mouth closed. A 'twisted' wedge technique is used. Two lateral fields are used, with wedges in the vertical and horizontal (one of which is therefore non-coplanar) planes and angled downwards using a couch twist of approximately 25° (Fig. 24.31).

Dose and energy

60 Gy in 25 daily fractions over 5 weeks (4–6 MV photons)

Posterior pharyngeal wall

Target volume

This includes (1) the entire hypopharynx with a 2 cm margin above and below macroscopic tumour and (2) the upper deep cervical nodes on both sides (Fig. 24.24). The posterior margin lies in front of the spinal cord.

Technique

Parallel-opposed lateral fields, wedged if necessary.

Dose and energy are as for postcricoid cancer.

Results of treatment

The outlook is poor for postcricoid and posterior pharyngeal wall cancer, with 15–20% 5-year survival for patients with involved nodes and 35% in rare early cases with negative nodes.

CANCER OF THE THYROID GLAND

Anatomy

The thyroid gland is composed of two lobes joined by a narrow isthmus, overlying the trachea (Fig. 24.25).

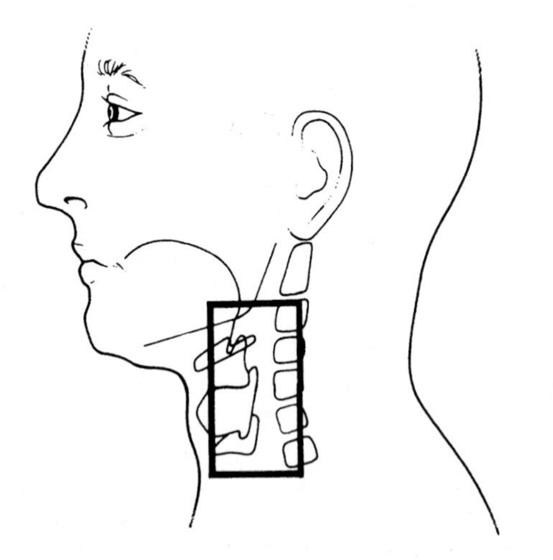

Fig. 24.24 Treatment volume for carcinoma of the posterior pharyngeal wall. (Redrawn from Dobbs & Barrett, Practical Radiotherapy Planning, 1st edn, Edward Arnold, 1985.)

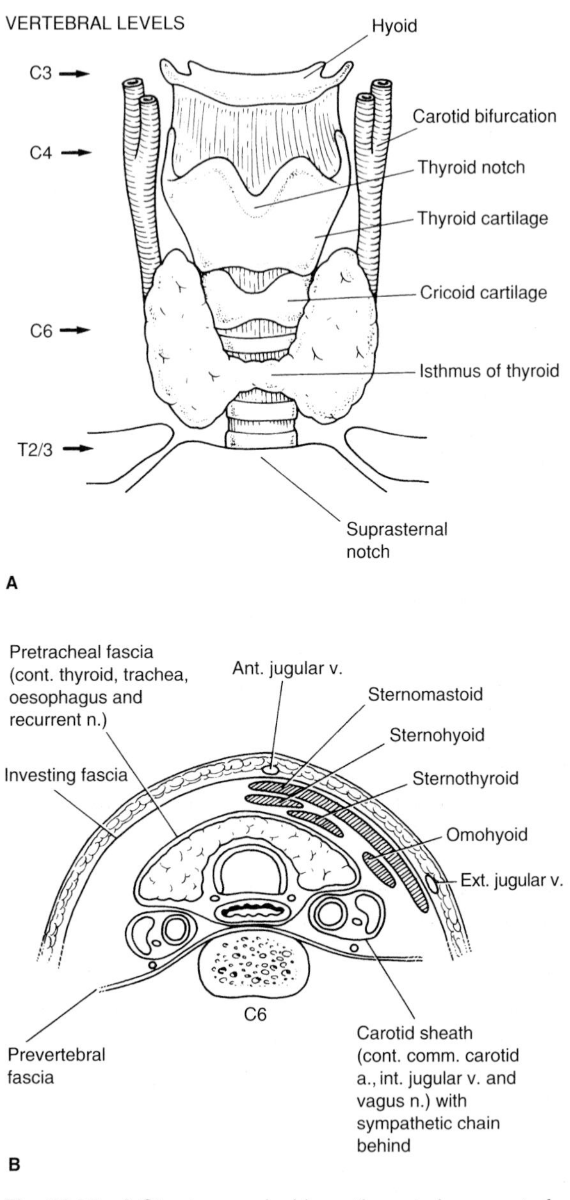

Fig. 24.25 A Structures palpable on the anterior aspect of the neck, together with corresponding vertebral levels. (Redrawn from Ellis, Clinical Anatomy, 5th edn, Blackwells, 1975). B Transverse section of the neck through C6 showing the relations of the thyroid gland. (Reproduced with permission from Ellis, Clinical Anatomy, 5th edn, Blackwells, 1975.)

To the right and left sides between the trachea and the oesophagus run the recurrent laryngeal nerves. The lymphatic drainage is to the deep cervical nodes, the pre- and paratracheal lymph nodes and downwards to the mediastinum.

Epidemiology

Thyroid cancer is rare, accounting for 0.4% of all cancers and 0.3% of cancer deaths. The incidence varies in differs parts of the world from 0.5–10 cases per 100 000 population. In the UK the incidence is 1 in 100 000. It can occur at any age but there is a minor peak between 5 and 20 years and a major peak between 40 and 65 years. Papillary and follicular cancer are rare in children. Their incidence rises with age in adults. Thyroid cancer is commoner in women, with a 2 : 1 sex ratio.

Tumours of the thyroid gland may be benign nodules (adenomas) or malignant. There are five malignant histological types:

- Papillary carcinoma
- Follicular carcinoma
- Anaplastic carcinoma
- Medullary carcinoma
- Lymphoma.

Papillary carcinoma is the most common. The incidence of thyroid cancer, particularly follicular carcinoma, is higher in areas of endemic goitre where iodine levels are low. By contrast, papillary carcinoma is commoner in areas rich in iodine (e.g. Iceland).

Papillary carcinoma is the commonest histological type induced by irradiating the neck in childhood. The latent period between exposure and diagnosis is at least 5 years. Risk is maximal at 20 years after irradiation, remains high for 20 years and then falls. The threshold dose to the thyroid for radiation-induced malignancy is as low as 10 cGy. At doses up to 1500 cGy, there is a linear relationship between dose and risk of cancer. At doses above 1500 cGy, the risk per cGy falls, probably because of cell killing. Young age of exposure is an important factor with the no increased risk after the age of 15–20. For children exposed to 1 Gy to thyroid the excess risk of thyroid cancer is 7.7. There is no increased risk among patients treated with iodine-131 for diagnostic or therapeutic purposes. There are too few children exposed to iodine-131 in childhood to exclude it being carcinogenic at this age. The increased incidence of papillary thyroid cancers among children exposed to radiation after the atomic tests in the Marshall Islands and more recently after the nuclear accident at Chernobyl in the Ukraine suggests, however, that both iodine-131 and short-lived isotopes are carcinogenic to the thyroid.

There is an increased incidence of thyroid cancer following mantle irradiation for Hodgkin's disease. Compensated hypothyroidism (normal serum thyroxine and free thyroxine index but elevated thyroid-stimulating hormone (TSH)) is common in these patients. It may be the persistent TSH drive that assists the carcinogenic properties of irradiation. Hashimoto's thyroiditis predisposes to thyroid lymphoma. The cause of anaplastic (undifferentiated) cancer is unknown but there is some evidence that it may arise from a differentiated form of cancer.

Genetic factors are important in the genesis of medullary carcinoma of the thyroid. It is inherited as an autosomal dominant; 20% of cases are familial. The familial form may occur in isolation, in association with a phaeochromocytoma or as part of multiple endocrine neoplasia. About 3% of papillary carcinomas are familial.

At a molecular level there are rearrangements of the tyrosine kinase domains of the *RET* and *TRK* genes with the amino-terminal sequence of an unlinked gene in some cases of papillary carcinoma. *RET* rearrangements are found in 3–33% of papillary carcinomas not associated with previous irradiation and 60–80% of those following exposure to radiation among children in Belarus after the nuclear accident at Chernobyl or among patients exposed to external beam irradiation in childhood. Much lower frequencies of *TRK* rearrangements are seen. *ras* mutations are common in thyroid adenomas and follicular carcinomas, implying that these mutations may play a part in the early pathogenesis of thyroid cancer. There are reports of activating mutations of the genes coding for the thyrotrophin receptor in some follicular carcinomas. Inactivating mutations of the *p53* tumour suppressor gene are frequently found in undifferentiated (anaplastic) thyroid cancer but rarely in well-differentiated thyroid cancer.

Pathology and clinical features

The main clinical features differentiating the various histological types are summarised in Fig. 24.26 and Table 24.2.

Papillary carcinoma is so-called because the characteristic microscopic picture has delicate finger-like cores of stroma lined by tumour cells. However, it is the cytology (and behaviour) of these cells that is the defining feature for diagnosis; they can be arranged in follicles in part or all of the tumour. It is characterised by overlapping cell nuclei which have a ground-glass appearance. There are often small specks of calcium (psammoma bodies) in the stroma. It is the commonest type of thyroid tumour, accounting for 60% of cases, including almost all of those in childhood and adolescence. Some cases present as a solitary mass in one lobe of the thyroid, but many show multiple foci throughout the gland. It is bilateral in about one-third. Metastasis is characteristically to the regional lymph

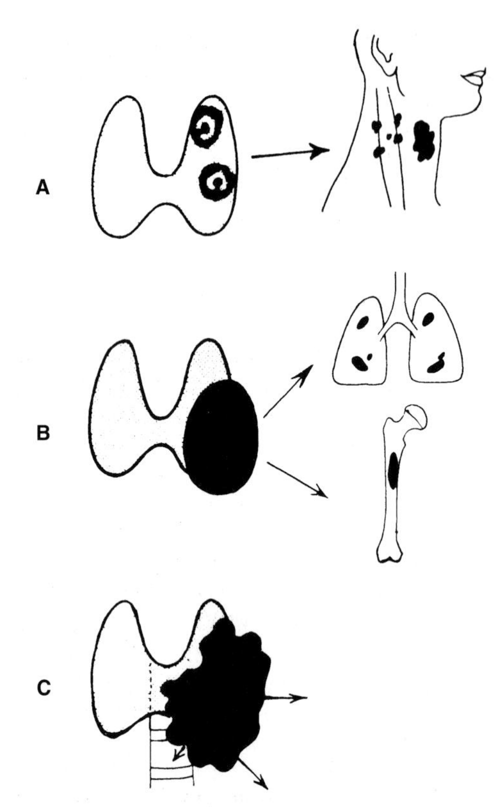

Fig. 24.26 Thyroid carcinoma: **A** papillary, metastases to lymph nodes; **B** follicular, metastases to lungs and bones; **C** anaplastic, local infiltration. (Reproduced with permission from Macfarlane, Textbook of Surgery, Churchill Livingstone.)

nodes, and enlargement of the latter is a frequent first symptom. Metastases to the lung are less frequent. Growth is usually very slow, and the long-term outlook remains good, even with established metastases.

Sometimes a tiny tumour is discovered incidentally during examination of a thyroid removed for other purposes (e.g. thyrotoxicosis). This occult sclerosing papillary carcinoma is usually ignored, and no treatment is necessary.

Follicular carcinoma is more variable in its behaviour; it characteristically spreads via the bloodstream to give metastases in bone and lung. It is usually a solitary, circumscribed mass; a very well-differentiated follicular carcinoma can be mistaken for a benign adenoma, the true diagnosis becoming apparent many years later when a metastasis is found. It is characterised by follicular differentiation. However, the nuclear changes typical of papillary carcinoma are not present. There are two forms identified by their pattern of invasion: minimally invasive and widely invasive. Multicentricity is less common than in papillary carcinoma. Moderately and poorly differentiated follicular carcinomas are more aggressive, and may show metastases at the time of diagnosis. Up to 10% of patients present with, for example, pathological fracture or dyspnoea from lung deposits.

An important feature of any well-differentiated thyroid tumour (papillary or follicular) is that some (about 50%) are capable of synthesising and secreting thyroid hormones. This feature is commoner in the

Table 24.2 Clinical features of thyroid cancer

Feature	Papillary	Follicular	Anaplastic
Typical age (years)	Under 40 including children and adolescents	40–50	60+
Growth rate	Slow (years)	Intermediate	Rapid
Presenting signs	Nodule in one lobe or secondary	Thyroid nodule for years or recent enlargement or secondary, e.g. pathological fracture	Large diffuse fixed swelling
Spread	Neck nodes	By blood, e.g. lung, bone	Lymphatic and blood
Primary treatment of choice	Total thyroidectomy or lobectomy	Total thyroidectomy	External radiation
Thyroxine therapy	Full (for TSH suppression)	Full (for TSH suppression)	Full (for replacement)
Radiosensitivity	Moderate	Low	?High
Radioactive iodine uptake	?Limited	Yes, ablation doses for residual thyroid tissue and functioning secondaries	None
Treatment of secondary neck nodes	Operable: surgery; inoperable: external irradiation	Ablation if iodine-131 uptake; if no uptake, surgery; if inoperable, external irradiation	External irradiation
Prognosis and 5-year survival	Good (80–90%); can be > 20 years (local or metastatic)	Intermediate (70%)	Poor (20%)

follicular than the papillary type. Even more striking is the fact that this capacity is also shown by their metastatic deposits. As in normal thyroid tissue, the hormones are built up from iodine removed from the blood and this enables radioactive iodine to be used in the treatment of these particular tumours. It is demonstrable in the metastases after oral administration of radioactive iodine, if all the normal thyroid tissue has been ablated (p. 124).

Anaplastic carcinoma. This undifferentiated tumour, often composed of giant or spindle cells, occurs typically in the elderly. Histologically it may be difficult to distinguish from a sarcoma or a high-grade non-Hodgkin lymphoma. In the absence of definitive histology, the distinction may only ultimately be made by the response to radiotherapy. Lymphoma usually responds quickly (often within 24 hours). Anaplastic carcinoma is relatively radioresistant. It grows rapidly, locally compressing the trachea, and may cause stridor and dyspnoea. The oesophagus may also be involved, causing dysphagia. Invasion of nerves may cause pain and, if the recurrent laryngeal nerve is involved, vocal cord palsy. It metastasises early to lung, bone and liver, but local growth in the neck is the main problem.

Medullary carcinoma. This arises from the parafollicular C cells, which make the hormone calcitonin. It is normally slow growing and may have amyloid in its stroma. Calcium may be present in the tumour and may be visible on X-ray. However, the absence of calcium, numerous mitoses, necrosis and spindle cells suggest more aggressive behaviour. Spread to lymph nodes and the mediastinum is common. Serum levels of calcitonin may be elevated but these are not specific to medullary carcinoma since calcitonin in secreted by non-thyroid tumours (e.g. lung, breast, colon and gastric cancer).

Malignant lymphomas. These are non-Hodgkin lymphomas of mucosa-associated lymphoid tissue (MALT) pattern, ranging from low- to high-grade malignancy. Many arise in association with Hashimoto's thyroiditis. Initially confined to the thyroid, they may spread to local lymph nodes or recur in the gastrointestinal tract.

Staging

The TNM staging classification is used (Table 24.3).

Table 24.3 TNM classification of thyroid cancer

T1	Tumour ≤ 1 cm
T2	Tumour > 1 cm
T3	Tumour > 4 cm
T4	Tumour extending beyond the thyroid capsule
N0	No lymph node metastases
N1	Lymph node metastases
M0	No distant metastases
M1	Distant metastases

Diagnosis and assessment

Management depends very much on history, examination and special investigations. The histological type strongly influences management so that a histological diagnosis is virtually essential for rational treatment. Assessment should be undertaken in a joint clinic between surgeon, physician and oncologist with specialised experience in the management of thyroid cancer.

A history should include a family history of thyroid or other endocrine disease, previous thyroid disease and irradiation of the neck. The neck should be examined for thyroid masses and a scar from previous thyroid surgery, which may have been carried out many years previously. Most differentiated thyroid nodules move on swallowing. Anaplastic carcinoma are commonly fixed. Nearly all patients with thyroid carcinoma are euthyroid. An indirect laryngoscopy should be performed to look for evidence of vocal cord paresis from involvement of or damage to the recurrent laryngeal nerve. X-ray of the neck may show (1) calcium as large irregular deposits or as a fine speckling (psammoma bodies in papillary carcinoma) in medullary thyroid cancer, and (2) widening of the prevertebral space (Fig. 24.27) or tracheal compression. Fine needle aspiration cytology is the most reliable test for distinguishing

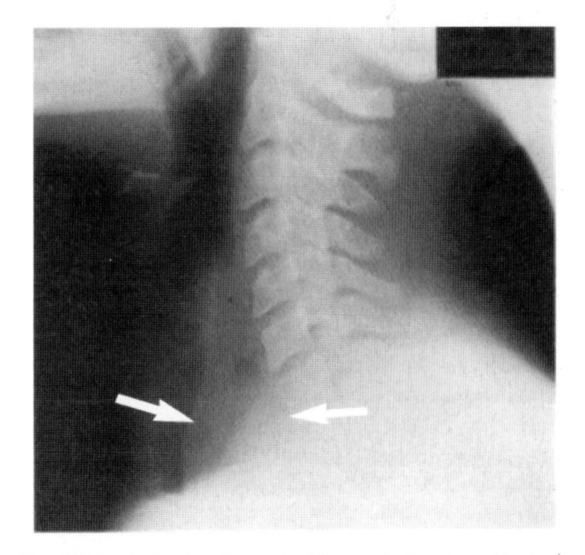

Fig. 24.27 Lateral radiograph of the neck showing widening of the prevertebral space (arrowed) due to carcinoma of the thyroid. (Courtesy of Dr R Nakielny, Sheffield.)

benign and malignant thyroid nodules. Ultrasound of the thyroid may assist in establishing the size of the nodule, diagnosis of other nodules and localisation for fine needle aspiration.

As a general rule, one of the first steps in investigating all thyroid masses is a radioactive iodine uptake test and scintiscan of the neck (p. 124). 'Cold' areas (Fig. 24.28A) are suspicious but not diagnostic of cancer; 'hot' areas (Fig. 24.28B) rarely prove malignant (see below).

There is least diagnostic difficulty in rapidly growing anaplastic tumours of the elderly, where the diagnosis is usually obvious. Benign enlargement of the thyroid can result in tracheal deviation. However, marked tracheal compression with symptoms of airway obstruction is usually due to malignancy. Tomograms of the larynx or trachea and a barium swallow may help to distinguish a tumour arising in the thyroid from one invading from an adjacent region such as the hypopharynx.

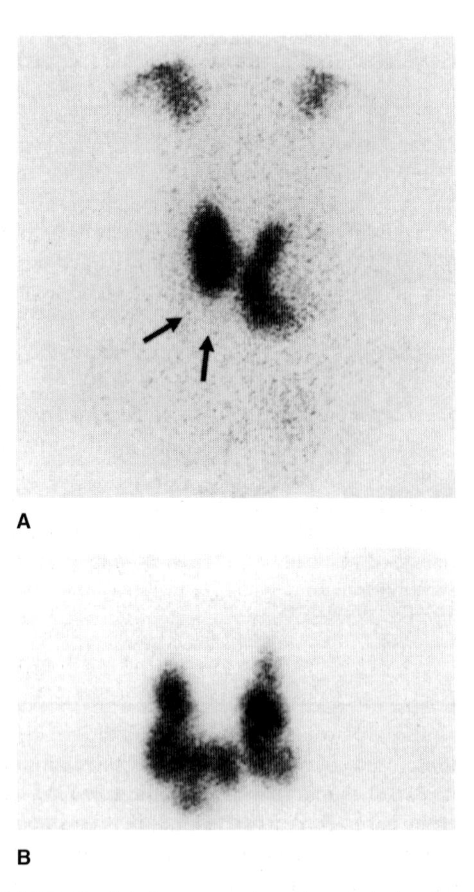

Fig. 24.28 Radioiodine scans (anterior view) showing **A** a 'cold' nodule in the right inferior pole of the thyroid gland and **B** toxic multinodular goitre. (Courtesy of the Department of Medical Physics, Sheffield.)

The only lesion with which it might be confused is one of the forms of thyroiditis (associated with the names of Riedel and Hashimoto); raised serum thyroglobulin and microsomal antibodies confirm thyroiditis. If medullary carcinoma is suspected, serum calcitonin should be measured.

Treatment

Surgery

If the patient is in good general condition and malignancy has been confirmed histologically, as much of the thyroid gland should be removed as possible (leaving no more than 2–3 g of thyroid tissue), ideally a total thyroidectomy and removal of any involved cervical nodes. For papillary carcinomas, many of which are multifocal, total or near total thyroidectomy results in a lower rate of recurrence than more limited thyroidectomy, and is preferable. It also facilitates ablation of residual thyroid tissue by iodine-131. The only exception to this principle is lymphoma. Some have argued for carrying out a complete lobectomy on the affected side and a subtotal removal on the other side to preserve one of the parathyroid glands. If all the parathyroid glands are removed, the production of parathormone is abolished. Hypocalcaemic tetany may result postoperatively. There are also risks of damage to the recurrent laryngeal nerve with total thyroidectomy.

Often enough, the diagnosis of malignancy and its type has to be awaited after partial thyroidectomy. It may even come as surprise. If it is of *papillary* type, a decision must be made as to whether to proceed to a further operation for complete removal of the thyroid gland. In favour of this is the fact that multiple foci are common. Arguments against further surgery are (1) papillary carcinomas grow very slowly and metastasise late; (2) second operations are always hazardous and carry increased danger of damage to laryngeal nerves and parathyroid glands. Practice varies. In the UK, surgeons are commonly recommended to carry out a near total or subtotal thyroidectomy. Lymphatic invasion in the thyroid specimen (as opposed to lymph node involvement) does not worsen the prognosis of papillary carcinoma. Hence prophylactic nodal dissection is not required. This operation can be carried out as and when nodal recurrence occurs.

If the nodule proves to be *follicular* carcinoma, the case for complete removal of the thyroid is stronger, since this type, in addition to being possibly multifocal, is more aggressive and more liable to metastasise, as well as being less radiosensitive. A second operation is therefore fully justified, even if there are metastases at presentation. Even if the decision is against a second operation, thyroid ablation by iodine-131 is carried out, as described below, to remove any remaining thyroid tissue. Prophylactic dissection of the lymphatics of the neck is not necessary, since the risk of recurrence following postoperative radioiodine treatment is low.

Urgent surgical relief of airway obstruction is commonly required for anaplastic tumours.

Hormone therapy

The activity of the thyroid gland, and therefore the production of the thyroid hormones, thyroxine (T4) and tri-iodothyronine (T3), is dependent on pituitary TSH. The production of TSH is in turn under the control of thyrotrophin-releasing hormone (TRH) from the hypothalamus. The amount of TSH produced is itself regulated by the amount of thyroid hormone produced by the thyroid, i.e. T4, T3 and TSH are in mutual adjustment by a feedback mechanism. Low circulatory T3 and T4 provoke more TRH, more TSH and so more thyroid activity. High T3 and T4 levels lead to less TRH, TSH and reduced thyroid activity.

All patients, after any form of thyroidectomy for malignancy (or even failing operation in anaplastic growths), should be given thyroxine tablets by mouth for the rest of their lives. The usual dose is 0.2–0.3 mg/day. This is for two good reasons: (1) after removal of the thyroid, replacement of the missing hormones is necessary, otherwise the patient would suffer all the effects of hypothyroidism (p. 546); (2) if there is any thyroid tissue remaining, it will be subject to stimulation by TSH, as will some well-differentiated thyroid cancers. Thyroxine in large doses removes the normal stimulus to the pituitary to secrete TSH. Low TSH results in low activity of thyroid cells, normal and malignant, and thus favours quiescence of any residual foci of tumour tissue in the neck or elsewhere.

In the case of anaplastic and medullary tumours, sufficient thyroxine should be given for replacement therapy, since this type of cell is unresponsive to hormonal factors. The adequacy of thyroxine therapy is assessed by measuring serum thyrotrophin 3 months after treatment is started. The aim is to maintain serum thyrotrophin at 0.1 microunit/litre and serum free T3 within the normal range.

Serum thyroglobulin. Normal or malignant follicular thyroid cells may produce thyroglobulin, a glycoprotein. It should not be measurable in patients with differentiated thyroid cancer if they have undergone total ablation of the thyroid. If present, it indicates persistent or recurrent disease. Serum thyroglobulin can be artificially altered by serum antithyroglobulin antibodies which occur in about 15% of thyroid cancer. Tests for the presence of these antibodies should be carried out each time serum thyroglobulin is measured. If serum thyroglobulin is detected during treatment with thyroxine, it will rise after thyroxine is stopped. Serum thyroglobulin after thyroxine has been withdrawn is a useful prognostic indicator. Patients with undetectable thyroglobulin levels after thyroxine has been withdrawn often remain disease free long term (e.g. > 15 years). On the other hand, patients who have serum thyroglobulin levels above 10 ng/ml while on thyroxine treatment and greater than 40 ng/ml after withdrawal of treatment have detectable foci of iodine-131 uptake in the neck or at distant sites after therapeutic doses of iodine-131 have been administered.

Treatment of neck nodes

Here again, treatment depends on the histological type. In *anaplastic* tumours, surgery is not helpful even if the nodes are operable, since distant metastases are virtually certain to be present. External irradiation is therefore the best option.

In *papillary* carcinoma, operable nodes may be removed but a full block dissection of the neck with its attendant morbidity is not necessary. This is because, although neck dissection may reduce the recurrence rate, there is no evidence that it improves survival. Inoperable nodes are treated by radiation. About two-thirds of patients will have lymph node metastases.

In *follicular* carcinoma, treatment again will depend on the ability of the nodes to take up iodine-131, as described below. If they cannot be induced to do so, block dissection is justified for operable nodes. If the nodes are not operable, external beam irradiation is given. About 35% of patients have lymph node metastases.

Radioactive iodine and functioning differentiated carcinomas

The differential uptake of iodine by the thyroid is described on page 123. Radioactive iodine, being clinically indistinguishable from stable iodine, is taken up in the same way, and thus is an ideal tool for internal—even intracellular—radiation. Well-differentiated carcinomas take up iodine not only microscopically but functionally, follicular more so than papillary. Iodine uptake occurs in about half of well-differentiated carcinomas. The degree of uptake may not be adequate for the purposes of radioiodine treatment. For this reason a tracer dose of iodine-131 is given and a scintiscan is taken 24 hours later (p. 124), which will reveal any functioning thyroid tissue. The scan can be extended to the rest of the body, and a 'profile' count obtained, with peaks opposite areas of above-normal uptake elsewhere, i.e. any functioning metastases. In practice it is very difficult to achieve complete surgical removal of the thyroid gland and some residual tissue in the neck is usually found on postoperative scan since some thyroid tissue is inevitably left behind by the surgeon to conserve the parathyroid glands. Only when an ablation dose has been given, destroying all normal thyroid tissue, can residual uptake in the neck or at distant sites be assumed to be due to presence of tumour. The decision to use radioiodine should therefore not be taken purely on histological grounds. Indications for radioiodine therapy are summarised in Table 24.4

Any remaining thyroid tissue after thyroidectomy of any degree, as revealed by the scan, should be eliminated as a potential danger. A *therapeutic ablation* dose of 3 GBq is given. The patient should be in a separate side-ward and full precautions taken against radiation hazards (Ch. 6). This dose will destroy remaining thyroid tissue. About 50% of follicular carcinomas will also take up iodine in the same way but if normal thyroid tissue is also present, then, as a rule, the normal tissue will take it up preferentially from the circulation, as it will be the successful competitor for whatever iodine is available in the circulation. The purpose of the ablation is to remove this competition. When all normal thyroid tissue has been destroyed by the iodine-131, the malignant tissue, stimulated by TSH, begins to function, to replace the missing thyroid.

Following the first ablation dose, a follow-up tracer scan should be carried out at intervals of 3–4 months, to detect any functioning tissue in the neck or elsewhere. Such tissue may be the focus for recurrence or metastases. If they take up worthwhile amounts of iodine-131 (i.e. 0.1% per gram of functioning tumour at 24 hours), they can now be destroyed by large therapeutic ablation doses of about 7 GBq. Assuming a biological half-life of 3 days, this will deliver a dose of 60 Gy to areas of tumour. If the degree of uptake is borderline, TSH (10 units intramuscularly) can be given daily for 3–5 days, before a therapeutic dose of iodine, to stimulate greater iodine uptake by the tumour. As long as there is adequate uptake, further therapeutic doses are given (bearing in mind the dose that can be given by external beam), unless there is a contraindication, such as low white cell count, or a maximum dose of 37 GBq has been reached. Beyond this dose, the risks of pancytopenia, aplastic anaemia and leukaemia increase. The investigation and treatment of patients with well-differentiated thyroid cancer is summarised in Figure 24.29.

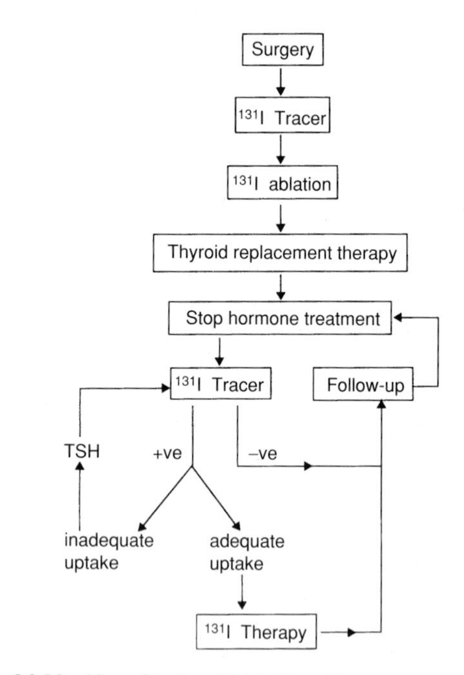

Fig. 24.29 Use of iodine-131 in thyroid cancer.

Table 24.4 Indications for ablation with iodine-131 for thyroid cancer (modified from Schlumberger 1998)

1. Incomplete excision of primary tumour
2. Complete excision of tumour but at high risk of recurrence and mortality
3. Complete excision of tumour but high risk of relapse due to:
   (a) age < 16 or > 45 years
   (b) histological subtype: tall cell, columnar cell or diffuse sclerosing papillary variants; widely invasive or poorly differentiated follicular subtypes; Hurthle cell carcinomas
   (c) extension beyond the thyroid capsule
4. Raised thyroglobulin more than 3 months after surgery
5. Distant metastases

Patients under the age of 35 with well-differentiated papillary or follicular carcinoma not penetrating the capsule (T1 or T2) and without lymph node or distant metastases have a particularly good prognosis. For this group of patients radioiodine therapy can be avoided.

Reactions to radioiodine. These large ablation doses can produce local and general reactions but these are usually mild.

In the gland itself there may be an inflammatory reaction with painful swelling and tenderness the next day, subsiding in the following week. If the swelling is severe, it may require a short course of oral or parenteral steroid therapy. If the thyroid remnant is large, treatment with steroids may be necessary for a few days to relieve local pain. There is also some excretion via the salivary glands (e.g. parotid) and a similar reaction may occur here (sialadenitis). The latter is usually mild and transient. Symptoms and signs of hypothyroidism do not usually develop until at least a month later and are usually mild.

General effects such as radiation sickness and lassitude are seldom troublesome and leucopenia is short lived (lowest at 3–6 weeks). The dose to the gonad is normally about half of the plasma dosage and sterility is unlikely to occur unless there is a pelvic bone metastasis close to the testis or an ovary. Pregnancy is an absolute contraindication to isotope therapy because of the risk of radiation damage to the fetus. There is a theoretical risk of mutagenic effects. It is advised that women delay conception for 1 year after treatment with radioiodine. There is no evidence that pregnancy influences tumour growth in women receiving adequate thyroxine therapy.

After radioiodine therapy men may experience a temporary reduction in spermatogenesis and women transient ovarian failure.

The risk of leukaemia and aplastic anaemia is largely avoidable if the total administered dose is limited to 37 GBq or if therapeutic doses are not repeated more frequently than once a year.

Painful swelling of the parotid glands may occur if the parotid duct becomes narrowed but this usually resolves spontaneously. Lung fibrosis may occur due to radioiodine uptake in lung metastases if high doses of iodine-131 (5500 MBq) are used or doses are given at short intervals (< 3 months).

Radical external beam irradiation

Indications

- All anaplastic tumours (regardless of any surgery performed).
- Inoperable thyroid tumour or neck nodes where iodine-131 is not appropriate.
- After incomplete thyroidectomy for papillary or follicular carcinoma (the alternative is a second operation to complete the thyroid removal) where iodine-131 has failed or is not appropriate.
- Lymphoma.

Target volume

This will depend on the pathological type, the loco-regional extent of the tumour and whether the nodes are involved. If all the regional nodes are included, the volume then extends from the hyoid bone above to the division of the trachea (carina) below. However, for well-differentiated cancers, only the thyroid bed and adjacent lymphatics need to be included. In this case the volume extends from the hyoid bone to the sternal notch. The posterior border lies parallel to the spinal cord and incorporates the anterior margin of the vertebrae. The anterior margin includes the skin of the neck.

Technique

External radiation of the thyroid presents technical difficulties. The contours are irregular, with rapidly changing dimensions from point to point. The treatment volume curves around the spinal cord. Careful planning is required to avoid exceeding the radiation tolerance of the spinal cord. A shell is necessary to immobilise the neck. The patient is treated supine with the head extended. Bolus is applied to the scar and any superficial tumour.

No nodes palpable. If only the thyroid bed and adjacent lymph nodes are treated, two anterior oblique wedged fields usually suffice (Fig. 24.30). Contours for computer planning are taken through the centre, top and bottom of the fields. Alternatively two lateral wedged oblique fields, angled down, are used. To compensate for

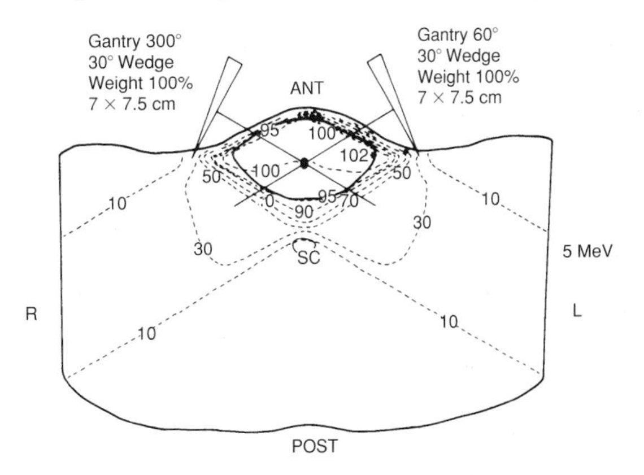

Fig. 24.30 Anterior oblique wedged fields used to treat localised carcinoma of the thyroid. (Reproduced with permission of Arnold from Jane Dobbs, Ann Barrett, Daniel Ash, *Practical Radiotherapy Planning*, 3/e, Arnold, 1999.)

the oblique incidence in the anteroposterior plane, a horizontal wedge is used for one field (Fig. 24.31). A vertical wedge is used for the other field. The wedges are interchanged after half the treatment to obtain homogeneous irradiation of the treatment volume.

Palpable nodes. Where the nodes are affected, a single direct anterior 20 MeV electron field with wax gives a suitable dose distribution (Fig. 24.32). An additional thickness of wax bolus can be placed over the central part of the field to bow the isodoses forward in front of the spinal cord.

For large anaplastic tumours and for lymphomas of the thyroid, simple anterior and posterior fields including all or most of the neck are satisfactory, with a downward tongue for the mediastinum (Fig. 24.33). The spinal cord dose should not exceed 40 Gy in 4 weeks.

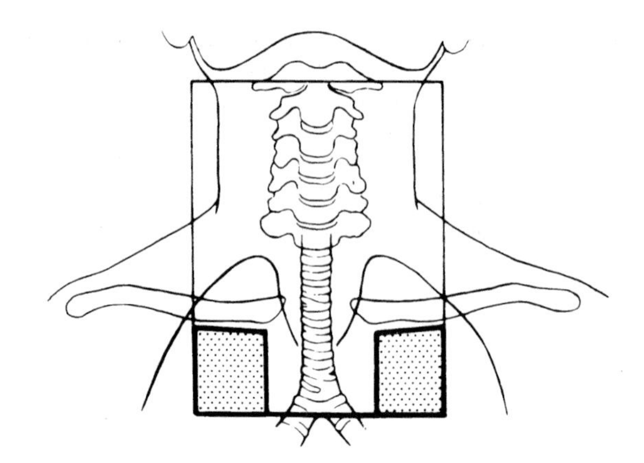

Fig. 24.33 Anterior and posterior fields used to treat anaplastic tumours. (Reproduced with permission of Arnold from Jane Dobbs, Ann Barrett, Daniel Ash, *Practical Radiotherapy Planning*, 1/e, Edward Arnold, 1985.)

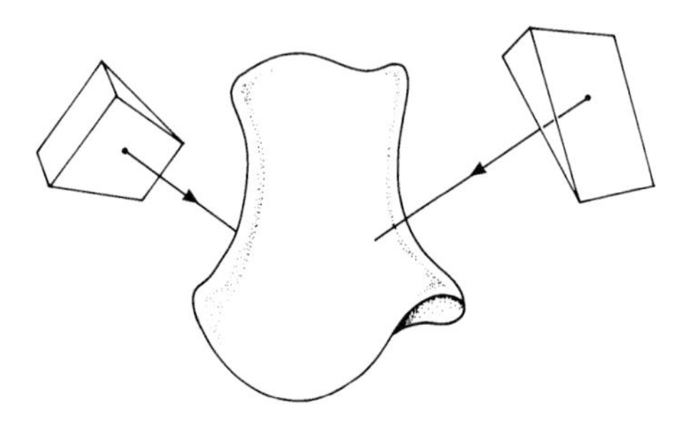

Fig. 24.31 Twisted wedge technique for treatment of postcricoid and thyroid carcinoma showing horizontal and vertical positions of the wedges. (Courtesy of Dr I Manifold, Sheffield.)

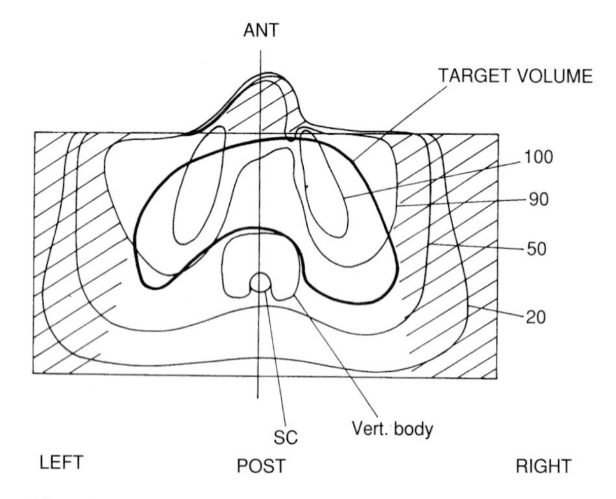

Fig. 24.32 Isodose distribution from an anterior 20 MeV electron field with additional bolus.

Dose and energy

Carcinoma

50–55 Gy TAD in 20–25 daily fractions over 4–5 weeks (4–6 MV photons)

Electrons may be used to boost residual masses.

Non-Hodgkin lymphoma

High grade

40 Gy in 20 daily fractions over 4 weeks (4–6 MV photons)

Low grade

35 Gy in 20 daily fractions over 4 weeks (4–6 MV photons)

Palliative radiotherapy

The indications for palliative external radiation are: (1) symptomatic neck nodes in patients not suitable for radical radiotherapy or surgery, and (2) bony metastases.

Dose and energy

22.5 Gy in 5 daily fractions (cobalt-60 or 4–6 MV photons)

The treatment of secondaries which take up iodine is described below.

Results of treatment

Survival times are extremely variable, as shown in Table 24.2. The anaplastic types fare worst and papillary best. Patients with papillary tumours may have strikingly long survival over many years, even in the presence of secondaries. Follicular carcinoma is not nearly as favourable. Overall 10-year survival for middle-aged adults is approximately 80–95%. Local or regional recurrences occur in 5–20% of patients. The main prognostic factors for recurrence and death are histological subtype and extent of disease. Radioactive iodine-131 offers excellent palliation in those patients who take it up in adequate concentration, including in secondary deposits.

Follow-up

Long-term follow-up is necessary and may include clinical assessment, and thyroglobulin (for well-differentiated carcinoma after complete ablation of the normal thyroid) or calcitonin as markers. The adequacy of thyroid hormone suppression should be monitored. Iodine-131 tracer scanning should be repeated as necessary. Hypocalcaemia may need treatment.

CHAPTER CONTENTS

25

Oesophagus, stomach, gastrointestinal tract, lung, thymus, pancreas, liver

Ian Kunkler

CANCER OF THE OESOPHAGUS

Anatomy

The oesophagus is a muscular tube which runs from the lower border of the cricoid cartilage at the level of the 6th cervical vertebra to the origin of the stomach at the level T10. For clinical purposes the oesophagus is divided into thirds: upper, middle and lower (Fig. 25.1).

The upper third (or cervical part) extends from its origin to the level of the bifurcation of the trachea at the junction of T4 and T5. At its origin, the oesophagus is in the midline and veers to the left as it descends. It is related to the trachea and thyroid gland anteriorly and the lower cervical vertebrae posteriorly. Laterally lie the common carotid arteries and the recurrent laryngeal nerves.

The middle third (or thoracic part) runs from the bifurcation of the trachea to the junction of T7 and T8. From lying slightly towards the left, it returns to the midline at T5 and then passes downwards, forwards and to the left. In front it is crossed by the trachea, the left main bronchus and the pericardium. Behind lie the thoracic vertebrae.

The lower third extends from the junction of T7 and T8 and passes forwards through the diaphragm to the opening of the stomach.

Lymphatic drainage. There is a rich lymphatic plexus around the oesophagus (Fig. 25.1), which drains into the posterior mediastinal nodes which in turn drain upwards to the supraclavicular nodes and downwards to the coeliac nodes close to the stomach. The importance of this interconnecting network of lymphatics is that cross-regional drainage is common. This explains why tumours of the upper third of the oesophagus frequently have abdominal nodal metastases at

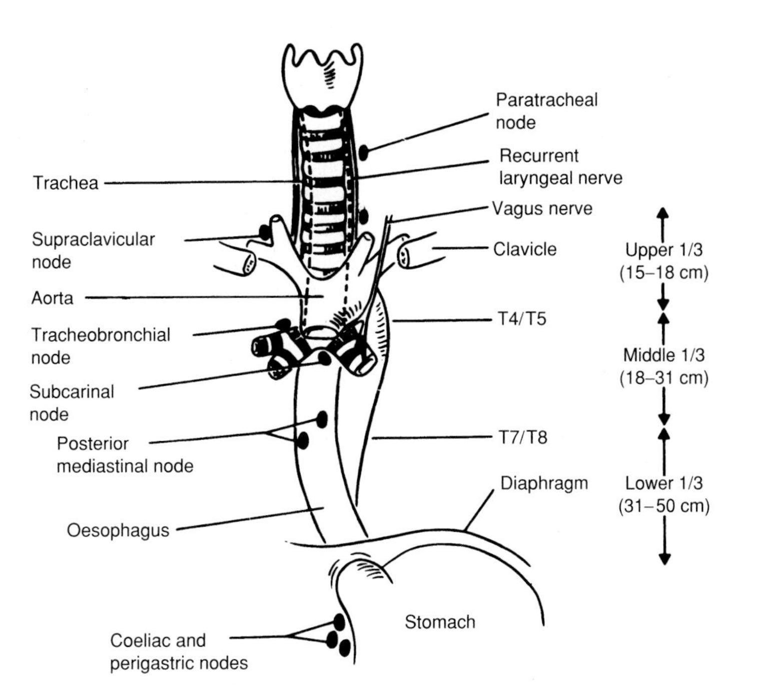

Fig. 25.1 Relations of the oesophagus and lymph node drainage. (Reproduced with permission of Arnold from Jane Dobbs, Ann Barrett, Daniel Ash, *Practical Radiotherapy Planning*, 3/e, Arnold, 1999.)

presentation. Overall, 70% of all patients have nodal metastases at the time of diagnosis.

Pathology

Cancer of the oesophagus accounts for about 1.9% of all cancers and 3.1% of cancer deaths. It is a disease of the elderly with a median age of about 65 years in both sexes. Overall it is commoner in men than women, with a sex ratio of 1.8 : 1. Cancer of the upper oesophagus is, however, commoner in women. There are areas of the world where the incidence is substantially higher, for example on the east coast of the Caspian sea in Turkmenistan and Iran, in Japan and parts of northern China. The reasons for the increased incidence are probably multiple. Dietary contaminants such as the nitrosamine group of chemicals and certain toxins from fungi (mycotoxins) have been postulated as aetiological factors. Alcohol and tobacco combine to increase the risk of oesophageal cancer. Tobacco smokers have a 5–10-fold increased risk. Heavy use of both alcohol and tobacco increases the risk by more than 100-fold compared to minor or non-users. Occupational exposure among rubber and asbestos workers increases risk, although to a minor degree. Hot beverages are a risk factor in Eastern countries. Conditions predisposing to the development of oesophageal cancer include: tylosis palmaris et plantaris, a scaling skin disorder of the palms and soles of the feet; Plummer–Vinson syndrome (upper third); achalasia of the cardia (mainly middle third); malnutrition; and Barrett's oesophagus (columnar metaplastic epithelium possibly associated from reflux and acidic damage).

15% of tumours arise in the upper third. The majority occur in the middle and lower thirds. 90% are squamous cell carcinomas. About 10% are adenocarcinomas, mainly in the lower third where they arise in the context of gastric reflux and glandular metaplasia (Barrett's oesophagus). The incidence of adenocarcinomas is rising. The degree of differentiation of the tumour is variable. Oat cell carcinoma (similar to oat cell carcinoma of the lung in its aggressive behaviour), adenoid cystic carcinoma and sarcomas of the oesophagus are rare. Because of the distensibility of the oesophagus, lesions often present with advanced disease when it causes obstruction.

It is important to appreciate that submucosal spread upwards and downwards is common and may extend several centimetres beyond the macroscopic limits of the tumour. 'Skip' lesions may occur elsewhere in the oesophagus several centimetres away from the primary tumour, owing to submucosal lymphatic and vascular spread. The oesophageal wall is thin and extraoesophageal spread to the aorta, trachea, pleura, pericardium and even vertebral bodies may soon follow. Blood-borne spread occurs early to the liver, and subsequently lungs and bones; 30% of patients have distant metastases at the time of diagnosis.

Clinical features

The cardinal symptom is progressive dysphagia, first for solids and later for fluids as well. There may be regurgitation and vomiting. If the oesophagus is obstructed, it can still cope with a large amount of contents, propelling small quantities of food past the obstruction in a series of waves of muscular contraction. Once the lumen of the oesophagus is reduced to a critical size, dysphagia becomes absolute. Discomfort and chest pain from extraoesophageal spread may follow. Malnutrition, loss of weight and dehydration will become serious if not relieved. As a result, the patient's general medical condition is often too poor to undertake either radical surgery or radiotherapy.

Diagnosis and staging

Staging is according to the TNM classification (Table 25.1)

It is necessary to establish the site of the tumour and obtain a biopsy.

The first investigation is a barium swallow. This may show the level of obstruction and narrowing. The upper level of the growth can be determined in this way, but the lower end may be difficult to discern. The movement of the diaphragm should be screened. Paralysis suggests compression of the phrenic nerve in the mediastinum.

Table 25.1 TNM staging of oesophageal cancer

Primary tumour (T)	
TX	Primary tumour cannot be assessed
T0	No evidence of primary tumour
Tis	Carcinoma-in-situ
T1	Tumour invades lamina propria or submucosa
T2	Tumour invades the muscularis propria
T3	Tumour invades adventitia
T4	Tumour invades adjacent structures
Regional lymph nodes (N)	
NX	Regional lymph nodes cannot be assessed
N0	No regional lymph nodes
N1	Regional lymph node metastases
Distant metastases (M)	
MX	Presence of distant metastases cannot be assessed
M0	No distant metastases
M1	Distant metastases

Next, instrumental oesophagoscopy is carried out under general anaesthesia. The tumour is inspected. Multiple biopsies are taken to give a good chance of establishing a histological diagnosis. The oesophagoscope should be passed downwards, if possible, to assess the length of the tumour. Temporary relief of dysphagia may be achieved by gentle dilatation to widen the lumen.

A bronchoscopy should be carried out at the same time as oesophagoscopy to exclude compression of the bronchi by the primary tumour or from involved mediastinal nodes.

A chest radiograph may show metastases in the lung fields or widening of the mediastinum due to nodal metastases. Endoscopic ultrasound is increasingly used because of its greater accuracy than CT scanning in assessing the T and N stage. Liver ultrasound is done to detect liver metastases. CT scanning of the chest and upper abdomen is often helpful in demonstrating nodal involvement (mediastinal and coeliac) and liver metastases. Positron-emission tomography (PET) does not have a routine place in staging but may do so in the future.

Treatment

Oesophageal cancer remains a major therapeutic challenge with a poor outcome in most cases. The situation is similar to that in lung cancer—surgery is possible for a minority. Surgery is contraindicated in many patients because of poor medical condition, invasion of the mediastinum, mediastinal nodes or distant metastases. Comparison of the relative merits of surgery and radiotherapy in clinical trials needs to be cautious, since patients treated with primary surgery tend to be at an earlier stage and those treated by radiotherapy more advanced. Surgical series often report their results on a small proportion of patients undergoing surgery or who are completely resected rather than all patients. Similarly, the direct comparison of more recent trials with historical controls may not be appropriate if recently treated patients have been more extensively staged with CT, endoscopic ultrasound and PET. Patients in older trials may have been understaged.

In general, adenocarcinomas, usually of the lower third, are best treated by radical surgery. Adenocarcinomas are relatively radioresistant. For this reason radical radiotherapy is not recommended. For squamous carcinomas of the upper third, radical radiotherapy is preferred, since laryngopharyngectomy can be avoided.

For the middle third either radical surgery or radical radiotherapy may be feasible. Attention to maintenance of general medical condition, e.g. correction of nutritional deficiencies and anaemia, is particularly important in patients undergoing radical treatment.

Radical surgery

Apart from age, poor general condition and evidence of spread beyond the oesophagus, radical surgery is contraindicated if the tumour is poorly differentiated or judged to be over 5 cm in length. The chances of finding a genuinely localised tumour are remote. Only about 40% of squamous cell carcinomas are operable. There are three main surgical procedures: transthoracic, total thoracic or transhiatal oesophagectomy. There is no definite survival advantage for any one of these procedures. The extent of lymphadenectomy is controversial with studies in Japan suggesting better survival with more extensive surgery.

Following oesophagectomy, the defect is replaced by transplanting part of the colon with its vascular supply between the proximal remnant of the oesophagus and the stomach. Operative mortality has fallen from in excess of 30% in the 1960s to 0–17% in most recent series.

Combined modality treatment

Combining surgery with radiotherapy seems a logical approach for a number of reasons. First, mortality from locoregional disease remains common after surgery. Secondly, surgical radial margins are narrow and difficult to evaluate and, thirdly, involved nodes are common at sites 10 cm or more away from the primary tumour but encompassed within radiation portals. Fourthly, some surgical procedures (transhiatal oesophagectomy) do not address regional lymph nodes. However, despite these theoretical benefits, adding radiotherapy to surgery does not seem to improve overall survival. In some of the trials locoregional failure was reduced.

Giving preoperative chemotherapy in locally advanced disease is able to achieve the cytoreduction needed to make the tumour operable. Response of locoregional disease often exceeds that of distant metastases. Phase II trials show response rates of 17–57%. Complete responses are, however, unusual. Median survival was 8–18 months, similar to surgery or radiotherapy alone. However, other trials using a combination of cisplatin, bleomycin and vindesine followed by resection or cisplatin and bleomycin showed no increased rates of resectability and no improvement in overall survival.

Combining chemotherapy and radiotherapy avoids the need for and risks of surgery and can be applied to a wider range of patients including those who are inoperable. It should address both locoregional and metastatic disease. Phase III trials with different drugs (e.g. 5-fluorouracil (5-FU), bleomycin, methotrexate, mitomycin C) alone or in combination show variable results. 5-year survival ranges from 6–30%. The best results were achieved using radiation therapy alone (64 Gy) compared to 50 Gy and two concomitant cycles of cisplatin and 5-FU, with a further two cycles following the completion of radiotherapy. Median survival was 9.3 months for radiotherapy alone and 14.1 months for combined treatment. 5-year survival was 0% for radiotherapy alone and 30% for combined treatment. The rate of locoregional failure, while lower in the combined arm, was still high.

Combining neoadjuvant chemoradiation preoperatively has also been assessed. Cisplatin has the advantage of acting as a radiation sensitiser. Although chemoradiation can produce a 25% pathological complete response rate, phase III trials have not consistently demonstrated a survival advantage.

Palliative surgery

Dilatation. Dilating the oesophageal lumen can provide short-term improvement in swallowing where only short lengths of the oesophagus are occluded. It can be carried out during diagnostic endoscopy and is repeatable.

Intubation. A very useful method when radical treatment is contraindicated is to insert a tube to maintain a free passage past the tumour and so ensure adequate swallowing for the remainder of life. Various types of tube are available. There are two main types, 'push-through' and 'pull-through'. Push-through types, such as the Souttar tube composed of flexible metal coils, are pushed blindly through the obstruction and are suitable for obstructions up to 10 cm in length in the upper or middle thirds of the oesophagus. Pull-through types, such the Mousseau–Barbin plastic tube or the soft rubber Celestin tube, are so called because they are pulled through the obstruction using a guidewire or string from above into the stomach where they are secured by a suture. They are most suited for tumours of the middle or lower thirds. The success rates for intubation vary from 40% to 85%, with an average duration of benefit of 4 months.

Intubation is not without hazard, carrying a mortality of up to 20%, usually from oesophageal perforation occurring during the procedure.

Gastrostomy and cervical oesophagostomy. This involves opening the stomach to insert a feeding tube which is brought out on the anterior abdominal wall. An opening is made in the cervical oesophagus to aspirate secretions from the upper airway and prevent aspiration. It may be valuable as a temporary measure while radical radiotherapy is carried out, but as a permanent procedure it is clearly objectionable. The patient is unable to eat or drink and personal hygiene is difficult to maintain.

Laser therapy. Debulking of the tumour by laser therapy can provide rapid relief of relatively short obstructing lesions. It is, however, only available in a limited number of centres in the UK.

Photodynamic therapy. Photodynamic therapy (PDT) involves the administration of a tumour-localising photosensitising agent which is activated by laser light of a specific wavelength. This entrains a sequence of photochemical and photobiological processes that damage tumour cells. The principles of PDT are shown in Figure 25.4. Since most photosensitising agents are fluorescent, drug localisation can be determined by fluorescence microscopy. Photodynamic damage to the plasma membrane can be seen within minutes of exposure to laser light. PDT can precipitate apoptosis. Among the early effects of PDT are the increased phosphorylation of tyrosine residues. The mechanism of apoptosis is not clear. It may be due to mitochondrial photodamage.

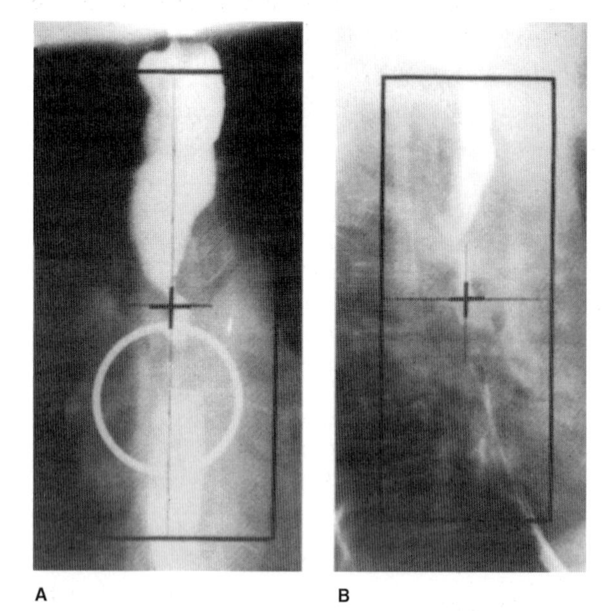

Fig. 25.2 Simulator radiographs showing field margins for carcinoma of the middle third of the oesophagus: **A** anteroposterior, **B** lateral. (Courtesy of Dr I Manifold, Sheffield.)

It seems likely that PDT may induce apoptosis without the need for intermediate signal transduction pathways that may be missing from drug-resistant tumour cells. It is thought the action of PDT on tumours depends on the state of the cell cycle or of genetic factors such as *p53*. The mechanism of selective uptake in tumours is not well understood. It may relate to the lower pH, increased numbers of low-density protein receptors and the presence of macrophages.

Photodynamic therapy (PDT) has been shown to provide comparable benefits to laser therapy in partially obstructing advanced oesophageal cancer. The response is slightly higher with PDT and the duration of response longer lasting (32% vs 20% at 1 month). In some subgroups responses were higher than laser therapy, e.g. in the upper and lower oesophagus and in tumours larger than 10 cm. There was no difference in median survival compared to laser therapy. About 19% of patients treated with PDT experienced mild sunburn reactions. PDT appeared to be better tolerated and easier to perform than laser therapy, particularly at sites where the morphology of the tumour or its site made laser therapy difficult.

Radical radiotherapy

Radical radiotherapy is applicable to a small proportion of patients with localised tumours of limited length in the middle and upper thirds of the oesophagus. Preoperative radiotherapy is an attractive concept with a view to sterilising the tumour and then resecting it but there is no convincing evidence that it improves survival compared with surgery alone.

There is little information on the value of postoperative radiotherapy following oesophagectomy. Surgeons are understandably reluctant to submit a patient to an additional major treatment procedure. Again, no convincing survival benefit over surgery alone has been demonstrated.

Criteria for selection for radical radiotherapy

1. Squamous cell carcinoma not greater than 5 cm in length
2. No mediastinal spread
3. No lymph node or distant metastases
4. Adequate general medical and nutritional state
5. Under the age of 70.

Advanced age is a relative contraindication. The prognosis for women with squamous cell carcinoma of the oesophagus is better than that for men. For this reason, if the first four criteria are fulfilled, a woman over the age of 70 with a squamous carcinoma may be treated radically. A man of the same age would be better treated by palliative radiotherapy.

Target volume

This should include the primary tumour, as defined by barium swallow and oesophagoscopy, with a margin of 5 cm above and below (Fig. 25.2). The length of the volume should not exceed 18 cm. The lateral margins should be sufficient to encompass the soft tissues of the oesophageal wall (usually 6 cm) or 8 cm if the adjacent nodes liable to invasion are included. In the older patient a reduction of a few centimetres in the margin above and below the tumour is advisable to limit the severity of the acute radiation reaction.

Technique

Anatomical factors constrain the delivery of a homogeneous dose of radiation to the oesophagus. The changing position of the oesophagus during its course and the variation in the contour of the body often require the plane of treatment to be inclined rather than parallel to the couch. It should be noted that the treated volume is cylindrical in shape. In addition, overdosage to the spinal cord and the lung must be avoided.

The technique for the upper third is described in Chapter 24 (p. 389). For middle and lower third lesions a three-field isocentric technique of an open anterior field and two wedged posterior oblique fields is used (Fig. 25.3). A CT planning scan is helpful in optimising the positioning of the fields and avoiding the spinal cord.

The patient is simulated supine with the hands resting behind the head. Thin barium is swallowed to identify the tumour and to choose the upper and lower limits of the field. Having defined the upper and lower limits and the width of the volume, the patient is simulated from the side to define the depth in the anteroposterior plane. Some inclination may be required to avoid inclusion of the spinal cord. Sometimes it is impossible to avoid the cord completely, if the tumour is to be adequately covered. However, not more than a 1 cm length should be included in the treated volume. The posterior oblique fields are viewed to confirm adequate coverage. Contours are taken through the top, middle and bottom of the volume. The positions of the target volume, spinal cord, heart and lungs are marked. A correction should be made for the greater transmission of radiation through the lungs (usually 3% per centimetre of lung traversed). A beam passing through the lung may give a 30–40% higher radiation dose to the oesophagus than the same beam through solid tissue. The dose to the spinal cord should not exceed 40 Gy in 20 daily fractions over 4 weeks.

Dose and energy

52.5 Gy given in 20 daily fractions over 4 weeks (9–10 MV photons)

Radiation reactions

Acute. Radical radiotherapy can be a severe strain and hospital admission, particularly for the second half of

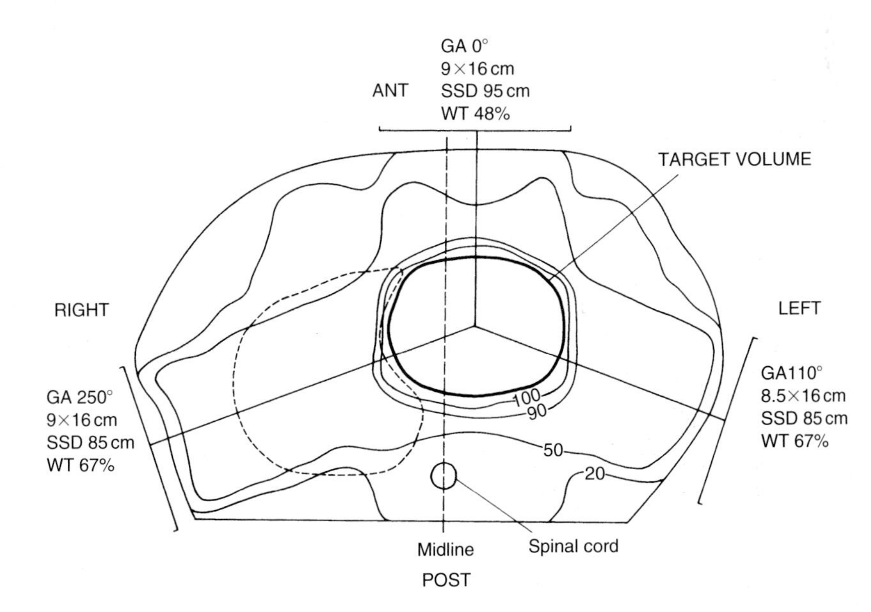

Fig. 25.3 Carcinoma of the middle third of oesophagus. Isodose distribution of anterior and two posterior oblique fields. (Courtesy of Dr J Bolger, Sheffield.)

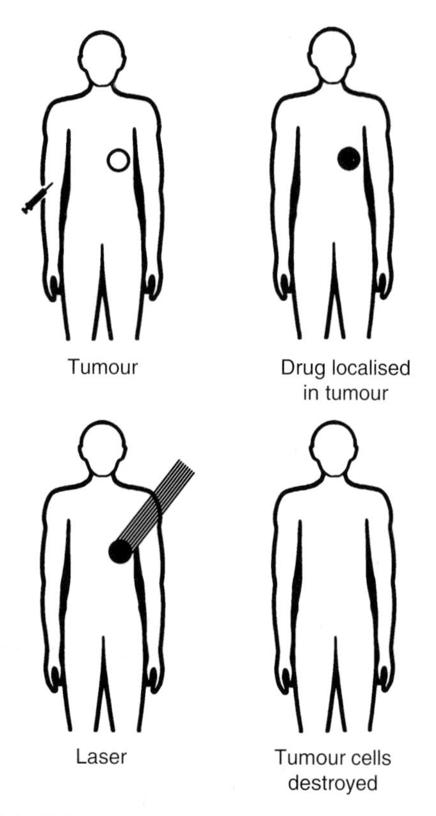

Fig. 25.4 Schematic diagram of clinical sequence of events in photodynamic therapy. (Reproduced with permission from Peckham, Pinedo & Veronesi, Oxford Textbook of Oncology, 1995 by permission of Oxford University Press.)

treatment, is recommended when symptoms of the acute reaction become more marked. General reactions with nausea and anorexia may occur and even interrupt treatment for a few days. Adequate fluid intake and nutrition must be watched. Radiation oesophagitis develops midway through the course and makes feeding even more difficult. Soft diet, high-calorie fluid supplements and mucaine are helpful. Nasogastric feeding with a fine-bore (Clinifeed) tube may be necessary if oral intake of calories is insufficient. Fungal infection of the oesophagus with candida is frequent and should be treated with antifungal therapy such as nystatin suspension.

Because of the thinness of the oesophageal wall, infiltration by the tumour in depth can soon occur and lead to perforation. This may even be precipitated by destruction of the tumour under radiation. Infective mediastinitis will follow, and is usually fatal. Similarly, a major blood vessel may be eroded, with rapidly fatal haemorrhage. Aspiration pneumonia is not uncommon and often fatal despite antibiotic therapy. Radiation pneumonitis (p. 426) is rare.

Late. Late complications are mainly oesophageal strictures. These can occur as early as 3 months after treatment, but patients rarely survive long enough to develop this complication. Treatment is by dilatation, repeated if necessary.

Palliative radiotherapy

Palliative radiotherapy is worthwhile considering to relieve dysphagia in patients for whom radical radiotherapy is contraindicated. This may be by external beam or single-dose intraoesophageal irradiation using a 'Selectron' containing a cobalt source. Suspected or proven tracheo-oesophageal fistula, a communication between the oesophagus and the trachea from tumoral invasion, is a contraindication to palliative radiotherapy.

External beam

Target volume
A small margin of 1–2 cm above and below the tumour is recommended to limit the severity of the acute reaction.

Treatment technique
A simple pair of parallel-opposed anterior and posterior fields is used.

Dose and energy
30 Gy given in 10 daily fractions or 25.5 Gy in 5 daily fractions (cobalt-60 or 4–6 MV photons)

Selectron

A single treatment of 15 Gy at 1 cm from the central axis of the cobalt-60 source.

Chemotherapy

Oesophageal cancer responds poorly to currently available chemotherapy. Agents such as cisplatin, bleomycin, methotrexate, 5-fluorouracil and doxorubicin have been used as single agents or in combination. Their toxicity makes their use difficult to justify since short-term partial responses in a minority of patients are all that can be achieved at present.

Results of treatment

The results of both radical surgery and radical radiotherapy in the UK are poor, with an overall 5-year survival of 5–10%. The best results of radical radiotherapy have been a 22% 5-year survival in a series from Edinburgh. Most series have been unable to match this. The prognosis is better in the upper third of the oesophagus (5-year survival 10–20%). Lower third tumours fare best with surgery, with a 30% 5-year survival.

CARCINOMA OF THE STOMACH

Pathology

Epidemiology and aetiology

The incidence of carcinoma of the stomach is declining in most countries including Britain but it still accounts for 10 000 deaths per year in England and Wales. It represents 7% of all cancers and 7.9% of all cancer deaths. It is the third commonest cause of death from cancer in men and the fourth most common in women. It is commoner in men than women, with a sex ratio of 2.2 : 1, and more common amongst manual workers than in professional groups. Its maximum incidence is in the sixth decade. There is a wide variation in the incidence in the UK. For example it is three times more common in the north-west of England than in the south-east. The highest incidence is in Japan (80 per 100 000), more than double the incidence in Britain.

The epidemiology of gastric cancer suggests diet as the main influence; Japanese who emigrated to the USA take on the local lower incidence. The precise factors are not clear; it is more frequent with higher carbohydrate consumption, and less common with higher consumption of green vegetables. Bacterial action on nitrates could produce carcinogenic nitrosamines; this reaction is inhibited by vitamin C. Bacteria may be more plentiful if gastric acid secretion is defective, and nitrites in the soil can enter the food chain.

Precursor lesions are rarely diagnosed, though cancer is more frequently seen in the context of chronic gastritis, or atrophy (as in pernicious anaemia), gastric polyps, post-gastrectomy stomach, gastric ulcer and familial polyposis syndrome. There is, however, no firm evidence that such conditions are predictable precursors of stomach cancer or are truly premalignant. Occasionally *dysplasia* can be identified as a precursor; in Japan, with its high incidence of gastric cancer, many tumours are picked up as early gastric cancer, i.e. superficial tumours with a good prognosis. Genetic factors may have a minor role, as the tumour is more common in blood group A than in group O.

It has been proposed that initial mucosal injury is caused by factors such as ageing or repeated exposure to aspirin, bile or alcohol. Nutritional deficiencies may impair the repair of the mucosa leading to chronic gastritis and proliferation of bacteria in the lumen. Bacterial nitrate reductases convert dietary nitrates to nitrites, which then subsequently react with dietary substances to produce nitrosamines. The latter may initiate a sequence of dysplasia, carcinoma-in-situ and eventually invasive carcinoma.

The diffusely infiltrating (*linitis plastica*) variant of gastric cancer varies less between cultures, so presumably has a different aetiology.

Molecular pathology

Overexpression of the protein p21 coding by the *ras* oncogenes, thought to be important in signal transduction, differentiation and proliferation, has been identified in gastric cancer and mucosal dysplasia. Mutations of the *p53* tumour suppressor gene are also frequent in gastric cancer. Higher levels of p53 correlate with the stage of the disease.

Macroscopic and microscopic features

Most stomach cancers are diffuse and infiltrating with a rolled edge and central ulceration; 95% are adenocarcinomas. 5% are lymphomas, leiomyosarcomas and rarely carcinoid. They occur mainly in the antrum/pylorus (50%), 20% involve the lesser curve, 5% the greater curve, 5% the fundus and 10% the cardia. Local spread occurs through the stomach wall to the pancreas and omentum. Lymphatic spread, present in 50% of cases, is to the regional nodes on the lesser and greater curves of the stomach, the coeliac and other abdominal nodes. From the coeliac nodes, metastases may reach the supraclavicular nodes via the thoracic duct. Spread may cross the peritoneum (transcoelomic) to the omentum and abdominal organs including the ovaries (the so called Krukenberg tumour). Blood-borne spread to the liver, lungs and bone is common.

Clinical features

The commonest symptoms are loss of appetite, weight loss and non-specific upper abdominal pain. If there is obstruction to the outflow of the stomach at the antrum, vomiting may occur. There may also be dysphagia, particularly if the tumour lies at the gastro-oesophageal junction. Common physical findings are a palpable upper abdominal mass and an enlarged left supraclavicular node (Virchow's node). The liver may be enlarged and masses may be palpable in the abdomen and pelvis.

Diagnosis and investigation

Barium meal or gastroscopy of the stomach is the initial investigation. Typically a barium meal shows a malignant ulcer with irregular walls. The stomach, if diffusely infiltrated, appears small and contracted (linitis plastica). The ulcer should be biopsied and gastric washings examined for malignant cells. An apparently normal barium meal or gastroscopy does not exclude gastric cancer. Gastroscopy should be considered if the barium meal is normal, or vice versa, since both investigations have a false negative rate of 20–30%. Additional investigations should include a full blood count and chest radiograph and liver ultrasound for lung and liver metastases respectively. In Japan, where the disease is common, it has been shown that earlier detection by screening, by means of a barium meal and gastroscopy, has increased the proportion of patients in whom surgical resection is possible. The mortality from the disease in Japan has fallen. The low and declining incidence of the disease in the UK would not justify a large screening programme for the disease but limited screening can successfully identify those at high risk of developing the disease. These would include patients with a history of previous gastric surgery, pernicious anaemia or blood group A.

Staging

Staging is based on the TNM classification (Table 25.2). Early gastric cancer is defined as cancer confined to the gastric mucosa and submucosa irrespective of its size or presence of nodal metastases. Such patients are potentially curable by surgery. Early gastric cancer accounts for 15% of gastric cancer in western countries and up to 40% of gastric cancer in Japan. The higher incidence of early gastric cancer in Japan is probably explained by their programmes of mass screening.

Table 25.2 TNM staging of stomach cancer

Primary tumour	
T1	Tumour invades lamina propria or submucosa
T2	Tumour invades muscularis propria or subserosa
T3	Tumour penetrates the serosa
T4	Tumour invades adjacent structures
Regional nodes	
N0	No regional lymph node metastases
N1	Metastases in perigastric lymph node(s) within 3 cm of the edge of the primary tumour
N2	Metastases in the perigastric node(s) more than 3 cm from the primary tumour or in lymph nodes along the left gastric, common hepatic, splenic or coeliac arteries
Distant metastases	
M0	No distant metastases
M1	Distant metastases (includes N3 and N4 nodal metastases)

Screening

Screening for gastric cancer is not recommended since there is no evidence to date that it reduces the mortality of the disease. Japan is well suited to the assessment of the value of mass screening by photofluorography, endoscopy with biopsy and cytology. The experience from Japan suggests that these investigations have led to increased recognition of early gastric cancer and reduced mortality from gastric cancer. However, similar trends have been observed in western countries that do not have screening programmes.

Treatment

Surgery

The only curative treatment is surgical resection. Unfortunately only 10–20% of patients present with disease limited to the stomach. In excess of 50% of patients have nodal metastases and direct invasion of adjacent structures. One-third of patients have distant metastases. Total gastrectomy is the most radical form of surgery.

For distal tumours (antral/pylorus) subtotal gastrectomy is recommended; high subtotal resections are carried out for smaller mid-gastric lesions and total gastrectomies for multicentric, mid-gastric or proximal gastric tumours. Such operations involve removal of the greater and lesser omenta, and the perigastric nodes along the lesser and greater curvatures. The Japanese have recommended the value of an extended radical lymphadenectomy to improve survival.

Where curative resection is not possible, palliative resection is preferable to bypassing distal obstructing lesions by gastrojejunostomy. The latter may be the only option to maintain nutrition and fluid requirements orally, which may allow discharge from hospital. Laser therapy can occasionally be of value in treating bleeding/obstructing tumours in some patients with advanced disease.

Chemotherapy

There is no established role for adjuvant chemotherapy.

Radiotherapy

Opinion is divided on the role of radiotherapy. Most radiotherapists feel that it has no useful role since stomach cancer is relatively radioresistant. Others believe useful palliation can be achieved in relieving dysphagia and haemorrhage, at least in proliferative tumours. Infiltrative tumours, however, tend not to respond and should not be treated.

Palliative

Technique

Parallel-opposed anterior and posterior fields are used.

Dose and energy

30 Gy in 10 daily fractions over 2 weeks (4–6 MV photons)

Intraoperative

Intraoperative radiotherapy (IORT), in which the residual disease is irradiated peroperatively, following tumour debulking, with high-energy electrons from a linear accelerator, is being evaluated. Sensitive surrounding structures are moved out of the radiation field to limit the morbidity of IORT. Initial results from Japan claim an improvement in 5-year survival in more advanced stages of disease. Late small bowel and neurological damage does, however, occur. It seems unlikely that this form of treatment will be widely practised because of logistical difficulties. Too few patients have been treated and followed up long enough to assess its real worth.

Chemotherapy

Chemotherapy has only a limited role in the treatment of stomach cancer. There is no evidence that it improves survival. Short-term palliation can be achieved in a few patients. The most suitable agent is probably 5-fluorouracil, which has a response rate of about 20% in advanced tumours. It has the advantage of limited toxicity. The optimum method of administration is uncertain. However, a continuous 5-day infusion of 750 mg/m^2 per 24 hours has the advantage of less toxicity than weekly injections. Acute stomatitis, joint pains and scaling of the skin may still occur.

Results of treatment

The best results of surgery have been achieved in Japan where 5-year survival of 80% has been obtained for tumours confined within the serosa and without nodal metastases, or 30–50% in patients with nodal metastases. It is not clear to what extent these excellent results are due to earlier diagnosis or better screening. Sadly, results in the UK remain poor with a 5-year survival of 4%. This only increases to 17% if a curative resection can be carried out.

COLORECTAL CANCER

Pathology

Epidemiology and aetiology

Tumours of the colon and rectum are the second commonest cause of death from cancer in the UK, causing 20 000 deaths per year in the UK and 200 000 in Europe. They represent 12.4% of all cancers and 12.5% of cancer deaths. The overall male to female ratio is 1.3 : 1. Colonic cancer, especially on the right side, is slightly commoner in women. However, males exceed females for rectal cancer by 2 : 1. Tumours of the colon outnumber those of the rectum by 3 : 2. Sites in order of frequency are rectum, pelvic colon, descending colon, hepatic and splenic flexures. The majority of colorectal cancers are thought to develop from preexisting benign polyps (adenomas). Adenomas are of three kinds: tubular, tubulovillous and villous. Of these, villous have the higher malignant potential as do large adenomas and those with high-grade epithelial dysplasia. It is estimated that approximately 5% of adenomas undergo malignant change over a period of 5–10 years. Polyps of < 1 cm have a lower (1%) risk of becoming malignant. Polyps over 2 cm have a 30% risk. Multiple polyps have an eightfold higher risk of malignancy than single polyps. Risk factors for recurrence following local excision include residual disease at resection margins and high-grade dysplasia.

Genetic and dietary factors are thought to play an important role in the aetiology of colorectal cancer. The disease is commonest in western countries and lowest in Africa, South America and Asia. It is thought that these differences are mainly explained by dietary factors. Western diets are low in fibre content and rich in animal fats and meat. By contrast, the African diet is associate with high fibre content and rapid bowel transit time. The exposure time of the bowel epithelium to carcinogens is likely to be shorter. The exact mechanism by which animal fats bring about the development of cancer is unknown. One hypothesis is that a change in the microbial flora is brought about by the ingestion of fat. This could result in a higher concentration of bile acids from the degradation of cholesterol. Bile acids are known to promote the action of carcinogens such as dimethylhydrazine under experimental conditions. Other evidence, however, has not supported this mechanism.

Genetic and molecular aspects

There are two principal predisposing genetic syndromes: familial adenomatous polyposis (FAP) and hereditary non-polyposis colorectal cancer (HNPCC). Other cases are considered to be sporadic.

A multistep model of carcinogenesis is widely accepted, based on the idea that a cell must accumulate four or five defects (mutational activation of oncogenes and inactivation of tumour suppressor genes) before malignant transformation occurs. In some individuals who have an inherited germline mutation, fewer subsequent germline mutations are needed to undergo malignant transformation. As a consequence, the phenotypic expression of the disease is earlier in life. Genetic changes that are thought to be important in the transition from dysplastic polyp to invasive cancer include K-*ras* mutation on chromosome 12p, *p53* loss on chromosome 17p, hypomethylation of DNA and *DCC* loss on chromosome 18q (Fig. 25.5).

The risk of malignant transformation in familial adenomatous polyposis is high (virtually 100% by the age of 40). The *APC* gene can be reliably detected in family members.

Hereditary non-polyposis colorectal cancer (HNPCC) has autosomal dominant inheritance. It is thought to account for 6% of cases of colon cancer. It is associated with other cancers (ovary, endometrium, skin and hepatobiliary tract) and mainly involves the right side of the colon. Criteria for the diagnosis are shown in Table 25.3. The disease is often histologically aggressive with high-grade mucinous tumours with a strong tendency for local invasion. 50–80% of patients with HNPCC will develop endometrial cancer. Despite its better prognosis than sporadic forms of colonic cancer, prophylactic subtotal colectomy is advised.

Table 25.3 Amsterdam criteria for hereditary non-polyposis colon cancer (HNPCC)

Three or more relatives with colorectal cancer
One affected case is first-degree relative of the other two
Cases over two or more generations
One or more case aged < 50

Other bowel diseases that predispose to colorectal cancer are ulcerative colitis and Crohn's disease. The risk of malignant change in ulcerative colitis is highest if the disease has been present for 10 years (10%) or has been present since birth. Other risk factors are schistosomiasis (a parasitic disease which also predisposes to bladder cancer; see Ch. 28) and previous surgery in which a ureter has been transplanted into the sigmoid colon (ureterosigmoidostomy).

Macroscopic and microscopic features

Colorectal cancers are usually polypoid masses, often with central ulceration and bleeding. Nearly all are adenocarcinomas. Direct spread may occur through the bowel wall into the pericolic and perirectal fat. The degree of penetration of the bowel wall is the basis of the TNM (Table 25.4) and Dukes' classification systems (see below). Lymphatic spread is to the regional nodes. These are involved in 50% of cases at the time of surgery. Blood-borne spread to the liver via the portal system is common (15% at the time of surgery).

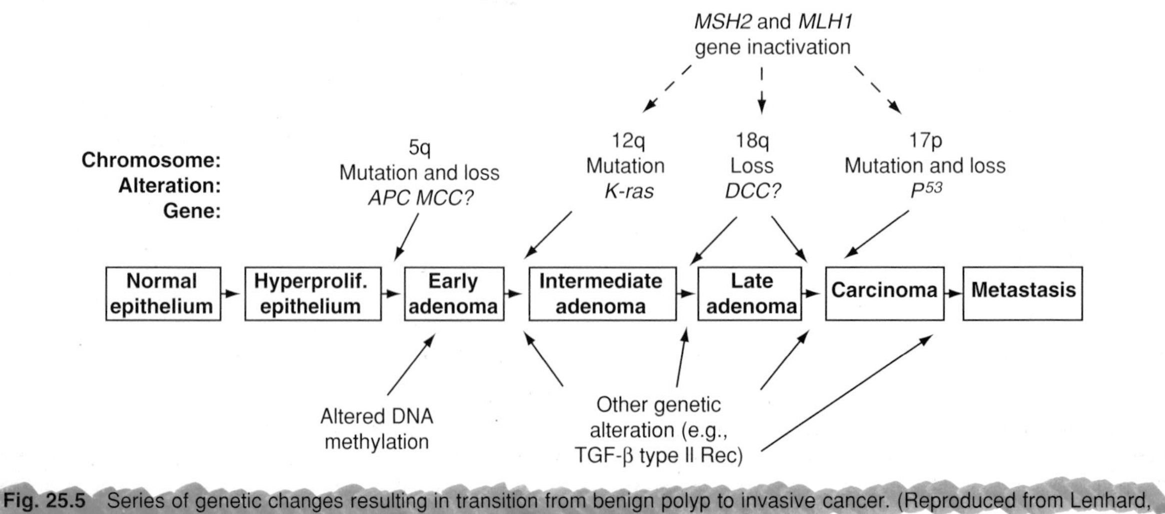

Fig. 25.5 Series of genetic changes resulting in transition from benign polyp to invasive cancer. (Reproduced from Lenhard, Osteen and Gansler, Clinical Oncology, American Cancer Society, 2000.)

Table 25.4 TNM staging of colorectal cancer

T: Primary tumour	
T0	Primary tumour cannot be assessed
T1	No evidence of primary tumour
Tis: Carcinoma-in-situ	
T1	Tumour invades the submucosa
T2	Tumour invades the muscularis propria
T3	Tumour invading through the muscularis propria into subserosa or in non-peritonealised pericolic or perirectal tissues
N: Regional lymph nodes	
NX	Regional nodes cannot be assessed
N0	No regional lymph node metastases
N1	Metastasis in 1–3 pericolic or perirectal lymph nodes
N2	Metastasis in 4 or more pericolic or perirectal lymph nodes
N3	Metastasis in any lymph node along the course of a named vascular trunk
M: Distant metastases	
MX	Presence of distant metastasis cannot be assessed
M0	No distant metastasis
M1	Distant metastasis

Screening for colorectal cancer

Studies have shown that faecal occult blood testing conducted annually between the ages of 50 and 80 can reduce the mortality of colorectal cancer by 33%. The Haemoccult test involves filter paper impregnated with guaiac, which undergoes oxidation in the presence of haemoglobin when hydrogen peroxide is added. The specificity is 90–99% with a positive predictive value of 2–50%. It has a 90% false-positive rate, one-third of which are due to adenomas. Routine screening for colorectal cancer is not yet conducted in the UK and its cost-effectiveness has yet to be established. The use of DNA markers targeted at recognised genetic alterations in colorectal cancer (e.g. mutant K-*ras*) is under investigation. However, K-*ras* may be originated from non-malignant sources (e.g. pancreatic hyperplasia). The specificity may be improved be targeting multiple DNA alterations such as mutational 'hotspots' on K-*ras*, *p53* and *APC* genes.

Screening by flexible endoscopy

Flexible sigmoidoscopy or flexible colonoscopy are possibilities for screening. Flexible sigmoidoscopy is highly sensitive and specific and is simple to perform. Its limitation is that only 65% of adenomas and cancers can be seen because of the limited extent of the colon and rectum which can be examined. A reasonable policy for screening may be to carry out flexible sigmoidoscopy every 3–5 years in men and women between the ages of 50–80. However, trials are needed to confirm this. Flexible colonoscopy has the advantage of enabling examination of a much greater length of the colon. This is more expensive and associated with significant morbidity but can reduce mortality by up to 70%.

Clinical features

Common symptoms are a change in bowel habit (constipation or diarrhoea), rectal bleeding, tenesmus (a feeling of incomplete evacuation of the bowel), mucoid discharge, unexplained anaemia and weight loss. Tumours of the right side of the colon rarely obstruct the bowel and tend to present with anaemia. Tumours of the sigmoid colon are more likely to cause obstruction. Rectal cancer typically presents with bleeding and tenesmus.

An abdominal or rectal mass may be palpable. Over 50% of rectal tumours are palpable on rectal examination. The liver may be enlarged by secondary deposits, with or without jaundice. Presentation may be with acute intestinal obstruction or perforation.

Diagnosis and staging

This should include inspection of the mucosa of the final 25 cm of the bowel by proctosigmoidoscopy. A flexible colonoscope can be used to look further down the lumen of the bowel. This should be followed by radiography of the bowel (barium enema). Contrast medium and air are instilled into the rectum. This provides a double-contrast image as strictures or masses indent the contrast. If the result is equivocal, the examination should be repeated or a colonoscopy performed. Accessible tumours should be biopsied. For inaccessible tumours the histological diagnosis is made at laparotomy.

Staging

The most commonly used staging system is TNM classification (Table 25.4) which is progressively replacing the Dukes' system based on the degree of invasion through the bowel wall and of lymphatic spread:

Dukes' classification

A—confined to the bowel wall

B—penetration beyond the muscularis propria to perirectal fat

C—draining nodes involved

Treatment

Surgery is the main curative treatment of colorectal cancer. Evidence suggests that better outcomes are obtained in units with surgeons specialising in the treatment of the disease. However, radiotherapy has been shown to have a useful role as an adjuvant treatment to surgery in rectal cancer and for palliation of recurrent (Fig. 25.6) or inoperable disease. Apart from palliation, there is no established role for radiotherapy in colonic cancer. Adjuvant chemotherapy plays an important role in reducing the risk of recurrence of Dukes' C colon carcinoma. Its role in Dukes' B disease is not yet established. It has no role in Dukes' A colon cancer.

Surgery

Radical surgical resection should include the affected segment of bowel and its local lymphatic drainage. This is followed where possible by anastomosis of the proximal and distal remnants of the bowel. The main vascular pedicle should be ligated and tumour-free margins obtained. The regional lymph nodes should be cleared for pathological assessment.

The role of prophylactic subtotal colectomy for patients is controversial. It is recommended for patients with FAP and HNPCC. Some surgeons have advocated it for patients under the age of 50 with a first colonic cancer because of the increased risk of a subsequent (metachronous) tumour elsewhere in the bowel. Other surgeons believe that this is unnecessary and early detection of second colonic cancers can be achieved by regular colonoscopy and removal of polyps when found.

In rectal cancer the type of operation will depend on the site of the tumour. The quality of surgery is particularly important in reducing the risk of local recurrence. The classical operation for rectal cancer is excision of the anus and rectum (abdominoperineal excision). Complete resection of the mesorectum is recommended, although the more extensive surgery does carry higher operative risks. Its benefit is the reduction in risk of local recurrence.

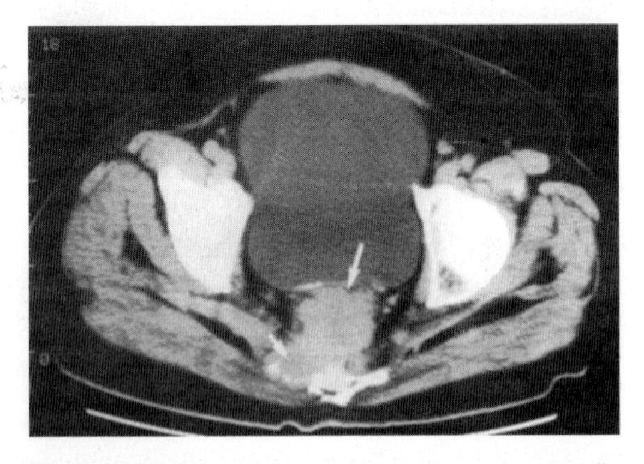

Fig. 25.6 CT scan showing invasion of the sacrum (small arrow) by recurrent carcinoma of the rectum (large arrow). (Courtesy of Dr R Nakielny, Sheffield.)

Sphincter-saving procedures have been developed to avoid the need for a permanent colostomy by lower anterior resection and colo-anal anastomosis. The operative mortality is similar for sphincter-saving surgery and abdominoperineal resection. Laparoscopic colectomy is being evaluated but its role has yet to be established.

In about 10% of rectal tumours the primary tumour can be removed and the continuity of the bowel restored (anterior restorative resection) if at least 5 cm of clearance below the tumour can be achieved. This avoids the need for a permanent colostomy and has a similar local recurrence rate to abdominoperineal resection.

Radiotherapy for rectal cancer

Local failure after surgery for rectal cancer is a major cause of morbidity and mortality. Local recurrence is rarely cured and therefore should be prevented if at all possible. The aims of surgery are to remove the bulk of tumour and for radiotherapy to sterilise residual disease. Because of the proximity of normal tissues, the surgeon often has to leave disease at the periphery of the dissection. The main cause of pelvic recurrence is lateral spread of microscopic foci. Surgical techniques aimed at reducing lateral spread have led to a reduction in local recurrence. In order to reduce the risk of local recurrence pre-, peri- and postoperative radiotherapy has been extensively investigated in clinical trials. These have demonstrated that if moderately high doses of radiotherapy are given preoperatively the risk of local recurrence is reduced to less than half. The proportional reduction is less with postoperative radiotherapy, even if higher doses are delivered. Improved survival has been shown in trials of postoperative radiotherapy but only when given in conjunction with chemotherapy.

Radiobiological considerations

Local control and acute and late effects on normal tissue are dependent on the volume, total dose, dose per fraction and overall treatment time. To achieve a high (90%) probability of sterilisation of microscopic disease, a dose of the order of 50 Gy in 25 fractions over 5 weeks is required. To reduce the overall treatment time between the start of radiotherapy and surgery, one either has to use multiple fractions per day or higher doses per fraction. With higher doses per fraction, the risk of late damage to normal tissues increases. In trials of preoperative radiotherapy 5 fractions of 5 Gy corresponds approximately to a dose of 42 Gy in 21 fractions of 2 Gy over 29 days.

Adjuvant radiotherapy

Whether radiotherapy should be given pre- or postoperatively has long been controversial. There is much evidence to indicate that higher doses of radiotherapy are needed postoperatively than preoperatively but there is no randomised trial to confirm it. Higher postoperative doses increase the risk of late morbidity. If the tumour is not operable or of borderline operability, preoperative radiotherapy is advised to see if the tumour can be rendered operable. Advantages of postoperative radiotherapy are that it may not be needed if the tumour is curable by surgery alone or if generalised intra-abdominal disease is found at surgery. Disadvantages of postoperative radiotherapy are that its initiation may be substantially delayed if there are postoperative complications. In up to half of patients, it is not possible to start postoperative radiotherapy within 6 weeks of surgery.

With preoperative radiotherapy for operable rectal cancer using short-course radiotherapy (e.g. 25 Gy in 5 daily fractions), the local recurrence rate in the irradiated group is between 11–16% compared to 37% for surgery alone. The difference is also significant for trials of postoperative radiotherapy but in fewer of the trials than when radiotherapy was given preoperatively. The relative reduction of local recurrence is generally higher with preoperative radiotherapy (22–65%) compared to postoperative radiotherapy (13–41%) despite the higher postoperative doses. In summary, preoperative is more efficient in reducing local recurrence than postoperative radiotherapy. A Swedish trial comparing patients treated by 5 × 5 Gy preoperatively showed a 5-year survival gain of 10% (58% vs 48%) compared to the non-irradiated group. A meta-analysis of randomised controlled trials of preoperative radiotherapy showed a more modest improvement in survival of 4.3%.

By contrast, none of the trials of postoperative radiotherapy alone has shown any improvement in overall survival. The only trials of postoperative radiotherapy which have shown a survival advantage have involved giving adjuvant chemotherapy in addition. The survival advantage may have been accrued by the chemotherapy alone.

The indications for radical radiotherapy for rectal cancer are:

1. Primary
   a. Inoperable localised disease
   b. Local recurrence of disease following surgery
2. Postoperative
   a. Peroperative tumour spillage
   b. Macroscopic residual disease
   c. Tumour at the resection margins (microscopic).

Increasingly, adjuvant chemotherapy is being given in conjunction with adjuvant radiotherapy.

Target volume

This includes the primary tumour or its bed, the local lymphatics and the presacral area (Fig. 25.7). The volume should ideally include the whole target volume while minimising dosage outside the target volume. The upper limit of the field is just above the top of the sacrum. Extending the upper margin beyond this level will include more small bowel in the field and increase the morbidity. Laterally, the pelvic side-walls and internal iliac nodes should be included. The inferior margin should extend 4–5 cm below the inferior limit of the tumour. The lower margin only includes the anal canal in low-sited tumours where rectal excision is planned. The posterior limit should encompass the presacral nodes and the sacral hollow.

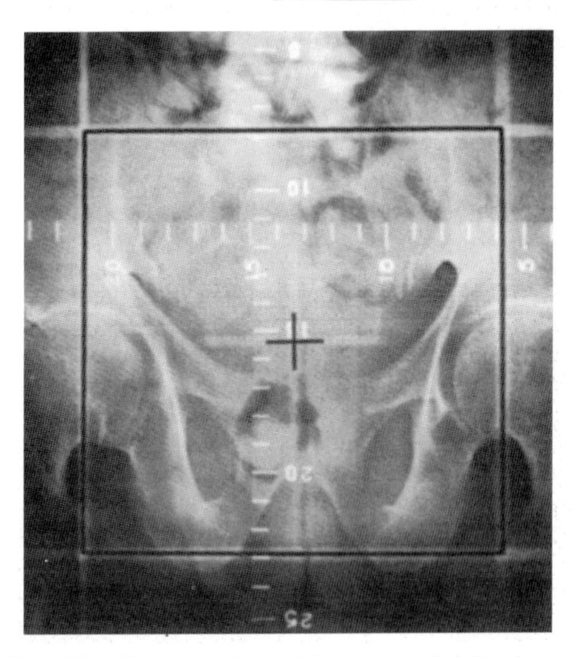

Fig. 25.7 Simulator radiograph (anteroposterior) showing radical treatment volume for carcinoma of the rectum. (Courtesy of Dr J Bolger, Sheffield.)

Anteriorly, a margin should be allowed in front of the anastomosis or the tumour and include, in women, the posterior vaginal wall. The tissues posterior to the sacrum and anterior to the anal orifice should be blocked on the lateral field (Fig. 25.8). The block on the caudal area anterior to the anal margin should be omitted if the tumour lies in the lower anterior part of the rectum.

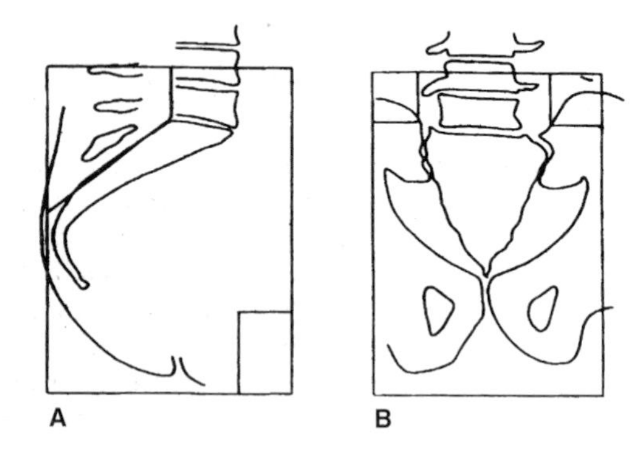

Fig. 25.8 Blocking tissues posterior to the sacrum and anterior to the anal margin. (Reproduced from Frykholm et al, International Journal of Radiation Oncology, Biology, Physics, 1996, 35: 1040; with permission from Elsevier Science.)

Technique

The patient is simulated in the prone position with the toes together and the heels apart, the head resting on the hands. A four-field box or three-field (direct posterior field and two lateral or posterior oblique fields) technique is recommended (Fig. 25.9). These have the advantage over a parallel-opposed pair of anterior and posterior fields that the dose to the bladder and small bowel is reduced. Lateral fields give a much sharper fall-off in dose anteriorly compared with posterior oblique fields. The latter give a more rounded dose distribution anteriorly. If the bladder or anterior abdominal wall is infiltrated, an anterior and posterior opposed pair of fields should be used.

For perineal lesions, a direct posterior field is preferred.

Dose and energy

50 Gy in 20 daily fractions over 4 weeks (9–10 MV photons)

Acute and late reactions. Proctocolitis and cystitis occur as described on page 475.

The risk of intestinal obstruction is dependent on total dose and volume irradiated. If the field is confined to the dorsal part of the pelvic cavity, the risk of

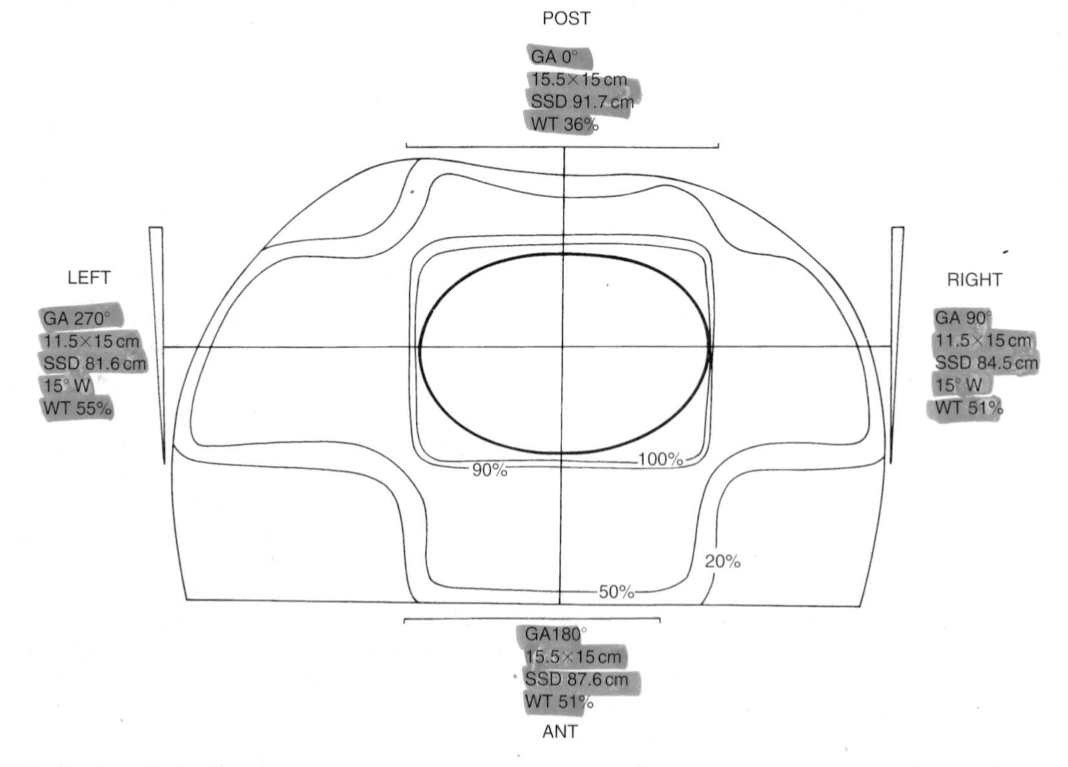

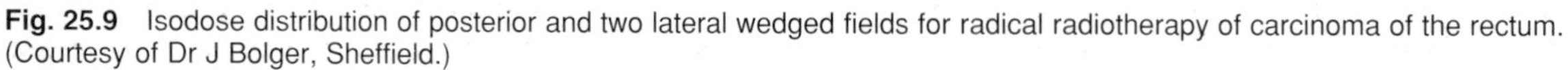

Fig. 25.9 Isodose distribution of posterior and two lateral wedged fields for radical radiotherapy of carcinoma of the rectum. (Courtesy of Dr J Bolger, Sheffield.)

small bowel obstruction is 5–10% compared to 30–40% where the beam extends further proximally into the abdomen. Chronic diarrhoea is common with radical postoperative radiotherapy.

Palliative radiotherapy

The indications for palliative radiotherapy are:

- Bleeding
- Pain
- Rectal discharge.

Target volume

This should include the primary tumour and the whole pelvis.

Technique

A parallel-opposed pair of anterior and posterior fields is used.

Dose and energy

20 Gy in 5 daily fractions or 30 Gy in 10 daily fractions (9–10 MV photons)

Chemotherapy

Adjuvant. Recurrences for colorectal cancer tends to occur in the liver, lung and bone. For this reason adjuvant chemotherapy has a good rationale. Although 80% of patient will have had a complete resection of the tumours, 50% of these patients will develop metastases. The aim of adjuvant chemotherapy is to eradicate micrometastases. The mainstay of adjuvant chemotherapy has been 5-fluorouracil. Its mechanism of action is discussed in Chapter 34 (p. 615). The administration of folinic acid with 5-fluorouracil is recommended since folinic acid increases the amount of inhibition of thymidylate synthase, reduces cellular thymidine and causes apoptosis. In principle, adjuvant chemotherapy should be started as soon as possible after surgery, since the removal of the primary may theoretically stimulate the growth of micrometastases inhibited by the presence of the primary tumour.

5-FU was initially combined with levamisole because of the latter drug's immunostimulatory properties.

A trial which randomised patients to surgery alone, surgery plus levamisole, or surgery plus 5-FU plus levamisole for colon cancer showed a 41% reduction of recurrence and 33% risk of mortality in patients treated by levamisole plus 5-fluorouracil compared to surgery alone. Subsequent trials have, however, shown no advantage of the addition of levamisole over 5-FU alone. Other trials have shown improved survival and reduced risk of recurrence by combining 5-FU with folinic acid, reducing the odds of death by 25–30% and improving survival by 5–6%. A meta-analysis of unconfounded randomised trials of adjuvant chemotherapy showed a 6–7% absolute survival advantage in adjuvant chemotherapy compared to surgery alone. Normally 5-FU is given as bolus infusion on 5 consecutive days every 4 weeks. Common side-effects are nausea and vomiting, mucositis and desquamation of the palms of the hands and soles of the feet. Optimum duration of therapy is uncertain but 6 months of therapy seems to be as effective as 12 months.

The value of adjuvant chemotherapy in patients at lower risk of relapse (e.g. Dukes' B carcinoma of the colon) is uncertain. There is inadequate evidence to support the use of chemotherapy except in Dukes' C carcinoma of the colon. It is possible that there may be benefits in subgroups of Dukes' B (e.g. patients with other risk factors for recurrence—vascular invasion, perforation or poorly differentiated tumours) but this has not been proven.

Rectal cancer. At present there is no good evidence of the value of adjuvant chemotherapy in carcinoma of the rectum.

For locally advanced and metastatic disease. 5-fluorouracil-containing chemotherapy provides better survival (by 3–6 months) compared to best supportive care, and better quality of life from early institution of treatment before symptoms developed. The addition of folinic acid doubles response but does not improve survival. High-dose infusional combinations tend to give better responses than bolus regimes. Infusional chemotherapy with 5-fluorouracil has marginal survival advantages over bolus therapy.

Ralidtrexed is a quinazoline antifolate that inhibits thymidylate synthase. At a dose of 3 mg/m^2 given 3- weekly, it shows similar response rates to bolus fluorouracil and folinic acid (daily for 5 days every 3 weeks) but causes less toxicity with less mucositis and neutropenia. Oxaliplatin is a platinum analogue which in combination with fluorouracil and folinic acid improves response rate and progression-free survival. The principal toxicity of oxaliplatin is neurotoxicity.

For colorectal cancer that is resistant to 5-FU, irinotecan, a DNA topoisomerase 1 inhibitor, has a response rate of 11% and a median duration of response of 6 months. In the absence of previous chemotherapy, the response rate ranges from 25–30%. Side-effects include diarrhoea, neutropenia and alopecia. It offers a modest 2–3 months' survival advantage over best supportive care.

Hepatic arterial chemotherapy for metastatic disease. Regional chemotherapy has been considered for patients who relapse in the liver alone after a resection with curative intent. Fluorouracil and its derivative fluorodeoxyuridine undergo significant arterial extraction and are therefore well suited for intra-arterial chemotherapy. However, while response rates are doubled by this form of treatment, there is only a slim survival advantage.

5-fluorouracil is currently the best choice since it is the least toxic and has a response rate of about 20%, which is as good as more toxic single-agent or combination chemotherapy.

Results of treatment

5-year survival is 80% for Dukes' A, 60% for Dukes' B and 25% for Dukes' C cancers of the colon and rectum.

About 30% of patients will obtain complete relief of their symptoms from palliative radiotherapy and a further 45% partial relief. Average duration of relief is 6–12 months.

Follow-up

Although about 3–10% of patients may have potentially surgically salvageable local relapse, routine screening tests for recurrence such as tumour markers (e.g. carcinoembryonic antigen [CEA]), chest radiograph and ultrasound do not show evidence of improving outcomes. However, larger trials are needed to compare more and less intensive policies of follow-up. 3-monthly follow-up in the first year and 6-monthly follow-up up to 5 years, and then discharge at 5 years seems a reasonable policy in the absence of more definitive data.

CARCINOID TUMOUR

Carcinoid tumours are neuroendocrine in origin deriving from enterochromaffin cells (also known as Kulchitsky cells). Embryologically they are thought to originate from the primitive foregut, midgut or hindgut. These are rare tumours with an incidence of about 10 per million population.

Pathology

These tumours are solid and yellow in colour owing to their high fat content. Microscopically the cells are uniform with granular cytoplasm and round nuclei with few mitoses. Enterochromaffin cells are so called because they stain with potassium chromate. They are also termed argentaffin cells because they take and reduce silver. The ability of the tumour to synthesise 5-hydroxytryptamine from tryptophan in the diet is pathognomonic. Carcinoid tumours are associated with multiple endocrine neoplasia type 1 (MEN-1) in approximately 10% of cases.

Clinical features

Carcinoid syndrome describes the clinical features related to the release of hormones directly into the circulation, usually due to metastases in the liver. Typical symptoms are flushing and diarrhoea and less frequently wheezing, pellagra and valvular dysfunction of the heart (mainly the tricuspid and less commonly the pulmonary heart diseases). Carcinoid crisis describes the occurrence of hypertension, tachycardia and arrhthymias, wheezing and CNS abnormalities. Such crises may be precipitated by anaesthetics or interventional procedures. The cause is thought to be the release of substantial quantities of amines into the bloodstream.

Investigation

The diagnosis can be made by measuring the 24-hour urine 5-hydroxyindoleacetic acid. Plasma levels of chromogranin A are raised in 80% of cases. Neuron-specific enolase, an isomer of a glycolytic enzyme originating in neuroendocrine cells, is increased in approximately 40% of cases but is less specific than chromogranin A.

The form of imaging depends on the site of the tumour. While carcinoid tumours in the stomach or intestine are best seen by endoscopy, endoscopic ultrasound is the most useful. CT and barium studies are helpful for polypoid lesions in the stomach and duodenum. CT and MRI can show thoracic carcinoids greater than 1–2 cm in size. Scintigraphy with labelled somatostatin can be used to detect the primary tumour or metastases, since carcinoid expresses a variety of neuroendocrine peptide receptors.

Treatment

Surgery is the sole means of curing carcinoid tumours. Resection of the tumour and clearance of the regional lymph nodes is the treatment of choice. Debulking surgery may be helpful to overcome mechanical obstruction and may improve survival. Liver transplantation for metastatic carcinoid can be successful. Actuarial 5-year survival for transplanted patients is 69%.

Patients should be advised to avoid alcohol, spicy foods and vigorous exercise which may precipitate symptoms. Expert advice should be sought to supervise treatment. Octreotide, a somatostatin analogue, is the most effective symptomatic treatment. It improves flushing in more than 70% of patients and diarrhoea in more than 60%. It may also achieve tumour shrinkage in some cases. The initial dose is 50 μg three times a week. This is gradually increased to 200 μg three times daily. Long-term use can cause steatorrhoea. Intravenous therapy can be used to prevent or treat carcinoid crisis. Lanreotide, a long-acting somatostatin analogue is given in a dose of 30 mg as an intramuscular injection. Chemotherapy is of limited value. The commonest regime is a combination of streptozotocin and fluorouracil or cyclophosphamide. It may result in tumour shrinkage in 30% of patients but responses are transient. Interferon given alone or in combination with fluorouracil may result in a biochemical response in 50%, but only in 10–20% does tumour regress.

Flushing and 5-hydroxyindoleacetic acid levels can be reduced by embolisation of the hepatic artery in patients with liver metastases in up to 80% of patients. Tumour bulk may be reduced and median survival in some reports may be up to 2 years. Hepatic artery embolisation may precipitate carcinoid crisis and should be prevented by prophylactic treatment by somatostatin. There is some mortality to the procedure but less than the 9% in early experience.

ANAL CANCER

Anatomy

The anal canal (Fig. 25.10) runs downwards and backwards to the anal orifice and is 3–4 cm long. The lower half is lined by squamous epithelium and the upper half by columnar epithelium. The walls are composed of an internal sphincter of involuntary muscle and an external sphincter of voluntary muscle.

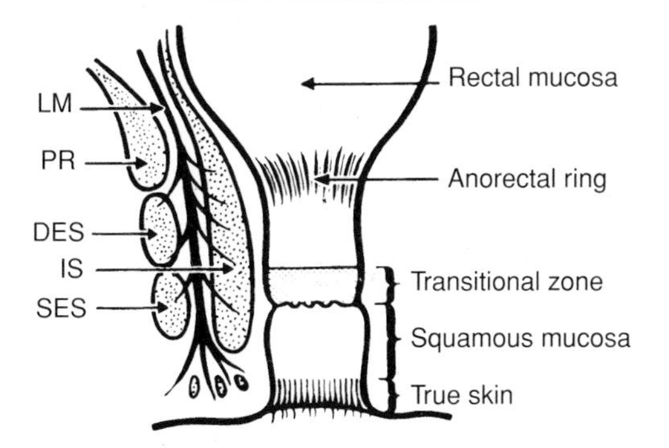

Fig. 25.10 Anatomy of the anal canal. LM = longitudinal muscle, PR = puborectalis, DES = deep part of the external sphincter, IS = internal sphincter, SES = superficial part of the external sphincter. (Reproduced with permission from Scott, An Aid to Clinical Surgery, Churchill Livingstone, 1977.)

Carcinomas of the upper half are adenocarcinomas and of the lower half squamous carcinomas. The lymphatic drainage of both halves is also different. The upper half drains to the lumbar nodes and the lower half to the inguinal nodes.

Pathology

Anal cancer accounts for only about 5% of large bowel cancer. The incidence seems to be rising in the UK. Although most cases occur without any obvious predisposing factors, a few develop in association with AIDS. There is a higher incidence in homosexual men, probably related to human papilloma virus infection. Most occur between the ages of 55 and 65. The majority of tumours of the anal margin are in men and of the canal in women. The tumour usually appears as an ulcer. It may extend up into the rectum or below to the perineal skin. The majority are squamous cell carcinomas (Fig. 25.11). A distinctive tumour of this area is the cloacogenic carcinoma; it has a lower metastatic potential than squamous carcinoma.

Clinical features

The commonest symptoms are bleeding, anal pain and itching (pruritus ani). Benign fistulae, warts and leucoplakia are commonly also present.

Diagnosis and investigation

An examination of the anus and pelvis under general anaesthesia determines the local extent of the tumour.

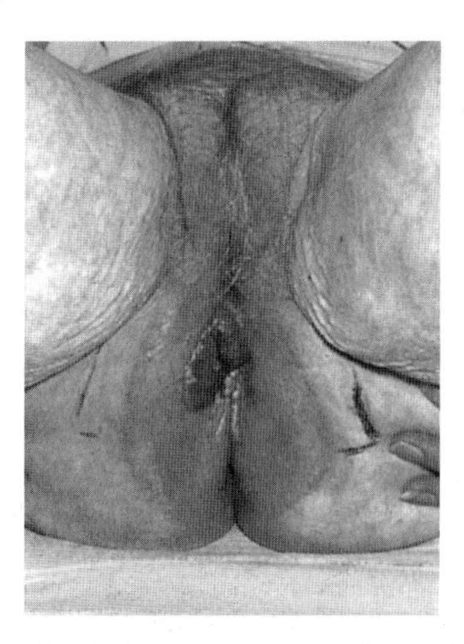

Fig. 25.11 Exophytic squamous cell carcinoma of the anal margin.

A biopsy is taken. A CT scan of the pelvis is helpful in determining the local extent and whether or not the presacral and iliac nodes are involved.

Staging

Staging is according to the UICC TNM classification (Table 25.5).

Treatment

The main treatments are radical surgery or radiotherapy, and, more recently, adjuvant chemotherapy. The management of this condition is controversial. Radical surgery (abdominoperineal excision) was the treatment for all squamous cell carcinomas except for superficial ones which could be implanted. It is increasingly appreciated that external beam irradiation and interstitial irradiation, alone or in combination, can be curative.

Table 25.5 TNM staging of anal cancer

Stage	Clinical findings
Anal canal	
Primary tumour	
T1	Tumour extending not more than one-third of the circumference or length of the anal canal and not infiltrating the external sphincter muscle
T2	Tumour occupying more than one-third of the circumference or length of the anal canal or infiltrating the anal sphincter
T3	Tumour extending to the rectum or skin but not to other neighbouring structures
T4	Tumour infiltrating neighbouring structures
Nodes	
N0	No involvement of regional nodes
N1	Involvement of mesorectal and/or inguinal nodes
Anal margin	
Primary tumour	
T1	Tumour 2 cm or less in greatest dimension, strictly superficial or exophytic
T2	Tumour greater than 2 cm and up to 5 cm in largest dimension or tumour with minimal infiltration of the dermis
T3	Tumour more than 5 cm in its greatest dimension or tumour with deep infiltration of the dermis
T4	Tumour with extension to muscle or bone, etc.
Nodes	
N0	No evidence of regional lymph node spread
N1	Mobile unilateral regional nodes
N2	Mobile bilateral regional nodes
N3	Fixed regional nodes

Surgery

Local excision is possible for superficial tumours less than 2 cm in diameter (10%). The local recurrence rate is, however, high at 40%. Abdominoperineal excision with a permanent colostomy is then required. Radical surgery can be used to deal with persistent or locally recurrent tumour following radical radiotherapy.

Radiotherapy

Radical radiotherapy using external beam with or without interstitial implantation offers a good alternative curative technique for selected tumours. It has the advantage over radical surgery that the anal sphincter can be preserved, with much lower morbidity and mortality. Treatment technique is influenced by the site, local extent and presence of regional lymph node spread.

Implantation alone is recommended for superficial T1 and T2 tumours fulfilling the following criteria:

1. Lie below the anorectal ring
2. Occupy less than 50% of the anal circumference
3. Are 1 cm or less in thickness
4. No involvement of regional nodes.

Because of the poor tolerance of the perineal region to radical doses (e.g. 50 Gy), a good compromise is to give a preliminary subradical course of external beam irradiation to the primary and posterior pelvis, followed by an interstitial implant.

An alternative is to give external beam alone to a radical dose, but there is a greater risk (10–20%) of causing an anal stricture requiring surgery than with implant alone.

Palliative radiotherapy for advanced anal carcinoma is not recommended since it is rarely effective.

External beam

Target volume

This should cover the primary tumour and the anal canal, the pararectal, hypogastric and obturator nodes (Fig. 25.12). The inferior margin should lie below the anal verge. The superior margin should be at the level of the bottom of the sacroiliac joints. The lateral margins allow coverage of the internal iliac nodes. The posterior margin includes the sacrum and the disease anterior to it.

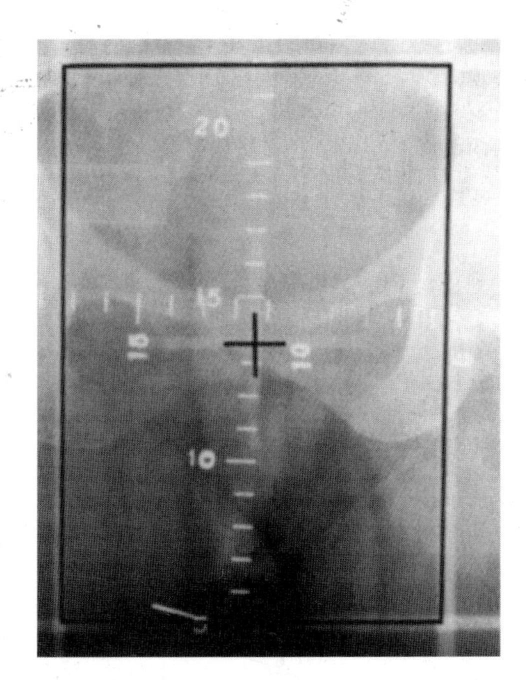

Fig. 25.12 Simulator radiograph (anteroposterior) showing radical treatment volume for carcinoma of the anal canal. (Courtesy of Dr J Bolger, Sheffield.)

Technique

The patient is simulated prone. Some barium is instilled into the rectum to outline the anus and lower rectum. In a first phase of treatment, the volume is irradiated by a parallel-opposed pair of fields. In the second phase a direct posterior perineal and two wedged posterior oblique fields are used (Fig. 25.13). Angles of less than 45° for the posterior oblique fields should not be used to avoid excessive skin reaction in the natal cleft. Bolus is applied over the perineum to bring up the dose to the skin. This technique gives less dose to the small bowel than would be the case with an anterior and posterior parallel-opposed pair of fields.

Dose and energy

Preimplant

30 Gy given in 15 fractions over 3 weeks (9–10 MV photons)

External beam alone

50 Gy in 20 daily fractions over 4 weeks (9–10 MV photons)

Interstitial implantation. Interstitial implantation alone with iridium-192 (Figs 22.10 and 22.11) wire is recommended for patients with T1 or T2 tumours of the anal margin or canal. The technique for implantation is described on page 342. The boost dose is 20–25 Gy.

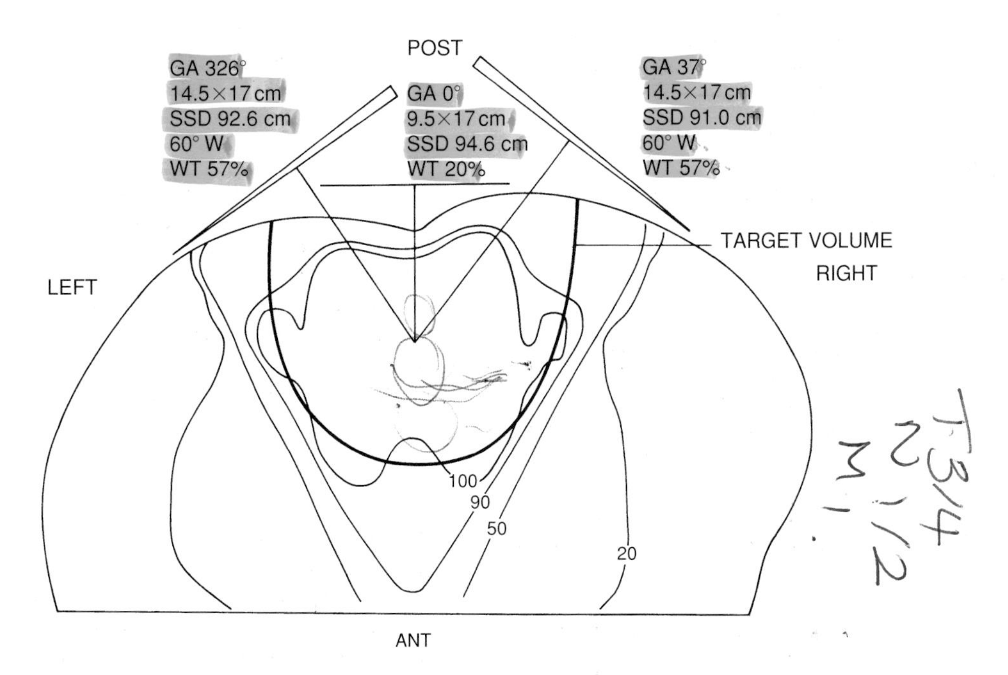

Fig. 25.13 Isodose distribution of direct posterior and posterior oblique wedged fields for radical radiotherapy of carcinoma of the anus. (Courtesy of Dr J Bolger, Sheffield.)

Radiation reaction

External beam. The acute reaction of moist desquamation is very uncomfortable. Analgesia is often required. Mucous rectal discharge is frequent. An antidiarrhoeal agent such as loperamide normally controls this. The acute reaction has normally settled by the third week after the end of treatment.

Implant. The acute local reaction of moist desquamation is mild and has normally settled within 3 weeks.

Complications

Radiation necrosis. Soft tissue necrosis usually settles with conservative measures such as the daily application of gentian violet. Excision is required for persistent necrosis. Anal stricture occurs rarely.

Inguinal nodes. If inguinal nodes are enlarged and mobile, the treatment is block dissection. Fixed nodes are inoperable and respond poorly to radiotherapy. Palliative radiotherapy should be reserved for pain and ulceration.

Technique

A direct field to the groin(s) with skin bolus.

Dose and energy

30 Gy in 10 daily fractions (cobalt-60 or 4–6 MV photons)

Chemotherapy

A UK trial has shown that combining radiotherapy concurrently with chemotherapy (intravenous 5-fluorouracil and mitomycin C) improves the local tumour response compared with radiotherapy alone. This chemoradiation approach is recommended for fit patients.

Results of treatment

The 5-year local control rate achieved by radical radiotherapy and radical surgery are similar. The results of radiotherapy are better in the anal canal, with a 5-year local control rate of 80%. 5-year survival following surgery is 50–60% for the anal canal and 65–75% for the anal margin.

CANCER OF THE LUNG

Lung cancer (bronchogenic carcinoma) is the commonest cause of death from cancer in men and the second commonest in women. There are 40 000 new cases in the UK per year and 175 000 per year in the USA. In Scotland the mortality from lung cancer exceeds that of breast cancer. The annual death rate of 40 000 in the UK indicates the scale of the problem. Overall it accounts for 35% of male and 15% of female cancer deaths. There has been a modest fall in the mortality in men but a continued rise in women. This rise is related to an increase in smoking among women. Over the last two decades there has been little change in the 5-year survival for lung cancer, with most patients dying within a year of the diagnosis. The highest age incidence is 45–65 years. The male : female ratio is 5 : 1.

Pathology

Aetiology

In the early part of this century lung cancer was relatively rare. Environmental factors (Ch. 16) are clearly at work in industrial situations, e.g. mining and factories with exposure, for example, to asbestos, nickel and chrome. There is overwhelming evidence that cigarette smoking is the main cause in up to 90% of cases of lung cancer. Cigars and pipes are much less dangerous. The risk is related to the number of cigarettes smoked. For example, the risk of developing lung cancer in a person who smokes 25 or more cigarettes per day is 25–30 times that of a non-smoker. Despite widespread antismoking campaigns in many countries, the incidence of lung cancer is likely to rise over the next half century with an increasing number of cases being caused not by smoking but by other environmental pollutants.

Molecular factors in the development of lung cancer

It is estimated that 10–20 genetic events are needed to transform a normal lung cell into a malignant one. These mutations result in the activation of oncogenes and removal of tumour suppressor genes. These genetic modifications lead to pathological changes initially with bronchial metaplasia proceeding successively to bronchial dysplasia, in situ carcinoma, invasive carcinoma and metastatic cancer. The development of cancer is not simply due to loss of growth control but to defects in the cell's control of programmed cell death (apoptosis). Factors which control apoptosis include growth factors, cytokines and hormones.

Prevention is an important element in the strategy to reduce mortality from lung cancer. Raising public awareness particularly among schoolchildren, restrictions on advertising cigarettes, banning cigarette smoking in public places and increased taxation of cigarettes all have a part to play. It is encouraging that if a smoker gives up the habit, the risk of developing lung cancer diminishes markedly, but the risk after stopping smoking for 20 years is still two to three times that of someone who has never smoked. Early onset of smoking, high tar content of the cigarettes and long duration of smoking all increase the risk of lung cancer. Passive smoking also increases the risk of lung cancer, albeit to a lesser degree, for example in the non-smoking wives of husbands who smoke.

Macroscopic and microscopic features

The majority of cancers (55%) arise near the root of the lung, close to a main bronchus; 40% are peripheral; about 5% are multifocal or indeterminate. If a bronchus becomes completely blocked, the lung beyond the obstruction will collapse and is prone to infection.

There are four main histological types. The commonest is squamous carcinoma (50%), with varying degrees of anaplasia. A special variety is oat cell carcinoma (20%): small slightly elongated, darkly staining cells with a fanciful resemblance to oat grains. In other respects these cells are anaplastic. 20% are large cell carcinomas (an unsatisfactory designation of undifferentiated tumours) and 10% adenocarcinomas.

Spread

Spread is local, lymphatic and blood-borne. Direct extension can occur to adjacent lung, pericardium and heart, oesophagus and chest wall including ribs. Pleural involvement may cause a pleural effusion, often blood-stained. Lymphatic spread is to adjacent nodes (Fig. 25.14) and later to nodes above the clavicle

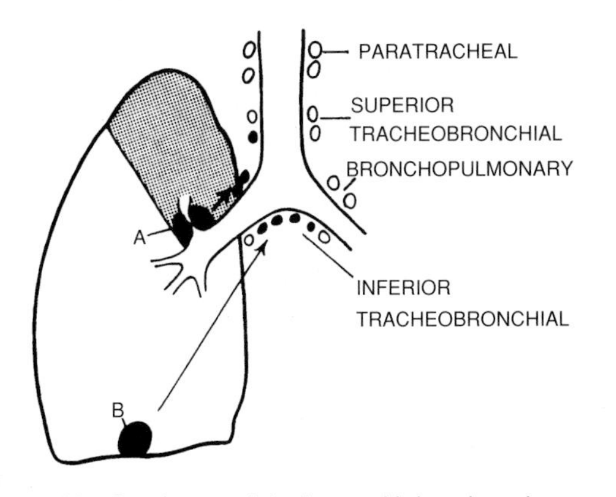

Fig. 25.14 Carcinoma of the lung, with lymph node distribution. **A** Central tumour causing bronchial occlusion and peripheral pulmonary collapse. **B** Peripheral tumour. (Reproduced with permission from Jayne, in Macfarlane, Textbook of Surgery, Churchill Livingstone.)

and occasionally to the axilla. Blood spread may be early and wide, to liver, skin, bone and brain. Metastatic spread is particularly common in small cell (oat cell) lung carcinoma, occurring in up to 80% at presentation.

Clinical features

The tumour may be silent for years and may only be discovered incidentally when a chest radiograph is taken for some other reason, or at mass radiography. Symptoms arise in various ways.

Respiratory

The commonest symptom is persistent cough. When the tumour ulcerates through the bronchial wall, the sputum becomes blood-stained (haemoptysis). Shortness of breath (dyspnoea) arises due to obstruction of the large or small airways, impairing lung function. Very severe dyspnoea and noisy main airway obstruction (stridor) may occur. Occasionally lung cancer may present as a chest infection which fails to resolve with antibiotic therapy. This is because infected material cannot be adequately cleared from beyond the blocked bronchus.

Invasion of adjacent structures

Pain may arise from invasion of the mediastinum or chest wall. Growths at the apex of the lung may cause pain radiating to shoulder and arm, classically in the distribution of the first thoracic nerve (T1) from involvement of the brachial nerve plexus. This clinical variety is the superior sulcus or Pancoast tumour (Fig. 25.15). This causes weakness of the hand grip and Horner's syndrome due to involvement of the sympathetic chain.

Involvement of the recurrent laryngeal nerve may cause vocal cord palsy with hoarseness.

Pressure on the great veins in the upper mediastinum, including the superior vena cava, leads to *mediastinal obstruction* (Fig. 25.19), with swelling of the head, neck and upper limbs, and engorgement of the veins of the neck. The veins of the chest wall become dilated due to the development of a collateral circulation. Pressure on the oesophagus can cause dysphagia.

Lymphatic and distant metastases

The first sign may come from a metastasis while the primary lung lesion is silent. Supraclavicular and axillary nodes may be palpable. Common sites of distant

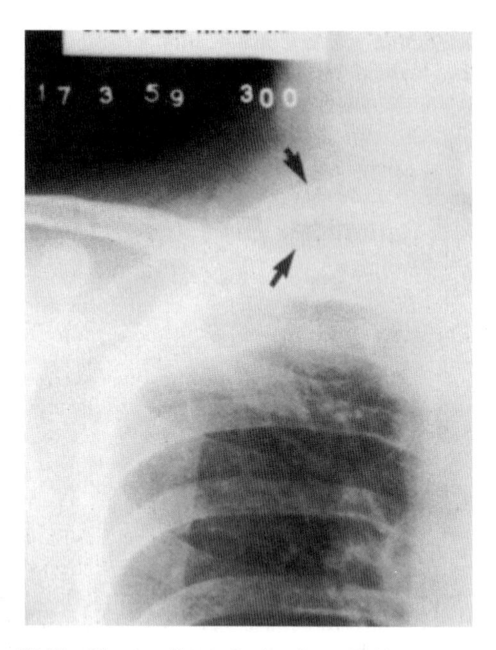

Fig. 25.15 Chest radiograph showing a Pancoast tumour of the right apex destroying the 1st rib (arrows). (Courtesy of Dr R Nakielny, Sheffield.)

metastases are the brain (raised intracranial pressure, change of personality), bone (pain, pathological fracture), liver (anorexia, weight loss, jaundice), skin (subcutaneous nodules). Metastases occasionally occur in the choroid of the eye (Plate 2.10).

General and non-metastatic effects

These include anaemia and lassitude. In addition certain non-metastatic effects may occur due to ectopic production from the tumour of chemical substances with endocrine effects. This occurs in all histological types but particularly with small cell lung cancer. These non-metastatic effects are described in Chapter 38.

Diagnosis and staging

Early detection of lung cancer is important but as yet no method of screening for lung cancer has been proven to reduced the mortality of the disease (see p. 267). Studies using chest radiographs have been ineffective. However, the availability of spiral CT scanning has changed the staging of lung cancer in several studies.

Basic investigations include a chest radiograph, sputum cytology, full blood count and liver function tests.

Chest radiograph. After full clinical examination, a chest radiograph almost always provides suggestive evidence. This may show a discrete tumour mass or enlarged nodes at the lung hilum or in the mediastinum. There is often a varying degree of lung collapse. Pleural effusions, rib metastases or a raised hemidiaphragm (due to phrenic nerve paralysis) are common. Central necrosis within the tumour is particularly associated with squamous cell carcinoma.

Tomography and CT scanning (see below) often define the tumour more precisely where the chest radiograph is equivocal.

Sputum cytology. Microscopy of the sputum (cytology) may show malignant or atypical cells. The latter are inadequate for a firm diagnosis of lung cancer.

Bronchoscopy. Flexible bronchoscopy under local anaesthesia is the next step. Tumour is visible in 60% of cases and a biopsy should be obtained. Bronchial washings from abnormal areas of the bronchial mucosa may show malignant cells.

Percutaneous biopsy. A direct percutaneous biopsy under radiological control may yield the diagnosis if bronchoscopy does not, particularly in peripheral tumours.

Mediastinoscopy. If there is a mediastinal mass and bronchoscopy is negative or radical surgery is contemplated, a mediastinoscopy to obtain tissue is advised. Involvement of mediastinal glands contraindicates radical surgery.

CT scanning and ultrasound. CT scanning may help establish the diagnosis when there are equivocal appearances on a chest radiograph (e.g. distinguishing a hilar mass from pulmonary vessels). It may also demonstrate mediastinal nodes. Nodes larger than 1.5 cm are likely to be malignant. Pulmonary deposits not visible on plain radiography may be demonstrated. Abdominal scanning may show lymphadenopathy, liver and adrenal metastases. When brain metastases are suspected, particularly in small cell lung cancer, CT is more reliable than isotope scanning.

Abdominal ultrasound is useful for the detection of liver metastases. If liver function tests are abnormal but a liver ultrasound is negative, a CT scan should be requested to exclude liver metastases.

Ultrasound is also helpful in determining the site of pleural effusions, especially if loculated, if initial aspiration has been unhelpful.

Positron-emission tomography

Positron-emission tomography (PET scanning) using 18-fluorodeoxyglucose provides greater sensitivity than CT in the detection of malignant lung lesions and mediastinal nodes (Fig. 25.16). Its availability is currently limited in the UK because of the need for a cyclotron to produce the short-lived isotope for the investigation. Selective use of PET scanning can be cost-effective, particularly for the assessment of mediastinal nodes (visible nodes < 1 cm in the short axis) where PET may result in upstaging the mediastinum in up to 50% of cases. The limitation of PET is that, despite its relatively high specificity for positive nodes (about 85%) it does not obviate the need for tissue sampling. A positive PET scan should be used in conjunction with CT scanning to guide tissue sampling of suspicious lesions. PET may detect extrathoracic metastases in 10–15% of patients. Transbronchial aspiration of regional lymph nodes guided by CT and/or PET can enable staging and diagnosis to be carried out at the same time. Use of these techniques should reduce the number of patients with unresectable cancers undergoing radical surgery and provide better selection of suitable cases for curative surgery.

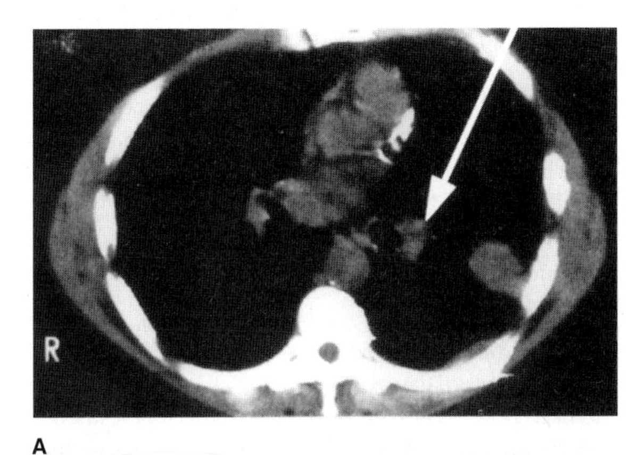

A

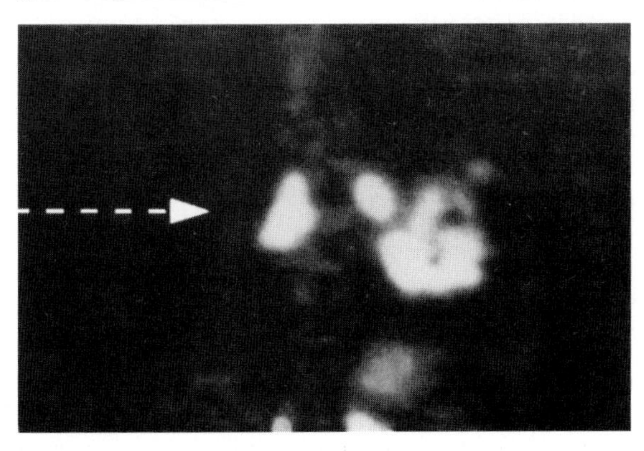

B

Fig. 25.16 **A** CT scan showing left lung mass with associated left hilar adenopathy (arrow). **B** Coronal positron emission tomography showing hypermetabolism indicative of tumour in left lung mass as well as right tracheobronchial nodes (broken arrow) due to large cell undifferentiated tumour. (Reproduced with permission from the Society of Thoracic Surgeons, from Lowe & Naunheim, PET in lung cancer, Annals of Thoracic Surgery, 1998; 65:1821–1829.)

Staging system

The TNM staging system (Table 25.6) is used for pathological types other than small cell (non-small cell lung cancer). These TNM stages are also grouped into the following stages:

Stage I: T1N0M0
T1N1M0
Stage II: T2N0M0
Stage III: Any T3
Any N2
Any M1

Small cell lung cancer. A separate and simpler staging system is widely used for small cell lung cancer since the survival of stages I–III on the TNM system is the same. Patients are divided into two categories: limited and extensive disease. Limited disease is defined as tumour confined to one hemithorax, mediastinum and ipsilateral supraclavicular nodes. Extensive disease is tumour more extensive than the limited stage, with distant metastases, e.g. liver, bone, bone marrow and brain.

Treatment

An important division is made between small cell lung cancer (SCLC)and non-small cell lung cancer (NSCLC)

Table 25.6 TNM staging of non-small cell lung cancer

Stage	Clinical findings
Primary tumour	
T0	Primary tumour not demonstrable
TX	Positive cytology but tumour not demonstrable
T1	Tumour less than 3 cm diameter without proximal invasion
T2	Greater than 3 cm or invading pleura or with collapse of less than a whole lung, more than 2 cm from the carina
T3	Tumour of any size with invasion of the chest wall; or less than 2 cm from the carina; or causing collapse of a whole lung or effusion
Regional nodes	
N0	No demonstrable metastases
N1	Ipsilateral hilar node metastases
N2	Mediastinal metastases
Distant metastases	
M0	No metastases
M1	Metastases present

since their treatments are different. The choice of treatment is based on histology, general condition and extent of disease. In general, surgery and radiotherapy are the mainstay of treatment for non-small cell lung cancer with a limited role for chemotherapy. For small cell lung cancer, chemotherapy is the principal treatment with a limited role for radiotherapy. In the future there may be a role for gene therapy to correct gene defects that lead to lung cancer. It is not certain whether correcting a single mutation in what is a multistage process of carcinogenesis will be adequate. The efficiency of gene transfer must be high to ensure that the genetic defect is corrected in all tumour cells. Currently adenoviruses can achieve gene transfer to just over 50% of cells exposed. Gene mutations which could be targeted include (a) oncogenes mutant epidermal growth factor receptor for NSCLC, and *myc* and *bcl2* for SCLC; (b) tumour suppressor genes (e.g. *p53* for NSCLC and SCLC). Other possible approaches include targeting the vasculature of tumours by creating antibodies to extracellular matrix proteins, so inhibiting new vessel formation.

Small cell lung cancer. Chemotherapy is the treatment of choice for fit patients with small cell lung cancer. Palliative radiotherapy to the primary reduces the incidence of local recurrence but does not increase survival. Surgery is not recommended because of the very high incidence of metastatic disease.

Non-small cell lung cancer. For non-small cell lung cancer, the choice is between radical surgery and radical or palliative radiotherapy. Non-small cell lung cancer is relatively resistant to chemotherapy. Chemotherapy is therefore not recommended for routine treatment.

After full assessment, two vital decisions have to be made:

1. Is the tumour operable?
2. If inoperable, is the patient suitable for radical or palliative radiotherapy or laser therapy?

Surgery

Radical. For non-small cell lung cancer radical surgery offers the best prospect of cure, but is only applicable to about 30% of patients. It should be considered for stage I disease. Removal of the whole lung (pneumonectomy) is necessary if the tumour arises in a mainstem bronchus, if the tumour involves more than one lobe or if the hilum is involved. A more limited removal of a lobe (lobectomy) may otherwise be performed. Adequate general medical condition and pulmonary function is required. Up to one-third of patients with resectable lung cancer are unsuitable for surgery because of concurrent disease or physiological impairment. The upper limits of resectability have been broadened by the use of lung-volume-reduction surgery to relieve dyspnoea and improve airflow in patients with advanced chronic airways disease. Trials have shown the applicability of this surgical technique to highly selected patients with lung cancer. However, the benefits of this technique on survival of patients with lung cancer is likely to be limited because those with severe underlying emphysema may well die of chronic obstructive airways disease rather than cancer.

Contraindications are mediastinal or distant metastases, pleural effusion, vocal cord or phrenic nerve paresis, mediastinal obstruction or tumours within 2 cm of the carina. Patients over the age of 70 are rarely operated on unless they are in very good medical condition.

The operative mortality for pneumonectomy is about 5% and for a lobectomy 2%.

Palliative. Palliative laser therapy can provide rapid relief of dyspnoea and haemoptysis if due to disease in the trachea or main bronchi. The patient is injected with a haematoporphyrin derivative 3 days before the laser source is applied. Local tumour destruction follows rapidly.

Radical radiotherapy

Radical radiotherapy should be considered in patients with localised disease if surgery is contraindicated or refused. It is suitable for less than 5% of patients. Criteria for eligibility are as follows:

- Tumour 5 cm or less in maximum dimension
- T1–3, N0, N1 and limited N2
- Good general medical condition
- Adequate pulmonary function (forced expiratory volume in 1 second at least 1 litre)
- Non-small cell histology.

Contraindications are:

- Recurrent laryngeal or phrenic nerve palsy
- Distant metastases

Target volume

The planned target volume should include the primary and (a) for N1 disease the ipsilateral mediastinal nodes with a 2 cm margin all round, (b) for minimal N2 disease the nodes involved on CT imaging and adjacent mediastinal nodes. The patient is rested for a month. Any patient who shows evidence of local progression, regional spread or metastases during the rest period is excluded from further treatment. In the second half of treatment, the treatment volume is reduced to cover the primary tumour and ipsilateral hilar nodes. For right-sided tumours the volume should include the lymphatics close to the right intermediate bronchus. The field should cross the midline to include the left paratracheal nodes, 1–1.5 cm lateral to the trachea. Left-sided tumours can spread to the contralateral paratracheal nodes, which therefore need to be included in the field.

Technique

The choice of technique will depend on the site of the tumour within the lung. A CT planning scan is helpful in accurate tumour localisation. Otherwise conventional simulation is carried out. Conformal radiotherapy techniques should be considered to limit the size of the target volume if this is likely to exceed 1000 cm^3.

Central tumours. For centrally placed tumours a three-field technique is used (Fig. 25.17) to reduce the dose to the spinal cord. The patient is simulated in the supine position, with the hands behind the head and elbows flexed. The anterior field is simulated and a radiograph taken; the patient is then screened from the side to determine the depth of the field and a lateral radiograph is taken. Care is taken to avoid the spinal cord. The posterior oblique fields are then viewed.

Peripheral tumours. Peripheral tumours in the mid and lower zones of the lung may be treated with a wedged pair of fields (Fig. 25.18).

Tumours at the lung apex of stage II and minimal IIIa should be considered for radical radiotherapy. A shrinking field approach in two phases is recommended. In phase I the volume should include the primary tumour with a 2 cm margin. The whole of the adjacent vertebral body should be included in the initial volume since subclinical infiltration of the neural canal is common. The volume is reduced to exclude the spinal cord after a dose of 40 Gy to give a further 20 Gy in Phase II.

Phase I: 6–10 MV photons 40 Gy midplane dose in 20 fractions over 4 weeks
Phase II: 6–10 MV photons 20 Gy midplane dose in 5 fractions over 1 week

Planning proceeds in the normal way (Ch. 12) with an outline drawing on which the target volume, heart, lungs and spinal cord are plotted. The presence of air in normal lung is a complicating factor in dosage calculation, since depth-dose tables and isodose curves are based on solid tissue. The presence of air decreases the absorption and scatter of radiation and increases the depth dose (on average 3% greater dose per centimetre of lung traversed) compared with solid tissue. If a beam passes through much aerated lung tissue, a correction has to be made to arrive at the true tumour dosage (see radical radiotherapy of the oesophagus, p. 405). For beams passing through the mediastinum, no correction is necessary.

Acute reaction. Both general and local reactions occur. They usually subside within 3–4 weeks of the end of treatment. General reactions are anorexia, nausea and vomiting. The last two symptoms can usually be controlled with simple antiemetics.

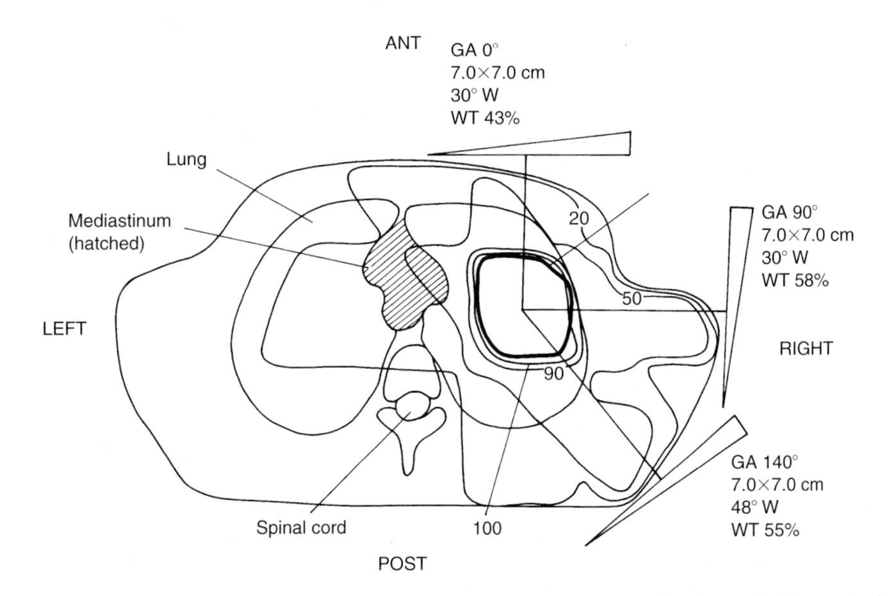

Fig. 25.17 Carcinoma of the right lung. Isodose distribution of three-field technique (9 MV photons). (Courtesy of Dr A Champion, Sheffield.)

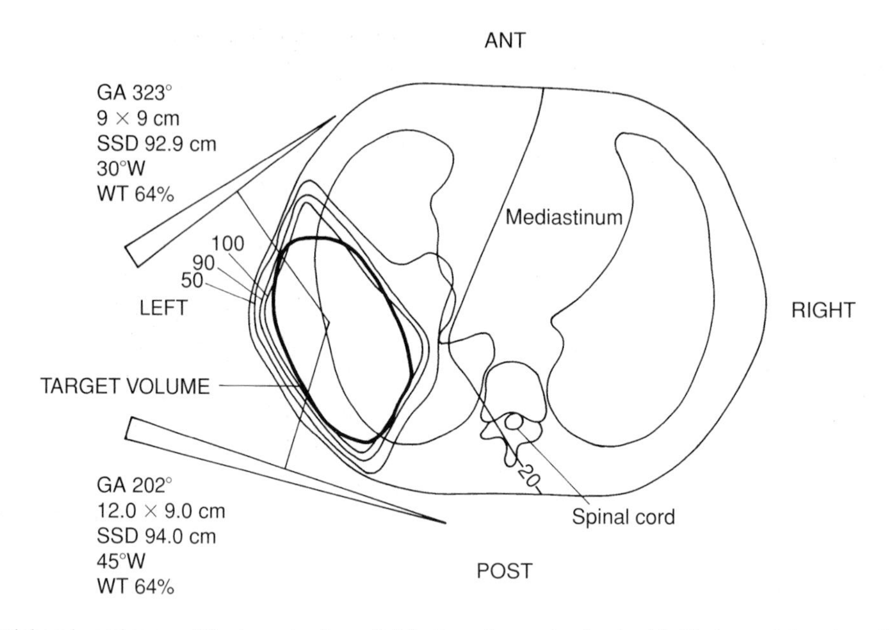

Fig. 25.18 Peripheral carcinoma of the lung. Isodose distribution of a wedged pair of fields for peripheral carcinoma of the lung (6 MV photons). (Courtesy of Dr A Champion, Sheffield.)

Local reactions include tracheitis causing a sore throat and expectoration of mucus and oesophagitis causing dysphagia.

Late reactions. An oesophageal stricture may occur several months after treatment. These rarely occur in patients with a previously normal oesophagus.

Radiation pneumonitis can occur 4–6 weeks after the end of treatment. There is the acute onset of dyspnoea, non-productive cough and chest tightness. There is commonly nothing abnormal to hear on auscultation of the lung fields. Chest X-ray may show a hazy appearance in the treated area. Treatment is with oxygen, broad-spectrum antibiotics and with steroids (prednisolone 60 mg per day). The dose of steroids can be tailed off gradually if there is a response or if there is no improvement within a fortnight. The outcome largely depends on the region and volume of lung irradiated. If the volume is large, the condition may be fatal. The apices of the lung tend to give rise to fewer symptoms since the ventilation and vascular perfusion of the upper lobes is normally less than that of the lower lobes.

Lung fibrosis within the treated volume occurs in virtually all patients but usually does not give rise to symptoms. The degree of fibrosis and the likelihood of dyspnoea is related to the total dose, secondary infection and pre-existing lung disease (e.g. chronic obstructive airways disease or industrial lung disease).

Occasionally there is transient radiation myelitis (Lhermitte's sign, see p. 514) but this usually recovers completely.

Palliative radiotherapy

For bulky stage IIIa, IIIb and IV, palliative radiotherapy is advised for superior sulcus tumours.

6–10 MV photons 3250 cGy midplane dose in 10 daily fractions over 2 weeks

Palliative radiotherapy for lung cancer

External radiotherapy is helpful in relieving symptoms from local and metastatic disease. An alternative is endobronchial irradiation with a single fraction of high dose rate brachytherapy from an afterloading machine (*microSelectron*, see p. 337). This seems to have equivalent efficacy to external beam but is currently available in only a limited number of centres.

In general, treatment should be withheld until symptoms develop since there is no evidence that palliative radiotherapy alters survival in non-small cell lung cancer. In practice some asymptomatic patients may find it difficult to accept that they will not immediately receive treatment. In these circumstances it may be helpful to reassure the patient that he or she can be seen at short notice if symptoms develop, and treatment promptly instituted, if appropriate.

Symptoms of local disease such as dyspnoea, haemoptysis, dysphagia and mediastinal pain usually improve during or within a few weeks of treatment. Haemoptysis is relieved in 80% of cases, and cough, dyspnoea and chest pain in 50% of cases. Pleural effusions and laryngeal and phrenic nerve palsy rarely respond. The treatment of pleural effusion is described in Chapter 38.

Mediastinal obstruction (Fig. 25.19) completely resolves in 50% of cases and partially in an additional 30%. No response is obtained in 20%.

Good symptomatic responses to external beam therapy can be obtained in most patients with bone, skin or brain metastases.

The response of *spinal cord compression* (p. 555) is influenced by the histological type and the degree and duration of pretreatment neurological deficit. Complete paraplegia with loss of bladder function, whatever the histology, rarely responds. Patients with small cell lung cancer respond better than those with non-small cell disease as long as there is moderate retention of motor power.

Target volume

For local disease, the tumour plus a generous margin of several centimetres should be included (Fig. 25.20). Typical field sizes are 12 × 10 cm. For treatment of bone metastases, see page 553; brain metastases, see page 540; spinal cord compression, see page 554; and skin nodules, page 334.

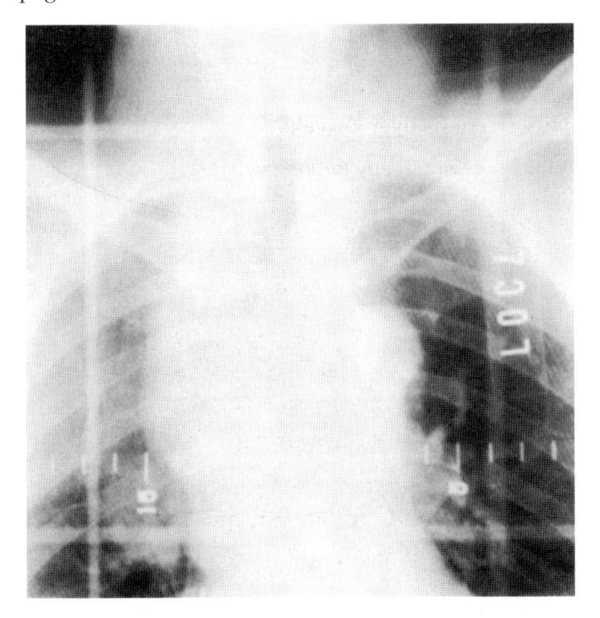

Fig. 25.19 Simulator radiograph showing field margins for palliative radiotherapy of superior mediastinal obstruction. Note widening of the superior mediastinum.

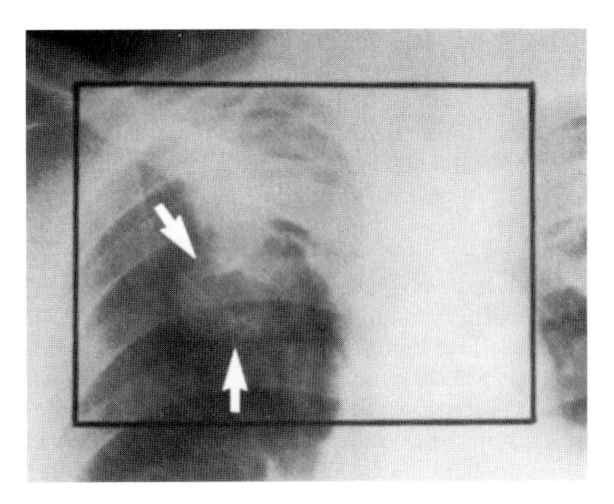

Fig. 25.20 Simulator radiograph showing typical field margins for palliative treatment of carcinoma of the right upper lobe.

Technique

For locoregional disease, anterior and posterior opposed fields are used. The techniques for brain and bone metastases are described on pages 556 and 580.

Dose and energy

1. *For patients with poor performance status (WHO grade 2 or greater)*

10 Gy midplane dose in a single fraction

2. *For patients with better performance status (WHO grade 0–2)*

39 Gy midplane dose in 13 daily fractions (limiting spinal cord dose to 35 Gy by introducing 2 cm wide block on posterior field for 4 of the fractions)

3. *For patients not suitable for 39 Gy in 13 fractions (volume too large or stage IV)*

17 Gy midplane dose in 2 fractions 6–8 days apart

Radiation reaction. Radiation oesophagitis develops after treatment. It is usually mild and transient.

Photodynamic therapy in palliation

Photodynamic therapy (PDT) has been shown to provide comparable benefits to laser therapy in partially obstructing advanced oesophageal cancer. The response is slightly higher with PDT and the duration of response longer lasting (32% vs 20% at 1 month). In some subgroups responses were higher than with laser therapy, e.g. in the upper and lower oesophagus and in tumours larger than 10 cm. There was no difference in median survival compared to laser therapy. About 19% of patients treated with PDT experienced mild sunburn reactions. PDT appeared to be better tolerated and easier to perform than laser therapy, particularly at sites where the morphology of the tumour or its site made laser therapy difficult.

Laser or photodynamic therapy may assist in palliative tumour debulking in both early and advanced non-small cell lung cancer.

PDT is well suited to the treatment of early stage lung cancer. In lung tumours measuring less than 2 cm the risk of lymph node metastases is low. It has the advantage that it preserves lung function and can be repeated if needed. Non-randomised studies show a complete response rate of the order of 95% for lesions less than 0.5 cm. Response rates are lower (37%) for lesions greater than 2 cm.

For locally advanced NSCLC, tumour response is similar with both modalities but relief of dyspnoea, cough and haemoptysis is superior with PDT than with laser therapy. Side-effects were similar with both treatments. If PDT is combined with radiotherapy, a higher rate of reopening of the airway (70%) was achieved compared to radiotherapy alone (10%).

Systemic therapy for advanced or metastatic disease

The role of chemotherapy for non-small cell lung cancer remains controversial. A meta-analysis shows that platinum-based chemotherapy improves outcomes at any stage of the disease. It is not known whether it should be given preoperatively in a neoadjuvant setting or after surgery or radiotherapy. This is the subject of a current UK trial.

Results of treatment

The results of treatment of non-small cell lung cancer are poor. The best results are obtained with surgery. Results of 'curative' resection are largely influenced by criteria for selection. Overall 5-year survival is 25–30%. For stage I disease it is about 55%, for stage II 25% and for stage III 15%. For photodynamic therapy of early stage lung cancer, 5-year survival is 65%.

For radical radiotherapy the 5-year survival is 6%. Average survival of patients treated palliatively is about 8 months.

SMALL CELL LUNG CANCER

Chemotherapy

Chemotherapy is the treatment of choice for small cell lung cancer. Combination chemotherapy (two to four drugs) is more effective than single agents in obtaining complete, though usually temporary, remissions, and in prolonging survival. Overall (complete and partial) response rates of 75–90% can be achieved. It must be stressed that these responses are normally of limited duration (about 10 months). No particular combination is optimal. However, platinum with etoposide is one of the most active regimes for limited stage small cell lung cancer, particularly when given concurrently with thoracic irradiation.Typical combinations with response rates of the order of 75% are shown in Table 25.7. Despite this, small cell lung cancer remains largely an incurable disease. Increasing the dose of individual drugs does not seem to overcome drug resistance,

Table 25.7 Chemotherapy regimes for small cell lung cancer

Regime	Day
PE	
Cisplatin: 60–90 mg/m^2 i.v. on day 1, given every 3 weeks	
Etoposide: 90–120 mg/m^2 i.v. on days 1–3	
ECMV	
Etoposide: 120 mg/m^2 i.v. infusion in 250 ml 0.9% saline over 30 min	Day 1
Cyclophosphamide: 1 g/m^2 i.v. bolus	Day 1
Methotrexate: 35 mg/m^2 i.v. bolus	Day 1
Vincristine: 1.3 mg/m^2 (max 2 mg) i.v. bolus	Day 1
Etoposide: 240 mg/m^2 orally	Day 2
Repeated every 21 days. Prophylactic antibiotics recommended	
EV	
Etoposide: 120 mg/m^2 i.v. infusion	Day 1
Vincristine: 1.3 mg/m^2 (max 2 mg) i.v. bolus	Day 1
Etoposide: 240 mg/m^2 orally	Day 2
Etoposide: 240 mg/m^2 orally	Day 3
Repeated every 21 days. Prophylactic antibiotics recommended	

Table 25.8 Poor prognostic factors in small cell lung cancer

Extensive disease
Poor performance status
Brain metastases
Marrow infiltration/anaemia
Abnormal liver function tests
Low serum sodium and albumin

which commonly develops after an initial response. High-dose chemotherapy and bone marrow transplantation confer no benefit.

Factors which influence the choice among no treatment, single agent and combination chemotherapy are prognostic factors such as age, general medical condition and performance status (Table 25.8). A balance has to be struck between the toxicity and clinical benefit of chemotherapy. Patients with extensive disease and low performance status may be suitable for single-agent oral or intravenous etoposide. Combination chemotherapy should be attempted in younger patients of good performance status.

It is recommended that three courses are given initially. Any useful clinical response usually occurs after one or two courses. Toxicity is cumulative and treatment beyond six courses is not recommended. If no response occurs after three courses, it is unlikely that a different combination is likely to be beneficial.

Symptoms such as anorexia, weight loss, haemoptysis, bone pain, cough, dyspnoea and dysphagia are relieved in 75% of cases after four courses of combination chemotherapy.

Radiotherapy

Radiotherapy to the primary tumour following chemotherapy is sometimes given in patients with limited disease. There is some evidence that relapse in the chest is reduced, with modest increases in survival, compared with radiotherapy alone. However, no firm conclusions can be drawn and routine thoracic irradiation is not recommended. Palliative radiotherapy may be needed for symptomatic relief of symptoms of locoregional and metastatic disease (see non-small cell lung carcinoma).

In patients who have obtained a complete response to chemotherapy, prophylactic cranial irradiation reduces the incidence of brain metastases to 8% compared to 22% following chemotherapy alone. It should only be given under these conditions. It is contraindicated in extensive disease. However, to date there is no evidence that prophylactic cranial irradiation prolongs survival. Late side-effects such as dementia and cerebellar dysfunction may occur in some of the few patients who survive beyond 3 years.

Results of treatment

Untreated, the median survivals of limited and extensive disease are about 3 months and 6 weeks respectively. Combination chemotherapy increases these to 9–12 months and 3 months respectively. The addition of radiotherapy to the site of the primary disease reduces the local recurrence rate and may increase survival.

Despite high response rates to combination chemotherapy, relapse at the primary site or at distant sites occurs in 75% within 2 years. In limited disease 15–20% of patients who obtain a complete response survive 2–3 years. Less than 5% survive 5 years and can probably be regarded as cured.

MESOTHELIOMA

Aetiology and pathology

Mesothelioma is a malignant tumour of the serosal surfaces. It can affect the pleura, pericardium and peritoneum. Involvement of the pleura is commonest. The main risk factor for its development is exposure to crocidolite, blue asbestos. Workers in the production of asbestos, shipyard workers, those in contact with insulation and boilers are occupationally at risk of developing mesothelioma. There is a long latent period between exposure and development of disease, usually in excess of 20 years. Asbestos exposure also predisposes to cancer of the lung. Histologically, pleural mesotheliomas are either epithelial, sarcomatous or mixed.

Clinical features

Presentation is often with progressive dyspnoea, nonproductive cough and aching pain in the chest. Clinically there are commonly signs of a pleural effusion.

Investigations

Plain radiographs may show pleurally based masses and/or a pleural effusion. Calcified plaques may be identified on chest radiograph. Open biopsy may be needed to confirm the diagnosis.

Treatment

Treatment of mesothelioma is essentially palliative. Neither surgery, chemotherapy nor radiotherapy make significant contributions to the treatment of this disease. Symptomatic tapping of pleural effusion and good palliative care are the most important aspects of treatment.

THYMOMA

Thymomas are rare epithelial neoplasms of the thymus gland in the anterior mediastinum. Mean age at presentation is 45–50 years. Children are rarely affected. Men and women are equally affected. The aetiology is unknown. In 50% of cases there is an associated paraneoplastic syndrome, of which the commonest is myasthenia gravis (30–40%). Pure red cell aplasia develops in 5% of patients. Presentation in 40–50% is with an abnormal chest radiograph in an otherwise asymptomatic individual, and in 30% with myasthenia gravis. Chest symptoms are uncommon. About 60% of thymomas are visible on plain radiographs. Distant metastases are rare. If they do occur they involve the pleural surfaces and the lung parenchyma.

Diagnosis and staging

CT scanning can help identify the tumour but cannot distinguish it from other mediastinal tumours (e.g. teratoma, seminoma). The majority of thymomas arise in the anterior mediastinum just above the pericardial sac. Pathologically, thymomas are divided into cortical, medullary or mixed types. Cortical thymomas have a longer survival compared to other subtypes. The Masaoka staging system is widely used (Table 25.9).

Treatment

Surgery and radiotherapy are the principal treatments for thymoma. Owing to its rarity, no randomised trials have been conducted to assess the relative merits of different treatments.

Table 25.9 Masaoka staging system of thymoma

Stage I	Macroscopically completely encapsulated with no microscopic extracapsular invasion
Stage IIa	Microscopic invasion through the capsule
Stage IIb	Microscopic invasion into mediastinal fat or pleura
Stage III	Invasion into adjacent structures (pericardium, great vessels or lung)
Stage IVa	Pleural or pericardial metastases
Stage IVb	Lymphatic or blood-borne metastases

Surgery

The treatment of choice is total surgical removal. This is feasible for the majority of thymomas. Biopsy prior to resection is not advised since it may cause capsular disruption and local spread of an encapsulated tumour. Approximately 30% of patients will be found to have invasive disease at the time of surgery. Incomplete resection is associated with poorer outcome. Local recurrence occurs in 28% of patient with invasive disease. Although most relapses occur within 5 years, late relapse up to 20 years after surgery has been reported.

Radiotherapy

Thymoma is relatively radiosensitive and long-term control with inoperable disease is common. Preoperative radiotherapy should be avoided to prevent unnecessary irradiation of the mediastinum. Primary radiotherapy has occasionally achieved long-term local control.

The role of postoperative radiotherapy is not well defined. There is no good evidence that radiotherapy is efficacious for non-invasive carcinoma. Its role for invasive cancer is well established. In the absence of postoperative radiotherapy for invasive thymoma, the relapse rate is 28% compared to 5% with radiotherapy. The local recurrence rate for encapsulated non-invasive thymoma is only 2%. In this circumstance, a policy of surveillance can be adopted, using radiotherapy for recurrence.

Primary radical radiotherapy is also recommended to delay tumour progression and to relieve local symptoms in inoperable disease.

Dose and energy

45 Gy in 20 daily fractions over 4 weeks is given (4–6 MV photons)

Technique

An anterior oblique wedged pair of fields is used, limiting the spinal cord dose to 40 Gy.

Chemotherapy

Thymoma is also chemosensitive. Patients should be considered for chemotherapy if surgery or radiotherapy fail or if they have metastatic disease. Short-term responses have been obtained with cisplatin, doxorubicin or prednisolone as single agents. Higher doses of cisplatin as a single agent and in combination have yielded better results (25–30% 5-year survival). A combination of cisplatin, doxorubicin and cyclophosphamide gives a response rate of 50% with a median duration of response of 12 months. An EORTC (European Organization for Research on Treatment of Cancer) trial of cisplatin plus etoposide showed an overall response rate of 56% with median duration of response of 3.4 years and median survival of 4.3 years.

Preoperative chemotherapy followed by surgical debulking of the residual disease is logical. Combined results from a number of studies showed an overall response rate of 89% to preoperative chemotherapy. Multimodality therapy with preoperative chemotherapy (cisplatin, doxorubicin, cyclophosphamide and vincristine), surgery and postoperative radiotherapy has shown a response rate of 77% in advanced thymoma; Longer-term follow-up is needed to assess the value of this approach. Patients who relapse after an initial response to platinum-based therapy can be successfully retreated with the same drugs if the disease-free interval prior to relapse is in excess of 12 months.

Results of treatment

10-year survival for non-invasive thymoma is 65% and for invasive tumour 30%.

CARCINOMA OF THE PANCREAS

The incidence of carcinoma of the pancreas has doubled over the last four decades. Its incidence increases with age, reaching 100 per 100 000 between the ages of 80 and 84 years. The aetiology is unknown but the incidence is doubled in cigarette smokers. Most (60%) of tumours occur in the head, 25% in the body and 15% in the tail of the pancreas; 90% are adenocarcinomas.

The tumour spreads locally to obstruct the common bile duct, causing jaundice, and to the duodenum, causing frank or occult gastrointestinal bleeding. Obstruction of the portal vein gives rise to ascites and portal hypertension.

Presentation is normally with jaundice, epigastric pain, diabetes mellitus, thrombophlebitis, anorexia and weight loss. In the presence of jaundice, 50% have a palpable gallbladder (unlikely to be due to stones, according to Courvoisier's law).

Ultrasound may show a pancreatic mass and can be used to guide a needle biopsy. Endoscopy is useful in showing extrinsic compression of the stomach or duodenum by a mass in the head of the pancreas and detecting tumours of the ampulla of Vater.

Treatment for most pancreatic cancer remains palliative since the disease is usually unresectable and is generally resistant to both chemotherapy and radiotherapy. In many advanced cases a palliative bypass procedure between the distended gallbladder and the jejunum is performed to relieve jaundice. A coeliac axis nerve block may help control pain uncontrolled by opiates.

The prognosis is very poor with virtually all patients dying within a year of the diagnosis.

LIVER

Primary liver cancer is rare. The vast majority of liver tumours are secondary deposits, particularly from cancers of the gastrointestinal tract and lung. The management of liver metastases varies with the extent of involvement and the chemosensitivity of the tumour. Surgical resection is rarely appropriate since isolated liver metastases are extremely uncommon. The role of chemotherapy is discussed under individual tumour sites.

Palliative radiotherapy can relieve the pain of hepatic distension in 80% of cases. A parallel-opposed pair of fields is used. If any part of the liver is irradiated, the dose is 30 Gy in 10 fractions over 2 weeks. If the whole liver is irradiated the same dose is given in 15 fractions over 3 weeks (cobalt-60 or 4–6 MV photons).

HEPATOCELLULAR CARCINOMA

Primary hepatocellular carcinoma is an aggressive disease, usually presenting with abdominal pain, weight loss and anorexia. A tumour marker, serum alphafetoprotein, is elevated in 80% of cases. Surgical resection or liver transplantation is the only curative treatment. Unfortunately few patients are suitable for surgery, because of cirrhosis of the liver, diffuse liver infiltration or metastatic disease. Radiotherapy and chemotherapy have no useful role. 5-year survival is poor (5–10%).

CHAPTER CONTENTS

26

Breast

Ian Kunkler

ANATOMY

Most of the breast tissue extends from the edge of the sternum to the anterior axillary line and from the second or third to the sixth or seventh costal edge. It overlies the second to the sixth ribs. Breast tissue can be found beyond these areas as high as the clavicle and laterally to the edge of the latissimus dorsi muscle. It is composed of lobules of glandular tissue lying in fat. The lobules are divided by fibrous ligaments (Cooper's ligaments) which run between the superficial fascia of the breast and the deep fascia overlying pectoralis major.

Lymphatic drainage

A knowledge of the lymphatic drainage of the breast (Fig. 26.1) is important. The principal lymphatic drainage of the breast is to the axillary nodes lying between the second and third intercostal spaces. Additional drainage occurs to the supraclavicular nodes through the pectoralis major and to the internal mammary chain adjacent to the sternum.

PATHOLOGY

Epidemiology

Breast cancer is the commonest form of malignancy in western countries and accounts for 12% of all cancers, 18% of all female cancers, 10% of all cancer deaths and 20–25% of all female cancer deaths. Worldwide there are approximately one million new cases annually. In the UK over 12 000 women die of the disease per year, and at least half a million worldwide. The risk of a woman developing the disease at some stage of her life is 1 in 12. The UK has the highest age standardised incidence and mortality for breast cancer in the world. The prevalence of breast cancer is 2%. Of every 1000 women aged 50, 15 will have had a diagnosis of breast cancer.

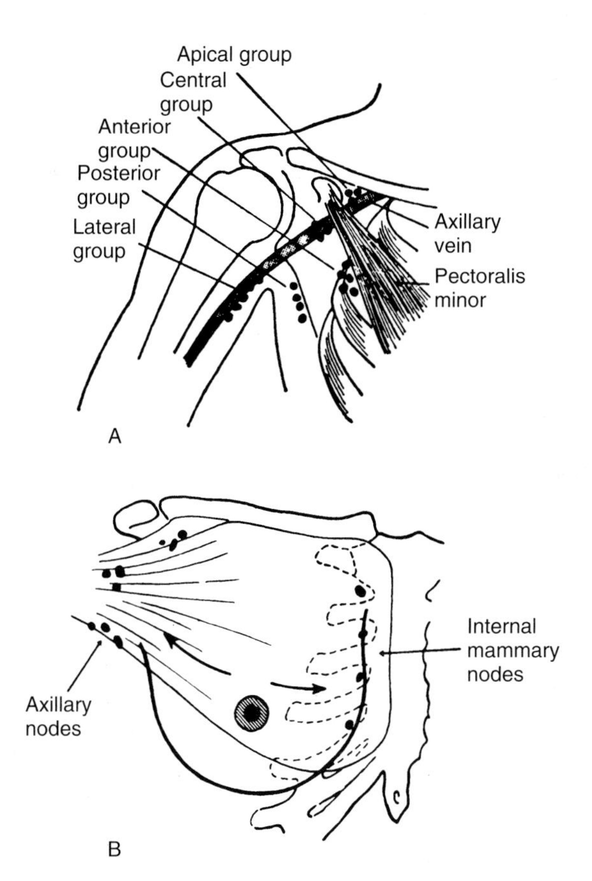

Fig. 26.1 **A** The lymph nodes of the axilla. **B** Diagram of the principal pathways of lymphatic drainage of the breast. These follow the venous drainage of the breast—to the axilla and to the internal mammary chain. (Reproduced with permission from Ellis, Clinical Anatomy, 5th edn, Blackwells, 1975.)

Breast cancer is rare below the age of 30. Male breast cancer is rare (1% of all breast cancer).

Aetiology

The aetiology of breast cancer is unknown in most cases but a number of predisposing factors have been identified. Both genetic and acquired factors are thought to play a part.

Genetic factors

It is estimated that up to 10% of breast cancers have a genetic basis. The sisters and daughters of a woman with breast cancer have a threefold increased risk of developing the disease. The risk of breast cancer for a woman whose sister is affected is doubled. This rises to 10-fold for women who have a mother and a sister affected. Women who have a first-degree relative with premenopausal or bilateral breast cancer are at particularly high risk. Two breast cancer predisposing genes, *BRCA1* and *BRCA2*, have been identified. The mode of inheritance is usually autosomal dominant with incomplete penetrance. It is important to note that the genetic susceptibility can be passed on by both males and females. Most cases of breast cancer with a genetic basis will have occurred by the age of 65. From a validated family history the risks of women at higher than normal risk of developing breast cancer can be identified. Those at very high risk will have four or more relatives affected with breast or ovarian cancer over three generations and one living affected relative. Those at substantial risk include women with:

- Three first- or second-degree relatives with breast or ovarian cancer
- One first-degree relative with bilateral breast cancer
- Two first- or second-degree relatives with breast cancer diagnosed under the age of 60 or ovarian cancer at any age on the same side of the family.

First-degree relatives are mother, sister or daughter. Second-degree relatives are grandmother, granddaughter, aunt or niece.

Acquired

Benign breast disease. A number of benign conditions (e.g. fibroadenomas, palpable cysts) in the breast increase the risk of breast cancer, although the effect is small. Overall the risk of breast cancer is raised by a factor of 1.5–3 for women with previous benign breast disease but rises to ninefold in women with severe atypical breast hyperplasia and a family history of an affected first-degree relative.

Menstruation. Breast tissue is subject to repeated monthly cyclical changes under hormonal stimulation. The epithelium of the breast proliferates during ovulatory cycles. This may be due to the stimulus of either progesterone or oestrogen. This causes temporary growth of the milk-secreting glandular tissue in preparation for possible pregnancy. The greater the number of years of menstruation, the higher the risk of breast cancer. If the menarche starts before the age of 12, the risk of breast cancer is nearly double that of women who begin to menstruate after the age of 13.

If menstruation continues above the age of 55, the risk of breast cancer is doubled compared with a normal menopause at 45 years. Furthermore, if a woman undergoes an artificial menopause (e.g. due to a hysterectomy and oophorectomy under the age of 40), there is a fourfold fall in the incidence of breast cancer.

Oral contraceptive pill and hormonal replacement therapy. The role of the ovarian oestrogens in the genesis of breast cancer is strongly suspected. Reductions in oestrogen levels may protect against breast cancer. Oral oestrogens, either as the contraceptive pill or as hormone replacement therapy, may accelerate the development of breast cancer. There is a small increased risk in women who are taking the oral contraceptive pill and for 10 years after cessation. However, type of oral contraceptive and duration of use do not influence risk of breast cancer. There is a small increase in risk among current users of hormone replacement therapy or those using it 1–4 years previously. Combined preparations of oestrogen and progestogen confer a higher risk.

Age at time of first pregnancy. The risk of breast cancer in a woman rises with her age at first pregnancy. It is three times higher in women who have their first baby over the age of 30, compared with those under the age of 18.

Lactation. Women who have breast-fed their children are slightly less prone to breast cancer.

Age at first full-term pregnancy. Pregnancy itself seems to have a protective role. Women who first become pregnant before the age of 30 have a lower risk of breast cancer than women who first give birth after the age of 30. This effect only applies to completed pregnancies.

Diet. A diet high in animal fats may promote the development of breast cancer. It is possible that the link between fat and breast cancer may be that many of the carcinogens acting on the breast are absorbed in the diet and are soluble in fat.

There is some evidence that a high intake of alcohol is linked to breast cancer.

Weight. In obese postmenopausal women, the risk of breast cancer is increased. This might be due to increased quantities of oestrogens stimulating malignant transformation of the breast.

Radiation. Exposure to ionising radiation increases the risk of breast cancer. This is true of women who underwent low-dose breast irradiation for benign mastitis. There is a linear relationship between dose and incidence of breast cancer up to 4 Gy. Beyond this the incidence plateaus. It has been calculated that one extra cancer per year after 10 years may be caused by radiation from a single mammogram among 2 million women over the age of 50. The risk is small compared to the incidence of breast cancer of 2000 per million women aged 60.

Children irradiated by the atomic bombs dropped on Nagasaki and Hiroshima showed an increased risk of breast cancer with dose.

Ductal and lobular carcinoma-in-situ

Premalignant in situ carcinoma may occur in the lobules (lobular carcinoma-in-situ (LCIS)) or ducts (ductal carcinoma-in-situ (DCIS)). With the advent of breast screening the diagnosis of DCIS has increased three to four times and now accounts for 15% of cases detected by mammography. Before screening, DCIS was mostly associated with symptomatic breast disease. Its natural history among asymptomatic women selected for screening is unknown and may differ. At post-mortem, the incidence of DCIS is much higher in women with breast cancer (40%) compared with those with normal breasts (5%). DCIS is associated with a substantial risk of progression to invasive carcinoma, with a mean delay of about 7 years.

LCIS is associated with an increased risk of tumour in both breasts, particularly infiltrating ductal carcinoma.

Malignant transformation from carcinoma-in-situ

When malignant cells are confined to the ductal–lobular system, they are termed *carcinoma-in-situ*. In situ carcinoma has the potential to become invasive cancer but it is not clear how often this transformation occurs.

Histology

A lump in the breast may be benign or malignant. Benign lesions include cysts, fibroadenomas and papillomas. Malignant tumours mainly arise from the glandular epithelium (adenocarcinomas). Breast cancers are classified as of no special type or of special type. The majority (80%) are of no special type. The histological types of breast cancer are shown in Table 26.1.

Invasive cancers have traditionally been classified by their microscopic appearance and by histological grade. Grading is based on nuclear pleomorphism,

Table 26.1 Classification of invasive breast cancer

1. No special type
2. Special type
   a. Tubular
   b. Mucoid
   c. Cribriform
   d. Papillary
   e. Medullary
   f. Classic lobular

degree of glandular formation and frequency of mitoses. Grading yields useful prognostic information; both disease-free survival and overall survival are shorter for high-grade cancers.

If in excess of 25% of the main tumour mass contains non-invasive (in situ) disease and in situ disease is present in the adjacent breast tissue, the tumour is described as having *an extensive in situ component*. Such patients are at risk of developing invasive cancer elsewhere in the breast and are not suitable for breast conservation.

Lymphatic or vascular invasion within the tumour confers an increased risk of local and distant recurrence.

Inflammatory carcinomas are typified by an enlarged warm breast, associated with an ill-defined underlying mass. Histologically, there is infiltration of the subdermal lymphatics. Prognosis is poor. In contrast, medullary carcinoma is slow growing and has a much better prognosis.

Lobular invasive carcinomas are often bilateral (40%) and multicentric. Paget's disease of the nipple is commonly associated with an underlying ductal adenocarcinoma.

Lymphatic spread

Most tumours develop within the ducts and spread along the ducts and fascia into the mammary fat, the lymphatic channels of the breast and into the peripheral lymphatics. Invasive tumour may infiltrate the dermal lymphatics of the breast, causing oedema of the skin (*peau d'orange*). Tumours of the upper outer quadrant are more likely to have involved axillary nodes. The larger the tumour, the higher is the incidence of involvement of the axillary nodes. The higher the level of axillary involvement, the worse is the prognosis. Palpable supraclavicular nodes reflect advanced disease (M1). In the presence of palpable axillary nodes there is a higher probability of involvement of the internal mammary nodes in tumours of the lower inner quadrant (72%), upper inner quadrant (45%) and central part of the breast (45%) compared with the lower outer quadrant (19%) and upper outer quadrant (22%).

Natural history

Tumours are commoner on the left side. Bilateral tumours are detected at the time of diagnosis (synchronous) in 1–2% of patients. A subsequent (metachronous) tumour in the opposite breast occurs in 7–8%.

Breast cancer shows a very wide range of behaviour, with great differences in rate of growth and tendency to metastasise. The majority of tumours (40%) originate in the upper outer quadrant of the breast. 30% occur in the central part of the breast, 15% in the upper inner quadrant, 10% in the lower outer quadrant and 5% in the lower inner quadrant. Although many tumours do progress locally and then regionally, blood-borne metastases do occur even when the primary is small or impalpable. A few, often young patients may die from rampant metastatic disease within a few weeks of the diagnosis. By contrast, particularly in the elderly, the disease may grow slowly and remain confined to the breast.

DIAGNOSIS

The patient may notice a lump herself on routine or casual self-examination. Sometimes it is detected by her general examination as part of clinical examination for other reason or as a result of routine examination in hospital. With the introduction of the breast-screening programme in the UK, asymptomatic breast cancer is being more frequently diagnosed among women routinely screened for breast cancer between the ages of 50 and 64. In 1998 75% of women (1.2 million) aged 50–64 were screened, detecting 7000 cancers, a yield of 0.6% (6 per 1000). With the extension of the breast-screening programme to older women up to the age of 69, the number of breast cancers detected through breast screening is likely to rise. Estimates of the cost per life saved range from 0.25–1.3 million pounds.

Patients should be referred to a specialist breast unit with multidisciplinary management from surgeon, oncologist, radiologist, pathologist and breast care nurse. There is evidence that patients managed in specialist breast centres have better outcomes than those in non-specialist centres.

Clinical assessment

A full history is required, including details of breast-related symptoms, particularly breast pain, nipple discharge, changes noted in the skin (erythema, dimpling) or shape of the breast, indrawing or distortion of the nipple, axillary lumps and systemic symptoms of weight loss, anorexia, nausea, vomiting, bone pain, breathlessness, headache or motor or sensory disturbance. A full menstrual history should be taken including onset of menarche, menopause, parity, age of first pregnancy, breast/bottle feeding and use of the contraceptive pill and hormone replacement therapy.

Mammography

Breast screening by mammography in the UK is recommended to women between the ages of 50–69 every 3 years. Not all women have access to routine breast screening. The age when screening should begin and the frequency with which it should be done is controversial. Interval cancers (cancers presenting between screens) are an index of the effectiveness of screening. Interval cancers are commoner in the year preceding the next due screen, suggesting that biennial rather than triennial breast screening would be preferable. In younger women the breast tissue is more radiodense and tumours may be difficult or impossible to identify. In older women the breast tissue tends to be more radiolucent and tumours easier to see. This suggests that breast screening may be particularly beneficial in older patients. In the UK two views of the breast are obtained (oblique and craniocaudal). Mammography requires compression of the breast and women often find the investigation painful. None the less, in the countries where it has been widely applied (e.g. in Sweden) its use has been shown to reduce the mortality of breast cancer by 30%. For such results to be achieved, high levels of compliance to invitations to attend (> 70%) has to be achieved and maintained. A strict quality assurance programme is essential to maintain the quality of a breast-screening service.

Features suggestive of malignancy are small microcalcifications, stellate opacities with 'legs' extending into the surrounding tissues (Figs 16.8 and 16.9) or distortion of architecture. Mammography may also show enlarged nodes in the axilla. About 15% of cancers are not detected by mammography and nearly 4% are neither palpable nor visible on mammography.

MRI scanning (Fig. 26.2) may have an important role in the assessment of (a) the local extent of the primary tumour and of multifocality in younger women where the density of the breast is often a limiting factor to the resolution of mammography and (b) recurrent disease in the irradiated breast 18 months or more after radiotherapy has been completed.

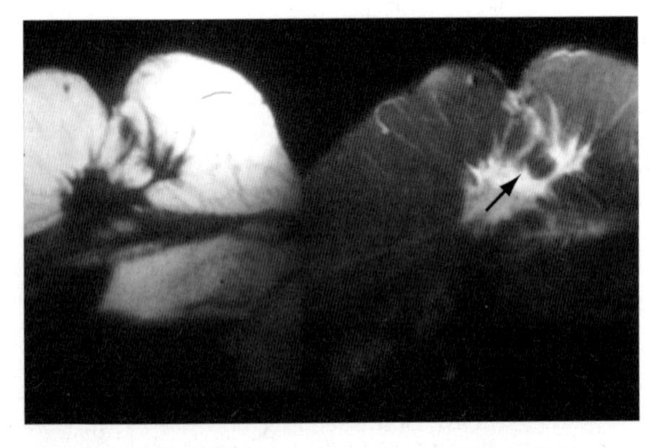

Fig. 26.2 MRI scan showing recurrent cancer in the breast. (Courtesy of Mr M. Dixon, Edinburgh Breast Unit.)

Breast ultrasound

Ultrasound of the breast has an important role in helping to distinguish benign from malignant lesions, particularly when mammography is normal or equivocal. Malignant tumours tend to show an abnormal echo pattern (Fig. 26.3). Colour Doppler ultrasound may show changes caused by increased tumour vasculature both in primary tumours and in lymph nodes.

Obtaining a histological diagnosis

It is important to obtain a histological diagnosis of breast cancer to confirm suspicious clinical or radiological features. If the tumour is palpable (usually 1 cm or larger), fine needle aspiration cytology (FNAC) is recommended as the initial method of confirming the diagnosis. Ideally this should be examined by a specialist pathologist to determine whether malignant cells are present. It should noted that FNAC does not remove sufficient tissue to determine whether invasion is present or the architecture of the tumour. Occasionally false-positive cytology may occur from what prove to be benign lesions such as a fibroadenoma. In view of this possibility, a decision to proceed to a mastectomy requires additional evidence of malignancy (such as a malignant mammogram).

Core biopsy under local anaesthetic for palpable lesions or stereotactic image-guided core biopsy for impalpable lesions is becoming increasingly popular as an adjunct to FNAC. If FNAC is negative or equivocal, core biopsy can be helpful since it provides more tissue available for histological analysis. Oestrogen receptor status can be established on FNAC or core biopsy.

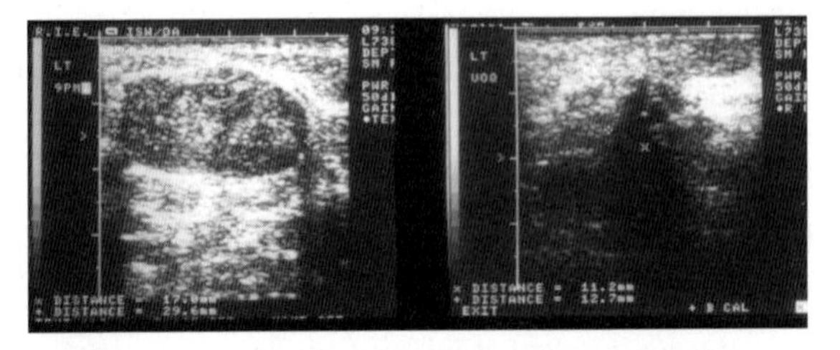

Fig. 26.3 Ultrasound of the breast showing indistinct outline of carcinoma (right) compared to well-defined margins of benign fibroadenoma (left). (Courtesy of Mr M. Dixon, Edinburgh Breast Unit.)

Unfortunately, lumps that appear to be clinically and radiologically benign (e.g. fibroadenomas) occasionally turn out to be malignant. For this reason there is an increasing trend for such lumps to be excised for histological analysis. If excision or core biopsy shows the lump to be benign, the patient can be reassured. Preoperative diagnosis is important since it enables the plan of management to be discussed with the patient by the surgeon and oncologist.

STAGING

Staging is important to assess the local, regional and metastatic spread of breast cancer since management may differ significantly depending on the extent of the disease. Staging involves clinical, radiological and laboratory assessment. The simplest staging system which is still in use in shown in Table 26.2. However, the TNM classification of the International Union Against Cancer (Table 26.3) has gained widespread acceptance. For the T and N classification, the size and mobility of the tumour and any tethering to the skin or underlying muscle or chest wall should be noted.

The regional lymph nodes are palpated (axillary and supraclavicular nodes) on both sides. Respiratory examination may show a pleural effusion.

Whether palpable nodes are histologically involved is often difficult to assess. Hard nodes, especially if they are tethered or fixed in the axilla, are usually malignant. Soft mobile nodes may be benign or malignant.

Staging investigations

For patients with T1–2N0M0 disease a full blood count, liver biochemistry and chest radiograph are recommended. For patients with (a) T3 or T4 tumours (b) N1–3 or MI, or (c) T0–2N0 disease with symptoms which could be due to metastatic disease (e.g. unexplained bone pain or weight loss), a liver ultrasound and a bone scan are recommended. Bone marrow aspiration and trephine biopsy should be performed if

Table 26.2 Clinical staging of breast cancer

Stage	Clinical findings
I	Freely movable (on underlying muscle). No suspicious nodes
II	As stage I but mobile axillary node(s) on the same side
III	Primary more extensive than stage I, e.g. skin invaded wide of the primary mass or fixation to muscle. Axillary nodes, if present, are fixed; or supraclavicular nodes involved
IV	Extension beyond the ipsilateral chest wall area, e.g. opposite breast or axilla; or distant metastases

Table 26.3 TNM classification of breast cancer

Stage	Clinical findings
Primary tumour	
Tis	Carcinoma-in-situ
T0	No demonstrable tumour in the breast
T1	Tumour less than 2 cm in greatest dimension confined to the breast
T1a	Tumour 0.5 cm or less in maximum dimension
T1b	Tumour more than 0.5 cm but not more than 1 cm in greatest dimension
T1c	Tumour more than 1 cm but not more than 2 cm in greatest dimension
T2	Tumour more than 2 cm but less than 5 cm in greatest dimension
T3	Tumour more than 5 cm in its greatest dimension
T4	Tumour of any size with direct extension to chest wall or skin
T4a	Fixation to chest wall
T4b	Oedema, infiltration or ulceration of the skin of the breast
T4c	Both of above
Regional lymph nodes	
N0	No palpable nodes
N1	Mobile ipsilateral nodes
N2	Fixed ipsilateral nodes, fixed to each other or to other structures
N3	Ipsilateral internal mammary nodes
Distant metastases	
M0	No distant metastases
M1	Distant metastases including skin involvement beyond the breast area and supraclavicular nodes

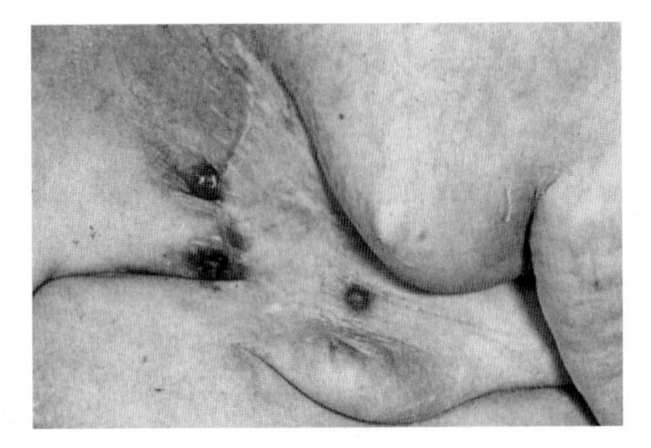

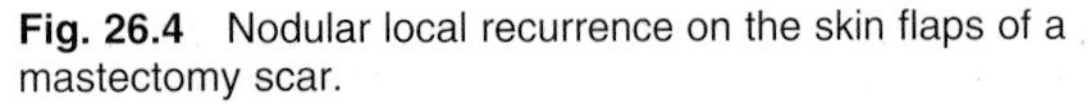

Fig. 26.4 Nodular local recurrence on the skin flaps of a mastectomy scar.

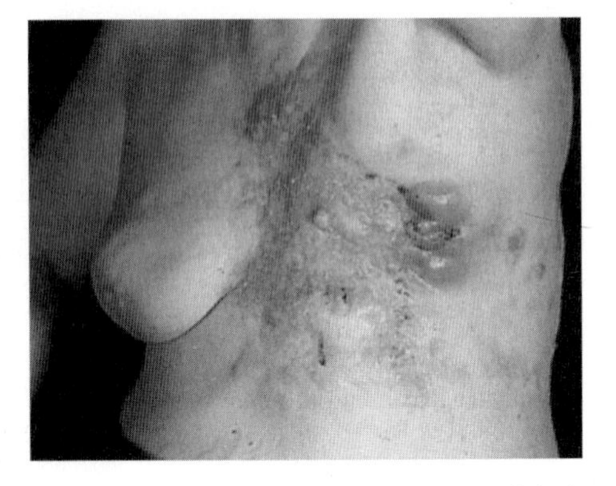

Fig. 26.5 Widespread nodular recurrence over left chest wall following mastectomy, extending to the other breast.

anaemia (typically leucoerythroblastic) from marrow infiltration is suspected.

All patients with locally recurrent disease following mastectomy (Figs 26.4 and 26.5) or breast-conserving therapy, regional or metastatic recurrence require bone scan and liver ultrasound in addition to full blood count, liver function tests and chest radiograph.

TREATMENT OF DUCTAL CARCINOMA-IN-SITU

Until the 1980s total mastectomy was the standard treatment for DCIS and still remains the most reliable curative treatment. Mastectomy remains the treatment of choice for multicentric DCIS and for large unicentric lesions. Regular mammography of the contralateral breast should be carried out, since there is an increased rate of contralateral breast cancer of approximately 7 per 1000. If the extent of the lesion is not more than 3–4 cm, then an attempt at conservative surgery may be made, aiming to achieve complete excision. The margins of clearance should be at least 1 cm. For patients with high-grade DCIS, postoperative whole-breast irradiation should be given, since it reduces the risk of local recurrence and of invasive cancer. For low- or intermediate-grade DCIS, the role of radiotherapy is less clear and still the subject of investigation. Randomised trials have shown that tamoxifen given in addition to radiotherapy following conservative surgery for localised DCIS reduces the cumulative incidence of invasive cancer from 7.2% to 4.1% at 5 years and of non-invasive cancer from 6.2% to 4.2%. The overall prognosis of DCIS is excellent with in excess of 97% of patients alive and disease free 10 or more years following diagnosis.

TREATMENT OF EARLY BREAST CANCER

The treatment of early breast cancer (usually defined as T0–3aN0–1M0) has always been controversial. Over the last decade there has been an increasing trend to offer women breast-conserving surgery rather than the more extensive operation of simple mastectomy.

Historical perspective

For the first half of the last century it was believed that regional lymphatic spread of breast cancer was the important route to systemic spread. The logical treatment was a radical mastectomy, an operation pioneered by an American surgeon, William Halsted. This involved removal of the breast in continuity with the local musculature (pectoralis major and minor) and a full axillary dissection. This was a very mutilating procedure with a high risk of lymphoedema and substantial psychological morbidity from the change in body image. That said, it was an operation that provided good local control. Patients who underwent a Halsted mastectomy are still seen disease free in breast follow-up clinics 30–40 years after surgery.

Radical radiotherapy was first employed as an alternative to radical mastectomy in the 1920s. A limited excision of the tumour was carried out and radium needles implanted throughout the breast. Although a crude form of interstitial implantation by modern standards, it was shown to provide comparable results (albeit not from a randomised trial) to radical mastectomy. In patients where the tumour was confined to the breast, the 5-year survival was about 70%. This conservative approach, introduced by Sir Geoffrey Keynes as early as 1924, did not fit in with the prevailing dogma of the locoregional spread of the disease and did not gain popularity until the 1960s when

Pierquin in France popularised the use of conservative surgery and breast irradiation.

In 1955 it was first demonstrated in a non-randomised study by McWhirter in Edinburgh that simple mastectomy with postoperative locoregional radiotherapy provided a less morbid form of treatment than radical mastectomy with postoperative radiotherapy but with comparable local control and survival.

In the early 1970s there was an increasing appreciation that breast cancer was often a systemic disease. This era saw the focus of breast cancer management shift to the development of adjuvant systemic therapy to treat subclinical systemic micrometastatic disease. More recently there is growing awareness that breast cancer is a heterogeneous disease with some patients with truly localised disease and others with systemic disease from the time of diagnosis.

Part of the difficulty in determining whether or not breast cancer is systemic is the limitation of the resolution of our current staging investigations. Bone marrow taken at the time of primary surgery and subjected to immunocytochemical analysis for tumour infiltration may show malignant cells. There is some evidence that the detection of bone marrow metastases by monoclonal antibodies may provide better discrimination as a prognostic factor than axillary node status. However, the biological significance of these marrow metastases is uncertain.

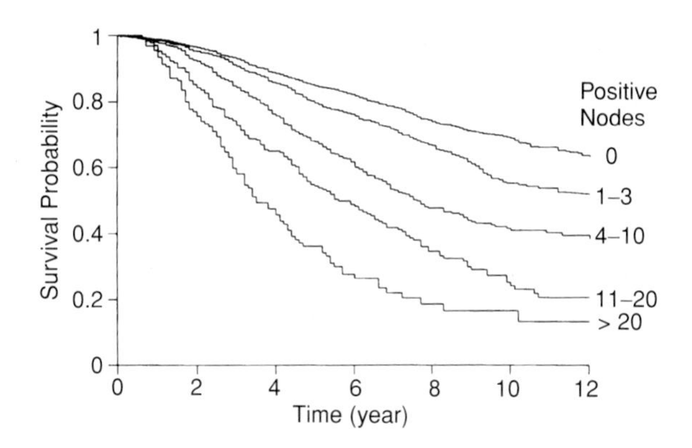

Fig. 26.6 Survival by axillary node status. (Reproduced with permission from Veronesi U (ed) Baillière's Clinical Oncology, 1988.)

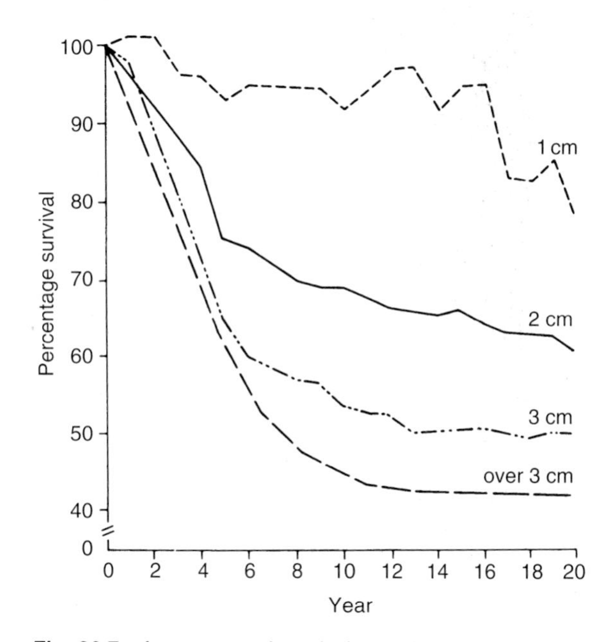

Fig. 26.7 Age-corrected survival rates by tumour size for patients treated for breast cancer apparently confined to the breast. (Reproduced from Halnan, Treatment of Cancer, 1st edn, Chapman & Hall, 1982.)

Prognostic factors

While there are a large number of biological prognostic factors for breast cancer, none has surpassed the value of assessing the number of histologically involved nodes and tumour size. There is a direct correlation between number of involved nodes and survival (Fig. 26.6). 10-year survival is about 40–65% with 1–3 positive nodes, and 20–42% for those with 10 or more positive nodes. 10-year survival is about 65–70% in women with negative nodes. By contrast, in excess of 50% of all women who are axillary node positive die within 10 years despite treatment.

Within any category of nodal status, tumour size is an independent prognostic factor. The decline in survival with increasing size of the primary tumour is shown in Figure 26.7. Less than 30% of patients with stage IIIb disease (T4) are alive at 10 years. Similarly survival declines with increasing tumour grade. 5-year survival falls from 80% for grade 1 to 25% for grade 3.

Oestrogen receptor (ER) status is predictive for disease-free and overall survival. Irrespective of stage, ER positivity predicts for longer disease-free (Fig. 26.8) and overall survival. Higher recurrence and lower survival rates are found in ER-negative patients. About 60% of ER-positive patients will respond to hormonal manipulation. Progesterone receptor (PgR) status may also help. Oestrogen stimulates PgR production in normal reproductive tissue and in human breast cancer cell lines. The highest response and disease-free survival rate is seen in ER+/PgR+ tumours. Very few tumours are ER–/PgR+, consistent with the production of progesterone receptors being dependent on oestrogen synthesis. Lowest

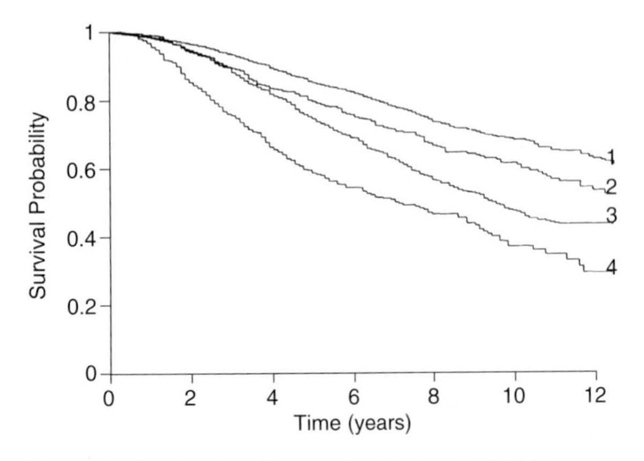

Fig. 26.8 Survival by axillary node status and oestrogen receptor status in 854 patients: 1 = negative nodes ER+; 2 = negative nodes, ER–; 3 = positive nodes, ER+; 4 = positive nodes ER–. (Reproduced with permission from Baillière's Clinical Oncology, International Practice and Research, 1988.)

response and disease-free survival rates are seen in ER–/PgR– tumours (Fig. 26.9).

Of the biological markers of prognosis including p53, cathepsin D, epidermal growth factor receptor and HER2/neu, HER2/neu is the most reproducible. Patients overexpressing HER2/neu have a higher risk of recurrence and shorter survival. There is evidence that tumours that overexpress HER2/neu are relatively resistant to chemotherapy with cyclophosphamide, methotrexate and 5-FU (CMF) and have greater responsiveness to anthracyclines.

Importance of locoregional control of breast cancer

Locoregional control of breast cancer is important for a number of reasons. First, there is evidence, at least from

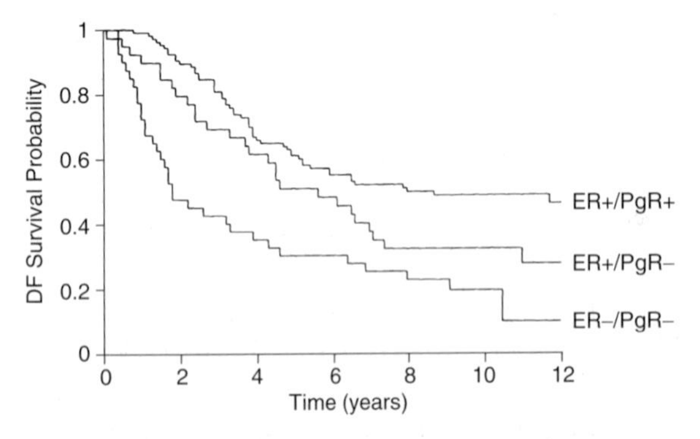

Fig. 26.9 Disease-free survival by oestrogen and progesterone receptor status in pathological stage II patients. (Reproduced with permission from Baillière's Clinical Oncology, International Practice and Research, 1988.)

patients at high risk of local recurrence after mastectomy, that local residual disease compromises survival. If the sole site of residual disease is locoregional, radiotherapy given to these areas in addition to systemic therapy may improve survival. If there is no residual local disease, survival is dictated by micrometastatic disease.

Secondly, uncontrolled local disease with its complications of persistent discharge, odorous infection and bleeding, and usually partial and transient responses to local or systemic treatment, causes immense distress to patients and a poor quality of life. A high quality of surgery (with or without radiotherapy as appropriate) is needed at the primary site and in the axilla to minimise the probability of residual locoregional disease.

Mastectomy or breast conservation

The decision as to whether to perform a mastectomy or breast-conserving surgery should be discussed preoperatively in a multidisciplinary clinic by surgeon and oncologist, once the results of staging investigations are available. A joint decision should be taken. In making this decision, due weight should be given to the patient's own preference. Breast care nurses acting as the patient's advocate may help provide additional information on the patient's views.

The technical feasibility of local surgery, suitability for radiotherapy, cosmesis and locoregional morbidity all need to be taken into consideration. In considering the possibility of breast-conserving surgery, the tumour size, the size of the breast and the mammographic appearance or histology from excision or core biopsy are important. As a general rule, most tumours in excess of 3 cm are unsuitable for breast-conserving therapy unless the breast size is sufficiently large not to result in a marked tissue defect marring cosmesis. Greater flexibility in offering breast conservation is possible with the availability of newer surgical techniques to fill the tissue defect from local excision by a graft. Tumours of 3 cm or greater, judged clinically or radiologically, are generally best treated by mastectomy and axillary node clearance. Patients who have clinical or radiological evidence of multifocal disease or have an extensive intraduct component (EIC) are not suitable for breast conservation.

Studies of patients who have undergone mastectomy show that invasive cancer and ductal carcinoma-in-situ are often present more than 2 cm from the primary tumour. It is therefore important to try to confirm radiologically that the tumour is localised if breast conserving surgery is to be recommended.

There is evidence that local recurrence rates following breast-conserving surgery are higher in younger women (under the age of 40). This may in part be due to the difficulty with mammography of identifying multifocal disease in the radiologically denser breast in young women. Women under the age of 35 have a two- to fourfold higher risk of local recurrence after breast-conserving surgery and radiotherapy.

Lobular cancer

Some histological forms of breast cancer, typically lobular cancer, are commonly multifocal but poorly imaged by mammography. If a core or excision biopsy of an apparently localised tumours shows lobular carcinoma, an initial wide local excision may be carried out. If the margins are involved or there is evidence of multifocal disease histologically, then breast conservation is not safe and mastectomy is advised. Where the margins are clear (by at least 1 mm superiorly, inferiorly, medially and laterally) then a breast-conserving approach for lobular cancer is feasible. Long-term follow-up of patients treated for lobular carcinomas with clear margins shows similar local control to other histological subtypes.

Reconstruction after mastectomy

Patients should be offered the possibility of immediate breast construction, often with the assistance of a plastic surgeon. Common reconstructive procedures include a latissimus dorsi flap to build up the breast mound and breast implants which are progressively inflated to the desired size postoperatively. Reconstruction of the nipple–areola complex is also possible. The main challenge is to match the ptosis and projection of the contralateral breast. Reconstruction using the rectus abdominis muscle (TRAM flap) is available in some specialist centres.

Patients not suitable for or declining a reconstruction should be offered a breast prosthesis.

Conservation therapy (limited surgery and postoperative radiotherapy)

In patients with T1 and small T2 tumours (up to 3 cm) some form of local surgery should be considered. The most popular choice is a wide local excision to obtain clear histological margins. This involves excision of the tumour with a margin of 1–2 cm. If the margins are found to be involved, a re-excision to clear the margins is recommended. If re-excision of the margins still shows tumour at the margin, breast conservation is not appropriate and a mastectomy is advised.

Alternatively, a more extensive local excision of the whole quadrant affected in the breast (quadrantectomy) may be carried out. The advantage of quadrantectomy is that local recurrence rates (about 1% at 5 years when combined with postoperative radiotherapy) are lower than after wide local excision and radiotherapy (about 5% at 5 years). The disadvantage is that the cosmetic result is generally poorer because of the asymmetry caused by the greater volume of tissue removed. Quadrantectomy or a very wide local excision may be considered in patients refusing or not fit for mastectomy or breast radiotherapy. This may be advisable in some older patients where comorbidity may compromise suitability for mastectomy. Criteria for breast conservation are summarised in Table 26.4.

Local recurrence after breast-conserving therapy. The treatment of choice of local recurrence after radical radiotherapy is a mastectomy.

Neoadjuvant therapy

In patients who are keen to avoid mastectomy with clinically and mammographically localised disease, preoperative neoadjuvant therapy with hormonal or cytotoxic therapy selected on the basis of oestrogen-receptor status may be considered. Experience to date suggests that rates of mastectomy can be reduced by neoadjuvant therapy. However, long-term data on local control and survival are not yet available. Until they are, neoadjuvant therapy should only be carried out in the context of a clinical study.

Management of the axilla

The management of the axilla is controversial. Some form of surgical procedure to obtain nodal histology is advised in all women with operable breast cancer. This needs to be decided jointly by the oncologist and the surgeon. For tumours 2 cm or less in diameter where the risk of axillary nodal involvement is lower than in larger tumours, a lower axillary node sample is advised. In this procedure, a minimum of four nodes

Table 26.4 Criteria for breast-conserving therapy

1. Tumours up to 3 cm
2. Satisfactory cosmetic result anticipated
3. Postoperative whole breast radiotherapy technically feasible
4. Medically fit for surgery
5. Clear histological margins at primary excision or re-excision
6. Able to attend for regular clinical and mammographic follow-up

are identified from the lower axilla. A randomised trial in Edinburgh showed that if the node sample is negative, then this is representative of the rest of the axilla (i.e. skip metastases are very uncommon). For patient with tumours >2 cm or with ipsilateral palpable nodes (N1) a level III axillary clearance up to the level of the medial end of the first rib is recommended. Normally there should be at least 10 axillary nodes in a level III clearance and commonly 20–30. The local control in the axilla from a level III clearance is similar to a policy of axillary radiotherapy for patients with a positive lower axillary four-node sample. With either policy the axillary recurrence rate is 5% at 5 years.

It is important that if the axilla is dissected rather than sampled it should not be irradiated unless there is macroscopic residual disease that the surgeon cannot clear (e.g. stuck around the axillary vein). In the uncommon circumstance that postoperative radiotherapy is required to residual disease in the axilla after axillary clearance, the patient should be informed of the greater risks of morbidity (see below).

Morbidity of axillary treatment

Side-effects of an axillary clearance include postoperative seroma and numbness in the upper limb. Lymphoedema occurs in 7–8% of cases. If axillary radiotherapy is added to the dissection, the risk of lymphoedema is substantially higher (between 30–40%).

With the risk of axillary clearance of causing lymphoedema, less-invasive methods of staging the axilla (sentinel node biopsy) are being explored.

After conventionally fractionated radiotherapy (e.g. 45–50 Gy in 20–25 fractions) to the axilla, the risk of lymphoedema is about 3–5%, i.e. lower than after axillary dissection. However, there is an increased risk of long-term restriction of shoulder movement and a small risk of brachial plexopathy (1% or less). This is a rare but serious complication and is usually irreversible. Very careful attention to radiotherapy technique with avoidance of overlap between axillary and breast/chest wall fields or moving the patient between the treatment of these fields is essential.

Sentinel node biopsy

Sentinel node biopsy is currently under investigation to see if it might avoid the need to carry out a full axillary dissection with its attendant morbidity. The sentinel node is the node most likely to drain the primary tumour. It is identified first by the injection of a vital blue dye (Plate 2.6) or a radioactive tracer, or a combination of both. In most patients the sentinel node is in the axilla but in a few medially placed tumours it may be in the internal mammary chain. The axilla is normally explored to identify the sentinel node either by the blue colour of the dye within it or by the high radioactivity scintillation count over it. If histology of the sentinel node shows no tumour, no further axillary surgery is needed. If the sentinel node biopsy is positive, the surgeon may proceed to a complete axillary dissection or refer the patient for axillary irradiation.

Sentinel node biopsy poses new dilemmas since it may detect micrometastases (≤ 2 mm). It is not clear how these should be managed. If the pathologist is asked to give the sentinel node special attention, the yield of positive sentinel nodes rises by 5–10%, and by a further 5–10% if the sentinel node is analysed by immunohistochemistry. If even more sensitive tests such polymerase chain reaction to a range of tumour antigens are carried out, the yield of positive sentinel nodes is likely to rise even further. The prognostic significance of these micrometastases is not certain.

The timing of the injection of the radionuclide and imaging by gamma camera needs to be carefully coordinated and requires the services of a nuclear medicine department. It is still not clear whether sentinel node biopsy will be generalisable to all cancer units undertaking breast surgery or should be confined to specialist centres. In specialist centres sentinel node biopsy has 97% accuracy.

An additional factor that has to be addressed is the pathology time needed to examine 40–50 slices of the sentinel node by stains for cytokeratin to detect tumour involvement. Such examination is likely to put significant pressures on pathology laboratories. If widely adopted and with adequate standards of quality assurance, sentinel node biopsy could significantly reduce the number of axillary dissections and attendant morbidity.

Trials of adjuvant postoperative radiotherapy

Historical aspects

Paterson in Manchester in 1948 conducted the first randomised trial of postmastectomy radiotherapy. He demonstrated that adjuvant irradiation given immediately postoperatively rather than delayed until the time of recurrence reduced the risk of local recurrence from 32% to 19% at 5 years. There was, however, no difference in overall survival. A Cancer Research Campaign trial in the 1970s in stage I and II disease with simple mastectomy with or without postoperative radiotherapy showed a reduction in local recurrence from 30% to 10% but similarly no difference in survival.

In 1987 an overview of randomised trials showed a 20% reduction in risk of death among patients who had not received adjuvant postoperative radiotherapy following radical mastectomy. The excess mortality of non-breast-cancer deaths was largely due to vascular causes related to irradiation of the heart. This was a particular risk of older radiotherapy techniques using orthovoltage where the divergence of the beam made unwanted cardiac irradiation difficult to avoid.

A reanalysis in 1994 confined to the more modern radiotherapy trials using megavoltage radiotherapy showed no adverse effect of radiotherapy. Indeed, there was a trend, albeit not statistically significant, to improved survival in irradiated patients. However, no particular subgroup could be identified in which survival was improved by radiotherapy.

Randomised trials in Denmark and Canada have shown a 9–10% survival advantage from the addition of locoregional radiotherapy to systemic therapy in high-risk premenopausal and postmenopausal women. However, the 2000 Oxford overview of randomized trials of adjuvant irradiation showed no difference in survival between irradiated and non-irradiated patients. If vascular damage from radiotherapy could be avoided, the Oxford overview predicts a small (2–4%) gain in 20-year survival from adjuvant irradiation. The possible reasons for the lower survival benefit in the overview compared to the Danish and Canadian trials is discussed later in this chapter.

1. After breast-conserving surgery

In general, postoperative whole-breast irradiation should be delivered following wide local excision or quadrantectomy as part of breast-conserving therapy. A number of randomised trials comparing wide excision alone with appropriate systemic therapy have shown a reduction in local recurrence from the addition of whole breast irradiation. A Scottish trial of patients with tumours up to 4 cm with or without involved nodes showed a 6% recurrence rate from the addition of breast radiotherapy to systemic therapy compared to 25% in the non-irradiated group. It is important that the whole breast is irradiated, since the recurrence rate is substantial if radical radiotherapy is confined to the primary site. A trial in Manchester confining radical electron beam irradiation to the tumour-bearing area alone showed a 16% recurrence rate at 5 years compared to 8% for whole breast irradiation. These findings are consistent with radiotherapy sterilising subclinical disease remote from the tumour-bearing area.

Is there a group of patients treated by breast conservation and adjuvant systemic therapy in whom radiotherapy can be omitted?

Most of the evidence from randomised trials shows a reduction in risk of local recurrence in patients treated by breast irradiation (Table 26.5). The extent of tumour margins is the most important factor influencing local recurrence rates. Where wide margins of normal tissue are taken (e.g. quadrantectomy) the risks of local recurrence without radiotherapy are smaller.

Whether breast radiotherapy is required in patients at low risk of local recurrence (e.g. node-negative patients with tumours of special type) after conservative surgery and systemic therapy is unclear. A number of randomised trials are currently addressing this issue. The need for breast irradiation in older patients is unresolved, largely because patients over the age of 70 were excluded from randomised trials. Older frailer patients may prefer to avoid prolonged attendance over 5–6 weeks for radiotherapy, particularly if this involves hospitalisation remote from their family. There is some evidence that recurrence rates fall in this older group of patients. However, until mature results of these trials assessing the role of breast radiotherapy in these subgroups of patients are known, most patients should be considered for breast irradiation. It needs to be borne in mind that breast conservation carries a constant risk of local recurrence (1%) per year up to at

Table 26.5 Results of randomised trials of breast-conserving surgery (BCS) with or without radiotherapy (RT) (modified from Wong J S and Harris J R 2001 Lancet Oncology 2: 11–17)

	Local recurrence (%)		Median follow-up (months)	Analysis
	BCS alone	BCS + RT		
NSABP B-06	10	10	144	12 years actuarial
Canadian	35	11	91	8 years crude
Scottish	25	6	68	5 years actuarial
Swedish	18	2	64	5 years actuarial
Milan III	18	2	52	5 years actuarial

least 15 years. However, in the older patient this needs to be balanced against the morbidity of radiotherapy and diminishing life-expectancy due to comorbidity. With the rising incidence of breast cancer among older patients, the determination of whether a more selective policy of breast radiotherapy can be adopted will assume even greater importance.

2. Following mastectomy

More than half of the locoregional recurrences following mastectomy occur on the chest wall. Where there are multiple sites of locoregional recurrence, the chest wall may be involved in 60–80% of patients. The mastectomy scar is the commonest site of recurrence on the chest wall. It is probable that secondary tumour emboli, particularly in the lymphatics, result in residual disease after mastectomy. This explanation is supported by the higher likelihood of locoregional recurrence where there is lympho-vascular invasion in the primary tumour or extensive axillary lymph node involvement.

The role of adjuvant radiotherapy following mastectomy remains controversial but is assuming greater importance with the evidence that it may confer a substantial survival advantage when given in addition to adjuvant systemic therapy in pre- and postmenopausal women at high risk of local recurrence.

In 1997, randomised trials in Denmark and Canada showed a 9–10% survival benefit from the addition of locoregional radiotherapy following mastectomy to adjuvant CMF chemotherapy. The much larger Danish trial (Fig. 26.10) of over 3000 patients led by Marie Overgaard showed that a significant advantage accrued to patients receiving adjuvant irradiation (10-year survival 54% vs 45%). A trial from the same group (Fig. 26.11) shows a similar 9% survival (45% vs 36%) benefit in high-risk postmenopausal women receiving locoregional regional irradiation in addition to adjuvant tamoxifen. However, the survival advantage only emerged late (i.e. at 10 years). In both the Danish and Canadian trials all of the peripheral lymphatics (axilla, supraclavicular and internal mammary chain) were irradiated. It is not clear whether irradiation of all of these areas, particularly the internal mammary chain is essential. A European trial is currently assessing the role of internal mammary irradiation. Internal mammary recurrences are uncommon in clinical practice despite the fact that if the axillary nodes are involved, the internal mammary nodes will be involved in 25% of cases. The radiotherapy technique in the Danish trial (Fig. 26.11) differed from the use of a pair of tangential fields in most UK centres to treat the chest wall. A combination

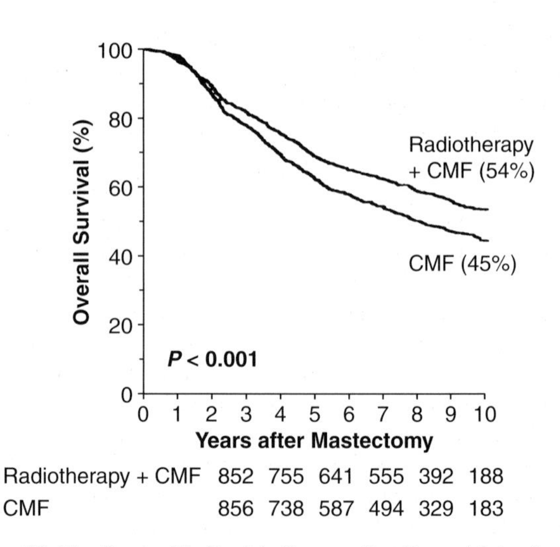

Fig. 26.10 Survival in Danish Cooperative Group trials of locoregional radiotherapy after adjuvant CMF in high-risk premenopausal women. (Reproduced with permission of the Editor, from Overgaard et al, 1997, New England Journal of Medicine 337: 949–955.)

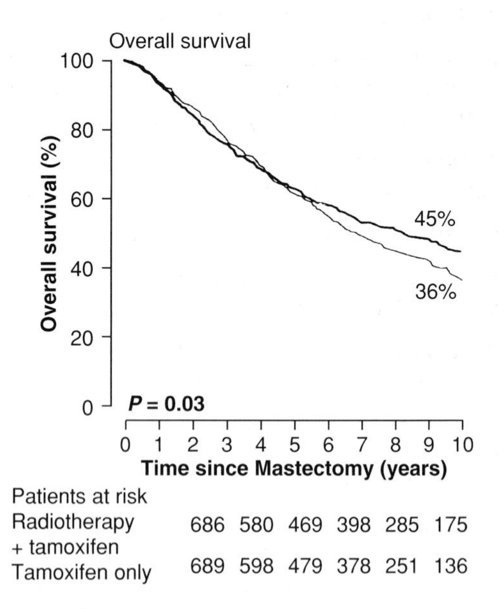

Fig. 26.11 Survival in Danish Cooperative Group trials of locoregional radiotherapy after adjuvant tamoxifen in high-risk postmenopausal women. (Reproduced with permission from Elsevier Science from The Lancet, 1999; 353: 1642.)

of electron beam with limited penetration beyond the chest wall was used to treat the medial part of the chest wall and matched with a photon field to treat the lateral half of the chest wall. 10-year follow-up data showed no excess of cardiac morbidity or mortality in the radiotherapy + systemic therapy group compared to those receiving systemic therapy alone. The results of the Danish trial emphasise the importance of good radiotherapy technique in minimising the dose to the heart.

In the 2000 update of the Oxford overview, postoperative radiotherapy reduced the risk of locoregional recurrence by two-thirds. Breast cancer mortality was reduced but non-breast-cancer mortality increased, particularly due to vascular causes. Overall 20-year survival was 37.1% with radiotherapy, compared to 35.9% for controls. The difference was not statistically significant. Patients irradiated over the age of 60 were particularly at risk of radiation-induced vascular mortality. The much lower estimates of a survival benefit from adjuvant radiotherapy in the Oxford overview are at variance with the much higher levels of benefit shown in the Danish and Canadian trials. In part this may be due to the inclusion within the Oxford overview of trials of radiotherapy using older treatment techniques where a survival benefit would have been reduced or negated by higher levels of radiation-induced cardiac mortality.

Indications for postmastectomy radiotherapy

International consensus supports the routine use of postmastectomy radiotherapy for patients who have a 20% or more risk of locoregional recurrence:

1. Tumours greater than 5 cm in diameter
2. Four or more histologically involved axillary nodes.

In addition radiotherapy is indicated for:

3. Close or involved surgical margins
4. Chest wall recurrence following mastectomy.

Cumulatively greater probability of local recurrence is conferred with the following risk factors:

1. Axillary nodal involvement
2. Grade 3 histology
3. Lymphatic/vascular invasion.

How these factors should be weighted in the selection of patients for postmastectomy radiotherapy is not clear. In the absence of definitive data, a reasonable policy is to offer radiotherapy to patients with two or more of these factors. Trials are ongoing to assess the role of postmastectomy radiotherapy in the group with 1–3 nodes positive and the value of other risk factors such as grade and lymphovascular invasion.

Target volume and techniques for locoregional irradiation

A wide variety of radiotherapy techniques are in use. In choosing a technique, guiding principles should be homogeneous irradiation of the target areas, avoidance of overlap of chest wall/breast with fields to the peripheral lymphatics, and minimising dosage to critical structures (lung, heart and the brachial plexus).

This is not an easy task because of the variation in shape and thickness of the chest wall and breast in the craniocaudal and transverse planes. In addition, the sternum slopes when the patient is lying flat. The proximity of the lung to the target volume means that some lung is commonly irradiated. As a result it is difficult to reduce the variation in dose distribution across the volume to the $\pm 5\%$ that is achievable by radical radiotherapy at other tumour sites. Dose inhomogeneity is exacerbated by lung effects due to scatter and lung transmission.

The aim should be to achieve a variation between the maximum and minimum dose of better than 15%.

Whatever technique is adopted, a careful audit needs to be kept of locoregional control, survival and morbidity in each centre.

CT simulation

Conventionally in UK centres most adjuvant irradiation has been planned without the benefit of CT planning or with only a single or limited number of CT slices. While modern simulators may give a better appreciation of the inclusion of part of the myocardium within the field, they are unable to give the volumetric assessment of the inclusion of these critical structures compared to multislice CT scanning.

Full CT scanning of the breast allows better selection of beam arrangements to minimise cardiac and pulmonary irradiation (Plate 2.7). CT scanning with a wider than the normal (70 cm) bore is usually needed to enable the patient in the treatment to be encompassed with the arm abducted to 90 degrees.

Radiotherapy technique

There are two main radiotherapy techniques adopted: multifield and 'en bloc'. Multifield treatment is preferable since it provides a more homogeneous dose distribution within the target volume with less unwanted irradiation of the lung and the heart than 'en bloc' techniques.

Immobilisation. Some form of immobilisation is essential to provide a reproducible treatment set-up. A variety of devices are in use. These may include a breast board (see Fig. 26.16) that fits onto the simulator and treatment couch, a custom-made foam mould from the head to the knees or a jig (Fig. 26.12). The patient is treated supine with the arm abducted to

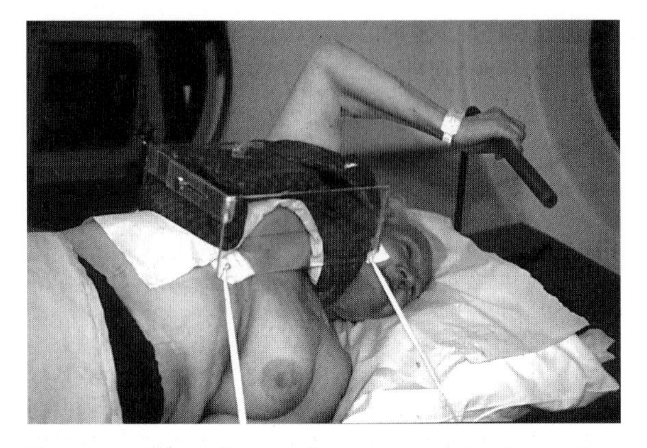

Fig. 26.12 Breast jig for radical treatment of patients with large or mobile breasts or for locally advanced disease. The jig is filled with bolus bags.

90 degrees. The breast board can be inclined to a range of angles to flatten the chest wall/breast.

This technique simplifies matching and avoids the need for rotating the collimator. The disadvantage is that it increases the volume of lung irradiated in the shoulder field.

Alternatively the patient can lie supine with the arm abducted to 90 degrees. Rotation of the collimator is needed to keep the posterior beam edge parallel to the slope of the contour. The disadvantage is difficulty in matching the chest wall to the shoulder field.

For the large or very mobile breast some additional form of immobilisation (shell or sling or jig [Fig. 26.12]) is needed. The very mobile breast tends to fall laterally, moving the posterior beam edge further back than the midaxillary point and increasing the volume of lung irradiated. The immobilising device will bring the breast medially and reduce the volume of lung irradiated.

Multi-field. Separate fields (Fig. 26.13) are planned to cover (1) supraclavicular fossa, axilla and, if desired, the upper internal mammary chain and (2) chest wall/breast and, if desired, the internal mammary

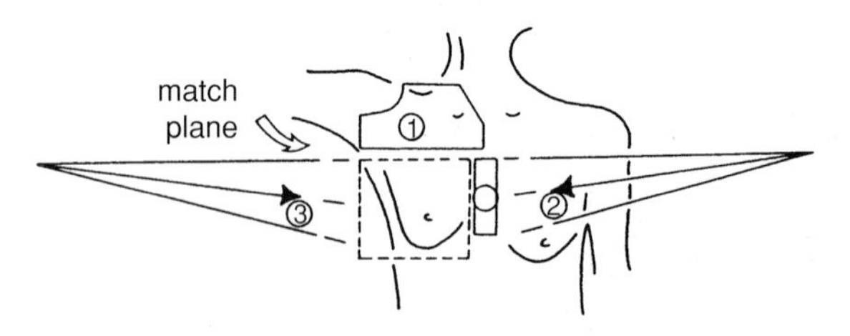

Fig. 26.13 Diagram showing fields to the chest wall/breast, axilla, supraclavicular fossa and internal mammary chain. (Reproduced with permission of the Editor of the British Journal of Radiology, 1984; 57: 736.)

chain. Whether it is necessary to irradiate the internal mammary chain is still controversial and most UK oncologists do not attempt to include it in the target volume. If the internal mammary nodes are to be irradiated, it is best to use a direct electron field of appropriate energy to cover them. Individualised CT planning is needed to ensure adequate coverage while limiting transmitted dosage to the underlying heart and lungs. Trying to include the internal mammary nodes within tangential fields is not recommended because of the greater risks of pneumonitis from the larger volume of lung irradiated and the uncertainty of adequate coverage. A computer plan of the dose distribution over the breast or chest wall should be derived from a manually or CT derived outline through the central plane.

With three-dimensional CT planning, beam entry and exit points can be adjusted to minimise dosage to these structures. The use of conformal radiotherapy techniques using intensity-modulated radiation therapy may improve the homogeneity of dose distribution within the breast while reducing the dose to heart, lung and contralateral breast.

Shoulder field. A direct anterior megavoltage field (Fig. 26.13) covers the supraclavicular fossa and axilla. The upper margin should be at the level of the thyrohyoid groove. The lateral margin should encompass the lateral border of the axilla. The length of the shoulder field should rarely exceed 10 cm, since the volume of lung irradiated rises as the lower edge of the treatment volume is extended inferiorly. This increases the risk of pneumonitis.

The shoulder joint and the part of the larynx within the field should be shielded by lead blocks. Some centres angle the shoulder field 15 degrees to exclude the spinal cord, although this is not essential as long as the dosage and fractionation are within cord tolerance. The lower border of the shoulder field should be non-divergent to avoid overlap with the tangential fields.

The axillary and supraclavicular nodes are commonly at the same depth and therefore a single anterior field may suffice. Some centres use a small direct posterior field (posterior axillary boost) to supplement the dose to the axillary nodes. The given dose to the posterior axilla is calculated to bring the mid axilla to the prescribed dose. With 6 MV photons, roughly 20% of the prescribed midaxillary dose is delivered from the posterior field. The posterior field is often treated on alternate days.

Supraclavicular field. Where the axillary clearance shows the nodes to be involved, irradiation of the ipsilateral supraclavicular nodes should be considered. There is no consensus on the threshold for medial supraclavicular fossa irradiation. This varies from any axillary involvement to a minimum of four involved nodes. If the axilla is to be cleared, the surgeon should be asked to place metal clips up to the medial extent of the axillary dissection to ensure that the lateral margin of the supraclavicular field abuts on, but does not overlap, the field of the axillary clearance.

Chest wall and breast. The chest wall or breast is treated isocentrically and can normally be encompassed in a pair of wedged tangential fields (Fig. 26.14) keeping the posterior beam edges parallel to minimise divergence into the lung. This should cover the scar of local excision or of the mastectomy. It normally extends from the level of the second costal cartilage down to 1–2 cm below the inframammary fold. The medial margin is the midline. The lateral margin is normally the midaxillary line. Occasionally the lateral margin may be slightly more posterior in the conserved breast for a laterally placed tumour or if the mastectomy scar extends beyond this point. Some

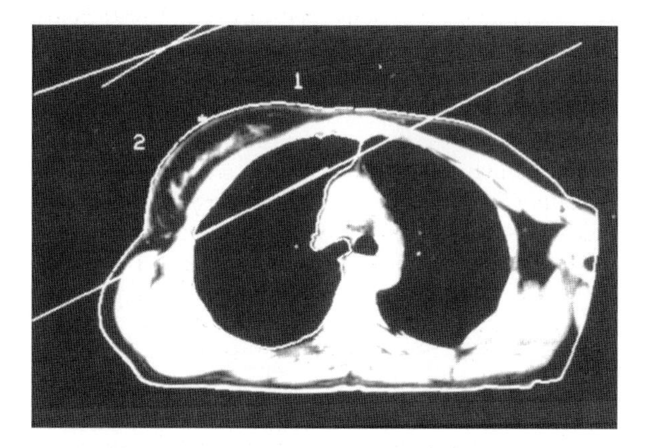

Fig. 26.14 Two tangential breast fields. By keeping the posterior beam edges parallel, irradiation of the lung is reduced.

compromise is necessary in defining these field margins, balancing adequate coverage of the target volume with the need to avoid excessive lung irradiation. A typical dose distribution in the breast is shown in Figure 26.15.

Internal mammary node irradiation. If the internal mammary nodes are to be irradiated, a separate direct electron internal mammary field should be used, which will need to cross the midline. This has the advantage of sparing excessive dosage to the heart. The internal mammary chain (IMC) lies deep to the midline and about 2–3 cm to each side of the midline. Part of the IMC field may be overlapped by the curved shape of the tangential field. This area of overlap should be blocked when the IMC field is treated.

Limitation of lung volume irradiated. At the time of simulation, the thickness of lung encompassed in the tangential fields should be measured (the central lung distance perpendicularly from the inner aspect of the chest wall to the posterior beam edge). The central lung distance should not exceed 3 cm. If it exceeds 3 cm, consideration should be given to using an internal mammary photon field to cover the medial part of the chest wall / breast and tangential fields to the lateral chest wall / breast or bringing the medial and / or lateral margins of the fields inwards, as long as this does not involve skimping on the coverage of the wide excision or mastectomy scars. To avoid divergence into the lung, the posterior beam edges should be kept parallel.

Skin bolus. To overcome the skin-sparing effect of megavoltage skin bolus (0.5–1 cm depending on the energy of photons) should be applied to the chest wall to ensure full skin dosage in patients where the skin is involved by tumour. Practice varies in the use of bolus for postmastectomy radiotherapy when the skin is not involved. Some centres apply bolus to a limited area above and below the scar (where recurrences are commonest) or to the whole of the chest wall, either for the

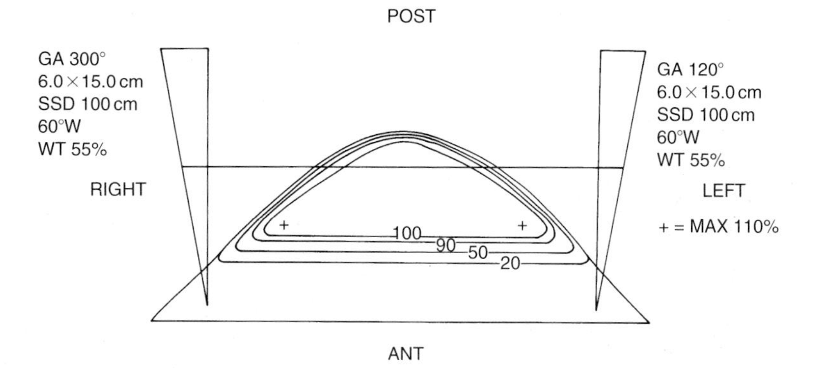

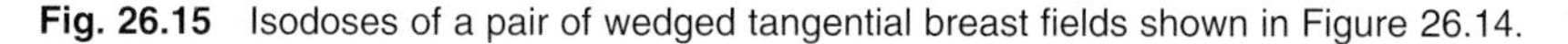

Fig. 26.15 Isodoses of a pair of wedged tangential breast fields shown in Figure 26.14.

whole or part of the course of radiotherapy. It is not clear which approach is optimal.

Field matching

One of the main challenges in breast/chest wall planning is to match the tangential fields to the shoulder field. Immobilisation should minimise movement between the treatment of fields to avoid the risk of over/underlap at the junction. Fields may be matched using the light beam and lasers by eye using couch rotation (usually 5–6 degrees) and some collimator rotation. Alternatively one can use:

1. A half beam block (Fig. 26.16A) to counteract beam divergence, allowing the field edges to be abutted. Asymmetric jaws facilitate this. The match plane can be vertical (Fig. 26.16B) or angled (Fig. 26.16C).
2. A vertical hanging block.
3. A single isocentre with blocks, avoiding the need for couch movement between fields.

Dosimetry

Planning is normally on a single CT slice. However, multislice CT scanning of the breast gives a better appreciation of the volume of lung and heart irradiated. 6 MV photons are adequate for most patients. Wedges are needed to compensate for missing tissue. Lung transmission increases the dose to the posterior breast. A correction factor of 10% may be needed. Variations in depth dose across the breast may be ± 20%, particularly in larger breasts. Build-up to 100% is 5–10 mm from the skin surface for 6 MV photons. The skin surface dose for tangential fields is 50–70% of the prescribed dose.

En bloc. An 'en bloc' technique is recommended for the very large or mobile breast or for a large primary tumour contiguous with the axillary node. The chest wall/breast and, if necessary, axilla and supraclavicular nodes are encompassed en bloc in a rectangular Perspex jig. The jig is filled with bolus (Fig. 26.12). No computer plan is used. The ipsilateral arm is placed behind the head, holding a horizontal bar, and the body rotated slightly to the opposite side and supported on a foam wedge.

The drawback of this technique is that when the peripheral lymphatics are irradiated some of the arm and shoulder are irradiated and cannot be satisfactorily blocked from the beam.

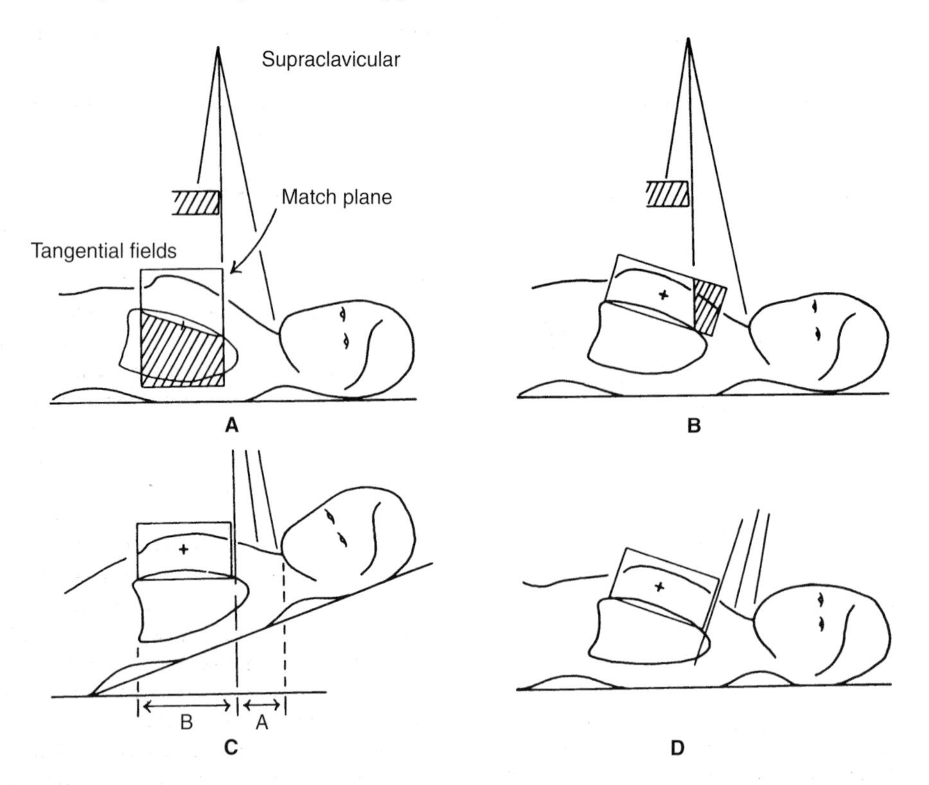

Fig. 26.16 Matching fields in a breast treatment. **A** Using a rotated half beam block to counteract beam divergence between cervico-axillary and breast fields. **B** Lead block to trim superior edge of the tangential fields to form a vertical match plane. **C** Match plane vertical on an inclined breast board. **D** Match plane angled in supine position. (Reproduced with permission of the Editor of the British Journal of Radiology, 1984, 57: 737.)

A mixture of photons to the supraclavicular and axillary region and anterior electron field to treat the internal mammary nodes and the medial chest wall (Fig. 26.17) was used in the Danish postmastectomy radiotherapy trials. Importantly, there was no excess of cardiac morbidity or mortality from postmastectomy added to systemic therapy compared to systemic therapy alone.

Conservation therapy

Boost to the tumour. Some form of boost of irradiation to the primary tumour is desirable to bring the tumour dose to 60 Gy in women under the age of 50. This is either given by electrons or by an iridium-192 implant (Fig. 22.9). Either form of boost will give comparable local control. However, the higher surface dose of electrons will cause telangiectasia on the treated skin. For implants, telangiectasia at the skin entry and exit points of the iridium wire can be avoided if the sources lie just beneath the skin surface. In general, the breast tissue tends to be thinner in the more medial and lateral parts of the breast. In these sites there may be inadequate tissue for an implant and electrons are preferable.

An iridium implant does enable a higher dose to be delivered than electrons for a similar level of morbidity. However, there is no compelling evidence that electrons are inferior to an implant in terms of local control in conservation therapy.

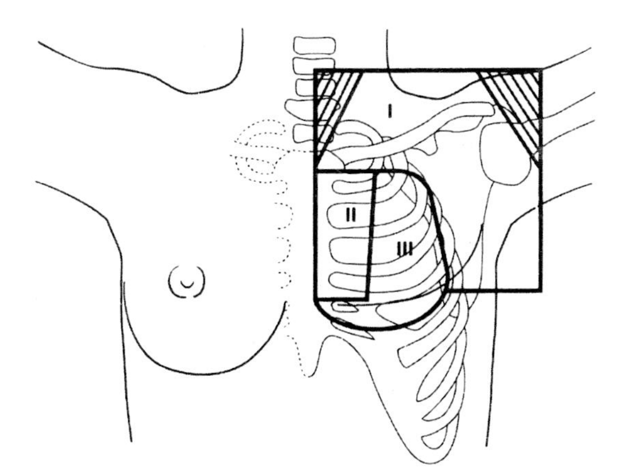

Fig. 26.17 Radiotherapy technique using mixed photon and electron beams for locoregional radiotherapy after mastectomy in the Danish Breast Cooperative Group trials. A direct photon field (I) treats the lateral chest wall and axilla and an electron field treats the medial chest wall (III) and internal mammary nodes (II). (Reproduced with permission from Elsevier Science: The Lancet, 1999, 354: 1426.)

Dose, energy and fractionation

Megavoltage irradiation (6 MV photons) is used for the tangential field to the chest wall or breast.

Radical radiotherapy schedules vary across the UK. The commonest regimes are 40 Gy in 15 fractions, 45 Gy in 20 fractions and 50 Gy in 25 fractions. The latter is the standard in the USA and most of continental Europe.

1. Multifield

a. Shoulder field (supraclavicular + axilla)

45 Gy maximum dose in 20 daily fractions over 4 weeks (6 MV photons)

(with posterior axillary boost brings midaxillary dose to 45 Gy treating alternate days)

b. Medial supraclavicular fossa

45 Gy maximum dose in 20 fractions over 4 weeks (6 MV photons)

c. Breast or chest wall

45 Gy target absorbed dose (TAD) in 20 fractions (6 MV photons)

2. En bloc (jig technique)

45 Gy maximum in 20 daily fractions over 4 weeks (6 MV photons)

Boost to the primary. It has been conventional to boost the site of tumour excision either with electrons of appropriate energy or temporary interstitial implantation using iridium-192. However, most of the data for both methods of boosting on which this policy was based were retrospective and subject to selection bias. A randomised trial in France using electrons (10 Gy) to the site of excision after whole breast irradiation (50 Gy) showed a slight but statistically significant reduction in local recurrence from 3.6% at 5 years compared to 4.5% with whole breast irradiation alone.

A much larger EORTC trial of over 5500 patients showed an overall 40% reduction in the risk of local recurrence with the use of the boost. Patients with clear margins after wide local excision were treated with whole breast irradiation (50 Gy in 25 fractions over 5 weeks) and randomised to either a boost (electrons—10 Gy) or implant. Age was an independent risk factor for recurrence. In women under the age of 40 the local recurrence with the boost was 10% compared to 20% without the boost. The absolute reduction in recurrence was smaller in women over the age of 40, but still statistically significant up to the age of 50. Similar benefits in local control were conferred whatever type of boost was used (external beam or implant). On this basis, for patients with clear excision margins, a boost is not recommended in women who are 50 or older. In patients for whom re-excision of positive margins is not possible, an electron or iridium-192 implant boost would still be indicated. Implantation can be carried out intraoperatively or postoperatively.

Electrons. The appropriate electron energy, usually 9–12 MeV, is chosen according to the depth of the breast tissue at the site of the tumour-bearing area. This is usually judged clinically but is more accurately measured by ultrasound or CT postoperatively. In order to avoid transmission of unwanted irradiation to the underlying lung, a Perspex degrader of appropriate thickness can be interposed between the electron applicator and the skin to attenuate the beam. The boosted volume should cover the tumour-bearing area with a margin of 1–2 cm (to take account of the inbowing of electron isodoses at depth) judged from clinical, mammographic and peroperative findings. Surgeons should be encouraged to place metal clips at the site of the excision, which assist the clinical oncologist in the identification of the tumour bed.

Electron boost dose

15 Gy maximum dose in 5 daily fractions over 1 week

Special situations

1. *Women with larger breasts*

In patients with larger breasts or following breast reconstruction, the same total dose may be given over a longer overall treatment time (e.g. 5 weeks rather than 4) to reduce the acute skin morbidity.

2. *Local recurrence after mastectomy*

If local recurrence occurs on the chest wall, 'spot' recurrence should be locally excised if feasible. For multiple 'spot' recurrences this is unlikely to be practical. Following radical chest wall irradiation, a boost with electrons should be considered to limited volumes of macroscopic recurrent disease. The same boost doses are used as for breast-conservation therapy.

Practical points in setting up the patient

1. Ensure that the patient lies in a comfortable and relaxed position at the time of simulation to ensure that the same position is maintained during treatment. Therapy radiographers have an important role in helping the patient to relax by explaining the planning process.
2. Take care to avoid overdosage and underdosage at field junctions.
3. Where irradiation of the breast or chest wall may include an excessive volume of the heart or lung to be irradiated, it may be necessary to limit the medial or lateral margins of the tangential fields. Where the tumour lies laterally in the breast, the medial margin can be reduced, and vice versa when the tumour is in the medial half of the breast.

General care

During treatment

- If the margins of the treatment fields are marked by a small number of tattoos, the patient can wash the treatment area during a course of radiotherapy. The only restriction is avoiding washing the electron boost area after whole breast irradiation in breast-conserving therapy since the margins of the treatment area are usually outlined by temporary skin marks.
- Apply proprietary baby powder to the treated area to keep it dry.
- If the skin becomes sore during radiotherapy, the application of cold air from a hairdryer may help.
- Shoulder exercises to keep the joint supple should be taught by a physiotherapist and practised by the patient during and after treatment

After treatment

- Apply an emollient cream, such as oilatum or aqueous cream to areas of dry desquamation. A small amount should be applied to the treated area twice daily.
- Apply antibiotic ointment (e.g. Graneodin) or Flamazine to areas of moist desquamation.
- Continue shoulder exercises indefinitely (particularly patients treated by axillary irradiation where restriction of shoulder movements may occur).

Morbidity of radical radiotherapy

Intact breast

1. Breast oedema is common, particularly in the first year after radiotherapy. It is commoner in patients who have had an axillary clearance. It tends to diminish after a year.
2. Subcutaneous fibrosis is common and may give rise to shrinkage of the irradiated breast over a period of years. The extent of fibrosis is clinically unpredictable. It tends to be more marked at the site of the breast boost.

Intact breast and postmastectomy

1. Skin—telangiectasia.
2. Lymphoedema of the ipsilateral arm.
3. Rib fractures. These occur in 1% of patients and are uncommon with conventionally fractionated radiotherapy. They tend to occur in the lateral 4th–7th ribs where the maximum dose points tend to occur from tangential breast or chest wall irradiation.
4. Pneumonitis and lung fibrosis. Virtually all patients will develop some degree of impaired lung function as an effect of radical breast or chest wall irradiation, especially if the peripheral lymphatics are irradiated. However, it is unusual for these changes to give rise to breathlessness unless there is pre-existing impairment of lung function or excessive volumes of lung have been irradiated. Occasionally transient cough occurs during radiotherapy but usually settles within a few weeks. Some degree of fibrosis is observed on chest radiograph.
5. Fibrosis of the shoulder joint can occur if the axilla is irradiated, restricting shoulder movement. Appropriate shoulder exercises should be taught to such patients during radiotherapy and continued indefinitely after treatment to minimise limitation of shoulder movements.
6. Cardiac morbidity. Patients, particularly if irradiated over the age of 60, are at increased risk of coronary artery disease and potentially of disease of other cardiac structures. Every effort should be made to minimise the volume of the heart within the irradiated volume by appropriate planning techniques.
7. Radiation-induced sarcoma. This is an extremely rare complication with a mean latency of 13 years from the time of radiotherapy. Prognosis is very poor. Mean survival is 15 months.
8. Hypothyroidism may occur because of inclusion of the thyroid gland in the shoulder or medial supraclavicular field.

Results of radical radiotherapy

Postmastectomy. Data from randomised trials and overviews of postmastectomy radiotherapy suggest that adjuvant irradiation reduces the local recurrence threefold. Typical recurrence rates at 5 years are 4% for stage I, 10% for stage II and 20% for stage III. Local recurrence after mastectomy is a poor prognostic factor with more than 90% of patients developing clinically overt metastases within 5 years.

Conservation therapy. The 5-year local recurrence rate for T1–2N0–N1M0 should be not more than 5% overall. The risks of local recurrence are higher in younger women and may approach 10–15% in women under the age of 40. The recurrence rates may be substantially lower in node-negative patients with small (< 2 cm) node tumours. Long-term follow-up of the British Association of Surgical Oncology trial (BASO 2) investigating the role of postoperative breast irradiation and adjuvant tamoxifen alone or in combination are still awaited. The survival of patients treated by breast-conserving therapy and salvage mastectomy for local recurrence is no different from that of patients treated by mastectomy ab initio.

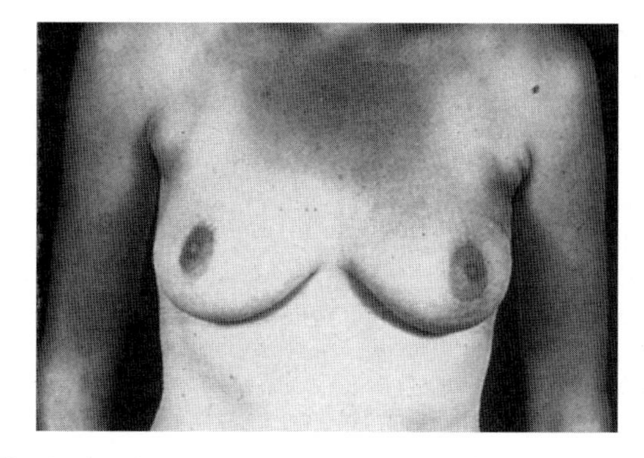

Fig. 26.18 Excellent cosmetic result of postoperative radiotherapy and iridium implant following lumpectomy for early carcinoma of the left breast. (Courtesy of Dr D Ash, Leeds.)

Cosmetic results are good in 87% of T1 and 54% of T2 tumours. An example of excellent cosmesis is shown in Figure 26.18. Cosmetic results tend to be poorer in patients with larger breasts. This may relate to the poorer homogeneity of dose distribution in larger breasts.

ADJUVANT HORMONAL AND CYTOTOXIC THERAPY

Rationale

It is generally accepted that a substantial number of patients with apparently localised breast cancer harbour systemic micrometastases. These are currently beyond the detection of the conventional staging. Axillary involvement has for more than three decades been the strongest prognostic factor for systemic relapse.

All patients should be considered for some form of adjuvant systemic therapy to try to eradicate micrometastases. The benefits have been determined from meta-analyses of the long-term follow-up of all randomised trials comparing women treated with or without adjuvant hormonal or cytotoxic therapy.

Who benefits?

The Early Breast Cancer Trialists' Group has provided a series of 5-yearly meta-analyses of over 75 000 women with early breast cancer. The advantage of this approach of meta-analysis is that it brings together large numbers of randomised trials. By virtue of the very large numbers of patients analysed it provides much greater power to detect significant effects of different treatments. The overview shows clearly that both hormonal (tamoxifen or oophorectomy) and cytotoxic therapy (CMF or anthracycline-containing combination chemotherapy) reduce the relative risk of relapse or death by up to 30% at 10 years. The overall survival benefits are more modest, with a 4–12% gain in overall survival. The benefits in overall survival are greater in premenopausal than postmenopausal women.

Following polychemotherapy, women aged 50–59 gain a 14% reduction in risk of death compared to 8% in women aged 60–69. The survival gains in the under 50 and 50–69 age groups are shown in Figure 26.19. Life expectancy is likely to be prolonged on average by 4 years for women under the age of 50 and by 1–3 years in women over the age of 50. Adjuvant chemotherapy reduces 10-year breast cancer mortality by 27%. For a woman who has a 50% chance of dying from breast cancer under the age of 50, the approximate reduction in risk of death is 13.5% (50% × 0.27). For a woman with a 10% risk of death at 10 years, the risk of death is about 8% (10% × 0.27 = 2.7%; 10% − 2.7% = 7.3%).

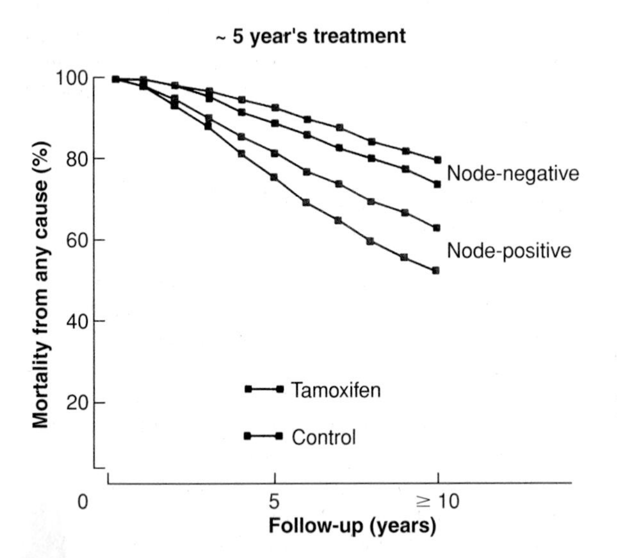

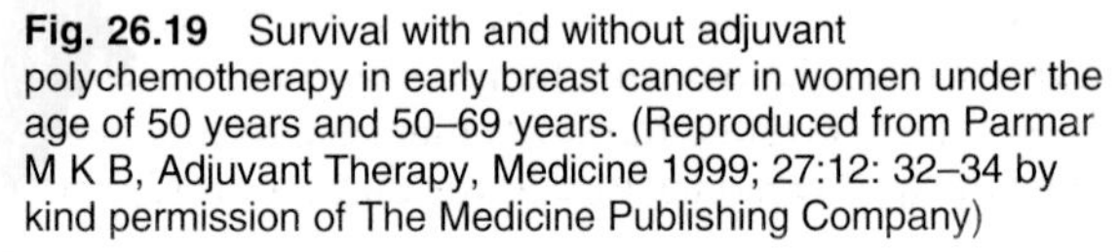

Fig. 26.19 Survival with and without adjuvant polychemotherapy in early breast cancer in women under the age of 50 years and 50–69 years. (Reproduced from Parmar M K B, Adjuvant Therapy, Medicine 1999; 27:12: 32–34 by kind permission of The Medicine Publishing Company)

Adjuvant tamoxifen

Adjuvant tamoxifen in a dose of 20 mg orally daily used to be given for life or until time of recurrence. The degree of benefit appears to depend on both the duration of treatment and whether the disease is node positive or negative.

Adjuvant tamoxifen reduces the annual risk of death by about 15%. The reduction in risk is 22% among women who have received 5 years of tamoxifen. The survival benefits of adjuvant tamoxifen are shown in Figure 26.20. Women with oestrogen receptor (ER)-rich tumours have 3–10 times the benefits of ER-poor patients. Life expectancy is increased by 2–3 years in women on tamoxifen for 2–3 years. If tamoxifen is

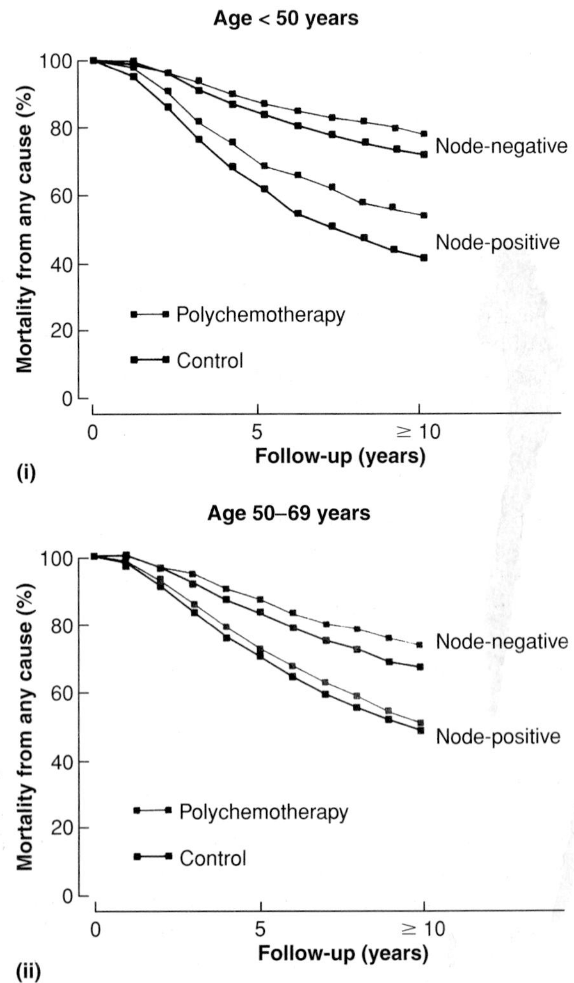

Fig. 26.20 Survival with and without 5 years of adjuvant tamoxifen in early breast cancer. (Reproduced from Parmar M K B, Adjuvant Therapy, Medicine 1999; 27:12: 32–34 by kind permission of The Medicine Publishing Company)

added to chemotherapy in ER-rich tumours, additional benefit accrues, as also happens when chemotherapy is added to tamoxifen. In addition, tamoxifen reduces the risk of contralateral breast cancer.

The optimal duration of administration of tamoxifen is not clear but most of the current evidence suggests that 5 years is probably optimal. There is good evidence that 5 years' duration is more effective than 2 years and that 2 years is superior to 1 year of therapy. Tamoxifen given for at least 2 years reduces the risk of recurrence by 28% and breast cancer mortality by 21%. 5 years of tamoxifen achieves a 22% reduction in odds of death.

Tamoxifen confers a similar reduction in risk of death in node-positive and node-negative women. However, the absolute reduction in risk is greater in node-positive women. The absolute gain in 10-year survival between 5 years of tamoxifen and no tamoxifen is 6% for node-negative and 11% in node-positive women. It confers benefit in both premenopausal and postmenopausal ER-positive women. Beyond 5 years the reduction in risk by tamoxifen is thought to decline and has to be balanced against the small risk of tamoxifen-induced endometrial cancer. In women less than 50 the benefits are less than in those over the age of 50.

Adding tamoxifen to chemotherapy in ER-positive patients confers additional benefit.

All patients who are ER positive regardless of their menopausal or nodal status should be considered for tamoxifen for 5 years.

Toxicity of tamoxifen

Postmenopausal symptoms of hot flushes, vaginal dryness and sexual dysfunction are experienced by 20–40% of patients. Cognitive deficits also occur (as they do after cytotoxic chemotherapy). These symptoms can significantly interfere with a patient's quality of life and should be regularly monitored at follow-up visits. Transient thrombocytopenia occurs in 5–10% and vaginal bleeding in 5%. Tamoxifen increases the development of benign endometrial changes such as hyperplasia. The risk of endometrial cancer, particularly in women who have been on tamoxifen for 5 years or more, is increased three- to fourfold, although the risk remains very small.

There appears to be some interaction between radiotherapy and tamoxifen with an increase in subclinical lung fibrosis when tamoxifen is given synchronously with radiotherapy.

It should be noted that tamoxifen also increases the risk of thromboembolism. Care should be taken to avoid giving tamoxifen concurrently with chemotherapy.

Adjuvant ovarian suppression

Suppression of ovarian function is one of the longest established of adjuvant therapies. It was Beatson, a surgeon in Glasgow, who in 1895 first showed that oophorectomy could reduce the activity of breast cancer. A small randomised trial conducted in Edinburgh comparing patients with operable breast cancer treated by adjuvant oophorectomy or CMF chemotherapy showed that oophorectomy had a significant advantage over CMF in ER-positive patients and CMF over oophorectomy in ER-negative patients. Until the Oxford overview in 1995 the value of adjuvant oophorectomy was not well supported because of the small numbers in individual studies. The Oxford overview showed a highly significant increase in recurrence-free survival (25%) in premenopausal women under the age of 50.

For node-positive premenopausal women the gains in recurrence-free and overall survival at 15 years were 10.5% and 13% respectively. Much smaller but still statistically significant benefits in both these parameters were seen in premenopausal node-negative women.

Medical ovarian suppression by goserelin (3.6 mg given subcutaneously monthly) provides a reversible means of stopping ovarian function. Goserelin is commonly given for 2 years. It has the advantage that if the patient finds the premenopausal symptoms intolerable (e.g. flushing and sweating) it can be stopped. If after 6 months of goserelin, menopausal symptoms are found still to be tolerable, the alternatives are to stay on goserelin or to proceed to an oophorectomy. If the patient prefers to stay on goserelin, it can be stopped after 2 years to check whether the patient is menopausal (raised LH and FSH with reduced oestradiol levels).

Adjuvant combination chemotherapy (polychemotherapy)

The 2000 Oxford overview shows no significant reduction in recurrence or risk of death comparing prolonged single-agent chemotherapy vs no chemotherapy. Prolonged combination chemotherapy (typically CMF) shows highly significant reductions in recurrence and death in women under the age of 50 and those aged 50–69. The reduction in risk of recurrence emerged in the first 4 years following treatment and the advantage in survival persists up to 15 years. There do not appear to be any large differences in effects between different types of combination chemotherapy. The age-specific benefits do not appear to be influenced by the ER status of the primary tumour, menopausal status or the administration of adjuvant tamoxifen. There did not appear to be any increase in non-breast cancer deaths from adjuvant chemotherapy. The proportional reductions in risk were similar in node-positive and node-negative patients. The absolute differences in 10-year survival are 11–12% for node-positive patients and 4–5% for node-negative disease. For the 50–59 and 60–69 age groups, combination chemotherapy improved 10-year survival by 4% and 2% respectively.

More recently the use of anthracycline-based chemotherapy (e.g. containing doxorubicin or epirubicin) has increased. The Oxford overview shows highly significant additional reductions in recurrence or death from anthracycline-containing regimes compared to CMF. The proportional reduction in risk did not appear to be affected by the age at diagnosis or by axillary nodal status. There were absolute gains of approximately 4% in survival, which persisted to 10 years.

Duration of treatment

The optimal duration of adjuvant cytotoxic therapy is not known. 6 cycles of adjuvant CMF chemotherapy (Table 26.6) are generally recommended or 4 cycles of epirubicin/doxorubicin followed by 4–8 cycles of CMF (Table 26.7). There is no evidence that more prolonged chemotherapy confers additional benefit at any age.

Choice of drugs

For patients at intermediate risk of recurrence (1–3 nodes positive) 6 cycles of CMF are recommended. With 4 or more positive axillary nodes, the anthracycline-containing regime is more intensive (Table 26.8) with 4 cycles of doxorubicin followed by 8 cycles of CMF chemotherapy. More recently, epirubicin has been used as an alternative to doxorubicin since it causes less nausea and vomiting.

Table 26.7 (a) Doxorubicin + CMF (Bonnadonna) adjuvant regime; (b) epirubicin + CMF

a. Doxorubicin + CMF
Doxorubicin 75 mg/m^2 i.v.
Repeated every 21 days for 4 courses
Followed by 8 cycles of CMF
Repeated every 21 days

b. Epirubicin + CMF
Epirubicin 100 mg/m^2 on day 1
Repeated every 21 days for 4 cycles
Followed by 4 cycles of CMF

Table 26.8 Palliative doxorubicin/epirubicin and cyclophosphamide

Doxorubicin 60 mg/m^2 or epirubicin 75 mg/m^2
Cyclophosphamide 600 mg/m^2
Repeated every 21 days

Morbidity

Morbidity of adjuvant cytotoxic therapy may be both physical and psychological. For CMF chemotherapy acute toxicity includes nausea and vomiting, temporary alopecia, lassitude, and soreness of the eyes (the latter due to secretion of methotrexate into the tears). Neutropenia-related infection is less common with CMF than with more intensive anthracycline-based chemotherapy. The anthracyclines (doxorubicin and epirubicin) cause complete, although reversible, alopecia. They are also potentially cardiotoxic, and cardiac function, judged clinically by electrocardiogram and cardiac ejection fraction, should be adequate before use. Otherwise congestive cardiac failure may result.

Anxiety and depression are common sequelae of treatment as a result of toxicity, change in body image and the cumulative emotional toll of the diagnostic

Table 26.6 Adjuvant CMF regimes

Classical		
Cyclophosphamide	100 mg/m^2 orally	Days 1–14
Methotrexate	40 mg/m^2 i.v. bolus	Days 1 and 8
5-fluorouracil	600 mg/m^2 i.v. bolus	Days 1 and 8
Repeated every 28 days		
Alternative		
Cyclophosphamide	750 mg/m^2 i.v. 3-weekly	
Methotrexate	50 mg/m^2 i.v. 3-weekly	
5-Fluorouracil	600 mg/m^2 i.v. 3-weekly	

pathway and prolonged treatment. It is important to recognise and treat them, if necessary referring for specialist advice to a psychiatrist or clinical psychologist.

MANAGEMENT OF LOCALLY ADVANCED BREAST CANCER (LABC)

Locally advanced breast cancer (T3 or T4 or N2 or N3M0) still presents a major challenge in management. It accounts for between 5% and 30% of patients presenting to the breast clinic. A typical example in shown in Figure 26.21. These are a very heterogeneous group of tumours with widely differing natural histories. While there have been substantial improvements in local response to a combination of systemic therapy and radiotherapy, the development of metastatic disease remains a major problem. Patients should be assessed by the multidisciplinary team.

Clinical features

The main features of LABC are skin nodules, peau d'-orange (T4b), inflammatory changes (T4d), ulceration and fixity to the chest wall (T4a), fixed axillary nodes (N2) or lymphoedema (N3). Local pain, bleeding, ulceration and infection are common symptomatic problems.

Principles of management

The main aim of management of LABC is to provide durable local control. The natural history of locally advanced disease varies widely. In some patients distant metastatic disease will rapidly supervene, in others the disease remains locoregional and relatively indolent. Some of the most difficult patients to manage are young with aggressive locoregional disease but who remain free of metastatic disease.

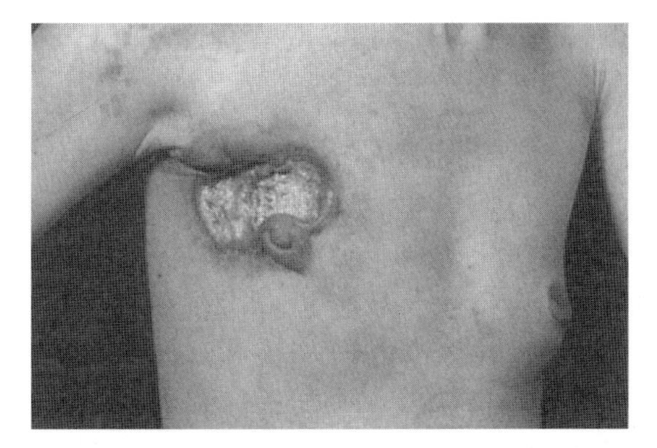

Fig. 26.21 Locally advanced and inoperable carcinoma of the right breast (T4).

Neoadjuvant therapy

The use of initial (neoadjuvant) systemic therapy is based on the observation that patients with LABC frequently develop metastatic disease. The aim of neoadjuvant therapy is to treat both local and micrometastatic disease and to downstage the disease prior to local therapy.

Initial treatment should be systemic with either hormonal or cytotoxic therapy depending on ER status. This should aim at maximum cytoreduction before proceeding to mastectomy (if skin oedema or inflammatory changes have settled) followed by radiotherapy, or by radiotherapy alone if skin oedema or inflammatory changes persist after systemic therapy.

Role of surgery

Surgery has a more limited role in the management of locally advanced disease. It encompasses: (i) initial core biopsy for diagnosis and ER status; (ii) mastectomy and axillary clearance in operable patients; (iii) mastectomy (ideally with myocutaneous flap reconstruction) for residual masses after chemotherapy and radical radiotherapy; and (iv) palliative debriding of infected and/or necrotic areas to reduce odour.

There are occasionally patients with small T4 tumours in the inferior part of the breast or inframammary fold who can be managed by standard breast-conserving surgery, postoperative radical radiotherapy and appropriate systemic therapy.

Systemic therapy

In general LABC in younger patients tends to be high grade and ER negative. For patients with inflammatory (T4d) disease irrespective of ER status initial treatment should, subject to general medical fitness, be with chemotherapy because of the aggressive nature of this form of the disease.

Combination therapy is more effective than single-agent therapy. A number of different combinations are possible. The optimal regime and scheduling has yet to be established. Doxorubicin and cyclophosphamide are an effective combination (Table 26.8). Between 4 and 6 cycles are given before local therapy depending on the response and 4–6 cycles after local treatment, again dependent on the initial response to neoadjuvant chemotherapy. If there is no response to chemotherapy after the first 2 cycles, chemotherapy should be abandoned and the patient should proceed directly to radical radiotherapy. Neoadjuvant therapy may debulk the tumour sufficiently for mastectomy or occasionally breast-conserving surgery to be made possible. Trials are assessing the benefits of using a different non-cross-resistant adjuvant therapy regime after local therapy in an attempt to eradicate residual tumour cells resistant to initial chemotherapy.

While the taxanes have an established role in the treatment of metastatic disease, their efficacy in locally advanced disease has yet to be established. Studies of dose intensification are in progress.

Concurrent chemoradiation

There are good theoretical reasons for giving chemotherapy and radiotherapy concomitantly since chemotherapeutic agents such as 5-FU are radiosensitisers and may increase the cytotoxicity of radiotherapy. An additional advantage is the shortened overall treatment time.

Concurrent chemoradiation, however, carries risks of enhancing complications of radiotherapy such as soft tissue necrosis, brachial plexopathy, radiation pneumonitis and cardiac failure. Until long-term data confirm the safety and efficacy of concomitant chemoradiation, sequential therapy is recommended.

Intra-arterial chemotherapy

Where local recurrence has occurred despite conventional chemotherapy and radiotherapy, intra-arterial chemotherapy has been successfully administered via the internal mammary artery. Although response rates in some centres are impressive, only small series of patients have been reported.

Radical radiotherapy

Technique

The principles of radical radiotherapy for early breast cancer apply also to locally advanced disease both for the intact breast or following mastectomy. The only difference is that 0.5–1 cm of skin bolus should be applied to the breast or chest wall to ensure that the skin receives a full dose (to overcome the skin-sparing effect of megavoltage radiotherapy). Axillary surgery is not normally carried out at staging and therefore the peripheral lymphatics will normally be irradiated. If mastectomy and clearance have been carried out, the axilla is not irradiated. Where there is macroscopic disease which would cross the conventional breast/shoulder field junction, it is best to use an 'en bloc' technique, treating both the breast and the peripheral lymphatics in a Perspex jig (see Fig. 26.12).

Dosage and fractionation

While there is evidence of a dose response effect in locally advanced disease, escalating dosage beyond 60–70 Gy is associated with an increased risk of major complications. Hyperfractionated radiotherapy may have advantages in reducing repopulation during radiotherapy. The long-term results of studies of hyperfractionated radiotherapy are awaited. Until there is convincing evidence of improved local control, conventional dosage and fractionation are recommended.

1. *Post-mastectomy*

45 Gy TAD in 20 fractions over 4 weeks (6 MV photons) (applying skin bolus)

2. *Intact breast*

45 Gy TAD in 20 fractions over 4 weeks (6 MV photons) (applying skin bolus)

Boost

15 Gy maximum dose in 5 daily fractions over 1 week with electrons of appropriate energy

To judge the appropriate choice of energy of electrons, an ultrasound scan should be carried out towards the end of the radical course of breast irradiation and the distance from the skin surface over the tumour to the maximum depth of the tumour measured. The other dimensions of the tumour should also be measured to help the selection of the appropriate electron field size.

Palliative radiotherapy

In some patients radical radiotherapy is not advised either because of poor medical condition, advanced age or evidence of metastatic disease elsewhere. Palliative radiotherapy can be very effective for symptomatic relief of local bleeding, ulceration, pain from axillary involvement and secondary upper limb lymphoedema. Responses are usually only partial but may be prolonged or short-lived. However, even some shrinkage can be worthwhile, improving the morale of the patient where chemotherapy or hormonal therapy has been unsuccessful.

Technique

This should be simple, either with parallel-opposed or tangential fields at megavoltage confined to the macroscopic area of tumour using a small Perspex jig, or, for flat limited areas of tumour, by a single electron field using a Perspex degrader to bring up the skin to full dose.

Dose

20 Gy in 5 daily fractions over 1 week (electrons or 4–6 MV photons)

Bone metastases

Patients with symptomatic bony metastases should be considered for up to 2 years of bisphosphonate therapy (e.g. pamidronate 90 mg monthly by intravenous infusion or oral clodronate 1600 mg daily) in addition to palliative radiotherapy. Patients at risk of pathological fracture should be referred to an orthopaedic surgeon for consideration of mechanical stabilisation (Fig. 26.22) followed by postoperative palliative radiotherapy.

Technique

Single or parallel-opposed fields are used. Single fields suffice for the thoracic, lumbar spine and sacroiliac joints. The cervical spine can be treated by a single posterior field but this will cause a sore throat due to the exit dose through the mouth. Lateral opposed fields reduce the dose to the mouth.

Dose

Single fractions of **8 Gy** are recommended at megavoltage.

Following surgical stabilisation, fractionated radiotherapy is given:

20 Gy in 5 fractions over 1 week at megavoltage

Palliative surgery

Where there is extensive ulceration and secondary infection causing distressing and offensive odour, surgical debridement of the affected area is often helpful in improving these symptoms. This can be repeated if necessary.

Cerebral or choroidal metastases. See Chapter 30 (pp. 551, 563) for treatment.

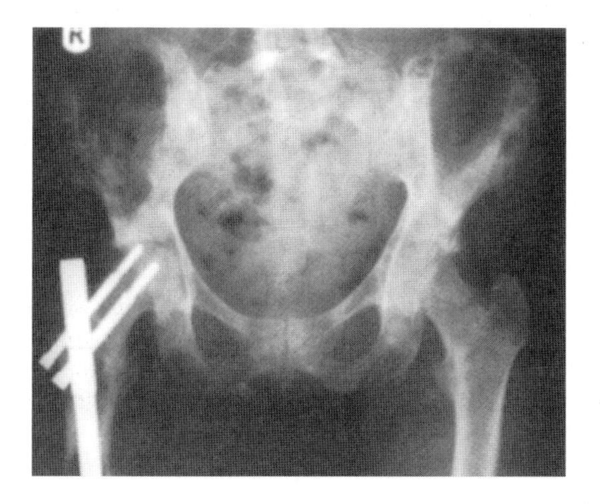

Fig. 26.22 Radiograph of pelvis showing pinning of pathological fracture of right hip due to extensive mixed and sclerotic disease from breast cancer.

Results of treatment

Overall the outcome of patients with locally advanced disease remains poor, largely because of the high incidence of development of metastatic disease. The only systemic therapy that improves long-term survival for LABC is tamoxifen. The main effects of systemic therapy and radiotherapy are on local control.

In general, response to neoadjuvant systemic therapy predicts survival. Preoperative neoadjuvant therapy can be very successful with response rates in excess of 50%. Response rates to systemic therapy combined with radiotherapy are of the order of 89%. About 75% of patients with ER-rich tumours will respond to hormonal therapy.

The size of the primary tumour (especially over 8 cm), high grade and axillary involvement are major prognostic factors for outcome. 5-year survival rates vary widely from 5% to 45% with the best results being achieved in patients achieving a complete response to neoadjuvant chemotherapy and the worst in patients with progressive disease despite neoadjuvant therapy. 5-year survival from radiotherapy alone is 20–25% with barely any survivors among patients with inflammatory disease. The addition of surgery to radiotherapy improves the 5-year survival to 40–50%.

MEDICAL MANAGEMENT OF METASTATIC DISEASE

Although about 90% of patients present with localised disease, about 50% of patients with involved nodes and 10% of those who are node negative will relapse within 5 years. This comes as a blow to most patients and psychological support from the breast care team is an important element in the care of such patients in addition to individualised medical management. Treatment is still essentially palliative since the average life expectancy from the time of diagnosis of metastatic disease is of the order of 18 months. None the less, durable and clinically useful disease control can be obtained by hormonal, and/or cytotoxic therapy. In addition, therapy with bisphosphonates can be useful in reducing the risk of complications of bony metastases.

Principles of management

The choice of treatment must take into account the age and general medical condition of the patient, menopausal status, oestrogen receptor (ER) status, sites of metastatic involvement and the tempo of the disease. It is important that all centres should have access to ER status, since responses to hormonal treatment in

ER-negative patients are virtually unheard of. There are two general forms of systemic therapy: hormonal and cytotoxic. In general, hormonal therapy is better tolerated than cytotoxic therapy and, in the absence of immediately life-threatening aggressive disease, is the preferred first line of treatment in ER-positive disease. For ER-negative disease, chemotherapy is the treatment of choice in fit patients. The general schema of systemic therapy for metastatic cancer is shown in Figure 26.23.

Age and general medical condition

In general, older patients and those in poor general medical condition require particularly careful assessment in selecting medical treatment. Some older patients tolerate chemotherapy well. Treatment should therefore be individualised and biological age given greater consideration rather than any arbitrary upper age limit for prescribing chemotherapy. Older patients, however, are more likely to have comorbidity such as impaired renal function or coronary artery disease. Selection of patients for chemotherapy therefore needs to be assessed carefully.

For older patients with adequate cardiac function, weekly doses of epirubicin allow sufficiently frequent surveillance to monitor tumour response and toxicity. Alternatively an oral form of doxorubicin (idarubicin 45 mg/m^2 as single dose or in divided doses over 3 days—maximum dose 400 mg/m^2) can be used. Fortunately, older patients tend to have ER-positive tumours, which can often be satisfactorily controlled by hormonal therapy.

Care has to be exercised in the use of megestrol acetate, which often causes fluid retention and may precipitate cardiac failure or angina in patients with coronary artery disease.

Menopausal status and hormone receptor status

In general, more postmenopausal than premenopausal patients are oestrogen receptor positive. Premenopausal patients tend to have more aggressive disease and are more commonly ER negative, especially under the age of 40. Patients with aggressive and/or ER-negative disease require chemotherapy.

Oestrogen and progesterone (PgR) receptor status is a useful guide to clinical response. ER+/PgR+ tumours have a response rate of 77%, ER+/PgR– of 27%, ER–/PgR+ of 46% and ER–/PgR– of 11%.

In premenopausal ER-positive patients, options include ovarian suppression by medical means

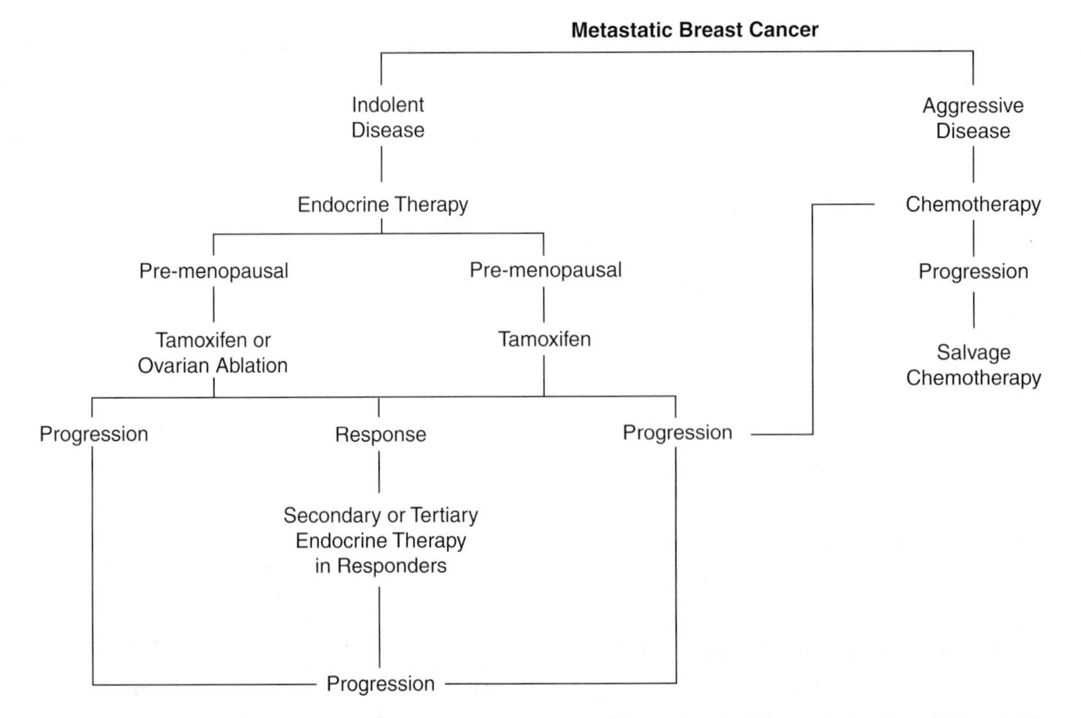

Fig. 26.23 Schema of systemic therapy for metastatic breast cancer. (Reproduced with permission from Holland J F, Frei E III, Bast R C et al (eds) Cancer Medicine, 4th edn. Vol 2, Williams & Wilkins, 1997.)

(goserelin 3.6 mg monthly subcutaneously), oophorectomy, radiation-induced menopause and tamoxifen. There is evidence in advanced disease that goserelin and tamoxifen have synergistic effects with higher response rate (but no additional survival benefit) and are best prescribed together.

The advantage of goserelin is that it is reversible once withdrawn. This has particular advantages in women who tolerate poorly the menopausal symptoms that it induces and wish to stop the treatment and continue tamoxifen alone. Oophorectomy is usually performed as a laparoscopic procedure.

In general, response to one hormonal agent predicts response to subsequent hormonal therapy. Overall, 50–60% of ER-positive patients will respond. The duration of disease control by first-line hormonal therapy is usually about 18 months. About 25% of patients who respond to first-line hormonal agent will respond to second-line hormonal therapy. However, only 15% of patients who fail to respond to first-line therapy will respond to second-line hormone therapy.

For first-line therapy in premenopausal ER-positive women with non-life-threatening disease a combination of tamoxifen (20 mg orally daily) and ovarian suppression with goserelin (3.6 mg subcutaneously monthly) is suggested; for second-line therapy anastrazole, an aromatase inhibitor, can be substituted for tamoxifen while continuing ovarian suppression with goserelin. If second-line hormonal therapy fails, cytotoxic chemotherapy should be considered.

For first-line therapy for recurrent disease in postmenopausal women the choice is between tamoxifen (20 mg per day), an aromatase inhibitor (anastrazole; 1 mg orally daily) or letrozole (2.5 mg orally daily); for second-line therapy, exemestane, an irreversible aromatase inhibitor (25 mg orally daily), is recommended; for third line therapy a progestogen, megestrol acetate (160 mg orally daily), is suggested. Megestrol acetate causes weight gain and should be avoided in patients with cardiac disease and/or thromboembolism.

Patients who are most likely to benefit from hormonal therapy for relapsed disease have one or more of the following characteristics:

- Disease-free survival over 2 years
- Soft tissue or bone disease
- Older postmenopausal.

Sites of metastases and impact on management

Visceral metastases (e.g. liver disease) tends to respond less well to hormonal therapy and more to cytotoxic therapy. However, durable responses to hormonal therapy are occasionally seen with ER-positive liver metastases.

Tempo of recurrent and metastatic disease

Both the site and rapidity of development of recurrent and metastatic disease are important factors in the choice of therapy. In general, slowly developing disease over a period of months allows hormonal therapy a chance to work. Between 6 and 12 weeks need to be allowed for a response to hormonal therapy to occur.

For rapidly evolving recurrent and metastatic disease, there is insufficient time for metastatic disease to respond to hormonal therapy even if the disease is ER positive. This is sometimes the case in patients with severe and progressive dyspnoea from pulmonary metastases. In the case of pleural effusions, which can cause a similar degree of breathlessness, aspiration of the effusions may rapidly alleviate symptoms, allowing the necessary time to respond to hormonal therapy. Further aspirations can if necessarily be carried out over the ensuing 6–8 weeks. If there is no evidence that reaccumulation of effusions has slowed or stopped at 8 weeks, a change to cytotoxic therapy should be considered.

Cytotoxic therapy

Breast cancer is moderately sensitive to chemotherapy. Response rates for single agents are shown in Table 26.9. The most commonly used agents are cyclophosphamide, doxorubicin, methotrexate and 5-fluorouracil.

More recently, the taxanes, paclitaxel and docetaxel (Table 26.10), have been approved as first- or second-line agents in metastatic breast cancer. Newer agents include herceptin and capecitabine.

Herceptin

Herceptin is a monoclonal antibody to the *HER2-neu c-erb2* oncogene. When amplified the *HER2* gene stimulates tumour growth. A transmembrane tyrosine kinase

Table 26.9 Single-agent response rates (not pretreated or not heavily pretreated)

Taxanes (taxol and taxotere)	50%
Doxorubicin and epirubicin	40%
Cyclophosphamide	36%
Mitoxantrone (mitozantrone)	27%
Methotrexate	26%
5-fluorouracil	25%
Vincristine	8%

Table 26.10 Palliative single therapy with docetaxel

Docetaxel 85–100 mg/m^2
Repeated every 21 days for up to 6 courses
Dose reduction to 75 mg/m^2 if liver function disturbed or toxicity

receptor is encoded by *HER2-neu* which is very similar to the epidermal growth factor receptor. Inactive receptor monomers are bound together to form active dimers. Once dimerisation has occurred, intracellular tyrosine kinase is activated and leads to signals which result in changes in gene expression and tumour growth. Herceptin is suitable for the 30% of patients who overexpress the cell surface antigen. Herceptin has a 13–16% response rate in heavily pretreated patients. Herceptin can be used in combination with cisplatin or paclitaxel. The addition of herceptin to anthracyclines or to a taxane (paclitaxel) increases median time to progression. The greatest addition to response rate came from combining herceptin with paclitaxel.

While it has cytotoxic activity when used alone (Table 26.11), its maximum effects are delivered in conjunction with conventional chemotherapy in terms of overall survival, progression-free survival and overall response rates. *HER2* testing is by immunohistochemistry or fluorescence in situ hybridisation (FISH).

Side-effects include allergic reactions and cardiac failure. Caution in the use of herceptin should be exercised in patients with a history of cardiac disease

Capecitabine

Capecitabine is an oral fluoropyrimidine with a slow release of 5-FU. It is well tolerated and effective.

Combination chemotherapy

The objective response to combination chemotherapy (60%) is generally higher than to single agents. Median time to response varies from 6–14 weeks. Median duration of response is 6–12 months. Response rates to second-line combination chemotherapy are generally much lower (about 20%) and to third-line therapy 5% or less. In only about 15–20% of patients is a complete response obtained.

Table 26.11 Treatment schedule for herceptin

Loading dose 4 mg/kg i.v. by infusion over 90 minutes
If loading dose is tolerated, subsequent weekly doses of 2 mg/kg i.v. by infusion over 30 minutes

It is important that the balance of symptomatic benefit and toxicity of chemotherapy is kept under regular review. In general, at least two courses of intravenous chemotherapy are required to demonstrate some evidence of response. If there is evidence of response, a further two courses can be given and the response reviewed again. If there is evidence of continued response, a further two courses can be given. A total of six courses is commonly given as long as response is maintained and toxicity is acceptable. Chemotherapy can be then be stopped and the patient kept under regular review.

There is evidence that increasing dose increases response rates but no evidence that dose intensity increases survival.

There are a wide range of palliative regimes of combination chemotherapy in use. For first-line treatment for relapse in patients who are fit for anthracycline therapy, doxorubicin/epirubicin and cyclophosphamide (Table 26.8) are suggested. If liver function is impaired, weekly epirubicin 20–30 mg/m^2 for 12–18 weeks can be tried. If patients are unfit for anthracylines, then cyclophosphamide, methotrexate and 5-fluorouracil (Table 26.12) are recommended. The response rate to CMF is 40–50%.

For second-line therapy, patients who have progressed on anthracyclines, should be considered for a taxane, e.g. docetaxel or paclitaxel. A reduction in dose or withdrawal of therapy may be needed in patients with impaired liver function. Alternative second-line regimes are mitomycin C and infusional 5-FU, mitomycin C + methotrexate + mitoxantrone (MMM) or classical CMF. The MMM regime may be suitable for frailer patients owing to its limited toxicity. In older patients an oral anthracycline (idarubicin) should be considered.

More recently a range of new agents have shown promise or sustained benefit in metastatic breast cancer. These include topoisomerase II inhibitors (see p. 616), antimetabolites and HER2 blockers. The most promising topoisomerase II inhibitor is liposomal doxorubicin with a response rate of 33% and without cardiotoxicity. Gemcitabine (see p. 616) is an antimetabolite with a response rate of 37% and a low level of toxicity. Capecitabine is an orally active prodrug of 5-FU with an objective response rate of 36%.

Table 26.12 Palliative CMF regime

Cyclophosphamide	600 mg/m^2 i.v. bolus	Day 1
Methotrexate	40 mg/m^2 i.v. bolus	Day 1
5-fluorouracil	600 mg/m^2 i.v. bolus	Day 1
Repeated every 21 days for up to 6 courses		

Bone marrow involvement

Bone marrow involvement complicates the delivery of cytotoxic therapy since the associated leucopenia and thrombocytopenia due to impaired marrow function may compromise the delivery of full-dose chemotherapy. Doses of chemotherapy have to be reduced to 50% or less of standard dosage. Weekly intravenous epirubicin or doxorubicin (25–30 mg/m^2) is generally well tolerated.

If chemotherapy is successful, haemoglobin, white count and platelet levels should eventually rise. Bone marrow involvement is not an absolute indication for cytotoxic therapy since responses are seen in ER-positive patients. However, rapidly evolving bone marrow infiltration will require chemotherapy.

Growth factor support

For patients who are experiencing treatment delays due to febrile leucopenia, treatment with granulocyte colony-stimulating factor (GCSF) is recommended. GCSF is given daily by subcutaneous injection, starting not less than 24 hours after chemotherapy and continuing until the predicated neutrophil nadir has passed and recovered into the normal range. Duration of treatment is normally up to 14 days depending on the drug regime, dosage and scheduling.

Common side-effects include pain and redness at the injection site and bone pain.

OVERALL SURVIVAL IN BREAST CANCER

As seen in Figure 26.24, the mortality of breast cancer exceeds that of the unaffected women, even up to 30 years or more after initial treatment.

Overall survival from the time of diagnosis of metastatic disease is about 18 months. The tempo of metastatic disease varies widely. It may be relatively indolent in bone with disease controlled for many years. However, the tempo of visceral disease is often more aggressive with survival often of 6 months or less.

FOLLOW-UP

Several groups of patients are followed up: (a) in remission following breast-conserving therapy or mastectomy

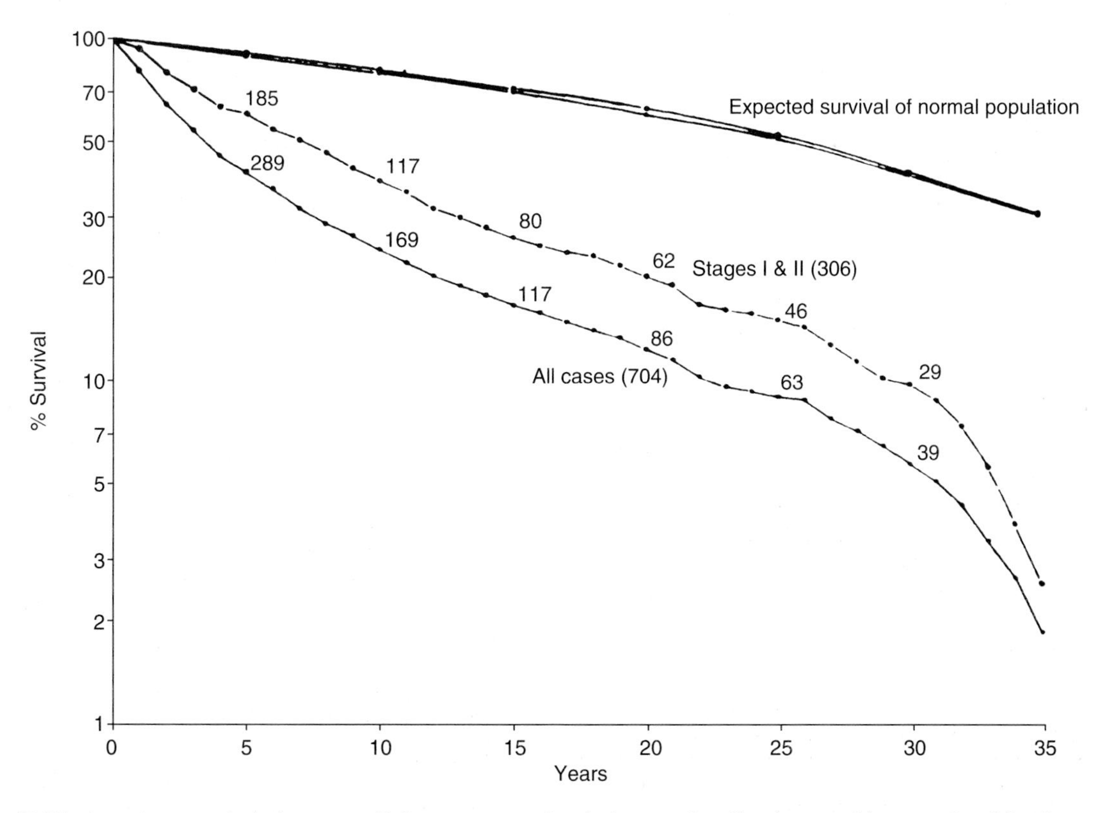

Fig. 26.24 Long-term survival of women with breast cancer. Survival curves for all patients and for stage I and II only. (Reproduced with permission from The Lancet, 1984.)

(b) in remission following treatment for locally advanced disease (c) recurrent or metastatic breast cancer. The approach to each group needs to be individualised.

Relatively few randomised data exist comparing different models and frequencies of follow-up despite the heavy usage of health resources that follow-up imposes. In general, most of the evidence, at least for patients managed by breast conservation, does not suggest that patients attending routine follow-up visits fare any better in terms of survival than those who re-present with symptoms at interval visits.

Traditionally most follow-up in the UK has been hospital based. However, community-based follow-up by general practitioners and/or nurse specialists may be as effective and acceptable to patients as hospital-based follow-up. With improvements in 5-year survival for breast cancer of 4.4% the number of women eligible for follow-up is steadily increasing.

The main goals of follow-up are to detect local recurrence and contralateral breast cancer, monitor response to treatment and treatment-induced morbidity and facilitate rehabilitation. From the patient's perspective, reassurance that there is no evidence of recurrence or of progressive disease is probably the most important. This has to be balanced by the anxiety caused to patients by anticipation of routine clinic visits, although anxiety levels normally fall a few weeks later.

Despite the rarity of recurrence being detected at routine hospital visits (1% of routine visits for breast-conserving therapy), patients' preference is still for hospital-based follow-up. They are often reluctant to be discharged, having become accustomed to regular clinic visits. Patients who are discharged need reassurance that rapid reassessment in the clinic is available if they develop new symptoms suspicious of recurrent breast cancer. Information leaflets on criteria for reassessment at the clinic may facilitate discharging patients from the clinic at the appropriate time.

Most of the evidence suggests, at least for women treated for operable breast cancer, that most recurrences whether after breast conservation or mastectomy present symptomatically. In practice the number of asymptomatic recurrences detected is very small (< 1% of clinic visits). Thus no significant abnormalities are detected at the majority of clinic visits.

It is probable that a policy of annual mammography to detect local recurrence in the conserved or contralateral breast and rapid access to the breast/oncology clinic for women with new symptoms would be much more cost-effective.

Alternative models of follow-up

Alternative models are specialist nurse-led follow-up in the hospital or in the community, or follow-up undertaken by the patient's general practitioner. There is scope for nurse- or general practitioner-led follow-up as long as they have adequate training in clinical assessment.

Unfortunately, there are few trials evaluating the clinical and cost effectiveness of these different models. However, there is evidence from one randomised trial that follow-up by the patient's general practitioner is as effective in detecting recurrence as hospital-based follow-up

In a trial comparing routine hospital follow-up to a policy of mammographic surveillance and referral to hospital with suspicious symptoms, there was no significant difference in the acceptability to patients of these two approaches. 94% found routine clinic attendance reassuring compared to 88% for annual mammography. The acceptability of mammographic surveillance was supported by the 93% acceptance of randomisation to mammographic surveillance alone. In addition, patients expressed a preference for less frequent follow-up.

Advantages of follow-up in primary care are convenience for the patient, and continuity of care. Potential disadvantages are the absence of a specialist breast cancer team in the community, delays in referral to specialist care and inadequate infrastructure for audit and research. Advantages of nurse-led follow-up include their skills in eliciting and addressing psychosocial problems commonly associated with the diagnosis of breast cancer or its treatment.

Frequency of follow-up

The frequency of follow-up needs to be tailored to the natural history of early breast cancer treated by conservation therapy or mastectomy or of advanced and metastatic disease and the effectiveness of therapy for recurrent or progressive disease. The detection of recurrence in the conserved breast and contralateral breast cancer are the main aims of follow-up. There is no good evidence that early detection of metastatic disease improves outcome. For most patients local recurrence after mastectomy is not curable, is often associated with metastatic disease and carries a poor outlook.

The optimal frequency of follow-up has yet to be determined for early breast cancer. There are wide variations in practice reflecting the paucity of good prospective studies.

Follow-up after breast-conserving therapy

For patients managed by breast-conserving therapy, the priorities are the detection of local recurrence which can be treated by mastectomy and of contralateral breast cancer. The risks of contralateral breast cancer is three to five times that of the normal population.

Recurrence rates within the treated breast remain constant at 1% per year up to 15 years. This argues that the frequency of follow-up does not need to be any more frequent in the early years after completion of treatment than in later years. Most studies of follow-up after breast-conserving therapy have been with annual mammography. The proportion of recurrences detected purely on mammography ranges from 24–35%. The optimal duration of clinical follow-up is uncertain. 5–10 years may be adequate screening, with rapid clinic access for reassessment of patients with suspicious clinical symptoms or signs. With such a policy, few local recurrences are likely to be missed. Patients discharged from clinical follow-up at 10 years and who are below the upper limit of age for breast screening (now 69 years in the UK) might reasonably be referred back to the breast-screening service for a 2-yearly mammogram.

Follow-up after mastectomy

For patients treated by mastectomy, local recurrence on the chest wall and contralateral breast cancer are the principal goals of follow-up. The pattern of local recurrence differs from that in patients undergoing breast-conserving therapy. Local recurrences on the chest wall are commonest in the first 2 years after mastectomy and 80% of chest wall and axillary recurrences occur within the first 5 years. The evidence-based guidelines of the American Society of Clinical Oncology recommend a careful history and clinical examination every 3–6 months for 3 years, then visits every 6–12 months for 2 years, and then annually thereafter. However, there is no firm evidence that this degree of intensity is any more effective than annual mammographic reassessment of asymptomatic patients. The optimal duration of follow-up is also not clear. Local recurrences are only detected at about 1% of routine visits. Most present symptomatically at interval visits. On this basis, annual follow-up with mammography of the remaining breast for 10 years with an optional follow-up visit at 6 months in the first year would be reasonable. As with breast conservation, patients may be discharged at 10 years and offered annual mammography of the remaining breast up to the age of 69. Mammographic follow-up of patients aged 70 and over should, as with breast conservation, be considered on an individual basis, depending on general medical condition and the patient's wishes.

Recurrent and metastatic disease

For patients with locally advanced or recurrent or metastatic disease, the follow-up schedules will need to be flexible, with more frequent visits for patients with symptomatic problems and when a change in systemic therapy is being assessed. Patients treated for locally advanced disease, especially if the tumour is inoperable, are likely to relapse in the first 2 years, often at distant sites. Where the tumour is inoperable, 3- to 4-monthly reviews are suggested in the first 2 years, then 6-monthly up to 5 years with annual mammography. For the limited numbers of survivors, annual clinical review and mammography between 5 and 10 years is suggested. Beyond 10 years the same policy of follow-up is suggested as for breast conservation and post-mastectomy.

Are routine investigations of value in follow-up?

Most recurrences (75–85%) are detected on history and clinical examination. 70% of recurrences are detected as a result of a patient developing symptoms. Biochemical abnormalities are the first sign of recurrence in only 1% of patients. An abnormal blood count is rarely the first indicator of recurrence. Regular chest radiographs will detect recurrence in 0–5% of cases. Less than 1% of bone scans will be positive in patients with no evidence of recurrence on history and clinical examination. Tumour markers such as carcinoembryonic antigen (CEA) and CA15–3 similarly have not established a useful role in following up patients. Mammography is commonly performed annually. However, whether less frequent mammography would be any less effective is unproven. Overall, with the exception of mammography, no routine follow-up investigations are recommended. However, women with clinical features suggestive of locoregional or metastatic disease should be fully restaged (full blood count, liver function tests, chest radiograph, liver ultrasound and bone scan).

BREAST CANCER IN PREGNANCY

The diagnosis of breast cancer in pregnancy is uncommon but presents difficult decisions for patient, oncologist and obstetrician. Close liaison between oncologist and obstetrician is essential. The interests of both mother and child need to be taken into account.

Management will be influenced by the stage of pregnancy and of the disease.

In the first trimester, termination is normally advised and followed by standard treatment. If a termination is declined, a simple mastectomy should be considered. No adjuvant radiotherapy or adjuvant systemic therapy is given until the delivery of the baby.

In the second trimester the choice is between simple mastectomy or termination of pregnancy followed by standard adjuvant therapy.

In the third trimester of pregnancy the breast becomes more vascular. Small tumours may be treated by size, with wide local excision followed after delivery by postoperative radiotherapy. For larger tumours, simple mastectomy with axillary node clearance is recommended. Elective induction or caesarean section at 36 weeks is followed, if indicated, by postoperative radiotherapy (same criteria as in the non-pregnant patient).

BREAST CANCER IN MALES

Breast cancer in men is rare, only representing 1% of breast cancer. Most cases occur in an older age group than in women, typically occurring over the age of 60. In some cases there is a genetic predisposition. A variable proportion of cases (3–20%) carry a mutation of the *BRCA2* gene. A family history of male breast cancer is a major predisposing factor to female breast cancer. In addition *BRCA2* mutations are associated with an increased risk of other cancers such lymphomas, laryngeal and kidney cancer.

Presentation is typically with locally advanced disease often affecting the nipple. Fixation to the chest wall is common. The advanced state of the local disease is in part probably due to the limited amount of breast tissue that the tumour has to invade and the lack of awareness among men that they can develop breast cancer.

Treatment where the disease is operable is by simple mastectomy and axillary node clearance. Postoperative radiotherapy is often needed because of skin infiltration. Although the rarity of the tumour means that there are no trials of adjuvant therapy, the same principles should apply as in female breast cancer. For ER-positive patients, tamoxifen is advised and for ER-negative disease, CMF chemotherapy. The outcome of the disease is usually poor with 5-year survival of about 40% reflecting the commonly advanced nature of the disease at presentation.

CHAPTER CONTENTS

27

Cervix, body of uterus, ovary, vagina, vulva, gestational trophoblastic tumours

David Radstone and Ian Kunkler

CANCER OF THE CERVIX

Anatomy

The cervix (Figs 27.1 and 27.2) projects into the vaginal vault. Adjacent are the anterior, posterior and lateral vaginal fornices. Anteriorly the cervix is related to the base of the bladder and posteriorly to the rectum and the pouch of Douglas. Laterally it is related to the ureters.

Lymphatic drainage (Fig. 27.3) is to the paracervical, obturator, presacral, external and internal iliac nodes and finally to the para-aortic nodes. The common iliac nodes extend up to the junction of the L4 and L5. Above this level lie the para-aortic nodes, which extend up to the junction of the T12 and L1.

Pathology

Epidemiology and aetiology

Cancer of the cervix is the second commonest gynaecological malignancy with an incidence of 13 per 100 000 in England and Wales. The average age at diagnosis is 50 years.

No immediate cause for cervical cancer is known. There is strong circumstantial evidence that it is a sexually transmitted disease. The disease is extremely rare in virgins. The incidence is higher in married than in single women and increases with the number of pregnancies. There is a fivefold higher incidence among prostitutes. It is commoner in women of lower socioeconomic groups. This is thought to be due to the early age of first intercourse. There is evidence of an association with human papillomavirus infection but

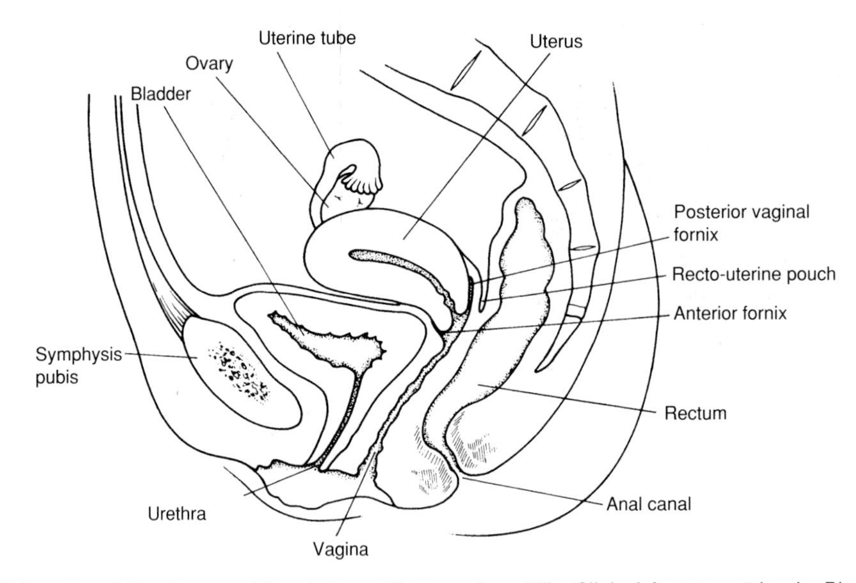

Fig. 27.1 Sagittal section of the uterus and its relations. (Redrawn from Ellis, Clinical Anatomy, 5th edn, Blackwells, 1975.)

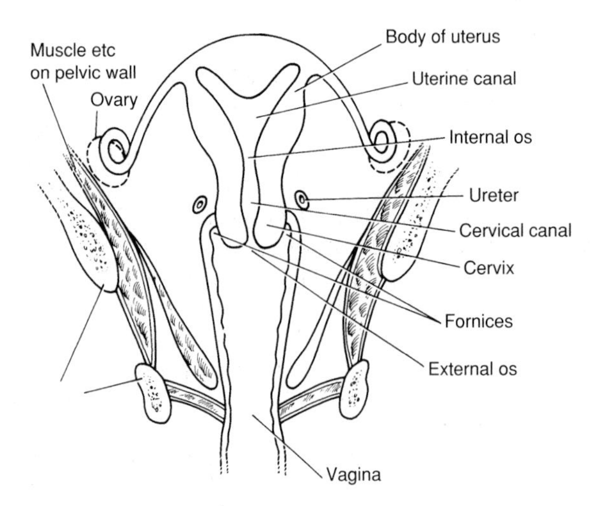

Fig. 27.2 Coronal section of the uterus and vagina. Note the important relationship of the ureter to the cervix.

no proof of its causative role. It is an AIDS-defining illness. Male factors may play a part. The 'high-risk male' is an itinerant worker who himself has a history of sexually transmitted disease. There is a slight increase in the incidence of the disease in the second wife of a man whose first wife died of the disease.

PREINVASIVE CARCINOMA

Cervical intraepithelial neoplasia (CIN III)

Cervical intraepithelial neoplasia (CIN) has now combined and replaced the previously used terms of carcinoma-in-situ and cervical dysplasia. CIN is graded according to the degree of histological abnormality. The features examined are (a) the degree of differentiation, (b) mitotic activity, and (c) the appearance of the cell nucleus. CIN III is the most abnormal grade. It corresponds to carcinoma-in-situ and is most likely to progress to invasive cancer. Minor degrees of CIN (I and II) may regress or go on to invasion. Overall about 30–40% of CIN will, if untreated, progress to invasive cancer. In one study 18% of CIN III had progressed to invasive malignancy at 10 years and 36% at 20 years.

Microinvasive cancer

Microinvasive cancer (stage Ia) is defined as a tumour measuring no more than 7 mm in diameter. It is classed as stage Ia_1 if invading to a depth less than 3 mm and stage Ia_2 if invading to between 3 and 5 mm. It requires an adequate biopsy (normally a cone biopsy, Fig. 27.4) for the diagnosis to be made.

Treatment

Cervical intraepithelial neoplasia is treated by laser therapy or cold coagulation (cryosurgery). Microinvasive carcinoma is treated by conisation (Fig. 27.4) in young patients and by hysterectomy in those who do not plan to have children.

INVASIVE CARCINOMA

Invasive cervical cancer appears as a warty growth or ulcer on the cervix; 90–95% are due to squamous cell

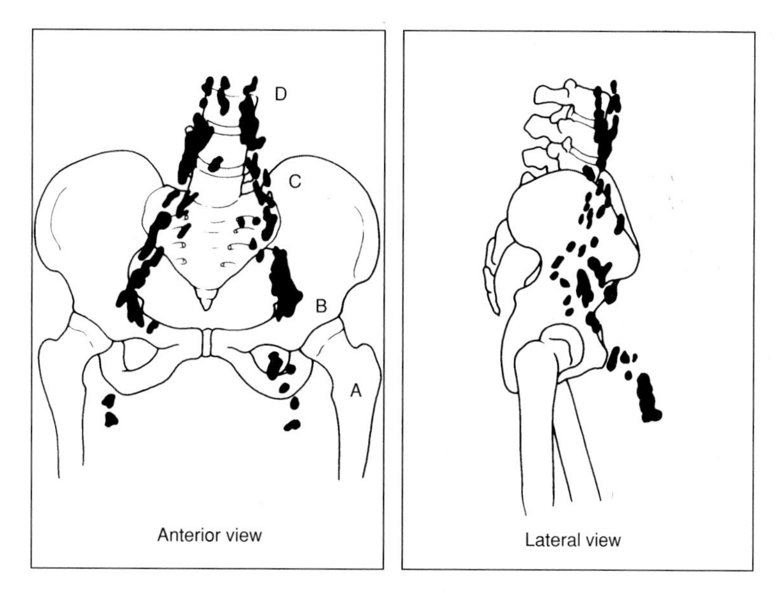

Fig. 27.3 Lymphatic drainage of the cervix: A, obturator; B, internal, external and common iliac; C, lateral sacral; and D, para-aortic. (Reproduced from Souhami and Tobias, Cancer and its Management, Blackwells, 1986.)

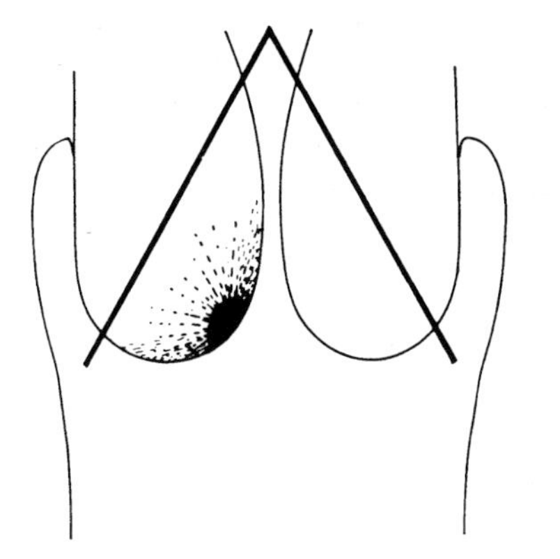

Fig. 27.4 The area of cervix removed by the operation of conisation. (Reproduced with permission from Jeffcoate, Principles of Gynaecology, Butterworths.)

carcinoma and about 5% are due to adenocarcinomas. Sarcomas, lymphomas, small cell carcinomas and melanomas are very rare.

Local spread is to the adjoining tissues (Fig. 27.5): vaginal vault, fornices, upward to the corpus, laterally to the parametria, anteriorly to the bladder and posteriorly to the rectum.

Clinical features

The cardinal symptom is vaginal bleeding or blood-stained discharge. This may occur irregularly between periods, after intercourse or after the menopause. Unfortunately, menstrual irregularities are common at the menopause and pathological bleeding may not be recognised, leading to delay in diagnosis. The growth may be obvious on clinical examination (inspection and palpation) but should be confirmed by biopsy. This will also establish the histological grade.

Pain is a late feature and indicates considerable spread beyond the cervix. Later invasion of the parametrial tissues and pelvic nerves causes lumbar aching, then pain radiating to the hip and thigh. In ulcerated lesions there will be associated infection, which will aggravate the symptoms.

Invasion of the base of the bladder will cause dysuria with urinary frequency and pain; destruction of the tissue between the base of the bladder and the vagina can cause a fistula allowing urine to leak from the bladder to the vagina (vesicovaginal fistula). The ureters pass through the parametria close to the cervix (Fig. 27.2). Compression of the ureters will lead to back pressure on the kidney and renal failure with uraemia. This is common in advanced or recurrent disease and is a common cause of death.

Staging and investigation

Clinical staging is carried out by an examination under general anaesthesia. Initially a colposcopy and curettage is performed by a gynaecologist. A cone biopsy is performed if the abnormal epithelium extends into the

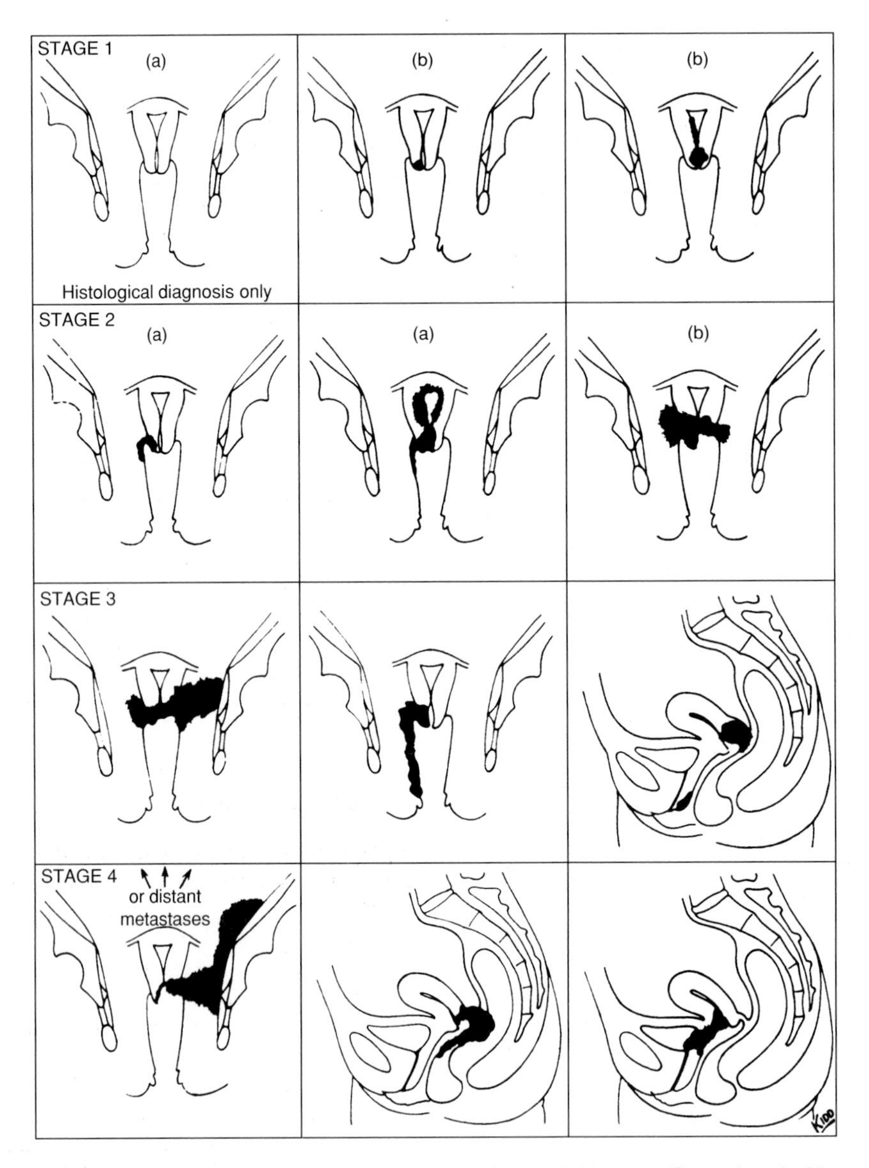

Fig. 27.5 Illustrations of the stages of cancer of the cervix. For details see Table 27.1. (Reproduced with permission from Jeffcoate, Principles of Gynaecology, Butterworths.)

endocervical canal. The tumour is inspected and palpated. Bimanual examination of the size, shape and mobility of the cervix is carried out. The presence and degree of parametrial or posterior extension is assessed by rectovaginal examination. Cystoscopy is performed to exclude involvement of the bladder. Bullous oedema of the base of the bladder is an appearance associated with invasion but unless there is tumour in the bladder, oedema itself does not change the stage.

Investigations

Essential investigations are a full blood count, serum urea, creatinine and electrolytes, chest radiograph and intravenous urogram (IVU) or a CT or MRI scan of the pelvis. IVU, CT or MRI may show hydroureter or hydronephrosis due to infiltration at the lower end of the ureters.

CT or MRI scans are used to demonstrate involvement of the pelvic and para-aortic nodes. The incidence of involved pelvic and para-aortic node rises with stage. For stages I–IV, pelvic nodes are involved in 15, 30, 45 and 55% and para-aortic nodes in about 5, 15, 35 and 40% respectively. However, the results of scanning may not necessarily influence treatment if the pelvic nodes are routinely irradiated with the primary tumour. Some radiotherapists irradiate the para-aortic nodes if the pelvic nodes are involved.

The FIGO clinical staging system is the most widely used (Table 27.1 and Fig. 27.5).

Treatment

Surgery and radiotherapy alone or in combination are curative in cervical cancer. Factors which influence the choice of treatment will include the age and general condition of the patient, the stage of the tumour, and the patient's own preference. For patients symptomatic of pelvic disease but not fit for radical radiotherapy, palliative intracavitary or external beam therapy should be considered. Palliative dosage is as for endometrial cancer (p. 479).

The general rule for radiotherapy in carcinoma of the cervix is that the intracavitary brachytherapy element is used to treat the primary cancer and external radiotherapy to the pelvis to treat the nodes. The balance of the doses given by these two elements is determined by the stage of the cancer and the risk of pelvic lymph node involvement.

Over the last few years most centres have combined the radiotherapy with weekly cisplatin chemotherapy.

Table 27.1 FIGO staging of carcinoma of the cervix

Stage	Clinical findings
0	Carcinoma-in-situ; also called preinvasive or intraepithelial carcinoma
I	Growth confined to the cervix. Upward spread to the corpus does not change the classification
Ia	Microinvasive carcinoma
Ib	Clinically invasive carcinoma
IIa	Spread beyond the cervix to the upper two-thirds of the vagina
IIb	Spread to parametrium but not as far as the lateral pelvic wall
IIIa	Spread to the lower third of the vagina
IIIb	Spread to the pelvic side-wall and/or hydronephrosis or non-functioning kidney due to ureteric compression by tumour
IVa	Spread to the bladder or rectum and/or extending beyond the true pelvis
IVb	Spread to distant sites outside the true pelvis

1. *Stage Ib*

For young women with non-bulky tumours who have a negative CT scan of the pelvic and para-aortic nodes, a radical Wertheim's hysterectomy is the treatment of choice. The latter includes removal of the uterus, tubes, ovaries, parametria and upper third of the vagina and a pelvic lymphadenectomy. This has the advantage that the ovaries can be preserved and avoids the fibrosis and drying of the vagina which pelvic irradiation induces. If at operation the para-aortic nodes are found to be involved, the operation is abandoned and treatment given by irradiation. Where many pelvic nodes are found to be infiltrated in the operative specimen, or the resection margins are very close to the tumour, post-operative pelvic irradiation should be given.

For patients who are older or have a positive scan or are not fit for or refuse surgery, radical radiotherapy with intracavitary therapy with or without pelvic external beam irradiation should be given. External beam is indicated if the tumour is bulky or poorly differentiated or the scan is positive. Many radiotherapists, however, treat all stage I cases with pelvic external beam in addition to intracavitary therapy.

2. *Stages Ib (bulky), IIa–IIIb*

Radical radiotherapy

Radical radiotherapy is the treatment of choice for bulky stage Ib, IIa–IIIb. This normally requires a combination of uterine and vaginal intracavitary therapy and pelvic external beam irradiation.

In patients with stage III disease, uraemia may be advanced at presentation if there is bilateral ureteric obstruction. Where the patient is in renal failure, particularly if young, the insertion of temporary nephrostomies (tubes placed in the renal pelvis under ultrasound control to drain the urine) should be considered to relieve renal tract obstruction prior to pelvic irradiation. Radical radiotherapy should only be started if renal function and general condition improve sufficiently. Since the prognosis with bilateral obstruction is very poor, it may be better to allow death painlessly from uraemia, particularly in those not too old and frail for radical radiotherapy.

General medical care. It is important to maintain patients in as good a medical condition as possible. Anaemia (Hb < 10 g/dl) should be corrected by blood transfusion before treatment since the prognosis of the anaemic patient is less good.

Combined surgery and radiotherapy

A combination of surgery and radiotherapy, if carefully combined, can achieve equally satisfactory cure rates in patients with stage Ib, IIa and early IIb disease. A colpohysterectomy and external iliac lymphadenectomy may be followed 2–6 weeks later by vaginal intracavitary therapy. In some cases this avoids the need for pelvic external beam irradiation and its associated morbidity in patients with no histological evidence of nodal involvement. Involved nodes or residual disease are indications for postoperative external beam irradiation.

3. Stage IVa

The outlook for this stage is grim and many patients are in poor medical condition. A vesicovaginal or rectovaginal fistula or both may be present, with or without renal tract obstruction. A preliminary colostomy or urinary diversion is desirable if radical radiotherapy is to be attempted. Intracavitary therapy may not be feasible because of fistula formation and treatment is limited to pelvic external beam irradiation alone. In some cases these patients may be salvaged by a pelvic exenteration. This major surgery involves a radical extended total abdominal hysterectomy combined with a cystectomy (an anterior exenteration) or the hysterectomy combined with an abdominoperineal resection of the rectum (a posterior exenteration) or both the hysterectomy combined with a cystectomy and an abdominoperineal resection (a total pelvic exenteration). Clearly such patients lose all their pelvic organs and end up with both a colostomy and a urostomy and need to be very motivated to get through this surgery.

Radical radiotherapy

Target volume

The aim is to treat the cervix, parametria and the pelvic nodes.

Because of the greater tolerance of the vagina to radiation it is possible to deliver a higher dose to it than to the rest of the pelvic tissues. The central disease is conventionally treated by uterine and vaginal intracavitary sources, usually caesium or cobalt. The sources provide a very high central dose. The isodoses from the uterine and vaginal sources are pear-shaped (Fig. 27.6). The dose falls off inversely with the square of the distance from the source (p. 226). External beam irradiation to a lower dose is used to treat the pelvic nodes and complement the dose to the distal parametrium where the intracavitary dose falls off rapidly. A specially designed wedge or shield may be placed over the central part of the pelvic field during external beam irradiation. The wedge reduces the dose of external beam to the central pelvis, which is heavily irradiated by intracavitary therapy.

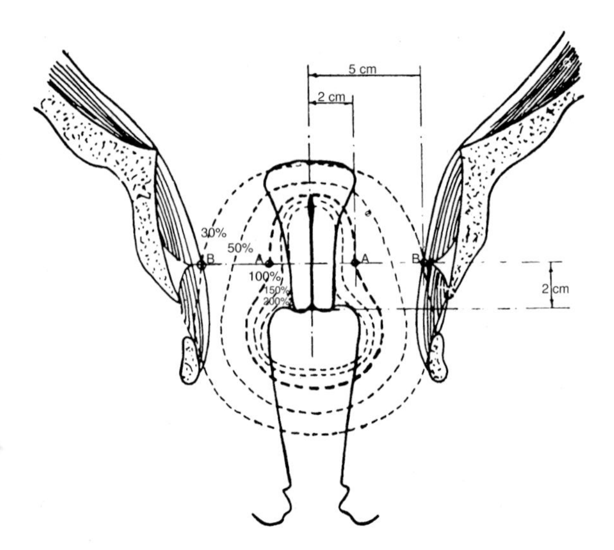

Fig. 27.6 Isodose curves in the pelvis for a typical radium distribution. The position of points A and B is shown. (Reproduced with permission from Tod, British Practice in Radiotherapy, Butterworths.)

Intracavitary therapy. A variety of techniques are in use. Previously the live sources used to be placed directly by the operator into the uterine cavity and vagina (e.g. the Manchester and Sheffield systems) or manually afterloaded in the ward by the nursing staff. This radiation exposure to medical and nursing staff is now unnecessary with the development of 'remote afterloading' (p. 228). Remote afterloading has replaced manual insertion of live sources in most centres in the UK.

Remote afterloading

Cathetron. The first high dose rate remote afterloading system using cobalt-60 was the Cathetron. The Cathetron has a number of advantages. Accuracy is high owing to the rigidity of the applicator system (two vaginal ovoids and a central uterine tube). Treatment times (a few minutes) and duration of hospital stay are short, allowing more patients to be treated than with lower dose rate systems. Drawbacks are the number of treatments required (commonly five), each under a general anaesthetic with its attendant risks.

Selectron. The most popular type of remote afterloading medium dose rate system in the UK is currently the Selectron (Fig. 14.3B). The Selectron uses caesium-137 sources for low and medium dose rate and cobalt-60 for high dose rate. The different dose rates are summarised in Table 14.2.

Many radiotherapists have adopted low dose rate remote afterloading machines to provide similar dose rates to the manually afterloaded systems with whose clinical effects they were familiar. Their aim has been to achieve similar pelvic dosimetry and cure rates without any increase in morbidity.

Intracavitary insertion. The insertion of the applicators is carried out in the operating theatre under general anaesthesia. The vagina, cervix and pelvis are assessed by inspection and bimanual examination. A cystoscopy should be carried out to exclude bladder invasion. A biopsy is taken for microscopy if not previously done. The cervical canal normally allows the passage of a very narrow 'sound' of about 3 mm diameter. To hold a uterine applicator the canal has to be dilated. This is done gently and gradually, by passing a series of long narrow metal sounds of increasing size until it is wide enough to admit a uterine applicator. Occasionally a growth begins inside the canal (endocervical) and there may be nothing obvious at first, until the canal is widened enough to give the operator access. An average uterine canal (cervix and body) is about 6 cm long.

Practical problems

Failure to identify the cervical os. If it is impossible to insert a uterine applicator because the cervical os cannot be confidently identified or because of local haemorrhage, a vaginal applicator alone may be inserted or the whole procedure deferred until more pelvic irradiation has been given to shrink the tumour and / or stop the haemorrhage. Intracavitary insertion may be possible once the tumour has shrunk (e.g. after 20 Gy in 10 daily fractions over 2 weeks (9–10 MV photons).

Perforation of the uterus. Occasionally, in error, the uterus may be perforated by the applicator, particularly if the external os is difficult to identify because the tumour has distorted it. If perforation has occurred, the applicator should be withdrawn and the patient started on antibiotics. A further attempt is made to carry out the insertion successfully a week later.

Verification of intracavitary insertion. After the insertion of the uterovaginal applicator, lateral and anteroposterior radiographs of the pelvis are taken to show the exact position of the applicators. This is best done in theatre itself, with a portable X-ray machine. Occasionally their position is found to be unsatisfactory. If positioning is seen to be poor, it can be corrected before the patient leaves the theatre.

The patient is returned to the ward and remains flat on her back for the period of insertion (typically about a day and half) to prevent displacement of the applicators.

Afterloading and care during intracavitary irradiation. Ideally a remote afterloading system is used to load the applicators from the source container (Fig. 14.3) in a specially protected ward. Essential nursing and medical procedures can be carried out by withdrawing the sources to their container for short periods of time.

In a manual afterloading system, the applicators are normally loaded by the nursing staff. A mobile lead screen 2.5 cm thick is placed at the bedside to reduce the dosage to staff and visitors. Nursing and medical procedures are minimised to avoid unnecessary radiation exposure.

For removal of the applicators at the appointed time, no anaesthetic is required. In a remotely afterloaded system the sources are pneumatically withdrawn into the source container before the uterovaginal applicator is withdrawn. Any vaginal packing is removed. Manually directly or afterloaded sources are placed at once in a lead box in a trolley which is then wheeled away to the isotope safe.

Dosimetry

Manchester points A and B. Most radiotherapists in the UK still prescribe intracavitary and external beam therapy to Manchester points A and B (Fig. 27.7). The position of point A is defined in relation to the midline but may vary according to whether the uterine cavity lies in the midline or is displaced to one side.

ICRU 38 recommendations. Many centres in Europe have adopted the ICRU 38 recommendations on dose

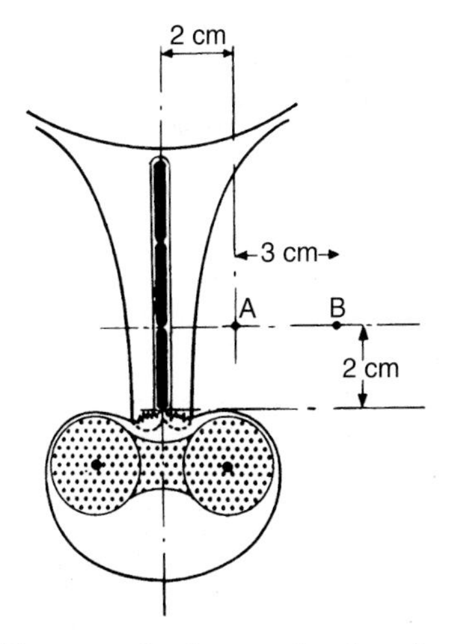

Fig. 27.7 Diagrammatic uterus and vagina, showing intrauterine tube, cross-sections of ovoids in lateral fornices, separated by spacer, and points A and B. (Reproduced with permission of Arnold from Ralston Paterson, *Treatment of Malignant Disease*, 2/e, Edward Arnold, 1963.)

prescription in gynaecological intracavitary therapy. These are summarised in Table 27.2.

The reference points for the measurement of doses to distal parametrium, bladder, rectum and to the pelvic and para-aortic nodes are shown in Figs 27.8 and 27.9.

The dosimetric points of the para-aortic and pelvic nodes are shaped like a trapezoid with the narrow end in the para-aortic region and the broad end at the level of the external iliac nodes. Computerised dosimetry based on radiographs taken with the unloaded uterovaginal applicator in situ allow the rapid calculation of the doses to these reference points.

The ICRU 38 reference points differ from the Manchester system. They exclude points A and B because, though valid when the uterus is in the midline position, the dose to the parametrium and pelvic side-wall may be underestimated if the uterus is deviated to one side and overestimated if it deviates to the opposite side. Instead the dose is prescribed to the 60 Gy isodose surrounding the uterine and vaginal sources (Fig. 27.10). This isodose has a more consistent position in the parametrium than point A since it is related to the actual position of the sources rather than to the midline. Whether or not these new reference points prove useful in setting dose limits to minimise rectal and bladder complications remains to be established.

Rectal probe. A further possible aid in avoiding rectal overdosage in directly loaded systems is a scintillation counter at the end of a narrow probe. This can be inserted at the end of the operation and the maximum dose rate at the rectal mucosa obtained by a series of readings at various distances along the rectal wall. If the dose is found to be excessive, the application must be adjusted.

Dosage. Cancericidal doses, e.g. 75 Gy at point A or to the 60 Gy isodose, from central sources can be safely

Table 27.2 ICRU 38 recommendations for dose and volume specification for reporting intracavitary therapy in gynaecology

1. The treatment technique must be completely described
2. The total reference kerma should be stated (p. 51)
3. The *reference volume* should be described in terms of the *height, width* and *thickness* of the volume enclosed in the 60 Gy isodose surface for low dose rate treatment of carcinoma of the cervix
4. The absorbed dose at reference points in organs at risk (*rectum, bladder*) should be determined (computed or measured) and expressed in well-codified ways to provide additional safety limits
5. The absorbed dose(s) at reference point(s) related to bony structures (*lymphatic trapezoid* and *pelvic wall* reference points should be reported)
6. The time–dose pattern should be completely specified

1. The **reference volume** is defined by three dimensions: (a) the height is the maximum dimension along the intrauterine source and is measured in the oblique frontal plane containing the uterine source; (b) the width is the maximum dimension perpendicular to the intrauterine source and is measured in the same oblique frontal plane; (c) the thickness is the maximum dimension perpendicular to the intrauterine source and is measured in the oblique sagittal plane containing the uterine source.
2. The **bladder reference point** (Fig. 27.9) is obtained by filling the balloon of a catheter in the bladder with 7 ml of radio-opaque fluid. The balloon is pulled down against the urethra. On the lateral radiograph the reference point is obtained on an anteroposterior line drawn through the centre of the balloon. The reference point is taken on this line on the posterior surface of the balloon. On the frontal radiograph the reference point is taken at the centre of the balloon.
3. The **rectal reference point** (Fig. 27.9) is located on an anteroposterior line drawn on the lateral radiograph from the lower end of the uterine source (or from the middle of the intravaginal sources). The point is on this line 5 mm behind the posterior vaginal wall.
4. **Lymphatic trapezoid** (Fig. 27.8A). A line is drawn from the junction of S1–S2 to the top of the symphysis pubis. Then a line is drawn from the middle of that line to the middle of the anterior aspect of L4. A trapezoid is constructed in a plane passing through the transverse line in the pelvic brim plane and the midpoint of the anterior aspect of the body of L4. A point 6 cm lateral to the midline at the inferior end of this figure is used to give an estimate of the dose rate to the mid-external iliac (R. EXT and L. EXT for the right and left external iliac, respectively).

At the top of the trapezoid, points 2 cm lateral to the midline at the level of L4 are used to estimate the dose to the lower para-aortic area (labelled R. PARA and L. PARA). The midpoint of a line connecting these two points is used to estimate the dose to the low common (labelled R. COM and L. COM) iliac nodes.

5. The **pelvic wall reference point** is intended to be representative of the absorbed dose at the distal part of the parametrium and at the obturator nodes. On an AP radiograph the pelvic wall reference point is intersected by a horizontal line tangential to the highest point of the acetabulum and a vertical line tangential to the inner aspect of the acetabulum (Fig. 27.8B). On a lateral radiograph the highest points of the right and left acetabulum in the craniocaudal direction are joined and the lateral projection of the pelvic wall reference point is located midway between these points.

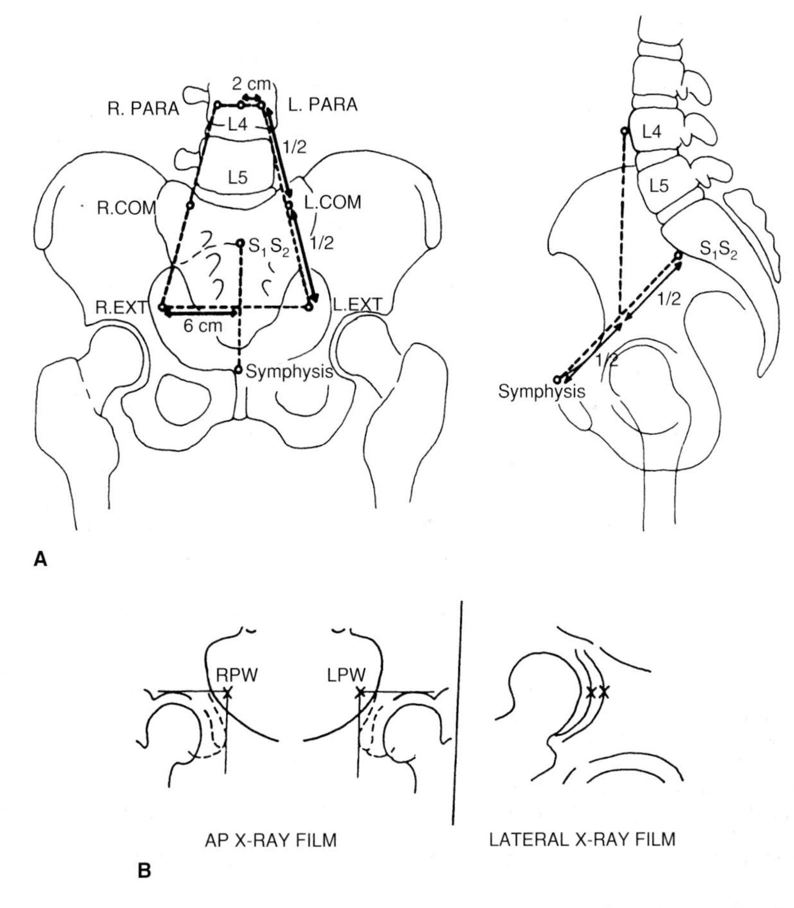

Fig. 27.8 Determination of **A** lymphatic trapezoid shown in anteroposterior view (left) and lateral view (right) and **B** the right (RPW) and left (LPW) pelvic side-wall reference points. (Reproduced with permission from ICRU Report 38: Dose and Volume Specification for Reporting Intracavitary Therapy in Gynecology, ICRU, 1985.)

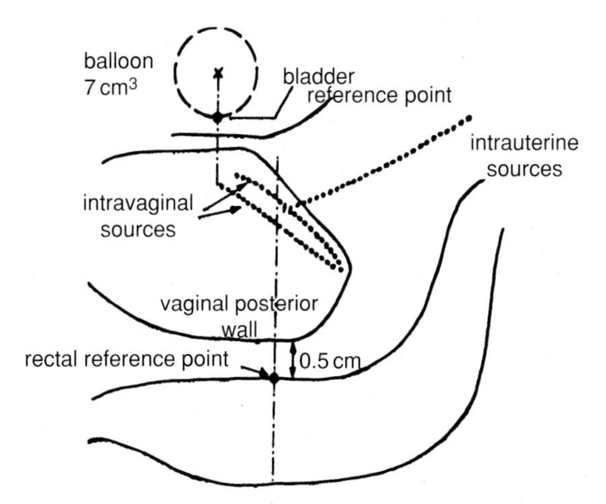

Fig. 27.9 Determination of the reference points for bladder and rectum. (Reproduced with permission from ICRU Report 38: Dose and Volume Specification for Reporting Intracavitary Therapy in Gynecology, ICRU, 1985.)

delivered. This would give point B about one-fifth of the central dose (15 Gy), much too low to deal effectively with disease in the pelvic lymph nodes. To achieve adequate dosage to B, e.g. 50 Gy, from the same sources would take about 10 days and involve 250 Gy at A. This would result in acute necrosis, early fistulae of rectum and bladder, and probable death from sepsis.

It is obvious from Figure 27.6 that the dose at the surface of the cervix and immediately adjoining is 200%, i.e. about 150 Gy. This is a very high dose, but this region is, fortunately, unusually tolerant and so permits an effective dose as far out as point A. If this were not so, treatment would be impracticable.

It is possible to make accurate dose calculations from the radiographs taken after the insertions, and some departments have done this routinely. Doing the calculations manually was very laborious and most

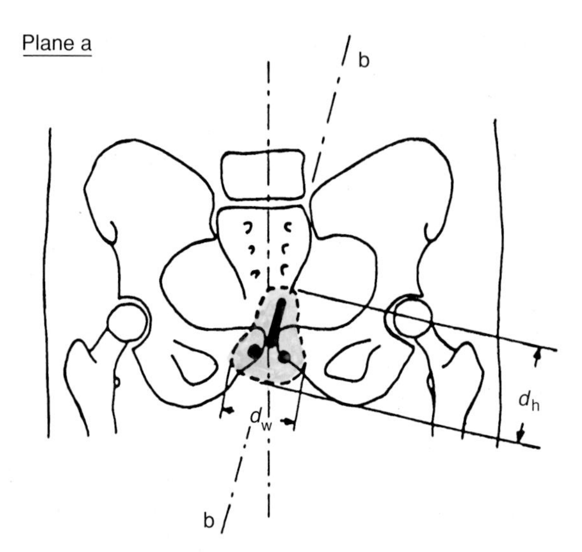

Fig. 27.10 Diagram showing the 60 Gy isodose and its dimensions in the frontal oblique plane surrounding the uterovaginal applicator: d_h, height; d_w, width. (Reproduced with permission from ICRU Report 38: Dose and Volume Specification for Reporting Intracavitary Therapy in Gynecology, ICRU, 1985.)

clinicians preferred to rely on simple inspection of the films, in the light of experience, to assure themselves that the source layout was reasonable. With the availability of a modern planning computer and remote afterloading these calculations are much faster and more accurate. Dose distribution can be individualised and optimised to fit the tumour and minimise dose to bladder and rectum.

External beam pelvic irradiation. For genuine stage I disease, intracavitary caesium alone is adequate, and capable of achieving a cure rate of 90% or more. However nodal metastases can hardly ever be ruled out with confidence. Most radiotherapists therefore supplement intracavitary therapy with megavoltage irradiation delivered to the lateral parts of the pelvis to bring this dosage to a tumoricidal level.

External beam can precede or follow intracavitary therapy.

Target volume

This should include the whole of the pelvis (Fig. 27.11). It will encompass the primary and any local spread, and the common, internal and external iliac nodes. The upper border of the field is the junction of the fourth and fifth lumbar vertebrae. The lower border is the bottom of the obturator foramina of the pubic bones. It may need to extend a few centimetres more inferiorly if there is involvement of the lower third of the vagina. The outer margin is 1 cm lateral to the pelvic brim.

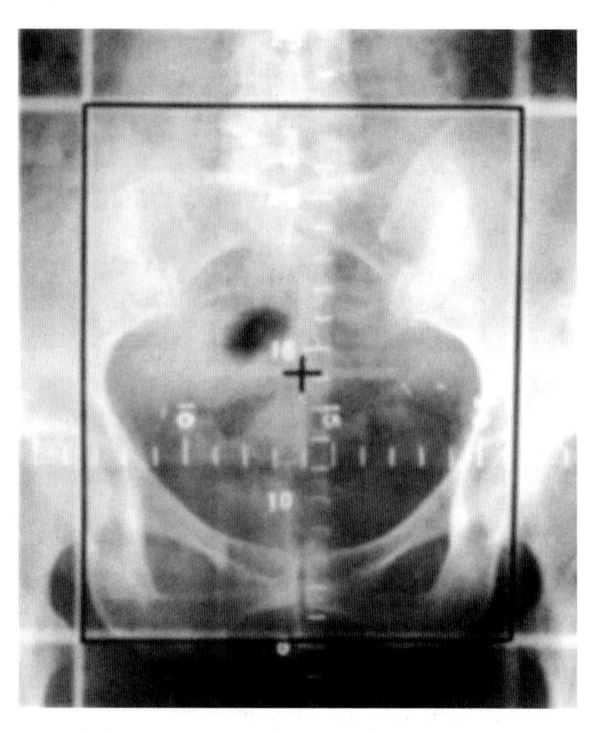

Fig. 27.11 Pelvic external beam field for carcinoma of the cervix and endometrium.

Technique

A pair of anterior and posterior opposed fields is planned on the simulator. There is a central wedge filter (4–5 cm wide) to protect midline structures (cervix, bladder and rectum). A typical field size is 16 × 14 cm. Alternatively an anterior field is supplemented by two lateral wedged fields to reduce the dose to the rectum.

If the para-aortic nodes are involved, a separate single direct 'spade' para-aortic field can be added at the end of pelvic irradiation. The width is normally about 8 cm. It extends from the T12/L1 junction to just above the upper border of the pelvic field. The length of the gap on the skin between the lower end of the para-aortic field and the upper end of the pelvic field is calculated so that no more than the 50% isodoses overlap at the depth of the spinal cord.

Energy and dose

Megavoltage therapy is advised. The aim is to give the desired dose at point B, additional to the dose already given from intracavitary therapy, while giving a much lower dose to A which is already heavily irradiated. There will be some photon dosage to A, if only from scattered irradiation. The dose to A can be varied while leaving the dose at B unchanged, by using different thickness of central filter, and changing them, if need be, during the course. In this way, the doses can be arranged to summate to the required levels. Table 27.3 summarises the intracavitary and external beam doses for different stages of the disease.

Para-aortic nodes

45 Gy maximum dose in 20 daily fractions over 4 weeks (4–6 MV photons)

Acute reactions. The cervix and body of uterus are unusually tolerant of high dosage (see above). The more vulnerable organs that are potential sources of trouble are the rectum, bladder and any loops of bowel trapped or adherent in the pelvis.

Bowel. As we have noted, special precautions are taken for rectal protection—packing or heavy metal filter. A minor degree of rectal irritation (tenesmus) and rectal bleeding, with perhaps slight diarrhoea, is usual after intracavitary caesium and settles rapidly.

During external irradiation diarrhoea is often troublesome, occasionally requiring treatment to be suspended for a few days. Treatment is with an antidiarrhoeal agent (e.g. loperamide), and a high-fibre diet, avoiding fruit and vegetables. The reaction has normally settled 3–4 weeks after the end of treatment.

Bladder. Irritation of the bladder with dysuria and frequency is both less common and less troublesome. The patient is advised to drink water regularly and cranberry juice can alter the acidity of the urine to a beneficial effect. An anticholinergic (e.g. propantheline) often relieves the discomfort. The time scale for resolution is the same as for the bowel.

Skin. Reactions are minor if megavoltage is used. Washing the treated area is permitted.

Infection. Cervical tumours are often infected. Manipulations involved in treatment, including dilatation of the uterine canal, may spread infection; hence the need for examination under anaesthetic and intracavitary insertions to be carried out under sterile conditions. Collections of pus in the uterine cavity (a pyometrium) behind a cervical tumour should be drained and antibiotics started.

Late reactions. The probability of developing late major pelvic complications following radical intracavitary and external beam therapy is about 5%. These mainly affect the bladder and bowel. Small bowel complications are predominantly related to external beam irradiation. Many factors play a part in the development of pelvic complications, including total dose, dose rate, treatment volume, and previous pelvic surgery or pathology.

Bowel. The bowel is most frequently involved because of the proximity of the rectum to the region of high dose from intracavitary therapy and the inclusion of small bowel in the pelvic radiation field. Normally the bowel is mobile. As a result the same segment of bowel may not consistently lie within the same part of the pelvic external beam field. However, previous pelvic inflammatory disease or surgery increases the likelihood of loops of bowel being trapped in the pelvis and irradiated to higher doses than mobile segments.

Large bowel. Large bowel complications develop earlier than in the small bowel, usually within 2 years of treatment. The average latent period is 6–18 months. Haemorrhage, rectal ulceration and fistulae occur. Symptoms are of colicky abdominal pain, rectal urgency, tenesmus, constipation and diarrhoea. The site of the ulceration is usually on the anterior rectal wall behind the posterior vaginal fornix where the intracavitary dose is high and the blood supply is meagre. Fistulae are usually confined to patients who

Table 27.3 Treatment of carcinoma of the cervix

Stage	Treatment	Point (Gy)	Cs (Gy)	Ext. beam (Gy)	Cs + ext. beam (Gy)
0	Conisation/hysterectomy	—	—	—	—
I	Hysterectomy (Wertheim's)/Cs + ext. beam				
		A	60	15	75
		B	15	35	50
IIa, b	Cs + ext. beam	Dosage as stage I			
IIIa, b	Cs + ext. beam or ext. beam alone	Dosage as stage I			
IVa	Defunctioning colostomy (rectovaginal fistula) or urinary diversion (vesicovaginal fistula). Then radical/palliative ext. beam	50 Gy in 25 daily fractions (whole pelvis) or 30 Gy in 10 daily fractions (whole pelvis)			
IVb	Palliative ext. beam ± chemotherapy or palliative Cs	30 Gy in 10 daily fractions (whole pelvis) 20 Gy to point A (one insertion)			

Cs, caesium; ext. beam, external beam

have had intracavitary therapy. Strictures are commonly seen on barium enema but only about 25% are symptomatic. The commonest radiological appearance is a long narrowed segment. Changes in the submucosa may give rise to a 'thumb-printing' pattern.

The treatment of troublesome proctocolitis is initially conservative, for example with Predsol enemas. If conservative measures fail, then surgery is required with either a temporary or permanent colostomy.

Small bowel. Symptoms of small bowel damage can occur within the first few months following radiation but are usually delayed on average until 1–5 years following treatment. Obstruction is the commonest complication, occasionally with perforation. Radiological examination of the small bowel with barium contrast (small bowel meal) may show straightening or narrowing of the bowel and filling defects or thumb-printing due to oedema and fibrosis.

Malabsorption is common and often accompanies other evidence of late pelvic morbidity. There may be no symptoms or there may be diarrhoea, weight loss and fatigue. If the ileum is extensively involved, the stools become fatty (steatorrhoea). If segments of the small bowel lose their contractility, its stagnant contents may encourage bacteria to proliferate (bacterial overgrowth), leading to malabsorption of vitamin B_{12}.

Bladder. The bladder is similarly vulnerable, lying just in front of the anterior vaginal wall. Up to 25% of patients may have severe symptoms of bladder dysfunction. This seems to be mainly due to damage to the detrusor muscle rather than to contraction of the bladder. Late effects tend to occur 1–10 years after treatment. Blood in the urine (haematuria) may result from telangiectasia at the bladder base. Cystoscopy is advisable, to exclude invasion of the bladder by tumour or an unrelated cause. Diathermy to the bleeding points is usually effective. The bladder may become contracted as a result of scarring and infection of the submucosal and muscle layers.

Vesicovaginal fistula is a major complication which results in continual leakage of urine from the vagina. The diagnosis can be confirmed by passing a blue dye (methylthioninium chloride (methylene blue)) through a urinary catheter and observing the dye escaping through the vagina. Treatment is by transplanting the ureters into the ileum (ileal conduit). The fistula will then usually heal. Urinary diversion may also be required if the intolerable urinary frequency occurs as a result of a contracted bladder. Occasionally ureteric obstruction may occur because of a 'frozen' pelvis. However, malignant disease is by far the commoner cause.

Results of treatment

The results of primary radical surgery or radiotherapy or a combination of preoperative caesium followed by surgery for stage Ib are excellent, with a 5-year survival of about 90%. Cure rates from radical radiotherapy decline with advancing stage: 80% (IIa), 65% (IIb), 45% (IIIa) and 35% (IIIb), and 15% (IV).

Follow-up

Most recurrences in the cervix or regional nodes tend to occur in the first 2 years after treatment. A suggested follow-up policy is 1 month after treatment and then 2-monthly for the first year, 3-monthly in the second year and 6-monthly from years 3 to 5. The likelihood of relapse beyond 5 years is small and routine follow-up is probably not essential. Early review for assessment of new symptoms can be arranged as required. Cervical cytology is not a reliable method of detecting recurrence since the cytological changes following radiotherapy are often difficult to distinguish from the presence of tumour.

Sexual rehabilitation

Sexual counselling should be given. Patients should be warned of vaginal dryness and stenosis. An oestrogen-containing cream, dienestrol, may reduce the dryness. The regular use of dilators to maintain the patency of the vagina should be encouraged.

Treatment of recurrence after radiotherapy

Sadly, recurrent disease is often too advanced for salvage surgery. Examination of the vaginal vault at follow-up is often limited by radiation-induced vaginal stenosis. Typical symptoms are of buttock pain, radiating down the back of the leg. There may be no palpable recurrence in the pelvis. An ultrasound may show enlarged pelvic nodes and/or a dilated ureter. MRI scanning can sometimes distinguish radiation fibrosis from pelvic recurrence. However, for recurrence confined to the central pelvis, radical surgery with removal of vagina and bladder (anterior exenteration) or rectum (posterior exenteration) may be possible. Long-term survival for recurrent disease is poor since recurrence is often inoperable (owing to extension to the pelvic side-wall) or associated with distant metastases.

CANCER OF THE CERVICAL STUMP

Subtotal hysterectomy, i.e. removal of the uterus above the level of the cervix (e.g. for fibroids), was a common operative procedure in former times, but is now rarely practised. Carcinoma may develop in the remaining stump. A distinction needs to be made between true stump carcinoma which has arisen on the cervical stump a year or more following surgery and coincidental stump carcinoma which is detected within a year of hysterectomy. In the latter case the cancer can be assumed to have been present but not suspected at the time of surgery. Intracavitary treatment is difficult, as the length of the canal left, about 2 cm, is rarely enough to hold a uterine applicator and space left by the removed uterus tends to be filled by less radiotolerant tissue such as small bowel. Vaginal applications can be made, supplemented, or replaced entirely, by external irradiation.

The results of radical radiotherapy for true cervical stump carcinoma seem to match those where the uterus is intact. However, the outlook for coincidental carcinoma is less favourable, probably because it represents cancer which has been inadequately treated by surgery.

CERVICAL CANCER IN PREGNANCY

Carcinoma of the cervix is fortunately rare in pregnancy, about 1% of cases. Management will depend upon the extent of the disease at the time of diagnosis, the stage of the pregnancy and the wishes of the patient. Most patients present with early disease (stages I and II).

In the first 3 months (trimester) of pregnancy, stage I disease is treated by a Wertheim's hysterectomy. In more advanced stages, a vaginal termination is followed by radical radiotherapy.

In the second trimester, for stage I the pregnancy is terminated by removal of the fetus from the uterus (hysterotomy) followed by a Wertheim's hysterectomy. For stage II or more advanced, the termination of the pregnancy is induced with prostaglandins, followed by radical radiotherapy. External beam is started first to allow time for the uterus to involute. Intracavitary therapy can then complete the treatment.

In the third trimester, with a viable fetus, a caesarean section is carried out at 34 weeks for stage I followed by a Wertheim's hysterectomy. For stage II or more advanced, radical radiotherapy is given following caesarean section. Treatment is started by external beam 10 days after delivery and completed by intracavitary therapy.

Occasionally at 24 weeks, a decision has to be taken whether or not to postpone treatment a short time until the baby is viable. The parents need to be aware of the risks to mother and child of doing so.

The outcome of treatment of cervical cancer occurring during pregnancy is not, stage for stage, different from the results in women who are not pregnant.

CANCER OF THE BODY OF THE UTERUS (CARCINOMA CORPUS UTERI)

Pathology

Endometrial cancer represents 1.9% of all cancers and 0.9% of cancer deaths. The internal surface lining of the uterine cavity is called the endometrium. It is a glandular epithelium. Tumours arising from it are adenocarcinomas and account for over 80% of cancers of the corpus (body); 70% are well-differentiated endometrioid adenocarcinomas. Papillary adenocarcinomas (5%) occur in an older age group and, like clear cell carcinoma (5%) have a less-favourable prognosis. Adenoacanthoma has squamous metaplasia, and has identical prognosis to other endometrioid adenocarcinomas. True adenosquamous carcinoma of the corpus is very rare and is much more frequent in the cervix. Sarcomas are rare (5%), arising from the muscular walls of the uterus.

Aetiology

Endometrial cancer is associated with nulliparity, diabetes mellitus, hypertension, obesity and polycystic ovarian syndrome. What these conditions have in common is excessive stimulation by oestrogenic hormone uninfluenced by progestogens. This results in endometrial overgrowth and eventual malignancy. Oestrogen-secreting ovarian granulosa tumours (p. 483) are a rare cause of the same phenomenon.

Oestrogens given as hormone replacement therapy at the menopause also cause endometrial hyperplasia and eventually endometrioid adenocarcinoma.

Spread

Spread of endometrial cancer may be downwards to the endocervix, and it may be impossible to say whether a growth arose in the cervix or the body. Such cases should be regarded as primary growths of the cervix. It may invade the uterine wall deeply and even penetrate into the parametrium. Secondary deposits in the ovaries are common, likewise in the vagina (the Bonney's nodule). The lower uterine segment and endocervical canal is involved in 5–10% of patients.

Lymph node metastases to pelvic and then to para-aortic nodes occur later and are less frequent than with cervical growths. The greater the depth of myometrial invasion and the less differentiated the tumour, the higher the incidence of nodal metastases and of vaginal recurrence. For example, if the tumour is confined to the endometrium the incidence of pelvic node metastases is only 3%. It rises to 8% if there is superficial myometrial invasion and to 45% if there is deep invasion (to the outer third).

Myometrial invasion occurs in less than 5% of well-differentiated tumours and about 30% of poorly differentiated tumours. Blood spread to lungs, liver and bone is relatively common in later stages.

Clinical features

Irregular bleeding, especially after the menopause, is the cardinal symptom. It is occasionally detected as an incidental finding in the cervical screening programme.

Diagnosis and investigation

The diagnosis may be established by hysteroscopy and biopsy, or dilatation and curettage (D and C) under general anaesthesia. The uterine canal is dilated and the cavity explored by a curettage to remove fragments of the lining tissue. The diagnosis may be immediately obvious, or only when confirmed by microscopy.

Staging

Staging is by the FIGO classification (Table 27.4).

Treatment

The standard treatment is surgical, i.e. total hysterectomy (removal of uterus, ovaries and tubes) in early operable cases where there are no contraindications such as hypertension, diabetes and obesity. Inoperable cases, e.g. appreciable extension outside the uterus, or cases technically operable but unsuitable for surgery, are treated by radical radiotherapy, either intracavitary, external beam or a combination of both.

Table 27.4 FIGO staging of endometrial cancer (T stages of TNM classification in parentheses)

Stage	Clinical findings
I	Carcinoma confined to the corpus (T1)
Ia	Uterine cavity 8 cm or less in length (T1a)
Ib	Uterine cavity > 8 cm in length (T1b)
II	Extension to the cervix (T2)
III	Extension beyond the uterus but confined to the true pelvis (T3)
IV	Extension beyond the true pelvis or involvement of the bladder or rectum (T4)

Radical radiotherapy

For a well-differentiated adenocarcinoma which is clinically stage I and penetrating less than a third of the myometrium, there is no need for supplementary pelvic irradiation.

The indications for postoperative radical radiotherapy are controversial and the subject of clinical trials but many centres would offer radiotherapy in the following cases:

- moderately or poorly differentiated histology
- stage II or III disease
- tumour at the surgical resection margins
- invasion of vascular spaces.

Target volume

For stage 1 disease, some workers prefer to confine the treatment volume to the vaginal vault using postoperative vaginal intracavitary caesium. This reduces the incidence of recurrence at the vaginal vault from about 10–25% to 4%. Others prefer to treat the whole of the pelvis by external beam since many of those patients at risk of recurrence at the vaginal vault are also at increased risk of pelvic nodal metastases.

The field margins for external beam irradiation of the pelvis are the same as for cervical cancer (p. 474).

Technique and dosage

Intracavitary therapy alone (postoperative). The principles are similar to those for the cervix, usually with a single insertion.

60 Gy to point A or to the reference isodose (Fig. 27.10)

Intracavitary combined with external beam (no surgery). Two intracavitary uterovaginal insertions are carried out. Dosage of intracavitary therapy and external beam is as for cervical cancer (Table 27.3).

The uterine cavity is usually on the large side, and will hold a longer applicator (e.g. 7.5 cm) than most cases of cervical cancer.

Vaginal applicators are of various types, as for the cervix. Some workers apply vaginal caesium at only one of the two insertions. The Manchester and Sheffield techniques are also applicable to the corpus.

In the Stockholm method (Fig. 27.12), the uterine cavity is packed with as many small caesium sources as it will accommodate—Heyman capsules, holding 8–10 mg each. Each capsule has an attached numbered thread, so that they can be removed in the correct sequence.

External beam alone (postoperative). A parallel-opposed pair of fields is used.

45 Gy in 20–25 daily fractions over 4–5 weeks (9–10 MV photons)

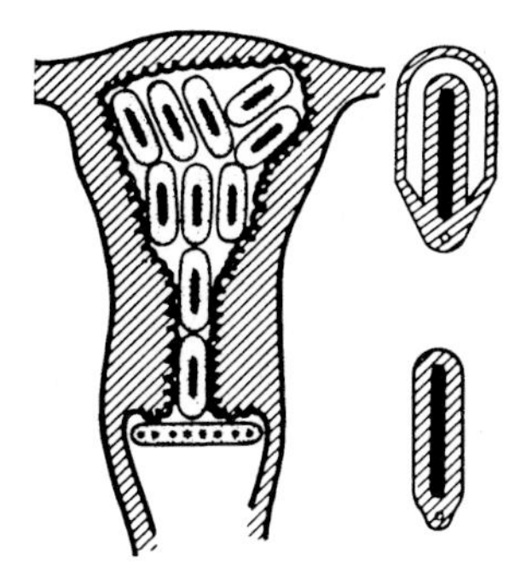

Fig. 27.12 Two types of Heyman applicators, and a uterine cavity packed with as many as it will hold. Note the flat box of caesium against the cervix, and the eyelets in the applicators for threads. (Reproduced with permission from Hulbert, Treatment of Cancer in Clinical Practice, Livingstone.)

External beam alone (no surgery). If the patient is unfit for a general anaesthetic or if there is any contraindication to intracavitary insertion, external pelvic irradiation alone is used.

A parallel-opposed pair of fields is used.

50 Gy in 25 daily fractions over 5 weeks (9–10 MV photons)

Vaginal recurrence. If vaginal recurrence occurs in a patient who has not received previous pelvic irradiation, intracavitary therapy is the treatment of choice. The aim is to give 100 Gy to the vaginal surface in two intracavitary insertions. It is the dose to the vaginal epithelium and not to point A that is important.

Palliative radiotherapy

Palliative radiotherapy is indicated for troublesome vaginal bleeding in patients who are not fit for radical surgery or radical radiotherapy. If the patient is fit enough for a general anaesthetic, a single uterine intracavitary insertion (20 Gy to point A or reference isodose) may be possible. If not, a simple parallel-opposed pair of fields is used (field margins as above).

Energy and dose

30 Gy in 10 fractions over 2 weeks or 20 Gy in 5 daily fractions over a week (9–10 MV photons)

Hormone therapy

Well-differentiated locally advanced or metastatic endometrial adenocarcinoma may respond to progestogens in about 30% of cases. Treatment is with medroxyprogesterone acetate 300–400 mg orally daily. Progestogens do not have a useful role as an adjuvant following primary treatment.

Results of treatment

Cancer of the corpus is one of the more favourable cancers, as most are well differentiated, slowly growing and metastasise late. For stage I disease 5-year survival is up to 90%, for stage II it is reduced to 50%, and to 20% for stages III and IV. 5-year survival falls with increasing depth of myometrial invasion (80% if no invasion, 60% if greater than half of the myometrium invaded). Similarly, increasing anaplasia impairs prognosis (5-year survival: 80% for well-differentiated, 75% for moderately differentiated and 50% for poorly differentiated).

UTERINE SARCOMAS

Uterine sarcomas are rare, representing less than 5% of uterine tumours. They may occur in young or in postmenopausal women. There are three principal histological types which, in order of frequency, are leiomyosarcoma, malignant mixed müllerian tumour and endometrial stromal sarcoma. Symptoms are of abnormal bleeding or of a pelvic mass. There is a high incidence of distant metastases, especially to lung. Treatment for stage I and II is a total hysterectomy and bilateral oophorectomy followed by postoperative pelvic external beam irradiation (50 Gy in 25 fractions over 5 weeks) for mixed müllerian and endometrial stromal sarcomas. For these two histological groups pelvic irradiation does reduce local recurrence and may improve survival. The exception is leiomyosarcoma which is highly radioresistant, and postoperative irradiation is palliative with only occasional responses. Chemotherapy with agents such as vincristine, DTIC and doxorubicin is palliative with only occasional responses. Overall 5-year survival is poor (20%).

CANCER OF THE OVARY

Anatomy

Each of the two ovaries is shaped like an almond and is attached to the back of the broad ligament on the side-wall of the pelvis (Fig. 27.2). In front lie the external iliac vessels and, behind, the ureter and internal iliac vessels. Along one of its attachments pass the ovarian vessels and lymphatics. Lymphatic drainage is to the para-aortic nodes.

Cancer of the ovary accounts for 20% of gynaecological malignancy and for about 4000 new cases per year in the UK and for over 2000 deaths. Overall it represents 2.3% of all cancers and 4.2% of cancer deaths. The average yearly incidence is 15 per 100 000 women and is rising. The peak incidence is between 40 and

60 years. The aetiology is unknown, though oral contraceptive use seems to have a protective role.

Pathology

There is a wide variety of histological types.

1. Primary malignant tumours
   a. Common epithelial tumours. Most ovarian tumours (90%) arise from the surface epithelium, or possibly its indentations, which produces the germ cells (ova, egg cells).
      Of these epithelial tumours, 10% are of 'borderline' malignancy (abnormal nuclei, increased mitotic activity, layers of tumour cells but no invasion). These borderline tumours may also be present as non-invasive implants on the omentum or on the pelvic side-wall.
      (i) Serous tumours (serous cystadenocarcinoma), often bilateral; so called because their fluid contents resemble serum in chemical composition. There are often papillary projections on the inner surface (papillary cystadenocarcinoma). This is the commonest type, amounting to about 42% of malignant tumours.
      (ii) Mucinous tumours (12%). Mucin is the viscid secretion of intestinal and other glands, and is also produced by the epithelium of these tumours. They are typically multicystic.
      (iii) Clear cell carcinoma (6%) (sometimes called mesonephroid).
      (iv) Endometrioid carcinoma (15%). This resembles its uterine counterpart, and may sometimes arise in endometriosis.
      (v) Undifferentiated carcinoma (17%).
   b. From germ cells (6%). These resemble tumours of comparable origin in the testis.
      (i) Dysgerminoma is a rare malignant tumour of children and young women. It is analogous to seminoma of the testis in males. It is highly sensitive to drugs and radiation.
      (ii) Teratomas differentiate the various embryonic layers. Most are benign.
      (iii) Choriocarcinoma.
      (iv) Yolk sac tumour (endodermal sinus tumour = old term).
   c. From specialised hormone-producing cells (2%).
      (i) Granulosa cell tumours secrete oestrogenic hormones and so cause precocious puberty in children or excess feminisation in adults, with menorrhagia or postmenopausal endometrial hyperplasia and bleeding. Most occur in postmenopausal women. Their malignancy is difficult to predict and variable, though they generally run a very long course over many years.
      (ii) Androblastomas are very rare and are usually benign. They may secrete androgenic hormones and so produce signs of virilism (hair growth and deepening of the voice).
2. Secondary tumours—uterus, breast, gastrointestinal tract. Krukenberg tumours are metastases in the ovary from a gastrointestinal primary cancer.

Staging is according to the FIGO staging system (Table 27.5).

Spread

Most tumours are cystic. Malignant change occurs within the cyst. As the tumour progresses, it spreads through to the outer peritoneal surface, or the cyst may rupture into the peritoneal cavity. Cells become attached to or invade adjacent structures—fallopian tubes, uterus, large and small bowel and bladder. Seeding may deposit them far and wide on peritoneal surfaces, and multiple small nodules with some ascites are commonly found at operation. The main sites of spread are shown in Figure 27.13.

Table 27.5 FIGO staging of ovarian cancer

Stage	Clinical findings
I	Tumour confined to the ovary
Ia	One ovary involved
Ib	Both ovaries involved
Ic	Tumour on the surface of one or both ovaries; capsular rupture; ascites containing malignant cells or positive peritoneal cytology
II	Tumour confined to the pelvis
IIa	Tumour extension to the adnexae
IIb	Tumour spread to other pelvic tissues
IIc	Tumour of IIa or IIb with tumour on the surface of one or both ovaries or capsular rupture; ascites containing malignant cells or positive peritoneal cytology
III	Tumour extending to the abdominal cavity, including peritoneal surfaces or the omentum
IV	Distant metastases

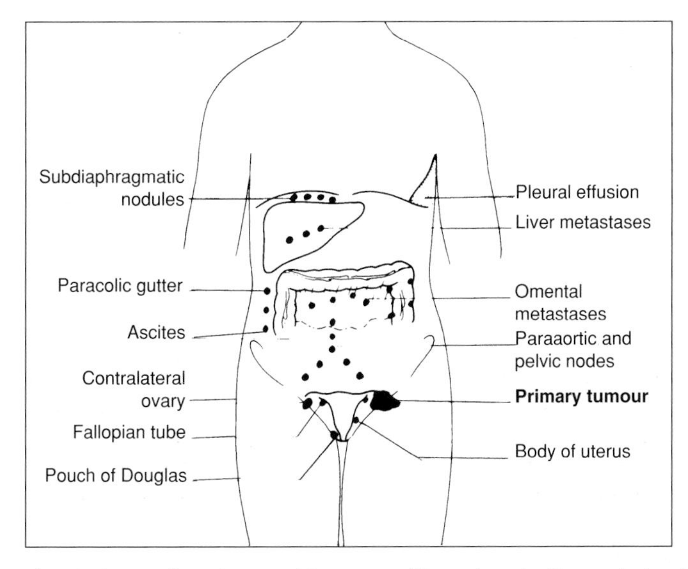

Fig. 27.13 Common sites of metastases of carcinoma of the ovary. (Reproduced with permission from Souhami & Tobias, Cancer and its Management, Blackwells, 1986.)

Spread to the para-aortic nodes occurs in 15% of stage I and II and 50% in stage III and IV disease. Blood-borne metastases occur late, typically to liver and lungs.

Natural history and clinical features

Ovarian tumours usually grow slowly and silently for some years and are usually advanced at the time of diagnosis; 60% have spread outside the pelvis at the time of presentation. In the uncommon hormone-secreting types the first signal may be from the effects described above. Benign tumours can attain enormous size, resembling advanced pregnancy. Eventually pressure symptoms from the enlarging mass occur: pain, swelling of the abdomen and lower limbs, dysuria from interference with the bladder. Anorexia and weight loss are common. Vaginal bleeding from uterine involvement or backache from para-aortic nodes may occur. Ascites and palpable pelvic masses, neck nodes or bowel obstruction may be present.

Staging and investigation

Current staging of ovarian cancer has become more accurate. Many patients with apparently early disease were previously understaged. The main staging classification (Table 27.5) is clinical and has a profound effect on prognosis. A laparotomy is required to assess the intra-abdominal extent of the disease. The whole of the abdominal cavity is examined for evidence of spread, particularly the subdiaphragmatic areas and the paracolic gutters. Additional investigations include full blood count, liver function tests, serum urea, creatinine and electrolytes, chest radiograph, abdominopelvic ultrasound and CT scan of the abdomen.

Tumour markers

There are no tumour markers specific to ovarian cancer. CA-125 is the most helpful tumour marker and is raised in about 80% of patients with advanced disease.

Treatment

The management of ovarian cancer requires a multidisciplinary approach. Surgery, radiotherapy and chemotherapy all have a part to play, although, sadly, more intensive treatment of advanced disease has not produced much improvement in survival.

Surgery

Surgery is central to the treatment of stages I–III ovarian cancer. If possible a total abdominal hysterectomy and bilateral salpingo-oophorectomy is carried out. It is essential to remove the other ovary in most cases since 20% of tumours are bilateral or have metastasised to the other ovary. Following removal of the uterus and ovaries and in the absence of visible residual disease, any peritoneal fluid is sampled for evidence of malignant cells. If there is no peritoneal fluid, peritoneal washings are taken for cytology, which may reveal malignant cells.

In young women who are keen to maintain their fertility, removal of the affected ovary alone may be justified. Such conservative surgery is only justified if the following criteria are met:

1. Unilateral, well-differentiated mucinous, endometrioid or clear cell tumours (not serous).
2. Negative peritoneal washings.
3. Negative wedge biopsy of the other ovary and the omentum.
4. Close surveillance is possible.

For stages Ia and Ib, where the capsule of the ovary is intact, there is no need for postoperative adjuvant therapy.

For stages II–IV the aim is to remove as much tumour as possible (a debulking operation) since the greater the amount of residual disease following surgery, the worse the prognosis. This requires an experienced surgeon. The best results are achieved if the size of the largest residual mass is less than 2.0 cm. About 75% of patients will be amenable to this form of surgery. In the remaining 25%, surgical debulking is not possible and only a biopsy is taken. A 'second-look' laparotomy may be used to assess the response to chemotherapy/radiotherapy following initial surgery and to remove any residual disease. However, this is not recommended routinely since it has not increased survival.

Radiotherapy

The role of radical radiotherapy in epithelial ovarian cancer remains uncertain. The whole of the abdomen is at risk of spread. This probably explains why pelvic irradiation alone for stage I and II disease is ineffective. For stages I–III where there is minimal residual disease, whole abdominal irradiation is advised. Contraindications are multiple abdominal operations (increased risk of late gastrointestinal morbidity) or impaired pulmonary function (risk of late pulmonary fibrosis).

Target volume

The volume should include the whole abdominal cavity. The upper border should be 2 cm above the diaphragm (in full expiration). The lower margin is the bottom of the obturator foramen of the pubis. The lateral margin extends to the outer border of the abdomen.

Technique

Anterior and posterior fields are used, simulated in the supine and prone positions. The kidneys are identified by an intravenous urogram (IVU) during planning and shielded from the front and the back by customised MCP blocks to limit the dose to each kidney to 20 Gy. A boost is given to the pelvis by parallel-opposed fields. The field margins are as for cervical cancer (p. 474).

Dose and energy

22.5 Gy is given in 20 daily fractions over 4 weeks to the whole abdomen (9–10 MV photons). The boost to the pelvis is 22.5 Gy in 10 daily fractions over 2 weeks at the same energy.

Monitoring of whole abdominal irradiation. Full blood count is monitored twice weekly since marrow impairment is normal after such wide field irradiation. Liver function tests become abnormal since the liver is irradiated. Full pulmonary function tests should be carried out before treatment since part of the lower lobes are included in the volume.

Acute reactions. Nausea, anorexia, vomiting and diarrhoea are normal during treatment but resolve usually within 3 weeks of the end of treatment. Antiemetics (e.g. metoclopramide), low-residue diet and antidiarrhoeal therapy (e.g. loperamide) are usually needed. Tiredness may last several months. White blood count and platelets fall and may require temporary suspension of treatment if they fall below certain thresholds (white count $< 2 \times 10^9/l$ or platelets $< 60 \times 10^9/l$). Liver function tests become abnormal but resolve following treatment.

Late reactions. Late complications are usually related to gastrointestinal toxicity (9%), particularly to small bowel. Stenosis and haemorrhage are the main risks, particularly if more than one abdominal operation has been carried out.

It is not recommended that radioactive isotopes (e.g. gold-198 or phosphorus-32) are introduced into the abdominal cavity to deal with residual disease. Dose distribution is uneven and loculation risks serious bowel damage.

Chemotherapy

Ovarian cancer is moderately sensitive to chemotherapy. Cures are extremely rare. Treatment is therefore essentially palliative. The most active drugs are cisplatin, its analogue carboplatin, the taxane paclitaxel, the topoisomerase inhibitor topotecan, and the alkylating agents (e.g. chlorambucil and cyclophosphamide). Care should be taken to balance toxicity of chemotherapy against the probability of symptomatic benefit. The response rates of combination chemotherapy especially carboplatin and paclitaxel, are greater than with single agents, although overall survival is no different. Since the toxicity of combination therapy tends to be more substantial, single-agent therapy is preferable.

Cisplatin (80–120 mg/m^2 3-weekly) has a response rate of 40–60% but is toxic, causing severe nausea and vomiting, renal impairment and deafness. Renal function and hearing should be carefully monitored. Carboplatin (400 mg/m^2 monthly) is preferred since it is much less emetic and causes no renal toxicity. Its limiting toxicity is to the bone marrow (leucopenia and thrombocytopenia). Both carboplatin and cisplatin are given intravenously.

Paclitaxel (135 mg/m^2 3-weekly) is usually given as a 3-hour infusion, combined with carboplatin. There is a high incidence of anaphylaxis associated with paclitaxel, which usually occurs within 10 minutes of giving the first or second dose. Prophylactic steroids and antihistamines are routinely prescribed and the patient is closely monitored during the infusion.

Chlorambucil has the advantages of oral administration on an outpatient basis and minimal toxicity (mainly leucopenia). A suitable dosage is 10 mg daily for 2 weeks out of every month, subject to satisfactory blood count. About 50% of patients respond. Similar response rates are achieved by oral cyclophosphamide. There is, however, an increased risk of leukaemia (usually acute myeloid) being induced by therapy with alkylating agents. Melphalan carries the highest risk. The cumulative incidence after 2 years of therapy with alkylating agents is of the order of 5%.

Results of treatment

Ovarian cancer has a poor prognosis, largely owing to its advanced state at the time of diagnosis. The overall survival rate is 50%. In patients who have had adequate surgery 5-year survival is 95% in stage I, 70% in stage II, 20% in stage III and 0–5% in stage IV. Where surgery has been inadequate, the survival for stages I–III is poorer (70, 60 and 10% respectively).

DYSGERMINOMA

This tumour occurs in a younger age group than do epithelial tumours. Average age is 20 years. Presentation is often with abdominal pain and a pelvic mass. Precocious puberty and abnormal menstruation may occur. Dysgerminoma does not normally produce tumour markers unless there are teratomatous elements (secreting beta human chorionic gonadotrophin and alpha-fetoprotein). A pregnancy test may be positive.

Staging

Staging investigations should include a chest X-ray and CT scan. If the CT scan is normal, a lymphangiogram is recommended. Most (75%) are stage I.

Treatment

Treatment for stage I is removal of the affected ovary alone (oophorectomy). The majority of patients with dysgerminoma have stage I disease and can be simply observed after surgery. For incompletely resected stage I disease or stage II or III disease, chemotherapy with a testicular regime such as BEP will prove curative in the majority of cases. For ill patients who are unable to tolerate chemotherapy, pelvic and para-aortic irradiation ('dog leg') as in testicular abdominal node irradiation (Fig. 28.14) or whole abdominal node irradiation is very effective, achieving a 5-year survival of 85%. Chemotherapy is the treatment of choice for stage IV.

GRANULOSA CELL TUMOURS OF THE OVARY

These tumours are rare. The majority occur in postmenopausal women although they may occur in girls before puberty. They often secrete hormones such as oestrogens, progestogens or androgens. Oestrogens are mainly derived from the cells of the theca and give rise to symptoms of menorrhagia, postmenopausal bleeding and breast tenderness. Precocious puberty occurs in young girls. 90% are stage I and are curable by abdominal hysterectomy and bilateral oophorectomy. The role of chemotherapy is uncertain. Recurrences may be suitable for further surgery or radiotherapy. Responses in recurrent disease may occur with chemotherapy.

Results of treatment

Prognosis is good: 5-year survival is 80%.

CANCER OF THE VAGINA

Most cancers in the vagina are secondary deposits from the cervix, uterus, rectum or ovary. Primary tumours of the vagina are rare with an incidence of less than 1 in 100 000 women. It usually occurs over the age of 60 years. The aetiology in most cases is unknown. However, there was an outbreak of adenocarcinoma of the upper third of the vagina in teenage children whose mothers had been treated with very high doses of diethylstilboestrol for threatened abortion. Most tumours occur in the upper vagina and may be difficult to distinguish from cervical cancers. Lymphatic drainage of the upper two-thirds is to the pelvic nodes, and of the lower third to the inguinal and pelvic nodes. Blood-borne metastases are rare. Over 90% are squamous cell carcinomas. Symptoms are of vaginal bleeding.

FIGO staging is shown in Table 27.6. To distinguish primary vaginal cancer from cervical cancer, the tumour must be sited in the vagina, not involve the cervix and not be a secondary deposit from a primary elsewhere. A biopsy is necessary to confirm the diagnosis. Staging investigations are as for cervical cancer.

Stage I and IIa squamous cell carcinomas in the lower third can be treated by interstitial implantation using iridium-192. For stages I–III in the upper third and stages IIb and III in the lower third, vaginal intracavitary and external beam are used often combined with weekly cisplatin (45 Gy in 20 daily fractions over 4 weeks; 9–10 MV photons) using an anterior and two posterior oblique fields. This is followed by vaginal intracavitary therapy delivering a further 25–30 Gy to the vaginal mucosa.

For stage IVa external beam alone is given (50 Gy in 20 daily fractions over 4 weeks; 9–10 MV photons).

Results of treatment

Prognosis is less favourable than for cervical cancer: 5-year survival following radical radiotherapy is about 75% for stage I, 60% for stage II and 20% for stage III.

CANCER OF THE VULVA

Cancer of the vulva is rare, one-fifth of the frequency of cervical cancer. It mainly occurs in elderly women.

Table 27.6 Modified FIGO staging of vaginal cancer

Stage	Clinical findings
I	Tumour confined to vaginal mucosa
IIa	Infiltration beneath the vaginal mucosa but not infiltrating the parametrium
IIb	Parametrial invasion but not to the pelvic side-wall
III	Parametrial extension to the pelvic side-wall
IVa	Spread to rectum or bladder
IVb	Distant metastases

Pathology

Aetiology

The aetiology is unknown. An association with viral infection (herpes simplex virus type 2, human papilloma virus) is suggested (but unproven), and vulval intraepithelial neoplasia (VIN) has been postulated. Viral vulval condylomata are also associated with vulval cancer. However, these condylomata rarely contain human papilloma virus (HPV) type 16, identified in invasive vulval cancer.

Macroscopic and microscopic appearance

Tumours may be exophytic or ulcerative. There is often associated leucoplakia.

Virtually all are squamous cell carcinomas. Adenocarcinoma is rare.

Spread

Local spread is to the surrounding skin, perineum, vagina and urethra. Lymphatic spread commonly occurs to the inguinal and femoral nodes and may be bilateral. Subsequent spread is to the external iliac nodes. Blood-borne spread is late.

Clinical features

Vulval itching is common (70%), often with a vulval mass or ulcer. Discharge and bleeding are less common. There is frequently a long delay between the development of symptoms and referral to a gynaecologist, often because the significance of the changes on the vulva has not been appreciated by other doctors.

Diagnosis and staging

The vulva, vagina and cervix should be carefully examined since multicentric lesions may be found elsewhere in the genital tract. A pelvic examination should be carried out under anaesthesia, noting the site, size and extent of the tumour. A biopsy is taken. A chest radiograph is necessary to detect lung metastases.

Treatment

Surgery

Surgery is the treatment of choice. Referral to a specialist gynaecological oncologist is advised since inadequate initial surgery may result in unsalvageable local and groin node recurrence.

In the few cases where invasion is less than 1 mm, a wide local excision may be adequate without groin node dissection. For all other cases of localised disease, a radical resection of the vulva and groin node dissection is recommended.

Radiotherapy

The role for radiotherapy is in the postoperative radical treatment of the pelvis for involved groin nodes and the palliation of local symptoms of advanced disease.

Involved groin nodes

Target volume
The groin and pelvic nodes bilaterally.

Technique
Parallel-opposed anterior and posterior fields.

Dose and energy
45–50 Gy midplane dose in 20 daily fractions over 4 weeks (9–10 MV photons)

Inoperable local disease

Target volume
The field should cover the tumour with a generous margin.

Technique
Direct field with bolus.

Dose and energy
30 Gy in 10 daily fractions over 2 weeks (9 MeV electrons)

Radiation reaction. The perineum is relatively intolerant of radiation owing to natural moisture and friction. Painful moist desquamation is inevitable. Analgesics and good nursing care are required.

Chemotherapy

There is no established role for chemotherapy in vulval cancer.

Results of treatment

If the groin nodes are free of disease, the 5-year survival is reasonable (70–80%). If the nodes are involved, survival falls to 20–50%. Involved pelvic nodes carry a very poor prognosis (20% 5-year survival).

GESTATIONAL TROPHOBLASTIC TUMOURS

Gestational trophoblastic tumours (GTTs) include hydatidiform mole, choriocarcinoma and its rare variant the placental site trophoblastic tumour. They affect women during and after their reproductive period. The unique feature of these tumours is that they are derived from the trophoblast of the placenta rather than from the patient's own tissues. Trophoblastic tumours retain the property of normal trophoblast to invade the muscular wall of the uterus (myometrium), and its vessels. Possibly because these tumours have paternal antigens they are very curable even in the presence of widespread metastases.

Hydatidiform mole is the simplest form of GTT. Histologically it is characterised by hyperplasia of the trophoblast and hydropic change in the placental villi. In the complete form there is no embryo since the conceptus has been abnormal from its beginning, containing only paternal genes. In the partial form there is an abnormal conceptus associated with an embryo. The latter dies early and the only residual evidence of the embryo is the presence of fetal red cells in the mole. Over 90% of moles degenerate spontaneously once the uterus has been evacuated. A further 8% do not settle and continue as persistent trophoblastic disease (such as an invasive mole), but are readily cured. A very small percentage transform to the highly malignant choriocarcinoma.

The remainder of gestational choriocarcinomas arise following about 1 in 50 000 pregnancies. They can develop from both normal and abnormal pregnancies (normal full-term pregnancy, an ectopic pregnancy, abortion or stillbirth). They contain both syncytiotrophoblast and cytotrophoblast. They are haemorrhagic tumours with a strong tendency to blood-borne spread, especially to the lungs.

Diagnosis

Clinical presentation of GTT is usually with a hydatidiform mole. Typically there is vaginal bleeding at the end of the first trimester. The uterus may be unduly large for the stage of pregnancy. The cystic trophoblastic villi give rise to multiple echoes on ultrasound. No fetus is present. Occasionally there is no immediate antecedent history and a woman may present several years following pregnancy. The diagnosis of choriocarcinoma should be borne in mind in any woman of reproductive age with disseminated cancer of unknown origin.

GTTs all secrete human chorionic gonadotrophin (HCG). This tumour marker is of great use in both establishing the diagnosis and monitoring the response to treatment. Current immunological assays can detect very small amounts of HCG in blood and urine (down to 2 iu/l). It is also detectable in the CSF in association with brain metastases. A baseline chest radiograph is taken to detect lung metastases.

Treatment

As soon as the diagnosis is suspected, the patient should be referred to a specialist centre for management. In the UK these centres are in Dundee, Sheffield and London.

The initial treatment of a GTT should be suction evacuation of the uterus. Serial blood HCG levels are measured before and after evacuation. In most uncomplicated hydatidiform moles, HCG levels fall to normal as the mole degenerates. Most GTTs are exquisitely chemosensitive, particularly to methotrexate. The following are indications for chemotherapy:

- Blood HCG levels over 20 000 iu/l for more than a month after evacuation of the uterus
- Rising levels of HCG
- Histological evidence of choriocarcinoma
- Presence of lung metastases greater than 2 cm in diameter or metastases in brain, liver or bowel
- Persisting uterine bleeding
- HCG detectable in body fluids 4–6 months after evacuation.

The choice of drugs depends on a variety of prognostic factors (e.g. age, sites and number of metastases, level of HCG). On this basis, patients can be divided into low-, medium- and high-risk groups.

Low-risk patients are treated with low-dose methotrexate and folinic acid; medium-risk with a combination of etoposide, methotrexate with folinic acid, 6-mercaptopurine and actinomycin D, and high-risk with actinomycin D, etoposide, high-dose methotrexate, vincristine and cyclophosphamide.

Patients with brain metastases should additionally receive intrathecal methotrexate. Isolated brain metastases should be excised if possible since chemotherapy may precipitate intracranial bleeding.

Results of treatment

Virtually all low- and medium-risk patients with GTT are cured. Even in the high-risk group, cure rates are about 90% in the best centres.

CHAPTER CONTENTS

28

Kidney, bladder, prostate, testis, urethra, penis

Duncan McLaren

KIDNEY

Anatomy

The kidneys lie retroperitoneally on the posterior abdominal wall. They are approximately 11 cm long and 6 cm wide in adults. The left kidney is 1 cm higher than the right. The right kidney is related in front to the liver, the second part of the duodenum and the ascending colon. In front of the left kidney are the stomach, the pancreas, descending colon and the spleen. On the top of each kidney lies an adrenal gland. Behind the kidneys lie the diaphragm and the 12th rib. On the medial side of the kidney there is an opening, the hilum, through which pass the renal artery and vein, and the ureter. The renal vein drains into the inferior vena cava. The lymphatic drainage is to the para-aortic nodes. The anatomical relationships relevant to the oncologist are shown in Figure 28.1.

Pathology

The three principal malignant tumours of the kidney are Wilms' tumour (nephroblastoma) in children (described in Ch. 32), renal cell adenocarcinoma (also called clear cell carcinoma, hypernephroma and Grawitz's tumour) and transitional cell carcinoma of the renal pelvis. Adenocarcinoma arising from the renal tubules accounts for 80% of tumours. Macroscopically the tumour appears as a yellowish vascular mass. Microscopically the tumour cells are large with a foamy or clear appearance to the cytoplasm. The nucleus is small, central and densely staining.

Renal cancer is uncommon, accounting for 3% of all cancers and 1.5% of cancer deaths. Over the last 10 years the incidence has risen by 23% in men and 29% in women within the UK, a pattern reflected throughout the world. Overall there is a 2 : 1 male to female

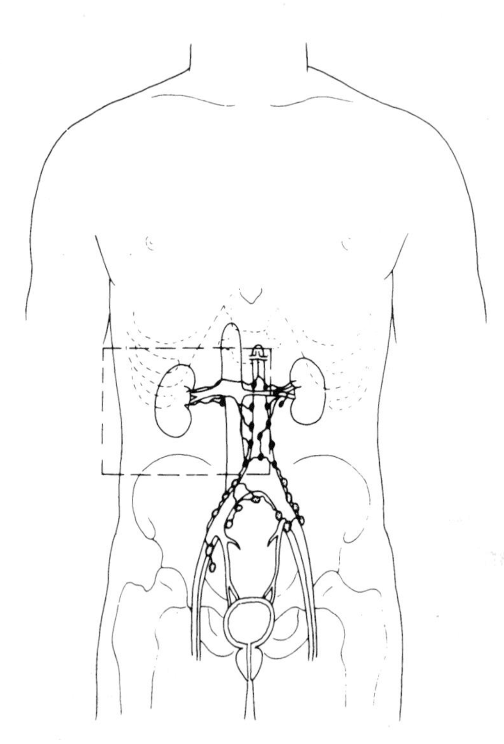

Fig. 28.1 Anatomical relationships of the kidney with lymphatic drainage pathways and typical treatment volume when irradiating the renal bed. (Reproduced with permission from Souhami & Tobias, Cancer and its Management, Blackwells, 1986.)

ratio in incidence and the disease occurs mainly in the 5th–7th decades of life. The aetiology of renal cell carcinoma is unknown, though smoking is a risk factor. 30% of patients present with metastatic disease.

Spread

There is direct spread through the renal substance and into the perinephric fat of the renal bed. The characteristic mode of spread is permeation along the renal vein and into the inferior vena cava. Tumour may rarely extend up to the right side of the heart, completely blocking the inferior vena cava. Lymphatic spread to local renal hilar and para-aortic lymph nodes and haematogenous metastatic spread to lung, bone and brain are common. The tempo of metastatic disease may be unpredictable; however, $< 10\%$ remain alive at 5 years from diagnosis. Rarely, spontaneous regression of metastases may occur following nephrectomy.

Clinical features

Presentation is usually with local symptoms. Painless haematuria is the commonest or colicky pain secondary to clots of blood. Other symptoms are aching or a mass in the loin which may be noticed by the patient. A coincidental finding following radiological imaging of the abdomen is an increasingly common presentation. Distant metastasis may be the first presentation —pathological bone fracture, haemoptysis from pulmonary metastases or symptoms of raised intracranial pressure from cerebral deposits. Systemic features such as anaemia, loss of weight and unexplained fever may occur. The kidney may be palpably enlarged.

Investigation and staging

The urine may contain frank or microscopic evidence of blood. Urine cytology may show malignant cells. The most important investigation is an intravenous urogram (IVU), which may show distortion of the calyces (the channels that drain urine to the renal pelvis and are outlined by the contrast medium) by the tumour. Calcification within the tumour may be visible on plain radiographs. Ultrasound and CT scanning (Fig. 28.2) are helpful in distinguishing between solid and cystic renal masses. Ultrasound may show extension of tumour into the renal vein or inferior vena cava. CT scanning of the chest, abdomen and pelvis may show direct tumour spread, venous and lymph node involvement and soft tissue metastases in liver and lung. Angiography is an invasive procedure and its use is diminishing. It still has a role in demonstrating the renal artery and new vessel formation when the kidney is to be embolised (i.e. material introduced into the renal arterial to cut off its blood supply and cause death of part or the whole of the kidney). Bone metastases are typically osteolytic (Fig. 28.3).

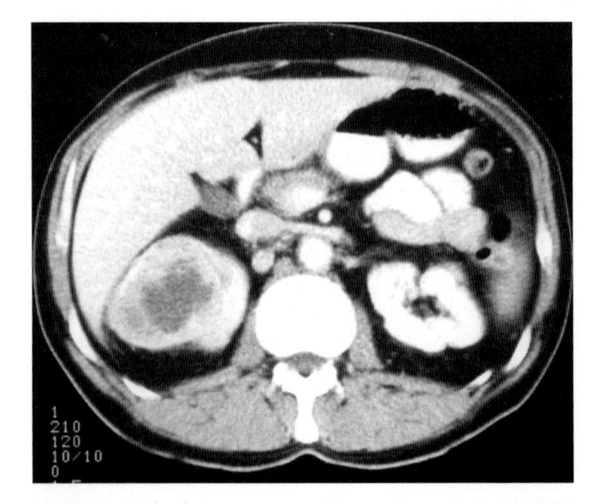

Fig. 28.2 CT scan showing a typical renal cell carcinoma in the right kidney.

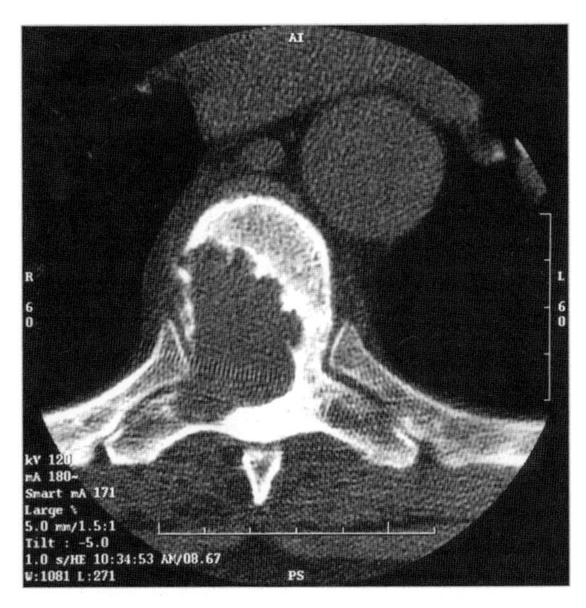

Fig. 28.3 Radiograph showing osteolytic metastasis of the vertebral body from renal cell carcinoma.

No staging system for renal cell cancer has universal acceptance. The UICC 1997 TNM classification is shown in Table 28.1.

Treatment

Surgery is the main treatment for localised renal cell cancer. Radiotherapy and embolisation have more limited roles. Chemotherapy is of unproven value. Immunotherapy is increasingly being utilised.

Surgery

Nephrectomy is indicated for tumours confined to the kidney and/or regional nodes. Extension into the inferior vena cava is not necessarily a contraindication to surgery. There is debate as to the role of nephrectomy in the presence of metastatic disease. In patients with good performance status suitable for subsequent immunotherapy, nephrectomy to reduce tumour bulk is increasingly utilised. In selected patients aggressive surgical removal of the primary tumour together with solitary metastases particularly in lung and bone may be followed by 35% 5-year survival. Palliative removal of the kidney may be required to control pain or haemorrhage or if a painful syndrome following embolisation occurs.

Embolisation

Embolisation of the kidney via a catheter inserted into the renal artery may be useful in both operable and inoperable cases. In operable cases embolisation is indicated where there is concern about blood loss at nephrectomy, e.g. in patients who refuse blood transfusion on religious grounds. In inoperable cases, it is effective in controlling renal pain and haematuria. A postembolisation syndrome with pain, ileus, and infection may complicate embolisation.

Radiotherapy

Renal cell carcinoma is relatively resistant to radiation. Pre- or postoperative radiotherapy does not reduce local recurrence where the tumour has spread locally outside the kidney. Its role is palliative to relieve symptoms from the primary tumour or from distant metastases.

Kidney

Target volume

The whole of the kidney and the regional nodes should be included (Fig. 28.1).

Table 28.1 TNM staging of primary renal tumours

Stage	Clinical findings
Tumour	
T0	No tumour
T1	Tumour 7.0 cm or less in greatest dimension, limited to the kidney
T2	Tumour more than 7.0 cm in greatest dimension, limited to the kidney
T3	Tumour extends into major veins or invades adrenal gland or perinephric tissues but not beyond Gerota's fascia
T3a	Tumour invades adrenal gland or perinephric tissues but not beyond Gerota's fascia
T3b	Tumour grossly extends into renal vein(s) or vena cava below diaphragm
T3c	Tumour grossly extends into vena cava above diaphragm
T4	Tumour extends beyond Gerota's fascia
Tx	Primary tumour cannot be assessed
Nodes	
N0	No regional lymph node metastasis
N1	Metastasis in single regional lymph node
N2	Metastasis in more than one regional lymph node
Nx	Regional lymph nodes cannot be assessed
Metastases	
M0	No distant metastases
M1	Distant metastases
Mx	Distant metastases cannot be assessed
Histological grading	
G1	Well differentiated
G2	Moderately differentiated
G3–4	Poorly differentiated/undifferentiated
Gx	Grade of differentiation cannot be assessed

Technique

A parallel-opposed anterior and posterior pair of fields is used.

Dose and energy

30 Gy in 10 daily fractions over 2 weeks (4–6 MV photons)

Distant metastases

Brain and bone metastases are treated by palliative radiotherapy, as described on pages 552 and 581 respectively.

Chemotherapy

Chemotherapy has little value in renal cancer. Single agent vinblastine with < 10% response rate is most extensively used. Oral progestogens have been claimed to benefit 20% of patients; however, in randomised clinical trials, this has fallen below 10%. Their major use is in the palliation of systemic symptoms such as anorexia. Phase II trials of new chemotherapeutic agents continue in the hope of improving response rates.

Immunotherapy

The observation that spontaneous regression of metastases may occasionally occur stimulated interest in immunotherapy. Interferon-alpha and interleukin-2, stimulate the body's immunological attack on tumours. Single-agent response rates of 15–20% are commonly reported. There is evidence of synergy if these agents are used in combination, with response rates approaching 27–38%. Toxicity is marked and the precise dose and scheduling of the combination for maximum benefit is yet to be decided. In those patients who respond, a few long-term remissions have been observed.

Results of treatment

The outlook depends on the stage at diagnosis. For tumours confined to the kidney, 5-year survival varies from 50 to 80%. Extrarenal local invasion, together with invasion into the renal vein lymph nodes and blood-borne metastases all confer a poor prognosis. Patients with metastatic disease at presentation have a median survival of only 12 months, with 20% remaining alive 2 years from diagnosis.

BLADDER

Anatomy

The bladder is related anteriorly to the pubic symphysis, superiorly to the small intestine and sigmoid colon, laterally to the levator ani muscle, inferiorly to the prostate gland and posteriorly to the rectum, vas deferens and seminal vesicles (see Fig. 28.7) in the male and to the vagina and cervix in the female. At cystoscopy the bladder mucosa and ureteric orifices can be inspected. Lymphatic drainage is to the iliac and para-aortic nodes.

Pathology

The bladder, ureters and renal pelvis are lined by transitional cell epithelium (urothelium). The same type of tumours may arise anywhere along the urinary tract but cancers in the renal pelvis and ureter are rare compared with those in the bladder. Prostatic adenocarcinoma and other pelvic tumours also sometimes secondarily involve the bladder.

Aetiology

In the majority of cases of bladder cancer, the aetiology is unknown. However, as discussed in Chapter 17, occupational exposure to certain carcinogens has accounted for some cases. The production of aniline dyes and processing of rubber are associated with 2-naphthylamine, now recognised as a procarcinogen. Workers in these industries are now offered regular cytological examination of urine to detect abnormalities or tumours at an early stage.

Smoking is perhaps the commonest factor that predisposes to bladder cancer. Bladder cancer is up to six times commoner in smokers than non-smokers and increases in frequency with the number of cigarettes smoked. Phenacetin formerly used as an analgesic drug and the cytotoxic alkylating agent cyclophosphamide may give rise to urothelial tumours. Squamous carcinoma tends to complicate chronic irritation of the bladder including a parasitic disease, schistosomiasis (formerly known as bilharziasis), which is common in Egypt and Central Africa. Adenocarcinoma occurs on the dome of the bladder in relation to embryological remnants of the urachus, and also from the trigone at the bladder base.

Genetic alterations in bladder cancer are common. Deletion of markers on chromosome 9 is an early event. Subsequent mutation in *p53* allows cells with DNA damage to proceed through the cell cycle, replicating genetic errors. Loss of the pRb (retinoblastoma) gene product disrupts cell cycling and increases the mitotic index. Patients with both mutations have higher-grade more advanced disease and a poor response to treatment.

Epidemiology

Bladder cancer is common and accounts for 4.4% of all cancers and 3.4% of cancer deaths. The male to female ratio is 3.8 : 1 and it has a peak incidence at the age of 65. The impact of smoking in women has seen a greater rise in incidence in this group over the last 10 years compared to men. It is twice as common in Caucasians as in Blacks. Over 90% are transitional cell carcinomas.

Macroscopic appearance

The chief types on inspection of the bladder are (1) papillary and (2) solid. Multiple growths are common.

Papillary carcinoma has a base with surface fronds. The tumours tend to be multiple and to appear in crops. Confined at first to the mucosa and submucosa, they eventually invade the submucosa, muscle coat and then outside the bladder.

Solid carcinoma is nodular, often ulcerated, grows more rapidly and infiltrates early.

From the point of prognosis a division can be made between superficial (papillary) and invasive (solid) bladder cancer. Superficial bladder tumours are the commonest (80%) and become invasive in 10–20% of cases. By contrast, invasive cancer, untreated, carries a very poor prognosis. The degree of invasion correlates with the risk of metastatic disease. Invasion of the lamina propria (the layer of tissue between the epithelium and the muscle layer of the bladder), superficial and deep muscle is associated with 20%, 30% and 60% incidence of lymphatic invasion.

Microscopic appearance

Benign tumours of the bladder are very uncommon. However, low-grade transitional cell malignant tumours are often erroneously referred to as papillomas.

Malignant tumours of the bladder include:

- Transitional cell carcinoma; papillary and solid variants
- Adenocarcinoma (uncommon)
- Squamous carcinoma (rare in the UK)
- Sarcomas (all very rare).

Transitional carcinoma accounts for 90% of bladder cancer and is classified histologically into grades 1–3 corresponding to well, moderately and poorly differentiated tumours. The degree of differentiation is important. High-grade tumours grow faster and infiltrate sooner.

After muscle has been invaded, lymphatic spread is to the pelvic and then para-aortic nodes. Blood-borne metastases are common to lung, liver and bone.

Clinical features

The presenting symptom is usually painless haematuria. Occasionally clots of blood are passed and are even more suggestive of the diagnosis. Papillomatous types grow slowly and may cause no other symptoms for a long time. When aggressive carcinomas invade muscle, there may be urinary frequency, dysuria and pain, especially when there is extravesical (i.e. outside the bladder) spread into the pelvic soft tissues. Bacterial cystitis may be associated with the tumour and may aggravate symptoms.

Obstruction of one or both ureters can occur at any time, with no symptoms at first. Later there may be upper urinary tract infection, pain in the flank(s) and eventual renal failure from backpressure. In localised bladder disease clinical examination is usually unremarkable.

Investigation and staging

Urine. The urine should be examined for red cells, pus cells and bacteria as well as undergoing cytology for malignant cells. Urine cytology is a valuable screening method for industrial workers at risk. Malignant cells are present in the urine of 60% of cases of bladder cancer, particularly the higher-grade tumours. However, negative cytology does not exclude malignancy.

Biochemistry. Serum urea, creatinine and electrolytes are measured for evidence of renal impairment.

Radiology. Radiology is important in the diagnosis and staging of bladder cancer. An intravenous urogram will determine the site of the tumour in the bladder and exclude a lesion higher up in the renal tract. Obstruction at the lower end of the ureter(s) will be shown by dilatation of the ureter and renal pelvis (hydroureter and hydronephrosis). Filling defects in the bladder can also be shown. A CT scan of the abdomen and pelvis may demonstrate extravesical spread or lymphadenopathy. MRI scanning may prove to be the staging investigation of choice.

Cystourethroscopy. This is the most important investigation of all. Under general anaesthesia the urethra and the whole of the bladder are inspected. The number, site, size and character of the tumours are noted and a biopsy taken. While the patient is relaxed under the anaesthetic, a bimanual examination of the pelvis is made, with a finger in the rectum and the other hand on the lower abdomen. In this way the tumour may be palpated and any extravesical spread assessed.

Clinical staging of bladder cancer is according to the 1997 TNM classification (Fig. 28.4 and Table 28.2).

Treatment

Treatment will depend on the stage, histology, size and multiplicity of tumours and the age and general medical condition of the patient.

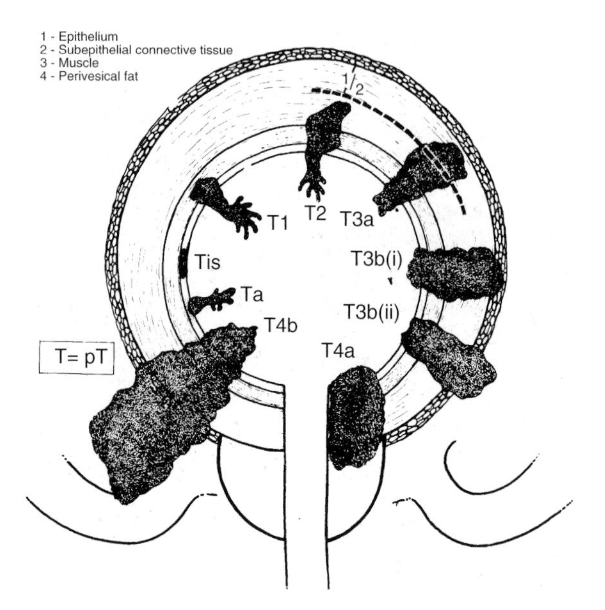

Fig. 28.4 T staging of bladder cancer—UICC classification. (Reproduced with permission from Hermanek P, Hutter R V P and Sobin L H (eds) 1997 International Union Against Cancer TNM Atlas. Illustrated guide to the TNM classification of malignant tumours, 4th edn, Springer-Verlag.)

Table 28.2 TNM staging of bladder cancer

Stage	Clinical findings
Tumour	
Tis	Carcinoma-in-situ
Ta	Papillary non-invasive carcinoma
T1	Invasion into submucosa but not beyond the lamina propria
T2a	Invasion into superficial detrusor muscle
T2b	Invasion into deep detrusor muscle
T3a	Invasion into perivesicular tissues microscopically
T3b	Invasion into perivesicular tissues macroscopically
T4a	Invasion of prostate or vagina
T4b	Invasion of pelvic side-wall or abdominal wall
Nodes	
N0	No evidence of nodal involvement
N1	Single node < 2 cm diameter
N2	Single nodal metastasis 2–5 cm diameter or multiple nodes none exceeding 5 cm
N3	Node > 5 cm
Metastases	
M0	No metastases
M1	Distant metastases

Superficial Ta and T1 tumours

Superficial tumours are biopsied and removed by transurethral resection (TUR) or diathermy at the time of cytoscopy. Random biopsies of the bladder are carried out to exclude carcinoma-in-situ. In the majority of patients these tumours tend to recur rather than invade (up to 60% recurrence rate). For this reason cystoscopic follow-up needs to be lifelong.

If recurrences are multiple or high grade, intravesical chemotherapy or BCG should be used to reduce the recurrence rate to 40%. Intravesical BCG may reduce the recurrence rates for carcinoma-in-situ from 80% to 40% and may also delay the rates of progression. Cystectomy is indicated if these measures fail.

Superficial tumours do respond completely to radical radiotherapy in over 75% of cases but there is recurrence in more than 50%. For this reason radical radiotherapy is rarely used in T1 lesions. 20% of patients present with T1G3 disease yet they constitute more than 50% of those patients who progress to more invasive disease. Radiotherapy may be more effective for this group of patients and is currently being evaluated in a clinical trial.

Invasive bladder cancer (T2 and T3)

Surgery and radiotherapy are the standard treatments for invasive bladder cancer.

T2 tumours. Endoscopic resection (TURBT) is inadequate to control these tumours alone. Additional radical treatment with either cystoprostourethrectomy (removal of the bladder and prostate with diversion of the ureters onto the abdominal wall) or radical radiotherapy is required. Local practice will determine treatment. Europe and America have favoured cystoprostourethrectomy as the treatment of choice. In the UK radical radiotherapy with salvage cystectomy for those patients with persistent or recurrent tumour is more commonly adopted. This policy has the advantage that the patient has a better chance of tumour control with the bladder intact. If radiotherapy fails there is a 30% chance of successful salvage by cystectomy. By contrast, if primary cystectomy fails, radical radiotherapy is rarely successful for recurrent disease. Each policy carries a similar 5-year survival of about 40–50%.

The use of neoadjuvant cytotoxic chemotherapy, to reduce tumour bulk and deal with microscopic lymph node metastases, followed by radical radiotherapy has failed to improve survival. Adjuvant chemotherapy following radical therapy has similarly yet to improve survival in a randomised controlled trial.

T3 tumours. If bimanual palpation and/or radiological imaging have demonstrated macroscopic extension of disease outside the bladder, cure rates fall to around 20% at 5 years. Such patients are more commonly treated with radical radiotherapy than with surgery. Preoperative radiotherapy followed by cystourethrectomy is an alternative approach; however, no survival advantage has been demonstrated. Combined modality treatment with concurrent chemotherapy (such as cisplatin) and radiotherapy remains under evaluation.

T4 tumours. A distinction must be made between T4a and T4b tumours. T4a means tumour penetration into the prostate or vagina. T4a includes both aggressive deeply invasive tumours infiltrating the prostate and less aggressive superficial tumours extending into the prostatic urethra and/or ducts. The latter has a much better prognosis than the former. T4a tumours should be treated radically. T4b tumours are fixed to neighbouring structures, are inoperable and should be treated with palliative radiotherapy.

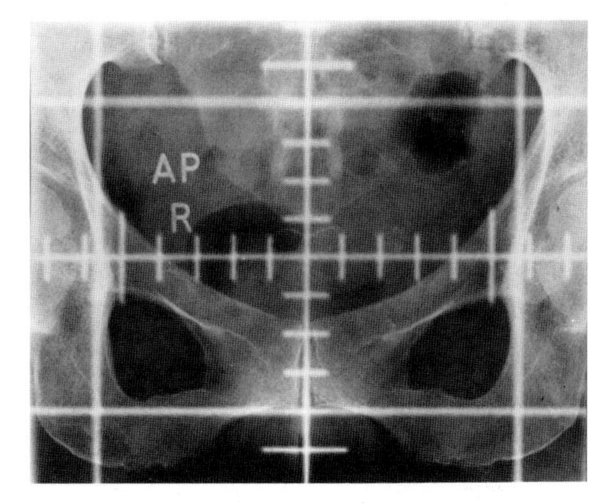

Fig. 28.5 Simulator radiograph showing anterior treatment volume for radical radiotherapy of a transitional cell carcinoma of the bladder.

Adenocarcinoma and squamous carcinoma of the bladder

Neither of these is very radiosensitive and they are better treated by cystectomy.

Radical radiotherapy

The following are criteria for accepting patients for radical radiotherapy:

- Age < 80 years
- Adequate general medical condition
- No inflammatory bowel disease or symptomatic adhesions
- Good bladder function
- Minimal or no CIS
- Transitional cell carcinoma
- Single tumour < 7 cm maximum diameter
- Recurrent T1G3, T2–T4a
- No metastases.

Target volume

The treatment volume is 1–2 cm around the tumour, judged by bimanual examination and CT scanning. The bladder is emptied before CT planning and before each treatment.

Radiation planning technique

The tumour is localised by intravesical contrast medium (cystogram) on a simulator (Fig. 28.5) or by a CT planning scan.

CT planning is preferable to conventional planning. It allows greater definition of the planning target volume (PTV). The patient is planned in the same position on the CT scanner as on the simulator and treatment couches (supine with feet in foot stocks and, hands by the side). On the planning computer the width of the target volume to encompass the tumour with a 1–2 cm margin is chosen. The superior and inferior target volume being 1 cm above and below the upper and lower limits of the bladder. It is common practice to cover the prostatic urethra in the PTV in view of the risk of local recurrence. The position of the rectum and femoral heads are marked on the computer and translated to the treatment plan. In our experience the treatment volume using CT planning tends to be larger than that using a cystogram. An open anterior and two lateral wedged or posterior oblique wedged fields are used, treating isocentrically (Fig. 28.6). A direct lateral field is preferred at our institution to reduce rectal doses in view of the sharp fall-off of the field. With high-energy photon beams such as

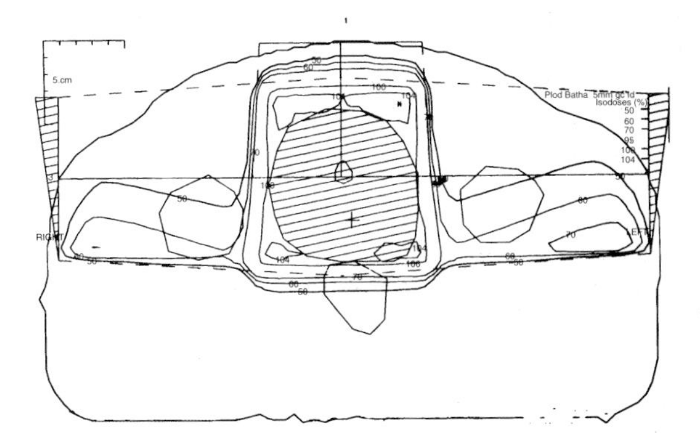

Fig. 28.6 Isodose distribution for radical radiotherapy of the bladder using anterior and two lateral fields.

16 MV femoral-head doses are kept below 50% of the tumour dose. The use of conformal therapy techniques may improve treatment-related morbidity in addition to possible dose escalation in the future.

Dose and energy

52.5–55 Gy in 20 daily fractions over 4 weeks (9–16 MV photons)

or

64 Gy in 32 daily fractions over 6.5 weeks (9–16 MV photons)

Radiation reaction. Before radiation begins, attention is paid to the patient's general condition and nutrition. The patient's haemoglobin level should be maintained over 12 g/dl, by blood transfusion if necessary, since anaemia will reduce the amount of oxygen available to the tumour. It is known that reduced oxygenation in parts of the tumour contributes to resistance to radiation. Urinary infection should be treated with antibiotics. The urine should be made sterile if possible before radiation begins, since inflammation has adverse effects on radiation response. However, with an ulcerated mass this may not be possible until the tumour has shrunk in response to radiation.

Acute reactions

1. Frequency and urgency, from radiation cystitis during and after the course, are common but not usually serious unless bacterial infection is gross. Painful spasm may require an antispasmodic drug. Fluid intake must be strongly encouraged. The patient should be warned that he or she might pass fragments in the urine (blood clot and tumour) and a little fresh blood.
2. Bowel reactions are also to be expected in almost every case—usually mild diarrhoea and tenesmus. If they are severe, treatment may have to be suspended or dosage reduced.

Late reactions

1. Fibrosis of the bladder. The bladder wall may be so contracted by fibrosis and the bladder volume so reduced that uncontrollable frequency may make life intolerable. Ureteric diversion may be required.
2. Telangiectasia on the bladder lining may develop, with repeated bleeding. It may be possible to seal them off with the diathermy point at cystoscopy. If they are uncontrolled by this means, cystectomy may be required.
3. Late bowel reactions are similar to those after the irradiation of cancer of the cervix (p. 475), though less common. Loops of bowel trapped in the pelvis by adhesions after previous surgery or inflammatory disease are especially at risk. There may be bleeding from telangiectasia on the bowel mucosa, ulceration, even necrosis and perforation. If conservative measures, e.g. steroid enemas, fail, a defunctioning colostomy may be required.

Palliative radiotherapy

Palliative radiotherapy should be considered in the following circumstances: age (> 80 years) or poor general condition with either significant local symptoms (e.g. haematuria) or symptomatic metastases, e.g. bone and skin.

Technique

A parallel-opposed pair or four-field 'box' technique of an anterior and posterior opposed pair of fields and a pair of lateral opposed fields is used. A cystogram is recommended for bladder localisation.

Dose and energy

30 Gy in 10 daily fractions over 2 weeks (9–10 MV)

Chemotherapy

Response rates of greater than 50% have been reported using cisplatin-based regimens such as CMV or MVAC for metastatic disease. Median survival, however, remains disappointing at 12 months.

Results of treatment

The 5-year survival for radical radiotherapy is 40–60% for T2 and 5–30% for T3 and T4 tumours.

PROSTATE

Anatomy

The prostate gland lies just below the base of the bladder and in front of the rectum (Fig. 28.7). It resembles a chestnut in size and shape. Through it passes the prostatic urethra. Into the urethra empty the ejaculatory ducts, which carry sperm from the seminal vesicles, which lie behind and to each side of the prostate gland. The prostate is divided into two lobes by a median groove. From a functional point of view it is divided into a peripheral zone, central zone and transitional zone. It is surrounded by a thin layer of fibrous tissue (true capsule) and a layer of fascia continuous with that surrounding the bladder (false capsule). Between these two layers lies the prostatic venous plexus. Part of the venous drainage is to a plexus of veins lying in front of the vertebral bodies. This may

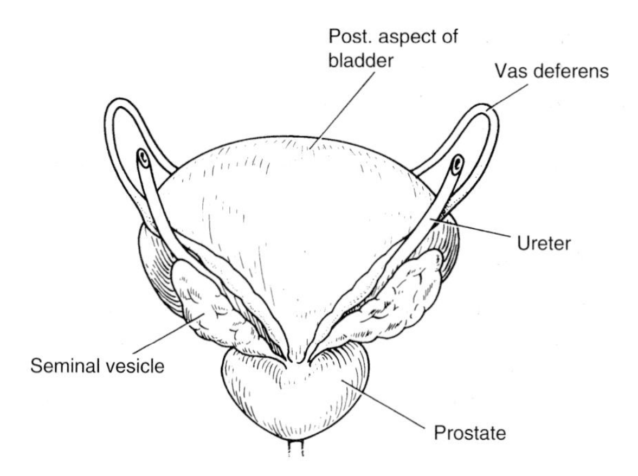

Fig. 28.7 Prostate, seminal vesicles and vas deferens in a posterior view of the bladder. (Redrawn from Ellis, Clinical Anatomy, 5th edn, Blackwells, 1975.)

account for the tendency of prostate cancer to spread to the vertebrae.

Pathology

Cancer of the prostate gland is the second commonest malignancy in men in the UK. In total 20 000 new cases and 10 000 deaths per annum are recorded. In Scotland a 48% increase in incidence between 1986 and 1995 was noted. Prostate-specific antigen (PSA) detection of incidental tumours and increased use of TURP account for much of this rise.

The exact aetiology of prostatic cancer is unknown. It is commonest in the seventh and eighth decades and rare under the age of 40. Marked worldwide variations in incidence exist. In particular, Japan has rates considerably lower than in the USA. A correlation with diet and in particular high fat consumption is directly implicated. Genetic factors have a role; siblings are at increased risk with a positive family history and USA Blacks have higher levels of disease noted compared to USA Whites. Environmental factors include exposure to radiation, heavy metals and chemical fertilisers although no definitive link has been determined.

Over 95% are adenocarcinomas, 70% arising from the peripheral part of the gland. The differentiation of prostate cancer is graded according to the Gleason grading system. It is based on the extent to which the tumour cells are arranged into recognisable glandular structures, grade 1 tumours forming almost normal glands while grade 5 tumours consist of sheets of cells (Fig. 28.8). Because of the heterogeneity in prostate cancer the two most common grades seen are added together to give a Gleason score.

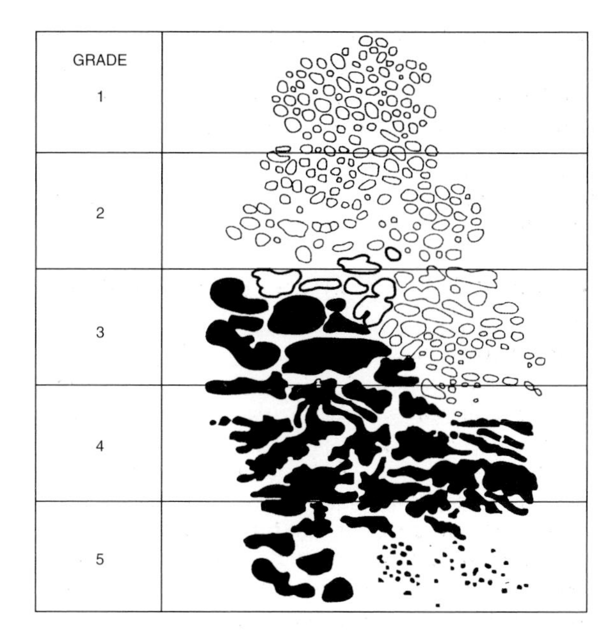

Fig. 28.8 Gleason grading system for carcinoma of the prostate. (Reproduced with permission from Kirby R S, Brawer M K and Denis L J (eds) 2001 Prostate Cancer Fast Facts, 3rd edn, Health Press.)

Before the advent of PSA testing and greater patient awareness, in 75% of cases the tumour had spread beyond the gland at the time of presentation, and 50% had distant metastases. The introduction of PSA screening in countries such as the USA, however, has dramatically reduced the numbers of patients presenting with advanced disease.

Prostate cancer may spread directly to the bladder, seminal vesicles and rectum. Lymphatic spread is to the obturator, presacral, internal and external iliac nodes. Further spread is to the common iliac and para-aortic nodes. It readily invades the pelvic veins and thence the pelvic bones and vertebrae. Bone secondaries are typically of sclerotic type, showing as an increased density on the radiograph because they induce new bone formation.

The natural history of the disease is very variable. It may be indolent in the elderly patient with a well-differentiated tumour and an incidental finding at post-mortem. The disease tends to run a more aggressive course in younger men particularly with poorly differentiated tumours.

Hormonal sensitivity

The prostate has analogies with the breast and is under hormonal control. Removal of male hormones by orchidectomy, or administration of female hormones (oestrogens), causes shrinkage of the normal gland, and of 80% of tumours.

PSA and screening

Prostate-specific antigen is a glycoprotein that liquefies semen. Approximately 20% of men with PSA levels above the normal range of 4 ng/ml have prostate cancer, and this risk increases to more than 60% in men with a PSA level above 10 ng/ml. PSA levels increase in proportion to the volume of disease and can be used to monitor the response to treatment and development of metastatic disease. PSA has largely superseded the use of an enzyme, acid phosphatase, secreted by normal and malignant prostate tissue, in the diagnosis and assessment of response to treatment.

The benefits of screening for prostate cancer are unproven. Increased case detection through PSA testing, however, is likely to continue.

Clinical features

The prostate often undergoes benign enlargement, and the early symptoms of cancer may be similar, i.e. increased frequency and difficulty of micturition. Haematuria and urinary obstruction can occur. Bone pain or pathological fracture may be the first presenting symptom. Back pressure on the kidneys may cause renal impairment. Sacral, sciatic or perineal pain may occur from infiltration of nerves in the pelvis. Clinical evidence of disease is rare under the age of 45.

Diagnosis and staging

The presence of a hard irregular gland on rectal examination suggests the diagnosis. This should be confirmed by a biopsy of the prostate. Usually six biopsies of the prostate (three from each lobe) are conducted under transrectal ultrasound guidance. Prostatic carcinoma is staged using the TNM classification (Table 28.3). The local stage of the disease is mainly based on rectal examination. This may be supplemented by ultrasound, CT or MRI scanning. MRI scanning in particular is helpful in showing extracapsular spread, enlarged pelvic nodes and local invasion of the bladder, seminal vesicles and rectal wall. Surgical dissection of the pelvic nodes to assess pelvic node involvement has not gained wide acceptance in the UK since it does not improve survival. A bone scan is recommended in view of the high incidence of bone metastases.

Table 28.3 TNM staging of prostate cancer 1992

Stage	Clinical findings
Tumour	
T1	Clinically inapparent tumour not palpable or visible by imaging
T1a	Tumour incidental finding in 5% or less of tissue resected
T1b	Tumour incidental finding in more than 5% of tissue resected
T1c	Tumour identified by needle biopsy (e.g. due to elevated PSA)
T2	Palpable tumour confined to the gland
T2a	Tumour involves half a lobe or less
T2b	Tumour involves more than half a lobe
T2c	Tumour involves both lobes
T3	Tumour extending beyond the capsule
T3a	Unilateral extracapsular extension
T3b	Bilateral extracapsular extension
T3c	Tumour invades seminal vesicle(s)
T4	Tumour fixed or invading adjacent structures
T4a	Tumour invades bladder neck, external sphincter, rectum
T4b	Tumour invades levator muscles and/or fixed to pelvic wall
Nodes	
N0	No nodes involved
N1	Single node metastasis < 2 cm in diameter
N2	Single node metastasis 2–5 cm in diameter or multiple nodes, none > 5 cm
N3	Node > 5 cm
Metastases	
M0	No distant metastases
M1	Distant metastases

Treatment

1. Clinically localised disease T1–2N0M0

There are no randomised-controlled trials to determine the optimum treatment for early prostate cancer. The clinical behaviour of the disease is unpredictable, a situation made worse by the lack of accurate prognostic indicators of disease behaviour. Aggressive treatment of indolent disease exposes patients to the toxicity of treatment, whereas undertreatment may lead to potentially curable disease causing significant morbidity or cancer-related death. Balancing these issues requires time and experience.

Treatment options include:

- Watchful waiting
- Radical radiotherapy
- Prostate brachytherapy
- Radical prostatectomy.

Factors that should influence the choice are the age and general condition of the patient, the likelihood of progression to symptomatic disease and the morbidity of treatment, particularly on sexual function. In general patients should have a life-expectancy of greater than 10 years before being treated radically. This is because untreated, it may take several years for there to be any symptoms from their disease, and several years beyond that before death ensues. Generally the higher the PSA, Gleason score and T stage the higher the chance of tumour progression and the need for radical treatment. Elderly, medically unfit men with less-aggressive histological features may be managed by watchful waiting (with deferred hormonal therapy and/or palliative radiotherapy for symptomatic progression).

There is evidence that radical therapy can cure localised prostate cancer, with survival curves flattening off between 10 and 15 years from treatment. The chance of local control with radiotherapy decreases with increasing PSA, grade and stage of disease. Neoadjuvant hormonal therapy for 3 months before radiotherapy has demonstrated improved local control and possibly survival over radiotherapy alone. The hormonal treatment reduces the size of the prostate by 30% and hence the treatment volume. It also reduces the number of tumour cells to irradiate, possibly through synergistic apoptotic mechanisms. Improving local control by dose escalation made possible by the development of conformal radiotherapy fields is currently being tested in a randomised controlled trial. Initial data, however, looks promising. Further refinement of radiotherapy technique with intensity-modulated radiotherapy may offer even greater gains.

Radical radiotherapy

Target volume

If the tumour staging demonstrates that the tumour is confined to the prostate and there is no obvious involvement of the pelvic nodes, the target volume is confined to the tumour and any local extension (e.g. seminal vesicles), with a 1 cm margin of normal tissue around it. At the rectal–prostate interface a margin of 0.6 cm is satisfactory. Pelvic radiotherapy in the UK is not commonly employed. By treating the nodes, morbidity is increased without significant gains in survival.

Technique

A three-field technique is used, either with one anterior and two posterior oblique fields at 120° to each other or one anterior and two wedged lateral fields. We tend to favour the later in view of the sharp rectal cut-off in dose. The patient lies supine. Localisation is done with a CT planning scan. The bladder should be full to displace the dome of the bladder and small bowel out of the field. CT cuts of 1 cm (0.5 cm if conformal treatment) are taken through the pelvis. A planning target volume with 1 cm margin around the prostate (0.6 cm at the rectum) is outlined. Difficulty in localisation of the prostatic apex and extension into the bladder are common areas of fault. The rectal outline and femoral heads are marked and a plan produced. With conformal treatment the volume is shaped to follow the prostate and in so doing shield as much of the normal tissues such as the rectum as possible (Fig. 28.9). A typical isodose distribution is shown in Figure 28.10.

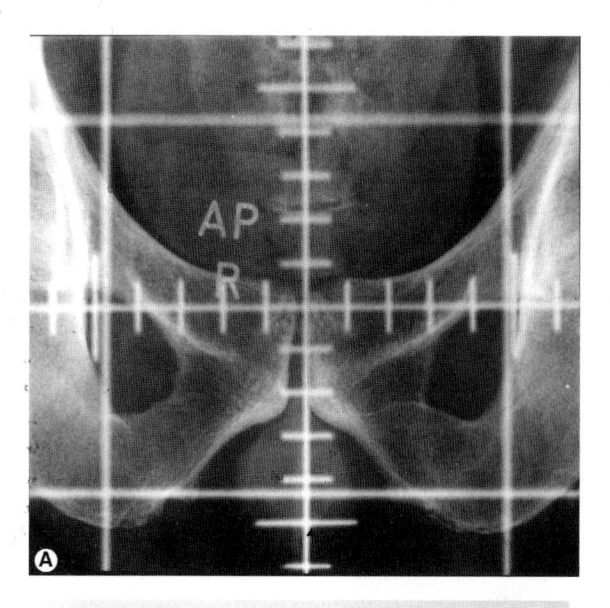

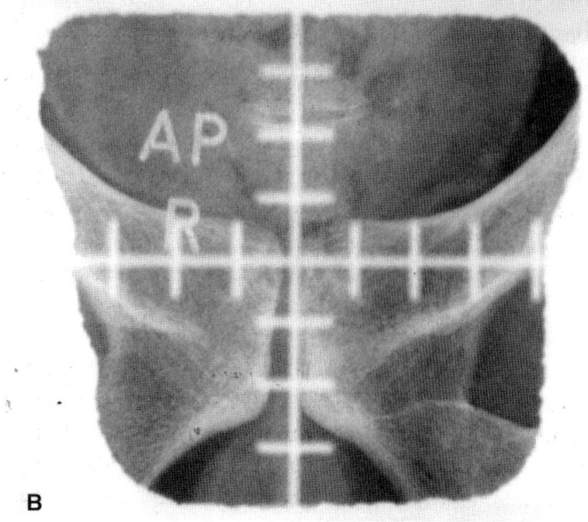

Fig. 28.9 Conformal radiotherapy for prostate cancer, anterior field without blocks **A** and with blocks **B**.

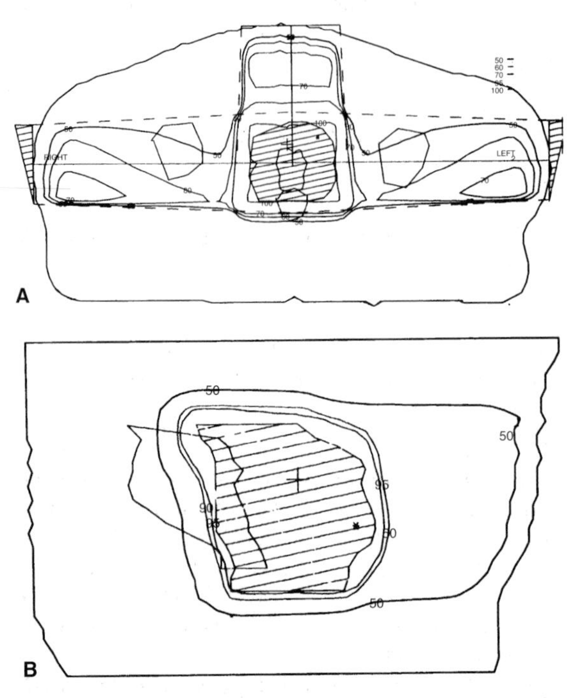

Fig. 28.10 Isodose distribution for radical radiotherapy of the prostate using anterior and two lateral fields. **A** Transverse section. **B** Sagittal section.

Dose and energy

52.5–55 Gy in 20 daily fractions over 4 weeks (9–16 MV photons)

or

64 Gy in 32 daily fractions over 6.5 weeks (9–16 MV photons)

Dose escalation: 74 Gy in 37 daily fractions over 7.5 weeks (9–16 MV photons)

Acute reactions. About half way through a radical 4-week course, urinary frequency and occasionally dysuria occur. These can often be relieved by mist. pot. cit. or an anti-inflammatory agent such as Froben 50 mg t.d.s. and normally settle within 4 weeks of the end of treatment. Diarrhoea and tenesmus from acute proctitis have a similar time course and are treated with a low-residue diet and Fybogel.

Late reactions. The main late urinary effects are chronic cystitis, urethral stricture or incontinence. Loss of sexual potency also occurs. Bowel morbidity includes rectal ulceration or stricture and small bowel obstruction. Symptoms are tenesmus, rectal bleeding or incontinence. Proctitis may respond to steroid (Predsol) enemas but ultimately a defunctioning colostomy is required in up to 2% of cases.

Results of radical radiotherapy. The 5-year survival for T1 and T2 is 78% and for T3 59%.

Prostate brachytherapy

Accurate delivery of radioactive iodine-125 or palladium-103 seeds directly into the prostate has led to a worldwide surge of interest in this treatment technique. The brachytherapist guides the implant needles directly into the prostate through a closed transperineal approach (Fig. 28.11). The position and number of seeds required is determined by computer in relation to the coordinates on a template grid and the distance from the base of the bladder as determined by the transrectal ultrasound. A dose of 145 Gy to a PTV of the prostate capsule plus 2–3 mm is delivered. The inverse square law determines that the dose to the rectum, bladder and neurovascular bundles is very low, with resultant decreased toxicity in comparison to external beam and surgery. The major toxicity is urethritis that may last some months. In carefully selected patients outcomes appear very good; however, randomised controlled trials have not been done.

Radical prostatectomy

Patients who are medically fit with organ-confined disease are suitable for surgery. A nerve-sparing radical prostatectomy has improved potency rates post-procedure. Severe incontinence is noted in < 5% but a higher proportion may have mild stress incontinence. Positive surgical margins in at least 30% of carefully staged patients are common.

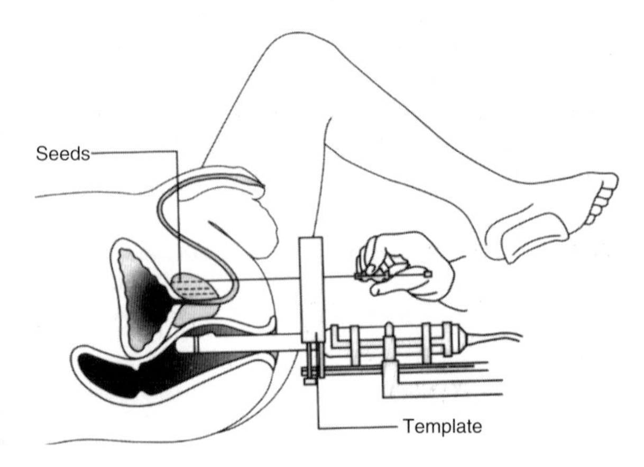

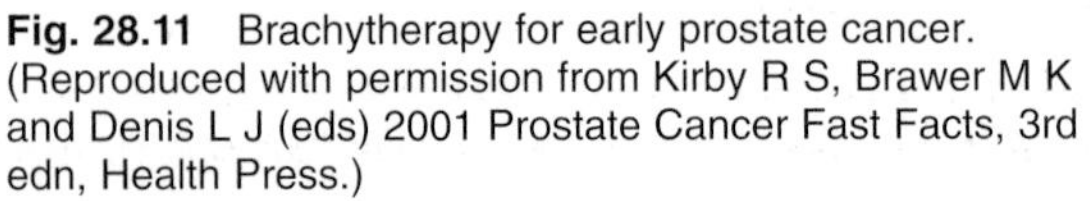

Fig. 28.11 Brachytherapy for early prostate cancer. (Reproduced with permission from Kirby R S, Brawer M K and Denis L J (eds) 2001 Prostate Cancer Fast Facts, 3rd edn, Health Press.)

2. Locally advanced T3N0M0, T4aN0M0

These patients have a greater risk of metastatic disease. If, however, staging investigations show no evidence of metastases then it is our policy to treat with radical radiotherapy following 3 months of neoadjuvant hormonal treatment. For those patients with particularly adverse features such as Gleason scores 8–10 additional adjuvant hormonal therapy may improve survival. Whether there are any benefits in survival because of the radiotherapy over and above hormonal treatment for locally advanced prostate cancer is under investigation.

3. Metastatic disease

Hormonal therapy

Most prostatic tumours contain elements sensitive to the androgenic hormone testosterone. Hormonal treatment is designed to reduce levels of testosterone circulating in the blood. This may be achieved in a number of different ways: (1) removal of the testes, which secrete testosterone (orchidectomy); (2) oral oestrogens, e.g. diethylstilbestrol; (3) chemical compounds, similar to luteinising hormone-releasing hormone (LHRH analogues), which diminish the pituitary production of luteinising hormone (LH) and thus reduce testosterone production—these are administered by monthly or 3-monthly depot injection; (4) oral agents which block the cellular action of androgens (e.g. cyproterone acetate, biclutamide).

About 80% of patients will respond to hormonal therapy. The median duration of response is 18–24 months. Early intervention with hormonal therapy reduces complications of the disease such as pathological fractures; however, it does not appear to improve survival. Median survival once patients become hormone refractory is 6 months. Maximum androgen blockade does offer a small survival advantage in the order of 2.5% at 5 years but at greater cost and toxicity. For this reason it has not gained uniform acceptance. Intermittent hormonal therapy is still under investigation.

Cytotoxic chemotherapy

Cytotoxic chemotherapy has proved disappointing to date. Mitoxantrone has been most extensively used, with some evidence of in improvement in quality of life and PSA response.

Palliative radiotherapy

Radiotherapy has a useful role in relieving pain from bone metastases. It can also shrink advanced local disease causing symptoms of outflow obstruction and pelvic nodes causing lymphoedema and nerve compression.

Technique

Parallel-opposed field or single fields.

Dose and energy

1. Prostate

30 Gy in 10 daily fractions over 2 weeks (9–10 MV photons)

2. Bone metastases

Confined to a limited area e.g. lumbar spine

Single fraction of 8 Gy or 20 Gy in 5 daily fractions (4–6 MV photons)

Widespread

Hemibody irradiation. Where there are widespread painful bony metastases, hemibody irradiation may be considered to encompass all the painful areas. Improvement in pain control tends to be prompt and may last the few months until death. Treatment of the lower half of the body is better tolerated because the side-effects are minimal.

Preparation. The patient is given intravenous fluids and fasted before treatment. Regular antiemetics are given before and after treatment.

Treatment volume

For the lower half, the field usually extends from the umbilicus to the knees and for the upper half from the top of the head to the umbilicus. Overlap with the lower field is avoided.

Acute reaction. Nausea and vomiting occur at the end of treatment and last for up to 6 hours. Lethargy is common. If the upper half is treated, hair loss starts at about 10 days. The mouth becomes dry and taste sensation is altered. The blood count reaches its low point at 10–14 days. Haemoglobin, white blood cell and platelet counts are all reduced (pancytopenia) and remain so for up to 8 weeks. Cough and shortness of breath occurring at 6 weeks are usually indicative of radiation pneumonitis. If both halves of the body are treated, an interval of at least 6 weeks is left after the first hemibody irradiation to allow the systemic effects to settle and the blood count to recover.

Technique

The patient is treated supine. Parallel-opposed anterior and posterior fields are used at extended FSD (140 cm).

Dose and energy

Lower half of body

8 Gy midplane dose in a single fraction (9–10 MV photons)

Upper half
6.5 Gy midplane dose in a single fraction (9–10 MV photons)

Strontium-89. Strontium-89 is a pure beta emitter with a half-life of 50 days. It is selectively taken up by bone metastases. After a 150 MBq dose, relief of bone pain may occur in 60–70% of patients, with little haematological toxicity. It is best avoided in those with a 'super-scan', as little benefit can be expected. If used early in the metastatic process, strontium can delay the onset of symptoms in new sites of bone disease.

TESTIS

Anatomy

Each testis (the diminutive form 'testicle' is also in common use, with its adjective testicular) lies within a fibrous capsule (tunica albuginea) within the scrotum (Fig. 28.12). In the embryo, the testes arise on the posterior abdominal wall and migrate downwards through the inguinal canal to the scrotum.

The testis is divided into 200–300 lobules. Each of these contains 1–3 seminiferous tubules. These drain into the epididymis, which lies on the posterior border of the testis. The lymphatic drainage of the testis is to the para-aortic nodes. It is important to note that the skin of the scrotum drains to the inguinal nodes. To avoid surgical contamination of the scrotal skin, the testis is surgically removed through an inguinal incision.

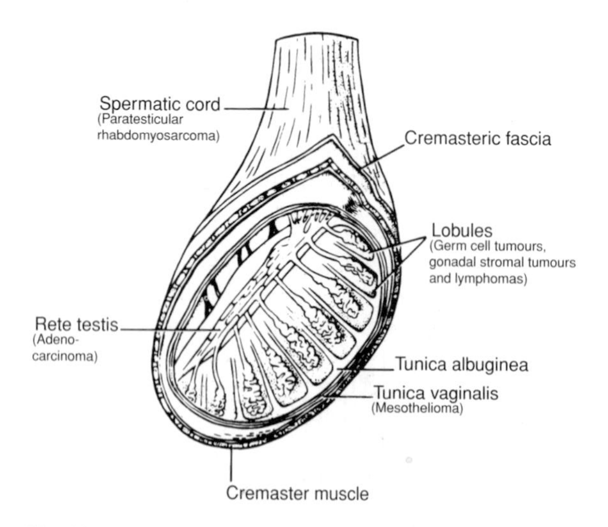

Fig. 28.12 Diagram of testis and spermatic cord indicating sites of tumour origin. Paratesticular rhabdomyosarcoma may arise from connective tissue of the cord or of adjacent structures. (From Textbook of Uncommon Cancers, Williams C J, Krikorian J G & Green M R, 1988, ©John Wiley & Sons Limited. Reproduced with permission.)

Pathology

Aetiology

The main factor predisposing to the development of germ cell tumours of the testis is an undescended testis. This accounts for 10% of cases. The risk is increased five-fold if one testis is maldescended and 12-fold if both are maldescended. However, even if one testis is maldescended, there is an increased risk of testicular cancer in the normally descended testis on the other side. Intratubular germ cell neoplasia or carcinoma-in-situ is a premalignant condition which gives rise to malignancy in 50% of patients within 5 years.

Testicular cancer is the commonest form of malignancy in men between the ages of 20 and 40. The incidence is rising, possibly through increased exposure to environmental oestrogens. Currently there are about 1100 new cases per year in the UK. It accounts for 0.1% of deaths from cancer. The types of common (germ cell tumours) and rarer tumours and their sites of origin in the testis are illustrated in Figure 28.12.

Germ cell tumours

There are two main tumour types that arise from the germ cells: seminoma and teratoma. Teratoma occurs mainly between the ages of 20 and 35, and seminoma between 25 and 40 years. Over the age of 50, tumours are more likely to be non-germ-cell tumours. These are non-Hodgkin lymphomas and tumours arising from other structures of the testis (Sertoli and Leydig cell tumours). Paratesticular rhabdomyosarcoma (Fig. 28.12) occurs in infancy and in young adult life.

Seminoma. Seminoma is the commonest type (60%). It arises from the cells of the seminiferous tubules. It is solid with a pale cut surface like a potato. There are two principal types: *classical* and *spermatocytic*. The characteristic histological feature of classical seminoma is its uniform appearance. The cells are rounded with a central nucleus and clear cytoplasm. The tumour is divided into lobules by a fibrous stroma, associated with a variable infiltration of lymphocytes.

Spread of seminoma may be local to the epididymis and to the spermatic cord, but lymphatic spread is more important. The first group of nodes to be invaded is the upper para-aortic, at the level of the renal hilum. Further lymphatic spread may be upward to the mediastinum and even the supraclavicular nodes through the thoracic duct, or downward to the lower para-aortic and pelvic nodes. If extratesticular tissues of the scrotum are invaded, including the scrotal skin, their draining inguinal lymph nodes may be invaded. Blood-borne spread is much less common.

Spermatocytic seminoma is uncommon and generally seen in older men. The tumour cells show differentiation to spermatocytes, and their behaviour is benign. Metastases are extremely rare.

Teratoma. Teratoma accounts for the remainder of germ cell tumours. Strictly speaking, a teratoma shows differentiation towards all three embryological germ cell layers of ectoderm (e.g. skin, neural tissue), endoderm (e.g. gut, bronchi) and mesoderm (e.g. fat, cartilage). In practice, the British classification applies the term more widely (while American terminology refers to this group as non-seminomatous germ cell tumours). Teratomas are subtyped according to their cell constituents as:

- Teratoma differentiated
- Malignant teratoma intermediate
- Malignant teratoma undifferentiated
- Malignant teratoma trophoblastic.

Teratoma differentiated (TD) shows cysts lined by various mature-looking epithelium surrounded by smooth muscle, with islands of cartilage and neural tissue. In infants its behaviour is benign, but in adults it is rare and can give rise to metastases. *Malignant teratoma undifferentiated* (MTU), by contrast, has no recognisable differentiated structures, but has undifferentiated rather than carcinomatous tissue. It often has tissue resembling yolk sac (YST), and there are frequently syncytiotrophoblast giant cells. These account for secretion of alpha-fetoprotein (AFP) and human chorionic gonadotrophin (HCG) respectively, which can be measured in the blood and are invaluable as markers of tumour load. It has an aggressive clinical behaviour with early metastasis via lymphatics to para-aortic lymph nodes, and blood-borne spread to the lungs. *Malignant teratoma intermediate* (MTI) has a mixture of differentiated and undifferentiated tissues. *Malignant teratoma trophoblastic* (MTT) has tissue resembling gestational choriocarcinoma (i.e. syncytiotrophoblast and cytotrophoblast), either throughout or in combination with features of other teratomas. Large amounts of HCG are secreted and the clinical course is very aggressive with widespread blood-borne metastases.

Tumour markers

The two tumour markers AFP and HCG are helpful in the diagnosis, staging and monitoring of response to treatment (Fig. 28.13). AFP has a half-life of about 5 days. It is produced by yolk sac elements but is not specific to teratoma. Elevated levels occur in the presence of liver damage. HCG is mainly a marker of trophoblastic neoplasms; it can, however, occur in seminoma. The half-life of HCG is 24 hours and of the beta subunit 45 minutes. Markers for the presence of seminoma are much less reliable. Serum placental alkaline phosphatase (PLAP) is often raised in the presence of seminoma, particularly if there is bulky disease. However, false-positive and false-negative results for PLAP are common. LDH is an important non-specific marker of disease volume and has been incorporated into the International Germ Cell Consensus Classification (Table 28.4).

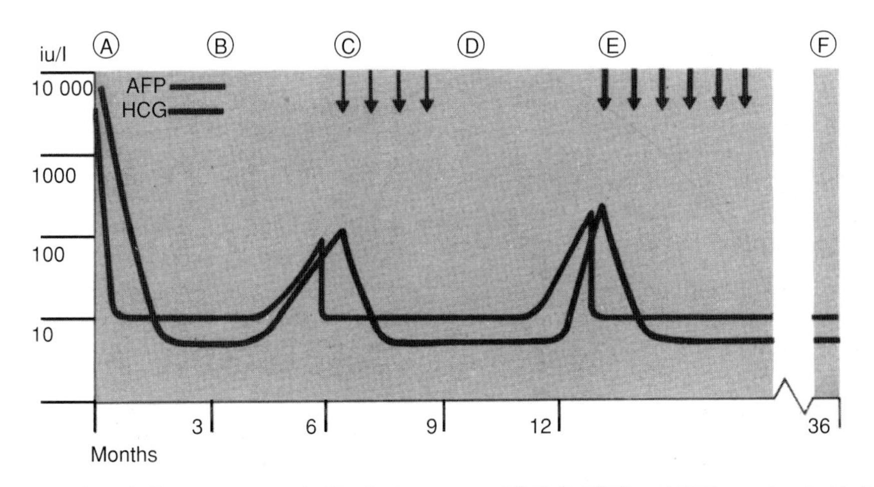

Fig. 28.13 Tumour markers in the management of testicular cancer. (A) Both HCG and AFP are elevated before orchidectomy but fall following operation (HCG more rapidly because of its short half-life). (B) No evidence of recurrence, followed by a rise in marker levels. (C) Combination chemotherapy for recurrence is followed by a fall in levels to normal (D). (E) A further rise in marker levels is treated more intensively and the patient is disease free at 3 years (F). (Reproduced with permission from Souhami & Moxham, Textbook of Medicine, Churchill Livingstone, 1990.)

Table 28.4 The IGCCC Prognostic Grouping

Teratoma	Seminoma
Good prognosis with all of:	
Testis/retroperitoneal primary	Any primary site
No non-pulmonary visceral metastases	No non-pulmonary visceral metastases
AFP < 1000 ng/ml	Normal AFP
HCG < 5000 iu/l	Any HCG
LDH < 1.5 upper limit of normal	Any LDH
56% of teratomas	90% of seminomas
5-year survival 92%	5-year survival 86%
Intermediate prognosis with all of:	
Testis/retroperitoneal primary	Any primary site
No non-pulmonary visceral metastases	Non-pulmonary visceral metastases
AFP ≥ 1000 and ≤ 10 000 ng/ml or	Normal AFP
HCG ≥ 5000 and ≤ 50 000 iu/l or	Any HCG
LDH ≥ 1.5 normal ≤ 10 normal	Any LDH
28% of teratomas	10% of seminomas
5-year survival 80%	5-year survival 73%
Poor prognosis with any of:	
Mediastinal primary or non-pulmonary visceral metastases	No patients classified as poor prognosis
AFP > 10 000 ng/ml or	
HCG > 50 000 iu/l or	
LDH > 10 normal	
16% of teratomas	
5-year survival 48%	

Clinical features

The usual presentation is a gradually enlarging painless testicular swelling, although atrophy of a testis may occur. The tumour feels hard. A third of patients describe pain in the testis, a third a dragging sensation, 10% give a history of trauma. The first symptoms and signs may be of metastatic spread (haemoptysis from lung metastases, back pain from para-aortic metastases, loin pain from ureteric obstruction or neck lymphadenopathy). Malignant teratoma trophoblastic (choriocarcinoma) may produce gynaecomastia (breast enlargement).

Diagnosis and staging

The diagnosis is made by surgical removal of the testis through an inguinal incision (inguinal orchidectomy) and histological examination. Immunocytochemical stains of the tumour for the presence of AFP and HCG may be positive. Blood levels of AFP and HCG are measured pre- and postoperatively. A chest radiograph is required (for overt lung metastases), together with a CT scan of the thorax (for small-volume lung and mediastinal metastases) and of the abdomen (abdominal nodal and liver metastases).

The Royal Marsden staging classification (Table 28.5), based on the extent of spread and bulk of disease, has been widely used for determining management. Although still useful for seminoma stage II nodal size subgrouping, it has been largely superseded by the IGCCC prognostic grouping.

Table 28.5 The Royal Marsden Hospital staging classification of testicular tumours

Stage	Clinical findings
Mk+	Rising serum markers with no other evidence of metastases
I	No evidence of metastases
II	Abdominal node involvement
a	< 2 cm diameter
b	2–5 cm diameter
c	> 5 cm diameter
III	Nodal involvement above the diaphragm
IV	Extralymphatic metastases
L1	Lung metastases three or less in number
L2	Lung metastases more than three in number (all 2 cm or less in diameter)
L3	Lung metastases more than three in number (more than 2 cm in diameter)

Treatment

1. Seminoma—good prognosis

Stage I and IIa

Postoperative abdominal node irradiation should be given routinely.

Target volume

For stage I and IIa uncomplicated disease, postoperative radiotherapy to the para-aortic nodes alone is recommended. The 2–3% of patients who will relapse in the pelvis following irradiation can then be salvaged with chemotherapy. The upper margin of the para-aortic field is at the level of the junction of the 10th and 11th thoracic vertebrae. The lower limit is the junction of the 5th lumbar vertebrae and the first sacral vertebrae. Where there has been previous inguinoscrotal surgery such as hernia repair, the field is extended to cover the ipsilateral pelvic and inguinal nodes (Fig. 28.14). This 'dog leg' shaped field is vertical in the para-aortic region and diverges at the level of the junction of the fourth and fifth lumbar vertebrae. The lower limit of the field is the bottom of the obturator foramina and should include the inguinal scar. Previous orchidopexy, removal of the testis through the scrotum or extension of tumour to the tunica vaginalis requires the ipsilateral scrotum to be irradiated in addition.

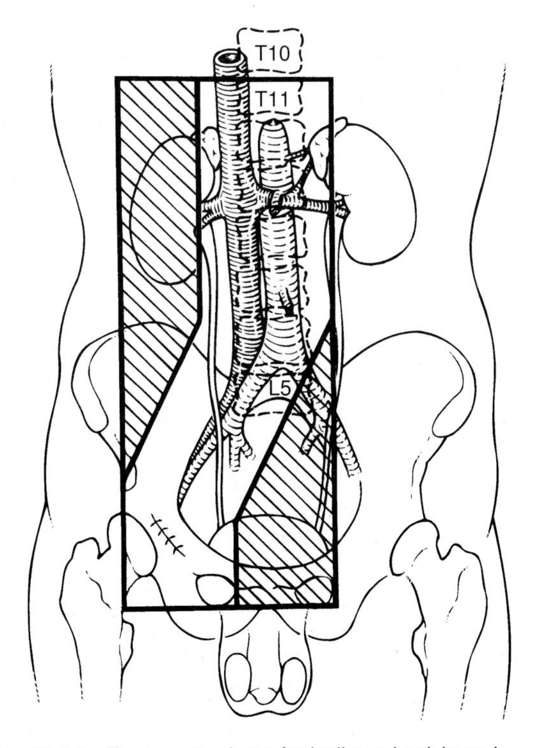

Fig. 28.14 Treatment volume for ipsilateral pelvic and para-aortic ('dog leg') irradiation for testicular seminoma.

Technique: PA strip

An anterior and posterior pair of fields is used. The patient is simulated supine at normal FSD. The width of the para-aortic field is normally 8–10 cm. Care should be taken not to include more than one-third of the renal substance within the para-aortic fields on either side. An intravenous urogram (IVU) during simulation is essential to verify the position of the kidneys.

Technique: dog-leg

An anterior and posterior pair of fields is used. The patient is simulated supine throughout, if treatment under couch at an extended FSD (about 140 cm) can be achieved. Ideally customised MCP blocks should be made to protect tissue outside the treatment volume. Care should be taken not to include more than one-third of the renal substance within the para-aortic fields on either side. An intravenous urogram (IVU) is used to verify the position of the kidneys. If there is involvement of the lower para-aortic nodes and risk of retrograde spread to the pelvic lymph nodes, then an 'inverted Y'-shaped field should be used to treat the para-aortic and pelvic nodes. If the hemiscrotum is to be treated, a direct electron field of appropriate energy or 300 kV X-rays may be used with shielding of the contralateral testis.

Dose and energy

Seminoma is one of the most radiosensitive of all cancers and can be cured with relatively modest doses. The present standard dose is:

30 Gy in 15 daily fractions over 4 weeks (9–10 MV photons)

Acute reaction. About 50% of patients will experience nausea lasting for 2–3 hours following treatment. Regular use of a 5-HT_3 antagonist is recommended.

Late reactions. Late side-effects are rare. Dyspepsia occurs in 5%, occasionally with evidence of peptic ulceration. Using the radiation technique and dosage described, the dose to the contralateral testis is very low (less than 0.5 Gy). None the less, this dose is sufficient to cause a moderate reduction in sperm count for 2–3 years, but it is not associated with permanent infertility.

Stage IIb, IIc, III and IV

In stage IIb disease, radiotherapy for small-bulk disease can still be used; however, there is a greater chance of relapse. In addition, in stage IIb and stage IIc disease, increasingly bulky abdominal nodes make it difficult to avoid irradiating more than one-third of the renal substance on both sides. Four cycles of combination chemotherapy with bleomycin, etoposide and cisplatin (BEP) (Table 28.6) are recommended for these stages. In good-prognosis seminoma in men over 40 or in those with previous chest irradiation EP may be used to decrease the risks of bleomycin lung.

Results of treatment

The results of treatment in early-stage seminoma are excellent, reflecting its radiosensitivity: 5-year survival rates by stage are 95% for stage I and 90% for stage IIa and IIb. For more advanced stages cure rates have improved with the availability of effective combination chemotherapy: 5-year survival for stages IIc and III is 75% and for stage IV 65%.

2. *Teratoma*

Stage I

Teratoma has a higher incidence of extralymphatic spread. In the presence of extralymphatic metastases, irradiating the para-aortic nodes prophylactically may compromise the ability to deliver subsequent combination chemotherapy at desired dosage and frequency. About 30% of patients with stage I disease following orchidectomy will have subclinical metastases and will relapse (80% of whom will relapse in the first 12 months). To avoid overtreatment of the majority of patients a policy of close surveillance with treatment at relapse is recommended. Patients with lymphatic or vascular invasion are at greater risk of relapse (40%) and are not suitable for surveillance. Such patients are best treated by two cycles of adjuvant combination chemotherapy.

Surveillance. For patients for whom a surveillance policy is adopted, tumour markers CXR and clinical examination are performed monthly in the first year with 3-monthly CT scans of chest and abdomen. In the second year, follow-up should be 2-monthly with CT scans at 18 and 24 months. Subsequent follow-up should be 3-monthly for the third year, 6-monthly to the fifth year and annually thereafter to 10 years.

Stages II–IV

These stages should be managed by combination chemotherapy (see below).

Table 28.6 BEP chemotherapy regime

Bleomycin	30 mg i.v. bolus	Days 1, 8, 15
Etoposide	100 mg/m^2 i.v. infusion	Days 1–5
Cisplatin	20 mg/m^2 i.v. infusion	Days 1–5
Repeated every 21 days		

Cytotoxic chemotherapy. The development of curative combination chemotherapy for advanced testicular cancer in the 1980s has been one of the most important advances in oncology.

The combinations of drugs used for treating seminoma are the same for teratoma. The most effective regimes contain cisplatin. Cisplatin was successfully combined with vinblastine and bleomycin (PVB). Now vinblastine is replaced by etoposide, which is less myelotoxic, without loss of efficacy. This regime is known as BEP (Table 28.6). An attempt to reduce toxicity by replacing cisplatin with carboplatin has proved to be less effective. Before each course of chemotherapy a number of investigations are carried out to assess fitness to treat, and to modify dosage, if necessary, because of the toxicity of the agents. A full blood count is required because of the myelotoxicity of etoposide.

Cisplatin is toxic to the kidney and to hearing. Renal function tests (serum urea, electrolytes and creatinine, 24-hour urine creatinine clearance or formal EDTA GFR) and hearing (audiometry) should be measured before, during and after treatment.

Bleomycin can be toxic to the lung (see below). Full lung function tests (including gas transfer factor) are carried out before treatment and repeated if toxicity is suspected.

Sperm storage, if available, is desirable for men wishing to father children following chemotherapy since sterility is commonly induced. Normally an initial sample is examined to count the number and motility of the sperm. If satisfactory, two additional samples are taken for sperm banking. However, chemotherapy, if urgently required, should not be delayed to await this procedure.

Dosage and scheduling. Normally four courses of BEP are given at 3-weekly intervals. Whether the number of cycles can be reduced to three for good-prognosis teratoma (see IGCC prognostic index) without compromising the 90% overall survival will be reported on completion of the MRC TE20 trial. For those patients in the intermediate- or poor-risk IGCC groups, survival is 40–70%. Efforts to increase the efficacy of chemotherapy schedules through dose intensification and new combinations are ongoing. As yet there has been no improvement over standard BEP.

Monitoring response to treatment. Clinical examination, chest radiograph, tumour markers, full blood count, and renal function tests are repeated before each cycle of treatment to monitor the response to and toxicity of treatment.

Following surgery, a fall in tumour marker levels in line with their half-lives usually indicates that there is no residual disease. A slower fall or rising levels suggest residual disease.

It may be necessary to delay the next cycle of chemotherapy or modify its dosage if blood count, renal function or hearing deteriorate below certain thresholds. Every effort should be made to deliver the chemotherapy on schedule and GCSF support may be required. Chemotherapy should not be given if the neutrophil count is below $1.0 \times 10^9/l$. CT scan of chest and abdomen is repeated after three cycles to confirm that the disease is responding. Rapid resolution of disease is usual after the first course. Residual 2–4 cm masses may, however, persist for several years.

Management of residual abdominal masses. Resection of residual abdominal masses following chemotherapy is only indicated for teratoma. Seminoma resection is difficult due to a lack of tissue planes and tumour infiltration beyond resection margins. A policy of observation only is recommended. Resection of residual masses after treatment for teratoma shows that most of them (44%) are due to differentiated (mature) teratoma or to fibrosis and necrosis (34%). Residual tumour is found in 22%. If recurrence occurs, as it does in 10–20% of patients, it is most likely to develop at a site of initial involvement. If surgical expertise is available, resection of residual masses is desirable. It serves both as a diagnostic and therapeutic procedure. Further chemotherapy is indicated if residual disease is found, but the outlook is poor, with less than 50% of such patients remaining free of disease.

Toxicity. In addition to renal damage and ototoxicity (impaired hearing), cisplatin causes severe nausea and vomiting and peripheral neuropathy. The 5-HT antagonists (ondansetron and granisetron) can reduce nausea and vomiting. Intravenous hydration is required 24 hours before cisplatin is given and for 24 hours afterwards to reduce the risk of renal damage. None the less, the majority of patients will experience renal damage. A 20–25% reduction in glomerular filtration rate is usual.

Etoposide causes alopecia and myelosuppression. The incidence of septicaemia with etoposide is less than with vinblastine since it is less myelosuppressive.

Bleomycin may cause pneumonitis. Presentation is with progressive dyspnoea. This complication may occur after relatively modest doses (e.g. 200 mg). It can be progressive, is irreversible and carries a 1% mortality. Other side-effects are fever, skin rashes, pigmentation and Raynaud's phenomenon.

Results of treatment

90% of patients with small-volume disease are cured following chemotherapy. For large-volume disease in extralymphatic sites, the probability of survival is reduced to 50–70%.

The 5-year survival is 90% for stages I and IIa, 70% for stages IIb and III, and 50–60% for stage IV.

TESTICULAR LYMPHOMA

Testicular lymphomas are rare (4% of testicular tumours). They are mainly non-Hodgkin lymphomas. Clinical features that help to differentiate them from germ cell tumours are bilaterality (20% at presentation or subsequently), older age group (over 50 years), different pattern of metastases, absence of maldescent and of gynaecomastia. They are usually of high grade (diffuse large B cell). Stages IAE and IIAE are only cured in 50% of cases with three cycles of CHOP chemotherapy and radiotherapy to the scrotum (IA) and involved nodes (IIA). For this reason six cycles of chemotherapy are recommended followed by radiotherapy. For stage III and IV disease CNS chemoprophylaxis is required in addition to scrotal irradiation.

Dose and energy

35 Gy in 20 daily fractions over 4 weeks (9–10 MV photons)

Results of treatment

The prognosis is poor. Overall 5-year survival is 20%. For stage IAE and IIAE it is 50%. Average survival with stage IV disease is about 8 months.

URETHRA

Tumours of the urethra are rare and are usually transitional carcinomas. Predisposing factors are as for bladder cancer (p. 490). Presenting symptoms and signs are pain and haematuria.

Female urethra

The tumour is twice as common in women as in men. In the proximal third transitional carcinoma predominates, and in the distal two-thirds squamous carcinoma predominates. The distal urethra drains to the inguinal nodes and the proximal urethra to the iliac nodes. Presenting features are offensive discharge, bleeding or a mass.

Treatment

For superficial squamous carcinoma of the urethral orifice, a permanent gold grain (gold-198) implant delivering 55 Gy at 0.5 cm is used. For more proximal lesions radical external beam irradiation using an anterior and two lateral wedged fields is used. A dose of 55 Gy is given in 20 daily fractions over 4 weeks at megavoltage.

Results of treatment

The cure rates with surgery and radiotherapy are similar at about 50%.

PENIS

Cancer of the penis is a rare tumour responsible for 0.4% of all cancers and 0.1% of cancer deaths. It occurs in older men, typically between 50 and 70 years old. The disease is commoner in South-east Asia, China and Africa.

Pathology

Aetiology

The disease rarely occurs among peoples who practise circumcision. There is a high incidence in Hindus, who are never circumcised. Phimosis is present in up to 50% of cases. Poor penile hygiene is thought to be an important predisposing factor. There is a strong association with human papilloma virus infections. There are several premalignant conditions, including viral warts (condyloma acuminata) and erythroplasia of Queyrat. The primary tumours are squamous carcinomas, usually well differentiated. Secondary deposits are rare but can occur from prostate and bladder cancer.

Clinical features

These tumours occur as warty growths or, more commonly, as indurated ulcers on the glans or the sulcus at the base of the glans. Symptoms have often been present for a year or more before presentation. The first sign may be an infected or bloody discharge from beneath the prepuce. Growth is superficial at first, then by invasion of the penile shaft. If the lesion is visible, the diagnosis is usually obvious. If phimosis hides it, the glans must be exposed by incising and peeling back the prepuce (dorsal slit) or by complete circumcision, under anaesthesia. A biopsy is taken at the same time.

Lymphatic spread occurs early to the inguinal nodes, though enlargement here may simply reflect infection. The nodes may eventually ulcerate. Blood-borne metastases are rare and late.

Staging

Both TNM and Jackson staging systems are in use (Table 28.7). If inguinal nodes are enlarged, needle aspiration to distinguish tumour from infection should be carried out. A CT scan of the pelvis may show the extent of abdominal lymphadenopathy.

Table 28.7 TNM and Jackson staging systems for penile cancer

Stage	Clinical findings
Tumour	
T1	Tumour invades subepithelial connective tissue
T2	Tumour invades corpus spongiosum or cavernosum
T3	Tumour invades urethra
T4	Tumour invades other structures
Nodes	
N0	No regional nodes
N1	Single inguinal node
N2	Multiple unilateral nodes or bilateral nodes
N3	Deep inguinal or pelvic nodes
Metastases	
M0	No distant metastases
M1	Distant metastases present
Jackson classification	
I	Tumour confined to the glans or prepuce
II	Tumour extending on to the shaft of the penis
III	Tumour with operable inguinal nodes
IV	Tumour with inoperable metastases

Treatment

Surgery and radiotherapy are the main treatments for penile cancer. Factors, which influence the choice of treatment, are the age and general condition of the patient, the extent of the disease, the desire to retain sexual function and the capacity to pass urine in the standing position for young males.

Surgery

Surgery involves amputation of part or the whole of the penis. Although curative in 70% if the inguinal nodes are not involved, the procedure is associated with considerable psychological morbidity, especially for young males.

Radiotherapy

Radical radiotherapy is the treatment of choice for early penile cancer since it permits the organ to be conserved. However, if there is deep invasion of the shaft, the chances of control by radiation are poor and surgery is preferable. Invasion of the urethra also favours surgery, since post-radiation fibrotic stricture is very liable to occur.

Treatment techniques and dosage

The choice of technique and energy will depend on the extent and site of the disease. For tumours confined to the glans or the prepuce, superficial, orthovoltage, electron beam or implants are possibilities. For infiltrating tumours or where the inguinal nodes are involved, megavoltage irradiation is required.

Implantation. A single or double plane implant with iridium-192 should include within the target volume a 2 cm margin around the tumour. Tumours greater than 4 cm in any dimension or invading the corpora cavernosa should not be implanted.

The implant (Fig. 22.6) is carried out under a general anaesthetic and following catheterisation. The penis is held upright and away from the testicles and thighs by foam padding secured by adhesive tape to the thighs. The dose to the testis is usually up to 3 Gy. This can be reduced by interposing 2–3 mm of lead shielding, if fertility needs to be conserved. The dose to the reference isodose using the Paris system should be 60–65 Gy. Duration of treatment is normally 6–7 days.

Superficial or orthovoltage therapy. For very small (T1) superficial tumours 100 kV or 250 kV X-ray therapy may suffice. A 0.5 cm margin of normal surrounding tissue is included in the treated volume. A dose of 50 Gy is given in 15 fractions over 3 weeks. Alternatively, low-energy (6 MeV) electrons can be used using an appropriate thickness of Perspex over the lesion to bring up the surface dose to 100%.

Megavoltage

Treatment volume

If there is evidence of spread on to the shaft of the penis, the whole of the penis should be treated.

Technique

A rectangular wax block with a central cylindrical cavity is made to encompass the penis and ensure homogeneous irradiation of the whole volume. The penis is treated en bloc by a parallel-opposed pair of lateral fields.

Dose and energy

50–55 Gy in 20 daily fractions over 4 weeks at megavoltage (4–6 MV photons)

Acute reactions. These are like skin reactions elsewhere but more marked and moist desquamation is commoner. The urethral reaction causes discomfort and dysuria. If very severe it may result in acute retention requiring catheterisation.

Late reactions. These include telangiectasia, skin atrophy, urethral stricture and necrosis. Urethral dilatation is required for stricture. Necrosis occurs in less than 10% of cases.

Management of regional nodes

If inguinal nodes are found to be histologically involved at presentation, a block dissection of the groin should be carried out, followed by radical radiotherapy to the primary. There is no value in giving prophylactic groin node irradiation. The only role for radiotherapy in the treatment of groin nodes is for palliation.

Palliative radiotherapy

Technique

A simple parallel-opposed pair of fields to the affected groin.

Dose and energy

30 Gy in 10 daily fractions over 2 weeks at megavoltage

Palliative chemotherapy

Cisplatin-based chemotherapy can be considered for fit patients. Response rates of 30–40% have been reported.

Results of treatment

Early superficial tumours have a high cure rate: 5-year survival for stage I disease is about 90%. This falls to 60% in stage II and 30–40% in stage III.

CHAPTER CONTENTS

29

Lymphoreticular tissues and bone marrow

Barry Hancock and Martin Robinson

MALIGNANT LYMPHOMAS

The term 'lymphoma' covers all the primary malignancies of lymph nodes. The two main types of lymphoma are Hodgkin's disease and non-Hodgkin lymphoma. The histological classification of Hodgkin's disease, known as the Rye classification, is widely accepted. In contrast, the classification of the non-Hodgkin lymphomas is more complex. This is due to the variety of cytological appearances and the capacity to identify different cell surface markers using immunohistochemical techniques. As a result there are several different classifications in use; more recently, however, the new World Health Organization classification is becoming universally adopted.

HODGKIN'S DISEASE

Pathology

Epidemiology

Hodgkin's disease is uncommon. It accounts for 0.7% of all cancers and 0.4% of cancer deaths. In the UK the incidence per 100 000 population per year is 2.65 for men and 1.81 for women. It has two age peaks. The first is between 25 and 34 years in and the second in old age. The disease is commoner in Jews in the UK, USA and Israel. The incidence is substantially lower in the Japanese and black Americans. The reasons for these ethnic variations are unclear.

Hodgkin's disease is commoner among the higher social classes. One hypothesis is that the disease is a rare sequel of a common infection in children (for nodular sclerosing but not other histological subtypes). Children in higher social classes who tend to be educated in a protected environment may be exposed to the infection later than children of lower social class. This may explain the later age of onset in children of higher social class.

Considerable differences in incidence occur between regions of the UK. No satisfactory explanation for these differences is available. There is no evidence that they are related to pollution from industrial plants.

Aetiology

The aetiological agent(s) responsible for Hodgkin's disease have not been identified. It seems likely that a number of factors may have to interact in order for the disease to develop. These include genetic susceptibility, infection and altered immunity.

The higher incidence in males and the slight excess of the disease in Jews suggest that genetic factors may be important. A genetic basis is also supported by the higher incidence in certain families. In Yorkshire 6% of all cases had one or more additional lymphoma or leukaemia sufferers among blood relatives; 50% of these were Hodgkin's disease.

Some time ago it was suggested that the disease had a different aetiology for each age peak. The peak in early adulthood (< 35 years) was postulated to be due to infection. Common viral infections were thought to be responsible. Part of the Epstein–Barr virus (EBV) was particularly commonly isolated in Hodgkin's disease. The link between EBV and Hodgkin's disease was thought to be similar to that between EBV and both nasopharyngeal carcinoma (p. 362) and Burkitt's lymphoma. The link between EBV and Hodgkin's disease is not a strong one. It may be that other agents, as yet unknown, are operating.

In addition, Hodgkin's disease has been associated with certain dusty (particularly wood dust) occupations thought to induce allergic reactions.

Microscopic features

Hodgkin's disease is characterised by the replacement of normal lymphoid tissue by atypical mononuclear cells, multinucleate Reed–Sternberg cells and a variable number of chronic inflammatory cells. Oddly for a neoplasm, malignant cells are in the minority. The majority are made up of cells such as lymphocytes, histiocytes, plasma cells, granulocytes and fibroblasts.

Reed–Sternberg cells are large. They have eosinophilic cytoplasm and often a perinuclear halo. The presence of Reed–Sternberg cells in an appropriate context is essential for the diagnosis of Hodgkin's disease.

Histological classification (Rye). There are four main types of Hodgkin's disease.

1. *Lymphocyte predominant (LP) < 10%.* This is uncommon. Reed–Sternberg cells are very scarce, and the tumour is dominated by lymphocytes and sometimes histiocytes. The new World Health Organization classification separates off nodular lymphocyte predominance from lymphocyte-rich Hodgkin's lymphoma.

2. *Nodular sclerosing (NS) 60%.* This is characterised by the division of the node into nodules. The nodules of tumour contain Reed–Sternberg (RS) cells; these often lie in little spaces or lacunae. Nodular sclerosing disease has been further subdivided into grades 1 (low grade) and 2 (high grade). Grade 2 shows depletion of lymphocytes or numerous Hodgkin's cells. All other cases are assigned to grade 1. These two grades have different prognoses (see later in this chapter).

Nodular sclerosing Hodgkin's disease has an equal sex distribution. It tends to affect the mediastinum and to occur in the young adult.

3. *Mixed cellularity (MC) 15%.* As the term implies, a variety of cells are present. These include Reed–Sternberg cells and non-neoplastic cells such as plasma cells, eosinophils, macrophages and lymphocytes.

4. *Lymphocyte depleted (LD) < 5%.* This is characterised by very atypical RS cells and few lymphocytes. Diffuse fibrosis is present.

Before accurate staging and curative chemotherapy was available, each histological subtype had prognostic significance. Prognosis was best for lymphocyte predominant and worst for lymphocyte depleted. Now the only histological type with definite prognostic significance is lymphocyte depleted. This carries a poor 5-year survival of 20%. All other subtypes have a similar survival, though grade 1 tends to have a better prognosis than grade 2.

Clinical features

The first symptom is usually painless enlargement of a group of nodes, most commonly in the neck (60%) (Fig. 29.1), but occasionally in the axilla (20%) or in the

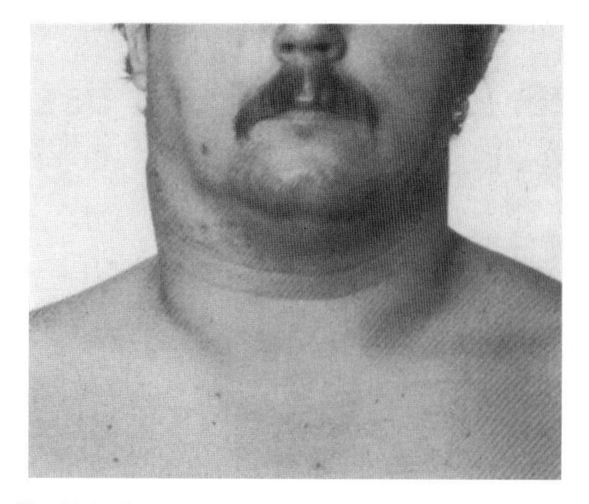

Fig. 29.1 Typical cervical lymphadenopathy in early Hodgkin's disease.

inguinal/femoral region (15%). The left side of the neck is slightly more commonly involved than the right. The size of the nodes may wax and wane. The spleen (10%) or liver (7%) may be palpably enlarged.

In 25–30% of patients, systemic or B symptoms are the presenting features. There are three B symptoms: fever (> 38°C), night sweats and weight loss (> 10% of body weight in previous 6 months). General malaise also occurs.

There may be a characteristic fever (Pel–Ebstein) in waves lasting a week or two separated by afebrile intervals. Itching (pruritus) occurs in 12% but is not a B symptom. Patients without systemic symptoms are designated as A (i.e. absence of systemic symptoms). The designation of 'A' or 'B' is always added as part of the Ann Arbor staging classification (see under Investigations).

A peculiar occasional symptom of unknown cause is severe pain in lymph nodes after taking even very small quantities of alcohol.

Investigations

The first step is usually lymph node biopsy to establish the diagnosis and the histological type. It is essential to establish the extent of the disease (staging) since this will influence the choice of treatment. The Ann Arbor staging classification is the most commonly used and is applicable both to Hodgkin's disease and non-Hodgkin lymphoma. It describes the anatomical distribution of lymph node involvement as well as of extranodal disease (Table 29.1).

The following basic tests should be carried out:

1. Full blood count and ESR (erythrocyte sedimentation rate)
2. Serum urea and electrolytes, calcium
3. Liver function tests
4. Chest X-ray (Fig. 29.2)
5. CT of chest and abdomen.

Radiological detection of intra-abdominal disease

At presentation, about 35% of patients will have disease below the diaphragm. Of these only 8% will have clinically detectable nodes. It is therefore of considerable importance to know whether the nodes are involved or not. CT scanning has largely replaced bipedal lymphangiography (Fig. 29.3) as the principal radiological investigation.

CT scanning can detect significant enlargement of nodes (> 1 cm) but cannot detect evidence of Hodgkin's disease in normal-sized nodes (≤ 1 cm).

Table 29.1 Ann Arbor staging classification of Hodgkin's disease

Stage	Clinical findings
I	Involvement of a single lymph node region (I) or of single extralymphatic organ or site (IE)
II	Involvement of two or more lymph node regions on the same side of the diaphragm (II) or localised involvement of an extralymphatic organ or site and one or more lymph node regions on the same side of the diaphragm (IIE)
III	Involvement of lymph node regions on both sides of the diaphragm (III) which may be accompanied by localised involvement of an extralymphatic organ or site (IIIE) or by involvement of the spleen (IIIS) or both (IIISE)
IV	Disseminated involvement of one or more extralymphatic organs or tissues with or without associated lymph node involvement

Clinical and pathological staging

There are two types of staging, *clinical* and *pathological*. Clinical staging is based upon the history, physical examination, blood chemistry, and radiological investigations. Pathological staging includes, in addition to

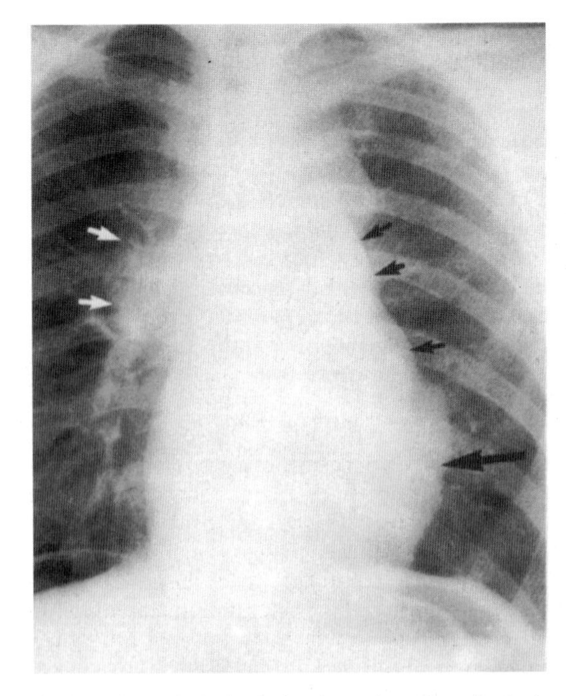

Fig. 29.2 Chest radiograph showing enlarged mediastinal nodes (small arrows) and pericardial nodes (large arrow) due to Hodgkin's disease. (Courtesy of Dr R Nakielny, Sheffield.)

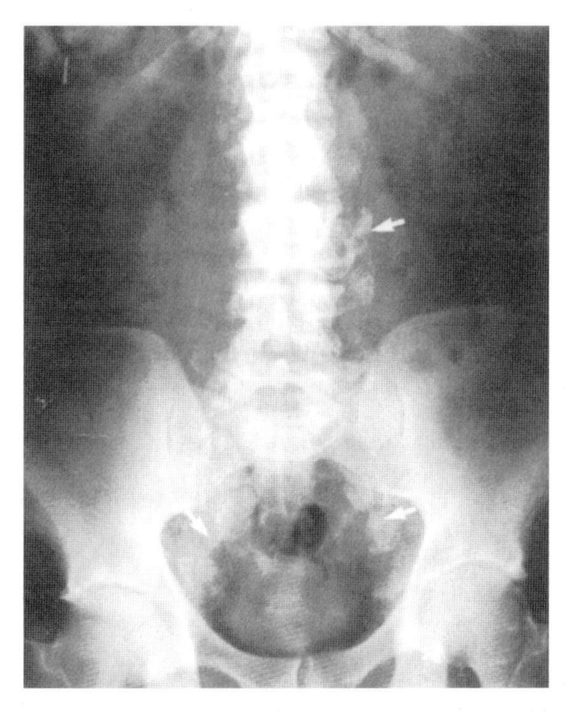

Fig. 29.3 Lymphangiogram showing typical enlarged 'foamy' pelvic and para-aortic nodes (arrowed) due to Hodgkin's disease. (Courtesy of Dr R Nakielny, Sheffield.)

the above, a staging laparotomy to establish the extent of intra-abdominal disease.

A staging laparotomy involves the careful inspection of the abdominal contents, a splenectomy and liver biopsy. In addition, the lymph nodes in the porta hepatis, coeliac axis and in the mesentery (none of which are demonstrable by lymphography), as well as the upper para-aortic, iliac and mesenteric nodes are biopsied. Any suspicious nodes on lymphography or CT scanning can also be sampled.

This operation has provided a great deal of information about the intra-abdominal extent of the disease. However, it is now no longer carried out as a routine procedure for a number of reasons.

1. Combination chemotherapy is able to cure a substantial proportion of patients who relapse after radiotherapy. Hence, knowing whether there is intra-abdominal disease at presentation is not essential.

2. A variety of prognostic factors (e.g. ESR, pathological grade and age) are able to predict with reasonable accuracy the probability of intra-abdominal involvement in an individual patient.

3. The morbidity and mortality even in skilled hands are not insubstantial. There is a major complication rate of about 8% (one half fatal). Serious infections (particularly pneumococcal) occur in 3% of patients. There is a minor complication rate of about 30% (e.g. wound infection).

4. The survival of patients who have not undergone staging laparotomy is similar to comparable patients who have.

Prognostic factors

A variety of prognostic factors have been identified in stage I and IIa Hodgkin's disease which appear to predict the outcome of therapy. The British National Lymphoma Investigation (BNLI) analysis shows the following to be adverse prognostic factors:

- Age over 60
- High ESR
- Male sex
- High-grade histology
- Multiple nodal sites
- Bulky disease
- Reduced lymphocyte count
- Low serum albumin
- Extranodal involvement.

More recently an International Prognostic Factors Project has defined risk categories for advanced Hodgkin's disease depending on how many of the following adverse features are present:

- Age ≥ 45
- Male sex
- Stage IV disease
- Low haemoglobin
- Low serum albumin
- High white blood count
- Low lymphocyte count.

Treatment of Hodgkin's disease

Radical radiotherapy was until recently the treatment of choice for early Hodgkin's disease, and chemotherapy for those with advanced disease (III and IV), systemic 'B' symptoms or poor prognostic factors.

Treatment of early Hodgkin's disease in adults (stages IA and IIA)

In the early 1980s locoregional radiotherapy was the treatment of choice for stage IA and IIA Hodgkin's disease. This approach has changed for two reasons: the recognition of prognostic factors for relapse and the occurrence of treatment-induced second malignancies.

Prognostic factors. First, it has been shown that some of these patients if treated by extended field irradiation (e.g. mantle or inverted Y) run a higher risk of relapse. They frequently require to be salvaged by chemotherapy. They include those with:

- Bulky mediastinal disease (tumour mass occupying a third or more of the internal diameter of the thoracic cage at the level of T5–6)
- ESR > 50 mm/h
- Unfavourable histology (nodular sclerosing grade 2, mixed cellularity, or lymphocyte-depleted histology)
- Three or more involved sites.

It seems logical to treat such patients primarily by chemotherapy. This has the additional advantage of avoiding the myelosuppressive effects of extended field irradiation which may limit the patient's capacity to tolerate subsequent chemotherapy in full dosage.

Even for patients with localised Hodgkin's Disease without adverse prognostic factors, some authorities would recommend 'minimal invasive therapy'—short-course chemotherapy followed by involved-field RT.

Choice of target volume. The terms 'involved' and 'extended' fields are commonly used in relation to the radiotherapy of Hodgkin's disease. 'Involved' field means one confined to the involved area of disease plus a small margin of surrounding normal tissue. 'Extended' field means encompassing the involved nodes plus all the other nodal areas above the diaphragm (mantle) or below the diaphragm (inverted Y). Both mantle and involved field radiation are in common use.

Radiation technique. Hodgkin's disease in lymph nodes tends to spread contiguously to adjacent lymph nodes. The inclusion of both involved and adjacent uninvolved nodes (extended-field irradiation) within the irradiated volume increases the cure rate compared to irradiating the involved nodes alone. 'Mantle' (Fig. 29.4) and 'inverted Y' (Fig. 29.5) radiotherapy are the techniques of extended-field irradiation for disease above and below the diaphragm respectively.

Mantle technique. The term derives from the similarity of the treatment fields to a cloak.

Target volume

The nodes of the neck, axilla, infraclavicular, paratracheal, hilar and anterior mediastinal regions are included (Fig. 29.4).

Technique

The patient lies supine. The chin is extended to exclude as much of the oral cavity as possible. The arms are slightly abducted with the hands on the hips. Anterior and posterior fields are used at extended SSD (120–140 cm).

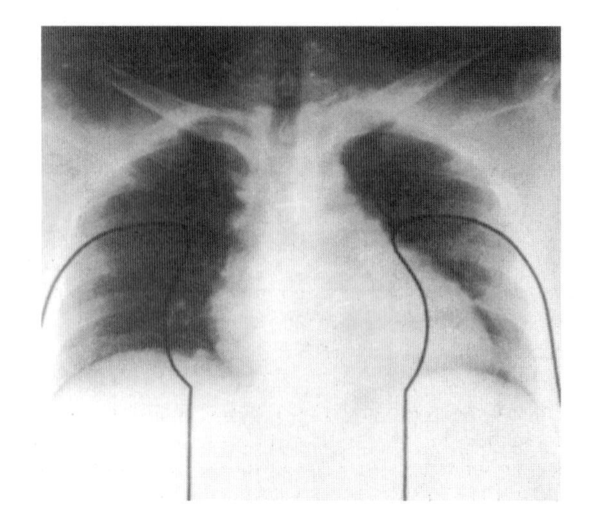

Fig. 29.4 Mantle field for Hodgkin's disease.

The upper limit of the field is on a line joining the chin to the external occipital protuberance. This line passes through the mastoid process. The occipital, submental and submaxillary nodes are included in the volume. However Waldeyer's ring, the preauricular and parotid nodes are excluded. If Waldeyer's ring is involved, the field should extend up to the base of the skull.

The lower limit is the junction of the 10th and 11th thoracic vertebrae. The lateral border runs along the lateral margin of the axilla through the acromioclavicular joint.

The width of the mediastinal field is usually 8–10 cm, depending on the size of the nodes. It can be shaped to encompass any nodal masses. These can be measured most accurately from a CT scan of the thorax. It is helpful to outline palpable lymph node masses with lead wire prior to simulation to ensure adequate coverage.

Shielding

1. The lung is shielded lateral to the mediastinum, a curved line running along the lower border of the fourth rib posteriorly (Fig. 29.4).

2. The larynx may be shielded for half of the treatment by lead on the anterior field. However, this should be avoided if there is adjacent lymphadenopathy, in case underdosage occurs.

3. Some clinicians also shield the cervical part of the spinal cord by a narrow 2 cm strip on the posterior field to limit the spinal cord dose to 30 Gy. However, so doing results in a small area of underdosage in the middle of the mediastinum. Although the incidence of transient Lhermitte's sign is probably commoner if the cervical cord is not shielded, there is no evidence that the incidence of chronic radiation myelopathy is increased.

Spinal shielding should be avoided particularly where the cervical nodes or mediastinum are involved.

It is important not to shield the axilla and the infraclavicular areas since these may be sites of recurrence.

Three points are tattooed on the front of the chest: (1) the centre of the field, (2) a point 10 cm below the centre of the field, and (3) a third point is made midway between the first two points and 5 cm lateral to the midline (to ensure there is no rotation of the thorax). Lead markers are placed on all three points and a radiograph taken. The clinician draws on the simulator films the outline of the lung blocks (Fig. 29.4). Lung blocks are then prepared (p. 173). A verification film is taken on the linear accelerator and compared with the simulator film. The medial ends of the clavicles and the spinous processes of the vertebrae usually provide useful bony landmarks on the portal film.

Dose distribution. The neck and the axilla are the thinnest structures in the anteroposterior plane. The midplane doses to the axillae and neck would be respectively 10–15% and 15–20% higher than the dose to the mediastinum, if no attempt were made to compensate for these variations in thickness. This can be overcome by applying Lincolnshire bolus bags in the axillae and over the upper chest for anterior and posterior fields. The superior level of the bolus should be at the topmost point of the chest wall. The effect of the bolus is to convert an irregular volume into a box-shaped volume of uniform thickness. The alternative is to adjust the dosage by shielding the areas of overdosage at an appropriate point during the treatment schedule.

CT planning techniques are now available which facilitate the use of the 3D dataset to outline the structures detailed above more accurately. With the increased use of chemotherapy, mantle treatments are reducing in number.

Dose and energy

35 Gy midplane dose in 20 daily fractions over 4 weeks at megavoltage (6–10 MV photons)

Boost to involved sites given on successive days after mantle treatment completed:

5 Gy in 3 daily fractions (orthovoltage or 6–10 MV photons)

The role of wide field radiotherapy has diminished over recent years with the recognition of serious long-term effects. For example in young women treated with Mantle radiotherapy there is an increased risk of breast cancer.

However, in initially bulky disease (particularly involving the mediastinum), where the response to chemotherapy is not complete, involved or extended field radiotherapy is given to locally persistent disease in a similar dosage and fractionation to that used in the Mantle technique.

Side-effects

Acute. The main acute side-effects of mantle radiotherapy are anorexia, nausea, vomiting, sore throat, dry mouth, dysphagia, impaired taste and hair loss in the occipital region. Apart from altered taste and dry mouth, the other side-effects have normally settled by a month after treatment. Mucaine 10 ml p.r.n. and before meals usually diminishes dysphagia.

Dry mouth and altered taste. Inclusion of the sublingual, submaxillary and part of the parotid gland results in reducing the output of saliva and making it more viscous. Taste is impaired but usually returns within a period of 3 months. Artificial saliva may help. Regular mouth washes are encouraged. A dental assessment before treatment is essential. Caries should be dealt with. Regular dental assessment is necessary following treatment since caries are more likely to occur once the protective effect of normal saliva is diminished.

Skin reaction. In the latter half of treatment skin erythema develops. This is followed by desquamation, dry in most areas but it may be moist in the axilla. Exposure to the sun should be avoided during treatment and until the acute reaction has settled. Simple analgesia may be necessary. An emollient cream such as E45 is applied to areas of dry desquamation and Flamazine to moist desquamation once treatment is completed.

Alopecia occurs over the occiput, and beard growth is inhibited. The hair in both areas normally regrows by 3 months after treatment. Dry shaving is recommended during treatment to protect the skin.

Inverted Y technique

Target volume

This includes the para-aortic, pelvic, iliac and femoral nodes (Fig. 29.5).

Technique

The patient is simulated supine and treated with anterior and undercouched fields at extended SSD.

The upper margin of the field is the junction of the 10th and 11th thoracic vertebrae or inferior to the gap calculated to allow overlap of the 50% isodose at the level of the spinal cord if a mantle field has been previously treated. This gap is usually about 2 cm on the skin. The lower border is the inferior margin of the obturator foramen. The width of the field is guided by the size of the nodes on lymphography and on CT scanning. It is normally 8–10 cm wide.

The abdominal cavity lateral to the nodal areas outlined above is shielded with individualised MCP blocks.

Kidney. The medial 1–2 cm of each kidney are necessarily included in the field. In the absence of

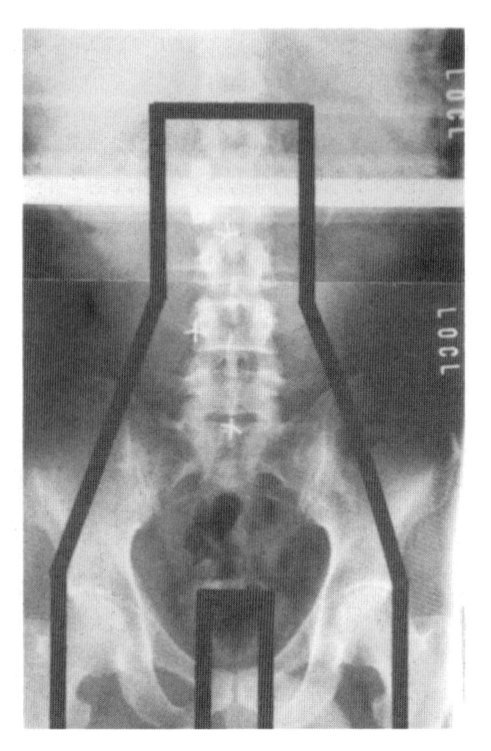

Fig. 29.5 Inverted Y fields for Hodgkin's and non-Hodgkin lymphoma.

pre-existing renal damage, up to a third of each kidney can be irradiated without compromising renal function. The position of the kidneys is verified by an IVU carried out at the start of simulation.

Ovaries. In young women the ovaries can be protected by transposing them at the time of surgery centrally to the inferior part of the body of the uterus (oophoropexy) and marking their position with clips. Lead blocks can then be placed over the new site of the ovaries. The only radiation that the ovaries then receive is from scattered radiation. This operation makes it possible for women to become pregnant while still receiving radical doses of radiation. Children born to such mothers do not show any evidence of impaired development.

Bladder and genitalia. A central rectangular block placed in the midline protects the ovaries (if transposed), the bladder and genitalia. Care should be taken not to shield involved nodes adjacent to the block. The block should be omitted if there is a risk of underdosage to these nodes.

The dose to the testis can be reduced by applying 1 cm thick lead cups around the testis. These can reduce the dose to the testis to 0.6 Gy out of a total dose of 40 Gy.

CT technique. CT techniques for the planning of inverted Y have been developed which facilitate accurate location of the kidneys and ovaries.

Acute reaction. Anorexia, nausea, vomiting, colicky abdominal pain and diarrhoea occur but should settle by 3 weeks after treatment. They can be reduced by use of a low-residue diet, particularly avoiding fruit and green vegetables.

Low blood counts are an inevitable consequence of wide field irradiation. The full blood count should be checked twice weekly on treatment. If the white cell count falls below 2×10^9/l or platelets to less than 60×10^9/l, treatment should be suspended for a few days until the blood count has risen above these levels. The blood count may need to be monitored more frequently thereafter.

Late effects. Late effects of radiation occur months or years after radiotherapy and tend to be permanent. These tend to be more marked in children because irradiation interferes with bone growth. Chemotherapy does not have this effect. It is therefore chosen in preference to wide-field irradiation. Radiotherapy, if given, is restricted to the site of involvement.

Most late effects occur after mantle rather than inverted Y irradiation. The organs mainly affected are the thyroid, lung and heart.

Thyroid. Abnormally low thyroid function (biochemically) develops in 40% of patients. Less than 10%, however, are clinically hypothyroid. This complication usually develops insidiously several years after radiotherapy. Low serum thyroxine levels are often associated with elevated TSH (thyroid-stimulating hormone). If the TSH level remains above normal, there is an increased risk of malignant transformation of the thyroid gland. Thyroxine should be given to suppress TSH. Thyroid function should be monitored intermittently.

Neurological. The most common syndrome is of numbness, tingling (paraesthesia) or an 'electric shock'-like sensation in the arms or legs following mantle or neck irradiation. It is often precipitated by flexion of the neck (Lhermitte's syndrome). It is thought to be due to transient demyelination of the spinal cord within the irradiated volume owing to damage to oligodendrocytes. It occurs 2–4 months after treatment. It is important to stress that it does not lead on to permanent spinal cord damage (transverse myelitis) but it may last up to 6 months.

Transverse myelitis should not occur if the above dose and fractionation schedule is observed. It may, however, occur if there is mismatching of supra- and infradiaphragmatic fields or retreatment of a previously treated area.

Lung. Radiation pneumonitis is an uncommon complication unless substantial volumes of lung are included in the mantle field. This is more likely to occur where the mediastinal disease is bulky. Lung function is minimally impaired in about a third of patients undergoing mantle therapy. Symptoms are of non-productive cough and dyspnoea, with or without fever. Chest radiography may show hazy shadowing in the central part of the lung fields. Treatment is with steroids (prednisolone 40–60 mg/day). Provided that sufficient normal lung lies outside the treated area, the symptoms usually settle.

Lung fibrosis usually develops within the irradiated areas of lung in the mantle field over 4–18 months. Most patients have no respiratory symptoms.

Cardiac. Radiation-induced cardiac disease occurs in less than 5% of patients. The incidence was higher in patients treated by a single anterior field rather than the conventional equally weighted parallel-opposed pair of mantle therapy. This is a technique which is no longer used. It usually presents with features of acute pericarditis (fever, chest pain, pericardial friction rub), asymptomatic pericardial effusion noted on chest radiograph or rarely (< 5%) with constrictive pericarditis and tamponade. Acute pericarditis usually settles with conservative management. Asymptomatic pericardial effusion usually resolves over several months. Constrictive pericarditis is more serious and may require surgery. In the long term there may be cardiomyopathy and premature coronary artery disease.

Bone. Avascular necrosis of the femoral head occurs in 2% of patients treated for Hodgkin's disease (Fig. 29.6). This is particularly likely following chemotherapy and intermittent steroid treatment. Inverted Y irradiation is also a contributory factor. Often, but not invariably, the patient has had the affected hip irradiated. Symptoms of hip pain develop on average about 2 years following the start of chemotherapy. If the condition progresses, total hip replacement may be necessary. Changes are not confined to the hips. The humeral head, for example, may also be affected.

Ovary and testis. Although the ovaries of younger women are more resistant to radiation, a dose of 1.2 Gy results in a high incidence of amenorrhoea, irrespective of pubertal status. Loss of ovarian function is rare if the dose to the ovary is 0.15 Gy or less. Transposition of the ovaries (see oophoropexy under Inverted Y) can achieve this.

The dose to the testes is determined by their relative depth and proximity to the edge of the beam during abdominopelvic irradiation. Little can be done to adjust the beam edge if pelvic nodes are to be adequately treated. With cobalt-60 the testicular dose may be up to 10% of the tumour dose (i.e. 3.5 Gy). This dose is sufficient to induce prolonged or permanent azoospermia and sterility. The dose can be reduced by 75% to 2.5% of the tumour dose (< 1 Gy) by a lead protective shield surrounding the testis.

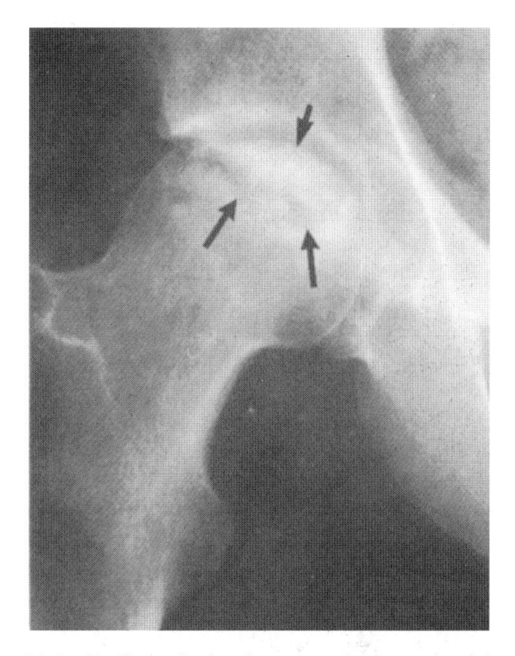

Fig. 29.6 Radiograph showing avascular necrosis of the femoral head in a patient treated with chemotherapy for Hodgkin's disease. (Courtesy of Professor B Hancock, Sheffield.)

Growth. Growth retardation with reduction in both standing and sitting height is common in children who have received mantle radiotherapy. Thinning of the neck muscles and shortening of the clavicles may occur. The appreciation of these complications has resulted in the avoidance of mantle irradiation in children where possible, and treatment by primary chemotherapy and/or limited field irradiation (see below).

Second malignancy. There is an increased risk of solid tumours (particularly breast and thyroid carcinoma and sarcoma) in young patients previously given radiotherapy; such tumours develop within radiation fields.

Chemotherapy

Combination chemotherapy has been outstandingly successful in obtaining complete and prolonged remissions. It is the treatment of choice for stages Ib, IIb, IIIa, IIIb, IVa and IVb. It is also indicated in bulky mediastinal Hodgkin's disease. Commonly used regimens are shown in Table 29.2. A prognostic score for advanced HD has been devised from an international collaborative project. Factors found to be predictive for poorer outcome were older age, advanced stage, male gender, raised white blood cell count, low haemoglobin and low serum albumin.

Initially most chemotherapy was with MOPP. The nitrogen mustard component is highly emetic and has largely been replaced by chlorambucil (as in LOPP) because it is not emetic. LOPP (ChlVPP) has been found to be as effective and less toxic than MOPP. ABVD is an alternative to alkylating agent combinations and may have superior efficacy without causing sterility and with a lower incidence of second malignancies. Alternating and hybrid regimens have given improved results in the UK. ChlVPP/PABlOE and ChlVPP EVA are popular here; in Europe and the US ABVD is favoured. More intensive but shortened combined modality schedules are being trialed. The role for radiotherapy after conventional chemotherapy is uncertain. An exception is bulky mediastinal disease where radiotherapy may be given after full-course chemotherapy. The average number of cycles of chemotherapy to achieve a complete response is three. Most patients require six to eight courses. Maintenance chemotherapy beyond eight courses has not improved survival.

Toxicity. MOPP has considerable toxicity. It causes hair loss, nausea, severe vomiting and peripheral neuropathy. Substitution of chlorambucil reduces some of the side-effects but these regimens render virtually all males and a substantial number of females sterile and second cancers are a problem.

ABVD causes nausea and vomiting and moderate myelosuppression. There is an increased risk of late

Table 29.2 Some typical chemotherapy regimens for Hodgkin's disease

MOPP	
Nitrogen mustard 6 mg/m^2 i.v.	Days 1 and 8
Vincristine 1.4 mg/m^2 (max. 2 mg) i.v.	Days 1 and 8
Procarbazine 100 mg/m^2 orally	Days 1–14
Prednisolone 40 mg/m2 orally	Days 1–14
Repeated every 4 weeks (minimum 6 courses)	
LOPP	
Chlorambucil (Leukeran) 10 mg orally	Days 1–10
Vincristine (Oncovin) 1.4 mg/m^2 (max. 2 mg) i.v.	Days 1 and 8
Procarbazine 100 mg/m^2 (max. 200 mg) orally	Days 1–10
Prednisolone 25 mg/m^2 (max. 60 mg) orally	Days 1–14
Repeated every 28 days (minimum 6 courses)	
ChlVPP	
Chlorambucil 6 mg/m^2 (max. 10 mg) orally	Days 1–14
Vinblastine 6 mg/m^2 (max. 10 mg) i.v.	Days 1 and 8
Procarbazine 100 mg/m^2 orally	Days 1–14
Prednisolone 40 mg orally	Days 1–14
Repeated every 28 days	
ChlVPP/PAB1OE	
Three courses of Ch1VPP (as above) alternating with three courses of PABIOE (minimum 6 courses)	
Doxorubicin 40 mg/2 i.v.	Day 1
Vincristine 1.4 mg/m^2 i.v.	Day 1
Bleomycin 10 000 units/m^2 i.v.	Day 1
Etoposide 200 mg/m^2 orally	Days 1–3
Prednisolone 40 mg/m^2 (max. 60 mg) orally	Days 1–10
Vincristine 1.4 mg/m^2 i.v.	Day 8
Bleomycin 10 000 units/m^2 i.v.	Day 8
ABVD	
Doxorubicin (Adriamycin) 25 mg/m^2 i.v.	Days 1 and 15
Bleomycin 10 000 units/m^2 i.v.	Days 1 and 15
Vinblastine 6 mg/m^2 i.v.	Days 1 and 15
Dacarbazine 375 mg/m^2 i.v.	Days 1 and 15
Repeated every 28 days (minimum 6 courses)	

cardiac and pulmonary damage. However, the risk of infertility and of second malignancies is reduced. Alternating or hybrid regimens may be less toxic (in the short and long term) but equally efficacious.

Second malignancy. An increased incidence of both leukaemia (usually acute myeloid) and solid tumours has been observed in patients treated by radiotherapy, chemotherapy or both. For example, the risk of patients developing acute myelogenous leukaemia is about 3–5% at 5 years in unselected cases of Hodgkin's disease followed for more than 5 years. The highest risk (10%) is in patients treated by a combination of chemotherapy (MOPP) and radiotherapy. The risk of leukaemia in patients treated with radiotherapy alone is thought to be small. It appears to be the chemotherapy, especially in regimens containing alkylating agents, rather than radiotherapy that is mainly carcinogenic. The risk of developing a solid tumour increases with time and is not associated with any particular form of treatment. A variety of tumours are seen.

Response and survival. Conventional chemotherapy can achieve complete response rates of 60–80% in advanced disease. Over half of those who achieve a complete response are cured.

Results of treatment

The prognosis of Hodgkin's disease has improved with the advent of effective combination chemotherapy and more accurate staging. The overall 5-year survival is 70–80%. The results of treatment by stage and grade of histology are summarised in Table 29.3.

Relapsed Hodgkin's disease

40% or more of patients treated with MOPP or LOPP will relapse. Failure to achieve a complete response is more likely in the following groups of patients:

- Prior chemotherapy
- Stage IV
- Multiple extranodal sites
- Systemic symptoms
- Age > 40 years
- Unfavourable histology types
- Bone marrow involvement
- Bulky disease.

Most relapses occur at the original site of disease, especially in nodes, and usually in the first 3 years after treatment. Relapse occurring within a year of the end of treatment has a particularly poor prognosis. Only a third of patients who relapse within a year of the end of treatment and who are retreated with the same drugs achieve a complete remission. They are rarely cured. If relapse is confined to the neck, axilla, mediastinum or to the para-aortic or pelvic nodes, mantle or inverted Y radiotherapy may be considered. If there is disease outside these sites, second line alternative (non-cross-resistant) chemotherapy is needed.

High-dose chemotherapy with autologous peripheral stem cell or bone marrow support may be the most

Table 29.3 Results of treatment of Hodgkin's disease (reproduced with permission from Souhami R L and Moxham J 1990 Textbook of Medicine, Churchill Livingstone, Edinburgh)

Stage	Symptoms	% total	Histological grade	CR rate (%)	5-year survival (%)
I	A	20	1	99	92
			2	98	83
	B	Very rare	—	—	—
II	A	21	1	96	94
			2	90	77
	B	7	1	74	78
			2	55	70
III	A	17	1	85	80
			2	70	71
	B	13	1	69	77
			2	60	55
IV	A	6	1	2	74
			2	44	56
	B	14	1	61	64
			2	43	46

CR = Complete response

likely hope of prolonged remission. About half of patients treated achieve a complete response, with prolonged remissions in about one-third.

Hodgkin's disease in children

Although the same histological subtypes occur in children, lymphocyte-depleted Hodgkin's disease is even less common than in adults. Lymphadenopathy is the presenting feature in 90%, of which 60% is cervical or supraclavicular.

CT scanning has the advantage of being non-invasive but may require sedation in young children.

Staging laparotomy used to be carried out if primary radiotherapy was the sole proposed treatment. The stage of the disease was altered in 30% of children undergoing laparotomy. However, severe life-threatening pneumococcal infection is a particular problem in up to 15% of children following splenectomy, with 2–5% mortality. It is now felt that the prognosis of childhood Hodgkin's disease is so good that the risks of staging laparotomy outweigh the benefits.

In view of the growth retardation, pneumonitis, pericarditis and hypothyroidism following mantle irradiation, limited involved-field irradiation with lower doses than in adults may be recommended in children for stage IA disease, e.g. unilateral isolated cervical or inguinal lymphadenopathy. Doses of 25 Gy to the vertebral column result in much less truncal shortening than doses of 35 Gy.

Chemotherapy and radiotherapy can be combined and tailored to the severity of the disease.

Combination chemotherapy with MOPP or ChlVPP results in complete remissions in 80%. Two-thirds of these children will have prolonged disease-free remissions. Relapse following chemotherapy carries a worse prognosis; high-dose chemotherapy offers the best chance of success.

Management of Hodgkin's disease in pregnancy

Most patients who develop Hodgkin's disease during pregnancy have localised disease. Patients with advanced symptomatic disease often have impaired ovulation and therefore are less likely to become pregnant.

One is concerned with the health of both the mother and the fetus. However, there is little evidence that pregnancy worsens the prognosis of Hodgkin's disease or that the disease adversely affects the fetus.

The management of Hodgkin's disease in pregnancy will depend upon the stage of the disease and of the pregnancy and the mother's wishes.

Radiotherapy is potentially teratogenic during the first trimester. Above a dose of 0.1 Gy to the fetus there is a risk of inducing a fetal abnormality.

It seems probable that chemotherapy is also potentially teratogenic. It is unknown if chemotherapy is carcinogenic to the fetus. There is no evidence that either radiotherapy or chemotherapy is teratogenic during the third trimester.

The staging of Hodgkin's disease in pregnancy should minimise exposure to ionising radiation. Thus initial investigations should include a chest radiograph, full blood count, ESR and liver function tests; magnetic resonance imaging is preferred to CT scanning.

In the first trimester or early weeks of the second trimester, if radiotherapy would deliver more than 0.1 Gy to the fetus or chemotherapy is indicated, therapeutic abortion should be considered. If the diagnosis is made later in the second trimester or in the third trimester, it may be possible to postpone treatment until after the child has been delivered by induced labour between 32 and 34 weeks. If urgent treatment has to be given because of advanced disease or therapeutic abortion is declined by the patient or is not feasible, combination chemotherapy is the treatment of choice. ABVD may be preferred because of its probable low risk of carcinogenicity and lower risk of reduced fertility in the child. Localised radiotherapy above the diaphragm can be safely given.

Patients who have been successfully treated for Hodgkin's disease should be advised to avoid pregnancy for 2 years after the end of treatment. This is because it is within this period that relapse is most likely. Beyond it the risk of relapse falls markedly. Patients can be reassured that subsequent pregnancy does not increase the risk of relapse of the disease.

NON-HODGKIN LYMPHOMAS

This group of tumours includes a very wide spectrum of malignancy, from almost benign to highly aggressive disease.

Pathology

Epidemiology

Non-Hodgkin lymphomas (NHL) are responsible for 1.4% of all cancers and 0.4% of cancer deaths. The peak incidence is in the fifth and sixth decades. Children in developed countries are rarely affected. The incidence among children in developing countries is higher, particularly of high-grade Burkitt's lymphoma. Males are slightly more commonly affected than females. The sex ratio is 1.7 : 1.

Aetiology

The cause of most NHL is unknown. The risk of developing NHL is increased in certain inherited genetic syndromes such as combined immunodeficiency syndromes and ataxia telangiectasia. Chromosomal defects have been identified in some types of NHL (14:18 translocation in follicular lymphoma and 8:14 translocation in Burkitt's lymphoma). However, these are acquired as part of tumour development, not inherited abnormalities.

Some NHL are associated with, though not necessarily caused by, viral infection. For example endemic Burkitt's lymphoma, originally described in East African children, is associated with infection by the Epstein–Barr virus (EBV). These children have evidence of antibodies to the viral antigen. EBV is unlikely, however, to be the sole causative agent of Burkitt's lymphoma since the virus is distributed worldwide, whereas the tumour is limited to areas where malaria is endemic. Malaria has therefore been suggested as a possible cofactor. Some NHL are caused by infection with the human T leukaemia virus type 1 (HTLV-1).

Conditions in which the body's immune system is impaired predispose to the development of NHL, particularly immunoblastic. Examples are rheumatoid arthritis, coeliac disease, hypogammaglobulinaemia and AIDS. There is a 60-fold excess of these tumours in patients who have undergone immunosuppressive drug therapy following organ transplantation.

Microscopic features

NHL are typified by the monoclonal proliferation, in order of frequency, of B lymphocytes or T lymphocytes.

The wide variation in histological appearance of NHL, and the difficulty in classifying many of them with certainty has led to a confusing variety of systems of pathological classification. The availability of modern immunohistochemical techniques to identify different cell types has contributed to the complexity. However, the basis of classification is to recognise the malignant cell, and name it according to its normal counterparts.

In the UK the British National Lymphoma Investigation (BNLI) group and the Kiel classifications have been most commonly used. The Working Formulation of the US National Cancer Institute and more recently the Revised European–American Lymphoma (REAL) classification are also popular. Much expertise is required to classify the NHL. High-grade NHL may be confused with a poorly differentiated carcinoma by the unwary. The management and prognosis of these two conditions is different. *Referral of all cases to a specialist histopathologist for review before taking a decision on management is recommended.*

BNLI classification. The BNLI classification is based on morphological appearances. Its attraction to the clinician is the division into grade 1 and grade 2 disease which provides a comprehensible and practical guide to decision making. The BNLI classification has the advantage of wide usage in the UK. The BNLI offers an excellent centralised service for review of pathology to centres participating in its studies.

Kiel classification. The Kiel classification is based on scientific principles and microscopic appearances. It also divides lymphomas into low- or high-grade malignancy. Both the Kiel and another classification (Luke–Collins) take account of the T or B cell origin of the tumour.

REAL classification. The Revised European–American Lymphoma classification lists lymphoid neoplasms which are distinctive biological entities and which can be reproducibly diagnosed by haematopathologists (Table 29.4). This has been accepted and updated in the new World Health Organization classification.

Low-grade tumours tend to behave in a less aggressive manner than high-grade tumours. However, this applies more to B cell than to T cell lymphomas. In general, low-grade tumours tend to have smaller cells with a closer resemblance to normal lymphoid cells. High-grade tumours usually have larger cells, often multinucleate with prominent nucleoli. Some tumours contain a mixture of cells, which can make them difficult to classify.

Table 29.4 Revised European–American Lymphoma Classification (simplified)

B cell	T cell
Precursor B cell	*Precursor T cell*
Lymphoblastic	Lymphoblastic
Peripheral B cell	*Peripheral T cell*
Small lymphocyte/CLL-like	CLL-like
Lymphoplasmacytoid	Mycosis fungoides
Mantle cell	Angioimmunoblastic
Follicular	Anaplastic large cell
Marginal zone	Unspecified
Diffuse large cell	Other
Burkitt	
Other	

Clinical features

NHL differ in several respects from Hodgkin's disease. These differences are simplistically summarised in Table 29.5. In contrast to Hodgkin's disease, very few patients (10%) have localised disease at presentation. Systemic B symptoms are common. A further difference is the frequency of presentation (20%) with involvement of extranodal sites. The most common of these are in the head and neck, particularly in the lymphoid tissue of the tonsil, nasopharynx and base of tongue (Waldeyer's ring). Second in frequency is the gastrointestinal tract (stomach > small bowel > large bowel). Less common sites are the skin, thyroid, CNS, bone, and testis. Epitrochlear and mesenteric nodes and the bone marrow are only rarely involved by Hodgkin's disease but not infrequently by NHL.

Investigations

The staging investigations for NHL are similar to those for Hodgkin's disease. An adequate biopsy is essential for proper histological examination and cell surface marker studies. There are, however, the following differences:

1. Surface markers. A number of monoclonal antibodies to cell surface proteins made by these tumours are useful in determining whether they are of B or T cell origin. Most (about 85%) lymphomas are of B cell origin. Individual subtypes can be identified using immunocytochemical markers. Staining with antibodies against epithelial cell components (e.g. cytokeratins) usually identifies undifferentiated carcinomas, separating them from lymphomas.

2. CT scanning. Since NHL tend to be more generalised than Hodgkin's disease, CT scanning of the thorax and the abdomen is preferred to lymphangiography. In those unfit for CT scanning of chest and abdomen because of advanced age or poor general medical condition, a chest radiograph and abdominal ultrasound provide simpler alternatives.

3. Bone marrow examination. A bone marrow aspirate and a small core of bone (trephine) should be examined for tumour infiltration. The trephine may be positive when the aspirate is negative. Marrow involvement is much commoner in low-grade (>60%) than high-grade (10–15%) NHL.

4. Staging laparotomy. This is not recommended since so few patients have localised disease. Many patients are elderly and unfit for surgery on medical grounds.

Table 29.5 Comparison of clinical features of Hodgkin's disease and non-Hodgkin lymphoma

Feature	Hodgkin's disease	Non-Hodgkin lymphoma
Localised	+++	+
Nodal spread		
Contiguous	+++	+
Non-contiguous	+	+++
Bone marrow infiltration	±	++
CNS involvement	±	+

The following standard staging investigations are recommended:

1. Haematology
   a. Full blood count and ESR
   b. Bone marrow aspirate and trephine
2. Biochemistry
   a. Liver function tests
   b. Serum immunoglobulins
   c. Serum urea, creatinine and electrolytes (including calcium)
   d. Serum uric acid
3. Radiology
   a. Chest radiograph
   b. CT scan of thorax and abdomen.

Principles of management

The management of NHL depends upon the age and general condition of the patient, the histology, the extent of the disease and whether the tumour is nodal or extranodal. NHL are generally very sensitive to radiation and to chemotherapy.

In general, widespread low-grade (BNLI grade 1, mostly REAL follicular B cell) tumours are treated with 'gentle' chemotherapy (chlorambucil with or without steroids) or slightly more aggressive combination chemotherapy (chlorambucil, vincristine (Oncovin) and prednisolone (CV(O)P); Table 29.6). Radiotherapy at modest doses is used for localised disease.

High-grade (BNLI grade 2, mostly REAL diffuse large B cell) tumours usually require more aggressive combination chemotherapy, e.g. with cyclophosphamide, doxorubicin, vincristine (Oncovin) and prednisolone [CHOP] (Table 29.7). Radiotherapy at higher dosage than for low-grade tumours is required for truly localised (stage Ia) disease or for masses failing to resolve completely on chemotherapy.

Table 29.6 CV(O)P regimen for low-grade non-Hodgkin lymphomas

Cyclophosphamide 750 mg/m^2 i.v.	Day 1
Vincristine (Oncovin) 1.4 mg/m^2 (max. 2 mg) i.v.	Day 1
Prednisolone 40 mg/m^2 orally	Days 1–5
Repeated every 21 days (minimum 6 courses)	

1. Localised disease (stages I and II)

Low-grade (grade 1)

For patients with localised stage I or II disease of low-grade histology local radiotherapy is generally recommended.

High-grade (grade 2)

Previously local radiotherapy alone was recommended for non-bulky (< 2.5 cm) stage Ia disease of high-grade histology. Nowadays, it is standard practice to give an abbreviated course of chemotherapy followed by radiotherapy. In view of the frequent failure of radiotherapy to control bulky stage I and stage II disease, full-course cytotoxic chemotherapy is advised and may be followed by radiotherapy to the initial site of involvement. Combination chemotherapy is most commonly with the CHOP regimen (Table 29.7) subject to response and patient tolerance.

Results of treatment. For low-grade stage I and II, local control is about 80% at 5 years; occasionally patients may be cured. For high-grade, local control of stage I disease is 65% at 5 years. Radiotherapy is less effective for high-grade bulky (> 2.5 cm) stage I or stage II (local control only 27% at 5 years). With chemotherapy before radiotherapy a 20% improvement is seen.

2. Widespread disease (stages III–IV)

Low grade

There is little evidence that treatment influences the natural history of stage III–IV disease of low-grade histology. Despite treatment, 75% of patients will relapse within 5 years. Since cure is unrealistic with current radiotherapy or chemotherapy, it is important to minimise the toxicity of treatment.

In general, in the absence of life-threatening disease (e.g. liver metastases, bone marrow failure, renal or cerebral involvement), asymptomatic patients should be kept under regular surveillance on an outpatient basis. Treatment is instituted with local radiotherapy or with chemotherapy if there is symptomatic progression or vital organs (e.g. kidneys) are threatened.

Chemotherapy. For symptomatic non-life-threatening disease, chlorambucil (0.2 mg/kg daily (max. 10 mg)) with or without prednisolone (10–40 mg daily) can provide good control. To reduce the risk of leukaemogenesis and preserve adequate bone marrow tolerance to subsequent chemotherapy, if needed, treatment with chlorambucil should usually be stopped 3 months after a response has been achieved. Total duration of treatment should not exceed 6 months.

If disease progresses despite chlorambucil and/or steroids, more aggressive treatment is necessary. Combination chemotherapy such as cyclophosphamide, vincristine and prednisolone (CV(O)P) is advised (Table 29.6) to a total of six courses if a useful clinical response is obtained. If not doxorubicin may be added.

New treatments are being evaluated especially in younger fitter patients, for example fludarabine (especially in combination chemotherapy), high-dose therapy with stem cell rescue and biological therapy (with interferon or anti-idiotypic antibodies such as rituximab).

High grade

Chemotherapy has been more successful in the control of high-grade than low-grade lymphoma. Combination chemotherapy is the treatment of choice. Of the available regimens, CHOP (Table 29.7) is still the gold standard (though more intensive forms of chemotherapy, such as high-dose chemotherapy, are currently being evaluated). Six courses are given, subject to response and patient tolerance. The most aggressive forms of high-grade disease (e.g. lymphoblastic) are often treated with leukaemia-type regimens and additionally with prophylactic CNS irradiation because of the high incidence of CNS involvement.

Results of chemotherapy for high-grade disease. Complete response rates of the order of 60% are achievable. Overall cure rate is about 40%.

Table 29.7 CHOP regimen for high-grade non-Hodgkin lymphomas

Cyclophosphamide 750 mg/m^2 i.v.	Day 1
Doxorubicin 50 mg/m^2 i.v.	Day 1
Vincristine 1.4 mg/m^2 (max. 2 mg) i.v.	Day 1
Prednisolone 50 mg/m^2 orally	Days 1–5
Repeated every 21 days (minimum 6 courses)	

Relapse

High-dose chemotherapy with or without autologous stem cell or bone marrow transplantation should be considered for patients failing to respond or relapsing after CHOP chemotherapy. However, the probability of cure is low.

Radiotherapy

Localised disease (low grade)

Target volume

Since NHL do not necessarily spread to contiguous nodes, local radiotherapy should be confined to the affected nodes, with a generous (e.g. 5 cm) margin. This is in contrast to regional (e.g. mantle) radiotherapy in Hodgkin's disease where the cervical, mediastinal and axillary nodes are treated, even if only one of these sites is involved.

Technique

For the treatment of neck nodes, patients should be immobilised using a plastic shell lying supine with the neck extended as much as possible. A direct anterior field is simulated with the nodal mass marked by use of wire. The medial border is usually placed lateral to the spinal cord. Where the disease is extensive, an opposed posterior field may be required.

Where both the pelvic and para-aortic nodes are involved, an inverted Y technique is used (as in Hodgkin's disease).

For involved mediastinal nodes, it is not necessary to include the cervical, infraclavicular or axillary nodes as in the mantle technique.

Dose and energy

The energy chosen will vary according to the site of involvement. For superficial nodes in the neck or the groin, orthovoltage (250–300 kV) is often adequate. For bulky nodes megavoltage is advised.

Dose 30 Gy in 15 fractions over 3 weeks is adequate for low-grade lymphoma

Localised disease (high grade)

Technique

This is similar to that for low-grade disease. Care should be taken to avoid delivering more than 40 Gy in 20 daily fractions to the spinal cord, either by excluding it from the field or shielding the cord with a central lead block placed over the spine.

Dose and energy

A higher dose is required than for low-grade disease.

40 Gy applied (250–300 kV) or midplane dose (4–6 MV photons) in 20 daily fractions over 4 weeks

Extranodal non-Hodgkin lymphomas

1. Gastrointestinal

Pathology. The stomach is the most common site (50%), followed by small bowel (30%). The large bowel is less commonly affected (10%). Most gastric lymphomas are of mucosa-associated lymphoid tissue (MALT) origin and aetiologically associated with the presence of *Helicobacter pylori*. These are commonly low grade. The majority of the others are of high grade (diffuse large B cell) type.

Clinical features. Clinical presentation is usually with abdominal pain, weight loss and anorexia, often associated, in small bowel tumours, with acute intestinal obstruction.

Diagnosis. A biopsy is needed. The diagnosis of gastric NHL is often a surprise finding made either at endoscopic biopsy of what was thought to be a benign gastric ulcer or at laparotomy for what appeared on naked-eye examination to be a gastric carcinoma. Small and large bowel tumours are often only discovered by laparotomy.

Management. The management of gastrointestinal extranodal NHL differs from that of nodal lymphomas in a number of ways. First, surgery may have a role in the resection of localised disease. Secondly, the gastrointestinal tract is a mobile structure which makes localisation for radiotherapy planning more difficult. Thirdly, the dose that can be delivered to large volumes of the abdomen is limited. Finally, there is a significant risk of intestinal haemorrhage or perforation following a response to chemotherapy or radiotherapy.

a. Localised. Many gastric (MALT) lymphomas regress with anti-helicobacter therapy; failing this, chemotherapy (the type depending on the grade) is appropriate. Nowadays surgery is much less often employed.

For intestinal lymphoma, surgery is often both diagnostic and therapeutic.

Staging. The same staging procedures should be carried out as for nodal NHL.

Postoperative management. Owing to the rarity of these tumours and the lack of prospective randomised studies, the role of postoperative radiotherapy and chemotherapy remains controversial.

For localised disease, there is probably no need for postoperative radiotherapy or chemotherapy if the following criteria are fulfilled:

1. Only one site of bowel is involved.
2. Surgical resection margins are clear of tumour.
3. Serosa is not penetrated.

4. Tumour is less than 10 cm in diameter.
5. There is no other evidence of intra-abdominal disease.

Postoperative chemotherapy. If there is high-grade residual tumour or the initial tumour was > 10 cm in diameter, postoperative chemotherapy is advisable. Doses may have to be reduced or cycles delayed because of poor general medical condition.

Postoperative radiotherapy. Radiotherapy is less frequently used as an adjuvant because of the difficulties in accurate tumour localisation and intolerance of the doses needed to eradicate disease (40 Gy) by normal tissues and the spinal cord.

Wide-field abdominal irradiation may be offered for low-grade residual disease where the necessary tumoricidal dose (35 Gy) can be delivered with acceptable morbidity while remaining within spinal cord tolerance.

Target volume

Localisation of the tumour-bearing area or operative site with barium is helpful. A generous margin should be allowed around the tumour-bearing areas to allow for the variability in the position of the bowel within the abdomen. In practice most of the abdomen is irradiated.

Technique

A parallel-opposed pair of anterior and posterior fields is used.

Dose and energy

It is rarely possible to deliver more than 30–40 Gy over 4–5 weeks to large areas of the abdomen because of gastrointestinal toxicity.

30–40 Gy midplane dose in 20–25 daily fractions over 4–5 weeks (9–10 MV photons)

Critical organs. The kidneys should be identified during simulation by intravenous urogram. Anterior and posterior MCP blocks should limit the dose to the whole kidney to 20 Gy. The dose to the spinal cord should not exceed 40 Gy in 4 weeks. CT technique may be used to define position of the kidneys and shielding blocks.

b. Advanced disease. This should be treated by chemotherapy appropriate to the type of tumour and provided that the patient's general condition will allow this.

2. Head and neck, bone, testis, brain and breast

Clinical features. Extranodal tumours in the head and neck commonly present in Waldeyer's ring, the thyroid gland and occasionally in the salivary glands, paranasal sinuses or in the orbit. In the tonsil they appear as smooth often vascular masses. Thyroid lymphoma typically presents as a rapidly growing painful thyroid mass and stridor from tracheal compression, sometimes with a previous history of Hashimoto's thyroiditis. In the orbit, pink fleshy conjunctival deposits (Plate 2.8) are seen. The lacrimal glands and retrobulbar area may also be affected. Bilateral involvement is common.

Primary NHL of bone is very rare. It mainly affects long bones, especially the humerus and femur.

Primary testicular NHL tends to occur in the elderly, typically between 60 and 80 years of age. Bilateral involvement occurs in 20% at some stage.

Primary NHL of the CNS usually involves the brain. The spinal cord is rarely affected.

NHL of the breast usually presents with a breast mass clinically indistinguishable from carcinoma.

Management. In general, stages IEA (grades 1 and 2) and IIEA (grade 1) are treated by local radiotherapy, which is preceded, in many cases, by an abbreviated course of chemotherapy. Stage IIEA (high grade), more extensive stages (grade 1 or 2) and those with B symptoms require full-course chemotherapy. The choice of drugs will depend on the grade of the tumour, as for nodal lymphomas. Following chemotherapy, radiotherapy may be required for residual masses.

a. Waldeyer's ring.

Target volume

For NHL of Waldeyer's ring the treatment volume should extend from the base of the skull to the clavicles, including the cervical lymph node chains on both sides of the neck.

Technique

For Waldeyer's ring down to the thyroid cartilage a parallel pair of lateral fields are used. An anterior neck field is matched onto the junction using an asymmetric diaphragm for optimal matching.

b. Thyroid.

Target volume

The thyroid gland and the cervical lymph node chains on both sides.

Technique

A parallel-opposed pair of anterior and posterior fields is used.

c. Orbit. (p. 558)

d. Bone

Target volume

The whole of the affected bone should be included in the initial volume. If possible the field should then be coned down to the site of involvement.

Technique
A parallel-opposed pair of fields is used.

e. Brain

Target volume
The whole brain should be treated.

Technique
A pair of lateral opposed fields is used (Fig. 27.5A).

f. Breast

Target volume
The breast, axillary and supraclavicular nodes should be included.

Technique
(1) A pair of medial and lateral glancing fields (en bloc technique) is used to cover the whole of the treatment volume or (2) a direct anterior field to cover the supraclavicular fossa and axilla and a glancing pair of fields to the breast are used (Fig. 26.15).

Dose and energy
Waldeyer's ring, thyroid, breast, brain.
40 Gy in 20 daily fractions over 4 weeks (4–6 MV photons)

Bone
Whole bone: 40 Gy in 20 daily fractions over 4 weeks (4–6 MV photons)
Tumour volume: 15 Gy in 10 daily fractions over 2 weeks (4–6 MV photons)

Testis

Target volume
Following orchidectomy, the para-aortic and pelvic nodes are irradiated. The value of adjuvant nodal irradiation to para-aortic and pelvic nodes for the treatment of testicular high-grade lymphoma is in doubt.

Technique
Inverted Y (Fig. 29.5).

Dose and energy
35 Gy in 20 daily fractions over 4 weeks (9–10 MV photons)

Mycosis fungoides

Mycosis fungoides is a malignant skin tumour derived from T lymphocytes. It may develop a leukaemic form (Sézary syndrome). In its localised form, groups of neoplastic cells aggregate in the epidermis. The average age of onset is in the fifth decade. It runs a long course, evolving typically over 10 years but occasionally up to 30 years.

There are three main stages: premycotic (erythematous), plaque (infiltrative) and finally tumour formation. Typically erythematous patches (Plate 2.9) start on the buttocks, upper thighs or breasts. Rarely the whole skin becomes involved and red (erythroderma or 'homme rouge' (literally, red man)). The latter is often associated with blood-borne spread (Sézary syndrome). Erythematous patches become thickened to form plaque, and finally fungating tumours, often likened to tomatoes. Local and systemic infection, depression (sometimes resulting in suicide) are common in advanced disease. Terminally, there is systemic spread with visceral involvement (e.g. liver and spleen).

Treatment

Treatment of mycosis fungoides is palliative. Care should be taken to avoid aggressive treatment in the early phases of the disease because of its long natural history. Death often occurs from an unrelated illness.

In the premycotic stage topical steroid or cytotoxic therapy (nitrogen mustard), photochemotherapy using long-wave ultraviolet light with psoralens (PUVA) or radiotherapy may control the disease. PUVA tends to be used first but is only appropriate for very superficial lesions. Systemic chemotherapy is indicated for visceral spread.

Nitrogen mustard is applied by the patient, wearing protective gloves. Often treatment has to be stopped because of sensitisation to the drug.

Photochemotherapy involves exposing the patient to ultraviolet light (UVA) after administering a photosensitising agent, psoralen, orally.

Radiotherapy may be to local areas or to the whole body surface by low-energy electrons (3 MeV) from linear accelerators or beta irradiation from a strontium-90 source (betatron).

1. Local
Dose and energy
10 Gy in 5 daily fractions (80–100 kV for superficial lesions, 250–300 kV or electrons of appropriate energy for plaque or tumour stage)

2. Whole body electron therapy. Four fields of approximately 45 cm in length can be used to cover the whole body at extended SSD (120 cm). Lead shielding is applied to protect the eyes and the finger nails. If the eyelids are involved by disease, a lead internal eye shield is used. If 5 or 8 MeV electrons are used, Perspex is needed to reduce the depth of penetration.

Dose

30 Gy in 6 fractions (once weekly) for 6 weeks

Side-effects. Temporary alopecia and loss of nails are followed by permanent skin atrophy, oedema and radiodermatis.

3. Chemotherapy. Combination chemotherapy with regimens such as CHOP (Table 29.7) is indicated for systemic disease. Complete response rates are low (20–25%) with high rates of relapse.

Results of treatment

Whilst the average survival is 5 years, patients with poor risk disease (with visceral involvement) fare much worse.

Overall results of treatment of non-Hodgkin lymphomas

The 10-year relapse-free survival is 50% for stages I and II low-grade NHL, and 30% for stages III and IV and those with patients with B symptoms. Cure is rarely achieved and relapse is common in all stages.

For high-grade stage Ia or IE NHL radiotherapy preceded by abbreviated chemotherapy is curative, with 80% 10-year relapse-free survival. For advanced disease a complete response is obtained in about 60% of cases, with long-term remission in 30–40%.

MULTIPLE MYELOMA

Multiple myeloma is a relatively common haematological malignancy, accounting for 0.9% of all cancers and 1.3% of cancer deaths. Its incidence is 3 per 100 000 per year. It tends to occur in late middle age. The median age at diagnosis is 62 years. The male to female sex ratio is 1.5 : 1 The aetiology is unknown. Genetic factors may play a significant role since in the USA the incidence of the disease in Blacks is twice that of Whites. Exposure to alpha particles may be a risk factor since myeloma developed in higher than the expected proportion of the survivors of the atomic bombs dropped on Japan in 1945.

Pathology

Myeloma is a plasma cell tumour of B lymphocyte lineage, usually originating in the bone marrow. Plasma cells are immunoglobulin-producing cells. Each immunoglobulin (Fig. 29.8) is composed of heavy and light chains. The neoplastic proliferation of plasma cells is thought to arise from a single cell (monoclonal). It leads to marrow destruction and failure and also to local destruction of bone. For this reason it is often classified with bone tumours.

There are four main types of myeloma:

1. Multiple myeloma (the commonest)
2. Solitary myeloma of bone (plasmacytoma)
3. Extramedullary myeloma
4. Plasma cell leukaemia.

Multiple myeloma is a generalised disease affecting many bones in its course. Rarely myeloma may be confined to one or two bones only (plasmacytoma). Extramedullary myeloma is even rarer and most often occurs in the upper respiratory tract, followed in decreasing order of frequency by the lymph nodes and spleen, skin and gastrointestinal tract.

Paraprotein production

Myeloma cells produce abnormal immunoglobulins (paraproteins) in 95% of cases. They are usually detectable in the blood as a monoclonal band on protein electrophoresis (Fig. 29.7). When light chains are produced in excess they are found in the urine as Bence Jones protein. These are parts of or whole immunoglobulin molecules (Fig. 29.8).

The incidence of the different types of these pathological immunoglobulins (Ig) is proportionate to that in the healthy subject (IgG 50–60%, IgA 20–25%, light chain only 20%, IgD 2%, IgE and IgM < 1%). The

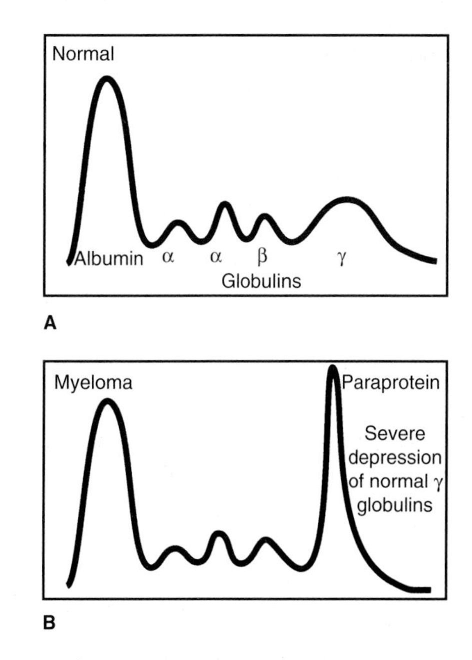

Fig. 29.7 Serum protein electrophoresis from **A** a normal individual and **B** a patient with myeloma. (Reproduced with permission from Souhami and Moxham, Textbook of Medicine, Churchill Livingstone, 1990.)

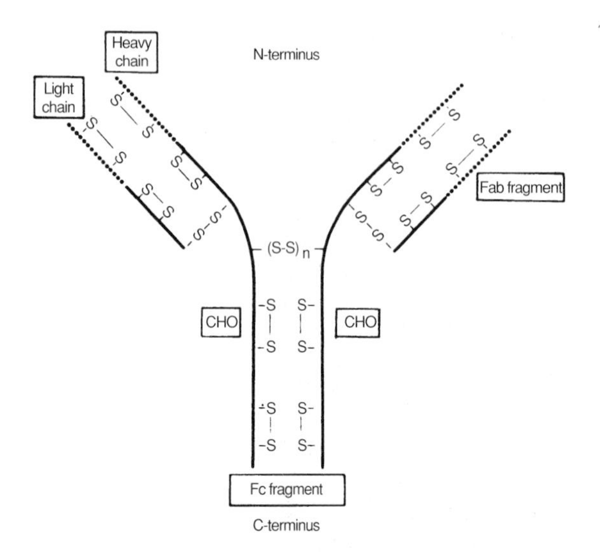

Fig. 29.8 Immunoglobulin molecule. (Reproduced with permission of Arnold from K. E. Halnan, *Treatment of Cancer*, 1/e, Chapman and Hall, 1982.)

paraprotein production can be quantified and changes measured in response to treatment.

In 5% of cases no paraprotein is detectable. This is the *non-secretory* type. In the rare cases in which there is abnormal production of immunoglobulins D and E, they may fail to be detected by conventional techniques.

Natural history

This is very variable. The first abnormality detected may be the presence of a monoclonal band on protein electrophoresis (Fig. 29.7) many years before any clinical or radiological abnormality. This may remain static or rise slowly over many years or rapidly over a 1–3 year period.

In some patients the disease may have an indolent course, remaining localised for many years to a single bone (solitary plasmacytoma). It may subsequently disseminate in about 50% of cases. In others the disease has a much more aggressive course with death within a year. High levels of paraprotein production result in plugging of the renal tubules and, if unresponsive to treatment, death within a few months from kidney failure.

Clinical features

The commonest presenting feature is bone pain (70%), usually from a rib or a vertebra. The destruction of cortical bone leads to pathological fractures in about 25% and hypercalcaemia in 30%. Fewer patients (12%) present with infection and with bleeding (7%). Spinal cord compression is occasionally the presenting feature. Most patients are anaemic. A third have evidence of myelosuppression with reduced white cell count and/or platelets.

If the paraprotein level is high enough a *hyperviscosity syndrome* develops. This is characterised by visual impairment, lethargy and coma.

Soft tissue lesions (lymph nodes, spleen or liver) are uncommon at presentation.

Diagnosis

Two or more of the following features must be present to fulfil the diagnosis:

- Serum or urine paraprotein
- Plasma cell infiltration of the bone marrow (> 20%)
- Typical radiological lesions (osteolytic deposits in the axial skeleton and ribs).

Occasionally the diagnosis is not clear cut. For example the patient may have a modest level of paraprotein, a small increase in plasma cells in the bone marrow (< 5%) and no radiological lesions. In such cases close observation is necessary to detect the development of other diagnostic features. Not all paraproteinaemias are malignant. The incidence of paraproteinaemias rises with age. It is 1% over 25 years, 3% over the age of 70 years and 25% over 90 years. For the most part they have a benign course. However, about 20–25% of cases of paraproteinaemia diagnosed in hospital will develop multiple myeloma if followed up for 10 years, and 40% at 15 years. Paraproteinaemia is a not uncommon feature of lymphoma.

Other investigations are designed to detect common sites of metastatic spread:

1. Full blood count (anaemia, leucopenia, thrombocytopenia from marrow infiltration)
2. Serum urea, creatinine and electrolytes (renal impairment from myelomatous infiltration, nephrotic syndrome, hypercalcaemia, amyloid)
3. Serum calcium (hypercalcaemia)
4. Serum electrophoresis (monoclonal paraprotein band) often accompanied by a reduction of immunoglobulins (immune paresis)
5. Bone marrow examination (excess plasma cells)
6. Skeletal survey (lytic lesions, especially skull (Fig. 29.9), ribs and vertebrae, or diffuse osteoporosis).

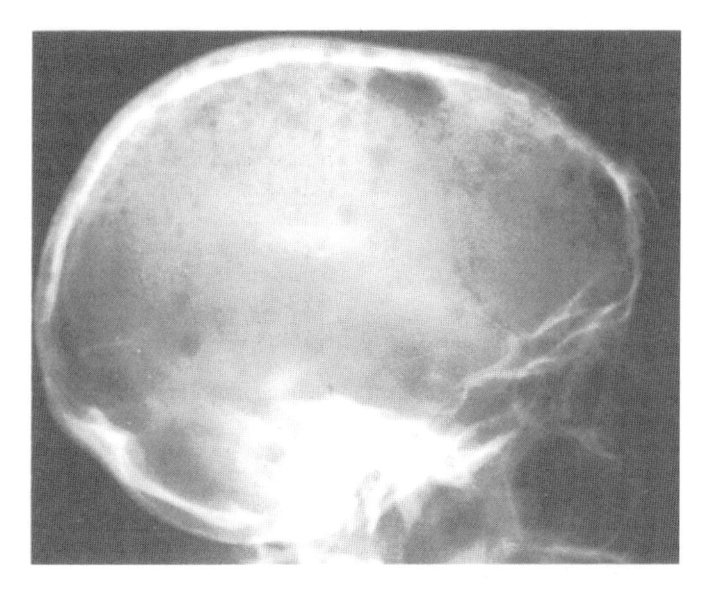

Fig. 29.9 Skull radiograph showing typical lytic lesions. (Courtesy of Prof. M Greaves, Aberdeen.)

Prognostic factors

Certain factors confer a poor prognosis in myeloma. These are:

1. Presenting haemoglobin < 8.5 g/dl
2. Hypercalcaemia (> 3 mmol/l)
3. Blood urea > 12 mmol/l (after correction of dehydration)
4. Poor performance status.

Treatment

Multiple myeloma

There is at present no curative therapy for the majority of patients with multiple myeloma. Treatment is aimed at alleviating symptoms, controlling the advance of the disease and preventing complications. The main forms of treatment are cytotoxic therapy and palliative radiotherapy. Recent trials have focussed on the role of high dose chemotherapy (usually melphalan) with peripheral blood stem cell rescue.

Cytotoxic therapy. Cytotoxic therapy is the only form of therapy known to prolong survival in multiple myeloma. One of the commonest initial regimens for multiple myeloma is:

Oral melphalan 7 mg/m^2 and prednisolone (1 mg/kg) daily for 4 days every 3 weeks

The addition of prednisolone to melphalan increases the response rate but survival is not improved. This combination of drugs results in approximately 50–75% reduction in the level of paraprotein in about half the patients treated. Average survival is 2–3 years.

Whether more aggressive combinations of chemotherapy prolong survival more than melphalan and prednisolone is debatable. Comparison of different combinations has been limited by different criteria of response. The Medical Research Council in its fifth myeloma trial showed that a combination (ABCM) of a 6-weekly regimen of: doxorubicin, BCNU, cyclophosphamide and melphalan had a significant survival advantage over intermittent melphalan alone. 2-year survival on ABCM is about 60%. The complete response rate is 7%; 20% of the complete responders will subsequently relapse. However, other studies have not shown unequivocal benefit of combination alkylating agent therapy over melphalan alone.

Higher doses of intravenous melphalan can achieve higher response rates (up to nearly 80%) but with greater treatment-related mortality and morbidity. Such treatment should only be undertaken in specialised units by experienced staff.

Supportive measures. *Pain* control is important. Opiates are usually required. Palliative radiotherapy, either localised or hemibody irradiation, is effective (see below).

Hypercalcaemia is treated by intravenous hydration and bisphosphonates.

Hyperviscosity, if causing significant symptoms and signs, is treated by plasmapheresis. In this process some of the patient's plasma is replaced by an appropriate colloid solution (usually albumin) to reduce the level of paraprotein.

Renal failure may require dialysis.

Infection due to neutropenia and immune paresis should be vigorously treated.

Criteria of response. The following criteria of a response are widely accepted. All should be fulfilled:

1. A reduction in paraprotein level to 50% or less.
2. If urinary paraprotein > 1 g/24 h, a reduction to 50% or less; if 0.5–1 g/24 h, a fall to less than 0.1 g/24 h.
3. Healing of radiological lesions.
4. More than 50% reduction of the plasmacytoma radiologically or by clinical measurement in the product of the two largest dimensions.

A complete response is defined as the absence of detectable paraprotein or urinary light chains and normalisation of the bone marrow with < 5% plasma cells.

Most patients reach a plateau of response. Maintenance therapy after a plateau phase of 6 months is unnecessary. Further response after 6–12 months of melphalan and prednisolone is uncommon. Complete response with disappearance of paraprotein is rare. Most patients improve symptomatically with chemotherapy, although lytic bone lesions do not usually heal. Of the 7% of patients who achieve a complete response to chemotherapy, 20% will relapse.

Relapse. If the disease does relapse after an initial period of a detectable but stable paraprotein level (plateau phase), a response may be obtained with further courses of melphalan. The paraprotein level may be stabilised again, but at a higher level. However, the duration of subsequent plateau phases tends to be short-lived. High-dose melphalan is less successful in relapsed disease than in untreated patients. Complete response rates of the order of 20% are obtainable but at the cost of considerable myelosuppression and gastrointestinal toxicity.

Allogeneic transplantation. The value and ideal timing of allogeneic transplantation in myeloma has yet to be established. Its applicability is limited by donor availability and the intolerance of the elderly of the morbidity of treatment. It is most effective when the tumour burden is small, for example when the first plateau phase has been reached. In future it may have a role at an early stage of the disease in selected patients with poor prognostic factors.

Interferon. Alpha-interferon appears to have some activity against myeloma, particularly in untreated patients. However, its efficacy is inferior to conventional cytotoxic therapy. Preliminary encouraging results of its combination with conventional chemotherapy still require confirmation. Lethargy is a common side-effect.

Palliative radiotherapy. Palliative radiotherapy has a useful role in the relief of pain from bony deposits, pathological fractures and spinal cord compression.

Bone deposits and pathological fractures. Patients may develop many painful bony deposits over the course of their illness. Pain often flits from one site to another, making the assessment of which sites to irradiate difficult. A new site of pain often emerges shortly after the last one has been irradiated. In addition, movement on and off the treatment couch may be limited by pain. For this reason prolonged fractionation should, if possible, be avoided. Single fractions using a single orthovoltage field or, for deeper-seated lesions, megavoltage is used. Longer fractionation is desirable in some circumstances, for example to the lower dorsal spine to avoid duodenal upset or for spinal cord compression.

Spinal cord compression. This may occur at any stage of the disease. It may be due to extradural disease rather than a collapsed vertebra. If the diagnosis of myeloma has been previously established surgical decompression is unnecessary since it is very radiosensitive. When, however, cord compression is the presenting feature of the disease, emergency laminectomy and biopsy are required to establish a histological diagnosis.

The management of spinal cord compression is as described in Chapter 30.

Dose and energy

Multiple myeloma

Rib deposits: 7 Gy single fraction at orthovoltage
Lower dorsal and cervical spine and pathological fractures: 20 Gy in 5 daily fractions over a week (250–300 kV or 4–6 MV photons)

Spinal cord compression: 20–25 Gy at the depth of the cord in 5 daily fractions over a week (4–6 MV photons)

Solitary plasmacytoma

For solitary myeloma, radical radiotherapy should be delivered to eliminate the local malignant plasma cell population. If the paraproteinaemia persists, chemotherapy should follow.

Target volume

Spine. The target volume should include the affected vertebral body and one normal vertebral body above and below. The scar from a laminectomy should be included.

Technique

This will vary with the site. For the spine a direct megavoltage field in the lumbar region (avoiding the kidneys) or a posterior oblique wedged pair (Fig. 29.10) in the cervical and thoracic region is usually adequate. Where there are multiple painful deposits in one or both halves of the body, hemibody irradiation may provide good palliation. The toxicity of treating the upper half of the body is greater, owing to radiation pneumonitis.

Dose and energy

Dose greater than 45 Gy over 4½ weeks using 4–6 MV photons should be used

Hemibody irradiation. Patients with progressive myeloma frequently develop widespread painful bony deposits, too numerous to encompass with single fields and often difficult to localise. In these circumstances, either the upper or lower half of the body can be encompassed in a single megavoltage field (9–10 MV photons) at extended SSD (e.g. 140 cm). This should be carried out on an inpatient basis.

Treatment of the other half of the body is carried out 4–6 weeks later, depending on general condition, response to treatment of the first hemibody irradiation and a satisfactory blood count (white cell count $\geq 2.0 \times 10^9/l$, platelets $\geq 60 \times 10^9/l$).

Preparation. To reduce radiation-induced nausea and vomiting, 5-HT_3 antagonists are administered shortly before treatment.

Target volume

1. *Lower half.* The field for the lower half extends from just below the 12th rib to just above the knee joints. The upper limit of the field should be tattooed to avoid overlap if the upper half is to be treated.

2. *Upper half.* The field extends from the vertex of the skull or the clavicles (if the eyes are to be avoided) to the level of the 12th rib in the midclavicular line. Because of the risk of pneumonitis, the dose to the upper half is less than to the lower half. If the skull is included the mouth should be shielded to avoid oral mucositis.

Dose and energy

Lower half: 8 Gy in a single fraction (9–10 MV photons)
Upper half: 6–8 Gy in a single fraction (9–10 MV photons)

Side-effects. About 30% of patients develop nausea and vomiting within a few hours of treatment. Regular antiemetics are necessary. When the lower half is treated, diarrhoea occurs in a third of patients 3–5 days after radiotherapy. This is controllable with antidiarrhoeal agents. Anaemia, leucopenia and thrombocytopenia are common. Blood transfusion may be required. The white count normally recovers by 6 weeks. The platelet count takes on average 10 days longer than the white count to recover.

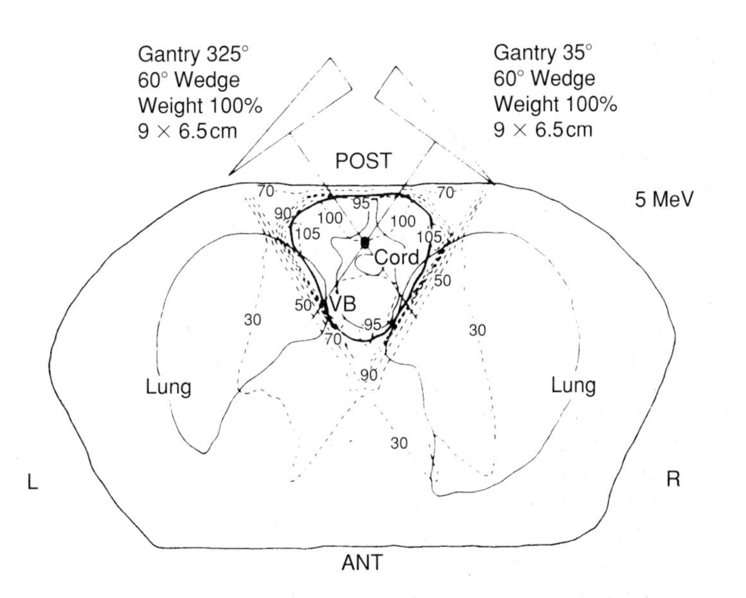

Fig. 29.10 Posterior oblique wedged pair of fields to treat tumour of vertebral body (VB). (Reproduced with permission of Arnold from Jane Dobbs, Ann Barrett, Daniel Ash, *Practical Radiotherapy Planning*, 3/e, Arnold, 1999.)

Response. Prompt pain relief is achieved in most patients.

Overall survival

About 50% of patients will survive 2 years. For patients with poor prognostic factors, 2-year survival is 10%, and, with a good prognosis, 75%.

LEUKAEMIA

Leukaemia encompasses a group of diseases characterised by the uncontrolled accumulation of malignant leucopoietic tissue in the bone marrow and peripheral blood. It accounts for 2.1% of all cancers and 2.6% of cancer deaths. The sex ratio is 1.5 : 1 in favour of males.

Pathology

Classification

Leukaemia is divided into two main subgroups, acute and chronic:

1. Acute
   a. Lymphoblastic (ALL)
   b. Myeloblastic (AML)
2. Chronic
   a. Lymphocytic (CLL)
   b. Myeloid (granulocytic) (CML).

Aetiology

In most cases the cause of leukaemia is not known; however, there are both acquired and genetic causes.

Acquired. With the exception of CLL, the other types of leukaemia can be induced by relatively high doses of ionising radiation. Typically this occurs 3–10 years following exposure. Evidence for this is:

1. Survivors of the atom bomb explosions at Hiroshima and Nagasaki showed a 20-fold increase as compared with the unirradiated population.
2. Patients irradiated for ankylosing spondylitis have a 10-fold increase in incidence.

One form of acute T cell leukaemia which occurs predominantly in the West Indies and in southern Japan is caused by the human T cell leukaemia virus (HTLV–1).

Some industrial chemicals, of which benzene is the main culprit, induce acute leukaemia (mainly AML).

Cytotoxic drugs, especially the alkylating agents, can induce leukaemia, particularly when given in conjunction with radiation. The risk at 10 years of developing leukaemia (mainly AML) in patients who receive MOPP chemotherapy for Hodgkin's disease varies from 3 to 13%. Current evidence suggests that there is no synergistic effect between chemotherapy and radiation in increasing the risk of leukaemia, except when the radiation fields are large.

Major chromosomal abnormalities in the form of deletions or translocations are seen in many cases of leukaemia.

Genetic. Children with Down's syndrome account for the majority of genetic cases. The increase in leukaemia is 20-fold. Much rarer causes, such as ataxia telangiectasia predispose to ALL and Fanconi's anaemia to AML.

White blood cells are either of lymphoid or myeloid origin. Any of them may undergo malignant change. Virtually all leukaemias are derived from a single clone of cells. In acute leukaemia primitive cells, blasts, are found in the bone marrow and in the peripheral blood. In the chronic forms more differentiated but still abnormal lymphoid and myeloid cells are seen.

The normal process of transformation from primitive stem cells into mature adult cells is somehow disturbed and arrested, so that immature cells accumulate in the marrow and enter the circulation in large numbers, to give the typical peripheral blood picture. The marrow becomes filled with leukaemic cells which displace other components—red cells (causing anaemia) and platelets (causing bleeding tendency).

Resistance to infection is lowered because of the immaturity of the white cells. Death is usually due to infection in association with bone marrow failure.

ACUTE LEUKAEMIA

Acute leukaemia may be of lymphoid, myeloid or other type, but the clinical picture is similar in all. ALL constitutes 80% of childhood cases and AML 80% of adult cases. AML may occur at any age but mainly in middle age and in the elderly. The clinical features of ALL and AML are comparable. They are described in Chapter 32.

Acute monocytic leukaemia

Acute monocytic leukaemia is a subgroup of acute myeloid leukaemia. It accounts for 10% of leukaemia. It is commonest over the age of 30. Swollen painful gums are more common in this form of leukaemia than in other types. Treatment is on the same lines as acute myeloid leukaemia.

Treatment of AML

Most current regimens consist of combinations of daunorubicin, cytosine, thioguanine and etoposide. Remission is achieved in approximately 80% of patients under the age of 40 and 50–60% over that age. Once a remission has been achieved, several further courses are given as *consolidation* therapy. *Maintenance* therapy is not considered to be of value.

Bone marrow transplantation

If the patient is below the age of 45 and has a histocompatibility antigen (HLA)-matched sibling as a bone marrow donor, bone marrow transplantation is an option. Unfortunately only 1 in 4 patients have such a match.

The rationale for bone marrow transplantation is as follows. It allows higher doses of chemotherapy and radiotherapy than the bone marrow would tolerate if unsupported. The bone marrow depression induced by chemoradiotherapy is compensated for by the infusion of donor bone marrow.

Bone marrow (and more recently peripheral blood stem cell) grafts are of two types. The first and commonest is *allogeneic* transplantation in which bone marrow is taken from an immunologically compatible (HLA-matched) sibling. Allogeneic transplantation is the treatment of choice for patients with AML and an HLA compatible donor.

The second is *autologous* transplantation. In this case when the patient is in remission his/her bone marrow or peripheral blood stem cells are harvested and stored before more intensive chemotherapy is given. It is then reinfused after chemoradiotherapy to sustain the marrow. The advantage of autologous transplantation is that there is no immunological rejection of the marrow since it belongs to the patient. There is, however, the potential hazard of reinfusing leukaemic cells that may repopulate the bone marrow.

Procedure. In the first phase, bone marrow (500–1000 ml) is aspirated from the donor's iliac crests under general anaesthesia. The patient then receives high-dose chemotherapy (cyclophosphamide 100 mg/kg over 2 days) with total body irradiation (10 Gy) (see below) to eliminate residual tumour. The stored bone marrow is freshly infused via a Hickman central venous line into the recipient. Following chemoradiotherapy, the white cell and platelet counts drop within 10 days. They recover 3–6 weeks after the marrow transplant. Over this period supportive antibiotics, red cell and platelet transfusions are given. Blood products are irradiated to kill T lymphocytes which may precipitate graft-versus-host disease (GVHD). Immunodeficiency due to defects of T cell and B cell functions occurs during the first 6 months and for longer in the presence of GVHD. Viral, bacterial and fungal infections may be fatal.

The main problem of allogeneic transplantation is the immunological reaction that the donor marrow elicits in the host. This is known as *graft-versus-host disease*. It may be acute or chronic. The acute effects take place in the first 8 weeks following the graft. The features of acute and chronic GVHD are as follows:

Acute

- Cholestatic jaundice
- Skin rashes
- Diarrhoea and weight loss

Chronic

- Arthritis
- Hepatitis and chronic liver disease
- Malabsorption and weight loss
- Oral mucositis and sicca syndrome
- Restrictive and obstructive lung disease
- Pericardial and pleural effusions
- Scleroderma
- Skin rashes

Prevention of GVHD. Since GVHD has a high mortality, its prevention is important. Ciclosporin, usually in combination with methotrexate, is very effective.

Total body irradiation (TBI)

Technique

A variety of techniques are in use. Some centres have dedicated machines for wide-field irradiation. Others use linear accelerators at extended SSD (about 4 metres) with the patient in a semi-sitting position. In Sheffield adults are treated seated and children supine on a specially designed mobile couch (Fig. 29.11). Extended SSD is necessary to enable the whole patient to be encompassed within the photon beam directed at 90′ to the long axis of the patient. Typical field sizes are 40 × 40 cm. After half the treatment the patient is turned through 180° and the other side is treated.

Careful dosimetry is needed using thermoluminescent dosimeters (TLD) positioned at regular intervals along each side and the midline of the body. The positions of the TLD probes and typical TLD values are shown in Figure 29.12. In general, doses to the thinner structures, the neck, lungs and the lower legs tend to be higher. To obtain a more even dose distribution (i.e.

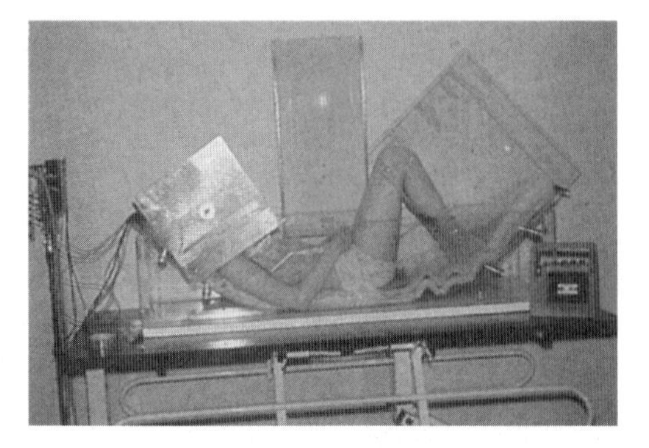

Fig. 29.11 Total body irradiation. Note tissue compensators over head and neck and below knee. (Courtesy of Dr K Dunn, Sheffield.)

less than 10% variation), compensators are placed lateral to the head and neck, thorax and lower leg. Typically, 8 mm, 1 mm and 6 mm brass compensators are placed over the head, neck and thorax respectively. Sheets of Perspex (3–10 mm) are placed lateral to the legs from the knees downward.

Dose and energy

14.4 Gy midplane dose in twice-daily fractions over 4 days (6 MV photons)

Side-effects

1. *Pneumonitis.* Since pneumonitis commonly occurs following bone marrow transplantation in the absence of radiation, the role of TBI in its causation is difficult to assess. In about half the cases there is an infectious cause. It is known, however, that lung damage is related both to total dose and to dose rate. Total doses above 8–9 Gy and dose rates above 0.05 Gy/min substantially increase the risk of lung damage. The incidence of pneumonitis is 50% for a total single TBI dose of 12 Gy given at low dose rate. This incidence is higher than might be predicted for the same dose given at higher dose rates. The explanation is probably that chemotherapy given at the same time reduces lung tolerance to irradiation.

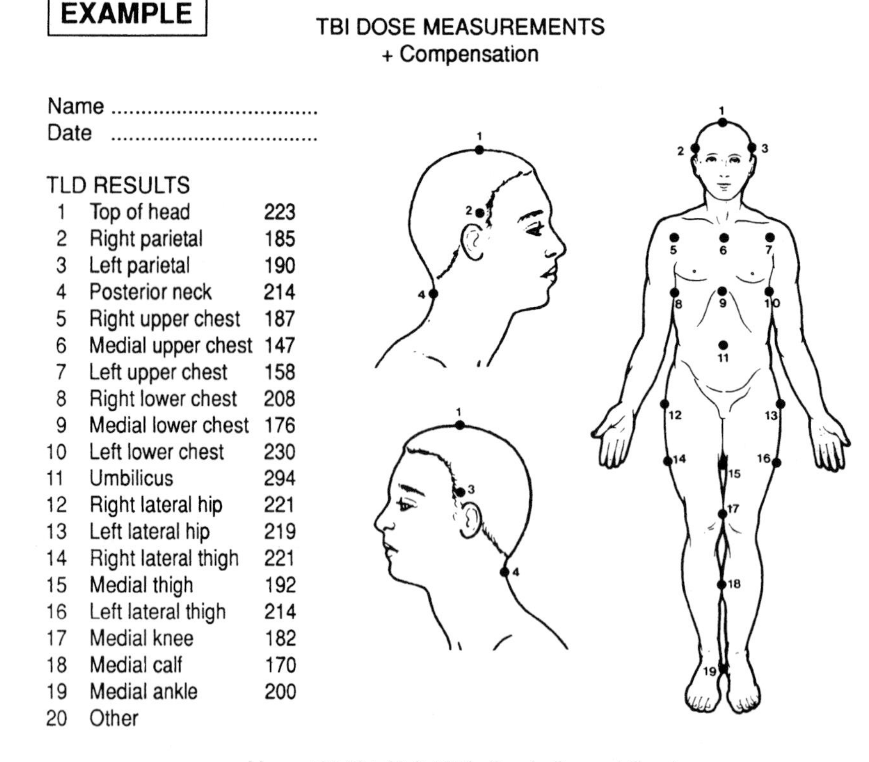

Fig. 29.12 Position for thermoluminescent dosimetry (TLD) measurements and typical doses for total body irradiation. (Courtesy of Dr J Conway, Sheffield.)

2. *Cataract*. The incidence of cataract varies with both dose and dose rate. At a dose rate of 0.02 Gy/min the incidence is about 20% between 3 and 6 years for single fraction irradiation. The incidence is similar for fractionated TBI. At 0.05–0.08 Gy/min for single-fraction TBI the incidence of cataract is 75% within 5 years. About 50% of patients with cataract need surgical treatment at some stage.

3. *Hepatic veno-occlusive disease*. Histologically confirmed veno-occlusive disease of the liver occurs in up to 25% of patients. In most patients symptoms are mild. However, the mortality of established disease is high (30%).

4. *Fertility*. In females the retention of ovarian function and fertility is related to age at the time of TBI and chemotherapy. Under the age of 25, periods are likely to return within 6 months of treatment. Over the age of 25, permanent sterility is likely.

In males puberty is delayed in two-thirds and most patients are rendered azoospermic. Sperm production is unlikely to recover. Sperm storage should be considered in all patients who are sexually mature.

5. *Hypothyroidism*. Hypothyroidism, of varying severity, occurs in up to 30% of patients. The commonest finding is compensated hypothyroidism (i.e. raised TSH and normal T4). Thyroid hormone replacement may be required.

6. *Growth delay*. Growth hormone secretion may be impaired, especially if previous cranial irradiation has been given.

7. *Second malignancy*. This may very rarely occur (0.2%).

Radiotherapy

Local radiotherapy is useful for relieving the pain of skin, bony or retro-orbital deposits.

Technique

Single fields are used for skin, retro-orbital and most bone deposits. Parallel opposed lateral fields are used for gums and some bone deposits.

Dose and energy

Megavoltage or cobalt-60 (eye, bone, gums); superficial (skin) or orthovoltage (skin, bone).

5 Gy in single fraction to bone and skin deposits and in two daily fractions to eye or gums

Results of treatment

About 25% of patients with AML who achieve a complete remission and undergo further intensive chemotherapy are cured. If relapse occurs during chemotherapy, the probability of achieving a second remission is small. However, if relapse occurs more than 6 months after treatment, a second remission can be induced in more than 50% of such patients.

CHRONIC MYELOID (GRANULOCYTIC) LEUKAEMIA

Chronic myeloid (granulocytic) leukaemia (abbreviated to CGL or CML) occurs mainly in the fifth and sixth decades. The incidence in the UK is 1 in 100 000. There is a slight male predominance (1.4 : 1).

A diagnostic feature is the presence of an abnormal chromosome 22, the *Philadelphia chromosome*. The long arm of chromosome 22 is translocated usually to chromosome 9 but occasionally to other chromosomes. It is present in over 90% of cases.

The typical picture is the insidious onset of progressive tiredness due to anaemia, with gross splenomegaly. The latter may cause a dragging sensation in the abdomen or acute pain if splenic infarction has occurred. The spleen may reach a huge size, filling the whole of the abdomen. Lymph nodes are not usually enlarged. Skin infiltration occurs rarely. The blood count shows a total white cell count typically between 100 and 500 × 10^9/1, of which 20–25% are myelocytes. Anaemia is often mild. The platelet count is normal or raised. The bone marrow is hypercellular.

The course of most of the illness is indolent (*chronic phase*). However, eventually it transforms, on average after 3.5 years, to an *accelerated phase* and death. The accelerated phase is characterised by the presence of immature blast cells in the marrow. In most cases these are of myeloid type but in 20% they are lymphoid.

Treatment

1. Chronic phase

The aim of treatment is palliative in most patients. No treatment is needed if the patient's general condition is satisfactory and haemoglobin and white cell count are at reasonable levels. Indications for treatment are:

- Anaemia
- High platelet count
- High white cell count
- Uncomfortable splenomegaly.

Allopurinol (300 mg daily orally) should be given to prevent gout, particularly if the serum urate is raised.

Chemotherapy with alkylating agents (e.g. busulfan) in low dosage is given to improve the blood count and reduce the size of the spleen. It is aimed to keep the white count at 10–15 × 10^9/1. Hydroxycarbamide (hydroxyurea) is an alternative to busulfan. The advantage of hydroxycarbamide is that its effects are reversible.

Dose: Busulfan oral 2–6 mg daily; hydroxycarbamide (hydroxyurea) oral 1–2 g daily.

Care must be taken not to overtreat, reducing the white count to dangerous levels where infection may be life-threatening. This is a particular risk with busulfan owing to its prolonged action (the nadir of the white count occurring at 4 weeks). For this reason busulfan is usually stopped when the white count reaches 20 × 10^9/1.

If clinical features of the hyperviscosity syndrome (p. 526) develop, leucopheresis is advised until chemotherapy has reduced the production of white cells.

Alpha-interferon has been shown to be effective in the control of a high white cell count and splenomegaly but whether it prolongs the chronic phase is as yet unproven.

Another promising agent is ST1571 (Glivec), a specific inhibitor of ABL tyrosine kinase.

Bone marrow (or peripheral blood stem cell) transplantation. Allogeneic transplantation should be considered for patients under the age of 45 with a compatible sibling donor.

2. Accelerated phase

The results of treatment of the accelerated phase in which myeloblasts appear are so poor that the clinician may decide not to offer chemotherapy. Hydroxycarbamide (hydroxyurea) or thioguanine may keep the blast cell numbers in check. For lymphoid transformation, the chances of obtaining a further remission with re-establishment of a second chronic phase are better. The drugs used are the same as for acute lymphocytic leukaemia (Ch. 32). If a remission is induced, craniospinal prophylaxis with intrathecal methotrexate and cranial irradiation are given.

Radiotherapy

CML is a very radiosensitive disease. In the past, radioactive phosphorus-32 was used but has been replaced by chemotherapy. Irradiation still has a useful role for: (1) uncomfortable splenomegaly uncontrolled by chemotherapy, (2) myeloblastomas (local tumours composed of acute myeloblastic leukaemic cells), and (3) prophylactic cranial irradiation (in lymphoblastic transformation).

Spleen

Treatment volume

Irradiation of the whole of the spleen is not necessary to achieve shrinkage and symptomatic benefit. Splenic irradiation can be repeated if necessary, but eventually resistance develops.

Technique

Direct anterior or lateral fields (e.g. 15 × 10 cm) are used.

Dose and energy

0.25 Gy per day, increasing by 0.25 Gy per day up to 1.5–2 Gy daily to a total dose of 3 Gy (cobalt-60 or 4–6 MV photons)

Myeloblastomas. Single fractions of 5 Gy or 10 Gy by single or parallel-opposed fields depending on site.

Prophylactic cranial irradiation. For patients who develop lymphoid transformation in the accelerated phase and achieve a second remission, prophylactic cranial irradiation is given. Technique and dosage are as described for ALL (Ch. 32).

Results of treatment

Average survival is about 3–4 years. With bone marrow transplantation in the chronic phase, 50% are disease free at 4 years. This figure falls to 12% for patients transplanted in the accelerated phase.

CHRONIC LYMPHATIC (LYMPHOCYTIC) LEUKAEMIA

This disease is grouped both with the leukaemias and with low-grade non-Hodgkin lymphomas. Its incidence in the UK is 2 per 100 000. The male to female sex ratio is 2 : 1. It is usually seen in middle age.

The onset is insidious with tiredness from anaemia. Rapid onset of anaemia often indicates the development of an autoimmune haemolytic anaemia. Enlargement of lymph nodes of the neck and other peripheral sites (including the epitrochlear nodes at the elbow), spleen and liver is common. The spleen does not reach the large size of the chronic myeloid variety. Infiltration of the skin rarely occurs. Sometimes the entire skin is reddened and thickened (generalised leukaemic erythroderma).

The white cell count is raised usually between 30–300 × 10^9/1; 5–99% are small lymphocytes. In about 25% the diagnosis is made as an incidental finding on a blood count done for other reasons. As the disease advances, CLL may undergo prolymphocytoid immunoblastic change. 'Smudge' cells, which are cells that have been ruptured when making the blood film, are commonly seen. The platelet count is only markedly reduced in the terminal phase of the illness. The bone marrow is hypercellular with 30–90% of the cells being of the lymphoid series. Biopsy of enlarged nodes shows infiltration with small lymphocytes.

The course of the disease is usually slowly progressive.

Treatment

Treatment is only indicated if the patient has symptoms or if critical organs are involved by the disease (e.g. renal tract obstruction from enlarged para-aortic nodes).

Chemotherapy

Chemotherapy with chlorambucil is normally the initial treatment.

Dose: 2–10 mg per day orally. It is not necessary to achieve a complete response and treatment may be discontinued after a few months.

Steroids are helpful if the patient is thrombocytopenic or has an autoimmune haemolytic anaemia. The dose is gradually reduced if there is a response and eventually discontinued.

Dose: prednisolone oral (5–40 mg daily).

Fludarabine is useful in relapsed disease.

Radiotherapy

If there is no response to chemotherapy, local radiotherapy to bulky tumour is indicated.

Technique

This will very with site. An anterior and posterior parallel-opposed pair of fields is suitable for axillary nodes. For the neck and groin, depending on the depth of the nodes, a single orthovoltage field may suffice.

Dose and energy

20 Gy in 4 daily fractions (250–300 kV, cobalt-60 or 4–6 MV photons)

Results of treatment

5-year survival of CLL is about 50% but patients presenting with advanced disease may live for less than a year.

POLYCYTHAEMIA RUBRA VERA, PRIMARY POLYCYTHAEMIA

Polycythaemia rubra vera (PCRV) is an uncommon disease of the bone marrow, occurring mainly between the ages of 50 and 65 years. It is slightly more common in men than women. There is hyperplasia of all of the marrow constituents—erythroblastic, leucoblastic and megakaryocytic—i.e. the precursors of red and white cells and platelets, which are all increased in the peripheral blood. The aetiology is unknown.

Clinical features

The clinical picture is dominated by the greatly increased number of red cells in the peripheral circulation (hence the name), but there may eventually be complete marrow exhaustion (aplastic anaemia), or the erythroblastic tissue may be exhausted first and the leucoblastic proliferation continue, leading to leukaemia.

The patient complains of headache, dizziness and tiredness, and has a cyanosed plethoric appearance. Pruritus occurs, particularly on exposure to heat or cold.

The spleen is palpable in 75% of patients at presentation. The increase in red cell volume increases the viscosity leading to thromboses (especially in brain, heart and limbs) and to haemorrhages. Other complications include peptic ulceration (10%), myelofibrosis, hyperuricaemia (30%) and gout (10%). Late leukaemic transformation develops rarely, either as a feature of the disease or due to treatment with radioactive phosphorus (see below).

Diagnosis

Typically the red cell count is raised (over 5.5×10^{12}/l in men and 5.0×10^{12}/l in women). The haemoglobin concentration is usually above 18 g/dl in men and 17 g/dl in women. The packed cell volume is normally in excess of 0.55 in men and 0.52 in women.

Other causes of polycythaemia must be excluded before making the diagnosis. Secondary polycythaemia can occur from the stimulus of hypoxia at high altitudes, in congenital heart disease and certain lung diseases (e.g. chronic obstructive airways disease and pulmonary fibrosis). It may also occur in association with renal lesions, especially renal adenocarcinoma.

True polycythaemia should be distinguished from spurious or stress polycythaemia in which raised haematocrit is due to a depleted plasma compartment. The mechanism is unknown, but it commonly occurs in overweight males who smoke and drink heavily.

Treatment

The aim is to produce prolonged reduction in the red cell volume to a fairly normal level. This may be achieved by (a) venesection (b) chemotherapy and (c) radiation.

Venesection

Venesection reduces the blood volume rapidly. 500 ml of blood may be removed initially and this affords quick symptomatic relief. A further 500 ml can be withdrawn 24 hours later and then every 48 hours until the packed cell volume reaches less than 0.50. The effect of venesection is temporary since it does not correct the defect in the bone marrow. It may be useful, e.g. before an operation, to reduce the risk of thrombosis. When the plasma viscosity has been controlled by venesection, treatment with chemotherapy (usually with busulfan) or radioactive phosphorus is needed.

Cytotoxic therapy

Cytotoxic therapy can be given in short courses. Busulfan in a dose of 4–6 mg daily for 4–6 weeks is recommended. Busulfan has a very prolonged action. Care is necessary to ensure that the drug is stopped if the platelet count falls below 120×10^9/l. Chlorambucil (4–10 mg daily) and melphalan (2–4 mg daily) are alternatives. However, they carry a higher risk of inducing leukaemia than busulfan or radioactive phosphorus. More recently, hydroxycarbamide (hydroxyurea) has been used extensively. This requires continuous oral therapy but may carry a lesser leukaemogenic risk.

Radioactive phosphorus (phosphorus-32)

Radioactive phosphorus (phosphorus-32) has the advantage that it is simple to administer and requires less frequent monitoring by blood counts than chemotherapy. It is given as an intravenous injection, usually as a phosphate salt. It is a beta emitter with a maximum energy of 1.7 MeV. Its physical half-life is 14.3 days and its biological half-life approximately 11 days.

Phosphorus is an essential constituent of all cells, especially of nuclei, and is therefore taken up to a greater extent in rapidly dividing than in slowly dividing cells.

It should be reserved for patients who are elderly or relatively immobile since the risk of leukaemogenesis is smaller and the likelihood of death from other causes greater in old age.

Phosphorus-32 is drawn up behind a Perspex protective screen (to absorb the beta rays). Protective goggles and gloves are worn. Absorbent paper lines the tray on which the phosphorus-32 is dispensed to minimise contamination from accidental spillage. The syringe used to draw up the phosphorus-32 is also protected by an additional outer covering of Perspex.

Dose

111–185 MBq as a single injection according to weight and the severity of the condition

A total dose of more than 1100 MBq is avoided to reduce the risk of inducing leukaemia.

Haematological effects

The maximum effect on the white cells and platelets occurs 3 weeks later. The red cell count falls at 6–8 weeks. The dose can be repeated if necessary at 3-monthly intervals depending on clinical and haematological findings. About 85% of patients go into remission, mostly after a single injection. A remission once achieved may last several years.

The risk of inducing acute non-lymphocytic leukaemia is 3–4% and rises with the total dose of phosphorus-32.

Results of treatment

Without treatment the average survival is about 5 years. With treatment this is doubled. The end comes with marrow failure, leukaemia, thrombosis, haemorrhage or heart failure.

CHAPTER CONTENTS

30

Central nervous system, eye and orbit

Ian Kunkler

TUMOURS OF THE CENTRAL NERVOUS SYSTEM

Anatomy

A knowledge of neuroanatomy (Fig 30.1) is important in appreciating the site of origin of different tumours of the central nervous system (CNS) (Fig. 30.2).

Epidemiology and aetiology

Tumours of the CNS are uncommon, accounting for 1.7% of all cancers and 1.8% of cancer deaths. They occur in both adults and children. The male : female ratio is 1.4 : 1. Benign tumours can be as clinically important as malignant ones, because, as space-occupying masses within the rigid skull, they can cause pressure symptoms and may be fatal if vital brain centres are compressed.

The only two definite aetiological factors in the development of brain tumours are exposure to ionising radiation and immunosuppression. Low dose irradiation given in the past to children to treat ringworm of the scalp (tinea capitis) increased the risk of meningiomas tenfold and gliomas threefold. Higher dose irradiation, e.g. for prophylactic cranial irradiation for acute lymphoblastic leukaemia, increases the risk of gliomas and sarcomas. Primary lymphomas of the CNS are increased in patients immunosuppressed by HIV disease or following T-cell-depleted allogeneic transplant.

A number of genetic conditions predispose to primary CNS tumours, including Von Recklinghausen's disease (type 1 neurofibromatosis), which is complicated by glioma in 15% of cases.

80% of CNS tumours are primary and 20% are secondary tumours from primary tumours elsewhere.

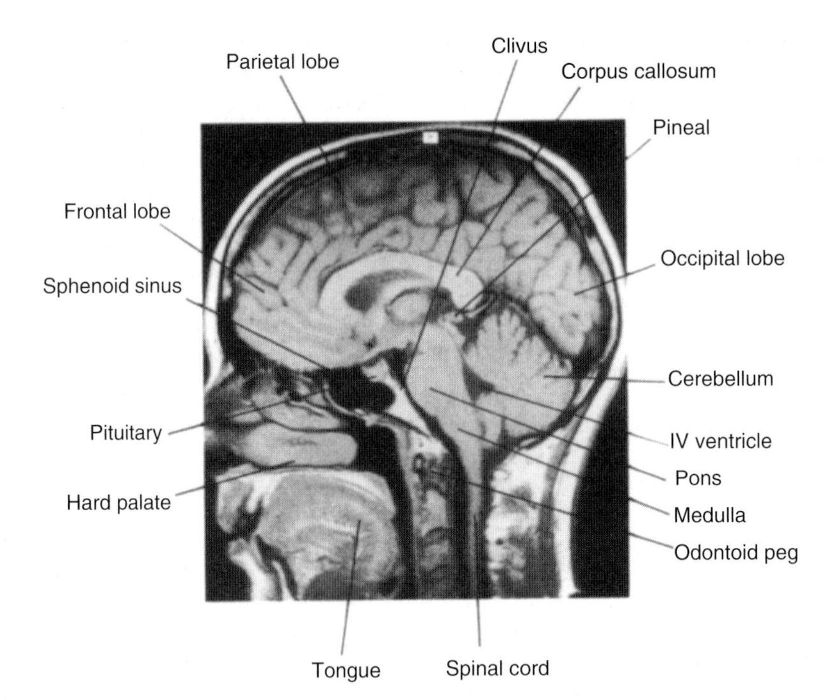

Fig. 30.1 Normal anatomy of the central nervous system. MRI midline sagittal section. (Courtesy of Dr L Turnbull, MRI Unit, Sheffield.)

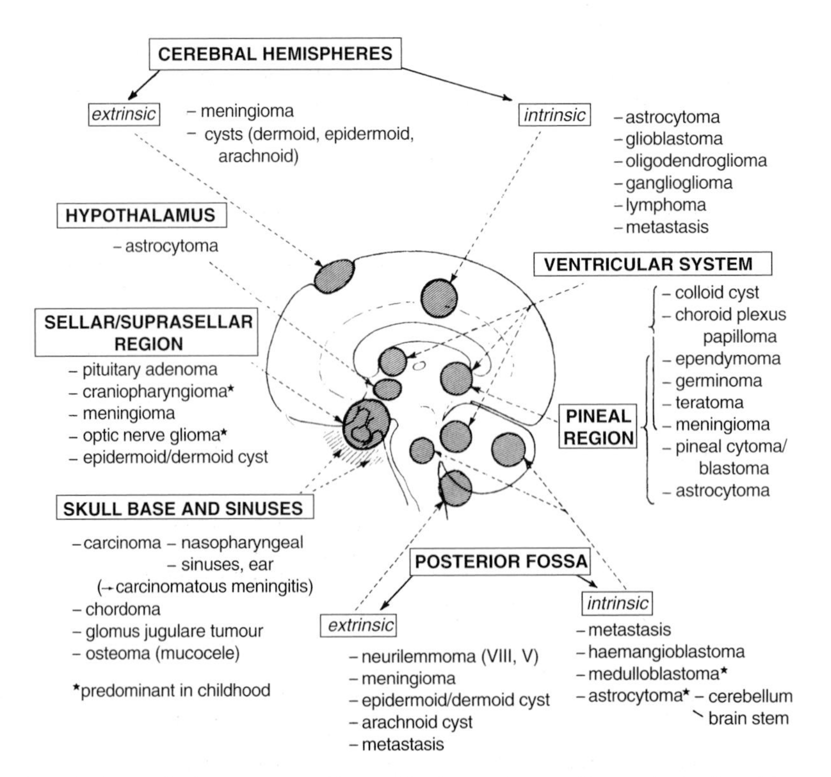

Fig. 30.2 Classification of intracranial tumours according to site. (Reproduced with permission from Lindsay et al, Neurology and Neurosurgery, Churchill Livingstone, 1991.)

Lung cancer accounts for 60% of metastases followed by breast (15%) and then a variety of tumours including urological (particularly kidney), colon, ovary, leukaemia and lymphoma. Metastases are usually multiple but occasionally solitary.

Pathology

Table 30.1 gives details of the chief histological types. It is noteworthy that none are tumours of actual nerve cells, but only of supporting tissues and glands. The central nervous system is composed of *neurons* and their processes surrounded by *glial cells*, composed of *microglia*, *oligodendrocytes* and *astrocytes*. In excess of 45% of intracranial tumours are *gliomas* (of glial origin). Gliomas are composed of *astrocytomas*, *ependymomas* and *oligodendrogliomas*. Microglial tumours are rare. *Astrocytomas* (75% of gliomas) have a wide spectrum of malignancy. The Kernohan grading system is commonly used. This ranges from relatively well differentiated (grades 1 and 2) to anaplastic (grade 3 and 4). The most malignant is *glioblastoma multiforme* (grade 4). Tumours can rarely occur in the choroid plexus as papillomas in the lateral ventricles in children and in the posterior fossa in adults. Gliomas may occasionally develop in the optic nerve, more commonly in children.

Oligodendrogliomas are less common (5% of gliomas) than astrocytomas. They occur almost exclusively in adults. Growth is slow but they may transform to a more aggressive tumour after many years. The frontal lobes are a common site. Calcification within the tumour is common and often seen on CT scanning. These tumours, unless anaplastic, tend not to enhance with contrast. The typical histological appearance is the presence of large round nuclei surrounded by clear cytoplasm, giving a 'halo' effect. Presentation is often with epilepsy, often many years before the development of focal neurological deficit.

Ependymomas are tumours arising from lining cells of the ventricles (typically the fourth ventricle), central canal of the spinal cord and the filum terminale. 50% are of low-grade malignancy. 60% of intracranial ependymomas are infratentorial. Tumours in the posterior fossa and high-grade tumours are more likely to spread to the CSF than are low-grade and supratentorial tumours. The most malignant ependymomas develop in children. There is a peak incidence at the age of 5 and a smaller peak at about the age of 35. The characteristic histological features are perivascular pseudorosettes (tumour cells lying radially around blood vessels) and ependymal rosettes (columnar cells lying around a central lumen). Definitive diagnosis can be made on electron microscopy when the cilia and microvilli of normal villi are found. Calcification is found in 15% of ependymomas, typically on CT scanning. Presentation is commonly with hydrocephalus due to obstruction of the fourth ventricle.

Medulloblastoma is a highly malignant tumour in children. It is rare in adults. It arises in the midline of the cerebellum from the floor of the fourth ventricle. The age of peak incidence is 4–10 years. The male to

Table 30.1 Tumours of the central nervous system

Tissue of origin	Histological type	Typical site and degree of malignancy	Incidence (%)
Neuroglia (connective tissue of CNS)	Astrocytoma	Commonest glioma Ranges from benign to highly malignant Adults: cerebral cortex Children: cerebellum	50
	Oligodendroglioma	Adults: cerebral cortex	
	Ependymoma	Children: ventricles, esp. 4th. Wide range of malignancy. Seeds via CSF	
Neuronal	Medulloblastoma	Children: cerebellum. Anaplastic, highly malignant. Seeds via CSF	
Meninges	Meningioma	Adults: benign. Malignancy rare	30
Pituitary gland	Chromophobe adenoma Eosinophil (acidophil) adenoma Basophil adenoma	Benign	12
Acoustic nerve	Acoustic neuroma	Benign, slowly growing	8
Pineal gland	Pinealoma	Mostly malignant, especially children Seeds via CSF	< 5
Blood vessels	Haemangioblastoma	Adults: malignant. Cerebellum	
Developmental anomaly	Craniopharyngioma	Benign (but can be fatal by pressure)	< 1

female ratio is 2 : 1. It may block the CSF pathway and cause hydrocephalus. It spreads to the cerebrospinal fluid and spinal cord. The typical histological appearance is of dense masses of small oval or round cells with a high number of mitoses. It may give rise to distant metastases, particularly to bone. Presentation is commonly with features of raised intracranial pressure, cerebellar signs and cranial nerve palsies.

Meningiomas are tumours, nearly always benign, arising from the arachnoid. They are attached to the meninges. Common sites are the parasagittal region, sphenoidal ridge and the olfactory groove. Peak incidence is at the age of 45. They may reach considerable size before they become symptomatic. They usually present with epilepsy before causing neurological deficit. Spread along the dura may result in cranial nerve deficit. They may stimulate an osteoblastic response in adjacent bone which can be seen on plain radiographs or CT scan.

Neurinomas are tumours arising from peripheral nerves. The commonest is the acoustic neuroma arising from the eighth cranial (acoustic) nerve. The main symptom is deafness.

There are some congenital tumours such as *craniopharyngiomas* and *chordomas*. Craniopharyngiomas are histologically benign tumours, developing from embryological remnants of Rathke's pouch in the area above the sella turcica (suprasellar), the recess enclosing the pituitary gland. They usually present in adolescence with endocrine dysfunction (diabetes insipidus, hypogonadism and visual failure). They commonly contain viscous fluid containing cholesterol.

Chordomas probably arise from the primitive notochord and occur at the upper or lower ends of the neuroaxis in the clivus or in the sacrum. Although histologically they look benign, they invade local structure but do not metastasise.

Tumours of the pineal region include malignant tumours such as *dysgerminoma* and *pineoblastoma*. Both have a tendency to spread to the CSF.

Spread of cerebral tumours

Spread is normally by local invasion, and metastasis outside the CNS is rare. The absence of lymphatic vessels helps to account for this. Spread of gliomas follows white matter pathways, particularly across the corpus callosum and via the anterior commissure. These are two routes which allow tumour to spread from one hemisphere to another. Sometimes tumour cells can be identified several centimetres away from the macroscopic tumour margin. Factors which facilitate local invasion include proteases, integrins, growth factors and the interaction between cells. The neural cell adhesion molecule (NCAM) stimulates cell adhesion. Its absence may encourage invasion. Similarly proteases such as metalloproteinases secreted by glioma cells may be important for local spread. Angiogenesis is also important for tumour spread. Tumour growth is dependent on an adequate blood supply. Vascular endothelial growth factor (VEGF) is important in stimulating capillary formation in glial tumours.

Metastatic spread is more likely if ventriculoperitoneal shunting has been carried out to relieve hydrocephalus. Local spread can occur from seeding of cells via the cerebrospinal fluid (CSF), giving rise to multiple deposits on the surface of the brain and spinal cord. This is characteristic of medulloblastoma, ependymoma and pineoblastoma.

Clinical features

Although the tumours listed in Table 30.1 are very diverse in nature and have individual natural histories, symptoms and signs arise in two distinct ways: (1) general effects from increased intracranial pressure and (2) local effects which can arise from local pressure and damage to adjacent nervous tissue. These can arise from any space-occupying lesion, whether neoplastic, inflammatory or traumatic.

1. There is a classical triad of headache, vomiting and papilloedema (oedema of the optic disc, the white patch on the retina where the optic nerve emerges).

It is important to recognise clinically that raised intracranial pressure can be present in an individual without each component of the triad being present.

Headache, often worse in the morning, is of a throbbing kind and gradually becomes worse if the intracranial pressure is not relieved. Papilloedema may be detected on ophthalmoscopy before the patient notices any disturbance of vision. Drowsiness, mental deterioration and personality changes may occur; with a tumour growing slowly, the behavioural disturbance may be considered to be of psychiatric origin.

2. Localising symptoms and signs depend very much on the site of the tumour. Some typical examples are:

Cerebellum:	loss of coordination of movement
Frontal lobe:	intellectual impairment and change in personality
Parietal lobe:	sensory or visual inattention
Occipital lobe:	visual field defects
Brainstem:	cranial nerve defects, involvement of motor and sensory tracts

Epileptic attacks are common with tumours of the cerebral hemispheres, especially slowly growing oligodendrogliomas. Epileptic fits occurring many years or months before the development of focal neurological deficit are typical of low-grade astrocytomas.

Diagnosis and investigation

A full history is taken. Information from the patient's family may indicate a change in personality or behaviour of which the patient may be unaware. The history and examination may suggest the site of the tumour. However, the diagnosis is most frequently made on CT or MRI scanning.

Plain radiographs of the skull may show calcification in a tumour (e.g. craniopharyngioma and some oligodendrogliomas), separation of the cranial sutures (between bones) from raised intracranial pressure in a child or erosion of the sella in pituitary tumours. Isotope brain scanning has largely been replaced by CT or MRI scanning.

CT scanning will show about 80% of tumours. It may show the tumour, associated oedema or hydrocephalus. It is usually carried out with the administration of contrast. For gliomas greater contrast enhancement tends to be seen in more malignant lesions. Figure 30.3 shows the typical appearance of a high-grade astrocytoma. Contrast enhancement is also seen in cerebral metastases and in meningiomas. MRI scanning gives better resolution of tumours in the posterior fossa and brainstem (Fig. 30.4).

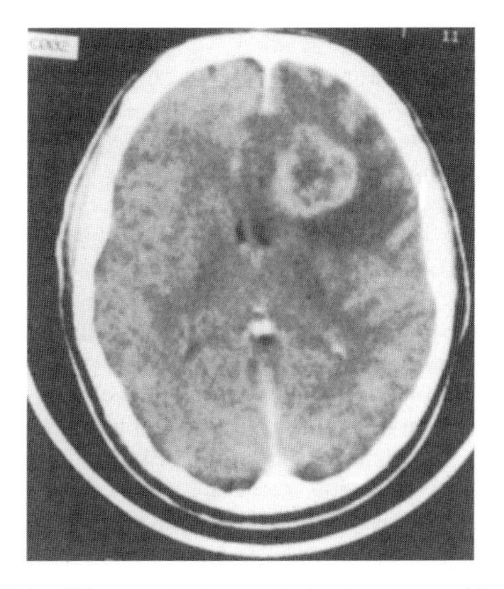

Fig. 30.3 CT scan showing grade 4 astrocytoma of the frontal lobe with surrounding oedema. (Courtesy of Dr T. Powell, Sheffield.)

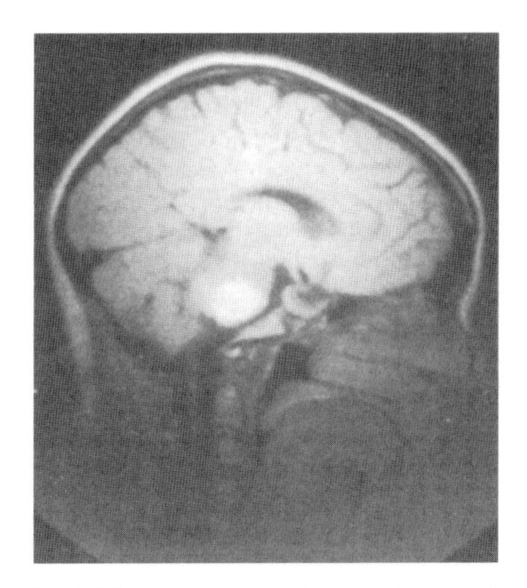

Fig. 30.4 MRI scan, sagittal section, showing brainstem glioma.

Other forms of imaging such as *positron-emission tomography* (PET) may assist in the diagnosis of non-enhancing lesions on CT scanning. If there is increased uptake of fluorodeoxyglucose in the lesion, this may guide the neurosurgeon in determining the site of biopsy. If there is no evidence of increased uptake on PET, a policy of surveillance may be adopted.

Cerebral angiography may complement CT or MRI scanning by showing the tumour circulation or by excluding a vascular lesion such as an arteriovenous malformation.

MRI spectroscopy, which measures biochemical differences between normal and malignant tissue, may help in the identification of gliomas and their histological grade but to date remains a research tool.

Principles of management

Surgery

Biopsy. Radiological investigations should in most cases be followed by a biopsy to confirm the diagnosis. A tissue diagnosis is important, despite the high degree of accuracy of modern neuroradiology. Biopsy is normally carried out under stereotactic control. In experienced hands the complication rate, mainly from bleeding or neurological deterioration, is normally around 1%. In some circumstances, e.g. for some brainstem tumours, it may be felt that the risks of biopsy are too great and that a diagnosis based on the appearance of the MRI scan will have to suffice.

One disadvantage is that the biopsy may only represent part of the tumour. This may be a problem for gliomas where different histological grades may be represented in the same tumour.

Craniotomy. Surgical removal of the tumour through a craniotomy incision should be considered in patients where the tumour is sited in silent areas of the brain such as the right frontal lobe. However, since malignant tumours often infiltrate the brain widely, only subtotal excision is possible in most cases. Some tumours such as those in the brainstem are usually not treated by surgery because of the critical structures which may be damaged, causing major neurological deficit. Similarly, very extensive tumours and older patients with major neurological deficit and poor performance status are not suitable for surgery.

Partial removal may be appropriate for moderately radiosensitive tumours such as decompressing the optic nerves from a pituitary tumour.

Tumours in the region of the corpus callosum are not suitable for even palliative surgery because of associated morbidity.

Palliative surgical procedures include relieving hydrocephalus by creating a drainage pathway for CSF between the atria of the heart or the peritoneum and the cerebral ventricles (ventriculoatrial or ventriculoperitoneal shunt). Aspiration of fluid from cystic tumours (e.g. craniopharyngioma) may relieve symptoms of raised intracranial pressure. An Ommaya reservoir can be inserted to relieve hydrocephalus or the delivery of cytotoxic drugs into the CSF (for example women with leptomeningeal metastases).

Radiotherapy

Radiotherapy may be radical or palliative in intent. For tumours such as medulloblastoma (see also Ch. 32) and pineal germinoma cure is achievable. For high-grade astrocytomas, only short-term palliation is possible even with radical doses. In vitro tests of radiosensitivity of high-grade gliomas suggest that intrinsic radioresistance is the major factor explaining treatment failure. By contrast, medulloblastoma shows greater in vitro radiosensitivity correlating with its better clinical outcome.

Megavoltage irradiation is the main form of radiotherapy for adult and paediatric brain tumours. It is usually given postoperatively following biopsy or debulking of the primary tumour. Intracavitary irradiation with radioisotopes such as yttrium-90 (for craniopharyngioma) or interstitial implantation with iridium-192 to boost high-grade gliomas or to treat recurrent disease after external beam are occasionally indicated.

The volume of the CNS irradiated will vary with the local extent and pattern of actual and likely spread of the tumour. There are three broad groups: (1) tumours treated by small-volume brain irradiation because they tend to remain localised, e.g. brainstem gliomas; (2) tumours treated by wide-field irradiation because of their tendency to infiltrate within the cerebral hemispheres, e.g. high-grade astrocytomas; and (3) tumours treated by whole CNS irradiation (e.g. craniospinal irradiation), e.g. medulloblastoma, ependymoma and pineoblastoma where seeding of tumour to the spinal cord via the cerebrospinal fluid may occur.

Steroid therapy

Steroids are used to reduce raised intracranial pressure. Dexamethasone in an initial dose of 16 mg per day in four divided doses is recommended. The dose should be reduced to a level that controls symptoms and, if possible, withdrawn completely, to avoid the development of steroidal side-effects. Of these, proximal myopathy of the lower limbs causes the most difficulty in mobility. Similarly, steroids should be tailed off after surgery or radiotherapy on an individualised basis. If there is no response to steroids after up to a week of treatment, they can be stopped without the need to taper off the dosage. It is advisable to prescribe an H_2 blocker (e.g. ranitidine 150 mg orally) to reduce the risk of steroid-induced gastrointestinal bleeding.

Rehabilitation and psychosocial support

Both patients and their families need support from the neuro-oncological team to help them cope with the psychological and physical effects of CNS malignancy and its treatment.

Radiation tolerance of the central nervous system

It is important to have an appreciation of the radiation tolerance of the central nervous system, since it influences the volume that can be safely irradiated.

The radiation tolerance of the CNS (brain and spinal cord) is of basic importance, in addition to the sensitivity of the actual tumour cells. Nerve cells are among the most resistant in the body. This is due to the fact that mature nerve cells never go into mitosis. Once destroyed they are not replaced. They are vulnerable to damage to their supporting tissues (neuroglia), and especially the small blood vessels on which they depend for oxygen and other nutrients. Obliterative endarteritis induced by radiation is the limiting factor in the tissue tolerance of the nervous system. The supporting glial cells can be renewed, albeit slowly. During the acute reaction to radiation, there is direct damage to nerve cells, blood vessels and glial cells. Damage to normal cells occurs by (1) impairment of renewal of glial cells and (2) narrowing of the small vessels of the arterial system leading to death of the tissues supplied. Typical late effects of brain irradiation are fibrosis, loss of cerebral white matter (demyelination), vascular damage and cell death (necrosis). The mechanisms are similar to those seen in other organs but the effects are more serious because of the irreplaceability of nerve cells.

The most sensitive parts of the central nervous system to radiation are the spinal cord (particularly the cervical part), the hypothalamus and the brainstem. The frontal, temporal and occipital lobes will tolerate higher doses.

Dose per fraction is an important factor in CNS tolerance. The tolerance to high doses per fraction is reduced. For this reason doses per fraction are conventionally kept to 2 Gy per fraction or less for radical treatment.

If the whole brain is irradiated, total dosage should generally not exceed 35 Gy in 10 daily fractions, 45 Gy in 20 daily fractions, 50 Gy in 25 daily fractions or 54 Gy in 30 daily fractions. For the brainstem 45 Gy in 20 daily fractions or 55 Gy in 30 fractions should not be exceeded.

Treatment of cerebral gliomas

Cerebral astrocytomas

The treatment of both low-grade and high-grade astrocytomas remains controversial.

Low-grade astrocytomas (grades 1 and 2). The optimal treatment for low-grade gliomas is uncertain. In general, low-grade astrocytomas in silent areas of the brain, e.g. the right frontal lobe, can be kept under surveillance without treatment. There is no conclusive evidence that early use of radical radiotherapy as opposed to delayed radiotherapy until the time of symptomatic progression has any advantage. Occasionally a tumour may behave more aggressively than is suggested by the low-grade histology. This sometimes reflects sampling from better-differentiated areas of a glioma which contains high-grade elements as well. In this circumstance it is reasonable to give postoperative irradiation on the presumption of high-grade tumour being present.

High-grade astrocytomas (grade 3 and 4). Surgical debulking should be carried out if possible, since it reduces the need for steroids and facilitates the delivery of postoperative radiotherapy. Where no debulking is carried out, postoperative radiotherapy may be accompanied by clinical deterioration due to radiation-induced oedema. Where a tumour lies in an eloquent area, e.g. the left parietal lobe, biopsy is often preferred to avoid damage to the speech area.

Radiotherapy

Opinions vary on the indications for postoperative radiotherapy. High-grade astrocytomas are relatively radioresistant. Cure is exceptional and local recurrence or persistent tumour the rule, even with radical doses. Treatment is therefore palliative, prolonging survival by only a few months compared to surgical debulking alone. Sadly the quality of life of many of these patients is poor as a result of both the disease and its treatment. With such limited benefits from postoperative radiotherapy, careful selection of patients most likely to benefit is particularly important. A discussion with the patient and his/her family about the realistic benefits of treatment may help the patient to decide whether or not to accept postoperative radiotherapy.

It is important not to irradiate patients who have a particularly poor prognosis. These include patients over the age of 60, those in poor medical condition or with a major neurological deficit (e.g. a hemiparesis) which fails to improve on steroids or with surgery.

Target volume

Since high-grade cerebral gliomas infiltrate widely, often well beyond the macroscopic limits of the tumour, the target volume should include a generous margin of normal tissue. Recurrence tends to occur at the primary site or close to it. On this basis it is a reasonable approach to treat the whole brain in the initial phase of treatment and then cone down with a boost to the primary tumour with a margin of 3–5 cm judged from CT or MRI scans. However, the only randomised trial comparing whole brain irradiation alone to whole brain irradiation plus a boost showed no difference in survival. For diffuse or bilateral tumours, whole brain irradiation without a boost is appropriate. There is no evidence that brachytherapy, hyperfractionated radiotherapy or radiosurgery confers any advantage over conventional radiotherapy.

Technique

For extensive diffusely infiltrating and all bilateral tumours, a parallel-opposed pair of fields is used covering the whole brain (Fig 30.5A).

For well-defined tumours a right-angled wedged pair may suffice. A third unwedged field between the

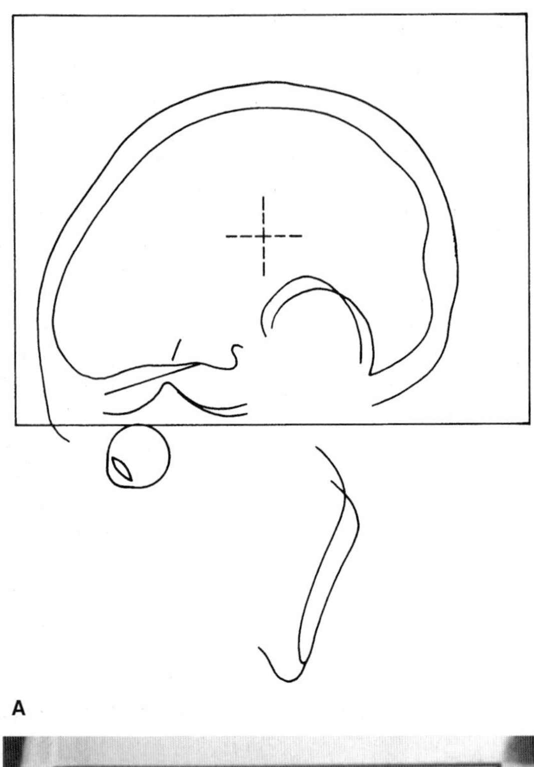

A

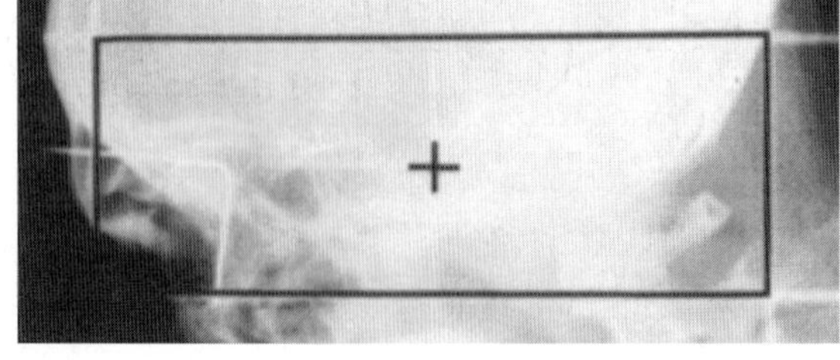

B

Fig. 30.5 **A** Field for whole brain irradiation. (Reproduced with permission from Perez & Brady, 1987.) **B** Field for palliative irradiation of the base of skull. (Courtesy of Dr J Bolger, Sheffield.)

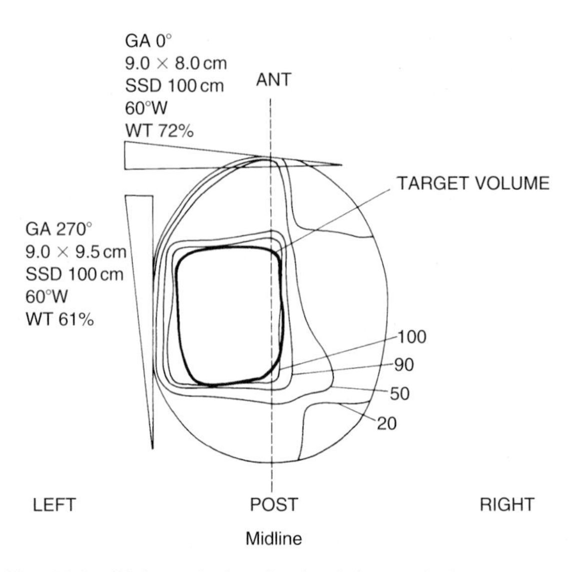

Fig. 30.6 Right-angled wedged pair for grade 4 astrocytoma of the frontal lobe.

wedged fields may be necessary to bring up the dose to the posteromedial part of the target volume (Fig. 30.6).

Dose and energy

Phase I whole brain irradiation

40–45 Gy midplane dose (MPD) in 1.7–2 Gy fractions (6 MV photons)

Phase II boost to tumour-bearing area

10–15 Gy target absorbed dose (TAD) in 1.7–2 Gy fractions (6 MV photons)

Side-effects. Acute side-effects are hair loss within the irradiated area, skin erythema, impaired hearing (if the ear is included in the volume) and somnolence. The most important late side-effect is radionecrosis.

Chemotherapy

Adjuvant chemotherapy has only been shown to add a modest survival benefit to surgery and radiotherapy (9% at 1 year and 3% at 3 years). Combination chemotherapy does not appear to offer any advantage over single-agent therapy. Adjuvant chemotherapy is not recommended routinely and should only be undertaken in the context of a clinical trial.

For recurrent disease following primary treatment, palliative chemotherapy may result in temporary growth restraint. CCNU, BCNU and procarbazine have been used, since they cross the blood–brain barrier. Responses rates are 20–40%. Temozolamide, a newer agent, has been shown to have a higher response rate than procarbazine in relapsed disease.

Results of treatment of cerebral astrocytomas

5-year survival is: grade 1 (60%), grade 2 (40%), grade 3 (10%) and grade 4 (2%).

Ependymomas

Low-grade supratentorial ependymomas should be treated by cranial irradiation alone. High-grade ependymomas and all infratentorial ependymomas should be treated by craniospinal irradiation.

Radical radiotherapy

Technique volume and dose are as for medulloblastoma (see Ch. 32).

Results of treatment of ependymomas

Overall 5-year survival for intracranial ependymoma is 50–60%. Survival is better for low-grade tumours (80%).

Oligodendrogliomas

Oligodendrogliomas tend to occur in young and middle-aged adults. They occur more commonly in the cerebral hemispheres, most commonly in the frontal lobes. Growth is normally slow. Presentation is commonly with epilepsy, often long before the development of focal neurological deficit.

MEDULLOBLASTOMA

The management medulloblastoma is described in Chapter 32.

PINEAL AND THIRD VENTRICULAR TUMOURS

Clinical features of tumours of the pineal and posterior end of the third ventricle are mainly due to CSF obstruction causing symptoms and signs of raised intracranial pressure. They are commonest between the ages of 15 and 25. Upward gaze may be impaired associated with nystagmus and reduced papillary responses (Parinaud's syndrome) due to compression of the midbrain. The cerebellum may also be compressed giving rise to an unsteady gait. Diabetes insipidus with absence of or delayed secondary sexual development in a teenager is typical of dysgerminoma.

Tumours of the anterior end of the third ventricle cause impaired vision and hypopituitarism.

Diagnosis and treatment

The management of intracranial germ cell tumours is described in Chapter 32.

BRAINSTEM GLIOMAS

Brainstem gliomas may occur anywhere in the midbrain, pons and medulla. The commonest site is in the pons. Most occur in children between the ages of 3 and 9. Presentation is often with ataxia, cranial nerve palsies, difficulty with swallowing and speech. Biopsy is hazardous and the diagnosis may have to be made on radiological and clinical grounds alone.

Treatment

The treatment of brainstem gliomas is described in Chapter 32.

PRIMARY CNS LYMPHOMA

Primary CNS lymphoma (PCNSL) is much less common than secondary intracerebral involvement. It typically affects the periventricular areas and the brainstem. Predisposing conditions are inherited immunodeficiency (Wiskott–Aldrich syndrome), acquired immunodeficiency syndrome (AIDS) and immunosuppression for transplantation. Age of presentation varies. For example, PCNSL due to Wiskott–Aldrich syndrome tends to present in childhood and AIDS-related lymphoma in the thirties. Sporadic PCNSL tends to occur later in the fourth and fifth decades.

The commonest histological type is diffuse large cell lymphoma. Seeding to the CSF may occur. Clinical presentation varies. For patients presenting with AIDS-related PCNSL loss of memory, confusion, epilepsy and focal neurological deficits are common. For the sporadic variety, headache, focal weakness and a change in personality are typical presenting features. Ocular involvement (slit lamp examination may show cells in the vitreous) occurs in 15%. Leptomeningeal disease at presentation or later in the course of the disease occurs in the majority of patients.

MRI scanning typically shows one or more poorly defined enhancing lesions without surrounding oedema. The diagnosis may be established by needle biopsy or, if there are leptomeningeal symptoms, by CSF cytology.

Treatment

While there may be dramatic clinical response to steroids, it tends to be short lived.

Radiotherapy

Radical radiotherapy is the principal form of treatment.

Target volume

Two phases of treatment are recommended if the tumour is localised:

Phase I

Whole brain irradiation by parallel-opposed fields.

40 Gy (MPD) in 1.6–1.8 Gy fractions

Phase II

15–20 Gy TAD to tumour with 2–3 cm margin in 1.6–1.8 Gy fractions (6 MV photons)

For multifocal disease whole brain radiotherapy alone is recommended.

45 Gy MPD in 1.6–1.8 Gy fractions (6 MV photons)

Craniospinal irradiation is recommended in patients who have proven leptomeningeal disease on CSF cytology.

Technique

The technique of craniospinal irradiation is described in Chapter 32.

Dose to spinal cord

30–35 Gy mean dose in 25 daily fractions over 5 weeks (6 MV photons)

Chemotherapy

PCNSL is sensitive to chemotherapy such as CHOP (cyclophosphamide, doxorubicin, vincristine and prednisolone). Treatment is recommended with chemotherapy initially followed by whole brain or craniospinal radiotherapy.

Results of treatment

The results of treatment of PCNSL remain poor. For patients with AIDS-related PCNSL average survival is about 4 months. For non-AIDS-related PNCNS complete plus partial response rates are 60–70%. Relapse is common and median survival is about 1 year.

MENINGIOMA

The principal treatment is surgical removal. If complete, no further treatment is needed. Radical radiotherapy is indicated for patients who have undergone partial removal or where the tumour is inoperable. Meningioma is not particularly radiosensitive so eradication of the tumour is extremely rare.

Target volume

Tumour plus 1–2 cm margin.

Technique

A two- or three-field technique with wedges is recommended.

Dose and energy

55–60 Gy TAD in 1.7–2 Gy fractions

Results of treatment

Radiotherapy reduces the risk of recurrence by about 50% for partially resected meningiomas to 15–20% at 5 years.

OPTIC NERVE GLIOMA

This rare tumour is normally slowly growing and of low-grade malignancy. It tends to occur in children under the age of 15. Clinical features include visual field defects, proptosis, nystagmus and optic atrophy. More than 50% involve the optic chiasm. The tumour is identified by CT or MRI. The diagnosis is established by biopsy. Surgical removal is hazardous. Treatment is normally by radical radiotherapy to arrest progressive visual loss or if there is intracranial extension.

Target volume

The tumour plus a 1 cm margin.

Technique

Supine position in a beam-directed shell. An open anterior field and two lateral wedged fields are used.

Dose

Adults
50 Gy TAD in 5–5.5 weeks (6 MV photons)

Children under the age of 15
45 Gy TAD in 4–4.5 weeks (6 MV photons)

Results of treatment

The results of radiotherapy are excellent. Radiotherapy improves vision in 40–50% of patients and stabilises the disease in the majority of those whose deficits are not improved. 5- and 10-year progression-free and overall survival is 80–90%.

CHORDOMAS

Presentation of chordomas in the clivus is with pain followed by neurological deficit from involvement of midbrain or brainstem or of other structures such as the pituitary, nasopharynx or sphenoid sinus. Sacral chordomas similarly cause local pain followed eventually by bladder and bowel dysfunction from compression of the cauda equina.

Treatment is by surgical debulking followed by radical radiotherapy to achieve palliation. In specialised centres, focal irradiation with proton and helium ions has achieved 50–70% control rates at 5 years but at the expense of considerable morbidity.

Results of treatment

5-year progression-free survival in patients treated by radiotherapy following partial resection or biopsy alone is 20–30%.

PITUITARY TUMOURS

Anatomy

The pituitary gland (Fig. 30.7) lies in the sella turcica, a recess in the base of the skull. The sella has a floor and

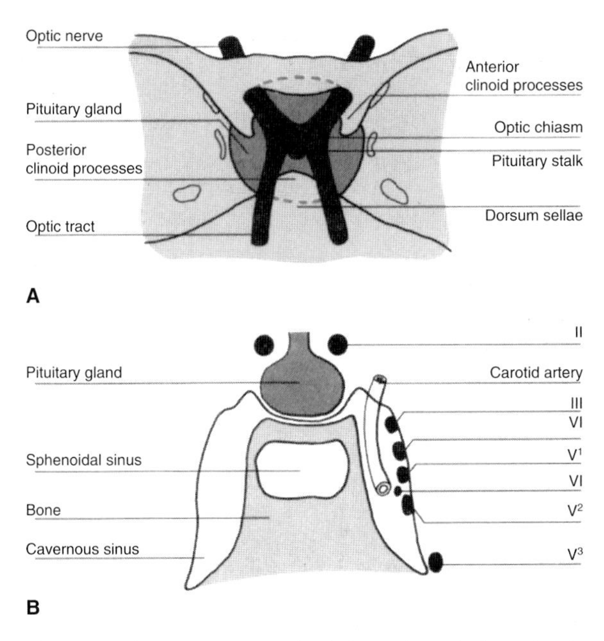

Fig. 30.7 Gross anatomy and relations of the pituitary gland. (Reproduced with permission from Souhami & Moxham, Textbook of Medicine, Churchill Livingstone, 1990.)

front and back walls bounded by anterior and posterior clinoid processes. It is composed of anterior and posterior lobes. It is connected structurally and functionally to the hypothalamus above. Above the pituitary gland lies the optic chiasm, where the visual pathways cross. To each side lie the cavernous sinuses through which pass the third, fourth and first and second divisions of the 5th cranial nerve, the 6th cranial nerve and the carotid artery. Below lies the sphenoid sinus.

The pituitary gland exerts control, through the hormones that it secretes, on the gonads, thyroid and adrenal glands and upon growth. The anterior lobe, under the influence of releasing factors from the hypothalamus, secretes the following hormones: prolactin, thyroid-stimulating hormone (TSH), adrenocorticotrophic hormone (ACTH), follicle-stimulating hormone (FSH), luteinising hormone (LH) and growth hormone (GH). The posterior lobe secretes antidiuretic hormone (ADH) and oxytocin.

Pathology

Tumours of the pituitary are relatively common, accounting for about 12% of tumours of the CNS. Virtually all arise from the anterior lobe of the gland. Histologically primary pituitary tumours are all benign. Their danger is due to the proximity of vital structures such as the optic nerves, compression of which can lead to partial or complete blindness. In addition to this local pressure, clinical syndromes due to underproduction or overproduction of hormones develop. Secondary tumours, of which breast cancer is the commonest, are rare. The principal clinical syndromes are described below.

It is the type and amount of hormone secreted rather than the staining characteristics (e.g. eosinophilic or basophilic) that correlate best with clinical features and behaviour of the tumour. A functional classification is therefore adopted. Tumours are classified as secretors or non-secretors and subclassified by the hormone they produce. Approximately 30% of large pituitary tumours (macroadenomas, i.e. > 1 cm in size) are non-secretory or functionless. The latter are normally chromophobe adenomas.

Hormone secretion

The commonest secretory tumours are prolactinomas, producing prolactin. They are usually eosinophilic. Occasionally tumours may secrete both prolactin and growth hormone. ACTH is most commonly secreted by basophilic tumours, causing Cushing's syndrome. Tumours which secrete TSH, FSH or LH are rare.

Clinical features

Local effects of pituitary and suprasellar tumours

- Pressure on the optic chiasm—visual field defects (blindness). Typically the upper visual fields are affected initially. A bitemporal hemianopia, in which the outer half of both visual fields is lost, may subsequently develop.
- Headache, often persistent.
- Extension into the cavernous sinus is rarely symptomatic unless extensive. If so, the 3rd, 4th and 6th cranial nerves and first and second divisions of the 5th nerve can cause pain in the eye, diplopia (double vision), closure of the eye (ptosis), sensory loss over the part of the same side of the nose and loss of the corneal reflex.
- Increased appetite and thirst.
- Pressure on the floor of the third ventricle (loss of recent memory).

Clinical syndromes

- Panhypopituitarism:
  —Children: failure of growth and of pubertal development.
  —Adults: non-specific malaise, pale 'waxen doll' skin complexion, cold intolerance (features of

hypothyroidism are rarely gross), amenorrhoea (women), loss of sex drive and potency, loss of secondary sexual hair, hypopituitary crisis (acute abdominal pain) and low blood sugar.
- Acromegaly, Cushing's syndrome.

Diagnosis and investigation of pituitary tumours

CT and MRI scanning are the investigations of choice. However, the initial diagnosis may be suspected from enlargement of the pituitary fossa on a lateral skull radiograph. CT scanning shows local extension, e.g. above the pituitary (suprasellar, Fig. 30.8) and into the cavernous sinus. Basal levels of the anterior pituitary hormones should be measured. Dynamic tests of pituitary function are performed in which the ability of the pituitary to secrete particular hormones in response to hypothalamic releasing factors is assessed.

Treatment of pituitary tumours

Surgery, radiotherapy and medical therapy are the treatments available for pituitary tumours. Close liaison is required between surgeon, oncologist and endocrinologist in choosing the appropriate combination of treatments.

Surgery

The surgical approach to the pituitary gland (Fig. 30.9) is most commonly through the nose (trans-sphenoidal) and less commonly through a craniotomy incision (transfrontal). Trans-sphenoidal surgery is used for small or medium-sized pituitary tumours with or without symmetrical extension above the sella (suprasellar). This approach allows small tumours (microadenomas) to be removed while leaving adjacent normal pituitary tissue intact. The morbidity of trans-sphenoidal surgery is low.

Transfrontal surgery is appropriate either to relieve compression of the optic nerves or to remove tumours which are (1) large, (2) have asymmetrical suprasellar extension, or (3) have spread laterally into the cavernous sinus. Removal of the tumour is subtotal and postoperative radiotherapy is required. The morbidity of transfrontal surgery is higher than that of trans-sphenoidal surgery and carries an operative mortality of 1%.

Hypopituitarism may occur, depending on how discrete the adenoma is and how radical the surgery needs to be. Hormone replacement is required (see below).

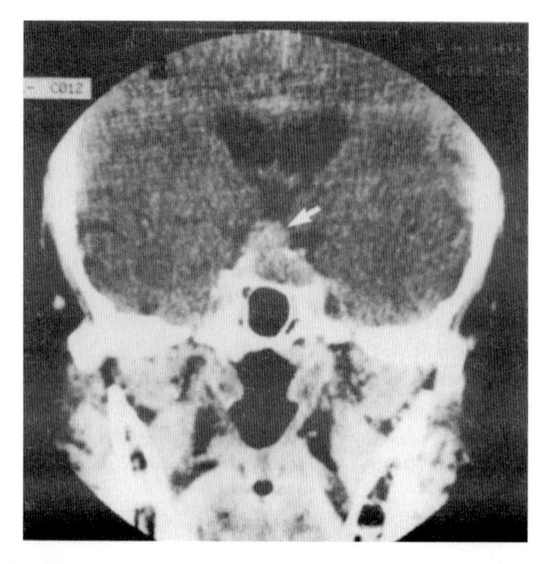

Fig. 30.8 Coronal CT scan showing pituitary tumour with suprasellar extension (arrowed). (Courtesy of Mr R Battersby, Sheffield)

Radical radiotherapy

There are a variety of ways of irradiating the pituitary gland. These are photons, yttrium implantation and proton beam therapy. Of these, photontherapy remains the most effective and, with appropriate dosage and fractionation, the safest. Yttrium-90 and gold-198 have been used to implant tumours confined to the sella. Although they can deliver a high dose to the pituitary gland, with more rapid effects than external beam, complications such as damage to the optic nerve and meningitis discourage use.

Target volume

This should include the pituitary tumour with a 1–2 cm margin. Postoperative field sizes normally range between 4–5 cm^2 (Fig. 30.10A).

Technique

A head mould is required. The patient is treated with the chin flexed to allow the anterior field to enter above the eyes. A three-field technique is commonly used (Fig. 30.10B). An alternative is a parallel-opposed pair of fields. A theoretical disadvantage of the latter is that the maximum dose is delivered to the temporal lobes. However, there is no clinical evidence of temporal lobe damage after conventional central tumour doses of 40 Gy over 4 weeks.

Dose and energy

40 Gy TAD in 20 daily fractions over 4 weeks (6 MV photons)

Operative approach

From BELOW:

1. *Trans-sphenoidal*

Through an incision in the upper gum the nasal mucosa in stripped from the septum and the pituitary fossa approached through the sphenoid sinus.

2. *Transethmoidal*

An incision is made on the medial orbital wall and the pituitary fossa approached through the ethmoid and aphenoid sinuses.

With the transethmoidal and trans-sphenoidal routes the pituitary gland can be directly visualised and explored for microadenoma. Even large tumours with suprasellar extension may be removed from below, avoiding the need for craniotomy.

From ABOVE

3. *Transfrontal*

Through a craniotomy flap the frontal lobe is retracted to provide direct acces to the pituitary tumour. approach is usually reserved for tumours with large frontal of lateral extensions.

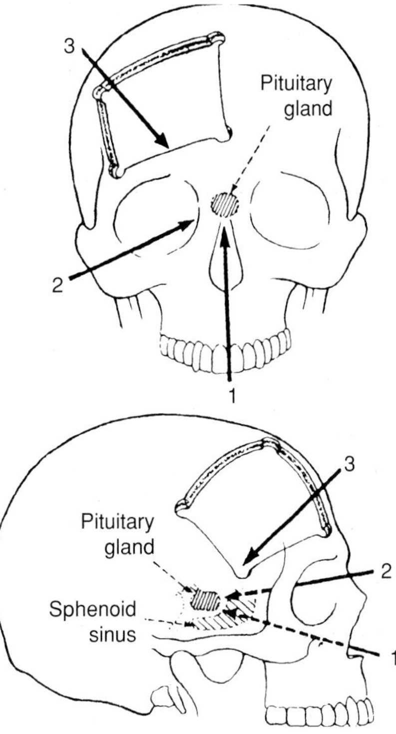

Fig. 30.9 Surgical approaches to the pituitary gland. 1, Trans-sphenoidal. 2, Transethmoidal. 3, Transfrontal. (Reproduced with permission from Lindsay et al, Neurosurgery and Neurology, Churchill Livingstone, 1991.)

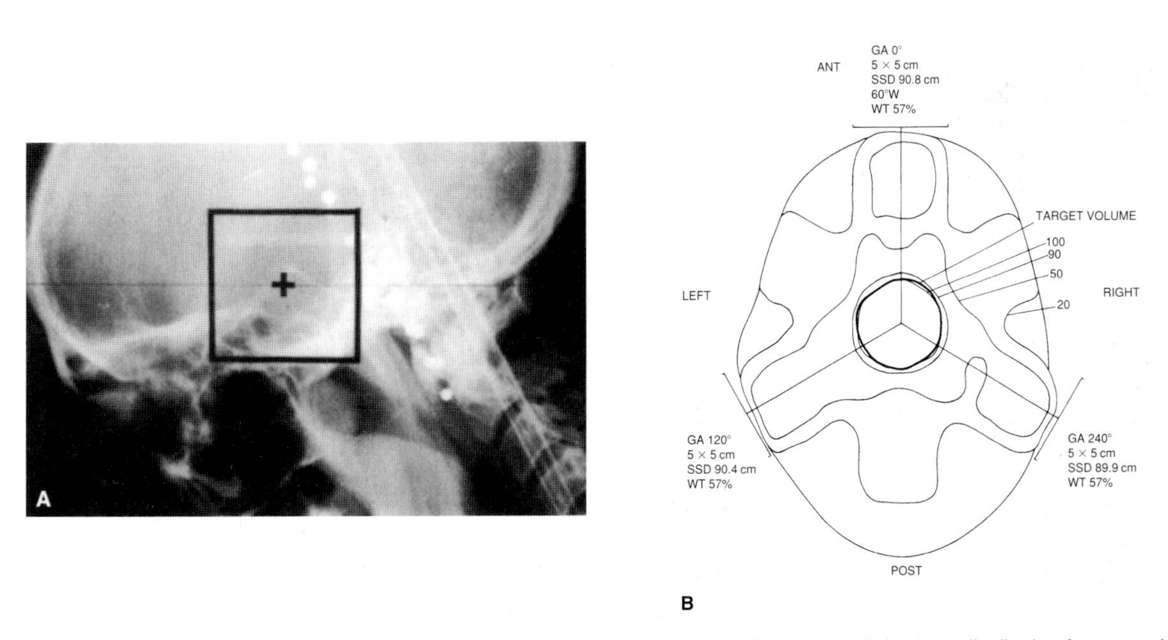

Fig. 30.10 **A** Lateral simulator radiograph showing treatment volume for pituitary tumour. **B** Isodose distribution from anterior and two posterior oblique fields for a pituitary tumour (6 MV photons).

Radiation reaction. Acute reactions are minimal. Erythema and hair loss occur. The commonest late effect is hypopituitarism, which is nearly universal. Hormonal replacement therapy is with thyroxine, hydrocortisone and the sex hormones (estradiol + progesterone as the oral contraceptive for women and testosterone for men). Using the doses and fractionation stated above, chiasmal damage should not occur.

Treatment of specific tumours

1. Prolactinomas

Large prolactinomas (macroprolactinomas) are greater than 1 cm in size. They behave differently from small prolactinomas (microprolactinomas, less than 1 cm). Large prolactinomas expand the pituitary fossa and compress the chiasm and require prompt treatment.

Macroprolactinomas. Bromocriptine is the initial treatment of choice for macroprolactinomas and can shrink very rapidly even large tumours compressing the optic chiasm. If bromocriptine fails to relieve chiasmal compression completely, surgical decompression is required. Postoperative external beam irradiation is advised to sterilise the tumour. If, however, a macroprolactinoma is untreated, there is a small risk that it may expand during pregnancy. For this reason normalisation of the serum prolactin with surgery or bromocriptine is advised before conception occurs. If bromocriptine is not tolerated, trans-sphenoidal surgical removal of the tumour should be carried out.

Microprolactinomas. Not all patients with an elevated serum prolactin have a prolactin-secreting tumour. In some patients there is no obvious cause. However, if the serum prolactin is in excess of 1000 mu/l, a microprolactinoma is likely to be present. The natural history of these tumours is more benign than that of macroprolactinomas. Treatment is not necessarily essential. Surgery is the only treatment which can effectively cure the disease. Bromocriptine may achieve temporary growth control.

Indications for treatment are: amenorrhoea, low oestrogen levels (which favour the development of osteoporosis), impaired sexual desire and function.

The risks of tumour expansion during pregnancy are smaller than for macroprolactinomas. Pregnancy may proceed with regular clinical assessment for signs of chiasmal compression.

Postoperative radiotherapy is only required if the serum prolactin is markedly raised preoperatively, fails to fall following surgery or the tumour is locally invasive.

2. Functionless tumours

These account for about a third of large pituitary tumours. Compression of the optic chiasm is common. Treatment is surgical, by trans-sphenoidal surgery if possible. Postoperative radiotherapy is given to reduce the rate of local recurrence. Medical treatment with bromocriptine is of little value.

3. Acromegaly and gigantism

Aetiology. Excessive secretion of growth hormone causes gigantism in a child who is still growing and acromegaly in an adult in whom skeletal growth is complete.

Clinical features. The effects of excess growth hormone in acromegaly are enlargement of the hands and feet and of the skeleton in general, coarsening of the facial features, prominence of the jaw, sweating, arthropathy, amenorrhoea and impotence. Impaired vision and headache are local effects of tumour extension. Nerve entrapment occurs due to overgrowth of the soft tissues, e.g. compressing the median nerve at the wrist (carpal tunnel syndrome). Arterial hypertension and diabetes mellitus are common. Untreated, the disease may be fatal, usually because of cardiovascular damage.

Diagnosis and investigation. The most useful test to make the diagnosis of acromegaly is to give an oral glucose load. In normal individuals this suppresses growth hormone levels to < 2 mu/l. In acromegaly, however, growth hormone levels are not suppressed.

Treatment. Treatment is required for virtually all patients with acromegaly. Cure of acromegaly is rare but control can commonly be achieved. Trans-sphenoidal removal of the adenoma is normally the first line of treatment and is urgent if vision is impaired. This is followed by postoperative radiotherapy (see radiation technique and dosage below) since it is often difficult for the surgeon to be confident that all the tumour has been removed.

Bromocriptine is the main medical therapy for acromegaly. It lowers growth hormone secretion from the pituitary in about 70% of patients but substantial falls in growth hormone levels are only achieved in 15–20% of patients. It is particularly effective in shrinking tumours that secrete both growth hormone and prolactin. It is used after surgery if growth hormone levels do not return to normal postoperatively or if the patient is unfit for or refuses surgery. Maintenance doses are normally 10–30 mg per day. Side-effects such as gastrointestinal intolerance may limit its use. A more recent drug, octreotide, derived from the hormone somatostatin, can considerably reduce growth hormone levels. Its role in the treatment of acromegaly is yet to be established.

Results of treatment. Cure of acromegaly, defined as a serum growth hormone level of less than 1 mu/l, is rare. The effects of radiotherapy on growth hormone levels are very slow. The average time to reach the normal range of growth hormone is about 7 years.

Cushing's disease. Cushing's disease (pituitary-dependent Cushing's syndrome) is treated by trans-sphenoidal surgical removal of the tumour. Metyrapone is used to block adrenal steroid production. Pituitary irradiation is employed for persistent or recurrent disease.

CRANIOPHARYNGIOMA

This is a congenital benign tumour arising from Rathke's pouch. Remnants of this may persist and form cystic tumours which may compress the pituitary.

Presentation is usually in early adulthood with endocrine dysfunction, with failure of growth and of sexual maturation, and diabetes insipidus. Visual impairment and signs of raised intracranial pressure are common.

Diagnosis and investigation

The presence of calcification above the pituitary fossa on a skull radiograph may suggest the diagnosis. CT scanning demonstrates both solid and cystic components.

Treatment

Surgical removal is the treatment of choice. This is often complete, especially in children, and no further treatment may be needed. Sometimes it is impossible to remove the whole tumour owing to its intimate relations with vital structures such as the optic chiasm or to the large size of the cyst. If the residual disease is predominantly cystic, the cyst can be drained under stereotactic CT guidance and a solution of radioactive yttrium-90 instilled. This reduces the likelihood of recurrence. If the disease is mainly solid, postoperative external beam is preferable. It is better not to delay irradiation until recurrence since the local control rate falls to 25%.

Radical radiotherapy

Target volume

This includes the tumour and a 1–2 cm margin of normal tissue.

Technique

A parallel-opposed pair of lateral fields or a three-field technique (as for the pituitary gland, see above) is used with a shell.

Dose and energy

45 Gy in 20 daily fractions over 4 weeks (4–6 MV photons)

Results of treatment

The prognosis is better in children than in adults. 5-year survival is nearly 100% for children and 95% for adults. Following external beam irradiation just over 50% of patients are free of disease at 5 years.

INTRACRANIAL METASTASES

Intracranial metastases may occur in the meninges, brain or the skull; 80% of brain metastases occur in the cerebral hemispheres and 16% in the cerebellum. Rarely deposits may occur in the basal ganglia, brainstem, pituitary gland and the choroid plexus. Metastases to the meninges may be isolated or part of carcinomatous meningitis where malignant cells are widespread in the CSF. Occasionally the source of the primary is not clinically evident. Two-thirds of metastases are multiple.

Clinical features

Presentation may be with raised intracranial pressure, epilepsy, or with a stroke. Frequently they develop in the context of advanced disease elsewhere and are often a terminal event. Lower cranial nerve palsies may indicate base of skull metastases.

Treatment

The treatment of brain metastases is virtually always palliative. Surgery, radiotherapy, chemotherapy and steroids are the treatments available. The choice is determined by the age, general condition, the number of metastases and the presence of disease elsewhere. If the patient is terminally ill, relief of intracranial pressure by steroids alone (dexamethasone 4 mg orally q.d.s.) may be all that is appropriate.

For those in better general condition the number of metastases is important. Isolated metastases may be amenable to surgical removal followed by postoperative radiotherapy. For multiple metastases surgery is inappropriate. Very occasionally it may be justified for two metastases if they are radioresistant and lie within the same operative field.

Palliative radiotherapy is helpful in relieving headache; 80% of patients obtain some symptomatic improvement and in about 50% relief is complete. Between 70 and 75% will have motor deficit improved, with complete resolution in 30–35%. The control of epilepsy requires anticonvulsant therapy.

Phenytoin 300 mg nocte is the initial treatment of choice in adults.

Chemotherapy is of little value in treating most cerebral metastases. Intrathecal methotrexate may be of benefit to patients with cerebral lymphoma, leukaemia or choriocarcinoma. A number of radiosensitisers such as gadolinium texaphyrin are under evaluation. Gadolinium texaphyrin is composed of a porphyrin ring with gadolinium at its centre. It is activated by external beam irradiation and is selectively taken up in the tumour. In Phase II studies it shows evidence of enhancing the effect of palliative cranial irradiation. Results of a phase III trial are awaited.

Palliative radiotherapy

Target volume

This includes the whole brain if there are supratentorial metastases. If the metastases are confined to the cerebellum, the infratentorial region of the brain need only be treated.

Technique

For whole-brain irradiation a simple parallel-opposed pair of lateral fields is adequate, using cobalt beam or megavoltage (see Fig. 30.5A). The same technique for base of skull metastases is shown in Figure 30.5B.

Simulation is not essential and anatomical landmarks of the base of skull (a line from the outer canthus to the external auditory meatus) can be used.

Dose and energy

30 Gy (MPD) in 10 daily fractions (6 MV photons or cobalt–60)

Results of treatment

The results of treatment of cerebral deposits are poor. With steroids alone average survival is 2 months. With palliative radiotherapy, it is between 3 and 5 months. In patients with isolated metastases treated by surgery and postoperative radiotherapy, median survival is about 6 months. Patients with an interval of more than a year between the diagnosis of the primary and that of cerebral metastases tend to have a longer survival.

Carcinomatous meningitis

Carcinomatous meningitis is an uncommon complication of a variety of tumours (e.g. lung and breast). Presentation is with headache which becomes progressively severe. Photophobia, neck stiffness and cranial nerve palsies are common. Diagnosis is confirmed on CSF cytology. However, several lumbar punctures may be needed to make a positive diagnosis. Associated features in the CSF are raised opening pressure (> 160 mmHg), lymphocytosis, increased protein and reduced glucose. CT or MRI may reveal enhancement in the periventricular areas and meninges. Treatment is palliative. Patients are rarely fit for more than palliative irradiation to the parts of the neuraxis causing symptoms, for example the base of skull (Fig. 30.5B).

Intraventricular methotrexate delivered via an Ommaya reservoir may provide symptomatic relief and is better tolerated than repeated lumbar punctures.

Palliative radiotherapy

Target volume

The base of skull is included. Typical fields sizes are 15 × 6 cm.

Technique

A parallel-opposed pair of fields is used.

Dose and energy

30 Gy MPD in 10 daily fractions over 2 weeks (4–6 MV photons or cobalt–60)

TUMOURS OF THE SPINAL CORD

Classification

Approximately 15% of tumours of the CNS develop in the spinal cord. They are classified according to whether they lie inside (intradural) or outside (extradural) the dura. Intradural tumours may lie within the cord (intramedullary) or outside it (extramedullary).

1. Extradural
   a. Primary
      (i) Chordoma
      (ii) Sarcoma
      (iii) Lymphoma
      (iv) Myeloma
   b. Secondary (e.g. breast and lung cancer)
2. Intradural
   a. Extramedullary
      (i) Meningioma
      (ii) Neurofibroma
   b. Intramedullary (gliomas)
      (i) Ependymoma
      (ii) Astrocytoma.

The majority of intramedullary tumours in the cervical cord are astrocytomas. In the thoracic cord, astrocytomas and ependymomas are equally common. In the lumbosacral region, ependymomas predominate. In the cauda equina virtually all are ependymomas. Astrocytomas account for a third of primary spinal cord tumours. They are mostly well differentiated.

Ependymomas represent the other two-thirds; 90% are well differentiated and rarely seed to the CSF.

Chordoma is a rare tumour arising from remnants of the notochord; 50% occur in the sacrococcygeal region, 35% in the base of the skull (e.g. clinoid process) and 15% at various levels of the vertebral column. It invades locally into the nasopharynx, pelvis, buttocks or retroperitoneal tissues. Metastases to lymph nodes, lung and liver occur in less than 10%.

Clinical features

Pain due to involvement of the nerve roots or vertebral body may precede signs of spinal cord compression (see below). Neurological function is lost at the level of and below the lesion. The loss may be motor and/or sensory. Upper motor neuron signs occur below the level of cord involved. Intramedullary tumours positioned laterally in the cord may give rise to hemisection of the cord (Brown–Séquard syndrome). In this syndrome there is loss of pain and temperature sensation on the opposite side of the body below the lesion, from compression of the lateral spinothalamic tracts, which enter and cross the spinal cord from the opposite side, and loss of motor function and vibration and joint position sense on the affected side, from damage to the pyramidal tracts and posterior columns respectively.

Chordomas may present as an intracranial space-occupying lesion with headache, cranial nerve palsies, spinal cord compression or pain, e.g. from destruction of the sacrum.

Treatment

Astrocytomas should be treated by surgical excision or maximal debulking. Ependymomas in the cauda equina cannot be treated by radical surgery because of the damage that would be done to nerve roots. In both tumours, surgery should be followed by postoperative radiotherapy to reduce the incidence of local recurrence.

Chordomas are best treated by surgical debulking followed by postoperative radiotherapy. Because of their site in the base of the skull or sacrum, complete surgical excision is usually impossible. Chordomas are relatively radioresistant. However, radiotherapy may relieve pressure symptoms.

Radical radiotherapy

Target volume

This should include the known extent of the tumour with a margin of 5 cm of normal tissue above and below the tumour.

Technique

Ependymomas and astrocytomas. The patient is treated prone in a shell immobilising the trunk. In the cervical and thoracic cord two posterior oblique wedged fields are used. In the lumbar region a direct field is used instead of posterior oblique fields to avoid overdosage of the kidneys.

Chordomas. Base of skull: a parallel-opposed pair of lateral fields. Pelvis: anterior and posterior pair of fields.

Dose and energy

45 Gy in 20 daily fractions over 4 weeks (4–6 MV photons)

Results of treatment

90% of well-differentiated ependymomas of the cauda equina are disease free at 5 years. For low-grade gliomas 5-year survival is about 50%. High-grade tumours respond poorly to treatment, with a survival similar to cerebral gliomas of the same grade.

Malignant spinal cord compression

Anatomy

The spinal cord runs behind the posterior margin of the vertebral bodies from the upper border of the atlas (C1) to the lower border of L1. It is important to know that the lower level may vary from the lower border of T12 to the upper border of L3 (Fig. 30.11). The spinal cord ends in a group of nerve roots, the cauda equina. The cauda equina is not part of the spinal cord but it is convenient to consider its management in conjunction with spinal cord compression because of their anatomical proximity.

The levels of the spinal cord segments are not at the same level as the correspondingly numbered vertebral bodies. In the adult, the spinal segment is about two segments above the corresponding vertebral level. For example, the sixth thoracic segment is opposite the 4th thoracic vertebra and the first sacral segment is opposite the 12th thoracic vertebra.

Aetiology and pathology

Epidural spinal cord compression (ESCC) complicates the course of about 5% of patients with solid tumours. The commonest primary sites are breast, lung and prostate. In 10% of patients the primary site is not found.

There are three main mechanisms of pathogenesis of ESCC: (1) arterial to the bone marrow from the primary

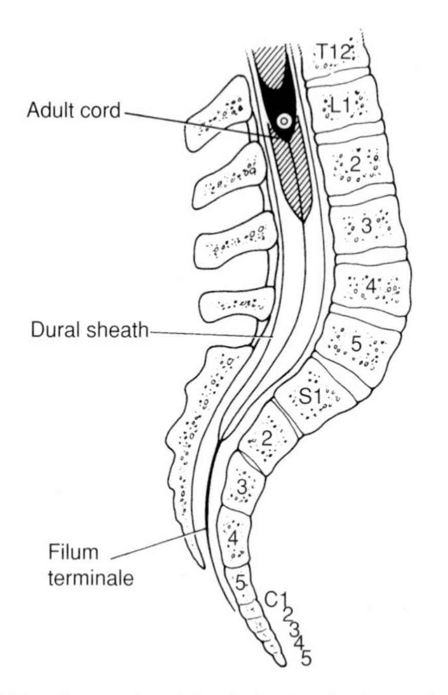

Fig. 30.11 Range of variation in the termination of the spinal cord. (Redrawn from Ellis, Clinical Anatomy, 5th edn, Blackwells, 1975.)

site (over 80% of solid tumours); (2) direct invasion through the intervertebral foramina (75% of lymphomas); (3) retrograde spread via Batson's vertebral venous plexus (rare). About 70% of ESCC occurs in the thoracic spine, 20% in the lumbosacral spine and 10% in the cervical spine.

Clinical features

Spinal cord compression may develop acutely or insidiously. Average age ranges between 53 and 63. Back pain is the commonest initial symptom (96%). Root pain is present in 90% of lumbosacral ESCC, 79% of cervical and 55% of thoracic epidural SCC. Root pain may precede neurological deficit by weeks or months. Since pretreatment neurological deficit predicts outcome, the detection of SCC before the onset of neurological deficit is important. Pain is typically constant and progressive and occurs at the site of compression. It tends to be worse on coughing, straining or on recumbency. Pain is commonly followed by limb weakness. This is usually bilateral. Urinary retention and incontinence are common. Sensory loss parallels the motor loss. Dermatomal sensory loss is a better guide than sensory level to localising the site of compression.

Diagnosis and investigation

Early diagnosis, ideally before the onset of neurological deficit, is important to achieve the best results of treatment. Once the diagnosis is clinically suspected, urgent magnetic resonance imaging of the whole spine should be carried out. MRI (Fig. 30.12) is preferable to myelography (Fig 30.13) because it is non-invasive and gives better definition of ESCC, vertebral metastases, intramedullary disease and multiple sites of compression. It also helps guide the neurosurgeon in assessing suitability for surgical stabilisation. Plain radiographs and bone scans are inferior guides to the site of compression and should not delay rapid access to MRI. Plain radiographs are abnormal in 85% of ESCC.

Pedicles may be absent ('winking owl' sign) or there may be evidence of vertebral collapse.

Where the source of the primary is not known, a chest radiograph, serum prostate-specific antigen assay, mammography and abdominal CT/ultrasound may help in its identification.

Treatment

The treatment of spinal cord compression remains controversial. Most published data on surgery and radiotherapy, the principal treatments, are retrospective, based on a variety of histologies and are subject to selection bias.

A major review in 1984 by Findlay, a British neurosurgeon, showed from pooled data that patients undergoing laminectomy were often neurologically

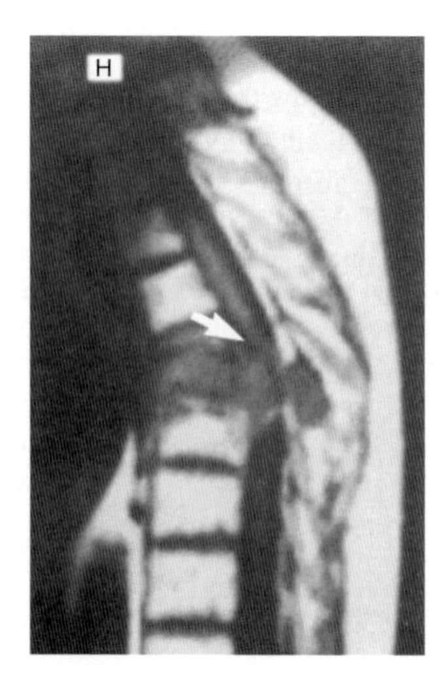

Fig. 30.12 MRI scan showing spinal cord compression (arrow) due to collapse of the 7th thoracic vertebra due to metastatic breast cancer (Courtesy of Dr L Turnbull, MRI Unit, Sheffield).

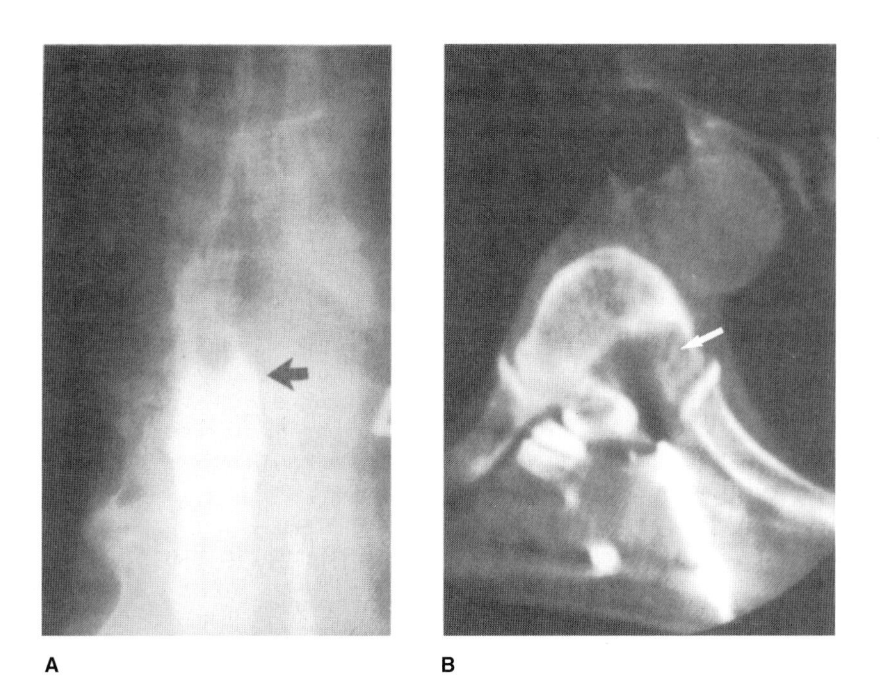

Fig. 30.13 **A** Myelogram showing complete block at T6 due to extradural compression from non-small cell lung cancer. **B** CT-guided biopsy of T6. Note destruction of the right side of the vertebral body (arrows). (Courtesy of Dr T Powell, Sheffield.)

worse compared to those who had primary radiotherapy. Increasingly, patients have been referred for palliative radiotherapy rather than surgery, and surgery has been reserved for patients where there is spinal instability, bony compression or paraplegia at presentation, deterioration during radiotherapy or in a previously maximally irradiated site. A systematic review by Loblaw and Laperriere suggested that radiotherapy should be the treatment of choice for ambulant patients except in the circumstances defined above.

Pain control with analgesia is a priority. Opiate medication may be required. Steroids should be started while awaiting definitive imaging, since the patient may have to be transferred to the cancer centre for treatment. 16 mg of i.v. dexamethasone can be given, followed by oral dexamethasone 4 mg q.d.s.

Unless there is evidence of spinal instability, patients may be mobilised. Physiotherapy to maximise recovery of ambulation is needed.

ESCC is a devastating complication of cancer for patients and their families. Support from palliative care specialists at home and in hospital is very valuable is helping patients and families to cope.

1. Palliative radiotherapy

Palliative radiotherapy is the treatment for the majority of patients with ESCC. It is most effective in radiosensitive tumours such as lymphomas, myeloma, breast and prostate cancer. It is advised in patients who can walk at diagnosis, have multiple sites of compression or who are unfit for surgery. Not surprisingly, the response of patients with purely epidural soft tissue disease is better than in those with bony collapse.

Target volume

Where MRI imaging is available, the site(s) of compression can be treated with a margin of one vertebral body above the below the highest and lowest sites of compression. Where MRI is not available, a wider margin is recommended of two vertebral bodies above and below the site(s) of compression judged from myelography. The lateral margin should encompass any associated soft tissue mass with a margin of 1–2 cm.

Technique

A single direct field is used. If there is more than one site of compression, then it may be possible to encompass these in a single field. Where the sites of compression are remote from one another, separate fields are recommended.

Dose

A variety of radiotherapy schedules are in use. Most centres use:

20–30 Gy in 5–10 fractions over 1–2 weeks (6 MV photons) prescribed at the depth of the spinal cord

There is no evidence that 20 Gy is any less effective than 30 Gy.

For solitary plasmacytoma causing cord compression, a higher dose is recommended to try to eradicate local disease.

40 Gy in 20 fractions over 4 weeks (6 MV photons)

Where the main aim of treatment is relief of pain and there is little prospect of neurological improvement, a single fraction of **8 Gy** may suffice.

Reirradiation of the spinal cord can be effective in relieving compression in a previously irradiated area which responded to the first course of radiotherapy.

2. Surgery

Surgery for spinal cord compression should be considered in the following circumstances:

- Radioresistant tumour such as sarcoma and melanoma
- Malignant spinal cord compression in a maximally irradiated site
- Progressive neurological deficit during radiotherapy
- Spinal instability
- Bony compression
- Rapidly evolving paraplegia.

Biopsy or laminectomy may be needed to establish a histological diagnosis in patients without a history of cancer. The role of surgery remains unclear. Certainly, maximal tumour debulking should be attempted to minimise the volume of disease to which radiotherapy is directed. Aggressive surgical management with vertebral body resection and insertion of Harrington rods above and below the compression can be effective in fit patients with reasonable life-expectancy in improving pain control and improving neurological deficit. In general, patients with lung cancer are not treated surgically because of their short life-expectancy. The significant morbidity and mortality of surgery also need to be taken into account.

3. Chemotherapy

Chemotherapy has a useful role in improving neurological deficit in conjunction with radiotherapy in chemosensitive tumours such as myeloma, lymphoma or teratoma.

Results of treatment

The major determinants of outcome are histology and degree of neurological deficit at diagnosis. Lymphoma, myeloma, breast and prostate cancer have an 80% initial response. Lung, melanoma and renal cancer respond in 25% of cases. The degree of weakness at presentation predicts outcome. Of those who are ambulant at presentation, 90% will remain so. About half of the patients with some degree of weakness will regain ambulation. However, only 13% of patients who are paraplegic with a radiosensitive tumour regain the ability to walk and none among those with radioresistant tumours. Recovery from paraplegia does occur, but rarely. Response may be slow over a period of weeks. In most patients any response that is likely to occur is likely to have occurred by a month after the end of radiotherapy. Assessment at a month after treatment is reasonable. Complete and durable responses may be seen in solitary plasmacytoma.

TUMOURS OF THE EYE AND ORBIT

Anatomy

The bony margins of the orbit contain the eyeball, the optic nerve and the recti and oblique muscles which move the eye. The optic nerve leaves the back of the globe and travels posteriorly, leaving the orbit via the optic canal. The eyeball is made up of three layers. The outer layer, the sclera, is fibrous. The middle layer, the uveal tract, is vascular and is composed of the choroid, the ciliary body and the iris. The choroid lines the inner surface of the sclera. The inner layer, the retina, is neural. The lens lies towards the front of the eyeball approximately 0.5 cm from the surface of the eye.

There are four rectus and two oblique muscles. The lateral rectus muscle moves the eyeball laterally and is supplied by the 6th cranial nerve. The other recti elevate, depress and move the eyeball inward, while the inferior oblique moves the eyeball upward and outward. These four muscles are supplied by the 3rd cranial nerve. The superior oblique moves the eye downward and outward and is supplied by the 4th cranial nerve.

The conjunctiva is a membrane lining the inner surface of the eyelids and is reflected over the anterior surface of the globe, terminating at the corneoscleral junction. The lacrimal gland lies in the upper lateral part of the orbit. Tears secreted by the gland drain into the nose through the nasolacrimal duct.

Pathology

Classification

Malignant tumours are best classified as orbital or intraocular. Orbital tumours may be primary or secondary. The principal sites of these tumours are shown in Figure 30.14.

1. Orbital tumours
   a. Primary
      (i) Lymphoma
      (ii) Rhabdomyosarcoma
      (iii) Lacrimal gland carcinoma
   b. Secondary
   Metastases (e.g. breast cancer, neuroblastoma)
2. Intraocular
   a. Primary
      (i) Retinoblastoma
      (ii) Malignant melanoma
   b. Metastases
      (i) Choroidal deposits (e.g. breast and lung cancer).

Frequency

In childhood retinoblastomas are the commonest neoplasms. They arise from the retina and may be bilateral. Uveal melanomas are the commonest primary neoplasms in adults. Most adult intraocular tumours occur in the choroid. Secondary tumour spread may occur by invasion of the orbit from tumours of the paranasal sinuses, nasopharynx and eyelids or as metastases from a primary tumour elsewhere. Of the latter, in order of frequency in adults are breast, lung, bowel and thyroid cancer. In childhood, neuroblastoma is the commonest tumour metastasising to the orbit, often bilaterally.

Radiation tolerance of the eye

The tolerance of different structures in the eye varies enormously. The most sensitive structure is the lens.

Lens

The probability of developing a cataract depends on the dose, the energy of radiation and the amount of the lens that has been irradiated. Cataracts may occur over a wide range of doses. Cataracts have been observed at doses as low as 2 Gy. However, normally doses of 5 Gy or more are required to cause clinically significant cataract. The tolerance of the lens to continuous low-dose-rate irradiation from an iridium-192 implant is greater, and doses of less than 20 Gy may not result in the formation of cataract. If cataracts are radiation induced, the period from treatment to the development of cataract is usually 2–3 years. Surgical removal of the cataract is usually possible.

Cornea and lacrimal gland

The acute effects of radiation on the cornea are normally temporary with pinhead-size erosions (punctate keratitis). Symptoms are local irritation and lacrimation.

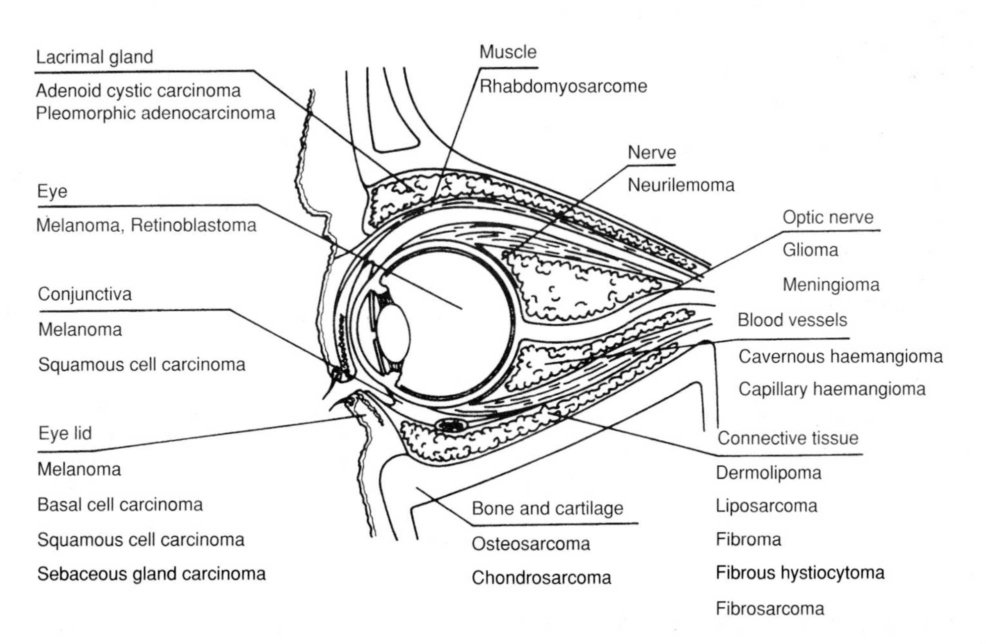

Fig. 30.14 Tumours of the eye and orbit. (Courtesy of Mr I Rennie, Sheffield.)

This normally occurs with doses of 30–50 Gy in 4–5 weeks and settles within a few weeks or months of irradiation. Topical steroids and antibiotics may alleviate the discomfort.

Megavoltage irradiation, because of its sparing of the superficial tissues, is less likely to cause acute keratitis than superficial and orthovoltage radiation.

The late effects are more serious. The lacrimal gland atrophies and tear production is impaired, if it has been irradiated to between 50 and 60 Gy. The result is a dry eye. At these dose levels, and those used for treating basal cell tumours at the inner canthus (e.g. 45 Gy in 10 daily fractions at 90–120 kV), the puncta and canaliculi of the lacrimal drainage apparatus may be occluded. As a result the eye may weep continuously (epiphora). In most cases epiphora following irradiation of basal cell carcinomas at the inner canthus is mild. However, surgical reconstruction of the duct may need to be considered if it is troublesome in a younger patient.

Most patients treated to doses of 30–40 Gy to the whole orbit do not develop marked symptoms of a dry eye.

The sensitivity of the cornea to painful stimuli is reduced. The absence of corneal pain may delay the diagnosis of corneal damage. The tolerance dose of the cornea is 50 Gy over 5 weeks. With doses in excess of 60 Gy, corneal ulceration occurs, usually following punctate keratitis and oedema, eventually healing with scarring and impairment of vision. Infection complicating the corneal radiation reaction increases the likelihood of corneal damage and should be treated with topical antibiotics.

Keratinisation of the cornea is a late complication. It tends to occur with doses in excess of 50 Gy. If the cornea is exposed to high doses of beta irradiation (e.g. 200–300 Gy from a strontium-90 applicator), secondary vascularisation and fatty infiltration may develop, causing blindness several years later.

Sclera

The sclera is rarely affected since it is avascular. Necrosis of the sclera is uncommon and doses of 100 Gy are needed to induce it. This may occur following irradiation with ruthenium-106 plaques for ocular melanoma.

Anterior chamber

Complications in the anterior chamber are rare. Rubeosis of the eye due to new vessel formation may follow cobalt-60 plaque therapy for retinoblastoma. Secondary glaucoma may follow.

Retina

No acute effects are experienced with conventionally fractionated external beam irradiation. Late effects are seen at doses in excess of 50 Gy. These changes are vascular. There are haemorrhages, exudates and degenerative changes. Optic atrophy may follow doses of 50–80 Gy over 4–8 weeks.

Principles of irradiation

It is difficult to irradiate the orbit uniformly while shielding the cornea and lens. A compromise is often necessary to enable adequate dosage to the tumour while limiting the dose to vulnerable structures, particularly the lens. It should be remembered that radiation-induced cataract can usually be removed surgically. Inadequate tumour dosage, however, may prove fatal. In these circumstances a higher risk of radiation damage may have to be accepted, if tumour cure is to be achieved. Ultimately the radiation-damaged eye may have to be surgically removed (enucleation).

Technique

For superficial tumours, for example lymphomas of the conjunctiva, a single anterior superficial (120 kV) or orthovoltage (250 kV) field may suffice. Treatment of basal and squamous cell tumours of the eyelids and inner canthus are described on page 329.

For deeper tumours (e.g. lacrimal gland carcinomas or rhabdomyosarcoma) an anterior and lateral wedged fields are used (Fig. 30.15). The front margin of the lateral field should lie at the outer canthus behind the cornea and lens. The lateral field is angled 5–10° posteriorly to avoid the lens of the opposite eye.

If there is forward displacement of the eye or involvement of the posterior or anteromedial part of the orbit, superior and inferior oblique fields give a better distribution of dose (Fig. 30.16).

RHABDOMYOSARCOMA

Pathology

The tumour is usually of embryonal type (see Ch. 31 on soft tissue sarcomas).

Clinical features

Rhabdomyosarcoma is a malignant tumour arising from the soft tissues. It is the commonest primary orbital tumour in childhood. The majority present under the age of 10 years, usually with rapidly progressive protrusion of the eye (exophthalmos). It may

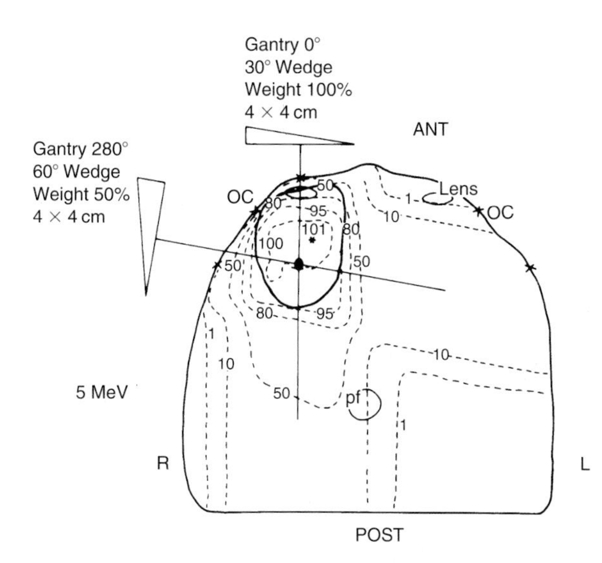

Fig. 30.15 Dose distribution for treatment of the orbit from an anterior and lateral field wedged pair of fields weighted 2 : 1. (Reproduced with permission of Arnold from Jane Dobbs, Ann Barrett, Daniel Ash, *Practical Radiotherapy Planning*, 3/e, Arnold, 1999.)

spread locally to the nasopharynx or ethmoid air sinuses. It metastasises to the cervical lymph nodes, lungs and occasionally bone.

Diagnosis and investigation

A biopsy should be carried out. Staging includes plain skull and chest radiographs, bone scan, orbital CT scan and bone marrow examination. Most patients are found to have localised disease.

Treatment

Treatment should be undertaken in a specialist centre. Initial cytotoxic chemotherapy is given to shrink the tumour (e.g. vincristine, actinomycin D and cyclophosphamide (VAC). This is followed by external beam irradiation to the whole orbit. Vincristine and cyclophosphamide are given during the period of radiotherapy. After radiotherapy, combination chemotherapy is continued for a further year.

Radical radiotherapy

Technique

An anterior and lateral wedged pair of megavoltage fields is used for posteriorly placed tumours. The eye is treated open to take advantage of the skin-sparing effect and reduce the severity of keratoconjunctivitis.

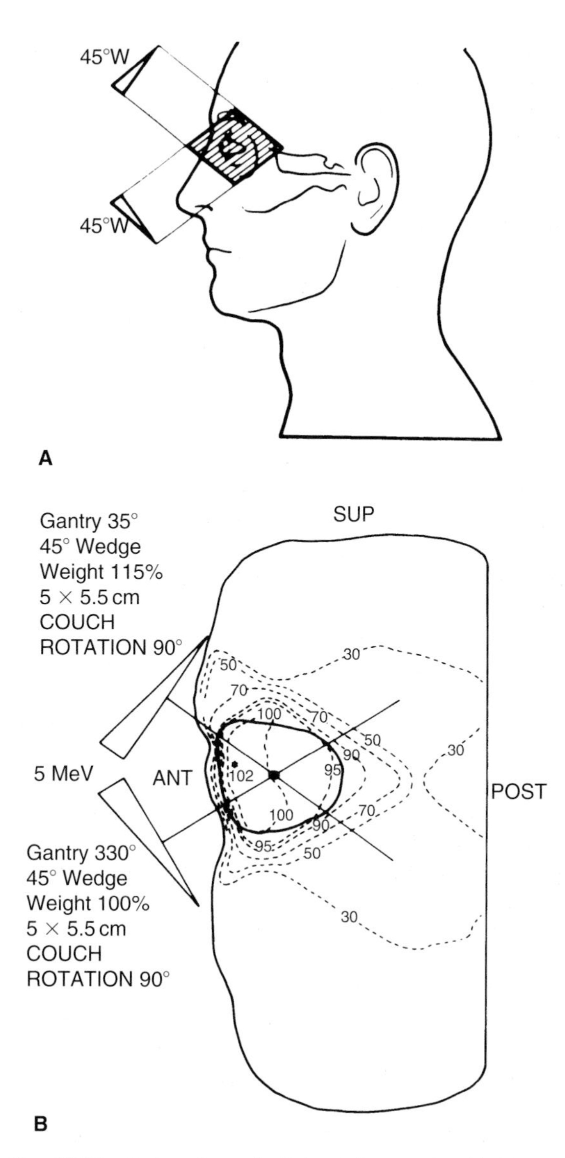

Fig. 30.16 **A** Superior and inferior oblique wedged fields for tumours displacing the globe. (Reproduced with permission of Arnold from Jane Dobbs, Ann Barrett, Daniel Ash, *Practical Radiotherapy Planning*, 3/e, Arnold, 1999.) **B** Dose distribution from **A**. (Reproduced with permission of Arnold from Jane Dobbs, Ann Barrett, Daniel Ash, *Practical Radiotherapy Planning*, 3/e, Arnold, 1999.)

For more anterior lesions an anterior electron field will suffice.

Dose and energy

40 Gy in 20 daily fractions over 4 weeks (6 MV photons or 16–20 MeV electrons)

Morbidity. The main acute reaction is painful keratoconjunctivitis. Cataract, impairment of bony growth of the orbit, and dry eye (xerophthalmia) are common late complications.

Results of treatment

The results of treatment are excellent, with over 90% of patients disease free at 5 years. Most relapses occur within the first 2 years. Careful follow-up by clinical and CT examination is essential.

OCULAR MELANOMA

Melanoma is the commonest primary intraocular tumour. In adults it most frequently affects the uveal tract, especially the choroid.

Clinical features and investigation

If the tumour arises on the iris, the patient or a relative may notice a pigmented spot. Melanomas more posterior in the eye are more difficult to diagnose and present with visual loss or symptoms of retinal detachment. Indirect ophthalmoscopy after dilating the pupil will reveal most tumours. Ultrasound is helpful in confirming the clinical diagnosis of choroidal melanoma (Plate 2.9). Fluorescein angiography is used to demonstrate tumour vascularity. MRI is superior to CT scanning in demonstrating involvement of the optic nerve or extraocular spread.

Natural history

Metastases are rarely present at the time of diagnosis but develop up to 15 years later in about 50% of patients, mainly in the liver, and are the main cause of tumour-related death.

Treatment

Iris melanomas

Melanomas of the iris are usually slow growing and can be kept under observation unless there is evidence that the tumour is growing, there is marked new vessel formation, impairment of vision or complications such as glaucoma. Small lesions can be locally excised. Removal of the eye (enucleation) is only very rarely indicated.

Choroid and ciliary body

The management of melanoma of the choroid and ciliary body is controversial. One of the main areas of disagreement is whether removal of the eye disseminates metastases. The aim of treatment is to preserve vision and to prolong survival.

For small melanomas of the choroid and ciliary body, the risks of a policy of observation alone are low. Laser therapy is suitable for very small tumours of the posterior choroid.

For medium-sized tumours (10–15 mm in diameter and 2–5 mm in height), the risks of observation alone are higher. The choice of treatment remains controversial. There is some evidence that the mortality of the disease is higher following enucleation. Radiotherapy does have a role in selected cases. Although melanoma is normally relatively radioresistant, brachytherapy to high doses with cobalt-60, ruthenium-106 or iodine-125 plaques and external irradiation with charged particles (protons and helium ions) have proved beneficial. It may be that radiation exerts its damaging effect on the tumour vasculature rather than by directly damaging tumour cells. Medium-sized tumours may also be locally resected.

Doses of protons 47–67 Gy in 5 fractions over 8–9 days have been well tolerated. Cobalt-60 or ruthenium-106 plaques are sutured to the sclera. Doses of 50–100 Gy are delivered to the apex of the tumour. Ruthenium-106 has the advantage of emitting predominantly beta radiation. The more limited penetration of ruthenium-106 is better suited to the depth of the tumour and requires less radiation protection than cobalt-60, which emits more penetrating gamma rays.

For large melanomas greater than 15 mm in diameter and 5 mm in height, local resection or enucleation is recommended.

Results of treatment

Iris melanomas metastasise in < 5% of cases and have a very good prognosis.

The prognosis of melanoma of the ciliary body and choroid is much poorer. Metastases usually occur within 5 years of diagnosis, typically first to the liver (60–70%). Most patients die within 6 months of the detection of metastases. Bad prognostic factors include large size, extrascleral extension, tumours arising in the ciliary body and old age. 50% of patients with large tumours die from melanoma. For small tumours of the choroid, the eye can be conserved, with useful vision in 75% of patients following proton irradiation.

RETINOBLASTOMA

Pathology

Retinoblastoma is a congenital tumour which develops from primitive cells in the retina. It is very rare

(0.5% of CNS tumours). Both inherited and sporadic (spontaneously arising) forms occur. The abnormal gene that is responsible for the inherited form lies on chromosome 13. However, only in about 10% of cases is a positive family history found, suggesting that spontaneous mutations account for the majority of cases. In the inherited form both eyes are affected (30% of cases).

Clinical features

Most (75%) of tumours present under 3 years of age and are sporadic. The presenting clinical features include an opaque light reflex (cat's eye reflex) in the normally dark pupil, or a squint. More advanced cases have raised intraocular pressure. Eventually there may be perforation of the globe. Local extension occurs within the orbit, often from tumour growth along the optic nerve. Metastases may occur to the central nervous system and the bone marrow.

Diagnosis and investigation

The management of children with retinoblastoma should be in specialised centres, in view of the rarity of the tumour and the good prospects of cure in the hands of an experienced ophthalmic surgeon and oncologist.

The diagnosis is made by indirect binocular ophthalmoscopy of both eyes under a general anaesthetic. The tumour is identified and staged according to a clinical classification (Table 30.2). It should be remembered that this classification relates to the prospect of retaining vision (falling with increasing stage) and not to survival. The diagnosis is clinical. Histological confirmation is not normally obtained unless the eye is removed. Additional staging investigations include a bone marrow biopsy, CSF examination and a bone scan to identify metastases.

Treatment

For small tumours every effort is made to conserve the eye and useful vision. Most unilateral non-inherited tumours present late and require enucleation. For advanced tumours or relapse following non-surgical treatment, enucleation is required.

1. Tumours up to 4 mm

Laser therapy is suitable for posteriorly placed tumours up to 4 mm in diameter. This form of treatment is not used for tumours just lateral to the optic disc because of the risk of damaging the macula. Cryotherapy (a method of freezing the tumour) is used for tumours lying more towards the front of the eye.

2. Tumours 4–13 mm in diameter

Tumours of 4–13 mm in diameter are treated with a radioactive plaque. Traditionally this was gamma--ray-emitting cobalt-60 or iodine-125. The external surface of the eyeball is exposed surgically and a specially prepared disc holding radioactive cobalt is sutured in position, overlying the tumour mass. The exact position of the growth must be determined by previous ophthalmoscopy. The disc is removed in a surgical operation a week later. A range of discs with diameters varying from 5–15 mm are available, each plaque forming part of a sphere that has an internal radius of 11 mm, corresponding to the radius of the eye.

Dose

A dose of 40 Gy is delivered to the apex of the tumour. The maximum dose at the surface of the eyeball is about 200 Gy.

3. Larger tumours

External beam irradiation is indicated for:

Table 30.2 St Bartholomew's Hospital modification of Reese staging of retinoblastoma

Stage	Clinical findings
I	Single or multiple tumours less than 4 disc diameters at or behind the equator (1 disc diameter = 1.5 mm)
IIa	Solitary lesion 4–10 disc diameters at or behind the equator
IIb	Solitary lesion larger than 10 disc diameters at or behind the equator
III	Lesions anterior to the equator
IVa	Multiple tumours, some larger than 10 disc diameters
IVb	Any lesion extending anteriorly beyond the limit of ophthalmoscopy
Va	Massive neoplasms
Vb	Vitreous seedlings
VI	Residual orbital disease or optic nerve infiltration

- Tumours in excess of 13 mm in diameter
- Two or more tumours which cannot be covered by a single plaque
- Vitreous seedlings
- Tumours close to the macula or optic disc.

Target volume
The whole of the eye should be treated.

Technique
Previously a direct anterior field was treated with cobalt-60 irradiation, shielding if possible the lacrimal gland and the nasolacrimal duct (Fig. 30.17). This ensured that the whole of the eye was treated to cover any vitreous seedling or second primary. The eyelid is taped to keep the eye open to spare the anterior part of the eye.

The technique using a lateral field illustrated in Figure 30.18 is recommended for single tumours lying at the back of the eye without vitreous seedlings. The child is sedated. A contact lens is placed over the cornea. The contact lens serves as a fixed point from which measurements can be made. The beam from a linear accelerator is split to reduce divergence so that the front of the beam edge is sharply defined. The depth of the back of the lens can be measured by ultrasound. The front of the lateral beam can then be positioned at this point. It is angled back to avoid the lens of the opposite eye.

Dose and energy
40 Gy in 20 daily fractions over 4 weeks (6 MV photons)

Morbidity. If the whole eye is irradiated, cataract will develop, usually 2 years after treatment. This may be removed surgically. Xerophthalmia (dry eye) and retardation of the growth of the orbit are common.

Chemotherapy

Chemotherapy is reserved for palliation and is of limited efficacy. Agents such as vincristine, cyclophosphamide and derivatives of platinum have been used.

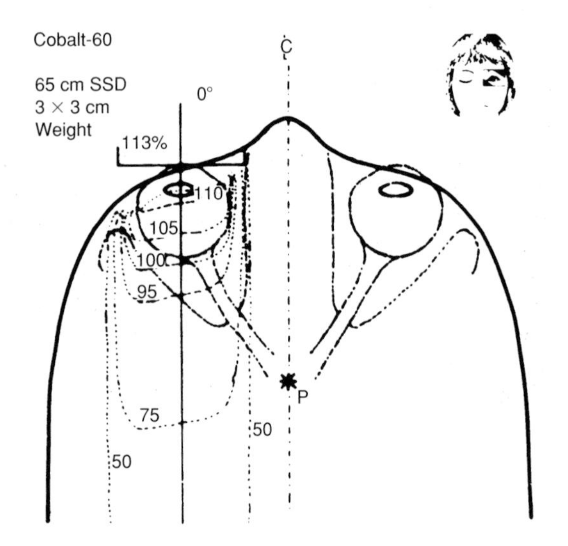

Fig. 30.17 A direct anterior megavoltage for treatment of the whole eye in retinoblastoma. The lacrimal gland and nasolacrimal duct may be shielded (see inset). (Reproduced with permission from Butterworth-Heinemann, a division of Reed Educational & Professional Publishing Ltd from Radiotherapy in clinical practice. Hope-Stone H F (ed) Textbook of Radiotherapy, 5th edn, 1986.)

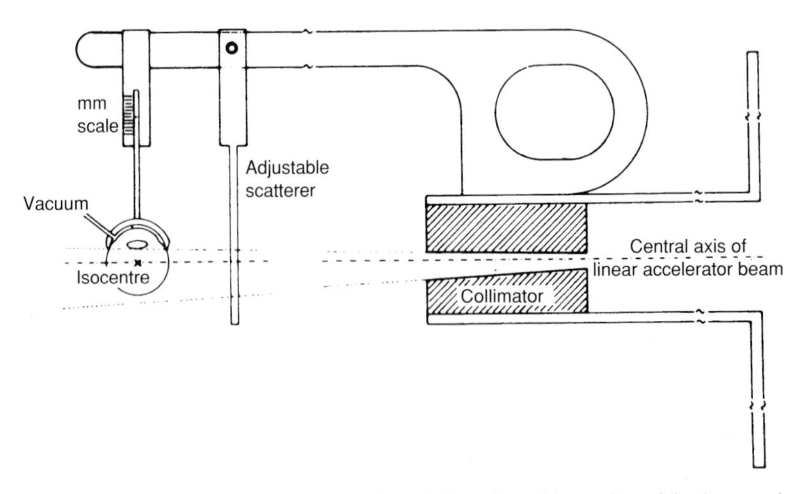

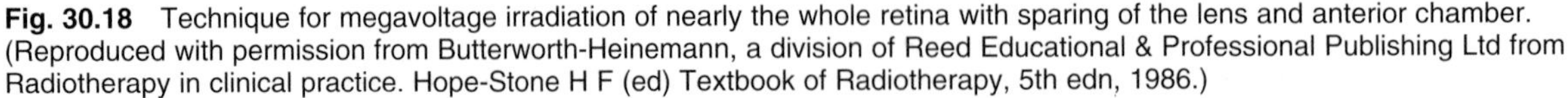

Fig. 30.18 Technique for megavoltage irradiation of nearly the whole retina with sparing of the lens and anterior chamber. (Reproduced with permission from Butterworth-Heinemann, a division of Reed Educational & Professional Publishing Ltd from Radiotherapy in clinical practice. Hope-Stone H F (ed) Textbook of Radiotherapy, 5th edn, 1986.)

Results of treatment

Many tumours present late with no prospect of useful vision. The eye is therefore removed.

Most posterior tumours can be controlled by radiation, with useful vision in up to 90%. This falls to 30% for multiple growths or those in the anterior part of the eye. About 50% of patients with extensive involvement of the optic nerve or residual disease in the orbit will die from metastatic disease.

CHOROIDAL DEPOSITS

Blood-borne metastases to the eye tend to lodge in the choroid, resulting in retinal detachment. Choroidal deposits generally present with sudden or rapidly progressive visual loss, usually in a patient with known breast or lung cancer. In 50% of cases, both eyes are affected. The typical 'honeycomb' appearance of the fundus is shown in Plate 2.11. Choroidal metastases usually imply a poor prognosis, with most patients dying within 1 year of the appearance.

Urgent radiotherapy is required to preserve vision.

Palliative radiotherapy

Target volume

The whole of the eye is included.

Technique

Choroidal deposits can be treated by a single anterior megavoltage photon or cobalt field or a lateral field angled 5–10° posteriorly. If an anterior field is used, the eye is taped open to take advantage of the skin-sparing effect of megavoltage to reduce the dose to the cornea and lens.

Dose and energy

30 Gy in 10 daily fractions over 2 weeks (6 MV photons or cobalt-60)

Results of treatment

Choroidal metastases are well worth treating, with improvement or at least conservation of vision in most patients.

CHAPTER CONTENTS

31

Sarcomas

Martin Robinson and Ian Kunkler

SOFT TISSUE SARCOMAS

Soft tissue sarcomas (Fig. 31.1) are malignant tumours arising from supporting connective tissues anywhere in the body. These structures (fibrous tissue, fat, blood vessels, smooth and skeletal muscle, tendons and cartilage) are derived embryologically from the mesoderm. Sarcomas of bone also occur and are discussed in this chapter under bone tumours. Tumours of peripheral nerves are generally included.

Despite arising from a wide variety of tissues, they have many similarities in pathology, clinical findings and behaviour.

Pathology

Soft tissue sarcomas are rare, representing 0.4% of all cancers and 0.3% of cancer deaths. The incidence is about 0.6 per 100 000 population per year. However, they constitute 6% of tumours in children under the age of 15. Most occur in the 40–70 age group. The sex ratio is virtually the same.

Their aetiology is largely unknown. In a minority of cases genetic factors are involved. There is, for example, an increased incidence of the tumour in association with certain genetically transmitted diseases, e.g. Gardner's syndrome, tuberous sclerosis, Von Recklinghausen's disease and Li–Fraumeni syndrome. Rarely soft tissue sarcomas may occur in the children of mothers with breast cancer of early onset.

Some sarcomas are radiation induced and occur within previously irradiated areas (especially for benign angiomas). The incidence of sarcomas among young people who have been treated with both chemotherapy and radiotherapy for Ewing's sarcoma may reach 18%.

Oncogenes may well have a role in malignant transformation, although the mechanism is as yet unknown. The *ras* gene has, for example, been identified in rhabdomyosarcoma, and there are chromosome 12 ab-

Table 31.1 Chromosomal translocations associated with sarcomas

Tumor type	Translocation	Fusion transcript
Ewing's sarcoma/peripheral neuroectodermal tumour (ES/PNET)	t(11;22)(q24;q12) t(21;22)(q22;q12) t(7;22)(q22;q12) t(17;22)(q12;q12) t(2;22)(q33;q12)	*EWS–FLI1* *EWS–ERG* *EWS–ETV1* *EWS–E1AF* *EWS–FEV*
Desmoplastic small round cell tumour	t(11;22)(p13;q12)	*EWS–WT1*
Myxoid liposarcoma	t(12;16)(q13;p11) t(12;22)(q13;q12)	*TLS–CHOP* *EWS–CHOP*
Extraskeletal myxoid chondrosarcoma	t(9;22)(q22;q12)	*EWS–CHN*
Clear cell sarcoma	t(12;22)(q13;q21)	*EWS–ATF1*
Synovial sarcoma	t(X;18)(p11.23;q11) t(X;18)(p11.21;q11)	*SYT–SSX1* *SYT–SSX2*
Alveolar rhabdomyosarcoma	t(2;13)(q35;q14) t(1;13)(p36;q14)	*PAX3–FKHR* *PAX7–FKHR*
Dermatofibrosarcoma protuberans	t(17;22)(q22;q13)	*COL1A1–PDGFB*
Congenital fibrosarcoma	t(12;15)(p13;q25)	*TEL–NTRK3*

normalities in tumours of fat. Many sarcomas have a demonstrable chromosome translocation (Table 31.1) with identifiable gene fusion products.

Rhabdomyosarcoma and soft tissue Ewing's sarcoma, although included in some lists of histological subtypes of soft tissue sarcomas, are quite different from the rest of the group, both in natural history and in being in general more chemo- and radiosensitive. Thus the principles of treatment outlined below do not apply to these two histological types.

The World Health Organization (WHO) classification is the most frequently used (Table 31.2). In some tumours it is not possible to be certain of the cells from which they originate (sarcoma not otherwise specified). Many others defy classification because they lack an obvious pattern of differentiation. From the point of view of management and prognosis the histological subtype is generally less important than the histological grading and the size of the tumour. Grading may depend in part on the tumour subtype, but more often is assessed by scoring the degree of necrosis and mitotic index. Low-grade tumours have a recognisable pattern of differentiation, relatively few mitoses, and no necrosis. High-grade tumours include all examples of certain subtypes (e.g. alveolar soft part), tumours with little or no apparent differentiation, and those with necrosis and a high mitotic rate. The tumour size is also important, and those over 5 cm are much more likely to recur locally or give rise to distant metastases.

Initial spread from the primary site is into adjacent tissue and along tissue planes between structures such as muscle bundles. Soft tissue sarcomas do not possess a true capsule but are often surrounded by a pseudocapsule of compressed surrounding tissues. This apparent encapsulation may tempt the surgeon to try to 'shell out' the tumour. Local recurrence from residual tumour at the periphery is then very likely (up to 90% within 2 years). Lymph node spread is infrequent, while blood-borne spread is common, giving rise to distant metastases, predominantly in the lungs.

Clinical features

Approximately 40% of soft tissue sarcomas occur in the upper and lower limbs. Of these about 75% occur at or above the knee. 10% of sarcomas arise in the upper half of the body. Of the sarcomas of the trunk, 10% occur in the retroperitoneum and 20% in the chest or abdominal wall. Presentation with advanced disease is common, particularly with intra-abdominal sarcomas, which may reach a very large size.

The history is usually of a painless lump developing over a few weeks or months and occasionally over years. Pain may occur from pressure on local structures, e.g. nerves and joints. Occasionally nonmetastatic effects are seen (e.g. hypoglycaemia in malignant fibrous histiocytoma).

Diagnosis and staging

Important features of local examination for limb or truncal sarcomas is the position of the lesion superficial or

Table 31.2 WHO histological classification of soft tissue tumours

I. Fibrous tumours
- A. Benign tumours
  1. Nodular fasciitis (including intravascular and cranial types)
  2. Proliferative fasciitis and myositis
  3. Atypical decubital fibroplasia (ischaemic fasciitis)
  4. Fibroma (dermal, tendon sheath, nuchal)
  5. Keloid
  6. Elastofibroma
  7. Calcifying aponeurotic fibroma
  8. Fibrous hamartoma of infancy
  9. Fibromatosis colli
  10. Infantile digital fibromatosis
  11. Myofibromatosis (solitary, multicentric)
  12. Hyalin fibromatosis
  13. Calcifying fibrous pseudotumour
- B. Fibromatoses
  1. Superficial fibromatoses
     - a. Palmar and plantar fibromatosis
     - b. Penile (Peyronie's) fibromatosis
     - c. Knuckle pads
  2. Deep fibromatoses (desmoid tumour)
     - a. Abdominal fibromatosis (abdominal desmoid)
     - b. Extra-abdominal fibromatosis (extra-abdominal desmoid)
     - c. Intra-abdominal fibromatosis (intra-abdominal desmoid)
     - d. Mesenteric fibromatosis (including Gardner's syndrome)
     - e. Infantile (desmoid-type) fibromatosis
- C. Malignant tumours
  1. Fibrosarcoma
     - a. Adult fibrosarcoma
     - b. Congenital or infantile fibrosarcoma
     - c. Inflammatory fibrosarcoma (inflammatory myofibroblastic tumour)

II. Fibrohistiocytic tumours
- A. Benign tumours
  1. Fibrous histiocytoma
     - a. Cutaneous fibrous histiocytoma (dermatofibroma)
     - b. Deep fibrous histiocytoma
  2. Juvenile xanthogranuloma
  3. Reticulohistiocytoma
  4. Xanthoma
- B. Intermediate tumours
  1. Atypical fibroxanthoma
  2. Dermatofibrosarcoma protuberans (including pigmented form, Bednar tumour)
  3. Giant cell fibroblastoma
  4. Plexiform fibrohistiocytic tumour
  5. Angiomatoid fibrous histiocytoma
- C. Malignant tumours
  1. Malignant fibrous histiocytoma
     - a. Storiform-pleomorphic fibrous histiocytoma
     - b. Myxoid fibrous histiocytoma
     - c. Giant cell fibrous histiocytoma (malignant giant cell tumour of soft parts)
     - d. Xanthomatous (inflammatory type) fibrous histiocytoma

III. Lipomatous tumours
- A. Benign tumours
  1. Lipoma
     - a. Cutaneous lipoma
     - b. Deep lipoma
       - (i) Intramuscular lipoma
       - (ii) Tendon sheath lipoma
       - (iii) Lumbosacral lipoma
       - (iv) Intraneural and perineural fibrolipoma
     - c. Multiple lipomas

Table 31.2 WHO histological classification of soft tissue tumours *(contd)*

2. Angiolipoma
3. Spindle cell or pleomorphic lipoma
4. Myolipoma
5. Angiomyolipoma
6. Myelolipoma
7. Chondroid lipoma
8. Hibernoma
9. Lipoblastoma or lipoblastomatosis
10. Lipomatosis
    a. Diffuse lipomatosis
    b. Cervical symmetrical lipomatosis (Madelung's disease)
11. Atypical lipoma

B. Malignant tumours
1. Liposarcoma
    a. Well-differentiated liposarcoma
        (i) Lipoma-like liposarcoma
        (ii) Sclerosing liposarcoma
        (iii) Inflammatory liposarcoma
    b. Myxoid liposarcoma
    c. Round cell (poorly differentiated myxoid) liposarcoma
    d. Pleomorphic liposarcoma
    e. Dedifferentiated liposarcoma

IV. Smooth muscle tumours
A. Benign tumours
1. Leiomyoma (cutaneous, deep and pleomorphic)
2. Angiomyoma (vascular leiomyoma)
3. Epithelioid leiomyoma
4. Intravenous leiomyomatosis
5. Leiomyomatosis peritonealis disseminata

B. Malignant tumours
1. Leiomyosarcoma
2. Epithelioid leiomyosarcoma

V. Skeletal muscle tumours
A. Benign tumours
1. Adult rhabdomyoma
2. Genital rhabdomyoma
3. Fetal rhabdomyoma
4. Intermediate (cellular) rhabdomyoma

B. Malignant tumours
1. Rhabdomyosarcoma
    a. Embryonal rhabdomyosarcoma
    b. Botryoid rhabdomyosarcoma
    c. Spindle cell rhabdomyosarcoma
    d. Alveolar rhabdomyosarcoma
    e. Pleomorphic rhabdomyosarcoma
2. Rhabdomyosarcoma with ganglionic differentiation (ectomesenchymoma)

VI. Tumours of blood and lymph vessels
A. Benign tumours
1. Papillary endothelial hyperplasia
2. Haemangioma
    a. Capillary (including juvenile) haemangioma
    b. Cavernous haemangioma
    c. Venous haemangioma
    d. Epithelioid haemangioma (angiolymphoid hyperplasia, histiocytoid haemangioma)
    e. Granulation type haemangioma (pyogenic granuloma)
    f. Tufted haemangioma
3. Deep haemangioma (intramuscular, synovial, perineural)
4. Lymphangioma
5. Lymphangiomyoma and lymphangiomyomatosis
6. Angiomatosis
7. Lymphangiomatosis

- B. Intermediate tumours
  1. Haemangioendothelioma
     a. Epithelioid haemangioendothelioma
     b. Endovascular papillary haemangioendothelioma (Dabska tumour)
     c. Spindle cell haemangioendothelioma
- C. Malignant tumours
  1. Angiosarcoma and lymphangiosarcoma
  2. Kaposi's sarcoma

VII. Perivascular tumours
- A. Benign tumours
  1. Glomus tumour
  2. Glomangiomyoma
  3. Haemangiopericytoma
- B. Malignant tumours
  1. Malignant glomus tumour
  2. Malignant haemangiopericytoma

VIII. Synovial tumours
- A. Benign tumours
  1. Tenosynovial giant cell tumour
     a. Localised tenosynovial giant cell tumour
     b. Diffuse tenosynovial giant cell tumour (extra-articular pigmented villonodular synovitis, florid tenosynovitis)
- B. Malignant tumours
  1. Synovial sarcoma
     a. Biphasic (fibrous *and* epithelial synovial sarcoma)
     b. Monophasic (fibrous or epithelial) synovial sarcoma
  2. Malignant giant cell tumour of tendon sheath

IX. Mesothelial tumours
- A. Benign tumours
  1. Solitary fibrous tumour of pleura and peritoneum (localised fibrous mesothelioma)
  2. Multicystic mesothelioma
  3. Adenomatoid tumour
  4. Well-differentiated papillary mesothelioma
- B. Malignant tumours
  1. Malignant solitary fibrous tumour of pleura and peritoneum
  2. Diffuse mesothelioma
     a. Epithelial diffuse mesothelioma
     b. Fibrous (spindled, sarcomatoid) diffuse mesothelioma
     c. Biphasic diffuse mesothelioma

X. Neural tumours
- A. Benign tumours
  1. Traumatic neuroma
  2. Morton's neuroma
  3. Multiple mucosal neuromas
  4. Neuromuscular hamartoma (benign Triton tumour)
  5. Nerve sheath ganglion
  6. Schwannoma (neurilemoma)
     a. Cellular schwannoma
     b. Plexiform schwannoma
     c. Degenerated (ancient) schwannoma
     d. Schwannomatosis
  7. Neurothekeoma (nerve sheath myxoma)
  8. Neurofibroma
     a. Diffuse neurofibroma
     b. Plexiform neurofibroma
     c. Pacinian neurofibroma
     d. Epithelioid neurofibroma
  9. Granular cell tumour
  10. Melanocytic schwannoma
  11. Ectopic meningioma
  12. Ectopic ependymoma
  13. Ganglioneuroma
  14. Pigmented neuroectodermal tumour of infancy (retinal anlage tumour, melanotic progonoma)

Table 31.2 WHO histological classification of soft tissue tumours *(contd)*

- B. Malignant tumours
  - 1. Malignant peripheral nerve sheath tumour (MPNST) (malignant schwannoma, neurofibrosarcoma)
    - a. Malignant Triton tumour (MPNST with rhabdomyosarcoma)
    - b. Glandular MPNST (malignant glandular schwannoma)
    - c. Epithelioid MPNST (malignant epithelioid schwannoma)
  - 2. Malignant granular cell tumour
  - 3. Clear cell sarcoma (malignant melanoma of soft parts)
  - 4. Malignant melanocytic schwannoma
  - 5. Gastrointestinal autonomous nerve tumour (plexosarcoma)
  - 6. Primitive neuroectodermal tumour
    - a. Neuroblastoma
    - b. Ganglioneuroblastoma
    - c. Neuroepithelioma (peripheral neuroectodermal tumour)
    - d. Extraskeletal Ewing's sarcoma

XI. Paraganglionic tumours
- A. Benign tumours
  - 1. Paraganglioma
- B. Malignant tumours
  - 1. Malignant paraganglioma

XII. Extraskeletal cartilaginous and osseous tumours
- A. Benign tumours
  - 1. Panniculitis ossificans and myositis ossificans
  - 2. Fibro-osseous pseudotumour of the digits
  - 3. Fibrodysplasia (myositis) ossificans progressiva
  - 4. Extraskeletal chondroma or osteochondroma
  - 5. Extraskeletal osteoma
- B. Malignant tumours
  - 1. Extraskeletal chondrosarcoma
    - a. Well-differentiated chondrosarcoma
    - b. Myxoid chondrosarcoma
    - c. Mesenchymal chondrosarcoma
  - 2. Extraskeletal osteosarcoma

XIII. Pluripotential mesenchymal tumours
- A. Benign tumours
  - 1. Mesenchymoma
- B. Malignant tumours
  - 1. Malignant mesenchymoma

XIV. Miscellaneous tumours
- A. Benign tumours
  - 1. Congenital granular cell tumour
  - 2. Tumoral calcinosis
  - 3. Myxoma
    - a. Cutaneous myxoma
    - b. Intramuscular myxoma
    - c. Juxta-articular myxoma
  - 4. Angiomyxoma
  - 5. Amyloid tumour
  - 6. Parachordoma
  - 7. Ossifying and non-ossifying fibromyxoid tumours
  - 8. Palisaded myofibroblastoma of lymph node
- B. Malignant tumours
  - 1. Alveolar soft part sarcoma
  - 2. Epithelioid sarcoma
  - 3. Malignant extrarenal rhabdoid tumour
  - 4. Desmoplastic small cell tumour

XV. Unclassified tumours

deep to the fascia at the primary tumour site and any involvement of bone, vascular or neural invasion. Regional nodes, although uncommonly involved, should be palpated.

A biopsy is required. In 90% of cases adequate histology can be achieved by needle core biopsy. Where an incisional biopsy is required, care should be taken to make the incision longitudinal so that any subsequent radical surgery or postoperative radiation fields can include it. This is particularly important where preservation of limb function is a major consideration. Appropriate siting of the biopsy is vital if the probability of local control is to be maximised. The biopsy should ideally be carried out by the surgeon who will undertake the definitive resection. There is otherwise the risk of tumour spillage, particularly after unplanned attempts to remove deep-seated lesions. If CT-guided biopsy is needed, for example for impalpable deep-seated lesions, there is also potential for needle track contamination. Close liaison with the surgeon and clinical oncologist is needed to plan the best route of biopsy. Specialist pathology review is essential in view of the complexity of these tumours and the need for careful assessment of the tumour margins.

A full blood count, liver function tests, chest radiograph, plain radiographs of the tumour-bearing region and liver ultrasound are the initial investigations. CT and MRI (Fig. 31.1) scanning are important in defining the local extent and operability of the tumour. MRI is the imaging modality of choice for limb sarcomas since it provides good contrast between the tumour and adjoining normal tissues. It also provides better multiplanar versatility in planning surgery and radiotherapy than CT. CT can be helpful in exclusion of cortical erosion of bone, albeit an uncommon finding. CT and MRI are also useful in confirming any subsequent local recurrence but should not be used for routine follow-up. CT of the thorax is advisable if chest radiography is normal and radical therapy is contemplated, since it may demonstrate small-volume lung metastases. The staging system commonly adopted includes grade, size, and presence/absence of metastases (Table 31.3).

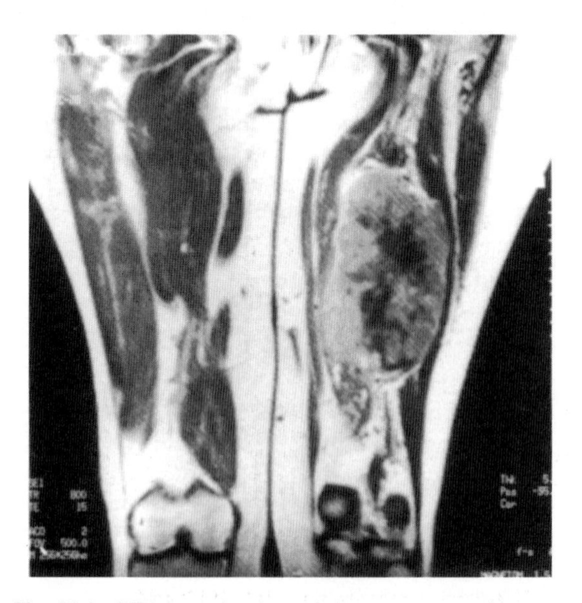

Fig. 31.1 MRI scan showing soft tissue sarcoma with central necrosis in the hamstring compartment of the thigh. (Courtesy of Dr L Turnbull, MRI Unit, Sheffield.)

Management

A multidisciplinary approach is required since surgery, radiotherapy and chemotherapy may all have a role to play, depending on the stage, site, grade and size of the tumour. A dedicated sarcoma unit allows treatment to be carefully coordinated and minimises the number of surgical procedures necessary. Correct procedures for biopsy, imaging and exclusion of metastatic disease are essential. Historically, amputation was the main treatment for limb sarcomas but in the 1970s it was appreciated that radiotherapy and surgery could provide comparable results. Limb-sparing surgery with postoperative radiotherapy achieved the same survival as amputation, albeit with a slightly higher local recurrence rate. In the past, sarcomas were regarded as relatively radioresistant tumours. It is now known that they are relatively radiosensitive, comparable to breast cancer.

Local control while maximising the probability of conserving limb function and long-term survival is of vital importance. For extremity limb sarcomas 90% local control at 5 years should be the standard. The management of soft tissue sarcomas is controversial. In part this reflects the limited number of randomised trials in this heterogeneous group of tumours. The relative rarity of non-extremity sarcomas makes the design of and recruitment to large randomised trials difficult. Few would dispute the primary role of radical surgery. If the surgical resections are clear, the 5-year local control for limb sarcomas is of the order of 90%. If the margins are involved, this falls to 60–80%. Involved margins are an independent risk factor for local recurrence. The extent of the resection will depend upon the site of the tumour. The more distal the tumour in the limb, the more difficult a complete excision becomes. Radical excision surgery of retroperitoneal sarcomas is also rarely feasible. The primary tumour should be resected with one anatomical plane clear of the tumour at all stages. The

Table 31.3 Staging system of soft tissue sarcomas

TNM	Clinical findings	Stage	
Tumour size		Ia	G1 T1 N0 M0
		Ib	G1 T2 N0 M0
T1	Tumour less than 5 cm in diameter	IIa	G2 T1 N0 M0
		IIb	G2 T2 N0 M0
T2	Tumour 5 cm or more in diameter	IIIa	G3 T1 N0 M0
		IIIb	G3 T2 N0 M0
		IIIc	Any G, T1–2 N1 M0
T3	Tumour invading bone, major vessels or nerves	IVa	Any G, T3, any N, M0
		IVb	Any G or T, M1
Nodes			
N0	No histologically verified metastasis to regional nodes		
N1	Biopsy-proven regional lymph node metastases		
Metastases			
M0	No distant metastases		
M1	Distant metastases		

G, histological grade (1, 2 or 3)

aim of the surgery is to achieve a wide local excision (margin ≥ 2 cm where possible) (Fig. 31.2). The resection should include all the skin and subcutaneous tissue near to the tumour, any previous excision or biopsy scars and areas containing blood clot from previous biopsies. The tumour itself should never be actively contacted during resection. Metallic clips at the margins of the excision are helpful in planning the limits of post-operative irradiation.

Amputation for extremity sarcomas is only indicated in the following situations:

1. When serious radiation-induced morbidity would result from attempting radical radiotherapy
2. In some distal limb sarcomas, where a below knee amputation may be more functional than a lower limb with the combined local morbidity of surgery and radiotherapy
3. When there is recurrent disease not suitable for limited resection or adjuvant radiotherapy.

Adjuvant therapy

For low-grade tumours less than 5 cm in size which have been widely excised with clear surgical margins, no further therapy is necessary in most cases. The same applies following an amputation. However, postoperative radiotherapy is indicated in the following circumstances to reduce the probability of local recurrence (see above):

- Limb-conserving or limited surgery (see below)
- Gross residual tumour or inadequate excision margins
- Grade 2 or 3 histology
- Tumours 5 cm or more in any dimension
- Virtually all tumours in the head and neck (because of the impossibility of adequate excision).

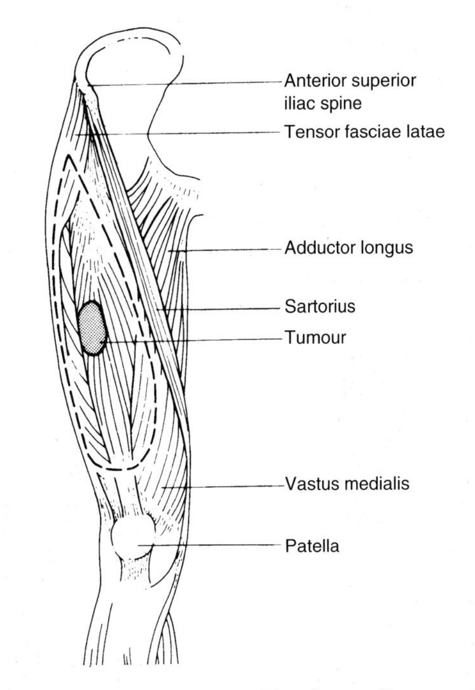

Fig. 31.2 Compartmentectomy. The diagram illustrates the wide surgical excision of soft tissue situated, in this case, in the rectus femoris. (Reproduced with permission from Souhami & Tobias, Cancer and its Management, Blackwells, 1986.)

Postoperative radiotherapy conventionally is with external beam (photons or particles—electrons, protons, pions or neutrons), although postoperative brachytherapy with iridium-192 (42–45 Gy over 4–6 days) had a high 5-year local control rate of 90% in a randomised trial compared to 65% for high-but not low-grade lesions. There are no randomised trials comparing brachytherapy with external beam irradiation. Brachytherapy should only be carried out in specialist units undertaking a substantial number of procedures. The reason for the ineffectiveness of brachytherapy in low-grade tumours is not clear. One possibility is that the long cell cycle in low-grade tumours may result in cells not entering the radiosensitive phase of the cell cycle during the period of brachytherapy.

The radiobiological effect of protons is similar to that of photons. The main advantage of protons is their capacity to configure the beam to limit doses to critical structures such as the spinal cord. Neutrons have the theoretical advantage over photons of reduced repair of radiation injury to tumour cells, radiosensitivity throughout the cell cycle and capacity to damage hypoxic tumour cells. Their major disadvantage is the increased risk of major late normal tissue damage. The use of neutrons is not recommended outside clinical trials.

Not all sites are suitable for radical radiotherapy. Pelvic, thoracic or abdominal sarcomas present particular difficulties because of the morbidity that would be caused by wide-field irradiation, dose-limiting critical structures (e.g. the spinal cord), tumour spillage in abdominal tumours, mediastinal shift after resection of thoracic tumours and pleural contamination.

Limb-conserving surgery

If limb-conserving surgery is undertaken (i.e. removal of the tumour mass with narrower excision margins), postoperative radiotherapy is given to deal with microscopic residual disease. In this way a more functional limb with a more satisfactory cosmetic result can be achieved. Conservative surgery is contraindicated where high-dose radiotherapy is poorly tolerated (see below).

Timing of radiotherapy

Preoperative radiotherapy has the advantage that the tumour is well oxygenated and intact. It may also allow coverage by smaller radiation fields and use of lower doses without reducing local control. These advantages have to be balanced against the disadvantages of difficulties in interpreting pathology following irradiation and an increase in risk of wound complications. Retrospective series of preoperative radiotherapy are subject to selection bias but have suggested that preoperative radiotherapy may be of value in lesions > 5 cm. A recent randomised trial comparing preoperative and postoperative radiotherapy was stopped because of increased wound complications in the preoperative arm. However, final limb function was still better in the preoperative group. Sites where preoperative radiotherapy may be considered within the constraints of normal tissue tolerance are the head and neck (paranasal sinuses, skull base, cheek and face), retroperitoneum, and extremity tumours.

Primary radical radiotherapy

Radical radiotherapy alone is indicated for patients unfit for surgery but otherwise in reasonable general condition, those who refuse surgery or where the anatomical site precludes it (e.g. retroperitoneum). Preoperative adjuvant radiotherapy is recommended for very large sarcomas.

Contraindications to radical radiotherapy. The high doses of radiotherapy required for sarcoma are poorly tolerated by highly stressed areas of the lower limb, e.g. Achilles tendon, or in the ribs where pathological fractures may occur. Radical radiotherapy to the Achilles tendon is inadvisable, especially in young and active patients, since rupture may occur.

Target volume

Definition of the target volume requires information from the surgeon, pathologist and radiologist. The surgeon should be encouraged to place radiopaque clips at the margins of the resection. The pathologist should comment on the adequacy of the resection. Very often it is necessary to ask the surgeon to carry out a further excision before postoperative radiotherapy is undertaken. The radiotherapist needs to discuss with the radiologist the position of the tumour, local extent and any residual disease as seen on CT and MRI.

Most sarcomas tend to spread in the axial plane of the limb (major fascial planes, bone and interosseous membranes). For this reason the margins of the radiation field must be generous in the craniocaudal directions. In the transverse plane, there can be greater confidence that local structures are not breached and field margins can be tighter. For non-extremity lesions the orientation of the fields should follow the planes of the local musculature, while including the local fascial planes.

For the purposes of planning, the gross tumour volume (GTV) should be defined, with a margin around it to include the tissues at risk of microscopic involvement, to create the clinical tumour volume (CTV). In practice, the GTV is defined radiologically on CT or MRI. Whether or not the peritumoral oedema should be included in the GTV is unclear (it is not known if the oedema contains tumour cells). Including the peritumoral oedema will significantly increase the CTV in most cases. Until we know whether or not peritumoral oedema contains tumour cells, its inclusion within the CTV is not recommended.

The target volume will vary with the grade of the tumour. For well-differentiated (grade 1) tumours a 5 cm margin above and below the site of the original tumour is adequate. For moderately and poorly differentiated tumours (grades 2 and 3), a 10 cm margin maybe considered. The margin required is another uncertainty in sarcoma radiotherapy. The target volume is reduced later in the treatment (see below) to include the length of the scar with a margin of security at either end of 2 cm for boosting with electrons. For brachytherapy, margins have been narrower (2 cm) with good local control rates (see above). It may be that the extent of margins for external beam irradiation is overgenerous. Until there is information to substantiate this, the guidelines for margins defined above for external beam irradiation should be followed.

Where there is macroscopic residual disease, the volume cannot be reduced in the same way as when the excision margins are clear. In this situation, a 5 cm margin around the tumour is sustained throughout treatment.

Three-dimensional treatment planning where available can assist in the delivery of a homogeneous dose throughout the treatment volume, while limiting the dose to normal tissues which may affect function and cosmesis. Intensity-modulated radiotherapy (IMRT) may have a role in the irradiation of sites where minimisation of dose to critical structures is particularly important, such as the skull base or the abdomen.

Technique

This will vary with the site of the tumour. For the limbs and retroperitoneum, a parallel-opposed pair of fields, often wedged, will provide a satisfactory dose distribution in most cases. In the shoulder region tangential fields may be needed to reduce the volume of lung irradiated. Tangential fields are also appropriate for superficial trunk lesions to spare the bowel. For tumours in the buttock, a direct posterior field and two wedged lateral fields will reduce the dose to the rectum. In the head and neck, the principles of planning and respect for the tolerance of critical structures such as the spinal cord are the same as for squamous carcinoma of the head and neck. Target volumes tend to be smaller than below the clavicles and so higher doses can often be delivered with acceptable morbidity. Computer planning is desirable to obtain a homogeneous distribution of dose within the target volume.

Stability of the limb is best assisted by a shell and appropriately positioned bolus bags. Bolus is applied to the scar to ensure it receives the maximum dose to minimise the risk of scar recurrence. Sagittal lasers are especially useful in lining up the limbs.

Care is taken to avoid irradiating the whole circumference of a limb to reduce the likelihood of lymphoedema as a late complication. This is achieved by adjusting the width of the field to leave a longitudinal strip of unirradiated tissue outside the target volume. In the proximal part of the limb, especially in the thigh, this strip occupies a large proportion of the limb.

When the retroperitoneum is irradiated, part or the whole of one kidney may need to be included in the target volume. Shielding of the other kidney by lead blocks on the anterior and posterior fields may be necessary, depending upon the site of the tumour.

Dose and fractionation

There is little information on total dose and response in sarcomas. Most centres tend to give 50 Gy to a wide volume, shrinking to a final boost of 10–16 Gy. There is limited information on the relationship between total dose and response. However, fraction sizes should be kept small (1.8–2 Gy) to minimise the risks of late damage to normal tissue. Hypofractionated and hyperfractionated schedules have shown no advantage over conventional fractionation.

Limbs

No gross residual disease

1. Large volume
   50 Gy in 25 daily fractions over 5 weeks at megavoltage (6–10 MV photons)
2. Boost volume
   10–16 Gy in 5–8 daily fractions over 1–1 ½ weeks

(1) and (2) deliver a total dose of 66 Gy in 33 fractions over 6.5 weeks to the tumour-bearing area.

Gross residual disease

66 Gy in 33 daily fractions over 6.5 weeks at megavoltage (6–10 MV photons) or up to 70 Gy in 35 fractions over 7 weeks, if volume permits in the boosted area

Implantation. Because of the low radiosensitivity of sarcomas, an implant may be used in appropriate circumstances to give a high dose to the boost volume, or to gross residual disease.

Retroperitoneum. Dosage is limited by small bowel tolerance.

45 Gy in daily fractions over 4 weeks

Head and neck

66 Gy in 33 daily fractions over 6 ½ weeks

Acute reactions. Skin reactions are often a problem. This is because very high doses are needed in the boost volume and are sometimes given to graft areas with surface bolus. Dry desquamation normally develops and is treated as for other skin reactions. Moist desquamation is more likely to occur in the axilla, groin and perineum and is treated with gentian violet.

Late reactions. Atrophy of the skin and subcutaneous tissues and fibrosis within the muscles are common. Stiffness of a limb may be partly due to fibrosis of the intermuscular septa and partly due to fibrosis in the joint capsule.

Osteoporosis of bone is common since bone is frequently included in the target volume. Occasionally, particularly if the bone is invaded by tumour, radionecrosis may occur. In the ribs this may cause pathological fractures.

Radiation-induced sarcoma is very rare. It has been estimated at 0.2% in patients who have been irradiated for breast cancer.

Palliative radiotherapy

Palliative radiotherapy is indicated for the relief of symptoms of local and metastatic disease.

Soft tissue disease

Technique

A single field or parallel-opposed pair of fields or direct electron field is used.

Dose and energy

30 Gy in 10 daily fractions over 2 weeks (4–10 MV photons or electrons of appropriate energy)

Alternatively weekly doses of 3–5 Gy can be given to enable some growth restraint.

Bone metastases. For dose see page 581.

Chemotherapy

There is insufficient evidence to support giving routine postoperative adjuvant chemotherapy to high-risk patients with high-grade or bulky tumours. For metastatic disease, chemotherapy has limited efficacy. The most active drugs are doxorubicin, ifosphamide and DTIC. Chemotherapy is rarely curative so it should be reserved for symptomatic metastases not relieved by radiotherapy. Toxicity should be minimised.

Results of treatment

In the best hands, conservative surgery and radiotherapy can achieve over 90% local control and 5-year survival in stage I disease. For stage II disease local control is 85–90% and survival 90% (IIa) and 65% (IIb). For stage III local control is similar to stage II but survival is lower, 85% (IIIa) and 45% (IIIb).

If there is only microscopic residual disease following surgery, overall survival is 65%, falling to 30% when there is gross residual disease.

BONE TUMOURS

Benign and malignant tumours may arise in bone. The pathological classification is shown in Table 31.4. Bone tumours represent 0.4% of all cancers and all cancer deaths. Primary bone tumours are rare, only 1% of bone tumours, compared with 99% which are secondary deposits. The main malignant tumour which forms bone is osteosarcoma; that forming cartilage is chondrosarcoma. Malignant tumours arising from the bone marrow are myeloma (Ch. 29), Ewing's sarcoma and lymphoma (Ch. 29).

OSTEOSARCOMA (OSTEOGENIC SARCOMA)

This is the commonest and most malignant primary bone tumour. It arises in bone-forming cells (osteoblasts) and is commonest between the ages of 10 and 20 years. There is a second peak incidence in the elderly, as a complication of Paget's disease of bone. The male to female ratio is 1.6 : 1.

The cause of the usual adolescent's tumour is unknown but both internal and external sources of radiation can cause osteosarcoma. However, there is also an increased incidence (400-fold) of osteosarcoma in patients with bilateral retinoblastomas, presumably because of the same genetic abnormality or mutation

Table 31.4 Classification of bone tumours

A. Tumours forming bone
   1. Benign—e.g. osteoma
   2. Malignant—osteosarcoma
B. Tumours forming cartilage
   1. Benign—e.g. enchondroma
   2. Malignant—chondrosarcoma
C. Giant cell tumour (generally benign)
D. Tumours of the bone marrow—myeloma, lymphoma and Ewing's sarcoma
E. Other tumours

of the Rb tumour suppressor gene developing outside the irradiated areas.

Pathology

Osteosarcoma is commonest near the knee in the metaphysis of the distal femur or proximal tibia. In the elderly, its distribution matches Paget's disease.

Macroscopically the tumour is usually haemorrhagic. It expands the bone, destroying both the cortex and the medulla. The periosteum is frequently raised giving rise to the radiological features of Codman's triangle where the raised periosteum meets the cortex. Extension into the soft tissue follows. Blood-borne metastases to the lungs occur early. Bone metastases, though less frequent, also occur. Microscopically, there are malignant osteoblasts laying down small pieces of irregular osteoid tissue. There are a variety of histological appearances. The two main varieties are osteoblastic and telangiectatic (containing irregular blood vessels). The third variety is parosteal sarcoma. It arises from the surface of the bone and does not involve the medullary cavity.

Clinical features

The commonest presenting feature is pain, usually with swelling and a limp. Sometimes pathological fracture may follow minor trauma. Rarely cough and dyspnoea may indicate lung involvement.

Diagnosis and staging investigations

Plain radiographs and CT scan (Fig. 31.3) of the affected part may show the typical features of bone destruction and soft tissue extension. The cortex may be raised with a 'sunburst' appearance. Full blood count, liver function tests and chest radiograph (for lung metastases) are required.

A CT or MRI scan is necessary if surgery is contemplated, to assess the involvement of the medullary cavity and the extent of soft tissue involvement. CT is also helpful in assessing whether the capsule of a limb joint has been breached. An isotope bone scan may show increased uptake at the site of the tumour, in the adjacent bone (due to increased vascularity), in bone metastases and in bone-forming metastases in soft tissues. A biopsy should be carried out to confirm the diagnosis. It is important that the position of the biopsy is chosen so that the whole biopsy scar can be excised with the tumour to include potentially surgically contaminated tissue along the track of the biopsy. The initial biopsy for histological confirmation and, in cases of high clinical and radiological suspicion, so-called 'clearance' biopsies to assess the distance of spread along the bone shaft, should be performed as the first procedure with a view to subsequent limb-sparing surgery. Ideally both biopsy and definitive surgery should be performed by the same surgical team. The limb prosthesis has to be planned several weeks ahead of limb-sparing surgery.

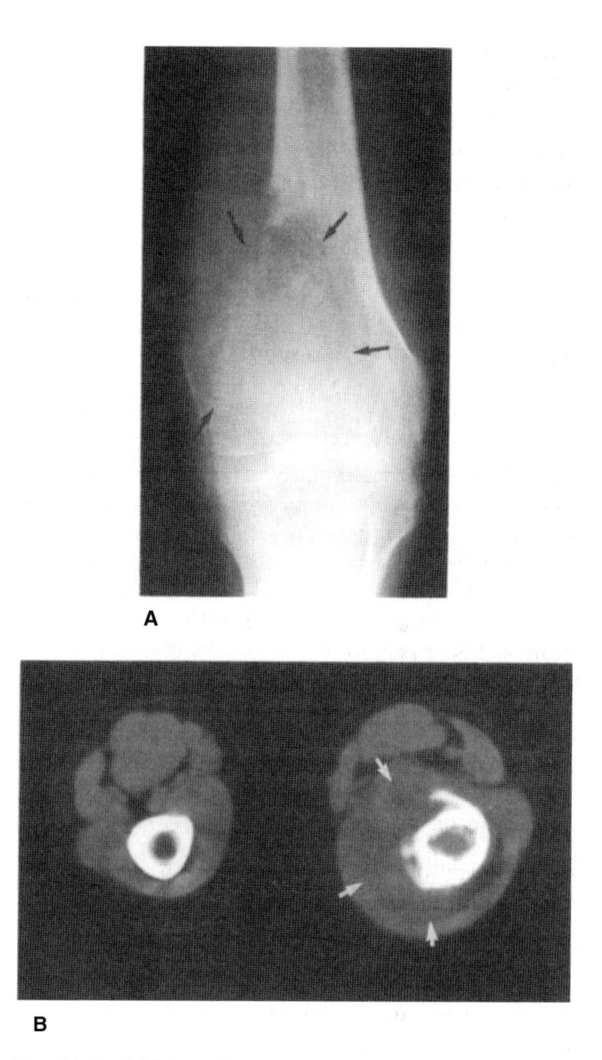

Fig. 31.3 **A** Plain radiograph and **B** CT scan of the femur showing bone destruction from an osteogenic sarcoma (arrows). Compare normal CT appearance on opposite side. (Courtesy of Dr R Nakielny, Sheffield.)

Treatment

The management of osteosarcoma requires a multidisciplinary approach including orthopaedic surgeon, oncologist, pathologist and physiotherapist.

Surgery

There has been an increasing trend since the early 1980s to conserve limb function as far as possible and avoid the mutilation of an amputation. Limb preservation involves removing the tumour and replacing the bone defect with a custom-made artificial prosthesis (Fig. 31.4). Careful preoperative assessment is necessary and referral to a specialist centre (Birmingham and London in the UK) is desirable. To obtain a margin of normal tissue above the tumour may involve removing the whole femur. However, it is now possible to carry out a total femoral replacement.

Contraindications to limb conservation are: (1) extensive soft tissue infiltration; (2) invasion of neurovascular bundles; and (3) involvement of the ankle joint. Similar principles apply to the upper limb.

Resection of lung metastases. Lung metastases are occasionally isolated and, in the absence of metastases elsewhere, surgical resection should be considered. Results are best in lung metastases of late onset. Surgery is contraindicated if there is pleural involvement.

Chemotherapy

Adjuvant chemotherapy is needed to deal with micrometastatic disease. Active drugs include doxorubicin, cisplatin, methotrexate and ifosphamide. Once the diagnosis has been established by the initial biopsy, a combination of doxorubicin and cisplatin is started to reduce and hopefully sterilise the tumour before radical surgery. Examination of the operative tumour may show extensive tumour necrosis. Prognosis is correlated with chemotherapy-induced necrosis. If chemotherapy seems to have achieved a response, then the same regime can be used postoperatively. If there is no response, an alternative regime may be chosen although there is little evidence that this improves outcome.

Radiotherapy

The indications for radiotherapy are: (1) use postoperatively where surgical margins are involved; (2) palliation of pain from the primary tumour in the presence of metastatic disease or of bony metastases; and (3) radical treatment of inoperable sites (e.g. skull, vertebrae, ilium and sacrum). However, proximity of critical structures, such as the spinal cord, often limits the dose that can be delivered.

Palliative radiotherapy of primary tumour

Technique

A parallel-opposed pair of fields is suitable for limb primaries.

Dose and energy

30 Gy in 10 daily fractions over 2 weeks (4–6 MV photons or cobalt-60)

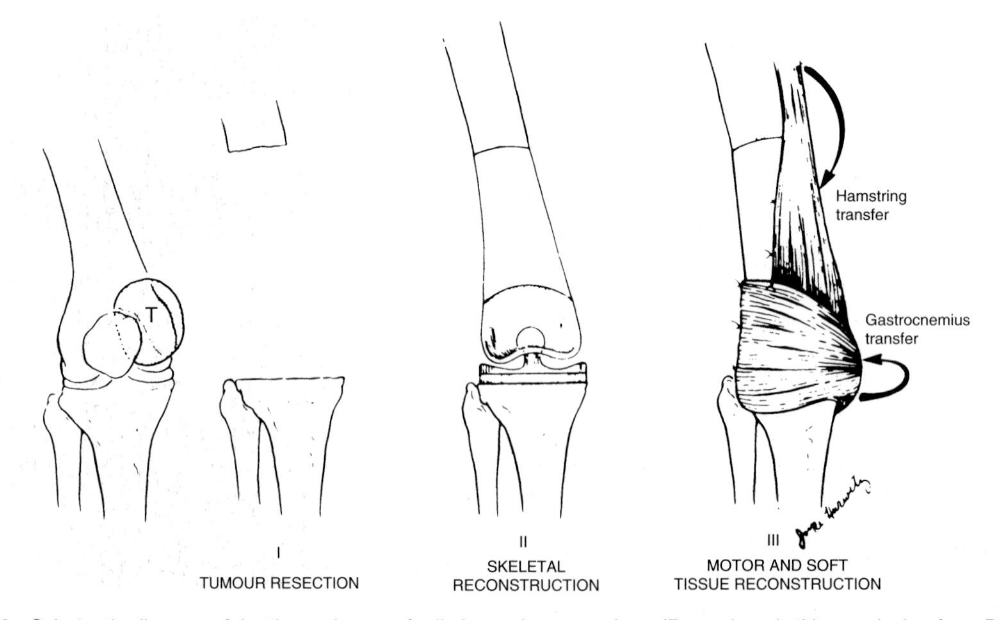

Fig. 31.4 Schematic diagram of the three phases of a limb-sparing procedure. (Reproduced with permission from DeVita VT, Hellman S, Rosenberg SA (2000) Cancer: Principles and Practice of Oncology, 6th edn. Lippincott, Williams and Wilkins, Philadelphia.)

Radical radiotherapy

Technique

This will very with the site of the primary. For tumours arising in a vertebra, a posterior oblique wedged pair (Fig. 29.10) with or without an unwedged direct posterior field provides a satisfactory dose distribution. For the ilium, parallel-opposed fields suffice.

Dose and energy

Megavoltage is required. The choice of dose will be determined by critical organ tolerance. In the spine above L2 it will be limited by spinal cord tolerance to **47.5 Gy in 25 daily fractions over 5 weeks.**In the ileum the dose delivered is limited by small bowel tolerance to a central tumour dose of **45 Gy in 25 daily fractions over 5 weeks**.

Results of treatment

The survival of osteosarcoma has improved with the development of more effective adjuvant chemotherapy. Average survival is 60% at 3 years. Osteoblastic and telangiectatic tumours have a similar prognosis. Parosteal sarcomas have a better prognosis and may be cured by surgery alone.

EWING'S SARCOMA

Ewing's sarcoma is the second commonest bone tumour. In the UK its incidence is 0.6 per million. The peak age is between 10 and 15 years. It is slightly commoner in males. It is very rare in blacks.

Pathology

Ewing's sarcoma probably arises from connective tissue within the bone marrow. The commonest sites in order of frequency are the pelvis, femur, tibia, fibula, rib, scapula, vertebra and humerus. In contrast to osteogenic sarcoma, a higher proportion of these tumours occur in the flat bones of the trunk. About 40% occur in the axial skeleton. Microscopically there are sheets of uniform undifferentiated, small, deeply-staining round cells. The tumour needs to be distinguished from other small-round-cell tumours, including non-Hodgkin lymphoma, Hodgkin's disease, neuroblastoma and metastatic carcinoma. 90% will absorb a special stain for the presence of glycogen (periodic acid–Schiff (PAS)). This stain is not specific for Ewing's sarcoma since it may also be positive in neuroblastoma. 90% have 11:21 chromosome translation.

There is local spread along the marrow cavity causing bone destruction. However, the epiphyseal plates are rarely breached. Blood-borne spread is early and common. About 50% will have lung metastases and 40% bone metastases and/or widespread bone marrow infiltration at presentation. Lymph node metastases are uncommon (less than 10%). Spread to the CNS may occur, usually late in the course of the disease.

Diagnosis and staging

Full blood count may show anaemia (leucoerythroblastic, if there is bone marrow infiltration) and a mildly raised white cell count. ESR is often moderately elevated. Liver function tests may be abnormal (raised lactate dehydrogenase (LDH) or alkaline phosphatase).

A biopsy of the tumour is required. As in osteogenic sarcoma, care is taken to ensure that the biopsy lies within the incision for any later proposed definitive surgical procedure. Plain radiographs of the primary are taken in two planes (usually anteroposterior and lateral). In long bones this may show the typical multi-layered 'onion-skin' (Fig. 31.5) appearance of the periosteal reaction and often a large adjacent soft tissue mass. Pathological fracture occurs in 5% (less frequently than osteogenic sarcoma). CT scanning gives more detail of the local extent of the tumour and is useful in planning the site for a biopsy and subsequent surgery. MRI is superior to CT in assessment of the extent of infiltration within the medullary canal. A bone scan is necessary to screen for bone metastases.

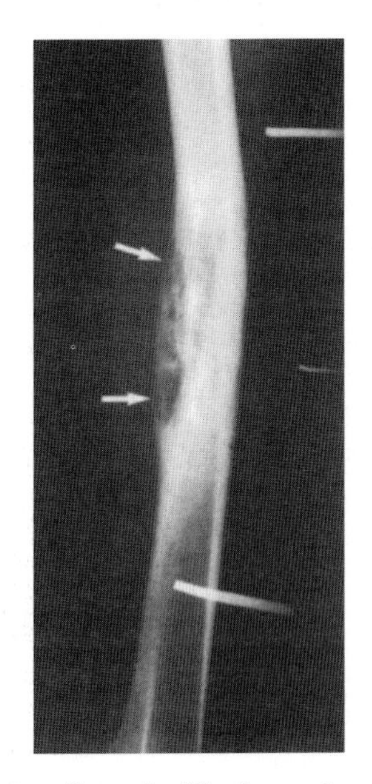

Fig. 31.5 Plain radiograph of the femur showing typical appearance of Ewing's sarcoma of bone. (Courtesy of Dr R Nakielny, Sheffield.)

A bone marrow and trephine are needed to exclude marrow infiltration.

Clinical features

Presentation is usually with a rapidly developing and painful swelling. Neurological symptoms may accompany this if there is nerve compression. Fever occurs in about 30% of patients.

Treatment

The choice of treatment will depend largely upon the site of the primary. Close liaison is required between orthopaedic surgeon and oncologist. Treatment should, as with osteogenic sarcomas, only be carried out by an experienced team.

Management differs from that of osteogenic sarcoma for three main reasons. First, Ewing's sarcoma is more chemosensitive. Secondly, Ewing's sarcoma occurs more frequently in the central than in the peripheral skeleton. Radical excision in the central skeleton is often not feasible because of limited access and the presence of adjacent vital structures (e.g. pelvic vessels). Thirdly, Ewing's sarcoma is more radiosensitive and can be controlled by radical radiotherapy when combined with adjuvant chemotherapy in about 75% of cases. However, the likelihood of local tumour control is less if the primary tumour is large (9 cm or more). In these circumstances, unless the soft tissue component is very substantial, radical surgical removal of the whole bone (e.g. rib or fibula) is advised. If there is a bulky soft tissue component, initial reduction of its volume should be attempted with several cycles of chemotherapy before proceeding to surgery. There is now a trend for more use of surgery, as local control is thereby improved.

Where radical surgery to a limb would cause major functional impairment, a conservative approach, as in osteogenic sarcoma, can be adopted. A customised artificial prosthesis can be inserted at the end of the resected long bone. However, amputation may be preferable for proximal tibial or distal femoral tumours in growing children because of reduced bone growth in the affected limb following local radiotherapy. The latter may give rise to limbs of unequal length and therefore a permanent handicap.

Radical radiotherapy

Target volume

It is not usually possible to deliver a radical dose uniformly to the whole bone unless it is very small, because of toxicity to normal tissue. For this reason a 'shrinking field' approach is adopted with two consecutive phases based on the pretreatment volume. The initial volume is the tumour and a 5 cm margin of adjacent tissue. In long bones, an unirradiated strip of normal tissue containing lymphatics outside the tumour- bearing area is left, if possible, to reduce the risk of lymphoedema as a late complication. In the second phase the volume is reduced to encompass the primary tumour with a 2 cm margin of normal tissue.

Technique

The choice of technique will vary with the site of the primary. For the limbs, a parallel-opposed wedged pair of fields usually suffices. A 'shrinking field' technique is used for limb tumours. For pelvic primaries, it may be possible surgically to displace the bowel out of the radiation field, by inserting an absorbable mesh. For rib primaries, electrons of appropriate energy may be used to diminish the dose to the underlying lung.

Dose and energy

A high local dose (of the order of 50–60 Gy conventionally fractionated) to the bulk of the tumour must be delivered at megavoltage, using photons or electrons as appropriate. Patients should be included in nationally agreed protocols. The following regime is illustrative:

Phase 1: 40 Gy in 22 daily fractions over 30 days (4–6 MV photons)

Phase 2: 15 Gy in 8 daily fractions over 10 days (4–6 MV photons)

Acute and late reactions. These are the same as for soft tissue sarcoma (p. 574).

Palliative radiotherapy

Whole lung irradiation is useful in relieving cough and dyspnoea from lung metastases.

Technique

A parallel-opposed pair of fields encompassing both lung fields is used.

Dose and energy

25 Gy in 20 daily fractions over 4 weeks (4–6 MV photons)

Chemotherapy

Adjuvant combination chemotherapy with agents such as vincristine, actinomycin D, doxorubicin, cyclophosphamide and more recently ifosphamide have proved effective. The search for the best combination is the subject of national and international studies.

Very intensive chemotherapy with autologous bone marrow transplantation for patients with poor prognostic factors is under investigation. Durable responses only seem to be obtained in patients in complete remission at the time of intensive treatment.

In the presence of metastases (e.g. in the lungs) cure can still be achieved in a small number of patients using the same agents as for adjuvant therapy.

Results of treatment

The outcome is better for patients with tumours of the peripheral rather than central skeleton. Up to 90% disease-free survival for peripheral tumours and 65% for central (axial) tumours has been achieved. Overall 5-year survival (and probably cure) is about 50%. Local recurrence occurs in about 10–15% of long bone primaries and 25–30% of pelvic tumours. The higher recurrence rate in the pelvis is probably due to the larger tumour size and the difficulty of irradiating the tumour homogeneously without damaging surrounding normal tissues.

CHONDROSARCOMA

Chondrosarcomas are malignant tumours of cartilage. They may arise in benign enchondromas or be malignant from the start. Adults aged 30–50 are affected. The commonest sites in order of frequency are the pelvis (50%), femur, humerus and scapula.

Macroscopically, the tumour is bulky, lobulated and semitranslucent. Microscopically, it is a sarcoma containing cartilage. Differentiation is variable. Poorly differentiated tumours (mesenchymal chondrosarcomas) behave more aggressively. In the well-differentiated form, spread is slow locally. Blood-borne metastases occur late to the lungs.

Clinical features

Presentation is usually with a slowly progressive painless swelling which eventually becomes painful.

Diagnosis and investigation

A biopsy is required. Plain radiography shows bone destruction and commonly abnormal flecks of calcification. CT scanning (Fig. 31.6) helps define the local extent.

Treatment

Radical surgery is the treatment of choice. Limb preservation may be possible. It is a very radioresistant tumour. Radiotherapy has only a palliative role for the relief of local symptoms, such as pain, and relatively high doses are required even for palliative effect.

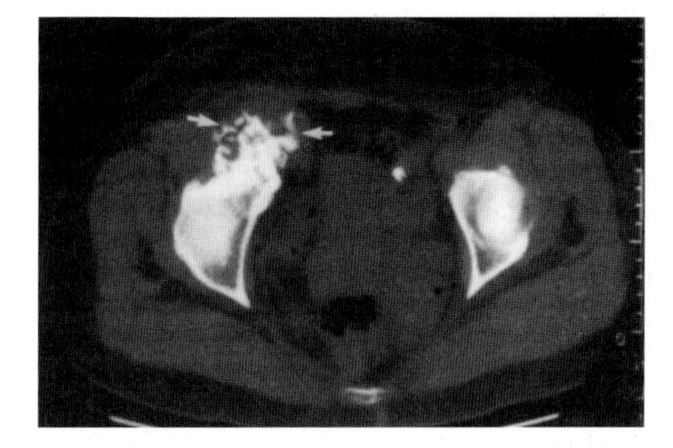

Fig. 31.6 CT scan of the pelvis showing a chondrosarcoma of the ileum (arrows). Note the flecks of calcification. (Courtesy of Dr R Nakielny, Sheffield.)

Radiotherapy

Technique

A parallel-opposed wedged pair of fields is suitable for the long bones. A three-field technique for pelvic tumours using anterior and posterior wedged fields with an open lateral field may limit the dose to the bowel.

Dose and energy

60 Gy in 30 daily fractions over 6 weeks at megavoltage (4–6 MV photons)

Results of treatment

5-year survival is about 50% over the age of 21 years but falls to 35% under that age. Younger patients tend to have tumours in the pelvis, where radical surgery is more difficult than in long bones. They also have more poorly differentiated tumours which metastasise more frequently.

OSTEOCLASTOMA (GIANT CELL TUMOUR OF BONE)

This is in most cases a benign tumour arising from osteoclasts. Occasionally it is malignant from the start or undergoes malignant transformation. It is commonest at the ends of long bones; 50% occur around the knee joint. Onset is usually between 20 and 35 years of age.

Macroscopically osteoclastomas are eccentric expanding tumours which destroy bone. Microscopically there are giant cells of osteoclast type and a stroma of mononuclear cells. Spread is local and may eventually penetrate the joint. Blood-borne metastases are late and to the lungs (15%).

Clinical features

Presentation is with the gradual onset of pain and swelling, and sometimes pathological fracture.

Diagnosis and investigation

Plain radiographs typically show bone destruction by a multilocular cystic lesion expanding the cortex. Diagnosis is confirmed by open biopsy.

Treatment

Surgical excision or curettage is the treatment of choice for accessible sites. Radiotherapy offers an alternative for centrally placed tumours, e.g. in vertebrae, and for tumours in long bones where amputation may be undesirable in a young person. Chemotherapy has not been proven to be of value.

Radical radiotherapy

Target volume

If the primary tumour is at the end of the femur or in the upper tibia, a margin of 4–5 cm normal bone proximally or distally, respectively, is needed. A smaller margin of 1–2 cm is given at the side of the tumour adjacent to the joint.

For tumours of a vertebral body, a margin of half a vertebral body above and below the affected vertebra is adequate.

Technique

For tumours in long bones, a parallel-opposed pair of fields is chosen. For vertebral tumours a posterior oblique wedged pair of fields is used to limit the dose to the spinal cord (Fig. 29.10).

Dose and energy

Relatively low doses (35 Gy in 15 daily fractions over 3 weeks) at megavoltage will control most tumours. If radiotherapy is the primary treatment, a higher dose is required (**50 Gy in 20–25 fractions over 4–5 weeks**). Care is taken to keep within spinal cord tolerance for vertebral tumours.

Results of treatment

Local recurrence following curettage is commoner, but following adequate excision prognosis is good, with 80% 5-year survival. Late sarcomatous change may occur, even at 15 years following radiotherapy. The role of radiotherapy in this malignant transformation is disputed.

SPINDLE CELL SARCOMAS

These include malignant fibrous histiocytoma (MFH), angiosarcoma and fibrosarcoma. They occur later (30–60 years of age) than osteosarcoma. Origin is both in the diaphysis and the metaphysis from the periosteum or the medullary cavity. Any bone may be affected. Microscopically there is variable collagen formation. Spread from the periosteum is to the soft tissues more than bone, and within the medullary cavity for endosteal tumours.

Clinical features

Pain and swelling are the main features.

Diagnosis and investigations

Plain radiography may show an area of bone similar in appearance to a bone infarct. A bone biopsy is necessary.

Treatment

Local excision is the treatment of choice with limb preservation if possible. Amputation may be necessary. Radiotherapy is only of palliative value. Adjuvant chemotherapy similar to that for osteogenic sarcoma is being evaluated.

Results of treatment

The prognosis is poor, with 5-year survival about 25%.

SECONDARY TUMOURS IN BONE

The great majority of bone tumours are not primary but are of metastatic origin. They represent 15–20% of the workload of a radiotherapy department. The most common primary sites are breast, lung, prostate, myeloma and kidney. The prognosis of bone metastases is generally poor, though the course of the disease may be relatively slow over a period of years, for example in some patients with breast cancer. Good symptomatic relief by a combination of analgesics and local radiotherapy can be achieved in most cases.

Clinical features and investigation

The usual presentation is with pain due to pressure on the periosteum or on nerve roots as they emerge from the spinal canal (Fig. 31.7). Early diagnosis is important before bone destruction has advanced so far as to cause pathological fracture or spinal cord compression.

Plain radiographs of the symptomatic area may show the deposits (osteolytic or osteosclerotic or both) or a pathological fracture. However, a metastasis in a vertebral body has to have reached a size of about 2 cm before it will be visible on a radiograph.

A radioisotope bone scan (p. 122) is helpful in detecting bone metastases too small to be visible on plain radiographs and to detect deposits elsewhere in the skeleton. Multiple bone metastases are common, predominantly in the spine, ribs, pelvis and upper femurs. CT scanning of areas of the spine and sacrum where plain radiographs and bone scan are equivocal or normal may show bone destruction. If there is no known primary site, a CT-guided biopsy may be necessary.

Treatment

The treatment of bone metastases includes analgesics, radiotherapy and occasionally surgery. Treatment is aimed at relieving pain as simply and quickly as possible. Analgesics are discussed in Chapter 36. The choice of treatment will depend on the site of the pain, its severity, complications such as spinal cord compression or pathological fracture, the underlying tumour and the general condition of the patient.

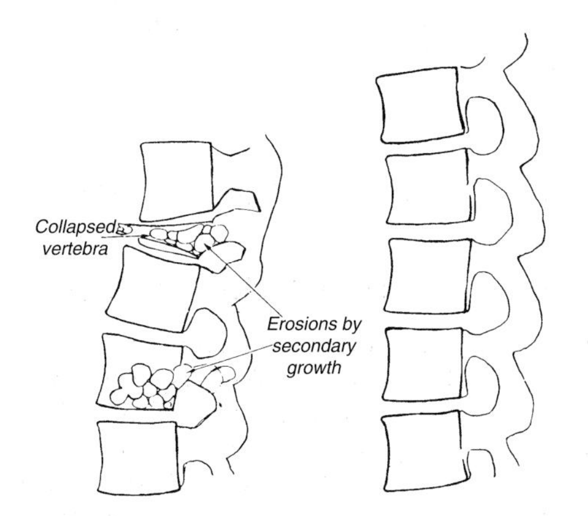

Fig. 31.7 Diagrammatic radiological appearances of normal vertebral column and secondary deposits from cancer (e.g. breast).

1. Site

Metastases in the spine are one of the commonest conditions that the radiotherapist irradiates. Careful clinical and radiological assessment is necessary to determine whether palliative radiotherapy is appropriate and, if so, which area is to be treated. Single fractions of 8 Gy to the affected vertebra and one normal vertebra above and below it are suitable for most thoracic and lumbar vertebrae (Fig. 31.8), with the exception of T12 and L1. The latter overlie the duodenum and fractionated doses (e.g. 20 Gy in 4 daily fractions) rather than single fractions may be preferred, to reduce the incidence of radiation-induced vomiting. Similarly, single fractions are not advised in the cervical spine owing to the greater sensitivity of the spinal cord in this region. Orthovoltage generally has adequate penetration for the ribs and cervical spine. For most other sites megavoltage irradiation with cobalt-60 or a linear accelerator is needed. A simulator or portal film should be taken as a record of the area that has been treated. This is helpful if the patient re-presents at a later date with metastases within or adjacent to the previously irradiated area. In general, it is wise to allow 2 years to elapse before reirradiating the spine and to fractionate the dose over a longer period of time (e.g. 20 Gy in 8 rather than 4 daily fractions).

Technique

Single fields are adequate for spinal (Fig. 31.8), sacral, rib and superficial skull deposits. For pelvic, long bone and base of skull deposits a parallel-opposed pair of fields is used.

2. Pathological fracture

If there is a pathological fracture of a long bone, an orthopaedic opinion should be sought on the feasibil-

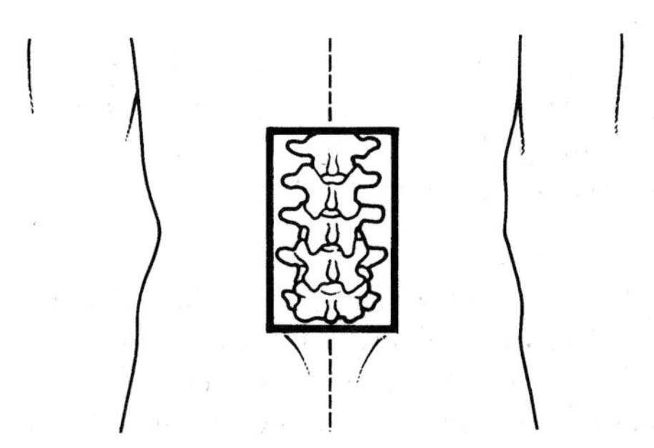

Fig. 31.8 Palliative single field (16 × 8 cm) to the lumbar spine (4–6 MV photons).

ity of reducing and stabilising the fracture (Fig. 26.22). Pinning a fracture usually provides prompt pain relief and a return to mobility.

If there is evidence of spinal cord compression, surgical decompression of the cord may be necessary prior to fractionated radiotherapy (p. 555). Steroids should be given to patients with pain from nerve root infiltration and spinal cord compression.

Hemibody irradiation

If there are widespread painful bone metastases and the tumour is relatively radiosensitive (e.g. myeloma and prostate cancer), hemibody irradiation in a single fraction can be considered (see page 529 for technique and dosage).

Hormonal therapy

Hormonal therapy should be considered for patients whose tumours may be hormone responsive, such as breast and prostate tumours (see Chs 26, 28 and 35).

Some patients are too unwell for even single fractions of treatment. Their pain should be controlled medically.

Results of treatment

About 75% of patients have worthwhile and often durable improvements in their pain following radiotherapy.

CHAPTER CONTENTS

32

Paediatric oncology

Roger E Taylor

INTRODUCTION

Cancer is rare in childhood. There are approximately 1400 cases each year in the UK. One child in 600 develops cancer before the age of 15. The range of tumours seen in childhood is very different from that in adults, and is given in Table 32.1. The evolution of the discipline of paediatric oncology has been one of the success stories of modern oncology. In the UK, treatment is coordinated by the network of 22 United Kingdom Children's Cancer Study Group (UKCCSG) paediatric oncology centres. In the last 40 years there has been a substantial improvement in survival for children with cancer and more than two-thirds can now expect to be long-term survivors. It was estimated that in the year 2000, 1 in 1000 of the adult population would have been a survivor of childhood cancer. This has been brought about largely as a result of the application of chemotherapy as part of a multimodality approach, including surgery and radiotherapy. However, for many children long-term survival comes at a price, namely the long-term effects of treatment. Long-term effects of radiotherapy include the neuropsychological effects of irradiation of the central nervous system (CNS), tissue hypoplasia, impaired growth and radiation-induced sarcoma. Long-term effects of chemotherapy include myocardial damage due to anthracyclines, nephrotoxicity due to ifosfamide or cisplatin, and secondary leukaemia related to drugs such as the alkylating agents. When planning protocols for the treatment of children, although the priority is to maximise the chance of cure it is also essential to consider the likely long-term effects of treatment. Continued vigilance for long-term effects of treatment is essential. This is carried out in dedicated long-term follow-up clinics.

Currently 40–50% of children with cancer receive radiotherapy as part of their initial treatment. It is

Table 32.1 Proportion of children with different cancers (UKCCSG registrations 1995)

Disease	Total number (percentage)
Acute lymphoblastic leukaemia (ALL)	379 (24.4%)
Acute non-lymphoblastic leukaemia (ANNL)	68 (4.4%)
Other leukaemias	20 (1.3%)
All leukaemias	**467 (30.1%)**
Ependymoma	38 (2.4%)
Astrocytoma	145 (9.3%)
Medulloblastoma/PNET	67 (4.3%)
Intracranial germ cell tumours	8 (0.5%)
Other CNS tumours	85 (5.5%)
All CNS tumours	**343 (22.1%)**
Osteosarcoma	44 (2.8%)
Ewing's sarcoma	28 (1.8%)
Peripheral PNET	13 (0.8%)
Hodgkin's disease	65 (4.2%)
Non-Hodgkin lymphoma	94 (6%)
Neuroblastoma	92 (5.9%)
Wilms' tumour	68 (4.4%)
Rhabdomyosarcoma	68 (4.4%)
Other sarcoma	41 (2.6%)
TOTAL	**1554**

important to provide the highest possible quality of radiotherapy. Careful planning and delivery are essential in order to achieve local tumour control with the minimum of irradiation of normal tissues to minimise long-term effects. It is extremely important that, as for the administration of chemotherapy, radiotherapy for children should be undertaken only in specialised centres associated with the United Kingdom Children's Cancer Study Group (UKCCSG) paediatric oncology centres. In a centre treating relatively large number of children with radiotherapy it is possible to establish a team including a specialist paediatric therapy radiographer and specialist nurse.

SEDATION/ANAESTHESIA FOR RADIOTHERAPY

Young children, particularly those under the age of 3–4 frequently find it very difficult to lie still for radiotherapy planning and delivery, particularly when a Perspex head shell is required. The assistance of an experienced play therapist can be very helpful in preparing the child for radiotherapy. Sedation sufficient to ensure immobilisation is difficult to achieve without it persisting for several hours. Because of the importance of immobilisation, short-acting general anaesthesia such as Diprivan (propofol) is sometimes essential. The daily fasting for this results in surprisingly little disruption to nutrition.

RADIOTHERAPY QUALITY ASSURANCE (QA)

Radiotherapy QA is particularly important in the treatment of children. Because of the high cure rate for most childhood cancers, it is important to achieve local control avoiding a 'geographical miss'. It is also important to avoid unnecessarily large field sizes, in order to minimise long-term effects.

Departmental QA

It is incumbent on all radiotherapy departments to deliver the highest possible standard of radiotherapy for all patients including children. Many radiotherapy departments have adopted a quality system according to the international standard ISO 9002.

QA in multicentre studies

The accuracy of delivery of radiotherapy contributes to improved tumour control, particularly for complex techniques such as craniospinal radiotherapy. In many of the North American paediatric multicentre studies, radiotherapy quality, including beam data, dose prescription, planning and verification films are reviewed in the Quality Assurance Review Centre (QARC) situated in Providence, Rhode Island. In most European multicentre studies QA is less well organised. Ideally, review of radiotherapy simulator or verification films by study coordinators should be sufficiently fast to provide feedback early in the course of radiotherapy so that the treatment plan can be modified if necessary. This is logistically difficult but has been achieved in Germany for radiotherapy for Ewing's sarcoma.

TOXICITY OF RADIOTHERAPY FOR CHILDREN

Acute morbidity

The side-effects of erythema, mucositis, nausea, diarrhoea, etc. occur in children as in adults, and are generally managed by the same means.

Subacute effects

Central nervous system

The 'somnolence syndrome' occurs in approximately 50% of children 4–8 weeks after 24 Gy prophylactic cranial irradiation for acute lymphoblastic leukaemia (ALL), and is probably related to temporary demyelination. Lhermitte's sign consists of an electric shock-like symptom radiating down the spine and into the limbs. It may follow radiation to the upper spinal cord, e.g. following mediastinal radiotherapy for lymphoma. Within the first 2 months following radiotherapy for brain tumours, children may experience a transient deterioration of neurological symptoms and signs.

Liver

A large proportion of the liver frequently has to be irradiated when treating Wilms' tumour. Radiation hepatopathy may occur 1–3 months following radiotherapy, and consists of hepatomegaly, jaundice, ascites, thrombocytopenia and elevated transaminases. A risk factor is the administration of actinomycin-D following hepatic irradiation. Long-term dysfunction is rare but the risk is dose related.

Lung

The whole lungs may require radiotherapy as part of total body irradiation, or in the treatment of pulmonary metastases from Wilms' tumour or Ewing's sarcoma. Mild radiation pneumonitis consists of a dry cough and mild dyspnoea. The risk of pneumonitis is dose and radiation volume related. Radiation pneumonitis is the dose-limiting toxicity for total body irradiation.

Long-term effects

Bone growth

Impairment of bone growth and associated soft tissue hypoplasia can be one of the most obvious and distressing long-term effects, particularly when treating the head and neck region. Abnormalities of craniofacial growth can cause significant cosmetic and functional deformity, including micrognathia leading to problems with dentition. The epiphysial growth plates are very sensitive to radiation, and are excluded from the radiotherapy field whenever possible. Age at time of treatment, radiation dose and volume are factors which have an impact on the severity of these orthopaedic long-term effects. There is evidence of a dose response effect, with a greater effect seen for a dose of >33 Gy compared with <33 Gy. Slipped femoral epiphysis and avascular necrosis have also been reported following irradiation of the hip. Laboratory evidence suggests a dose response effect between 5 Gy and 35–40 Gy, and an effect of dose per fraction. Careful consideration of the late orthopaedic effects of radiation is extremely important whenever planning radiotherapy for children.

Central nervous system

Radionecrosis is rare below 60 Gy, and generally occurs with a latency of 6 months to 2 years. It results from a direct effect on glial tissue. It is very unusual to have to deliver a dose of 60 Gy to any part of the CNS for a child. It occurs in approximately 50% of patients treated by interstitial implantation for recurrent brain tumours following prior radical external beam radiotherapy. The clinical effects of radionecrosis vary according to the site within the CNS and are most devastating in the spinal cord. Radionecrosis of the spinal cord in children has been seen as a consequence of the interaction between radiation and cytosine arabinoside given intrathecally for metastatic rhabdomyosarcoma.

Necrotising leucoencephalopathy may be seen when cranial irradiation is followed by high-dose methotrexate for the treatment of leukaemia. The clinical features include ataxia, lethargy, epilepsy, spasticity and paresis.

Neuropsychological effects. The effects of cranial radiotherapy are now well established. When compared with siblings, children given 24 Gy prophylactic cranial irradiation show an approximate fall in IQ of 12 points. Following higher radiation doses given for brain tumours, an increased risk of learning and behaviour difficulties is seen. An important risk factor for the incidence of neuropsychological long-term effects is the age at diagnosis.

Kidney

Long-term effects on renal function are usually seen 2–3 years following a course of radiotherapy. The risk increases following a dose of greater than 15 Gy to both kidneys. The severity is related to the dose received, and when mild consists of hypertension. When more severe, following a higher dose, renal failure may ensue.

Endocrine

Endocrine deficiencies following radiotherapy are common. Of particular concern is the risk of growth hormone and other pituitary hormone deficiencies following pituitary irradiation for tumours of the CNS.

Table 32.2 Normal tissue tolerance doses

Tissue/organ	Tolerance dose (Gy)
Whole lung	18
Both kidneys	15
Whole liver	20
Spinal cord	50

Following radiotherapy to the thyroid, the incidence of elevated TSH is 75% after 25–40 Gy.

Reproductive

In boys the germinal epithelium is very sensitive to the effects of low-dose irradiation. In adult males transient oligospermia is seen after 2 Gy, but slow recovery can occur after 2–5 Gy. In girls the oocytes are also sensitive. Subsequent pregnancy is rare but has been reported after 12 Gy whole body irradiation.

TOLERANCE OF CRITICAL ORGANS TO RADIOTHERAPY

The tolerance of critical organs frequently limits the dose of radiation that can be given. The critical organs and their 'tolerance doses' are listed in Table 32.2.

CHEMOTHERAPY/RADIOTHERAPY INTERACTIONS

Interactions between radiation and chemotherapy are complex and poorly understood. Interactions can be exploited in order to attempt to improve disease-free survival. The most frequently employed mechanism in paediatric oncology is 'spatial cooperation' whereby chemotherapy and radiotherapy are combined to exploit their differing roles in different anatomical sites. Examples are the use of radiation for local control of a primary, with chemotherapy for subclinical metastatic disease such as in the treatment of Ewing's sarcoma, and the use of radiotherapy for the treatment of 'sanctuary sites', e.g. CNS prophylaxis for the treatment of ALL. Chemotherapy and radiotherapy may be combined with the aim of increasing tumour cell kill without excess toxicity. An example is the use of combined chemotherapy and radiotherapy for children with Hodgkin's disease. It may be possible to reduce the intensity of both treatment modalities and hopefully reduce long-term morbidity. When using combined modality therapy the aim is to improve the therapeutic ratio. Many protocols for children involve the use of concurrent chemotherapy and radiotherapy.

It is essential to be vigilant for additional early or long-term morbidity. Clinically important chemotherapy–radiotherapy interactions are often unpredictable and their mechanisms are poorly understood. Actinomycin-D and cisplatin increase the slope of the radiation dose–response curve and actinomycin-D inhibits the repair of sublethal damage (SLD). Clinical interactions include:

- Enhanced skin and mucosal toxicity when radiation is followed by actinomycin-D (the 'recall phenomenon')
- Enhanced bladder toxicity when chemotherapy is combined with cyclophosphamide
- Enhanced CNS toxicity from combined radiation and methotrexate or cytosine arabinoside
- Enhanced marrow toxicity from wide-field irradiation and many myelotoxic chemotherapeutic agents.

In the case of the effect of combined radiation and anthracyclines such as doxorubicin on the heart, doxorubicin has its effects on the myocytes and radiation on the vasculature.

LEUKAEMIA

The leukaemias account for the largest group (approximately 30%) of paediatric malignancies. Approximately 80% have acute lymphoblastic leukaemia (ALL). The remainder have acute non-lymphoblastic leukaemia (ANLL), usually acute myeloid leukaemia (AML) or rarely chronic myeloid leukaemia (CML). The improvement in survival of children with ALL was one of the early successes of paediatric oncology. Currently more than 70% are long-term survivors. The four phases of treatment are:

1. Remission induction, usually with vincristine, corticosteroids and asparaginase.
2. Consolidation or intensification with multidrug combinations.
3. CNS prophylaxis.
4. Maintenance, usually based on a continuous low-dose antimetabolite drug such as 6-tioguanine.

Since the 1960s the routine use of whole brain radiotherapy and intrathecal methotrexate for CNS prophylaxis had reduced the risk of CNS relapse to less than 10%.

When planning prophylactic whole brain radiotherapy, it is important to include all the meninges usually down to the lower border of the second or third cervical vertebra. Great care is taken to include the cribriform fossa, temporal lobe and base of skull. Although the lens is shielded, as much of the orbit as possible is included, as ocular relapses occasionally occur (Fig. 32.1).

Because of the neuropsychological consequences of whole brain radiotherapy, CNS prophylaxis with cranial radiotherapy has been superseded by the routine use of intrathecal methotrexate. A UK trial for patients with a presenting white count of greater than $50 \times 10^9/l$ being randomised to either intrathecal and high-dose intravenous methotrexate, or intrathecal methotrexate with cranial radiotherapy has recently closed.

Boys who suffer a testicular relapse are treated with testicular radiotherapy. The field includes the scrotum and lower spermatic cord (Fig. 32.2), and the dose given is 24 Gy in 12 fractions.

For ANNL the basis of therapy is intensive multidrug chemotherapy, which can achieve a survival rate of 60%. As for adults, bone marrow transplantation is frequently employed for children who have an HLA-matched sibling. A survival rate of 65% can be achieved for children in first complete remission given a bone marrow transplant as consolidation therapy for acute myeloid leukaemia.

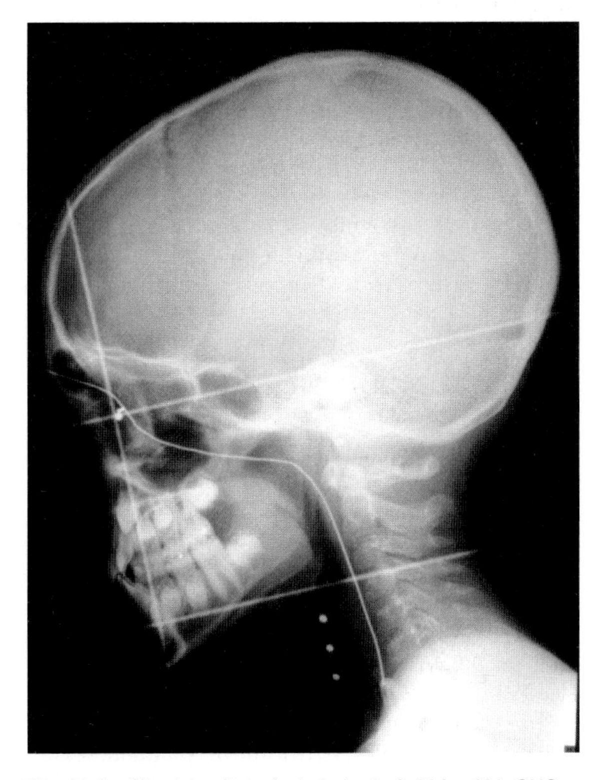

Fig. 32.1 Simulator film of whole brain field for ALL CNS prophylaxis.

Total body irradiation (TBI)

As in the treatment of adults with haematological malignancies, TBI is an important technique used together with high-dose cyclophosphamide (Cyclo-TBI) as the conditioning regimen prior to bone marrow transplantation (BMT). BMT has been routinely available for more than 15 years. Bone marrow donors are generally HLA-matched siblings, but the increasing availability of volunteer unrelated donors is resulting in a significant increase in the number of children for whom BMT can be considered.

For children the 'standard' radiation dose employed in the UK for TBI is 14.4 Gy in 8 fractions of 1.8 Gy given twice daily. As the dose-limiting toxicity is pulmonary toxicity, this dose is specified to the point of maximum lung dose. The aim is to irradiate the target volume, which in this case is the whole body, to a uniform dose. For such a large and complex target volume it is not feasible to adhere to the ICRU 50 guidelines of a range of –5% to +7%, and a range of –10% to +10% may be more realistic. Individual techniques for TBI have evolved in different departments. Dosimetry is usually based on in vivo measurements performed at a 'test dose' prior to the TBI. Modern linear accelerator design and field sizes allow the use of large anterior and posterior fields (Fig. 32.3). For children with ALL many centres advise a cranial boost in addition to the TBI with the aim of reducing the risk of CNS relapse. Planning for the cranial boost is the same as for prophylactic cranial irradiation (see above). The prescribed dose varies but typically would be 5.4 Gy in 3 daily fractions.

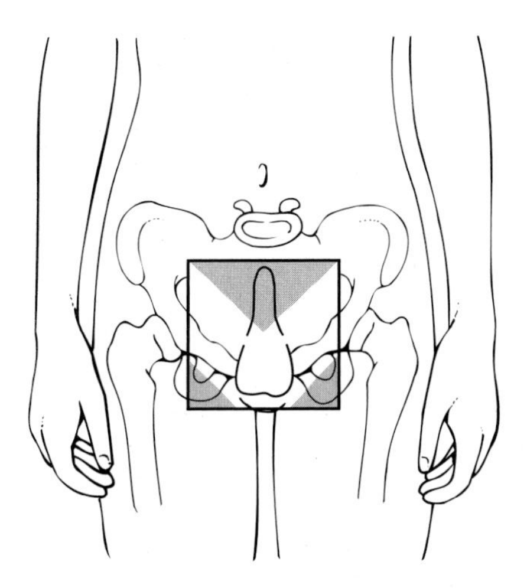

Shaded areas = position of shielding

Fig. 32.2 Diagram of field for testicular radiotherapy.

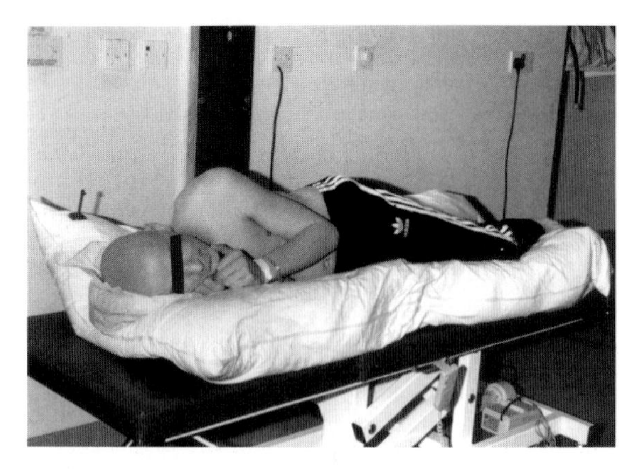

Fig. 32.3 TBI technique.

Indications for BMT/TBI in children

Children with AML are selected for BMT and TBI based on risk status at presentation. Those with an HLA-matched sibling are selected for BMT if they fall into the intermediate- or high-risk category, whereas those with low-risk disease, i.e. those with chromosome mutations t(8;21), t(15;17) or Inv 16 do well with standard chemotherapy. Children with ALL selected for BMT and TBI include relapsed patients and those presenting with features indicating a high risk of failure with standard chemotherapy. This 'hazard ratio' is based on age (prognosis worse for older children), sex (prognosis worse for boys), and presenting white cell count (prognosis worse for those with a higher white cell count). Other indications include those with Philadelphia chromosome-positive disease, and a 'near haploid' phenotype. Other conditions considered for BMT where TBI is sometime employed include severe aplastic anaemia, thalassaemia and immunodeficiency syndromes. Long-term effects of TBI include impaired growth owing to growth hormone deficiency, and a direct effect from irradiation of epiphyses. There is also a possibility of cataract, hypothyroidism and in some studies the possibility of renal impairment. TBI is generally not considered for children under the age of 2, and instead a conditioning regimen with two drugs busulfan and cyclophosphamide (Bu-Cy) is used.

HODGKIN'S DISEASE

The survival rate for children with Hodgkin's disease is approximately 90%. In current protocols the aims are to maintain this good overall survival rate and reduce long-term effects. These include infertility from alkylating agents and procarbazine, and the orthopaedic long-term effects of radiotherapy. Wide-field radiotherapy such as the 'mantle' technique used widely in adults is avoided in children. Many North American and European protocols employ low-intensity chemotherapy and low-dose involved-field radiotherapy with the aim of avoiding infertility and serious orthopaedic effects. In the UK single modality therapy is used. Children aged 10 or older with disease high in the neck will generally receive involved-field radiotherapy. The dose prescribed is 35 Gy in 20 fractions. Both sides of the neck are irradiated to avoid asymmetric cervical spine growth, and the clavicles are shielded. With this approach, approximately 70% of children with stage I disease remain disease-free and 30% relapse, requiring chemotherapy. For children aged less than 10 and for those with more extensive disease, including all stages II–IV and children with stage I disease low in the neck, chemotherapy is used.

NON-HODGKIN LYMPHOMA (NHL)

Compared with adults, a different spectrum of NHL is seen in children. The majority have either T cell lymphoblastic lymphoma, Burkitt's, Burkitt-like, or anaplastic large cell lymphoma. Diffuse large B cell lymphoma and follicle centre cell lymphoma, which are common in adults, are uncommon in childhood. Survival rates have continued to improve in recent years, and currently more than 80% are cured. Therapy is based on intensive multiagent chemotherapy including CNS prophylaxis with intrathecal chemotherapy. There is no routine role for radiotherapy in the management of NHL in childhood. However, children with T cell lymphoblastic lymphoma, which is managed according to the same principles as ALL, may be considered for BMT with TBI.

WILMS' TUMOUR (NEPHROBLASTOMA)

Wilms' tumour is an embryonic renal tumour, being the most frequent abdominal tumour in childhood. The median age at diagnosis is between 3 and 3.5 years. In 4–8% of cases Wilms' tumour is bilateral. Wilms' tumour may be genetically associated with aniridia (congenital absence of the iris) and other inherited syndromes such as the Beckwith–Wiedemann syndrome. The *WT1* gene is located on chromosome 11, and is a tumour suppressor gene. If both copies of the gene are lost by mutation, then Wilms' tumour may arise.

The current long-term survival rate for Wilms' tumour is 80%. Current treatment programmes are aimed at maintaining this high survival rate while attempting to reduce the long-term side-effects. The

North American series of National Wilms' Tumour Study (NWTS) protocols have as their basis immediate nephrectomy. Staging is based on histological examination of the primary tumour. Postoperative chemotherapy is given using the drugs vincristine, actinomycin D and doxorubicin, the number of drugs and duration depending upon the staging. Postoperative radiotherapy is given to the flank for stage III patients, i.e. those with incompletely resected primary tumours, and whole lung radiotherapy for patients with pulmonary metastases at presentation.

In Europe the series of International Society of Paediatric Oncology (SIOP) studies have been based on preoperative chemotherapy to 'downstage' the primary, reducing the number who have tumour rupture at surgery, and the number who require flank radiotherapy. Radiotherapy is given to the flank for those with stage III disease, 14.4 Gy in 8 fractions for those with favourable histology and 25.2 Gy in 14 fractions for those with unfavourable (e.g. anaplastic) histology. Care is taken during planning to include the full with of the vertebral body to avoid asymmetric spinal growth and scoliosis (Fig. 32.4). The clinical target volume includes the tumour and kidney with a margin of 2 cm. Occasionally whole abdominal radiotherapy is employed. However, this has considerable acute and long-term morbidity and should probably be reserved for those who present with extensive intra-abdominal tumour spread. For children presenting with pulmonary metastases, whole lung radiotherapy is given. The fields have to include the costophrenic recess and the lower border generally extends to the lower border of the 12th thoracic vertebra (Fig. 32.5). The humeral heads are shielded. The dose prescribed is 12 Gy in 8 daily fractions of 1.5 Gy specified to the midplane of the central axis without lung correction or 15 Gy in 10 fractions with a lung density correction.

NEUROBLASTOMA

Neuroblastoma usually occurs in very young children and one-third are aged less than 1 year. It arises in neural crest tissue in the autonomic nervous system, usually in the adrenal area, but can arise anywhere from the neck to the pelvis. Children frequently present with widespread metastases. Current survival rates are generally poor, approximately 45% overall. However, the prognosis varies considerably and is related to several prognostic factors. Prognosis is better for children aged less than 1 at presentation, and is worse for children whose tumours have amplification of the oncogene N-*myc*. Deletion of

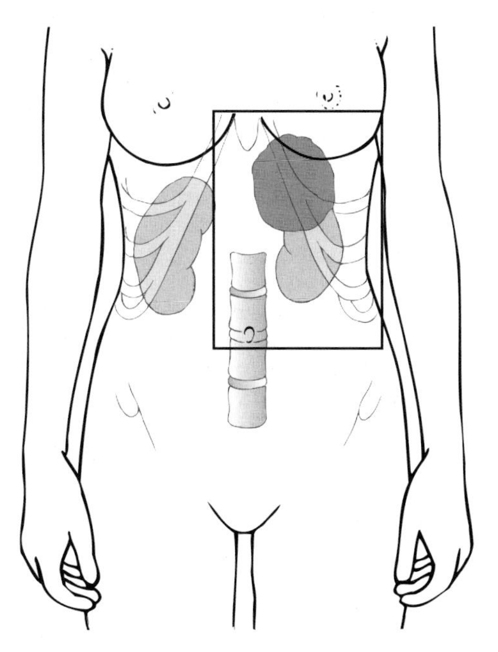

Fig. 32.4 Diagram of flank radiotherapy field for Wilms' tumour.

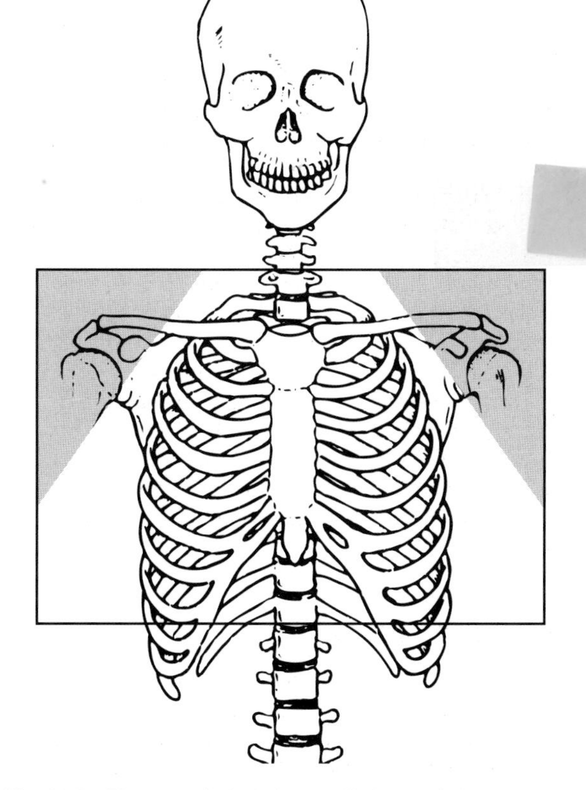

Fig. 32.5 Diagram of whole lung radiotherapy field.

the short arm of chromosome 1 has emerged as an important prognostic factor, with a worse prognosis for those with 1p deletion. Tumours which are hyperdiploid have a better prognosis. Management is now stratified according to risk grouping. Patient in the best risk group with a survival rate of greater than 90% can be managed with surgery alone. The majority are treated with intensive chemotherapy with drugs such as vincristine, cisplatin, carboplatin, etoposide, and cyclophosphamide. Currently, external beam radiotherapy does not have a clearly defined role in the management of children with neuroblastoma. For 'good-risk' patients, radiotherapy is unnecessary and for poor-risk patients the predominant relapse pattern is metastatic rather than local. Postoperative radiotherapy to the tumour bed (21 Gy in 14 fractions) may have a role in patients whose metastatic disease responds well to chemotherapy and who proceed to resection of their primary tumour.

The majority of neuroblastomas take up the guanethidine analogue meta-iodobenzyl guanidine (MIBG). MIBG can be conjugated with iodine radionuclides for imaging and 'targeted radiotherapy' of neuroblastoma. ^{123}I-MIBG is used for diagnostic imaging. High-activity ^{131}I-MIBG (typically 3.7–7.4 GBq) can be used for therapy. For children with residual disease after chemotherapy, a response rate of 30% can be achieved. The use of therapeutic MIBG together with chemotherapy as part of first-line treatment is being explored.

RHABDOMYOSARCOMA

These arise in striated muscle. Although these may arise at any site, they have a predilection for sites in the head and neck region such as the orbit and nasopharynx, and urogenital tract such as bladder, prostate and vagina. Currently the long-term survival rate is approximately 65%. The challenges are to continue to increase the survival rate but also to try to do this with acceptable long-term morbidity. The sequelae following radiotherapy to the head and neck in young children may be considerable.

In many European countries including the UK, children are treated according to the International Society of Paediatric Oncology (SIOP) MMT 95 study. The basis of the European MMT series of trials has been the use of intensive chemotherapy, with the aim of improving the survival and reducing the use of local therapy with surgery and/or radiotherapy and thus minimising long-term effects. The strategy for the current MMT 95 study includes stratifying patients within risk groups based on histological subtype, stage of disease and primary tumour site. Patients in the 'low-risk' category, i.e. those with localised tumours which are microscopically completely resected, are treated with chemotherapy using actinomycin D and vincristine for a duration of 9 weeks. Standard-risk tumours are those which are locally more extensive but at selected favourable sites, the vagina, uterus or paratestis, and are treated with ifosfamide, vincristine and actinomycin-D. Poor responders switch to a six-drug combination. High-risk tumours include other incompletely resected tumours, including all those arising in parameningeal sites (nasopharynx, middle ear) and those with involved lymph nodes. These are treated with chemotherapy involving a randomisation between three drugs (ifosfamide, vincristine, actinomycin-D) and six drugs (carboplatin, epirubicin, vincristine, ifosfamide, etoposide, and actinomycin-D).

In the MMT 95 study, radiotherapy is used for patients who fail to achieve a complete response following chemotherapy and surgery. Thus radiotherapy is used to convert a partial response into a complete response. The tumour volume following a response to chemotherapy is used to define the target volume. The standard dose is 45 Gy in 25 daily fractions with a 'boost' of 5–10 Gy to sites of residual macroscopic disease evident at the start of radiotherapy. For high-risk parameningeal disease (skull base erosion or cranial nerve palsy) the target volume is based on the pre-chemotherapy extent of disease. For those who require RT following relapse after initial treatment with chemotherapy alone, the target volume is based on the tumour extent at the time of relapse and before second-line chemotherapy. For children with initially involved nodes, these are included in the target volume if they require radiotherapy. It is now recognised that patients presenting with primary tumours in the orbit or limbs have a high risk of recurrence and they now routinely receive radiotherapy in the current European protocol.

Planning of radiotherapy demands careful attention to detail, avoiding excessive field sizes particularly in the head and neck region (Fig. 32.6), because of the major morbidity from hypoplasia in this area.

Brachytherapy may be considered for selected children with limited tumours arising in the head and neck, vagina, bladder or prostate. Brachytherapy may provide a means of local control with reduced morbidity compared with external beam RT. However, very few children are suitable for this approach.

EWING'S SARCOMA/PERIPHERAL PRIMITIVE NEUROECTODERMAL TUMOUR (PPNET)

Ewing's sarcoma of bone has its peak incidence in the early teenage years. Approximately 60% occur in the long bones of the limbs, and 40% in the flat bones of

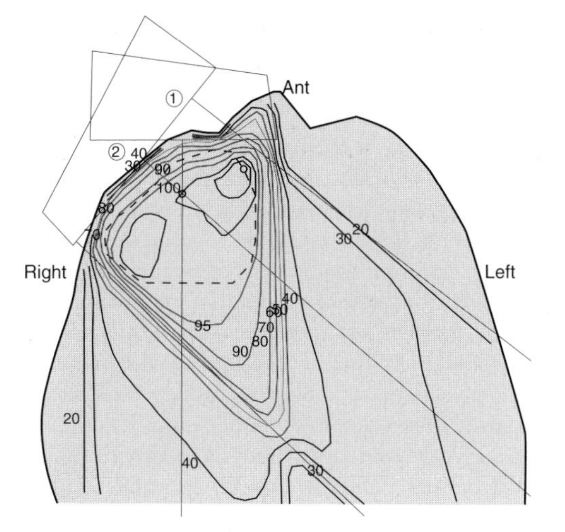

Fig. 32.6 Orbital rhabdomyosarcoma radiotherapy plan.

the ribs, vertebrae or spine. Soft tissue extension is common. Peripheral primitive neuroectodermal tumour (PPNET) has become more frequently recognised recently. PPNET arises in soft tissues. The original subtype of PPNET recognised was the 'Askin tumour' of the chest wall. The majority of Ewing's sarcomas of bone and PPNET share a common chromosomal translocation, t(11;22) (q24;q12). It is now recommended that Ewing's sarcoma and PPNET are treated according to common protocols. Current survival rates are reported to be between 55% and 65%.

Managing children with Ewing's sarcoma and PPNET involves a multidisciplinary team approach. Initial treatment is with chemotherapy, with the appropriate use of local therapy, either surgical resection, radiotherapy, or both. Protocol development for Ewing's sarcoma / PPNET is in a state of evolution, with current discussions in the UK centred around the forthcoming European Ewing's Tumour Working Initiative of National Groups (Euro-E.W.I.N.G. 99). In this study, patients will be stratified according to primary tumour volume. For patients with small tumours (< 200 ml), and those with a good histological response to initial chemotherapy with ifosfamide, doxorubicin and vincristine, chemotherapy will continue using doxorubicin and vincristine and a randomisation to either cyclophosphamide or ifosfamide. For those with a poor histological response, there is a randomisation between conventional chemotherapy and high-dose chemotherapy with busulfan and melphalan.

The decision as to whether surgery, radiotherapy or both should be employed for the primary tumour demands on careful multidisciplinary discussion. In previous series of patients, survival has been better following local treatment with surgery, compared with radiotherapy alone. However, these series are confounded by selection bias, with patients with smaller tumours selected for surgery.

In common with planning of radiotherapy for adult sarcomas, planning of radiotherapy for Ewing's sarcoma or PPNET is technically challenging. All available technical radiotherapy planning developments including CT planning (Fig. 32.7), and in future three-dimensional planning, may need to be employed in order to achieve a uniform dose within the target volume, which is frequently large and adjacent to critical organs. 'Multidisciplinary radiotherapy planning' involving radiologists, physicists, specialist therapy radiographers and mould room technicians is important at the outset.

'Definitive radiotherapy' is given for inoperable tumours to a dose of 54 Gy. Selected patients may require a higher dose up to 64 Gy. For postoperative radiotherapy, the prescribed dose depends on the extent of surgery and histological response of the primary to initial chemotherapy. Following 'intralesional surgery' or 'marginal surgery' with poor histological response to chemotherapy (> 10% residual tumour cells), 54 Gy is prescribed. For 'marginal surgery' with good histological response (< 10% residual tumour cells) or 'wide surgery' with poor histological response, 45 Gy is prescribed. Radiotherapy planning is based on the principle of using the pre-chemotherapy tumour extent, with a 5 cm margin where possible for the initial 45 Gy followed by a 2 cm margin for a second phase of radiotherapy. For patients who present

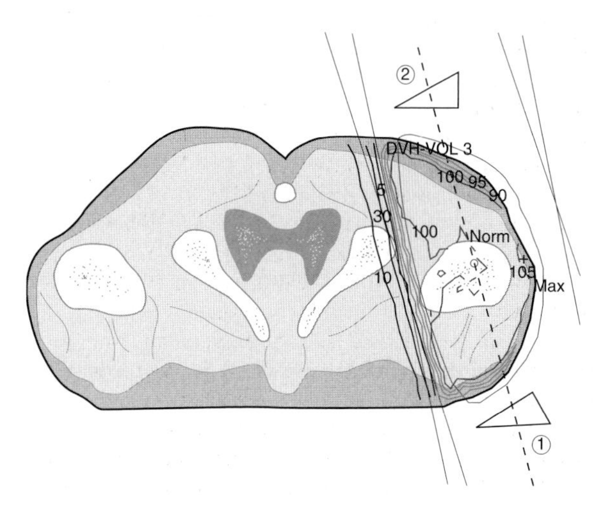

Fig. 32.7 CT plan of radiotherapy for pelvic Ewing's sarcoma.

with pulmonary metastases, whole lung RT is employed: 15 Gy for patients aged less than 14 and 18 Gy for those aged over 14, with these doses corrected for reduced attenuation in lung.

Care must be taken when combining chemotherapy and radiotherapy to avoid excessive morbidity from enhanced radiation reactions. Actinomycin-D is avoided during radiotherapy and doxorubicin avoided if there is a significant amount of bowel or mucosa in the treated volume.

OSTEOSARCOMA

This is the most common bone tumour in childhood, with the majority arising in teenagers. Approximately 65% arise around the knee in the lower femur or upper tibia. Less common sites are humerus, fibula, sacrum, spine, mandible and pelvis. Prior to the advent of effective chemotherapy 80% of patients died with pulmonary metastases. Currently a survival rate of approximately 55% can be achieved with the use of intensive chemotherapy. The majority of primary tumours can be resected and the affected bone replaced by a titanium endoprosthesis, thus avoiding the need for an amputation. The most frequently employed chemotherapy regimen is the combination of cisplatin and doxorubicin. The current European Osteosarcoma Intergroup (EOI) study is a randomised study comparing the efficacy of 6 cycles of cisplatin and doxorubicin given either every 3 weeks or every 2 weeks, using granulocyte colony-stimulating factor (GCSF) to accelerate recovery of the blood count.

Radiotherapy has only a minor role in the management of osteosarcoma. However, it is not as radioresistant as previously thought. Radiotherapy is sometimes employed for the treatment of an unresectable tumour such as a spinal vertebral primary. In this case the dose has to be as high as normal tissues will tolerate, i.e. 60 Gy if possible. In selected patients after insertion of an endoprosthesis, postoperative radiotherapy may be employed for those felt to be at a high risk of local recurrence, i.e. those with tumour at a resection margin. Radiotherapy can be employed for the local palliation of metastases. Using a relatively high dose, e.g. 40 Gy in 15 fractions, many tumours will regress with relief of symptoms.

TUMOURS OF THE CENTRAL NERVOUS SYSTEM (CNS)

Although tumours of the central nervous system (CNS) account for over one-fifth of malignant childhood tumours, individual tumour types are uncommon and experience is limited. Approximately 350 children develop CNS tumours each year in the UK. The overall 5-year survival rate is approximately 50%, which is inferior to that reported for many other paediatric tumours. Many of the survivors experience sequelae from either the tumour or therapy or both. In contrast to most other paediatric malignancies, the use of chemotherapy has not yet resulted in significant improvements in survival. The relative frequencies of paediatric brain tumours are given in Table 32.1.

Problems experienced by children with CNS tumours and their families are complex and multifaceted. It is essential that patients and their families are managed by a specialised paediatric neuro-oncology multidisciplinary team. The recent UK publication 'Guidance for Services for Children and Young People with Brain and Spinal Tumours' describes the elements of a comprehensive multidisciplinary service.

In the last decade there have been important advances in surgical techniques, anaesthesia and intensive care support. There have also been improvements in technique as a result of the development of the operating microscope and ultrasonic surgical aspirator. It is now possible to biopsy tumours in most areas of the brain using stereotactic techniques.

Radiotherapy for children with CNS tumours is technically challenging. Many children require craniospinal radiotherapy, one of the more complex techniques employed in most radiotherapy departments.

Long-term effects of radiotherapy for CNS tumours

For many children the hypothalamic/pituitary axis has to be included in the irradiated volume. This may lead to endocrine deficiency, usually growth hormone deficiency but other endocrine deficiencies such as TRH or ACTH deficiency may occur.

Of great concern are the long-term neuropsychological effects of radiotherapy to the CNS particularly for very young children. Other factors include effects of the presence of the tumour itself, both direct and indirect such as the effect of hydrocephalus and also the effects of surgery. The most important factor which predicts for long-term neuropsychological outcome is the age at treatment. For children aged less than 3 at diagnosis, radiotherapy is delayed if possible by the use of chemotherapy.

Chemotherapy for CNS tumours

For many paediatric CNS tumours, chemotherapy does not yet have a well established role. An exception is in the treatment of intracranial non-seminomatous germ cell tumours. The role of chemotherapy is being evaluated in other clinical settings, e.g. prior to radiotherapy for medulloblastoma. The role of chemotherapy for the treatment of relapse following standard therapy with surgery and RT is being evaluated in many programmes.

LOW-GRADE ASTROCYTOMA

These form the most frequent group of CNS tumours in childhood. The most frequent types are WHO grade I (pilocytic) or grade II (usually fibrillary). Other varieties such as ganglioglioma and oligodendroglioma are much less frequent. The presence of neurofibromatosis type I (NF1) predisposes to the development of these tumours. Modern management is based on the recognition that low-grade gliomas may undergo long periods of 'quiescence', even when not completely resected. It is now also clear that low-grade gliomas are not chemoresistant. The current 5-year survival rate is 85%, but late relapse is not uncommon.

Treatment is initially with surgical resection, as complete as is considered safe. This may be relatively more straightforward for tumours arising in the cerebellum than for those arising from the optic tract or optic chiasm. There have been recent attempts to standardise the management of low-grade gliomas. The current International Society of Paediatric Oncology (SIOP) study sets out a strategy for managing these tumours. Following maximal surgical resection patients undergo a period of observation. Those with clinical or radiological evidence of progression receive non-surgical treatment. In the current study, those over the age of 5 are treated by radiotherapy. Those under the age of 5 receive chemotherapy with carboplatin and vincristine with the aim of delaying radiotherapy.

Radiotherapy for low-grade gliomas is based on careful imaging for target volume definition. Generally the T2-weighted MR image is employed. Careful planning is important to avoid irradiation of non-target structures. In the current SIOP study the radiotherapy dose is 54 Gy in 30 fractions of 1.8 Gy. The technique will usually be a two- or three-field technique, depending upon anatomical location (Fig. 32.8). Techniques for 'merging' MR and planning CT imaging can be very useful for target volume definition. Three-dimensional conformal planning can reduce the amount of normal brain within the irradiated volume, and has the potential for reducing long-term effects, an important priority for this group of patients who have a high chance of long-term survival.

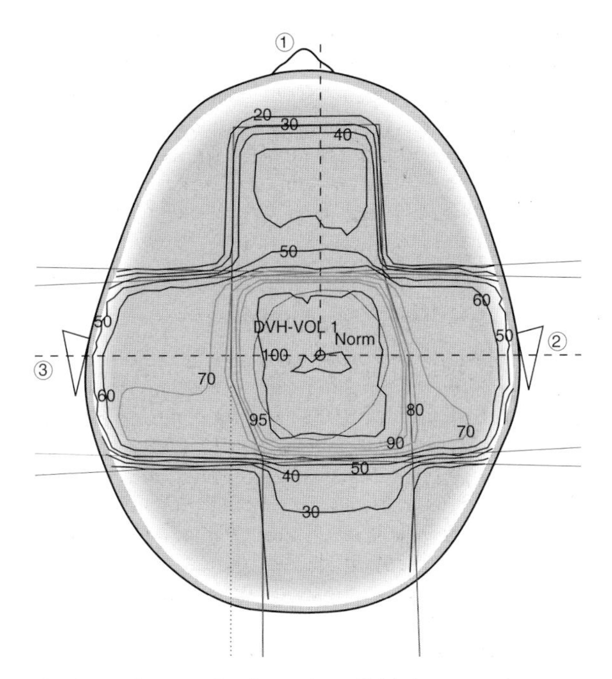

Fig. 32.8 Low-grade glioma three-field plan.

HIGH-GRADE ASTROCYTOMA

Unlike in adults, high-grade astrocytomas are uncommon in childhood. However, the outlook, in common with that in adults, is generally poor. Survival is currently approximately 20% at 5 years. Current management is based on surgical resection and postoperative radiotherapy (54 Gy in 30 fractions). There is no definite routine role for chemotherapy, and recent studies have examined chemotherapeutic agents given prior to radiotherapy in the form of a 'window' phase II study.

EPENDYMOMA

Ependymomas are uncommon and there are very few randomised studies on which to base management strategies. Historically, management was with surgical excision, followed by radiotherapy, which was generally craniospinal for those with posterior fossa primaries or high-grade histology. It is now recognised that although there is a risk of CSF metastases, this risk is not influenced of by the use of craniospinal radiotherapy. The risk of CSF metastases is related to the probability of primary local control. There is currently no evidence to support the routine use of craniospinal radiotherapy. The overall 5-year survival rate is approximately 50%.

The current European SIOP ependymoma study recommends that for completely resected tumours postoperative focal radiotherapy (54 Gy in 30 fractions) should be given, and for incompletely resected tumours, a trial of chemotherapy using vincristine, cyclophosphamide and etoposide.

MEDULLOBLASTOMA/PNET

Medulloblastoma is a primitive neuronal tumour which arises in the cerebellum. It is notable for its propensity for metastatic spread via the CSF, and its radiosensitivity. Primitive neuroectodermal tumour (PNET) arises elsewhere in the CNS, usually the supratentorial cerebral cortex but sometimes the pineal area (pineoblastoma). Although histologically identical to medulloblastoma, supratentorial PNET has a significantly worse prognosis (approximately 20% compared with 50% 5-year survival).

Standard therapy for medulloblastoma/PNET is initial maximal surgical resection followed by craniospinal radiotherapy and a 'boost' to the primary site.

Until recently in the UK, the 'standard' dose for craniospinal radiotherapy was 35 Gy with a 20 Gy 'boost' to the primary site. The recently closed European SIOP/UKCCSG PNET-3 study employed craniospinal RT, 35 Gy in 21 daily fractions of 1.67 Gy with a 'boost' of 20 Gy in 12 daily fractions of 1.67 Gy. There was a randomisation to this radiotherapy alone or preceded by four cycles of chemotherapy employing vincristine and etoposide, with alternating cyclophosphamide and carboplatin. This study has shown an advantage for chemotherapy, and has also demonstrated the importance of avoiding gaps in the radiotherapy schedule. For the last 4 years in North America it has been standard practice to employ adjuvant chemotherapy (vincristine, CCNU, cisplatin) following radiotherapy and this has now also become standard practice in Europe. Because of the poor survival of patients with CSF metastases, all these children receive chemotherapy and radiotherapy. Promising results have been reported from small North American studies of hyperfractionated radiotherapy employing craniospinal radiotherapy, 36 Gy in 36 fractions of 1 Gy twice daily, and a total dose of 72 Gy in 72 fractions of 1 Gy twice daily to the posterior fossa. The use of twice-daily fractionation allows an increase in the total dose delivered, and should hopefully result in an improvement in the therapeutic ratio. The use of hyperfractionated radiotherapy will be evaluated further in multicentre European studies.

Craniospinal radiotherapy (CSRT)

CSRT is one of the most complex radiotherapy techniques delivered in oncology departments. The target volume for CSRT is complex and has to include the whole of the CSF and meninges (Fig. 32.9). CSRT involves the use of large lateral whole brain fields, whose lower borders are carefully matched to the upper border of one or more spinal fields. Individual departments' CSRT techniques vary in detail but are generally based on standard principles. Meticulous attention to detail in the planning and delivery of craniospinal RT is essential and contributes to the cure of medulloblastoma/PNET.

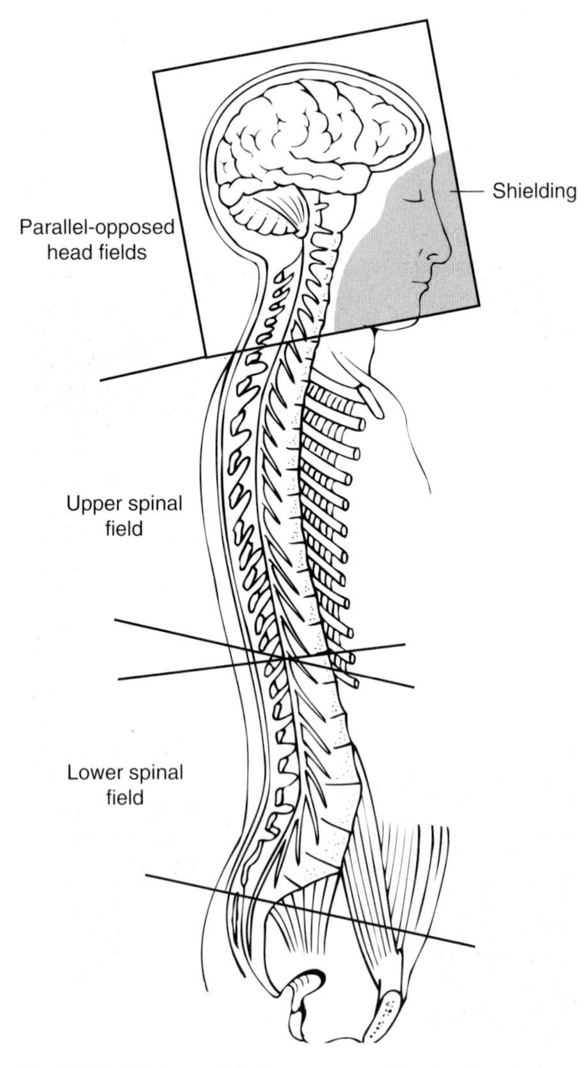

Fig. 32.9 Diagram of field arrangement for craniospinal radiotherapy.

Accurate immobilisation is essential and involves the use of a prone head shell, and also body immobilisation. It is essential to avoid areas of underdose at field junctions and partial shielding of any area of meninges. It is standard practice to employ a 'moving junction' between the head and spine field. This is a 'safety measure', which reduces the risk of underdose or overdose in the cervical spinal cord if a systematic error develops during CSRT. When planning the shielding blocks which are used to shield the lenses, nasal structures and dentition from the whole brain fields, it is important to take care to avoid shielding meninges at the cribriform fossa, temporal fossa, and base of skull (Fig. 32.10). In children the cribriform fossa frequently lies between the lenses (Fig. 32.11), making planning difficult. The lower border of the spinal field has generally been placed at the lower border of the second sacral vertebra. However, there is evidence that the lower border of the thecal sac varies and planning of the lower border of the spinal field should be based on MR scanning. The spinal field should be wide enough to encompass the extensions of the meninges along the nerve roots, and therefore wide enough to encompass

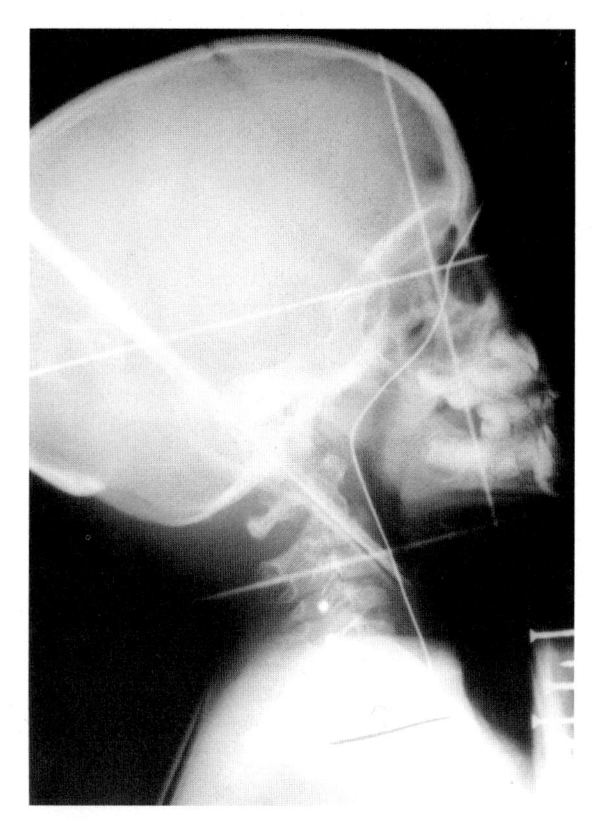

Fig. 32.10 Simulator film of whole brain field for medulloblastoma.

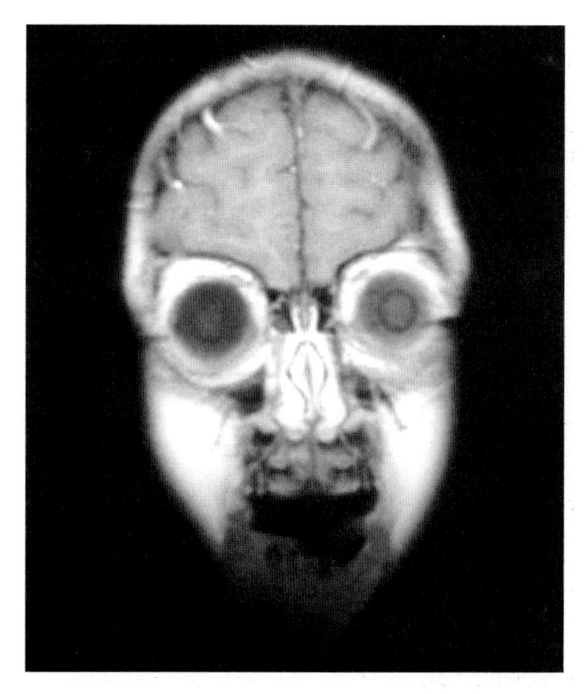

Fig. 32.11 MRI scan showing position of lens and cribriform fossa.

the intervertebral foramina in the lumbar region. The spinal field will typically be 5–6 cm wide.

When planning the posterior fossa 'boost' for medulloblastoma, it is generally accepted that the whole cerebellum should be included in the target volume, because of the risk of local meningeal spread of the primary. It has been standard to employ a standard field arrangement (Fig. 32.12), with a parallel-opposed pair of fields. However, to avoid a higher dose in the neck, it is usually necessary to employ wedges as tissue compensators.

CSRT techniques are continuing to evolve, and need to incorporate technical developments in radiotherapy immobilisation, planning and treatment delivery. For the posterior fossa 'boost' it is possible to employ three-dimensional conformal planning to reduce the radiation dose to non-target structures such as the hypothalamus and middle ear. 'Virtual simulation' has been used to define the target volume for CSRT in critical areas such as the cribriform fossa.

INTRACRANIAL GERM CELL TUMOURS

Intracranial germ cell tumours account for approximately 30% of paediatric germ cell tumours. Germinomas are the histological equivalent of testicular seminoma. They generally arise in the suprasellar region but may occur in the pineal region. Non-germi-

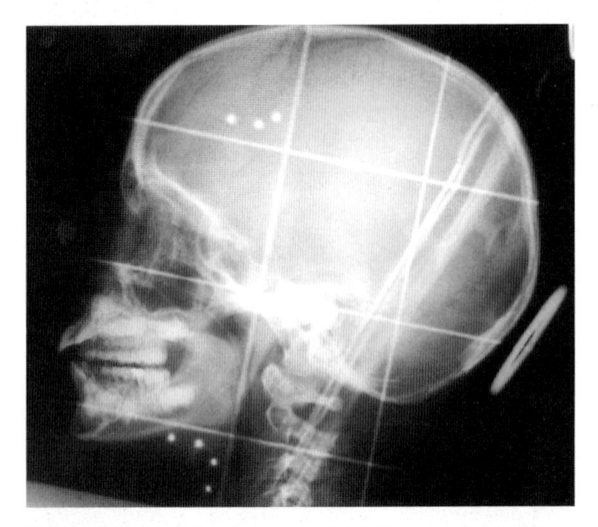

Fig. 32.12 Posterior fossa boost field for medulloblastoma.

nomatous germ cell tumours are the histological equivalent of testicular non-seminomatous germ cell tumours, i.e. embryonal carcinomas, yolk sac tumours or choriocarcinomas. They generally arise in the pineal region and may secrete alpha-fetoprotein (AFP) and/or human chorionic gonadotrophin (HCG). More than 90% of germinomas are cured with radiotherapy. Because of the risk of meningeal metastases, craniospinal RT is used. However, as with testicular seminoma there has been a gradual reduction in both the CSRT dose and the dose used for the 'boost' to the primary tumour in an attempt to minimise long-term effects. In the current International Society of Paediatric Oncology (SIOP) protocol the CSRT dose is 24 Gy in 15 fractions of 1.6 Gy and the boost dose to the primary is a further 16 Gy in 10 daily fractions of 1.6 Gy. Germinomas have a tendency for subependymal spread, which has to be taken into account when planning the boost volume, with a margin of 2 cm around the gross tumour volume. For non-germinomatous tumours the prognosis is worse. Initial treatment is with chemotherapy followed by radiotherapy, either focal for non-metastatic tumours or craniospinal for those with meningeal metastases. In the current SIOP protocol the chemotherapy used is a combination of cisplatin etoposide and ifosfamide followed by radiotherapy. The total radiotherapy dose is 54 Gy to the primary tumour, with 30 Gy to the craniospinal axis for patients with meningeal metastases.

BRAINSTEM GLIOMA

This includes tumours arising in the midbrain, pons and medulla. Historically they were regarded as a single entity. However, it is now clear that they can be subdivided into focal (5–10%), dorsal exophytic (10–20%), cervicomedullary (5–10%) and diffuse intrinsic tumours (75–85%). Focal, dorsal exophytic, and cervicomedullary tumours are usually low-grade astrocytomas. Surgical excision is the treatment of choice with radiotherapy reserved for inoperable tumours.

The majority of children with brainstem gliomas have diffuse pontine tumours, which are usually high-grade astrocytomas. They are diagnosed by their typical MR appearance, and biopsy is dangerous and contraindicated. Their prognosis is very poor with a median survival of approximately 9 months and very few long-term survivors. The management of these children remains a major challenge, and domiciliary palliative care usually has to be introduced at a relatively early stage.

The standard radiotherapy approach is to treat the tumour with a 2 cm margin around the gross tumour volume on MR scan using parallel-opposed fields and a dose of 54 Gy in 30 daily fractions of 1.8 Gy. Chemotherapy has been of no benefit. Conventional radiotherapy provides useful palliation for approximately 75% of children. However, the progression-free survival is short, usually less than 6 months. Neither hyperfractionated nor accelerated radiotherapy has improved outcome for these patients. Current protocols are evaluating novel chemotherapy approaches.

CONCLUSIONS

Patients treated by the multidisciplinary paediatric oncology team present with a wide variety of diseases, which pose many different problems. Management is aimed not just at the patient, but the whole family. Prognosis varies considerably from those where treatment failure is rare, namely intracranial germinoma to those where cure is rare, such as intrinsic pontine glioma. Management in specialised centres is essential, according to national or international protocols. Radiotherapy plays an important role in the management of many of these children. They deserve the highest standard of radiotherapy planning and delivery, incorporating all technical developments. When planning radiotherapy, consideration of the long-term effects of treatment is always of paramount importance. Therapeutic developments initially investigated in adults, such as hyperfractionation, also require investigation for childhood cancers. With the increasing use of concurrent chemotherapy and radiotherapy, constant vigilance for interactions is required.

33

Non-malignant disorders

Ian Kunkler

CHAPTER CONTENTS

Cancer is not the only disease process in which radiation can be useful. It was inevitable that such a powerful form of energy should be widely explored in the early days before its dangers and limitations could be and were appreciated. X-rays were discovered in 1895 by Konrad Röntgen. Radiation was delivered to a very wide range of non-malignant conditions by enthusiasts in the pioneer days. The first application was described by Freund for treating a benign disease—a 'hairy mole' which disappeared after treatment with X-rays. Ionising radiation is known to be effective in the treatment of inflammatory conditions. Unfortunately a great deal of damage, some of it fatal, was done unwittingly before the serious consequences emerged. For example, irradiation of the enlarged thymus gland in infancy used to be practised and it caused gratifying shrinkage. Years later, however, carcinoma of the thyroid developed in some cases, undoubtedly induced by the effect of the rays on the immature thyroid cells. Similarly, some patients who received spinal irradiation to relieve spinal discomfort from ankylosing spondylitis, a chronic rheumatic disorder, later developed leukaemia and other tumours. The development of leukaemia in these patients discouraged many radiotherapists from treating this and other benign conditions with radiotherapy.

Where treatment appeared to be useful, e.g. in many non-malignant skin disorders, repeated dosage was commonly given for recurrent disease, since the cumulative effects of even low doses were for long not appreciated.

At present the indications for the use of radiotherapy for non-malignant conditions are much more limited. To a large extent this is due to the appreciation of radiation-induced malignancy but it also reflects the availability of more effective non-radiotherapeutic treatments. None the less, there is considerable variation in the use of radiotherapy for benign disease between radiotherapy departments in the UK.

In general, the use of ionising radiation for the treatment of benign disease should be discouraged and alternative therapies sought.

ENDOCRINE DISORDERS

Pituitary

Radiation is commonly used postoperatively following the surgical removal or debulking of pituitary tumours (see page 547 for detailed description).

Ovary

The ovary, beside producing the ova or egg cells which unite with the sperm to form the next generation, secretes female sex hormones (e.g. oestrogen) which control secondary sexual characteristics and the various changes in the female organism. Towards the age of the menopause ovarian function may become irregular and cause intermittent excessive uterine bleeding (menorrhagia). If medical treatment fails, surgical hysterectomy is often advised. An alternative is to suppress ovarian hormonal secretion by radiation. This can be applied in two ways: internal and external.

Internal therapy

An intrauterine tube containing caesium, as used in uterine cancer, will irradiate and inhibit both the endometrium and the ovaries. A 50 mg tube applied for 40–48 hours will deliver about 5–10 Gy to the ovaries. General anaesthesia is needed, and this provides the essential opportunity for a thorough pelvic examination, uterine curettage and biopsy, to exclude malignancy as the cause of bleeding. This technique is very effective and still used, though it can lead to some degree of endometritis and uterine discharge. It is contraindicated in patients who are not fit enough for general anaesthesia, usually because of poor cardiorespiratory function.

Induction of an *artificial menopause* in this way involves sterilisation of the patient. In almost all cases, this causes no problems and is in fact desirable. It is wise, however, to obtain the written informed consent of the patient, who should be asked to sign a form stating that the effects of the treatment have been explained, understood and accepted.

In the past, radiation was used to treat dysmenorrhoea and pelvic inflammatory disease. Such practice is to be condemned because of the risk of gene mutations affecting succeeding generations.

External therapy

External beam irradiation is the commonest means of inducing an artificial menopause. It is suitable for patients where general anaesthesia is contraindicated.

Target volume

The target volume is the true pelvis. A typical field size is 15 cm wide and 10 cm long.

Technique

A parallel-opposed pair of anterior and posterior fields is used.

Dose and energy

There is some variation in the dose required to ablate ovarian function, which is related to age and to individual factors. A larger dose is needed at and beyond the age of 35 years.

Under the age of 35: **12.5 Gy midplane dose in 5 daily fractions (9–10 MV photons)**

Aged 35+: **4.5 Gy midplane dose in a single fraction (9–10 MV photons)**

Radioactive iodine and the thyroid gland

For the physical and technical aspects relating to this section reference should be made to Chapter 8.

The thyroid gland synthesises the hormones thyroxine (T4) and tri-iodothyronine (T3) which are essential for the maintenance of normal metabolism, utilising iodine from the diet. As with other endocrine function, the activity of the thyroid gland is controlled by the pituitary through the thyroid-stimulating hormone (TSH) (p. 395). By substituting radioactive iodine, this unique affinity for the chemical provides a useful method of producing a high dose of radiation within a very small volume of tissue.

Thyrotoxicosis (hyperthyroidism)

This is a clinical state associated with raised levels of circulating T4 and/or T3. As a result there is an increase in the body's metabolism, manifested by agitation, palpitations, profuse sweating and weight loss. In some cases there is protrusion of the eyes (exophthalmos). The disease affects females more commonly and usually occurs in the 25–45 year age group. It is sometimes associated with a significant enlargement of the thyroid gland (goitre). Occasionally when a large gland extends behind the sternum (retrosternal extension) there may be evidence of compression of the trachea.

The high affinity of the thyroid gland for iodine forms the basis of both diagnosis and treatment.

Myxoedema

Myxoedema (hypothyroidism) is a state of thyroid hormone deficiency, causing sluggish metabolism. Clinical features include tiredness, weight gain, hair loss, slow pulse and slow relaxing reflexes.

Investigation of thyroid function

The important in vivo tests of thyroid function are those associated with the uptake of radioactive iodine (iodine-131) or other isotope (technetium-99m). These may provide a measure of the physiological activity of the gland (tracer techniques) or of its size and position (imaging or scanning). Both of these tests require sophisticated apparatus and are in vivo. Blood levels of T4 and T3 and, if hypothyroidism is suspected, TSH are measured.

The tracer investigation. This can be carried out on an outpatient basis. The patient attends the isotope laboratory before breakfast and takes a very small dose of iodine-131 (0.55 MBq) through a straw. 4 hours later the patient returns and lies on a couch and a counter above the neck measures the radiation emitted from the gland. This gives a measure of the amount of iodine-131 which has been absorbed by the cells of the thyroid from the test drink, following its passage from the gut into the bloodstream. The count is repeated at 48 hours when a blood sample is taken and the iodine-131 content of the blood proteins is measured.

Interpretation of the tracer test. The main relevant details are given in Chapter 8 and Figure 24.28B.

1. Gland. Normally the measured radioactivity rises gently to a plateau, reached soon after 24 hours, but the toxic gland removes iodine from the blood at such a rapid rate that the iodine-131 curve rises to a sharp peak in a few hours and then falls. Thus the measured uptake at 4 hours will identify most thyrotoxic cases.

2. Plasma. Normally the blood is cleared of iodine gradually and at 48 hours very little is left. However, in the toxic cases there is a secondary rise due to secretion of newly formed hormone, incorporating some of the iodine-131. The 48-hour figures for protein-bound iodine give almost conclusive evidence in most cases.

The thyroid scan. An image of the gland may be obtained by giving the patient a small quantity of radioactive iodine or technetium (see above) and using a special detector called a rectilinear scanner. The latter will measure the activity within the gland at automated 1 cm intervals and produce a composite picture of the size and shape of the gland with areas of high and low activity clearly defined. The typical appearance of toxic multinodular goitre is shown in Figure 24.28B. Variation in shape and activity are easily detected and the test is invaluable in revealing retrosternal goitre, and particularly in the investigation of thyroid cancer (p. 394). The latter usually appears as a 'cold' area (Fig. 24.28A).

In vitro tests

1. Measurement of circulating T4 and T3 by chemical means (as distinct from the radioactive test).

2. Measurement of TSH. The level is low in thyrotoxicosis, as other mechanisms of thyroid stimulation are in operation in this disease, and increased in hypothyroidism.

3. T3 resin uptake. This reflects the amount of hormone binding to TBG (thyroid-binding globulin). A resin is mixed with the patient's serum. There is competition between the resin and the infilled binding sites on TBG. The amount of T3 retained in the resin after washing reflects the concentration of the unoccupied binding sites.

4. Free thyroxine index. This is calculated as: serum T4 × T3 resin uptake.

5. TRH test. When TRH (thyroid-releasing hormone), one of the hypothalamic hormones, is given intravenously in the euthyroid person, it stimulates a rise in serum TSH levels. In hyperthyroidism there is little or no rise in TSH. Thus a positive response rules out primary hyperthyroidism.

In vitro tests are more important than tracer studies so that the administration of radioactive material can very often be avoided altogether.

Treatment of thyrotoxicosis

A small proportion of patients with thyrotoxicosis will improve spontaneously but active treatment is required in most patients. Essentially, treatment is concerned with the reduction of circulating thyroxine, either by partial destruction of the gland or by interrupting the synthesis of the hormone.

Destructive therapy may be achieved by surgery (removal of most of the gland) or by using the specially radioactive iodine in carefully measured doses. Both methods have a place in the management of hyperthyroidism, but radioactive iodine therapy has the advantage of being relatively simple and devoid of serious side-effects and complications.

Medical control is achieved by antithyroid drugs such as carbimazole and propylthiouracil. Serious side-effects may occur (e.g. agranulocytosis with carbimazole). Drug therapy is usually used to render the patient euthyroid prior to surgery. It may be especially important where surgery or iodine-131 cannot be used because of other medical conditions, poor general condition or pregnancy.

Radioactive iodine therapy

The technique is simple. A dose calculated from the size of the gland and the uptake of radioactive iodine (in the tracer test) is given to the patient under the same conditions as for the diagnostic test. Unless the patient is ill, this can be arranged on an outpatient basis, although the patient should stay at the hospital for a few hours until the possibility of vomiting and other side-effects has subsided. The size of the therapeutic drink is of the order of 74–296 MBq which is usually sufficiently low to avoid the need for special precautions to prevent contamination and ensure the safety of staff. If the disease is not controlled by a single treatment, then more doses may be necessary, having allowed up to 12 months to elapse in order to assess the full effect of the first dose.

The drawback of this treatment is the progressive effects of the irradiation, which frequently leads to increasing atrophy of the gland with a slow decrease in the amount of circulating hormones, which can ultimately produce hypothyroidism.

This treatment is usually restricted to patients over the age of 40 because of the theoretical risk of inducing leukaemia or thyroid cancer. There is also the possibility of gene mutations in the reproductive cells of the ovary and testis.

RHEUMATIC DISORDERS

Ankylosing spondylitis

This is a disabling process, mostly in young men, with pain and stiffness, leading to 'poker back' rigidity, It usually begins in the sacroiliac joints, spreading later to the small joints between the vertebrae, and the costovertebral joints (where the ribs attach to the spine). The chronic inflammation leads eventually to ossification of ligaments, fusion of joint surfaces and bony ankylosis. Radiation gives dramatic pain relieve and enables the patient to return to work.

Until 1955, deep X-ray therapy was widely and successfully used as the mainstay of treatment directed at either the sacroiliac joints alone or the whole spine. Total doses up to 30 Gy were applied. Then it was discovered that 10% of treated patients developed leukaemia, undoubtedly a late radiation effect. This led to the abandonment of the treatment by most radiotherapists, in favour of general measures, physiotherapy and drugs. There are still a few cases (e.g. a peripheral painful joint or boggy plantar fasciitis) where, if other methods fail, localised radiotherapy can be justified. The slight risks should be fully explained to the patient to whom the final choice is left. A full blood count should be taken before treatment to ensure no cellular abnormality is present.

Technique

A simple field or parallel-opposed pair is suitable for peripheral joints.

Dose and energy

2 Gy twice weekly to a total dose of 10 Gy (4–6 MV photons or cobalt-60)

Rheumatoid arthritis

Radiotherapy is rarely indicated. Occasionally instillation of yttrium-90 (185–277.5 MBq) is used to treat one or two large joints (e.g. the knee) if medical therapy including steroid injections has failed to control synovitis. It can be repeated once only. Because of the potential induction of secondary malignancy, patients under the age of 45 years should not be treated.

Villonodular synovitis

Yttrium-90 is also instilled into the knee joint to treat residual synovium in the posterior part of the knee joint, which is difficult to remove by synovectomy. The dose is the same as for rheumatoid arthritis.

DISORDERS OF THE EYE AND ORBIT

Radiotherapy is rarely indicated in benign conditions of the eye. It is occasionally used in pterygium, corneal vascularisation and for thyroid eye disease. Care must be taken to avoid irradiating the lens and so avoid cataract formation. Similarly, the drainage of the aqueous humour must not be obstructed or glaucoma may occur.

Pterygium

Pterygium is a growth of fibrovascular tissue on the cornea. It is rare in the UK. It is related to exposure to ultraviolet light. The incidence is 3% in Northern California. It tends to grow slowly as a fleshy expansion of the bulbar conjunctiva across the cornea, nearly always on the medial side of the globe. Its pathogenesis is not known. It may impair visual acuity as it does so. Surgical excision is the treatment of choice for visual loss, local irritation and limitation of lateral gaze. Beta irradiation from a radioactive strontium-90 applicator (60 Gy in 6 weekly fractions) is occasionally used immediately or a few days post-operatively to prevent the formation of episcleral vessels which may give rise to granulation tissue and recurrent pterygium. Beta irradiation is effective, although there are widely differing reported levels of benefit. The risk of radiation-induced scleral damage is up to 4%. Local recurrence rates with and without radiotherapy vary from 3–16% to 8–50% respectively.

Dose

7 Gy at the surface of the cornea once weekly for 3 treatments

Corneal vascularisation

The normal cornea is completely devoid of vessels. Ulcers or infection may lead to abnormal extension of tiny vessels from the surrounding conjunctiva to heal the lesion (Fig. 33.1). The new vessels are liable to persist, even if their purpose has been served, and with them any corneal scar is also liable to persist. If they can be obliterated, fading of the corneal opacity is encouraged. The aim of localised irradiation is to produce a reaction that seals the vessels. Small leashes of vessels are treated.

Dose

5 Gy weekly to a total of 4–5 treatments

Graves' ophthalmopathy

Graves' disease is an autoimmune disease. Its clinical features are hyperthyroidism, ophthalmopathy and pretibial myxoedema. Graves' ophthalmopathy complicates 20–40% of cases of Grave's disease. It is normally bilateral but is unilateral in 20%. Hyperthyroidism occurs in 90% of cases of ophthalmopathy. The pathogenesis of Graves' ophthalmopathy is not known. Close liaison is needed in management between endocrinologist, ophthalmologist and clinical oncologist. Treatment may involve surgery, steroids or surgery. Radiotherapy can be effective in treating moderate to severe ophthalmopathy but the benefits have to be balanced against potential late side-effects such as damage to the retinal vasculature or late carcinogenesis, although these are rare. However, without radiation, there is a risk of visual loss and side-effects from steroids. Radiotherapy is contraindicated in patients with pre- existing retinopathy, diabetes mellitus, and women under the age of 40. Patients should be euthyroid before radiotherapy is contemplated. 10–30% will experience a transient increase in inflammation of the soft tissues.

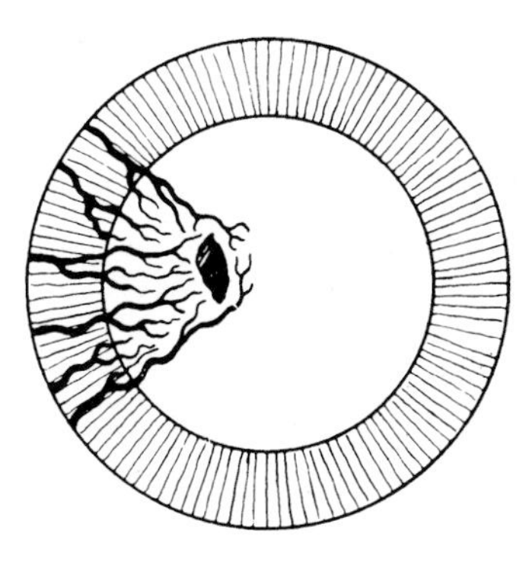

Fig. 33.1 Vascularisation in corneal ulcer.

Target volume

This covers the swollen extraocular muscles.

Technique

Parallel-opposed lateral fields with beam splitting aims to reduce the dose to the contralateral lens to about 4% of the prescribed dose. If beam splitting is not used, angling the beams posteriorly increases the dose to the contralateral lens. A beam-directed shell is used.

Energy

4–6 MV photons (cobalt should be avoided because of the penumbra and scatter).

Dose and fractionation

20 Gy midplane in 10 daily fractions over 2 weeks

Pseudotumour of the orbit

Pseudotumour of the orbit is an idiopathic inflammation of the orbit. It may involve any part of the orbit including the lacrimal gland. It is normally unilateral. Both eyes may, however, be affected. It may occur at any age. Pseudotumour of the orbital apex is also termed the Tolosa–Hunt syndrome. Clinical and radiological features are non-diagnostic. While the condition may be self-limiting, steroids are normally the first line of treatment. However, responses are only durable in one-third of cases after one course of steroids. Radiotherapy may achieve long-term local control or good response rates in 66–100%.

Technique

CT planning using a beam-directed shell in the supine position.

If unilateral with retrobulbar involvement, a single photon field which is beam split or angled posteriorly to minimise the dose to the contralateral lens is used. If there is superficial involvement of the anterior orbit only, an electron field may suffice.

Energy

4–6 MV photons (or electrons of appropriate energy).

Dose and fractionation

20 Gy to 100% isodose in 10 fractions over 2 weeks (with 95% covering the target volume)

Late effects of irradiation on the eye

With doses of 14–16.5 Gy to the eye, the majority will develop a cataract. Visual acuity may be impaired at a dose of about 15 Gy. Retinopathy, dry eye or optic neuropathy should not be seen at doses less than 30–40 Gy. To date, no cases of radiation-induced tumours have been reported after irradiation for Graves' ophthalmopathy.

KELOID SCARS

Keloid scars are sometimes irradiated following excision to reduce the incidence of recurrence. Therapy is usually given 7–10 days postoperatively once the wound is no longer at risk of dehiscence. Care should be taken not to irradiate keloid scars on the neck of children in case thyroid cancer is induced.

Target volume

The target volume is limited to the keloid scar without a margin of normal tissue.

Technique

Single direct field.

Dose and energy

10–12 Gy in 1–3 fractions (90–120 kV)

CEREBRAL ARTERIOVENOUS MALFORMATION AND ACOUSTIC NEUROMAS

Cerebral arteriovenous malformations (AVMs) are composed of a network of arterial and venous channels. The AVM itself does not contain normal brain tissue. AVMs account for 1–2% of all strokes. 50% present with intracranial haemorrhage. Other clinical features are headache, epilepsy, cranial nerve palsies, hydrocephalus and raised intracranial pressure. The risk of bleeding from an untreated AVM is 2–3% per year.

Acoustic neuromas are benign tumours of the acoustic nerve. They are often bilateral. Progressive deafness and facial palsy are common.

Cerebral arteriovenous malformations

Superficial AVMs can be removed surgically. Smaller AVMs, especially if deep-seated, e.g. in the brainstem, are best treated by stereotactic focal irradiation. This can be delivered in a single fraction using a cobalt-60 gamma (Leksell) unit (Fig. 33.2) or fractionated using a linear accelerator or proton beam from a syncyclotron. This form of radiation treatment is known as 'radiosurgery', a term reflecting the original development of this technique by a neurosurgeon.

The treatment head of the Leksell unit contains a hemispherical array of 201 cobalt sources. The beams from each source are collimated and focused to provide a small high-dose volume. The fall-off in dose beyond the high-dose volume is steep, allowing normal brain tissue surrounding an AVM largely to be spared. Different collimators are used (4, 8, 14 and 18 mm) sometimes in combination, depending upon the size and configuration of the AVM.

Treatment involves the fixing of a stereotactic frame to the head of the patient under local anaesthesia. An angiogram (or occasionally a CT scan) is performed to identify the AVM. One or more collimators are selected to ensure the 50% isodose covers the fistulous component of the lesion (Fig. 33.3). With larger and irregularly shaped AVMs (> 3 cm) some normal brain tissue is almost inevitably included in the treated volume. The dosimetry and coordinates of the centre of each treatment field are calculated by computer. The patient is treated prone or supine, depending on the optimal position of the collimator to cover the AVM. The coordinates in the vertical (z) and sagittal (y) planes are set on the stereotactic frame. The frame is secured within the treatment machine and the x axis set in the horizontal plane (x). Treatment is given in a single fraction. Treatment time is normally 15–30 minutes per field, depending on the activity of the sources. A process of progressive thrombo-obliteration within the AVM is established.

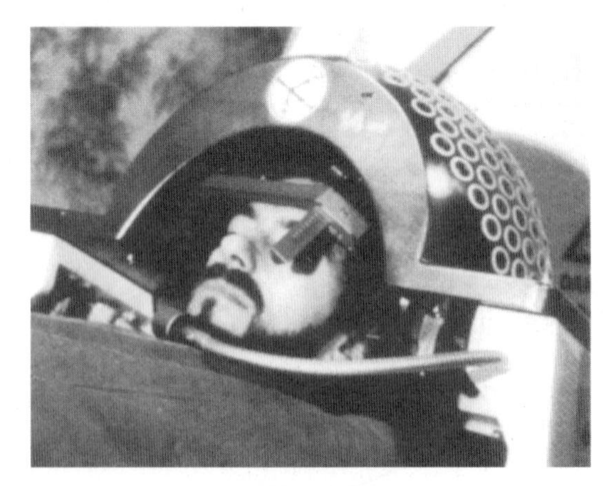

Fig. 33.2 Patient in treatment position in Leksell unit. (Courtesy of Mr D Forster, Radiosurgery Unit, Sheffield.)

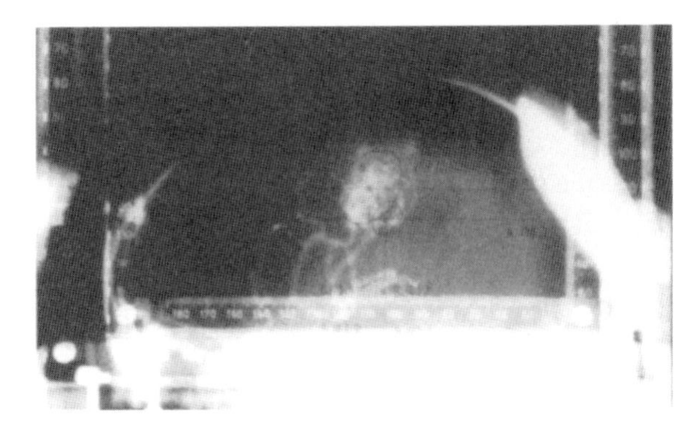

Fig. 33.3 Lateral view of planning angiogram showing temporoparietal arteriovenous malformation (AVM) and horizontal (y) and vertical (z) axes on the stereotactic frame. The AVM is encompassed by 50% isodose curves of 18 mm (anterior) and 8 mm (posterior) collimators. (Courtesy of Mr D Forster, Radiosurgery Unit, Sheffield.)

Dose

20–25 Gy is given to the 50% isodose (peak dose 40–50 Gy) in a single fraction

Acoustic neuromas

The Leksell gamma unit can also be used to treat acoustic neuromas to avoid the need for surgery. A CT scan is performed with a stereotactic frame in place to identify the tumour.

Dose

16–18 Gy to tumour margin in a single fraction.

Morbidity

Acute morbidity with gamma (Leksell) unit therapy is minimal. Major side-effects of treated AVMs (mainly focal neurological defects) occur in 3–4% of patients. Some of these deficits may be due to radionecrosis of normal brain included with the treatment volume. Eloquent areas of the brain seem particularly prone to radiation damage.

Trigeminal or facial nerve damage occurs in about 30% of patients irradiated for acoustic neuromas.

Experience with proton beam radiosurgery suggests higher morbidity (16%).

Results of treatment

About 50% of AVMs treated by a gamma unit are completely or almost completely obliterate 1 year after treatment and 84% by 2 years.

In selected acoustic neuromas (i.e. 3 cm or less) reduction in tumour size and preservation of hearing can be achieved in about 50% of patients.

Stereotactic multiple arc radiotherapy

Stereotactic multiple arc radiotherapy (SMART) can be used to treat AVMs. A relocatable frame is secured on a base plate on the treatment couch to a dental impression of the patient's jaw. Early experience with SMART suggests that obliteration rates are comparable to gamma (Leksell) unit treatment.

Since the frame is relocatable, SMART can be fractionated. Fractionation is likely to improve the tolerance of normal brain to irradiation and tumour cell killing. Its applicability to small-volume intracranial tumours is being evaluated.

RADIATION INHIBITION OF ARTERIAL RESTENOSIS

The use of ionising radiation to prevent the restenosis of coronary arteries after balloon angioplasty (a procedure in which the aperture of a narrowed coronary artery is expanded to improve blood flow) is perhaps one of the most important developments of radiotherapy for the treatment of benign disease.

Angioplasty has been shown to provide an effective alternative to coronary artery bypass graft. However, restenosis occurs in 30–50% of cases, typically within 6 months. In the USA 500 000 transluminal angioplasties are carried out per year. It can be easily seen that any treatment that reduced the rate of restenosis could have considerable clinical and economic implications. Stents have been inserted into vessels to maintain their patency. None the less, abnormal healing processes, 'in-stent stenosis' and especially neointimal hyperplasia occurs and may be accelerated. Intimal stenosis is also a cause of obstruction to flow and ischaemia of limbs, brain, kidney and liver and compromise of patency of vascular shunts or fistulas in patients on haemodialysis.

The initial stenosis is thought to be due to the development of atherosclerosis. However, restenosis seems to occur by a different mechanism. The critical cell in the restenotic process is either the smooth muscle cell and/or the fibroblast. The balloon causes damage to the intimal and media layers and internal elastic membrane of the coronary artery. A mural thrombus occurs because of the deposition of platelets and fibrin; 3–7 days later, cells migrate into the intima and proliferate. A process of fibrosis ensues causing restenosis. Studies of the restenosis in rats and pigs showed that brachytherapy, the insertion of radioactive sources (iridium-192) into the blood vessels could inhibit intimal proliferation. Alternative techniques involve using lower-dose-rate endoluminal radioactive stents inserted at the time of angioplasty. There is some experimental evidence that whether a dose of 20 Gy can permanently prevent or simply postpone the development of restenosis depends to a major degree on the proliferative capacity of damaged normal tissue.

The clinical studies on the use of radiation to prevent restenosis suggests that there is a therapeutic window between the radiation dose that would inhibit stenosis and the dose that would be needed to induce vascular stenosis.

Radiation to prevent stenosis of peripheral vascular access

Both endovascular brachytherapy and external beam with electrons are currently being investigated to assess their role in preventing postangioplasty dialysis access restenosis. At present such treatment should be regarded as investigational since there remain unresolved issues around the sources and dosimetry for brachytherapy, studies are small and follow-up short.

34

Cancer chemotherapy

Ian Kunkler

CHAPTER CONTENTS

INTRODUCTION

'Cancer chemotherapy' refers to the subject of cytotoxic (cell-poisoning) drugs. Hormonal anticancer therapy is described separately in Chapter 35. Chemotherapy has made important contributions to the treatment of the common cancers such as breast, bowel and small cell lung cancer and to rarer malignancies such as Hodgkin's disease, ovarian cancer, the leukaemias, testicular teratoma and choriocarcinoma. However, the role of chemotherapy in the treatment of advanced and metastatic stages of solid tumours such as bowel, breast and lung cancer remains essentially palliative and the intense research effort for curative treatment for these stages of disease has yet to be rewarded. Drug resistance remains a common problem and methods of overcoming it elusive. The uses of chemotherapy are summarised in Table 34.1. Chemotherapy commonly forms part of multimodal therapy in conjunction with surgery and radiotherapy, for example in breast cancer.

The cancer specialist responsible for the delivery of chemotherapy varies in different parts of the world. In the UK, Clinical Oncologists, Medical Oncologists and Haematologists are trained in the use of chemotherapy. The responsibility for its supervision in any individual centre will depend on referral patterns and the experience and number of cancer specialists. Increasingly in the UK there is specialisation in the management of cancer on a cancer-site-specific basis within multidisciplinary teams. In addition, specialist cancer nurses are increasingly involved in the administration of chemotherapy.

General indications for chemotherapy

Chemotherapy is used in three main situations. First, it is used in the adjuvant setting after surgical removal of the primary tumour in breast, ovarian or colorectal cancer in an attempt to eradicate subclinical

Table 34.1 Uses of chemotherapy

Curative
Testicular teratoma and seminoma
Acute leukaemia
Hodgkin's disease
Non-Hodgkin lymphoma (high grade)
Wilms' tumour
Moderate survival benefit
Breast cancer
Colorectal cancer
Small cell lung cancer
Myeloma
Ovarian cancer
Cervical cancer
Non-Hodgkin lymphoma (low grade)
Limited or uncertain survival benefit
Gastric cancer
Oesophageal cancer
Bladder cancer
Nasopharyngeal cancer
Non-small cell lung cancer
Sarcoma
Pancreatic cancer
Head and neck cancer
No survival benefit
Melanoma

micrometastatic disease and reduce the risk of recurrence. Secondly, it is used to treat inoperable, residual or metastatic disease. Thirdly, it is used as neoadjuvant therapy to debulk the primary tumour prior to surgery. An example of this cytoreductive therapy is the neoadjuvant therapy of large breast primaries so that conservative local surgery rather than mastectomy is made possible (p. 455).

Historical development of chemotherapy

The major developments in cancer chemotherapy are relatively modern, dating from the 1940s. However in the 17th and 18th centuries, belladonna, antimony and arsenic were used to treat cancer. In the 19th century, in the 1860s, potassium arsenite was used without success to treat leukaemia.

The turning point came during the Second World War from the investigation of poison gases. Even during the First World War, sulphur 'mustard' gas was noted to have a severe depressant effect on the bone marrow, and leucopenia was noted in those dying of mustard gas poisoning. In the 1940s the nitrogen mustards were found to cause gene mutations and chromosomal damage, leading to cell death at subsequent mitosis, in a manner similar to radiation. These agents were termed *radiomimetic* (i.e. imitating radiation). Profound effects on the bone marrow were observed. In 1942 a brief clinical remission was achieved in a patient treated with nitrogen mustard for lymphoma. The demonstration of some antitumour activity by nitrogen mustard prompted the development and testing of many thousands of agents. In 1948 an analogue of folate, aminopterin, was shown to cause remission in children with acute lymphocytic leukaemia. Despite the careful testing of many agents, only a very small proportion have been sufficiently effective to be adopted into clinical practice. Though small in total number, some agents (e.g. doxorubicin) have activity against a wide variety of malignancies.

Development and testing of anticancer agents

New cytotoxic agents are developed in four main ways. First, their efficacy may be detected from random screening for activity in tumour cell lines. Secondly, they may be synthesised as modifications (analogues) of cytotoxic agents which are known to be effective. Thirdly, they may be created *de novo* to a specification which should confer particular anticancer properties. The second and third categories represent an increasing trend in the development of chemotherapeutic agents. Fourthly, there are chance discoveries of anticancer activity in drugs.

Once an agent has been shown in its preclinical assessment to have sufficient activity against animal tumours, with acceptable toxicity, it can be considered for clinical evaluation. In the UK approval of local ethics committees is required before clinical testing can begin. There are three phases of clinical assessment.

Phase I studies

In *phase I* studies the main aim is to establish the maximum tolerated dose and the safety, but not the efficacy, of the agent under investigation. Such studies, usually on up to 30 patients, are performed with the informed consent of patients whose advanced disease has failed to respond to standard therapy. The starting dose is determined by preclinical data where evidence of tumour response has been shown in human tumour cell lines. In phase I studies, pharmacokinetic studies (how the body handles the drug, for example by metabolism) and pharmacodynamic studies (assessing the impact of the drug on the physiology of the body) are conducted.

Phase II studies

If the agent shows acceptable toxicity in phase I studies, it may proceed to *phase II* studies designed to assess its antitumour activity. These are carried out on groups of patients with the same type of tumour. The selection of the tumour type will be guided by the response rates in different animal tumours and in phase I studies. The number of patients in each tumour category that need to be recruited in phase II studies will depend on the level of response of the best established agent. The new agent will need to show a higher response rate than established agents (or less toxicity for the same degree of response) to justify further testing. Usually at least a 20% response rate is required in a phase II trial to justify proceeding to a phase III trial.

Phase III trial

In *phase III* studies the new agent is compared with an established treatment in a randomised trial with survival as the main endpoint. A group of patients with tumours against which the agent has shown activity in phase II studies is selected. The allocation of patients to the new or established treatment should be random. The response of the primary tumour, regional or metastatic spread is carefully documented in addition to data on toxicity, quality of life and cost-effectiveness. With the increasing costs of new anticancer agents, a careful review of data from phase III trials is needed before such agents are routinely prescribed, to ensure that the quality and duration of clinical responses justify the costs.

Assessing tumour response

A *complete response* is defined as eradication of all known disease based on two assessments at least 4 weeks apart. A *partial response* represents a reduction of at least 50% in measurable disease maintained for at least 4 weeks in the absence of any progressive or new lesion. *Stable disease* represents < 50% reduction in measurable disease or < 25% increase in measurable disease. *Progressive disease* represents an increase of 25% or more in an area of measurable disease or the development of new lesions.

PRINCIPLES OF CYTOTOXIC THERAPY

To understand the rationale of cytotoxic chemotherapy it is important to understand the features of tumour growth. Most tumours grow exponentially in the early phase. With further increases in size, growth is slower. By the time that is it clinically detectable, the majority of its growth has already occurred. The asymmetric sigmoidal growth curve (Fig. 34.1) which describes this natural history is known as Gompertzian, named after an English actuary who created a mathematical model to explain the relationship between age and expected time of death. It is estimated that most human cancers begin less than 2 years from the time of clinical presentation. In the early exponential phase of growth, the rates of tumour cell growth and tumour cell loss are proportional to the tumour cell burden at any point. Since most anticancer agents are more toxic to proliferating cells and most tumours are in a relatively slow phase of growth when diagnosed (i.e. they lie high on the Gompertzian growth curve), this explains the limited effectiveness of chemotherapy for many cancers. The rationale for tumour cytoreduction (e.g. by surgery) before chemotherapy is to bring the tumour to a lower point on the growth curve when the growth fraction of the tumour rises. The concept of moving the tumour down the Gompertzian curve underpins the rationale of adjuvant chemotherapy.

Unfortunately it is not only the proliferating cells that must be eradicated by chemotherapy but also the small population of clonogenic cells mainly in G_0 phase. The stem cell model of tissue growth developed for stem cells of the bone marrow is applicable to tumour growth since virtually all cancers arise from a single pluripotential cell. Each dose of chemotherapy should produce the same proportional reduction in number of tumour cells. At the same time, small differences in drug dose may have a significant effect on cell survival. For a tumour containing 10^6 cells and

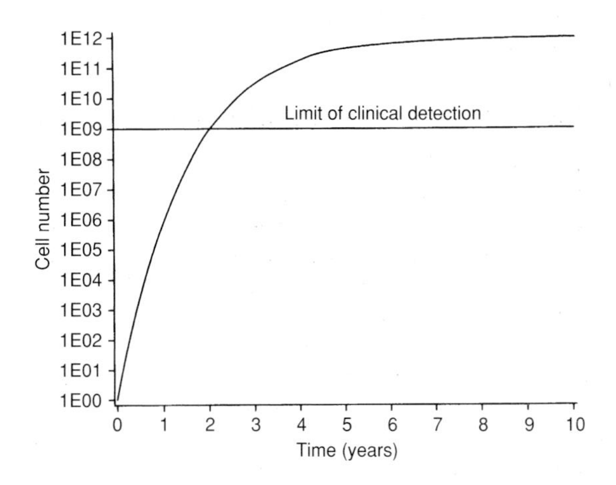

Fig. 34.1 The Gompertzian growth curve. During the early stage of development, growth is exponential. As a tumour enlarges, its growth slows. By the time it is clinically detectable, most of its growth has already occurred, and the exponential phase is complete. (Reproduced from Lenhard, Osteen and Gansler, Clinical Oncology, American Cancer Society, 2000).

death of 99.9% of cancer cells at each course, if 1 log of cell growth occurs between courses, five courses of treatment will be needed to eradicate the tumour in its entirety.

Cytotoxic drugs act by interfering with the process of cell division (mitosis). Unfortunately these agents are not specific in acting against malignant cells, and damage both normal and malignant proliferating cells. As with radiation, a careful balance has to be kept between toxicity to the tumour and to the patient's normal tissues. What distinguishes normal and malignant cells is the failure of the malignant cell, unlike normal cells, to recover from cytotoxic damage.

Selection of chemotherapy agents

It would be ideal if cancers could be eradicated by treatment by a single agent. However, experience shows that this is rarely curative, although it may achieve useful symptomatic benefit. For curative purposes chemotherapeutic agents with proven anti-cancer properties against a particular tumour but with different mechanisms of action and as far as possible non-overlapping toxicities are combined. This is known as *combination chemotherapy*. For example in treating breast cancer three agents—cyclophosphamide, methotrexate and 5-fluorouracil (known as CMF)—all have activity against breast cancer as single agents. However, their response rate as a combination (around 40%) is two- to threefold that of their response rates as single agents.

Predicting chemosensitivity

Unfortunately, to date, methods of predicting chemosensitivity of an individual patient's tumour have not been successful, largely because of the failure of experimental systems to recreate the complex host–tumour micro-environment in tumour vasculature. In addition host immunity play an important role. At present one can only recommend a combination of drugs for an individual patient on the basis of the probability rather than the certainty of them working.

Dose and frequency of administration

Initially single cytotoxic agents were given *continuously* in low dosage. Their administration was suspended when a response was obtained. When the tumour recurred, a second agent was administered in a similar manner. It was soon appreciated that this was relatively ineffective in controlling many tumours. In addition, with continuous administration there was no opportunity for the normal tissues to recover. In many cases tumour regression and eradication were improved by administering the drug *intermittently* (e.g. 3–4-weekly) in much higher dose and allowing an interval for the normal and often dose-limiting tissue to recover. Intermittent pulses or courses of treatment take advantage of the growth kinetics of malignant and normal tissues. In Figure 34.2 the effects of pulsed chemotherapy on a tumour and on the normal bone marrow can be seen. After each pulse, the normal and malignant cell populations decline due to killing of cells in mitosis. The lowest level of the blood count is known as the *nadir*. However, whereas the bone marrow recovers to its previous level, the malignant cell population does not. With each subsequent course this difference is accentuated. Larger doses per pulse than would be feasible with continuous treatment increase the fraction of tumour cells that can be killed per treatment.

The advantages of pulsed therapy may be summarised:

1. Maximum tumour cell killing occurs, while minimising toxicity.
2. Larger total dose maximises chance of cure.

It would be misleading to suggest that the 3–4-weekly schedules commonly used for the delivery of cytotoxic agents are necessarily optimal. However, these frequencies have been derived from extensive assessments of different schedules. There is an increasing trend towards intensive weekly treatments.

If the interval between pulses is too short, toxicity may prevent the delivery of further pulses on schedule

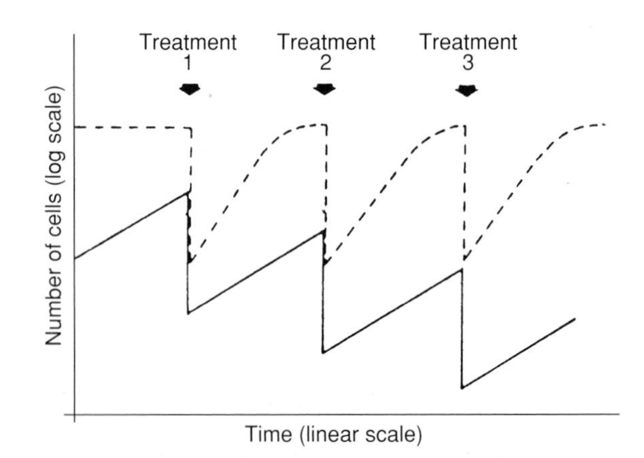

Fig. 34.2 The effect of multiple courses of cytotoxic therapy on normal and tumour cell populations: - - -, normal cells; —, tumour cells. (Reproduced with permission from Springer-Verlag: from Priestman T J. Cancer Chemotherapy: An Introduction, 1989.)

(Fig. 34.3). If the interval is too long, tumour may regrow between courses (Fig. 34.4).

The total dose that can be administered is limited by the tolerance of normal tissue. Toxicity is often cumulative and may be irreversible. For example the major dose-limiting toxicity of the anthracyline, doxorubicin, is cardiotoxicity.

High-dose chemotherapy

Higher than conventional doses of chemotherapy can be delivered if the primary organ toxicity is to the bone marrow and there is minimal toxicity to other organs. Dose intensity is recognised to be important, particularly in chemosensitive tumours. Bone marrow toxicity can be overcome by autologous bone marrow transplantation. Normal bone marrow is harvested from the patient before high-dose chemotherapy. It is returned to the patient at the time of chemotherapy to support the bone marrow through the period of neutropenia and thrombocytopenia. High-dose melphalan has been used, for example, to treat advanced cases of melanoma. A similar approach is under evaluation in young women at high risk of relapse with operable breast cancer. Results of trials to date do not suggest a survival advantage. The dose–response curve of tumour cells plateaus at higher dose. This means that even if higher doses can be delivered with acceptable toxicity, it is unlikely that all tumour cells will be eradicated.

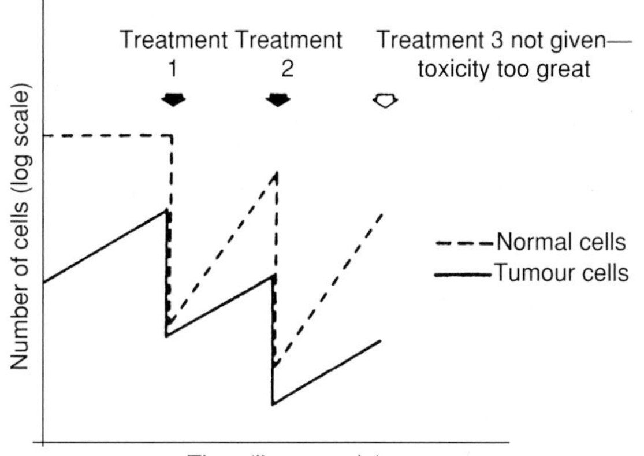

Fig. 34.3 The effect of multiple courses of chemotherapy with too short an interval for normal cell recovery: - - -, normal cells; —, tumour cells. (Reproduced with permission from Springer-Verlag: from Priestman T J. Cancer Chemotherapy: An Introduction, 1989.)

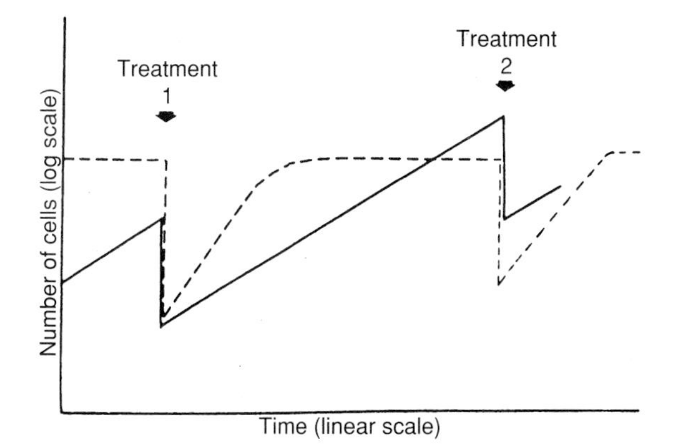

Fig. 34.4 The effect of multiple courses of chemotherapy with too long an interval, allowing increases in tumour cell population between courses: - - -, normal cells; —, tumour cells. (Reproduced with permission from Springer-Verlag: from Priestman T J. Cancer Chemotherapy: An Introduction, 1989.)

Route of administration

The route of administration is governed by the solubility, chemical stability and local irritant properties of the agent.

Oral. This is the simplest and most convenient route of administration. Examples are chlorambucil, cyclophosphamide, capecitabine and etoposide. Patients can take their tablets at home with intermittent outpatient visits to monitor treatment.

Unfortunately many cytotoxic drugs are unstable and inactivated in the stomach, rendering them ineffective.

Subcutaneous or intramuscular. injection is avoided where possible since it can be painful, cause bruising in thrombocytopenic patients, requires hospital attendance and absorption may be unreliable. Bleomycin is often given by the intramuscular route.

Intravenous injection is the commonest route of administration of cytotoxic agents since it gives direct access to the systemic circulation. It can be done by delivery of a bolus dose or by infusion. Continuous infusions can be given (e.g. 5-fluorouracil) linked to a battery-operated pump worn around the patient's waist. The risks of intravenous administration are the introduction of infection and damage to the tissues around the site of administration if extravasation occurs. For this reason the antecubital fossa is best avoided. At this site extravasation is often difficult to detect. If it occurs, severe ulceration and contractures with major functional impairment may follow. Plastic surgery is often needed. Injections should be given into a vein on the back of the hand or on the radial side of the wrist.

Where very intensive chemotherapy is given (e.g. acute leukaemia in children) or prolonged infusional chemotherapy peripheral venous sites may soon become thrombosed. The insertion of a catheter into the superior vena cava, usually under general anaesthesia, and tunnelled subcutaneously allows comfortable and convenient access (Fig. 34.5).

Intrapleural chemotherapy is given to reduce the likelihood of recurrence of a pleural effusion. The effusion is tapped to dryness before the cytotoxic agent is instilled. It produces a chemical irritation of the pleura causing the two layers to become adherent to one another to prevent reaccumulation of the effusion. Bleomycin is most commonly used.

Intraperitoneal chemotherapy has been given in diseases predominantly confined to the abdomen such as ovarian cancer. Higher concentrations within the peritoneal cavity can be achieved without causing severe systemic toxicity. It is only suitable for tiny microscopic foci of peritoneal disease. Its use is limited because of the variability of drug absorption from the peritoneal surface and complications such as pain and bowel obstruction.

Intra-arterial administration is rarely used. It has the advantage of delivering the drug in high concentration to the tissue supplied by the artery. Its limitations are the complexity of administration and the difficulty in identifying correctly the arterial supply of the tumour. Its main use is in the infusion of chemotherapeutic agents into the hepatic artery of patients with liver metastases from colorectal cancer. Other examples are isolated limb perfusion for melanoma or rarely internal mammary artery access for chemotherapy for locally advanced breast cancer.

Intrathecal injection is used to deliver drugs in high dose into the CNS. Many cytotoxic drugs do not cross the blood–brain barrier and are therefore unable to kill tumour cells within the CNS. Methotrexate is the agent most commonly given by this route, e.g. in preventing CNS relapse in acute lymphoblastic leukaemia in conjunction with prophylactic cranial irradiation (Ch. 32).

Topical administration of cytotoxic agents is effective in a small number of tumours (e.g. nitrogen mustard in mycosis fungoides (Ch. 29) and 5-fluorouracil in Bowen's disease, a premalignant disease of the skin, and some superficial basal cell carcinomas).

Intravesical chemotherapy involves the instillation of cytotoxic therapy through a catheter into the bladder. In view of the limited depth of absorption, it is only appropriate for superficial tumours (Ch. 28). The drug (commonly thiotepa or mitomycin C) is left in the bladder for 1–2 hours before being drained. The main side-effect is a mild, short-lived chemical cystitis.

Factors influencing the efficacy of chemotherapy

A variety of host factors influence the response to chemotherapy, in addition to the intrinsic chemosensitivity of the tumour and drug scheduling. These include the growth fraction of the tumour, the availability of the drug to the tumour and drug resistance.

Drug resistance

Resistance to chemotherapy may be intrinsic or acquired. Some tumours are intrinsically chemoresistant and show no response to treatment *de novo*. In other tumours there is an initial response followed by relapse due to acquired resistance. Acquired resistance may have a variety of mechanisms. These include

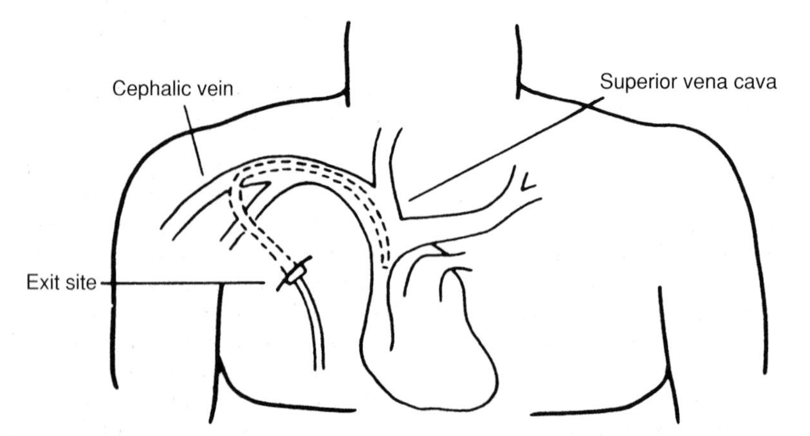

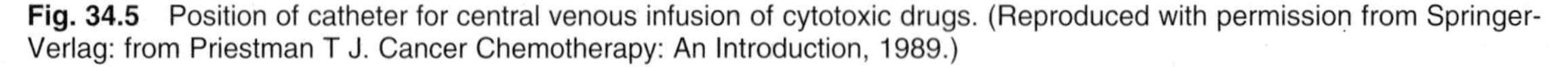
Fig. 34.5 Position of catheter for central venous infusion of cytotoxic drugs. (Reproduced with permission from Springer-Verlag: from Priestman T J. Cancer Chemotherapy: An Introduction, 1989.)

(1) changes in the cell membrane impeding drug transport (e.g. of methotrexate), (2) DNA repair of drug-induced lesions (e.g. caused by alkylating agents), (3) utilisation of alternative metabolic pathways (e.g. 5-fluorouracil), (4) increased production of a target enzyme (e.g. dihydrofolate reductase binding to methotrexate), or (5) modification of the target enzyme, enabling it to recognise the difference between true and false metabolites. Irreversible binding between enzyme and cytotoxic drug (e.g. 6-mercaptopurine) is thus avoided.

The multiple drug resistance gene (*MDR1*) encodes P-glycoprotein. The latter is a membrane-associated efflux pump which serves to protect normal cells in the testis and kidney from drug-induced damage. Cancer cells may overexpress *MDR1* so conferring resistance to a variety of chemotherapeutic agents. In addition *p53*, the 'guardian' of the genome and an important mediator of apoptosis (programmed cell death) may be mutated and give rise to chemoresistance in a number of solid tumours.

The reasons for drug resistance are not fully understood. It is common to find that a tumour responds to a particular drug or combination of drugs for a period of time and then ceases to do so. It is thought that within many tumour populations there are genetically determined drug-resistant cells. When the chemosensitive cells have been killed, the resistant population may proliferate.

Drug resistance to repeated exposure to a single agent will usually result in cross-resistance to other compounds of the same class of drugs. This is probably due to common transport mechanisms and pathways of metabolism and intracellular cytotoxic targets. However, cancer cells which have become resistant to one class of drugs may retain sensitivity to another class of drugs.

Some drugs may have a variety of mechanisms of drug resistance. The anthracyclines (e.g. doxorubicin) is thought to derive some of its cytotoxicity from the formation of free radical intermediates. One of these free radicals, the superoxide anion, gives rise to the highly reactive hydroxyl radical, which damages DNA directly. One of the mechanisms of resistance to anthracyclines may be impaired superoxide anion levels in the tumour owing to poor tumour vascularity. Alternatively, enhanced repair of peroxidative damage to DNA may account for some of the resistance to anthracylines.

Reduced accumulation of a drug may be due to reduced influx (e.g. of methotrexate), impaired membrane transport (resistance to nitrogen mustard), increased drug efflux (multidrug resistance). Resistance may result from changes in drug metabolism, inactivation of a drug or of cofactors.

Resistance to cisplatin is considered to be mediated by increased DNA repair. The cytotoxic action of cisplatin is known to be due to lethal intrastrand DNA crosslinks. It is known that DNA synthesis increases in ovarian cancer cells resistant to cisplatin. Inhibitors of DNA polymerase, which is involved in DNA repair, are under investigation to try to overcome resistance to cisplatin.

Some drugs which show excellent cell kill in vitro fail to do so in vivo. Sometimes this is due to a sanctuary site of tumour in the CNS where the drug does not cross the blood–brain barrier. Occasionally the tumour outstrips its vascular supply so that inadequate concentrations of drug reach the tumour. There is also some evidence that some tumours exhibit drug resistance that is in part due to host factors which modify the pharmacokinetics of the anticancer agent in vivo.

Chemotherapy, as radiotherapy, is most effective in killing proliferating cells. While the growth fraction is high in many chemosensitive tumours, such as the lymphomas and testicular teratomas, it is relatively low in many common tumours, e.g. colorectal cancer.

In parts of the tumour the blood supply tends to be poor. As a result concentrations of drug reaching the tumour may be inadequate. In addition, as a result of the hypoxia induced by a poor blood supply, the growth fraction is reduced.

A number of approaches are being pursued to try to overcome drug resistance. These include giving very intensive initial chemotherapy to try to eradicate the whole tumour cell population. Attempts are being made to develop anti-P glycoprotein antibodies either bound to toxins or to complement which can target P glycoprotein-positive cells.

Adjuvant and neoadjuvant chemotherapy

Even when the primary tumour appears to be localised, clinically undetected metastases (micrometastases) may already have seeded to distant sites. The classical example is breast cancer where the lungs, liver and bone may be infiltrated by metastases. This is particularly so if the axillary nodes are involved at the time of primary surgery. Chemotherapy aimed at eradicating these micrometastases is called *adjuvant*. Other tumours in which the elimination of micrometastatic spread by adjuvant chemotherapy may be possible include colon cancer, ovarian cancer, osteogenic sarcoma and Ewing's sarcoma of bone.

Adjuvant therapy is normally given shortly after surgical treatment of the primary. The rationale for early postoperative therapy is that (1) the growth fraction of metastases falls as they grow, (2) the probability of drug-resistant cells emerging increases with time, and (3) areas of necrosis and hypoxic cells develop, due to impaired blood supply, and limit access to drugs.

Adjuvant combination cytotoxic chemotherapy confers a moderate but clinically useful survival advantage in women with operable breast cancer. More impressive have been the improvements in survival in Wilms' tumour, Ewing's sarcoma and osteosarcoma in children.

Neoadjuvant therapy refers to delivering chemotherapy before surgery in order to reduce the tumour burden. By reducing the size of the primary tumour, the extent of surgery may be diminished. For example, a large breast tumour that would require a mastectomy might, if reduced by chemotherapy, be amenable to local excision. An additional potential advantage is the killing of micrometastases at an earlier stage than with conventional adjuvant therapy. However, if the tumour proves chemoresistant, toxicity will have been inflicted without any benefit. As yet neoadjuvant therapy is at an early phase of assessment and it is uncertain whether it will confer benefit in long-term survival.

CLASSIFICATION OF CYTOTOXIC DRUGS

The available agents may be divided into a few broad groups:

- Alkylating agents
- Antimetabolites
- Natural products
- Random synthetics
- Hormones (Ch. 35).

Some cytotoxic drugs act only on particular phases of the cell cycle (cell cycle specific), while others act throughout the cycle (cell cycle non-specific). These differences are summarised in Figure 34.6.

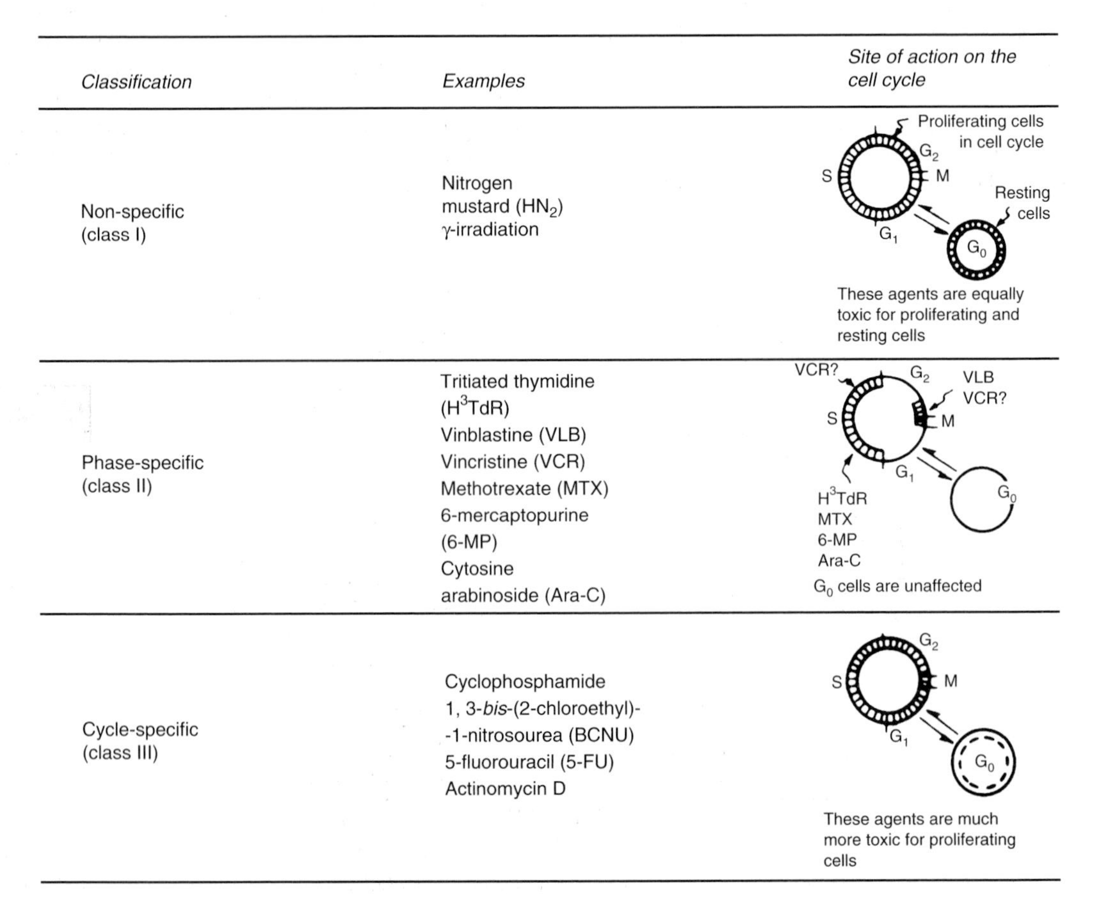

Classification	*Examples*	*Site of action on the cell cycle*
Non-specific (class I)	Nitrogen mustard (HN_2) γ-irradiation	These agents are equally toxic for proliferating and resting cells
Phase-specific (class II)	Tritiated thymidine (H^3TdR) Vinblastine (VLB) Vincristine (VCR) Methotrexate (MTX) 6-mercaptopurine (6-MP) Cytosine arabinoside (Ara-C)	G_0 cells are unaffected
Cycle-specific (class III)	Cyclophosphamide 1, 3-*bis*-(2-chloroethyl)--1-nitrosourea (BCNU) 5-fluorouracil (5-FU) Actinomycin D	These agents are much more toxic for proliferating cells

Fig. 34.6 Classification of anticancer agents according to action in cell cycle. (Modified from Calman, Smyth & Tattersall, Basic Principles of Cancer Chemotherapy, The Macmillan Press, 1980 reproduced with permission of Palgrave.)

For specific dosage and scheduling and guidance on administration, specialist advice should be sought from an oncologist/haematologist.

Cytotoxic agents may interfere with precursors of nucleic acid synthesis, with DNA or RNA, or with specific proteins (Fig. 34.7).

Alkylating agents

Mechanism of action

The main antitumour action of alkylating agents is the binding of an alkyl chemical group ($R\text{-}CH_2$) to DNA, so inhibiting its synthesis. They also bind to RNA and other cell proteins but these reactions are much less cytotoxic. The majority of alkylating agents have two available alkyl groups with which they can bind with DNA. Crosslinking may occur between a single strand of DNA or between two separate strands. Alkylating agents (e.g. nitrogen mustard) with this capacity to crosslink are called *bifunctional* and are more cytotoxic than alkylating agents with only one available alkyl group for binding to DNA. Alkylating agents have relatively steep dose–response curves and are therefore favoured for trials of high-dose therapy.

Nitrogen mustard (chlormethine [mustine]). Nitrogen mustard was the first of the alkylating agents to be used. It was developed originally as a gas for chemical warfare. It was incidentally noted to be toxic to lymphoid tissue. It is chemically unstable and has to be given by rapid intravenous injection via a fast-running drip.

Side-effects. Like mustard gas, it is a strong vesicant and is intensely irritant to the skin and other tissues. If it extravasates into the skin and subcutaneous tissues, it may cause painful thrombosis and phlebitis. In severe cases, this may lead to tissue necrosis requiring excision and skin grafting.

General effects are severe nausea and vomiting within the first 3 hours following injection but rarely lasting for more than 8 hours. Vomiting can usually be reduced by prior antiemetic therapy. White blood count and platelets fall over 6–8 days with a nadir at 14–18 days. Hair loss and temporary amenorrhoea occur.

Main uses. It was formerly used in the treatment of Hodgkin's disease but is now seldom used.

Cyclophosphamide (Endoxana). Cyclophosphamide has the advantage that it is chemically stable and can be given orally in addition to intravenously. It is activated by the enzyme P450 in the liver. It is converted there to two active metabolites, acrolein and phosphoramide mustard. It is excreted solely in the urine. Dose adjustments are therefore necessary if kidney function is impaired.

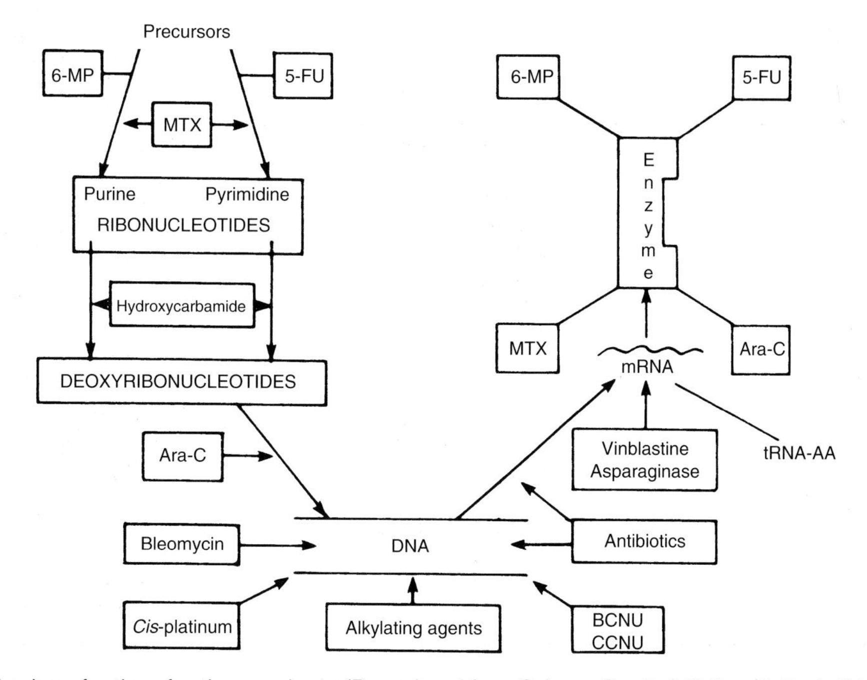

Fig. 34.7 Mechanism of action of anticancer drugs. (Reproduced from Calman, Smyth & Tattersall, Basic Principles of Cancer Chemotherapy, The Macmillan Press, 1980 with permission of Palgrave.)

Side-effects. Anorexia, nausea and vomiting are, unless high doses are used, much less severe than with chlormethine (mustine). Myelosuppression is the main dose-limiting toxicity. The nadir is 5–10 days. Recovery occurs 10–14 days following administration. Platelets are less affected.

An acute haemorrhagic cystitis may occasionally occur at higher doses, or at lower doses if patients have renal impairment for any reason. Of these, dehydration is probably the commonest. The severity of cystitis varies from mild to severe. The cystitis is due to the irritant effects of urinary metabolites of the drug, particularly acrolein and 4-hydroxycyclophosphamide. Bladder fibrosis may follow.

Adequate hydration is essential before, during and after the administration of cyclophosphamide.

Rarely pneumonitis develops, similar to busulfan pulmonary toxicity. The onset is insidious. Typically this develops after prolonged therapy or continuous low-dose treatment. Pathologically this is an alveolitis and may proceed to pulmonary fibrosis, respiratory failure and death. Steroids may help.

Cardiac damage may occur at high dose, ranging from asymptomatic minor abnormalities of the electrocardiogram to severe cardiac failure.

Other side-effects are alopecia, inappropriate antidiuretic hormone (ADH) secretion, oligo- or azoospermia and amenorrhoea. Both male and female infertility is usually permanent.

Mesna is used, reducing bladder toxicity at high dose (see below, under ifosfamide).

Drug interactions. Hepatic enzyme inducers (phenobarbital, phenytoin and chloral hydrate) increase the metabolism of cyclophosphamide and reduce its efficacy.

Cyclophosphamide potentiates the hypoglycaemic effects of sulphonylureas.

Main uses. Cyclophosphamide is useful against a wide range of malignancies including non-Hodgkin lymphomas, small cell lung cancer, ovarian cancer and soft tissue sarcomas.

Ifosfamide. Ifosfamide is structurally an analogue of cyclophosphamide. As with cyclophosphamide, it requires activation in the liver and is excreted in the urine. Unlike cyclophosphamide it cannot be given orally. It is always given intravenously with adequate hydration. Weight for weight, ifosfamide is less myelosuppressive than cyclophosphamide.

Side-effects. Nausea and vomiting occur within a few hours of injection and last for about 3 days. It is dose related and can be very severe if high doses are used. Bone marrow suppression is moderate, affecting both white count and platelets. The nadir of the white count is at 5–10 days with recovery after 10–14 days. Alopecia is virtually universal. Central nervous toxicity may occasionally occur, particularly in patients who are inadequately hydrated, have impaired renal function or low serum albumin. The clinical features are of an encephalopathy with confusion, somnolence, lethargy and in severe cases coma and death. A sterile phlebitis may occur at the injection site. Necrosis may occur if there is extravasation.

Mesna in reducing bladder toxicity. In patients receiving ifosfamide therapy or, rarely, high-dose ($> 1 g/m^2$) cyclophosphamide, the risk of bladder toxicity can be minimised by giving oral or intravenous mesna. The sulphydryl group of this agent binds to metabolites (including acrolein) responsible for bladder toxicity. It converts them to compounds which do not damage the bladder.

Drug interactions. Hepatic enzyme-inducing drugs have the same effects as on cyclophosphamide (see above).

Main uses. Soft tissue sarcomas, cervical cancer, testicular teratoma.

Chlorambucil. Chlorambucil has the advantages of oral administration and little symptomatic toxicity. It is predominantly excreted in the urine. The dose may need to be reduced if there is renal impairment. It is normally given intermittently (e.g. 10 mg orally daily, alternate fortnights) or continually in a low dose (e.g. 2–5 mg orally per day).

Side-effects. The main dose-limiting toxicity is to the bone marrow, causing leucopenia and thrombocytopenia. The nadir of the white count is normally at 14 days. Gastrointestinal toxicity, alopecia, pulmonary fibrosis and liver damage are uncommon. Hair is usually retained. Sterility, irreversible marrow damage and second malignancies occur.

Main uses. Hodgkin's disease, low-grade non-Hodgkin lymphoma, ovarian cancer.

Melphalan (L-phenylalanine mustard). Melphalan may be given orally or intravenously. Oral absorption may be erratic. Like chlorambucil it has few side-effects. It is the classical drug for high-dose chemotherapy because of the absence of second organ toxicity (see under Principles of cytotoxic therapy).

Side-effects. The main dose-limiting toxicity is bone marrow suppression, mainly affecting white count and platelets. The nadir is at 28 days. Nausea, vomiting and alopecia occur with higher doses.

Main uses. Multiple myeloma.

Thiotepa (triethylene thiophosphoramide). Thiotepa may be given by oral, intravenous or intracavitary routes. It has limited indications. It is mainly instilled into pleural effusions or ascites as a palliative procedure.

Side-effects. Bone marrow toxicity is dose limiting (leucopenia and thrombocytopenia). Nausea and vomiting and local pain at injection sites are the other most frequent side-effects.

Main uses. Intracavitary or high-dose chemotherapy.

Busulfan. Busulfan is only given orally. It is selectively active against granulocytes. Its inactive metabolites are excreted in the urine.

Side-effects. Bone marrow depression. At low dose, granulocytes are depressed with relative sparing of platelets. At higher dose, platelets are also depressed. The nadir is at about 28 days and is prolonged. Recovery is slow, from 24 to 54 days.

Lung fibrosis may develop after prolonged treatment. Regular chest radiographs should be taken and pulmonary function regularly monitored. The drug should be stopped at the first signs of lung fibrosis and steroids commenced. Otherwise, irreversible respiratory failure and death may occur.

Skin pigmentation occurs over pressure areas, axillae, skin creases and nipples, in a similar distribution to Addison's disease. Adrenal failure and cataract formation are rare.

Main uses. Chronic myeloid leukaemia, polycythaemia rubra vera.

Procarbazine. Procarbazine is a derivative of the hydrazine chemical group. It is a pro-drug which is oxidised to form alkylating species. It seems to be cell cycle phase-specific, with its main cytotoxic effect on S phase (DNA synthesis). It is given orally and crosses the blood–brain barrier. The main route of excretion of its metabolites is in the urine.

Side-effects. Bone marrow suppression is the main dose-limiting toxicity. The nadir of the platelet count is at 4 weeks followed by that of the white and red cell counts. The blood count has normally recovered by 6 weeks. Nausea, vomiting and diarrhoea start within a few days of administration. CNS toxicity has a wide variety of symptoms including dizziness, ataxia, headache, nightmares, hallucinations, somnolence and depression.

Interactions. (1) Tricyclic antidepressants, monoamine oxidase inhibitors, and tyramine-rich foods (e.g. cheese, wine and bananas) may precipitate hypertensive crisis. (2) CNS depressants (narcotic analgesics, phenothiazines and antihistamines), and hypotensive agents (e.g. methyldopa) accentuate CNS depression. (3) Alcohol may increase gastrointestinal toxicity.

Main uses. Hodgkin's disease, brain tumours.

Antimetabolites

Mechanism of action

Antimetabolites are structurally similar to normal metabolites involved in nucleic acid synthesis. They are divided into three groups: folate, purine and pyrimidine antagonists. They substitute for their normal purine and pyrimidine counterparts in metabolic pathways, resulting in abnormal nuclear material that fails to function normally, or bind to enzymes, so inhibiting protein synthesis. They generally act on S phase of the cell cycle.

1. Folate antagonists

Methotrexate is the classical example. A number of cofactors are necessary for the synthesis of purines and pyrimidines. The reduction of folic acid is essential for the production of these cofactors. A key reaction in this process is the reduction of dihydrofolic acid to tetrahydrofolic acid by means of an enzyme, *dihydrofolate reductase*. This is the main site of action of methotrexate. Methotrexate is structurally similar to folic acid and has a much greater affinity for dihydrofolate reductase than does folic acid. Methotrexate therefore binds preferentially to dihydrofolate reductase and inactivates it. As a result, tetrahydrofolates cannot be made and purine and pyrimidine synthesis is inhibited.

Methotrexate can be given orally, intravenously or at low dose intrathecally. About 50–60% of the drug in the serum is bound to protein. In conventional doses, it is excreted unchanged in the urine. It is widely distributed in body fluids. This is of importance because it may be retained in pleural effusions and ascites, causing abnormally prolonged systemic toxicity. Such fluid collections should, if possible, be drained before methotrexate is administered.

High-dose therapy. Methotrexate is one of the drugs for which there is evidence of increased effectiveness with higher doses in some sensitive tumours (e.g. small cell lung cancer and osteosarcoma).

Folinic acid 'rescue'. The metabolic block on the activity of dihydrofolate reductase can be bypassed by administering an intermediate metabolite, folinic acid (also known as citrovorum factor or leucovorin). Folinic acid is a tetrahydrofolate which provides an alternative source for continuing nucleic acid synthesis. It is also possible that folinic acid may act by displacing methotrexate from its binding to dihydrofolate reductase. In both these ways the cytotoxic action of methotrexate and its toxicity can be diminished. Folinic acid is only required when high doses (> 100 mg) of methotrexate are used. It is delivered by the oral or intramuscular route 24–36 hours after the administration of methotrexate until the serum concentration of methotrexate is $< 10^{-7}$ mol/l. This is timed to allow the methotrexate to have its necessary cytotoxic action but to prevent further toxicity associated with persistently high blood levels of methotrexate. Starting folinic acid 40 hours or more after methotrexate has been given is ineffective. When high-dose methotrexate is given, urine alkalinisation to pH 6.5–7.0, with oral or intravenous sodium bicarbonate or oral acetazolamide, and fluid hydration should be started beforehand.

Side-effects. The main side-effects of methotrexate are on the bone marrow and on the gastrointestinal tract. Anaemia, leucopenia and thrombocytopenia may develop rapidly. The nadir of the white count is at 10 days. Anorexia, nausea and vomiting are the first symptoms, followed 4–6 days later by oral and pharyngeal mucositis and diarrhoea. Skin rashes are common. Conjunctivitis may occur as a result of accumulation of the drug in tears. Renal failure may complicate high-dose therapy. Liver damage (ranging from elevated liver enzymes to cirrhosis), lung injury (mainly fibrosis) and osteoporosis may complicate prolonged therapy. Alopecia is uncommon.

Drug interactions. (1) Drugs which are protein bound (e.g. salicylates, phenytoin, sulphonamides) may displace methotrexate from its binding with plasma protein, causing the serum levels of methotrexate and the risk of toxicity to rise. (2) Methotrexate potentiates the effects of anticoagulants such as warfarin.

Main uses. Non-Hodgkin lymphoma, acute lymphoblastic leukaemia, breast cancer, soft tissue and osteogenic sarcomas, head and neck cancer, choriocarcinoma.

2. Purine antagonists

6-mercaptopurine. 6-mercaptopurine is a purine antagonist. It has to be metabolised to an active form. It inhibits a number of enzymes involved in the synthesis of the purines, adenine and guanine. It is strongly bound to plasma proteins, metabolised in the liver and its metabolites are excreted in the urine.

It is normally given orally.

Side-effects. The main toxicity is on the bone marrow (leucopenia and thrombocytopenia) and the liver. The nadir for white count and platelets is at 15 days.

Raised serum bilirubin is the commonest feature of liver toxicity. This normally returns to normal on withdrawing the drug.

Interactions. Allopurinol inhibits the metabolism of mercaptopurine. If given concurrently the dose of mercaptopurine has to be reduced.

Main uses. Leukaemia, especially acute lymphoblastic.

6-thioguanine. 6-tioguanine is also a purine antagonist and is an analogue of guanine. It requires activation to an active form and may be given orally or intravenously.

Side-effects. The main dose limiting toxicity is to the bone marrow and is more marked when given intravenously than orally. Gastrointestinal intolerance is uncommon. Liver toxicity is less frequent than with mercaptopurine.

Drug interactions. If allopurinol is given with tioguanine the dose of thioguanine does not have to be reduced because its metabolism is not inhibited as it is with mercaptopurine.

Main uses. Acute and chronic myeloid leukaemia.

Fludarabine. Fludarabine is a more recently developed antipurine.

Side-effects. Its main toxicity is bone marrow depression. Autoimmune haemolytic anaemia may occur in the absence of any previous history or Coombs' test status.

Main uses. B cell chronic lymphocytic leukaemia.

3. Pyrimidine antagonists

5-fluorouracil. 5-fluorouracil is a fluoropyrimidine (a combination of a uracil and fluorine) which inhibits DNA synthesis by inhibiting the main enzyme in pyrimidine synthesis and thus the formation of cytosine and thymine. In addition it is incorporated into RNA instead of uracil and inhibits RNA synthesis. 5-FU is metabolised intracellularly to fluorouridine monophosphate and subsequently to fluorouridine triphosphate (FUTP) and fluorodeoxyuridine monophosphate (FdUMP). FUTP becomes erroneously incorporated into RNA inhibiting its function. FdUMP forms covalent bonds with thymidylate synthase and its cofactor 5,10-methylene tetrahydrofolate, creating a complex which inhibits the formation of thymidine from deoxyuridine monophosphate (dUMP), so inhibiting DNA synthesis. One problem with 5-FU is that elevated dUMP may overcome the inhibition of thymidylate synthase. Thymidylate synthase inhibitors, e.g. ralitrexed, have been developed. Ralitrexed appears to be active against colorectal cancer and is better tolerated than bolus 5-FU and folinic acid.

Absorption of 5-FU by the oral route is unpredictable and the drug is normally given intravenously. It can also be applied topically. Most of the drug is rapidly metabolised in the liver and excreted in the urine.

Side-effects. The main toxicity is to the gastrointestinal tract (diarrhoea, nausea and vomiting). Stomatitis occurring 5–8 days after treatment is usually an early sign of severe toxicity. Myelosuppression also occurs, with a nadir at 10 days. Less common side-effects are alopecia, skin rashes, and rarely an acute cerebellar syndrome.

Cytosine arabinoside. Cytosine arabinoside is an analogue of deoxycytidine. It is a competitive inhibitor of the enzyme DNA polymerase. Its principal action is as a false nucleotide competing for the enzymes which are responsible for converting cytidine to deoxycytidine and for incorporating deoxycytidine in to DNA. It is a cell cycle-specific drug, only acting on proliferating cells.

It can be given by intravenous or subcutaneous routes. Most of the drug is excreted in the urine.

Side-effects. Bone marrow suppression, nausea, vomiting and diarrhoea, and oral ulceration are common. Reversible hepatotoxicity also occurs.

Main uses. Acute leukaemia (especially myeloid).

Gemcitabine. Gemcitabine is a second-generation pyrimidine analogue. It is metabolised by nucleotide kinases intracellularly to the active diphosphate and triphosphate. It inhibits DNA synthesis. It is cell phase-specific, mainly killing cells in S phase. It is given by intravenous infusion and is excreted in the urine.

Side-effects. Nausea and vomiting, myelosuppression, flu-like symptoms, rashes and oedema occur.

Interactions. There is enhancement of radiation toxicity when given with concurrent radical radiotherapy.

Main uses. Non-small cell lung cancer, breast cancer, pancreatic cancer.

Natural products

These include mitotic inhibitors, antibiotics and enzymes.

1. Mitotic inhibitors

There are three valuable alkaloids from the periwinkle plant (*Vinca rosea*): vincristine, vinblastine and vindesine.

Mechanism of action

The vinca alkaloids inhibit the formation of the small tubules (microtubules) which make up the spindle on which the chromatids line up in metaphase. Cell division is therefore prevented.

Vincristine. Vincristine is given intravenously. It is excreted mainly via the bile and the faeces. Its toxicity may be enhanced in obstructive liver disease.

Side-effects. It is vesicant locally. Neurotoxicity is the main dose-limiting toxicity. This is in the form of a sensorimotor peripheral neuropathy (paraesthesiae in fingers, muscle cramps, paralytic ileus, constipation). Vincristine should be stopped if there is any evidence of motor neuropathy. Less common is inappropriate antidiuretic hormone (ADH) production. Alopecia is rare.

Main uses. Lymphoma, leukaemia, breast cancer, sarcoma.

Vinblastine. Vinblastine is given intravenously. It is partly excreted in the bile and urine. The dose should be reduced in obstructive liver disease.

Side-effects. It is a sclerosant, causing a cellulitis if extravasation occurs. Bone marrow depression is the main dose-limiting toxicity. The nadir for myelosuppression is 10 days. Neurotoxicity is less severe than with vincristine. Abdominal cramps, pain and constipation are common.

Main uses. Lymphoma, head and neck cancer, testicular teratoma.

Vindesine. The pharmacokinetics of vindesine are similar to those of the other vinca alkaloids.

Side-effects. Bone marrow suppression is the main dose-limiting toxicity (leucopenia with sparing of platelets). Neurotoxicity is milder than with vincristine. Alopecia occurs.

Main use. Malignant melanoma, lung cancer.

Topoisomerase inhibitors

Topoisomerases are enzymes involved in the coiling and uncoiling of DNA. There are two types. Topoisomerase I inhibitors bind to double-stranded DNA and cause a single strand break in DNA. Topotecan and irinotecan are topoisomerase I inhibitors. Topoisomerase II exists as alpha and beta isoenzymes. They undergo covalent bonding to complementary strands of DNA and cleave both strands. Topoisomerase II inhibitors repair these breaks.

Epipodophyllotoxins. Epipodophyllotox topoisomerase II inhibitors, are analogues of podophyllotoxin, an extract of the May apple. Podophyllotoxin is a spindle poison, binding to the microtubular proteins. It arrests cell division in the premitotic phase of the cell cycle (late G_2 and S). Etoposide (VP16) is the most widely used of this group. It is a good example of a schedule-dependent drug. It is more effective given over 5 days than on 1 day. It can be given orally or intravenously. It is mainly excreted in the urine.

Side-effects. The dose-limiting toxicity is bone marrow suppression. The nadir is at about 16 days with recovery at 20–22 days. Nausea, vomiting and anorexia are relatively minor but more marked if etoposide is given orally. Alopecia is common. Mucositis and a mild peripheral neuropathy occur occasionally.

Note. Care should be taken not to give etoposide intravenously over less than 30 minutes, to avoid hypotension.

Main uses. Hodgkin's disease, non-Hodgkin lymphoma, leukaemias, small cell lung cancer, testicular teratoma, Ewing's sarcoma.

Taxanes

Paclitaxel and docetaxel are tubulin-binding drugs which inhibit the disassembly of microtubulins.

In vitro docetaxel breaks up the microtubular network necessary for interphase and mitotic cellular function. It is given by intravenous infusion 3-weekly. It is eliminated by renal and biliary routes.

Side-effects. Hypersensitivity reactions, myelosuppression, rashes, fluid retention, nausea, vomiting, diarrhoea, abdominal pain, neurosensory changes, alopecia.

Administration should be under steroid cover because of the risks of hypersensitivity reactions.

Uses. Breast and ovarian cancer.

2. Antibiotics

Anthracyclines

Daunorubicin, doxorubicin (Adriamycin) and epirubicin are the principal anthracycline antibiotics. They are produced from different strains of fungi (streptomyces). The mechanisms of their cytotoxic action are not fully understood. They include insertion between opposing strands of DNA (intercalation), altering membrane permeability, alkylation, free radical formation and forming cytotoxic complexes with metals such as iron, copper and zinc. Their main effects are exerted during S phase of DNA synthesis.

Doxorubicin and epirubicin are given intravenously. Excretion is mainly via the liver. Reduction in dosage is essential in patients with liver dysfunction.

Side-effects. The toxicity is to the bone marrow, gastrointestinal tract and to the heart. The nadir of the white count is at 10 days. Epirubicin causes slightly less vomiting than the other two anthracyclines.

Daunorubicin and doxorubicin and, to a much lesser extent, epirubicin cause cumulative cardiotoxicity. The maximum recommended total dose of doxorubicin is 450–550 mg/m^2 and for daunorubicin 20 mg/kg. If cyclophosphamide, which is also cardiotoxic, is given at the same time as doxorubicin and daunorubicin, the total anthracycline dose is reduced to 450 mg/m^2. Acute cardiac toxicity is manifest by arrhythmias and abnormalities of electrical conduction. The chronic effect is a cardiomyopathy (pericarditis and congestive cardiac failure). Anthracyclines should be avoided if there is previous history of cardiac failure or ischaemic heart disease.

Interactions. Cyclophosphamide (see above).

Main uses. Lymphoma, breast cancer, sarcomas, lung cancer, Wilms' tumour, neuroblastoma. Acute myelogenous leukaemia (daunorubicin).

Non-anthracycline antibiotics

Actinomycin D. Actinomycin is only given intravenously. Its metabolism is minimal and its excretion slow in faeces and urine.

Side-effects. The dose-limiting toxicity is myelosuppression. Oral ulceration, nausea, vomiting, diarrhoea, alopecia and skin rashes are common. It is very irritant if extravasation occurs.

Main uses. Wilms' tumour, rhabdomyosarcoma, osteogenic sarcoma, teratoma, Hodgkin's disease.

Mitomycin C. Mitomycin C is activated to an alkylating agent and forms crosslinkages with DNA. In addition it gives rise to free radicals. Both DNA and RNA are inhibited. It is mainly eliminated by metabolism in the liver. It is given intravenously or instilled into the bladder via a catheter.

Side-effects. The dose-limiting toxicity is myelosuppression. The nadir is delayed, with nadir of white count and platelets at 3–8 weeks after administration. Anorexia, nausea and mild vomiting develop within 1–2 hours. Renal toxicity occurs, particularly if total dosage exceeds 100 mg. This is normally reversible if the drug is withdrawn. Interstitial pneumonitis is uncommon. Mitomycin C is highly irritant if it extravasates.

Main uses. Gastrointestinal, bladder and breast cancer.

Bleomycin. Bleomycin intercalates with DNA strands causing single and double strand breaks. It inhibits DNA synthesis, and, to a lesser degree, RNA synthesis. It is a cell cycle-specific agent (Fig. 34.6) with its main effects on G_2 and M phases. It is rapidly inactivated in the liver and kidney. Excretion is mainly in the urine. It is given intramuscularly, subcutaneously, intravenously, intrapleurally (for pleural effusions) and, rarely, intraperitoneally (for ascites).

Side-effects. The main toxicity is to the lung and is most likely to occur if the total dose exceeds 300 mg. Progressive fibrosis occurs. Presentation is with a non-productive cough and dyspnoea. A chest radiograph initially shows pulmonary infiltrates which may proceed to fibrosis. Pulmonary function tests show a restrictive defect and reduced gas (carbon monoxide) transfer. Respiratory complications of general anaesthesia are increased.

Occasionally there may be an immediate life-threatening anaphylactic reaction. Fever and chills are common. Hypotension, renal failure and death may result from associated sweating and dehydration. These signs may not develop until several hours after administration.

Skin changes are common: pigmentation, erythema, and thickening of the nail bed. Alopecia is uncommon.

Myelosuppression is minimal.

Main uses. Head and neck and cervical cancer, teratoma, lymphoma, malignant pleural effusions.

3. Enzymes

Asparaginase. Asparagine is an essential amino acid for protein and nucleic acid synthesis. Asparaginase is an enzyme produced from bacteria which degrades asparagine. Tumour cells, unlike their normal counterparts, have no or little asparagine synthetase, the enzyme necessary for making asparagine. When asparagine levels fall, both protein and nucleic acid synthesis are inhibited. Asparaginase remains largely confined to the vascular compartment, probably owing to its large size. Urinary or biliary excretion is minimal.

A test dose is advised because of the risk of anaphylaxis. If the patient is found to be hypersensitive, an alternative preparation is available.

Side-effects. Nausea and vomiting are generally mild. Hypersensitivity reactions are common but life-threatening anaphylaxis is rare. Pancreatitis, hypoglycaemia, encephalopathy, abnormal liver function and clotting defects also occur.

Use. Acute lymphoblastic leukaemia.

Random synthetics

Cisplatin, carboplatin. Cisplatin and carboplatin and inhibit DNA synthesis. Both act in a similar way to alkylating agents by forming crosslinkages between a pair of their chlorine atoms and the guanine molecules of opposing DNA strands (interstrand linkages), but differ in that they also bind to bases on the same DNA strand (intrastrand linkages) Both drugs are administered intravenously and are predominantly excreted in the urine.

Side-effects. Cisplatin causes severe nausea and vomiting (Table 34.2). This can be substantially reduced by giving high doses of intravenous metoclopramide. Cisplatin causes ototoxicity and renal impairment. Pre- and post-treatment hydration is always used (with or without mannitol). Hypomagnesaemia is common and tetany sometimes occurs. Magnesium supplements are often required. Hearing is also reduced because of damage to the auditory nerve, with characteristic high-tone loss. Peripheral neuropathy also occurs.

Carboplatin has the advantage of much less emesis, ototoxicity, nephrotoxicity and neurotoxicity. The dose-limiting toxicity is to the bone marrow, particularly to platelets.

Main uses. Cisplatin and carboplatin are used in testicular teratoma and seminoma; ovarian and head and neck cancer.

Dacarbazine (DTIC). The mechanism of action of dacarbazine is uncertain. It is metabolised to products which have alkylating properties and these probably account for its cytotoxic properties. It is given intravenously.

Side-effects. Myelosuppression is the principal dose-limiting toxicity. The nadir is at 21 days. Acute nausea and vomiting occur commonly in the first 12 hours following administration. A flu-like illness may occasionally develop 7 days after administration and last 1–3 weeks. Facial flushing, paraesthesiae and liver toxicity also occur.

Interactions. Phenytoin and phenobarbital may induce the metabolism of DTIC, reducing its efficacy.

Main uses. Malignant melanoma, sarcoma, lymphoma.

Hydroxycarbamide (hydroxyurea). Hydroxycarbamide is an analogue of urea. It inhibits the ribonucleotide reductase enzyme system that converts ribonucleotides to deoxyribonucleotides, inhibiting DNA synthesis (Fig. 34.7). It is given orally. It is mainly metabolised in the liver and excreted in the urine.

Side-effects. The main side-effect is bone marrow depression. Nausea, vomiting, diarrhoea or constipation, skin atrophy and dryness and erythema are common.

Interactions. Hydroxycarbamide potentiates the effects of irradiation. Radiation recall reactions may also occur (erythema and irritation in previously irradiated areas).

Main uses. Chronic granulocytic leukaemia.

Nitrosoureas (CCNU, BCNU, methyl-CCNU and streptozotocin). The nitrosoureas are a group of analogues whose main mechanism of action is thought to be alkylation. BCNU is the only member of the family with two alkylating groups and can crosslink DNA. In addition, the nitrosoureas inhibit a number of important enzymes in the synthesis and repair of DNA. They can be given orally or intravenously. Their high lipid solubility allows them to cross the blood–brain barrier into the CNS. They are extensively metabolised in the liver. Urinary excretion is slow.

Side-effects. (1) CCNU, BCNU, methyl-CCNU: nausea and vomiting frequently occur 4–6 hours after

Table 34.2 Summary of short- and medium-term toxicity of cytotoxic drugs (Reproduced with permission from Springer-Verlag: from Priestman T J. Cancer Chemotherapy: An Introduction, 1989)

	Myelosuppression	Gastrointestinal toxicity	Neurotoxicity	Alopecia	Pneumonitis and/or lung fibrosis	Cardiotoxicity	Renal damage	Hepatotoxicity	Skin changes	Endocrine abnormalities	Haemorrhagic cystitis	Acute allergic reactions
Nitrogen mustard	3	2	1	1					1			
Cyclophosphamide	2	2		2	1	1		1	1	1	2	
Ifosfamide	2	2	2	2	1			1			3	
Melphalan	3	2		1	1				1			
Chlorambucil	2	1		1	1			1				
Thiotepa	2	1										
Hexamethylmelamine	2	2	2									
Busulfan	2				2				1	1		
Nitrosureas	3	2		1	1			1	1			
Methotrexate	2	2	2	1	1		1	1	1			
5-fluorouracil	2	2	1	1	1				1			
Cytosine arabinoside	2	2	1				1	1				1
6-mercaptopurine	2	1						2				1
6-tioguanine	2	1						1				
Vincristine	1	2	3	1						1		
Vinblastine	2	1	1	1					1			
Vindesine	2	1	2	1					1			
Doxorubicin	3	2		3		3			1			
Daunorubicin	3	2		2		3						
Epirubicin	2	1		2		2						
Actinomycin D	2	2							1			
Mitomycin C	2	2			1		1					
Bleomycin		1		2	3				1			1
Cisplatinum	2	3	2				3					1
Carboplatin	3	2	1				2	1				1
Mitoxantrone (mitozantrone)	2	1		1		1		1				
Dacarbazine	1	2	1	1				1	1			1
Procarbazine	2	2	1					1				
Etoposide	3	2		2								1
Asparaginase	2	2	2	1	1		2	2		2		1
Amsacrine	3	2	1	1		1		1				
Hydroxycarbamide (hydroxyurea)	2	1							1			

1. Occasional or minor side-effect
2. Common or moderately severe side-effect
3. Invariable or dose-limiting side-effect

administration. Myelosuppression is dose limiting and delayed. The nadir of the white count is at 28 days. Alopecia and transient abnormalities of liver function are common. Kidney and lung damage are rare. (2) Streptozotocin: renal and gastrointestinal toxicity are dose limiting. Bone suppression is less marked compared with the other nitrosoureas.

Interactions. Hyperglycaemic action of streptozotocin is increased by steroids.

Main uses. Brain tumours, lymphoma, carcinoid (streptozotocin).

SIDE-EFFECTS OF CYTOTOXIC CHEMOTHERAPY

The main normal tissues damaged by cytotoxic therapy are those with rapidly dividing cell populations: the bone marrow, the gastrointestinal epithelium, the hair and the germ cells of the testis. By contrast there is little effect on non-proliferating tissues such as skeletal muscle and nervous tissue. The short- and medium-term side-effects of commonly used cytotoxic drugs are shown in Table 34.3.

Bone marrow

The bone marrow contains stem cells from which develop red cells, white cells and platelets. Cytotoxic therapy exerts its inhibitory effects on cell division on the stem cell population. It has little effect on mature red cells, white cells or platelets.

The time of onset of anaemia, leucopenia and thrombocytopenia reflects the life spans of different mature cells. Leucopenia tends to occur first since the survival of white cells is about 5 days. Thrombocytopenia occurs next. Platelets survive 9–10 days. Anaemia occurs last since the red cell life span is considerably longer at 120 days.

The main risk of leucopenia is the increased susceptibility to infection. Septicaemia may be life-threatening. Any infection should be promptly treated. Growth factors are now available for red cells and white cells to reduce toxicity. Recombinant human granulocyte colony-stimulating factor (GCSF) is indicated in patients undergoing chemotherapy associated with febrile neutropenia. It is administered daily starting 24 hours after the administration of chemotherapy and continued until the nadir has passed and the neutrophil count has returned to the normal range, usually within 8–14 days of chemotherapy. It should not be used in patients with myeloid malignancy.

Gastrointestinal tract

The nausea and vomiting caused by many cytotoxic agents are multifactorial in origin. They are mainly due to stimulation of receptors in the gut (principally the small bowel). Other stimuli come from the cerebral cortex, the vestibular apparatus of the inner ear and an area of the brainstem (chemoreceptor trigger zone).

Drugs causing severe vomiting are:

- cisplatin
- nitrogen mustard
- doxorubicin
- actinomycin D
- dacarbazine.

Treatment. Nausea and vomiting can be reduced or abolished by a variety of agents (Table 34.3). Among the most effective are the 5-hydroxytryptamine ($5\text{-}HT_3$) antagonists such as ondansetron and granisetron.

Oral mucositis is commonly caused by methotrexate, 5-fluorouracil and doxorubicin.

Treatment. The probability of mucositis from methotrexate can be reduced by folinic acid rescue (see under Methotrexate).

Diarrhoea may be caused by 5-fluorouracil and mitomycin C.

Hair

Hair loss (alopecia) is due to damage to hair follicles and is a reversible side-effect. Thinning of the hair is usually confined to the scalp. It usually begins about a month after the first dose of chemotherapy. The probability of alopecia varies from agent to agent and sometimes with

Table 34.3 Agents used in the treatment of nausea and vomiting

Agent	Dose
Corticosteroids (dexamethasone)	12–16 mg i.v.
Metoclopramide	10 mg/kg i.v. per 24 hours (high dose for cisplatin)
Domperidone	10–20 mg 4–8-hourly oral/p.r.
Phenothiazines	5–10 mg oral/i.v./i.m./p.r. 8-hourly
Chlorpromazine	25 mg oral/i.v./i.m. 8-hourly
Cannabinoids	
Nabilone	1–2 mg oral 12-hourly
Butyrophenones	
Haloperidol	1–2 mg oral/i.v. 3–6-hourly
Benzodiazepines	
Lorazepam	2–4 mg oral 4-hourly
$5\text{-}HT_3$ antagonists	
e.g. ondansetron or granisetron	8 mg i.v./oral, then 8 mg oral twice daily 3 mg i.v., then 1 mg twice daily

dose (e.g. cyclophosphamide). Regrowth starts about 2 months after the end of treatment. New hair may differ in colour and texture.

Scalp cooling may limit the amount of hair loss with anthracylines at conventional dosage. At high dosage, its value is uncertain.

Complete loss of scalp hair is likely with:

- doxorubicin
- etoposide
- epirubicin
- ifosfamide.

It is unlikely with:

- cisplatin
- chlorambucil
- mitomycin C.

Alopecia occasionally occurs with:

- methotrexate
- mitoxantrone (mitozantrone).

Germ cells of the testis

The germinal epithelium becomes depleted following chemotherapy with many agents. It is most common in prepubertal boys. The sperm count falls. Sperm cells may disappear completely (azoospermia). Damage to the germinal epithelium is often cumulative. Combination chemotherapy is more likely to result in azoospermia with lower doses of drugs than is single-agent therapy. Recovery of sperm production is difficult to predict. The higher the dose the lower and slower is the probability of recovery.

In contrast to the ovary (see below) male endocrine function (i.e. testosterone production) is rarely affected.

Hodgkin's disease. Most men treated with MOPP or similar regimes (e.g. MVPP) for Hodgkin's disease are sterilised permanently. The ABVD regime has a much lower incidence of azoospermia (30%).

Testicular cancer. In patients undergoing combination chemotherapy with cisplatin, vinblastine and bleomycin, the probability of active spermatogenesis is about 80% 18 months after treatment. Spermatogenesis does not resume during the first 12 months of treatment.

Germ cell depletion is likely with:

- chlorambucil (especially > 400 mg)
- cyclophosphamide (especially > 6 g)
- nitrogen mustard
- procarbazine
- busulfan.

It is unlikely with:

- methotrexate
- vincristine
- 6-mercaptopurine
- 5-fluorouracil
- etoposide.

Prevention. Infertility may be overcome in some patients by sperm storage and cryopreservation before starting chemotherapy. Referral to an infertility clinic for counselling and sperm collection is necessary. Usually 2–3 specimens of semen are required over a 1–2 week period. Only if there are adequate numbers of motile sperm is banking worthwhile. Unfortunately many patients with germ cell tumours of the testis or Hodgkin's disease are infertile as a complication of their disease.

Female fertility

Female infertility is less likely than male infertility to be induced by chemotherapy. This is mainly because the number of ova is fixed before birth, in contrast to sperm which are continuously produced throughout adulthood. Chemotherapy may none the less be toxic to the ovaries, causing ovarian fibrosis, amenorrhoea, hot flushes and infertility. The probability of this occurring increases with age.

Single-agent therapy

Ovarian function is more likely to be conserved in women under the age of 35–40, for a moderate dose of chemotherapy, than above this range. Periods are more likely to return within 6 months of chemotherapy under the age of 40 (e.g. in 50% of women after cyclophosphamide) than over 40.

Drugs most likely to cause infertility are:

- cyclophosphamide
- busulfan
- melphalan
- chlorambucil.

Drugs unlikely to cause ovarian failure are:

- methotrexate
- 5-fluorouracil
- 6-mercaptopurine
- etoposide.

Combination chemotherapy

Hodgkin's disease. Most information has been collected on patients undergoing MOPP for Hodgkin's disease.

Ovarian failure occurs in 40–50% of women receiving this regime. Most women over the age of 30 will be sterilised. However, under the age of 20 most will retain fertility. For example, 50% of women receiving alkylating agents (e.g. chlorambucil, cyclophosphamide) as part of combination chemotherapy are likely to be sterilised. Combination chemotherapy is more likely to induce sterility than single-agent therapy.

Breast cancer. Women undergoing CMF chemotherapy for breast cancer are commonly sterilised.

Choriocarcinoma. Most women (over 85%) will retain their fertility after chemotherapy. This is because methotrexate, the main agent used, rarely causes ovarian failure.

Cardiac damage

Cardiac damage is uncommon, with the exception of doxorubicin and daunorubicin. The pathogenesis is unclear. It may be due to the toxic effects of free radical formation, damage to cardiac membranes or intercalation of DNA base pairs. Previous cardiac disease and irradiation predispose to cardiotoxicity. The mortality of this form of toxicity is as high as 60%. No morphological change is completely predictive of doxorubicin-induced heart failure.

Lung damage

Pulmonary toxicity is uncommon but is associated with:

- bleomycin
- cyclophosphamide
- busulfan
- methotrexate.

The toxicity is usually cumulative and irreversible. Presentation is normally with non-productive cough and progressive dyspnoea. Chest radiography may show lung infiltrates progressing to fibrosis.

Neurological damage

The vinca alkaloids (particularly vincristine) are the commonest causes of neurotoxicity. This is in the form of a peripheral neuropathy (see under Vincristine).

Methotrexate may cause central nervous toxicity (dementia) if given by the intrathecal route, particularly if cranial irradiation is given concurrently (e.g. in the treatment of acute lymphoblastic leukaemia). 5-fluorouracil may cause ataxia, and ifosfamide encephalopathy.

Damage to the fetus

This is a very serious concern. Little information, however, is available about the effects of chemotherapy on pregnant women since chemotherapy is avoided if at all possible in these circumstances. In the few cases that have been reported, the evidence for a causal relationship is not firm. Most data on teratogenicity are derived from animal testing of anticancer agents. if chemotherapy has to be started during the pregnancy, the pregnancy may have to be terminated, depending on the medical condition and wishes of the patient and her partner.

Contraception. Care should be taken to ensure that patients are not or do not become pregnant during chemotherapy. Barrier contraceptive methods are advised.

Teratogenicity. The most serious risk of inducing a major, and often lethal, fetal abnormality (teratogenic effect) is during the first 8 weeks of pregnancy when the organ systems are developing. Examples of teratogenic effects are limb deformities and retinal defects. At the end of this period the organs have formed. Fetal growth is then the major change. The risks of fetal damage diminish. The teratogenicity of methotrexate is best documented and it is contraindicated during the first trimester.

Fetal growth retardation. Chemotherapy after the eighth week of pregnancy may cause fetal growth retardation. Anticancer agents can pass from the maternal circulation via the placenta to the fetus and cause the same side-effects as in the mother.

Premature delivery and low birth weight. These have been reported in some but not all pregnant women treated for leukaemia.

Genetic damage. Chromosomal damage by cytotoxic therapy is a theoretical risk but there is no clinical evidence to show that congenital abnormality in the offspring of patients who received chemotherapy is any greater than in the normal population. Studies of children born to women treated with chemotherapy for choriocarcinoma show no increased risk of congenital defects. Since the true risk is unknown, firm guidelines to couples on when they can safely attempt to have children after the end of chemotherapy cannot be given.

Advice to patients. Avoiding pregnancy for a year after the end of chemotherapy is a reasonable guideline.

Interaction with irradiation (radiation recall)

Patients who have been exposed to previous irradiation, when given certain cytotoxic agents (e.g. actinomycin

D), may experience a repeated radiation reaction within the irradiated volume.

Psychological effects

Psychological difficulties may be related to malignant disease or a pre-existing psychological or psychiatric disorder. This applies to patients undergoing any form of conventional treatment for cancer. These are dealt with in Chapter 37.

The diagnosis of cancer, uncertainties about the future and the physical side-effects of chemotherapy frequently give rise to anxiety and depression. In extreme cases, suicide may be attempted. In women, change in body image (e.g. alopecia, weight gain or loss) can be very distressing. Marital and family disharmony are common. A normal sex life may be interrupted because of loss of libido on the part of either patient or partner. Loss of self-esteem from prolonged periods off work with loss of earning capacity and fear of redundancy are also frequent.

Prevention and treatment. A clear explanation of the diagnosis and treatment and continuing counselling during and after treatment may allay many anxieties. Clinical staff need to be alert to the development of symptoms of an anxiety or depressive state. Referral to a clinical psychologist or psychiatrist is desirable for advice on management. Anxiolytic or antidepressant therapy may be helpful. Patients who are cured may still fail to rehabilitate psychologically to a normal working and home life. Constant reassurance is required, reinforced if necessary by investigations objectively confirming remission.

Day-care units or self-help groups. of patients with and previously treated for cancer may help maintain morale and encourage rehabilitation. Sometimes patients with the same tumour (e.g. young men with testicular cancer) may provide mutual support during and after treatment, from the common experience of coping with chemotherapy.

Second malignancy

From the long-term follow-up of both adults and children treated with single-agent and combination chemotherapy for malignant disease, there is clear evidence of a carcinogenic effect of chemotherapy.

Agents known to be carcinogenic in man

1. Alkylating agents—busulfan, chlorambucil, cyclophosphamide, melphalan, treosulfan, methyl-CCNU
2. Antimetabolites—azathioprine.

Some agents are carcinogenic in laboratory animals but not in man (e.g. bleomycin, doxorubicin, vinca alkaloids and cisplatin).

Mechanism of carcinogenesis. The exact mechanisms of carcinogenicity by anticancer agents are not known. The most likely is DNA damage. Alkylating agents bind to DNA and somehow interfere with its function, resulting in abnormal mitosis. This explanation is supported by the fact that agents which do not bind DNA (e.g. methotrexate) are not carcinogenic.

Effect of drug dosage. With some drugs the carcinogenic risk rises with total dose. For this reason chlorambucil is commonly discontinued after 6 months of treatment to reduce the likelihood of leukaemogenesis.

There is some evidence that prolonged low-dose chemotherapy is more carcinogenic than higher doses given intermittently.

Type and incidence of second tumours

Acute non-lymphocytic leukaemia. The risk of developing leukaemia at 10 years following MOPP chemotherapy is 5–10%. It is maximal when chemotherapy is combined with radiotherapy. Prognosis is poor (< 10% remission rates). Leukaemogenesis also occurs following melphalan and cyclophosphamide for ovarian cancer and multiple myeloma. Melphalan is more leukaemogenic than cyclophosphamide.

Non-Hodgkin lymphomas. These are commoner after treatment of Hodgkin's disease. The risk at 10 years following combination chemotherapy for Hodgkin's disease is 4%. If the patient has also received radiotherapy the risk is even higher (15%).

Solid tumours (e.g. sarcomas, bowel and lung cancer). These are also increased after MOPP chemotherapy for Hodgkin's disease. The cumulative risk of a solid tumours at 10 years is 7%.

Time of onset. The latent period for the development of acute leukaemia is 5.5 years and for solid tumours 9.5 years.

Prevention. Where two agents are equally effective against a particular tumour, the least carcinogenic should be chosen (e.g. cyclophosphamide rather than melphalan in ovarian cancer), but the chances of cure should not be compromised.

CHAPTER CONTENTS

35

Hormones and oncology

Ian Kunkler

The removal of certain of the body's own hormones or the addition of synthetic hormones can either stimulate, control or eradicate tumour growth. Hormonal therapy plays a major role in breast and prostate cancer.

HISTORICAL DEVELOPMENT

The relationship between hormones and cancer is an old one. An early milestone was the work of a Scottish surgeon, George Beatson, who in 1896 removed the ovaries of two young women with breast cancer and found that the tumours subsequently regressed. It was thought at the time that the mechanism involved removal of some 'ovarian irritation' responsible for the breast lesions, but recurrence soon occurred. Although others repeated the procedure, the results were unpredictable and improvements only temporary. As a result the operation fell into disuse and its full significance was not appreciated until much later. Ovarian ablation by irradiation was first carried out in 1922. However, it was 30 years after the original observation of Beatson that the hormone oestrogen was isolated, whose source in the ovary Beatson had removed and which explained the temporary regression of the breast cancer.

Later, animal work again drew attention to hormonal factors, e.g. the incidence of spontaneous breast cancer was reduced by removing the ovaries (ovariectomy or oophorectomy). Other striking experiments produced breast tumours in mice by prolonged administration of ovarian hormones. Clinical interest revived in 1941 when Huggins in the USA reported favourable results of removing the testes (orchidectomy) in cancer of the prostate (p. 499). Much of the early work on endocrine therapy in cancer was empirical, involving the surgical or radiotherapeutic ablation of different endocrine glands. Such hormonal sensitivity is observed in a substantial number of patients with cancers of the breast, prostate and endometrium.

OESTROGEN RECEPTORS

In the latter part of the 1960s the presence of *oestrogen receptors* was demonstrated in a number of breast tumour cells. It subsequently emerged that a response to endocrine therapy in some patients with breast cancer corresponded with the presence of these receptors. We now know that oestrogen receptors (ER) are steroid receptors predominantly found in the nucleus of target cells. Similarly, the absence of oestrogen receptors corresponded with a low probability of a response to endocrine therapy. Subsequently the presence of receptors for progesterone (PgR) has been demonstrated on breast tumour cells. Some cells may have receptors for oestrogen or progesterone alone or a combination of both. The highest level of response (about 50–60%) is seen in patients whose breast tumours contain both receptors. However, not all ER-positive tumours will respond to antioestrogens. The cause of endocrine resistance in ER-positive tumours is in the process of being elucidated. Mutant or variant oestrogen receptors may be a major part of the explanation. These receptors can impede the activity of normal oestrogen receptors by competing with the normal wild-type receptor for binding sites. Variant forms of oestrogen receptor might explain less common forms of receptor which contain ER but no PgR (e.g. ER+, PgR-). About 10–30% of breast cancers have undetectable or very low levels of oestrogen receptors. They are also associated with other poor prognostic factors such as the presence of c-erb B-2 and epidermal growth factor.

More recently it has been suggested that tumours control their own growth by producing their own (paracrine) growth factors. Some breast tumour cells have surface receptors for both oestrogen and for growth factors, e.g. epidermal growth factor (EGF). There is an inverse relation between EGF and oestrogen receptors. Cells with large numbers of EGF receptors generally have low numbers of oestrogen receptors and vice versa. In addition it has been shown that EGFs reduce the number of oestrogen receptors within the cell.

When an oestrogen receptor is stimulated, the result may be the synthesis and release of further growth factors which stimulate cell division and tumour growth. Alternatively, it may result in the synthesis of progesterone receptors which inhibit cell division and stimulate cell differentiation away from malignant development. It is not clear what determines the choice between these two responses. It may relate to relative hormonal levels. The production of growth factors is favoured by low oestrogen concentration and of progesterone receptors by higher oestrogen concentrations.

Tamoxifen stimulates breast cancer cells to produce transforming growth factor beta (TGFβ), an inhibitory growth factor which inhibits the production of stimulatory growth factors such as TGFα and platelet-derived growth factor (PDGF). There are probably also oestrogen receptor-independent actions on protein kinase C and NK (natural killer) cell activity.

Paradoxically responses to endocrine therapy are occasionally seen when hormonal therapy is withdrawn. These withdrawal responses tend to be seen in patients who have responded and then progressed on endocrine therapy for breast cancer. This paradox may be explained by tamoxifen and other additive endocrine therapies having the capability of being tumour agonists. Breast cancers may contains populations of cells with heterogeneous sensitivity to tamoxifen. If a breast cancer which is regressing on tamoxifen contains small-volume clones of cells which respond to tamoxifen as a tumour agonist, they may come to dominate and the net effect will be tumour progression. There are other mechanisms by which tamoxifen can exert a tumour agonist effect. One of its metabolites, a weak oestrogen, is converted to a more potent oestrogen which may promote tumour cell growth.

Oestrogen at least from in vitro experiments can stimulate the growth of breast cancer cells. For this reason oestrogen-containing hormone replacement therapy is advised against once breast cancer has been diagnosed. It is thought that oestrogen exerts its stimulatory action on tumour cell growth through a variety of pathways including the production of proteins which participate in cell cycle control (e.g. jun, fos, myc), cyclin-dependent kinases and cyclins (see p. 293).

Surgical ablative therapy still plays a part in endocrine therapy for breast and prostate cancer. Orchidectomy, the removal of both testes, and oophorectomy reduce the main source of sex steroids to very low levels. However, they do not eliminate the source of sex steroids from the adrenal glands. Bilateral adrenalectomy was effective in achieving some responses in postmenopausal women with endocrine-sensitive disease. However, it was soon replaced by medical means of suppressing the adrenal sex steroids such as aminoglutethemide, which non-specifically inhibits the cytochrome P450 enzyme that catalyses the conversion of adrenal androgen to oestrogens. Similarly, hypophysectomy (ablation of the pituitary gland) was once used in premenopausal women to reduce oestrogen synthesis by cutting the source of gonadotrophins to the ovaries and ACTH to the adrenal gland. Hypophysectomy is now no longer practised.

GONADOTROPHIN-RELEASING HORMONE (GnRH) ANALOGUES

Downregulation of the gonadotrophin-releasing hormone (GnRH) receptors in the pituitary is achieved by the application of continuous secretion of gonadotrophin-releasing hormone analogues implanted subcutaneously and replaced on a monthly basis in premenopausal women (e.g. goserelin 3.6 mg). These analogues of the naturally occurring hypothalamic luteinising hormone- releasing hormone (LHRH) initially cause a transient surge of gonadotrophin (LH) secretion. However, with continuous exposure to these analogues, the LHRH receptors in the pituitary become desensitised, resulting in reduction in the secretion of gonadotrophins. The advantage of medical suppression of ovarian function with GnRH analogues is that the process is reversible. Thus a trial with these agents can be undertaken in a premenopausal woman to assess the tolerability of menopausal symptoms before proceeding to a surgical and irreversible oophorectomy. Once the agent is withdrawn, periods and the reproductive potential should return. It should be noted that GnRH analogues have no role in postmenopausal patients.

AROMATASE INHIBITORS

Aromatase inhibitors play an important role in the endocrine management of advanced and recurrent ER-positive breast cancer. It is possible that this may extend into the adjuvant situation if trials of these agents against the standard therapy of tamoxifen suggest greater efficacy or equivalent efficacy with reduced acute and late toxicities. The earliest of these aromatase inhibitors was aminoglutethimide, which inhibited the enzyme 20,22-desmolase, which cleaved the cholesterol side-chain. Aminogluthemide replaced bilateral adrenalectomy in postmenopausal women. It had response rates similar to those of tamoxifen. However, about 10% of patients had to discontinue treatment because of rashes, fever and lethargy. At high doses aminoglutethemide inhibits the production of cortisol and aldosterone. For this reason both mineralocorticoid and glucocorticoid replacement was required. When initially used in full dose (250 mg q.d.s. orally) steroid replacement was required with hydrocortisone. However, in low doses (125 mg b.d.) per day similar response rates were seen but steroid replacement was unnecessary. Aminogluthemide does not, however, suppress aromatisation of ovarian oestrogen and therefore has no useful role in premenopausal women with breast cancer.

A number of selective aromatase inhibitors have been developed. These include 4-hydroxyandrostenedione (formestane), anastrazole and letrozole.

ANDROGEN RECEPTORS

In contrast to breast cancer where oestrogen receptor levels play an important role in management, the role of the androgen receptor (AR) in the management of prostate cancer is not established. ARs have been demonstrated both in benign prostatic hyperplasia and in prostate cancer. There is no good evidence that the presence of androgen receptors predicts response to endocrine manipulation in prostate cancer although there are suggestions that AR-positive tumours do have a better survival. It is known that castration (orchidectomy) reduces ARs to much lower levels (10% of normal) compared to other hormonal treatments such as flutamide.

GnRH analogues such as goserelin are a key aspect of the hormonal manipulation of prostate cancer. They provide equivalent androgen suppression to orchidectomy and avoid the need for a surgical procedure that many men find unacceptable, symbolising the definitive loss of manhood. Even after orchidectomy levels of intracellular dihydrotestosterone may remain elevated, even though serum testosterone levels are low. It is possible that this is due to the conversion in peripheral tissues of adrenal androstenedione. If antiandrogen (e.g. flutamide) is combined with a GnRH analogue, greater adrenal suppression may be achieved. However, although duration of progression-free survival is enhanced, combined therapy is associated with greater side-effects, particularly diarrhoea.

HORMONES AS THERAPEUTIC AGENTS

There are a limited number of human cancers where hormone therapy is of value. These are in organs in which hormonal stimulation and control are known to be important, mainly prostate, breast, thyroid, and body of uterus. Quantitative and qualitative variation in clinical response is very wide. Remissions rarely last for more than a few years but symptomatic benefit may be substantial, and even dramatic, during this period.

While the administration of hormones avoids the morbidities particular to surgery, radiotherapy and cytotoxic chemotherapy, it is often accompanied by side-effects, which are sometimes unacceptable (e.g. masculinising effects of androgens in women with breast cancer) and can be dangerous (e.g. cardiovascular morbidity from diethylstilbestrol for prostate cancer). A careful balance has to be struck between toxicity and benefit in tumour control.

Addition of hormones

Female hormones (oestrogens and progestogens)

Oestrogens. Synthetic rather than naturally occurring oestrogens are used since the naturally occurring are metabolised in the liver.

Action in females. Oestrogens are responsible for the enlargement of the breasts at puberty and during menstrual cycles, and for maturation and maintenance of secondary sexual characteristics and sexual organs.

Action in males. Oestrogens (1) inhibit the release of luteinising hormone (LH) from the anterior lobe of the pituitary gland, leading to a fall in testicular androgen production, and (2) possibly have a direct effect on the prostate gland.

Preparations

1. Diethylstilbestrol
   Indication: prostate cancer
   Dose: 1–5 mg orally daily
2. Ethinylestradiol
   Indication: prostate cancer
   Dose: 0.1–0.5 mg t.d.s. daily
3. Phosphorylated methylestradiol (Honvan)
   Indication: prostate cancer
   Dose: loading dose of 500–1000 mg daily for 5 days i.v., then 100–600 mg daily orally as maintenance.

Side-effects

- Nausea and vomiting (50%)
- Fluid retention, sometimes leading to oedema, hypertension and cardiac failure
- Enlargement of the breasts
- Deepening pigmentation of the nipple and areola
- Uterine bleeding, from stimulation of the endometrium, even long after the menopause. This is also liable to occur if the oestrogen is stopped abruptly. Dosage should be tailed off gradually. The patient should be warned of possible bleeding to avoid alarm
- Thromboembolism
- Hypercalcaemia may be induced at the start of therapy.

In men:

- Loss of libido
- Shrinkage of the genitalia
- Enlargement of breast tissue (gynaecomastia).

Progestogens. The *corpus luteum* of the ovary secretes progesterone towards the end of each menstrual cycle. The main action of progesterone is the maturation of the endometrium ready for the implantation of the fertilised ovum. The mechanism of action of progesterones in breast and endometrial cancer is unclear. Probably the most important effect is its *antioestrogenic* action:

1. Increases the enzymatic conversion of oestradiol to the less potent oestrone, so reducing the level of available oestradiol to stimulate oestrogen receptors.
2. Reduces the number of oestrogen receptors.
3. Increases the number of progesterone receptors and cellular differentiation and inhibits cell division.
4. It seems to inhibit directly ovarian and adrenal production of sex hormones and has an important indirect action by inhibiting pituitary gonadotrophin production.
5. It may have a direct cytotoxic effect.

Side-effects

- Weight gain
- Sweating, muscle cramps, tremor (adrenergic effects)
- Fluid retention
- Increased blood clotting and risk of thrombosis (medroxyprogesterone acetate)
- Nausea, urticaria, carpal tunnel syndrome, thrombophlebitis, alopecia (megestrol acetate)
- Vaginal bleeding, amenorrhoea.

Preparations

1. Medroxyprogestone acetate
   Dose: 200 mg t.d.s. or 500 mg b.d. orally (breast cancer)
   Dose: 100 mg t.d.s. orally (endometrial cancer)
2. Megestrol acetate
   Dose: 160 mg once daily orally (breast cancer).

Antioestrogens

Tamoxifen is the most important synthetic antioestrogen preparation. It has two main actions:

1. Antioestrogenic: competitive binding to oestrogen receptors (ER).
2. Weak oestrogenic action, raising levels of sex hormone binding globulin, which binds to freely circulating oestrogen and so reduces the amount of free oestrogen available to bind to oestrogen receptors. The

binding of oestrogen to the oestrogen receptor reduces the synthesis of growth factors and stimulates the production of progesterone receptors. As a result cell division is arrested at the G_1 phase of the cell cycle (p. 294).

Lowering the free oestradiol levels stimulates the production of follicle-stimulating hormone (FSH) from the pituitary. FSH then stimulates the ovarian production of oestrogen. In theory this latter effect of tamoxifen should contraindicate its use in premenopausal women with breast cancer because of the risk of oestrogen-induced tumour growth. This theoretical risk has not been borne out in practice.

Indications

1. Adjuvant therapy in early breast cancer in pre- and postmenopausal women.
2. Recurrent and advanced breast cancer.

Preparations
Tamoxifen.
Dose: 20 mg orally daily.

Side-effects
These are infrequent. The following may occur:

- Nausea
- Hot flushes
- Dizziness
- Vaginal bleeding
- Fluid retention
- Mild transient thrombocytopenia
- Retinopathy
- Acute hypercalcaemia in patients with bone metastases
- Endometrial cancer.

Antiandrogens

Flutamide. This is a non-steroidal antiandrogen and is a pure androgen antagonist. One of its important metabolites, hydroxyflutamide, is thought to be responsible for its cellular action. It blocks the binding of dihydrotestosterone to its receptor, so inhibiting the action of androgen. When administered with medical or surgical castration, both testicular and adrenal androgen activity are suppressed.

Indications: locally recurrent and metastatic prostate cancer.

Dose: 250 mg t.d.s. orally.

Side-effects

- Gynaecomastia and/or breast tenderness
- Nausea and diarrhoea
- Insomnia
- Abnormal liver function
- Tiredness.

Bicalutamide. Bicalutamide (Casodex) is a non-steroidal antiandrogen. It binds to androgen receptors and therefore inhibits androgen stimulation.

Indications: treatment of advanced prostate cancer in conjunction with LHRH analogue or castration.

Dose: 50 mg orally daily.

Side-effects

- Hot flushes
- Pruritus
- Abnormal liver function and cholestasis
- Somnolence
- Heart failure
- Anorexia, dry mouth, dyspepsia.

Cyproterone acetate. This is a progestogenic antiandrogen. It has two actions. First, it reduces the production of testosterone in the testis by inhibiting the secretion of the pituitary gonadotrophins. Secondly, it competes with androgen receptors, from which it displaces testosterone.

Indications: (1) to suppress flare with initial LHRH analogue therapy; (2) long-term palliative treatment where LHRH analogues are contraindicated or poorly tolerated.

Dose: 200–300 mg orally daily.

Side-effects

- Liver dysfunction
- Impotence
- Fluid retention
- Depression
- Gynaecomastia.

Luteinising hormone-releasing hormone (LHRH) analogues

LHRH is a protein which binds to receptors in the anterior pituitary and stimulates the production of luteinising hormone (LH) and follicle-stimulating hormone (FSH). The initial response is an increase in FSH and LH levels but within a few days there is a reduction in the number of pituitary LHRH receptors. The LH and FSH levels fall and correspondingly the levels of androgens and oestrogens produced peripherally fall.

Preparations

1. Goserelin acetate (Zoladex)
   Indications: recurrent and metastatic prostate cancer
   Dose: 3.6 mg subcutaneously every 28 days

2. Buserelin (Suprefact)

   Indications: recurrent and metastatic prostate cancer
   Dose: 100 μg by intranasal application six times a day.

Side-effects

- Hot flushes
- Loss of libido
- Gynaecomastia
- Nausea.

An initial increase in testosterone may cause transient deterioration. Cyproterone acetate is sometimes given to prevent this during the first 2 weeks of treatment.

Adrenal hormones

The adrenal cortex produces three main groups of corticosteroid hormones: mineralocorticoids (regulating sodium balance), glucocorticoids (controlling carbohydrate and protein metabolism) and sex hormones (oestrogens, androgens and progesterone). The amount of glucocorticoid production is controlled by the levels of adrenocorticotrophic hormone (ACTH) from the anterior lobe of the pituitary gland. The naturally occurring glucocorticoids are cortisone and hydrocortisone. Synthetic glucocorticoids are prednisone, prednisolone and dexamethasone. Of these, dexamethasone has the highest glucocorticoid potency, 25 times that of hydrocortisone. The relative glucocorticoid and mineralocorticoid potencies and common dosages are shown in Table 35.1.

Glucocorticoids have cytotoxic properties against specific tumours (e.g. lymphomas, breast cancers and leukaemias). Some of these tumours have been found to have *glucocorticoid receptors*. In acute leukaemia, better responses are seen in patients with higher levels of receptors than those with lower levels. However, the levels of glucocorticoid receptors do not seem to correlate with tumour response when cytotoxic agents are combined with steroids. Factors other than steroid receptor status may be important in mediating tumour response to steroids in breast cancer. It may be that steroids work by feedback inhibition on ACTH, so reducing circulating oestrogen levels. They reduce the production of androgens from which oestradiol is derived. In addition, steroids act as anti-inflammatory agents, reducing the oedema around secondary tumour deposits. At a cellular level, steroids inhibit glucose transport and phosphorylation, inhibit protein synthesis and retard mitosis.

Glucocorticoids are of benefit for complications of malignant disease—cerebral oedema, chemotherapy-induced vomiting, nerve root and spinal cord compression.

Side-effects are important and potentially life-threatening, especially after prolonged therapy, when adrenal suppression has developed. Sudden withdrawal of steroids for any reason or increased steroid requirements (e.g. due to infection or the stress of an operation) may result in acute adrenal insufficiency. For this reason all patients on steroids should carry a blue *steroid card* detailing their name, address and telephone number and that of their medical practitioner and their current steroid preparation and dosage. This card or a permanently worn bracelet or neck chain indicating that the patient is on steroids should alert medical staff in the event of the patient being too unwell to report that he or she is on steroids.

Side-effects

- Adrenal insufficiency
- Sodium and water retention (low serum potassium, fluid retention and cardiac failure)
- Cushingoid appearance (mooning of the face, 'buffalo' hump on upper back)

Table 35.1 Relative potencies of natural and synthetic glucocorticoids (modified from Priestman 1989)

Drug	Relative potency		Typical dose (mg/day)
	Glucocorticoid	Mineralocorticoid	
Hydrocortisone	1	1	10–20*
Cortisone	0.8	1	10–20*
Prednisone	4	0.8	15–60†
Prednisolone	4	0.8	15–60†
Dexamethasone	25	0	2–16†

* Dose for replacement therapy where adrenal insufficiency is treatment induced, e.g. by aminoglutethimide
† Dose for active treatment of malignancy

- Gastrointestinal upset (dyspepsia, peptic ulceration with or without perforation)
- Increased risk of infection
- Osteoporosis
- Hyperglycaemia
- Modification of tissue reactions (resulting in spread of infection, poor wound or ulcer healing)
- Skin changes (thinning of skin, bruising, acne)
- Psychosis
- Cataract formation
- Muscle weakness (especially thighs).

Aromatase inhibitors

Anastrazole. Anastrazole is a selective aromatase inhibitor which binds to the active site of the aromatase enzyme. It blocks the binding of androstenedione and testosterone to the active site of aromatase and prevents oestrogen synthesis. It is a reversible inhibitor which competes with androgens for binding to aromatase.

Indications: first-line hormone therapy for endocrine-sensitive recurrent breast cancer.

Dose: 1 mg orally daily.

Side-effects

- Hot flushes
- Vaginal dryness
- Hair thinning
- Anorexia, nausea, vomiting and diarrhoea.

Letrozole. Letrozole is a reversible highly specific inhibitor of aromatase, inhibiting oestrogen biosynthesis. It does not impair steroidogenesis.

Indications: first-line hormone therapy for endocrine-sensitive recurrent or advanced breast cancer.

Dose: 2.5 mg orally daily.

Side-effects

- Hot flushes
- Hair thinning
- Musculoskeletal pain
- Headache
- Dyspnoea.

Exemestane. Exemestane is an irreversible inhibitor of aromatase which binds to its catalytic binding site. It blocks the binding of the natural substrates androstenedione and testosterone to the active site of aromatase and prevents oestrogen biosynthesis.

Indications: second-line therapy for endocrine-sensitive recurrent or advanced breast cancer.

Dose: 250 mg orally daily.

Side-effects

- Hot flushes
- Nausea
- Fatigue
- Sweating
- Dizziness.

Formestane. Formestane is a selective and irreversible inhibitor of the aromatase enzyme which converts androgen to oestrogens. It inhibits oestrogen biosynthesis.

Indications: third- or fourth-line for endocrine sensitive recurrent and advanced breast cancer especially where compliance with oral medication is difficult.

Dose: 250 mg by intramuscular injection every 2 weeks.

Side-effects

- Pain or painful lump at injection site
- Hot flushes
- Nausea and vomiting.

Aminoglutethimide. Aminoglutethimide was the first aromatase inhibitor but is not selective and has largely been replaced by selective aromatase inhibitors.

Indications: locally recurrent or metastatic breast cancer in postmenopausal women.

Dose: 125–500 mg orally b.d. and hydrocortisone 10–20 mg b.d.

At a dose of 125 mg b.d. the degree of adrenal suppression is insufficient to require hormone replacement with hydrocortisone. However, steroids do reduce the incidence of side-effects from aminoglutethimide and their use is therefore recommended but not mandatory.

Removal of hormones

Ovaries. The chief source of the female hormone, oestrogen, may be removed surgically (oophorectomy / ovariectomy). This is usually carried out laparascopically under general anaesthesia, necessitating only a few days in hospital. Alternatively the ovaries can be irradiated by a pelvic radiation field to stop them functioning (as for menorrhagia, see p. 598). Castrate hormonal levels are reached by 6 weeks.

Testes. The male hormone testosterone can be abolished by bilateral subscapular orchidectomy.

Adrenals. The glands may be removed by surgical adrenalectomy. This used to be done for advanced breast cancer but, because of the morbidity of the procedure, has been replaced by selective aromatase inhibitors such as anastrazole and letrozole.

Pituitary. This is the master endocrine gland, as it controls all the others by its various secretions. Ablation may be achieved by surgical removal of a large part of the gland (transnasal hypophysectomy) or by radiation. Pituitary ablation for advanced breast cancer is now practised extremely rarely because of the development of antioestrogens (tamoxifen) and aromatase inhibitors. The best responses tend to be seen in patients with bone metastases.

HORMONE THERAPY IN BREAST, PROSTATE, ENDOMETRIAL AND THYROID CANCER

The hormonal management of these tumours is discussed in Chapters 26, 28, 27 and 24 respectively.

CHAPTER CONTENTS

36

Palliative and continuing care

Ian Kunkler and David Radstone

In a regional oncology centre at least 50% of the work is concerned with palliative care for advanced disease. For such patients the main aim is the relief of physical and psychological distress. The period of *palliative and continuing care* incorporates the time from the diagnosis of incurable malignancy to death. The life expectancy of terminally ill patients may be a matter of a few days or weeks. Some patients with slow-growing but incurable tumours such as breast cancer, soft tissue sarcomas and gliomas may survive months or even years.

Some patients may be in the terminal phase of their illness at the time of diagnosis. In others, curative therapy may have been attempted and failed or incurable local recurrence or metastases supervened.

The radiotherapist and oncologist should form part of a multidisciplinary team including general practitioners, specialists in palliative medicine, community nurses, anaesthetists, surgeons, medical social workers, dieticians, physiotherapists and clergy.

'NO PLACE LIKE HOME'

Most patients prefer to be cared for in their own homes where they are in familiar surroundings and close to family and friends. Every effort should be made to keep the patient at home and to support the family and friends in caring for the dying patient.

Professional help from the general practitioner, MacMillan or Marie Curie nurses or other support nurses, and voluntary workers can ensure a comfortable and dignified death at home for most patients. If this is not possible, admission to a hospital or hospice is required. Admission of terminally ill patients whose symptoms are not controlled at home should be accorded a high priority. Uncontrolled pain is distressing for both the patient and family.

A short period of hospital treatment may bring symptoms under control, or defuse a difficult situation at home. This may allow the patient to return home for the last days of life.

ORGANISATION OF PALLIATIVE CARE

The provision of palliative care and continuing care should be suited to the needs of each community. Of nearly 135 000 patients dying per year of malignant disease in the UK, 60% will die in an acute general hospital. Medical and nursing staff in general hospitals should receive training in symptom control. Specialist advice is available from visiting consultants in oncology or from anaesthetists in most general hospitals. Hospital palliative care support teams, modelled on home care teams, have been established to work both in the general hospital and in the community. A typical team would include a specialist in palliative medicine, a medical social worker, occupational therapist, secretary and chaplain.

Hospices

Since the early 1980s there has been a rapid expansion of the provision of purpose-built hospices to care for the terminally ill. Hospices provide both inpatient and outpatient facilities, predominantly for adults. Most terminally ill children are managed by paediatric oncologists. At present there are two hospices in the UK specifically for children.

The hospice is often the base for a palliative home care team. Hospices are staffed by doctors and nurses experienced in palliative care. They care for about 30 000 patients per year, or a quarter of all patients who die from cancer and other terminal diseases. It is estimated that 40–50 hospice beds are required per million population. This figure has not yet been reached.

The provision of hospice care is not just a question of bricks and mortar. Some communities may feel that a home care service suits their needs better than a building. Geographical, financial and social factors are decisive. If patients and their relatives have to travel long distances to a regional oncology centre, a local hospice or home care service may be more appropriate.

Health authorities have taken over the running costs of many hospices. Health authorities and charitable bodies must ensure long-term funding of any hospice or home care service before it is inaugurated. A high nurse-to-patient ratio is needed to enable a high standard of patient care to be delivered. 25 beds is regarded as an economic size. Close links are needed with various departments in a general hospital to provide specialist advice and facilities.

Hospices provide a more informal, less institutional and quieter environment than the noisy, busy surgical, medical or oncology ward. A high staff-to-patient ratio gives more time for the patients to talk to staff about their illness.

Palliative care medicine is now recognised as a separate speciality with specific training requirements. This should improve the provision of high standards nationally, and should encourage research into palliative care.

Admission of a patient for respite care may provide relatives with an opportunity for a much-needed holiday and enable them to continue to care for a dying relative at home. Volunteer staff may visit to sit with the patient by day or night to give relatives an additional break.

Home care teams

About a third of patients will die at home. Teams of home care nurses trained in palliative care, commonly MacMillan nurses, provide additional support to the established services of the general practitioner and community nurses.

Day care centres

Many patients appreciate the support of others in a time of stress. Day centres may provide company and psychological and nursing support. In many such centres patients may attend whilst they are recovering from radiation reactions.

Family members may share care for some of the week with the day care centre. This may allow some patients to remain at home who would otherwise require hospitalisation.

SYMPTOM CONTROL

Pain, anorexia, nausea, vomiting, weight loss, dysphagia, dyspnoea and lack of energy are common symptoms in patients with advanced cancer. Patients with advanced cancer often have multiple symptoms.

Principles of management

As in any other branch of medicine the cause of symptoms should be established to provide a rational basis for treatment. While most symptoms will be caused by cancer, even a patient with advanced cancer may have a benign headache.

A careful history, clinical examination and limited investigations will establish the cause of most symptoms. Investigations should only be performed if their result is likely to influence management.

Symptoms are what the patient says they are. Whilst a bone scan may show multiple bony metastases in ribs and spine, the patient may only be complaining of pain in one rib. One treats the symptoms, not the scan.

The priority is to establish which areas are really troubling the patient. Each symptom will need addressing in order of priority.

Pain is the most pressing symptom. Pain interferes with mobility and sleep and lowers morale in the whole family. However, 80–90% of pain can be successfully controlled by oral analgesia and adjuvant medication. About 10–20% of patients have pain which is difficult to control and relatively resistant to opioid analgesia.

Some complications such as spinal cord compression require urgent assessment and treatment if neurological function is to be improved or retained (p. 553). Symptoms are often multiple. Each will need addressing in order of priority. Since the patient's life expectancy is short and symptoms are unpleasant and frightening, prompt assessment and treatment is required.

The patient should be constantly reviewed, as symptoms may change daily in nature, site and severity. Experienced nursing staff, seeing the patients frequently and monitoring their physical and mental state, are the backbone of good palliative care.

Guidelines for treatment

Treatment should be aimed at specific goals, without upsetting the patient or attempting to prolong life inappropriately. The patient and family should be given a straightforward explanation of these aims, and of the reasons for a change in treatment.

Pain

Pain is a presenting feature in 30–45% of patients with cancer and occurs in 70% of those with advanced disease. In two-thirds of patients the pain is caused by the cancer itself.

Multiple sites of pain are common, with 80% of patients having more than one site. In one hospice the three commonest causes of pain were bone, nerve compression and soft tissue disease. The types of treatment for cancer pain are summarised in Figure 36.1.

Assessment. Pain has both physical and psychological components. Anxiety or depression may accentuate the perception of pain and lower the pain threshold. Conversely, elevation of mood may raise the pain threshold. In addition to monitoring the physical attributes of pain, especially the site, character, frequency and intensity, the psychological state of the patient needs to be assessed and frequently reviewed.

Principles of analgesic treatment. The following guidelines should be followed:

1. Establish the cause of the pain.
2. Give a suitable analgesic on a regular and prophylactic basis.
3. Start with simple non-opioid analgesia and progress, if necessary, to opiates.
4. Use the oral route if possible.
5. Choose the minimum dose that controls the pain.
6. Increase the dose of opioid analgesia until the patient is pain free.

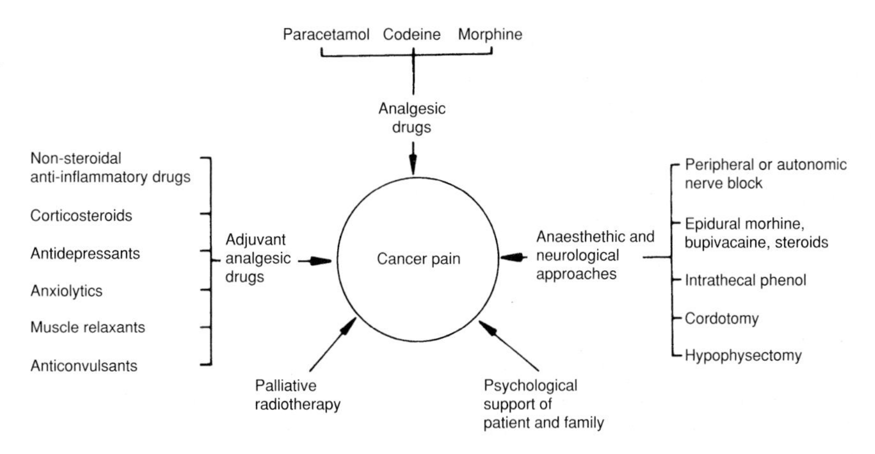

Fig. 36.1 The treatment of cancer pain. (Reproduced from Baines, British Medical Journal, 1989 with permission from the BMJ Publishing Group.)

7. Deal with psychological factors which may be influencing the pain.
8. Consider the use of coanalgesics such as non-steroidal anti-inflammatory drugs (NSAIDs), steroids, and antidepressants.
9. Consider non-drug treatments, such as radiotherapy, nerve blocks, splints and physiotherapy.
10. Regularly review the situation.

Escalation of analgesia

Mild and moderate pain

1. Paracetamol (1 g 4-hourly) and aspirin (300–1200 mg 4-hourly) are suitable for mild pain.

2. Aspirin or another NSAID such as flurbiprofen (50 mg t.d.s. or q.d.s.) is useful for moderate pain.

3. NSAIDs often cause gastric upset which may be relieved by an oral antacid or an H_2-receptor blocker such as ranitidine (150 mg b.d.) or cimetidine (400 mg b.d.).

4. A low-efficacy opioid such as codeine or dihydrocodeine (30–60 mg 4-hourly), sometimes usefully in combination with an NSAID, may be sufficient for moderate pain.

Severe pain

1. Strong opioids such as morphine or diamorphine are indicated for severe pain. Morphine or diamorphine are often usefully combined with NSAIDs in this situation.

2. Inexperienced practitioners may be reluctant to prescribe morphine for fear of psychological or physical dependence. If morphine is used appropriately, psychological dependence is not a problem. If the pain becomes less severe or subsides completely it is possible to wean the patient off morphine without precipitating the symptoms of physical dependence.

3. The dose of oral morphine sulphate may vary from as little as 5 up to over 100 mg 4-hourly. Long-acting preparations of morphine sulphate, such as MST Continus tablets, enable dosage to be given twice daily only. Pain control is generally achieved more quickly if analgesic opioid requirements are established by titrating the dose of oral morphine sulphate every 4 hours.

4. Suggested increments are: 2.5, 5, 10, 15, 20, 30, 45, 60, 90, 120, 180, 240 and 320 mg. Doses beyond 320 mg 4-hourly are unlikely to achieve better pain control. Some forms of pain are intractable to usual doses of opioids. The role of psychological factors should be considered where escalating doses of morphine are not controlling the pain.

5. A larger dose of morphine at bedtime, one and a half to twice the daytime 4-hourly dose, may enable the patient to sleep through the night without being woken by pain, or by a nurse.

6. Once the daily total morphine requirement has been determined, the patient's dosage may be converted to a b.d. regime of a long-acting oral morphine preparation. For example a patient controlled on 20 mg 4-hourly has a daily morphine requirement of 120 mg, which could be given as 60 mg of MST b.d.

7. A regular laxative is necessary to prevent the inevitable constipation caused by morphine.

8. With the exception of children and the elderly, approximately 80% of patients are controlled on 20 mg of morphine 4-hourly. For patients with bone metastases, 60–90 mg 4-hourly are often needed, often combined with an NSAID.

9. Choice between morphine and diamorphine:

a. The actions and side-effects of morphine and diamorphine (heroin) are similar. Diamorphine is metabolised to morphine and another active metabolite very quickly and before it reaches the central nervous system.

b. Although diamorphine is more potent than morphine, the efficacy of both drugs is the same. Diamorphine is preferred for injections (intravenous/subcutaneous/intramuscular) because it is more soluble than morphine.

c. For oral use, the conversion factor is 1.5, so that 10 mg of diamorphine is equivalent to 15 mg of morphine. For injection, 5 mg of injected diamorphine is equivalent to 15 mg of oral morphine, a conversion factor of 3.

10. Other routes of administration:

a. If a patient is unable to swallow, then sublingual, subcutaneous, intramuscular and rectal routes are alternatives.

b. The sublingual route is suitable if the patient has adequate saliva. Buprenorphine, an opioid, 0.2–0.4 mg 8-hourly may be a useful equivalent to 60–240 mg of morphine daily. Both morphine and another potent opioid, phenazocine, may also be given by this route.

c. A continuous subcutaneous infusion of diamorphine via an indwelling butterfly needle, usually placed into the abdominal wall, is useful when oral medication is not possible because of nausea and vomiting, dysphagia, weakness or unconsciousness. Regular injections can largely be avoided. Diamorphine is delivered via a syringe driver, with most syringe drivers being calibrated in millimetres per 24 hours. With a standard 10 ml syringe a rate of 2 mm per hour is typical. The syringe can be topped up in hospital or, if qualified staff are available, at home. The infusion site usually has to be changed every 3 days.

d. Other drugs can be given via a syringe driver, in addition to diamorphine. These include antiemetics such as haloperidol, levomepromazine (methotrimeprazine) and cyclizine; and hyoscine for a 'death rattle'.

e. Intramuscular injections are sometimes necessary for the same indications as for the subcutaneous route. Diamorphine injections are given regularly every 4 hours if they are the sole form of opioid analgesia.

f. Morphine (10, 15, 30 and 60 mg suppositories) and oxycodone (30 mg and 60 mg) are strong analgesics that can be given by the rectal route. Oxycodone acts for longer (6–8 hours) than morphine (4 hours).

g. In patients who become very sedated on high doses of oral morphine required to control their pain, the insertion of an epidural catheter to deliver morphine may be considered. These are usually inserted by an anaesthetist.

The central tranquillising effect of morphine is absent and an anxiolytic may be needed. There is a lack of constipation normally caused by oral morphine.

Complications include dislodgement or blockage of the catheter requiring reinsertion. However, some catheters have remained in situ for up to 250 days.

h. Nerve blocks are appropriate in a limited set of circumstances. The advice of an anaesthetist should be sought. When very high doses of narcotics are ineffective, or when the pain is very localised, nerve blocks may be helpful. The solution injected normally includes phenol and alcohol.

(i) Intercostal blocks are useful for rib metastases, chest wall infiltration and pathological fractures.

(ii) A brachial plexus block may relieve the pain of a Pancoast tumour or malignant infiltration of the plexus, commonly by breast cancer.

(iii) Coeliac axis block. Pain from pancreatic cancer can be relieved in up to 75% of cases. This procedure is associated with a risk of hypotension, and hospitalisation is required for 24–48 hours after the procedure.

(iv) A pudendal block is helpful for perineal pain.

Pain that is difficult to control with opioid analgesia. There are a small group of patients whose pain responds poorly to opioid analgesia. Much higher doses are required and this may result in severe unwanted side-effects such as drowsiness. Neuropathic pain falls into this category. It is due to direct infiltration of nerves by tumour. Patients sometimes find it difficult to describe the character of the pain but burning or aching are common descriptors. Initial treatment is with a tricyclic antidepressant such as amitriptyline. If this fails, an anticonvulsant, e.g. sodium valproate, can be tried (starting at 200 mg b.d. and increasing to a total dose of 1600 mg per day). Some patients may benefit from the use of a transcutaneous nerve stimulator. Steroids (dexamethasone 8 mg per day) may help by reducing local oedema at the site of tumour infiltration.

Nausea and vomiting

Nausea and vomiting trouble about 40% of patients who are terminally ill. The causes of these symptoms are legion and treatment should depend on the cause. They may be due to the cancer, its treatment or concurrent medical or surgical conditions. Common causes are summarised in Table 36.1. Stimuli to vomiting may act at the level of the cortex or the gut. In this process neurotransmitters play an important role. Many of the drugs effective in treating emesis are neurotransmitter blockers.

Drug-induced vomiting is common. Haloperidol is the treatment of choice. In addition it has anxiolytic and antipsychotic properties. A dose of 1–1.5 mg is given stat

Table 36.1 Causes of nausea and vomiting in malignant disease (reproduced with permission from Twycross & Lack, 1990)

Due to cancer	Due to treatment
Irritation of the upper gastrointestinal tract	Radiotherapy
	Chemotherapy
Gastrointestinal obstruction	Drugs, e.g.
Constipation	Opioids
Hepatomegaly	NSAIDs
Raised intracranial pressure	Aspirin
Anxiety	Antibiotics
Pain	Carbamazepine
Hypercalcaemia	Steroids
Hyponatraemia	Oestrogen
Uraemia	Iron
	Expectorant mucolytics
Other conditions	
Peptic ulceration	
Infection	

and nocte. If the night dose is inadequate, it is increased to 3–5 mg. For radiation-induced vomiting 5 mg is suggested. For chemotherapy or metabolic causes of vomiting, 5–20 mg nocte or in divided doses is often necessary. Its side-effects are anticholinergic (e.g. dry mouth, constipation), extrapyramidal reactions and sedation. For further discussion of chemotherapy-induced vomiting, see Chapter 34.

Metoclopramide (10 mg 4-hourly oral/intramuscular) is suitable if nausea and vomiting are due to physical or chemical irritation of the stomach. It increases gastric emptying, upper gastrointestinal peristalsis and contracts the lower oesophageal sphincter.

Prochlorperazine (5–10 mg 4–8-hourly), a phenothiazine, is preferred if the patient is anxious, since it is also sedative. Chlorpromazine (25 mg 6–8-hourly) is an alternative phenothiazine.

Dexamethasone (4 mg 6-hourly) is used to relieve nausea and vomiting due to raised intracranial pressure (Ch. 30). If this fails, cyclizine 50 mg b.d. is often helpful.

With severe vomiting an initial intramuscular injection should be given followed by a subcutaneous infusion linked to a syringe driver.

For chemotherapy-induced vomiting (e.g. cisplatin or anthracyclines) a 5-HT_3 antagonist such granisetron 1 mg or ondansetron 2.5 mg is advised, combined with dexamethasone 8 mg as an i.v. bolus.

Dysphagia

Dysphagia encompasses any problem in moving liquids or solids from the mouth to the stomach. The process requires a normal mucosa, intact 5th, 7th and 9th–12th cranial nerves and coordinated function of smooth and skeletal muscle. The causes (Table 36.2) may be related to the tumour, treatment, neurological damage or intercurrent illness, or a combination of these factors.

Treatment will depend on the cause. If the patient is able to swallow liquids but not solids, a liquidised diet is advised. If even fluids cannot be swallowed, an endo-oesophageal tube is needed. If the oesophageal aperture is 1 cm or more, a Clinifeed tube can usually be passed through the nose into the stomach using a guidewire. If this is not possible, insertion of a Celestin tube into the oesophagus under general anaesthesia should be considered. Intravenous fluids are often needed to correct the initial dehydration.

Oropharyngeal candidiasis is treated by oral antifungal agents (e.g. nystatin, 100 000 u/ml, 1–5 ml 4-hourly). Treatment of the tumour by surgery, radiotherapy or chemotherapy or debulking by laser therapy may relieve obstruction.

Table 36.2 Causes of dysphagia in malignant disease (reproduced with permission from Twycross & Lack, 1990)

1. Caused by cancer
   - (a) Intraluminal
     Tumour in mouth, pharynx or oesophagus
   - (b) Intramural
     Infiltration of the pharyngeal or oesophageal wall
   - (c) Extraluminal
     External compression by mediastinal nodes or tumour
2. Neurological
   e.g. damage to brainstem or disruption of motor (5th, 7th, 9th–12th) or sensory (5th, 9th, 10th) pathways of cranial nerves
3. Caused by treatment
   - (a) Radiation
     Loss of saliva; acute oral, pharyngeal or oesophageal reaction; radiation fibrosis in mouth/pharynx/oesophagus (stricture)
   - (b) Chemotherapy
     Oral mucositis
   - (c) Surgery—radical resections, e.g. tongue flap repairs
4. Intercurrent conditions
   Benign oesophageal stricture; oral/pharyngeal/oesophageal candidiasis

Benign or radiation-induced strictures can be dilated. Dilatation may have to be repeated if dysphagia recurs.

Anorexia

The origin of anorexia is often multifactorial. Causes include the underlying malignancy or its complications (e.g. bowel obstruction or pain), treatment by radiotherapy or chemotherapy, alteration in taste, oral ulceration, depression and anxiety. Anorexia is closely linked to cachexia. It is thought that the presence of a cancer stimulates the release of cytokines from the immune system such as cachectin-tumour necrosis factor and interleukins 1 and 6. In addition, tumours can secrete products which induce lipolysis, induce anorexia and net loss of nitrogen.

The advice of a dietician familiar with the dietary problems of patients with cancer should be sought. Such advice can have a very positive effect on a patient's morale. Guidance is needed on the amount of liquid food (e.g. Buildup or Complan) required to supplement the normal diet in order to maintain body weight. Nasogastric feeding (see above) may be necessary if the patient is unable to swallow.

Treatment of the cause, alteration of diet and appetite stimulants may all help.

Loss of taste may be improved by adding seasoning to foods. Fish, poultry or eggs may provide protein when appetite for meat is lost. Flexibility and imagination in presentation and in the frequency, content and volume of meals are needed.

A trial over 7–10 days of oral steroids (prednisolone 15–30 mg mane) or dexamethasone 2–4 mg is worthwhile and sometimes improves the appetite. However, the benefits only last 3–4 weeks and are purely subjective with no improvement in caloric intake or nutrition status.

Medroxyprogesterone acetate and megestrol acetate are progestational agents which do improve caloric intake and nutritional status. There are, however, unwanted side-effects of oedema and an increased risk of thrombosis.

Dyspnoea

Dyspnoea occurs in 50% of patients who are terminally ill. It is a frightening symptom. The anxiety that it generates (will I suffocate or stop breathing?) exacerbates the symptom. In many cases treatment of the underlying cause (e.g. tapping pleural effusion, relieving bronchial obstruction by radiotherapy (Ch. 25), correction of anaemia) is effective. Where anxiety is a factor, an anxiolytic (diazepam 10 mg stat or 5–20 mg nocte) may help. To break the cycle of anxiety and increasing breathlessness, relaxation exercises are encouraged (remain calm, purse lips, relax shoulder, back and arms and concentrate on breathing slowly). In the acute situation lorazepam 0.5–2 mg sublingually may help, since it has a rapid if short-lived action. By contrast diazepam is long acting (half-life 15–20 hours) and can be given as a single night-time dose.

Morphine depresses both the respiratory rate and the sense of distress (2.5–5 mg orally 4-hourly). Where the patient is already on morphine for pain, the dose should be increased by 50% to relieve dyspnoea. Oxygen by mask or nasal spectacles reduces hypoxia. It is helpful in acute dyspnoea. Reassurance from staff, relaxation and breathing exercises can all assist.

For wheezing due to bronchial obstruction or lymphangitis carcinomatosa, steroids are worth a trial (prednisolone 10 mg orally q.d.s.).

Anxiety and depression

It is said that anxiety and depression are experienced by at least a quarter of patients undergoing treatment for cancer. This is almost certainly an underestimate. The diagnosis is made more commonly by staff who have received psychiatric or psychological training. Since medical or psychological therapy may often help, close liaison with a clinical psychologist or psychiatrist should be established.

Patients often do not mention mental symptoms, owing to a sense of shame or because they think that the staff are only interested in physical symptoms. Alternatively, they may not realise that their symptoms are psychological rather than physical. Patients may reveal these symptoms to any member of staff, often to a dietician or physiotherapist, who is seen as an impartial confidant(e). Good communication between staff is needed to ensure that such information is passed on to medical and nursing staff.

Clinical features

The symptoms of anxiety may be divided into psychological and somatic. Psychological symptoms include weakness, dizziness, feelings of illness, insecurity and irritability. Somatic symptoms include palpitations, breathlessness, chest pain, headache, paraesthesia, fatigue, sweating, flushing, dry mouth and urinary frequency.

The main symptom of depression is low mood. This is commonly accompanied by loss of appetite and of sexual interest, inability to enjoy pleasurable events, insomnia, loss of energy and interest in work, slowing of movement and reduced facial expression, loss of self-esteem, anxiety, reduced ability to think and concentrate, suicidal thoughts, and bodily complaints including constipation, nausea and vomiting.

Distinguishing between the normal feelings of sadness and disappointment and clinical depression is often difficult. This again emphasises the need for access to expert psychological advice.

Fear induced by the diagnosis of cancer. The diagnosis of malignancy still induces widespread fear, irrespective of whether cure is possible. Most adult patients know someone who has died of malignancy. The experience understandably colours their own expectations of cancer treatment and of prognosis. Fears about unpleasant treatment, separation from family, change in body image, loss of job and income and career advancement are common. The loss of these aspects of normal life is like a bereavement reaction. This starts with a sense of disbelief and is followed by mental agonising, dejection and finally but not invariably an acceptance of the reality. Some patients cope by denying their illness.

Many of these fears can be overcome by a clear explanation of investigations, treatment and the prospects of cure or palliation. It is important to consider the whole patient and not simply the patient's symptoms. An interest expressed in a patient's life (family, job or interest) may have a very positive effective on morale.

Prognosis. In regard to prognosis, it is often helpful to ask the patient how specific an answer he or she requires. Some patients find the knowledge of their probability of 5-year survival reassuring if it is high but depressing if it is low.

Financial worries. Concerns about the consequences of time off work for family and personal finances can often be alleviated. Guidance from a medical social worker can be given on eligibility for disability or attendance allowances or for help for relatives with travelling expenses to and from the hospital.

Efficient delivery of services. The management of cancer frequently involves a multiplicity of appointments for investigation and treatment. Delays incurred in waiting for investigations and uncertainties as to when tests or treatment will be carried out all contribute to the patient's anxiety. Prompt, courteous and informed answers from clinical and clerical staff all help to allay anxiety.

Communication with the general practitioner. The patient's general practitioner needs to be regularly briefed about his or her patient's progress, prognosis and plans for further management. The anxious patient may well have forgotten what the oncologist said in the initial consultation and often looks to the family doctor for explanation and reassurance. If the general practitioner is concerned about new symptoms in a patient, an early outpatient appointment should be arranged. If the patient is not well enough, a domiciliary visit can be arranged. Such visits are reassuring to patient, family and general practitioner, even if no change in therapy is considered appropriate.

Medical treatment

Anxiety. Time spent discussing a patient's concerns about the diagnosis, investigation, treatment, prognosis or other issues can substantially reduce anxiety. Relief of physical symptoms such as pain, vomiting or constipation reassures the patient that clinical staff have the medical condition under control.

If the patient still remains anxious, anxiolytics, e.g. diazepam, a benzodiazepine, 2–20 mg orally nocte may be needed. If the patient also has pain of a severity to justify morphine, the anxiolytic effect of morphine may avoid the need for a benzodiazepine.

Depression. If depressive symptoms do not lift with explanation and reassurance, medical treatment is indicated. The most widely used are the tricyclic and related antidepressants. The choice of antidepressant will depend upon the clinical features of depression. The starting dose should be small and built up over 3–4 weeks to a maintenance dose. Clomipramine initially in a dose of 10 mg orally nocte and increased to 50–150 mg is useful in patients with associated obsessional features. It has some anticholinergic effects. Amitriptyline 25 mg orally nocte and increased to 50–75 mg has more sedative and anticholinergic effects.

Palliative surgery

Palliative surgery has a variety of useful roles. The decision to operate will take into account the severity of symptoms, the general condition of the patient, life expectancy and probability of benefit.

Operations include: (1) stabilising painful pathological limb fractures and restoring mobility; (2) toilet mastectomy for malodorous or bleeding advanced breast tumours; (3) decompression of spinal cord compression if pretreatment neurological deficit is not marked; (4) debulking of brain tumours or aspiration of cystic tumours to relieve raised intracranial pressure; and (5) colostomy for bowel obstruction or rectovaginal fistula.

CHAPTER CONTENTS

37

Quality of life

Ian Kunkler and Jane Kunkler

In the last decade there has been a rapid expansion of interest in the nature and measurement of the quality of life of patients with cancer. Cancer touches a wide range of aspects of life: psychological, physical, spiritual and cultural. It is widely accepted that the diagnosis and treatment of cancer have a major disruptive effect on most patients' lives. The influence of psychological factors on patients with cancer is discussed in an earlier chapter (p. 639).

The concept of quality of life is not a new one. It is enshrined in the Hippocratic oath taken by doctors to do no harm to their patients. Clinical staff are well aware that surgery, radiotherapy and chemotherapy can have both transient and long- term unpleasant side-effects. There is increasing public awareness of quality of life as an issue in the choice of anticancer treatment.

Traditionally the outcomes of cancer treatment have been measured in terms of survival alone. However, quality of life is increasingly being included in the assessment of outcome in clinical trials, although there is less agreement on its definition and measurement. Routine incorporation of quality of life (QOL) measures into clinical practice has yet to be achieved. However, the development of computer-based acquisition of QOL in the outpatient setting may facilitate the much wider acceptance of measurement of QOL.

IMPORTANCE OF QUALITY OF LIFE AND ITS MEASUREMENT

The need for objectivity

Why is more objective, time-consuming and potentially costly assessment necessary? First, if quality of life is sufficiently important to influence treatment decisions and policies, it is worth the effort of measuring it as accurately as possible. Secondly, subjective impressions may result in capricious and misleading results. Thirdly, it helps to identify what aspects of health, illness and treatment do and do not concern patients. A knowledge of the important factors in a patient's quality of life may clarify the care and support that he or she needs.

Already quality of life assessments are included in the evaluation of the efficacy of a variety of trials of cancer therapy. Only 4% of cancer trials included a measurement of quality of life in 1975–1976. Now most trials of new anticancer therapies will incorporate some form of quality of life assessment. This is likely to increase further if quality of life assessments are found to be practical, valid and reliable. To date there have been fewer quality of life assessments in radiotherapy and surgery than in chemotherapy. However, they are very relevant to the assessment of all forms of cancer therapy.

Assessment of toxicity

With increasing survival following curative treatment for cancer, the importance of long-term sequelae are increasingly being appreciated. This is particularly pertinent to children where growth, intellectual function, mobility and endocrine function may all be affected.

Where the therapeutic intent is cure, patients will generally endure substantial side-effects (e.g. severe vomiting from cisplatin in the treatment of testicular teratoma). However, many treatments for advanced stages of common cancers (e.g. breast and colon) are still palliative. None the less, some therapies, particularly chemotherapy, inevitably cause toxicity if useful regression of disease is to be achieved. Toxicity is less of a problem with well-planned palliative radiotherapy.

The toxicity (morbidity) of treatment is inextricably linked to quality of life. One of the principles of good palliation (p. 307) is that minimal upset should be caused to the patient. Where two palliative treatments for cancer offer equal probabilities of disease regression, the one offering the patient the best quality of life is clearly preferable.

Choosing between alternative anticancer therapies

The initial focus of quality of life was in terminal care and advanced disease. However, quality of life assessment has a much broader application to the comparison of both curative and palliative treatments in cancer and to other diseases. For example, where cure rates of two treatments are similar (e.g. for stage I carcinoma of the cervix by surgery or radical radiotherapy), the quality of life of the patients on each treatment should strongly influence both patient and clinician in the choice of treatment.

A MODEL OF QUALITY OF LIFE

Calman has stated that: 'the quality of life can only be described and measured in individual terms, and depends on past experiences and future hopes and dreams and ambitions.' Life is of good quality when expectations are matched by their achievement. For poor quality of life the converse is true. Quality of life may vary over time, influenced by personal and therapeutic successes or failures. Calman's model provides a useful representation of quality of life (Fig. 37.1). The upper line represents the hopes, ambitions and dreams of the individual. The lower line represents reality. Quality of life is measured by the gap between the two lines. Quality of life improves the closer each line is to the other and deteriorates the further apart they are.

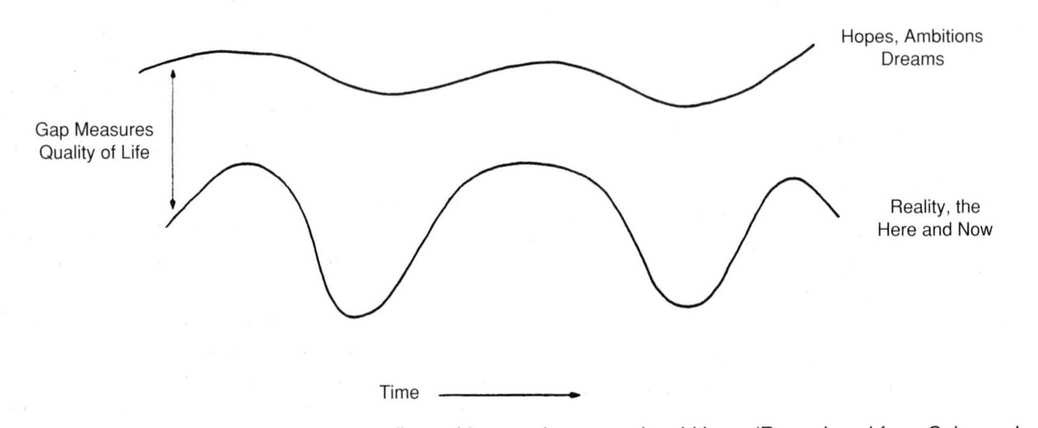

Fig. 37.1 Representation of the gap between reality and hopes, dreams and ambitions. (Reproduced from Calman, Journal of Medical Ethics, 1984 with permission from the BMJ Publishing Group.)

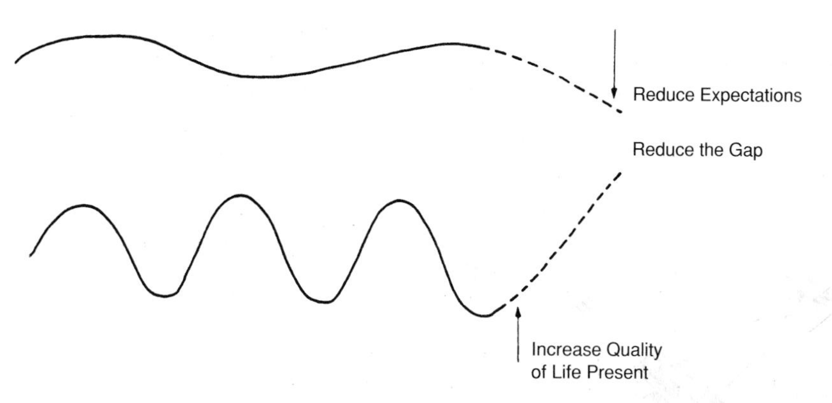

Fig. 37.2 The improvement in the quality of life represents either a reduction in expectations or a change in reality. (Reproduced from Calman, Journal of Medical Ethics, 1984 with permission from the BMJ Publishing Group.)

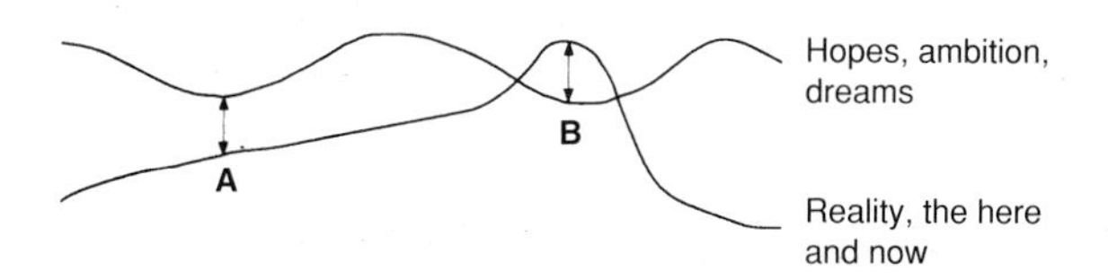

Fig. 37.3 Modification of Calman's model, showing expectation (top line) falling short of reality (lower line) at A and exceeding it at B.

To narrow the gap, and so improve the quality of life, one has to modify either expectations or reality (Fig. 37.2). If reality exceeds expectation, the lines will cross (Fig. 37.3).

To illustrate this model: if a terminally ill patient anticipates, unrealistically, returning from hospital to live at home, quality of life will be poor if he or she remains in hospital. If the patient accepts that he or she is unable to go home but can realistically expect to be ambulant about the ward, quality of life may be higher. In terminal illness the patient needs limited but achievable goals for quality of life to be maintained at a reasonable level.

DEFINITION OF QUALITY OF LIFE

Ever since Aristotle wrote in his *Ethics* 'When it comes to saying in what happiness consists, opinions differ', there has never been a universally agreed definition of quality of life. Its definition will vary with the emphasis that each individual puts on each of its components.

Although definitions of quality of life vary, most would agree that it should include the following areas:

- Psychological functioning
- Physical and occupational functioning
- Social interaction
- Physical symptoms.

Psychological functioning

Stress and coping

It has long been thought that there is an association between an individual's life and illness or maladjustment. It is not possible to say what constitutes good coping behaviour in a given situation but there are indications of patterns of behaviour associated with poor coping (e.g. rumination, anger with oneself, alcohol abuse).

There is a growing body of evidence that factors such as the number and characteristics of major life events may influence the natural history of cancer.

Life events. A person's experiences can make an individual vulnerable to stress. This in turn may make the person more prone to feeling unable to cope. The physiological responses of anxiety may then influence, via the pituitary–adrenal axis, the patient's susceptibility to certain hormone tumours (e.g. breast cancer). Additional factors include not only the more major life events (e.g. bereavement and moving house) but the minor irritations of daily living (e.g. finding a parking place).

Social support. The degree of social support that the person perceives as being available can also affect the degree of stress and coping, and thus the quality of life.

Personality and cognitive processes. The psychological make-up of an individual (which is influenced by the person's own genetic make-up or experiences) has a considerable impact on the capacity to cope with major life events, such as cancer, and minor daily stresses. Individuals vary in the ways in which they cope with these stresses. Some may deploy problem-solving skills and weigh up the advantages and disadvantages before deciding on any particular course of action. Others find themselves paralysed by the seriousness of the diagnosis of cancer. Still others may cope by avoiding thinking about the diagnosis or denying its existence. The coping strategies used by individuals may vary over time, even though they may tend generally to have preferred styles of coping.

Patients' appraisal of the situation will depend on their thinking (cognitive) processes and their resources and options for coping. Their response to the diagnosis may be influenced by the probability of cure given by the clinician. If there is a reasonable prospect of cure, it may be possible to concentrate one's energy on achieving that outcome. If the tumour is incurable, 'fighting' the cancer may seem pointless.

Locus of control. Patients' perception of their quality of life also depends on whether they feel that they have any influence over their lives and treatment (*internal locus of control*) or feel that they are controlled by it or that what happens is entirely due to chance (*external locus of control*). Those who feel they can have some influence may take a more active role in complying with treatment regimes. They may, for example, do exercises to avoid postoperative complications of immobility (e.g. deep venous thrombosis or chest infection) which can reduce quality of life. Some may respond with fighting spirit, while others respond with little or none. Personality factors (feelings of mastery, self-esteem, strong commitments, religious beliefs and values) may also play a role.

Anxiety and depression. Anxiety and depression commonly affect patients with cancer and impair their capacity to cope. Worries about the effects of unemployment on the ability to meet personal and family financial commitments add to the anxiety generated by diagnosis, treatment and prognosis.

Physical and occupational functioning

Physical functioning

The local, regional and metastatic spread of cancer may result in considerable functional impairment and change in body image. Brain tumours may result in paralysis of one side of the body (hemiparesis) such that the patient is unable to walk and is confined to a wheelchair. Tumours of the frontal lobes may cause urinary incontinence due to interference with cortical control of continence. Bowel or bladder tumours may require a colostomy or urostomy, resulting in loss of normal control of bowel and bladder emptying, respectively.

Regional lymphatic spread to the axilla from breast cancer may result in a swollen, heavy and useless arm owing to lymphoedema. Lymphoedema of the legs because of para-aortic node metastases or spinal cord compression (p. 553) may limit the patient's mobility.

Mutilating head and neck surgery may interfere with eating and swallowing. Mastectomy may be perceived as resulting in reduced femininity. Both pelvic radical radiotherapy and surgery may limit the normal sexual functioning of the vagina.

Occupational functioning

Cancer and its treatment may limit both the physical and mental capacity of a patient to carry out his or her previous job. Confusion or impaired memory because of brain disease may preclude the carrying out of the simplest tasks at work. Visual field defects or epilepsy may prevent the patient from driving. The patient may lose his or her job if dependent on a car to fulfil work commitments. Impaired sensation in the fingertips from the neurotoxicity of vinca alkaloids may prevent work requiring manual dexterity. Any impairment of the capacity to walk may limit access to places of work, particularly where stairs have to be climbed. Sometimes it is loss of energy from the effects of the disease or treatment, inability to concentrate, anxiety or depression, or lack of confidence which limit a return to work.

Social interaction

For most people interpersonal relationships are essential to their happiness. The support of family, friends and health care professionals can be of inestimable value to patients in enabling them to cope with cancer.

However, their previous ability to socialise, whether as a spouse or parent or in peer groups, may be altered by their illness. This may result in loss of self-esteem. Marital dysharmony, breakdown and divorce are not uncommon results.

Patients may be reluctant to attend social gatherings because of embarrassment from disfiguring facial or breast surgery, weight gain or loss, or odour from a fungating tumour. Lack of physical energy and loss of earning capacity may also limit attendance and participation.

Members of the general public may believe that the cancer itself is contagious. As a result the company of the patient may be shunned. Refusing to eat or drink from cutlery or crockery used by the patient or to use bedclothes in which the patient has slept is not uncommon. Such behaviour reinforces isolation.

Physical symptoms

Symptoms such as nausea, vomiting, pain and immobility have a major impact on the quality of life. These may be features of the disease (e.g. pain from bone metastases) or of the treatment (nausea from chemotherapy or radiotherapy or difficulty swallowing from radical surgery for oral cancer). Chronic pain, for example, can dominate a patient's consciousness, making him or her a virtual prisoner. Nevertheless, it should be stressed that good quality of life is more than just the absence of symptoms.

ASSESSMENT OF THE QUALITY OF LIFE

Problems in assessment

There are many difficulties in assessing quality of life. There are the usual problems of designing questionnaires. These include ordering and weighting the questions to avoid response bias and 'halo' effects. There are also difficulties particular to assessing quality of life. These include separating out factors due to the illness, its treatment or psychological factors (which are themselves influenced by the illness and its treatment) such as anxiety and depression. A further complication is that psychological factors such as stress and coping are difficult to define and therefore to assess. The design of assessment measures and the analysis and interpretation of results need to be carried out by staff with training in questionnaire design, research methodology and analysis and a good understanding of psychological assessment and of the physical effects of the illness and its treatment. Clinical psychologists have appropriate training in these areas and are well placed to collaborate with clinical oncologists in assessing quality of life.

There are interactions between all of the areas outlined above. For example a depressed psychological state may influence physical (retardation), social (isolation) and occupational functioning (unemployment). Both the disease and its treatment and the patient's response to them and the reactions of others may influence physical, psychological and social well-being.

Questionnaires and rating scales

The assessment of quality of life can be based on casual observations or on a more formal structured basis. At the simplest level the patient can be asked whether the quality of life is the same, better or worse than it was before treatment. However, comparison between patients is impossible without some agreement on what elements of quality of life are being assessed and how they are defined and quantified. This has led to the development of more structured measures of assessment, which include questionnaires and rating scales.

Choice of test

The choice of assessment method for measuring the quality of life will depend on the aim, the aspects of quality of life considered most relevant and the time and personnel available to carry out the assessment. There are, for example, well-established scales of toxicity following chemotherapy. The most widely used is the WHO grading system. The performance status of the patient is commonly assessed using the Karnofsky or International Union Against Cancer (UICC) scales (Table 37.1) before, during and after treatment.

Psychological assessment: linear analogue scales

Psychological assessment is an important part of assessing quality of life. One of the most frequently used methods of assessing this has been to use rating scales. Of these, the *linear analogue scale* is perhaps the most popular. It can be used as a self-rating scale (i.e. it is the subject and not the observer who completes the scale). The subject is asked to make a mark along a 10 cm line joining two extreme descriptions, for example:

Table 37.1 Karnofsky and UICC performance status scales

Karnofsky	
100	Normal, no complaints
90	Normal activity, minimal signs or symptoms
80	Normal activity with effort, some symptoms
70	Caring for self, unable to work
60	Needs occasional assistance, but able to cater for most of needs
50	Needs considerable assistance and frequent medical care
40	Disabled, needs special care
30	Severely disabled, needs hospital care
20	Very ill, in hospital, needs supportive care
10	Moribund
0	Dead
UICC	
Grade	
0	Able to carry out normal activity
1	Able to live at home, with tolerable symptoms
2	Disabling symptoms, but less than 50% of time in bed
3	Severely disabled, greater than 50% of time in bed but able to stand
4	Very ill, confined to bed
5	Dead

Table 37.2 Format of the Rotterdam Symptom Checklist

In this questionnaire you are asked about your symptoms. Would you please, for any of the symptoms mentioned, indicate to what extent you are bothered by it, by circling the answer most applicable to you. The questions are related to the past 3 days (the past week).

Have you, during the last 3 days (week) been bothered by:

Lack of appetite:	not at all	a little	quite a bit	very much
Irritability:	not at all	a little	quite a bit	very much
Tiredness:	not at all	a little	quite a bit	very much
Worrying:	not at all	a little	quite a bit	very much

'I feel sad most of the time'—'I feel happy most of the time'.

The mark represents how the patient is feeling at the time of or shortly before completing the scale. Linear analogue scales have been found to be a reliable and valid method of assessing mood and mood change in depressed patients. They allow small changes in rating to be recorded and are therefore applicable to situations where, as in cancer therapy, repeated assessments are required.

Questionnaires

A variety of questionnaires are available. Some focus on the physical and psychological symptoms. Others measure health more generally, encompassing physical, emotional and social factors. They are based on the concept that health is not simply the absence of illness. Important factors are the selection of the appropriate questionnaire to measure the appropriate endpoint, timing and compliance. If the frequency of administration is excessive, patient interest and compliance will wane. If the questionnaires are not administered frequently, important changes in QOL may be missed.

Questionnaire on QOL fall into three main groups. The first group tend to be short and focused on symptoms, e.g. breathlessness for lung cancer. An example is the daily diary card, which has been successfully applied to patients with lung cancer. This type of questionnaire is well suited to patients whose symptoms are changing over a short-term period. The second group are of medium length and cancer-site specific. An example is the Lung Cancer Symptom Scale. Symptoms of treatment and of disease are treated separately and graded on 10-point analogue scale. The third group of questionnaires are longer and incorporate both cancer-site-specific symptoms and general aspects of QOL. The Functional Assessment of Cancer Therapy (FACT) includes over 40 questions including 33 general questions. Answers are graded on an analogue scale of 0–5 from 'not at all' to 'very much'. The domains covered include: (1) physical; (2) social; (3) emotional; and (4) functional well-being. These domains do not correlate with symptoms, which need to be assessed separately. In this category of questionnaires are included the EORTC (European Organization for Research on Treatment of Cancer) site-specific modules, e.g. for breast cancer. These have been validated and have the advantage of foreign language versions.

If a comparison is being made between cancer and a different disease or a cost–benefit analysis is being attempted, the *Nottingham Health Profile* or *Sickness Impact Profile* is suggested.

Table 37.3 Symptoms (34) included in the Rotterdam Symptom Checklist (modified from de Haes J C J M, Van Knippenberg F C E, Neijt J P 1990 British Journal of Cancer 62: 1034–1038)

Lack of appetite	Feeling lonely
Irritability	Tension
Tiredness	Crying spells
Worrying	Abdominal aches
Sore muscles	Anxiety
Depressed mood	Constipation
Lack of energy	Diarrhoea
Low back pain	Heartburn/belching
Nervousness	Shivering
Nausea	Tingling hands or feet
Desperate feelings about the future	Difficulty concentrating
Difficulties sleeping	Sore mouth/pain when swallowing
Headaches	Loss of hair
Vomiting	Burning (or sore) eyes
Dizziness	Deafness
Decreased sexual interest	Shortness of breath
Itching	Dry mouth

If comparison is being made between cancer patients, a cancer-specific test is needed. Of the cancer-specific tests, the *Rotterdam Symptom Checklist* (RSCL) (Tables 37.2 and 37.3) is currently well regarded in terms of appropriateness, format, administration, scoring structure, clinical usage, reliability and validity. It is intended to measure psychological and physical distress and takes about 8 minutes to complete.

If levels of anxiety and depression are to be included, the *Hospital Anxiety and Depression Scale* (HADS) is recommended. Both RSCL and HADS have the advantages of being relatively quick to complete and being acceptable to patients.

CHAPTER CONTENTS

38

Medical complications of malignant disease

Robert Coleman

Cancer can cause a huge variety of medical and metabolic problems. These can be due to the physical presence of the tumour causing obstruction of, for example, the bile duct or a ureter, secretion of fluid into a body cavity such as the pleura (an effusion) or local invasion of adjacent structures. In addition, cancers frequently predispose the patient to infection and may cause constitutional disturbances which are not due to the local effect of the tumour but are collectively known as paraneoplastic syndromes. The problems of invasion into neighbouring structures are discussed in Chapter 17. In this chapter we discuss the problems caused by effusions, infection and paraneoplastic syndromes (Table 38.1) in malignancy.

EFFUSIONS SECONDARY TO MALIGNANT DISEASE

Normally, the pleural, pericardial and peritoneal spaces contain only a few millilitres of fluid to lubricate the inner and outer surfaces. However, in cancer the normal capillary and lymphatic vessels can become damaged and the hydrostatic pressures which regulate the transfer of fluid from one compartment of the body to another are disturbed. A build-up of fluid at any of these three sites can cause unpleasant symptoms which require treatment. Although effusions are usually a sign of advanced malignancy and treatment is only palliative, intervention is worthwhile and can provide useful benefit and improvement in quality of life.

Pleural effusions

The commonest malignancy to cause a pleural effusion is carcinoma of the bronchus. In addition, metastasis from carcinoma of the breast, other adenocarcinomas and lymphoma may also quite frequently cause pleural

Table 38.1 Endocrine and paraneoplastic manifestations of malignancy

System	Manifestation
Endocrine	Hypercalcaemia due to parathyroid hormone related peptide Water retention due to inappropriate ADH secretion Cushing's syndrome due to ACTH Hypoglycaemia due to insulin-like proteins/somatomedins Gynaecomastia due to human chorionic gonadotrophin Thyrotoxicosis due to human chorionic gonadotrophin
Neurological	Peripheral neuropathy Cerebellar ataxia Dementia Transverse myelitis Myasthenia gravis Eaton–Lambert syndrome
Haematological/vascular	Anaemia Polycythaemia Thrombophlebitis Red cell aplasia Thromboembolism Disseminated intravascular coagulation Non-bacterial endocarditis
Musculoskeletal	Polymyalgia rheumatica Arthralgia Clubbing Hypertrophic pulmonary osteoarthropathy
Dermatological	Pruritus Various skin rashes
Renal	Nephrotic syndrome

effusions. Clinical detection is not possible until at least 500 ml has accumulated, and typically the effusion comprises 1000–4000 ml of fluid. This is usually straw coloured but may be blood-stained and will cause increasing shortness of breath, a dry cough and sometimes pain as it increases in size.

Drainage of the fluid is required for relief of symptoms. This can be performed through a needle inserted into the pleural space, which provides good emergency management, but, to prevent recurrence of the effusion, either effective treatment of the underlying cancer is required or the effusion must be drained to dryness. To achieve this, a flexible drainage tube needs to be inserted into the pleural space and the fluid allowed to drain via a sealed drainage system which prevents air from replacing the fluid. Drainage should be relatively slow as sudden removal of large volumes of fluid causes distress to the patient due to shift of the mediastinal structures, and this may also precipitate pulmonary oedema. After 24–48 hours, when the effusion has drained to dryness, it is usual to inject a drug or chemical into the pleural space to effect a pleurodesis. This will inflame the pleural surfaces to encourage sticking together of the two layers and the development of fibrosis. Tetracycline and bleomycin are the most commonly used agents and will prevent recurrence of the effusion in 50–75% of patients. If recurrent effusions remain a problem after this approach, referral to a thoracic surgeon may be worthwhile to drain the fluid under general anaesthetic and insufflate talcum powder, a more effective method of achieving a pleurodesis.

Pericardial effusions

Pericardial effusions are much less common than pleural effusions. Again the same tumour types are usually responsible but probably less than 1% of cancer patients will develop a symptomatic collection of pericardial fluid. When this does occur the build-up of fluid restricts normal cardiac function and produces symptoms and signs of cardiac failure, first affecting the right ventricle, which as it worsens subsequently impairs left ventricular function, a condition known as cardiac tamponade.

Patients with tamponade are unable to lie flat, have chest discomfort, oedema and breathlessness. When cardiac tamponade develops, urgent drainage of the pericardial fluid can be life-saving and is indicated if the patient is otherwise in reasonable health.

Pericardial drainage is technically more difficult than pleural drainage and is best performed by a cardiologist with ultrasound control to ensure safe placement of the drainage catheter. Treatment of the underlying malignancy will usually prevent recurrence but, if this is not possible, injection of sclerosants into the pericardial space is occasionally advised. However, to prevent recurrent pericardial effusions, the formation of a pericardial window by a thoracic surgeon is preferred if the general condition of the patient makes this a realistic option.

Peritoneal effusions (ascites)

In cancer, ascites is usually caused by widespread peritoneal seedling metastases which exude protein-rich fluid. Liver metastases may contribute to the problem through hypoalbuminaemia or portal hypertension. Ascites is most commonly caused by advanced carcinomas of the ovary, gastrointestinal tract, breast and pancreas. Patients present with abdominal distension which becomes progressively uncomfortable, limits food intake and splints the diaphragm, making breathing difficult. Diagnosis is by clinical examination and is confirmed by ultrasound and aspiration cytology.

Treatment is by tube drainage (paracentesis) and should be performed relatively slowly, generally not exceeding a rate of 500 ml/hour. Drainage to dryness is not realistic and therefore sclerosants are less effective for ascites than for pleural effusions. Diuretics are commonly prescribed to prevent reaccumulation but are rarely effective in relieving established ascites. Intraperitoneal radioactive colloids or chemotherapy are sometimes of benefit and agents such as thiotepa, mitoxantrone (mitozantrone) and carboplatin have been used with some success. For recurrent ascites, surgical procedures should be considered if medical treatments have failed to control the underlying disease. A peritoneovenous shunt can be inserted, which drains the fluid through a one-way valve into the venous system. Interestingly, despite drainage of large numbers of malignant cells into the circulation, metastatic disease in the lungs and other sites do not appear to be more common.

METABOLIC AND ENDOCRINE MANIFESTATIONS OF MALIGNANCY

Hypercalcaemia

Hypercalcaemia is a complication in around 5% of patients with advanced malignancy, and is particularly common in patients with carcinomas of the breast, lung and multiple myeloma. Three mechanisms are involved. Firstly, metastatic cancer cells in bone stimulate osteoclasts, the normal bone cells which break down bone, to destroy bone faster than the osteoblasts, the normal bone cells which build bone, can repair the damage. Secondly, the tumour may secrete proteins into the circulation which have similar destructive effects on bone but also promote the kidney to reabsorb more calcium from the urine than is appropriate. Finally, dehydration or damage to the kidney, as commonly occurs in multiple myeloma, can be important.

Hypercalcaemia causes many symptoms including lethargy, nausea, thirst, constipation and drowsiness. Because the symptoms are non-specific and commonly encountered in many patients with advanced cancer, the diagnosis can be easily missed. Treatment, however, will rapidly improve the patient's condition and relieve the unpleasant symptoms. This can be reliably achieved without side-effects by rehydration of the patient and inhibition of bone breakdown by one of the class of drugs called bisphosphonates. A single short infusion of one of the potent bisphosphonates that are now available will restore the serum calcium to normal in around 90% of patients.

Inappropriate secretion of antidiuretic hormone (ADH)

This syndrome results in retention of fluid by the kidney and is characterised by a low serum sodium. This causes weakness and confusion, occurring most commonly in patients with small cell lung cancer. Treatment is by fluid restriction, drugs such as demeclocycline which inhibit the action of ADH, and chemotherapy for the underlying malignancy.

Other endocrine manifestations of malignancy

Many cancers produce hormones and peptides with biological activity. These include ACTH, which may result in the features of Cushing's syndrome, hypoglycaemia from production of insulin-like substances and gynaecomastia from tumour production of human chorionic gonadotrophin (HCG).

Hyperuricaemia and tumour lysis syndrome

An acute metabolic disturbance may result from the rapid destruction of a tumour following chemotherapy. This is particularly likely to occur in childhood leukaemia and rapidly growing lymphomas. As chemotherapy kills the cancer, the cells release products of nitrogen metabolism, especially urea and urate, plus large amounts of potassium and phosphate into the circulation. The high urate concentration may result in urate crystal formation in the kidneys and lead to acute renal failure. High potassium levels can cause cardiac dysrhythmias, and increased phosphate may cause tetany. The syndrome can be prevented by prescribing allopurinol to prevent the production of large amounts of urate and intravenous fluids to encourage the kidneys to excrete the products of cell breakdown.

INFECTION

Infections are a major cause of death in cancer. Not only do they occur frequently but they are often more severe than in other patients, less responsive to therapy and sometimes are produced by organisms which in normal health would not cause any problem. The susceptibility of cancer patients to infection results from suppression of host defence mechanisms produced by the disease and its treatment. Infections are particularly frequent when the neutrophil count is suppressed by chemotherapy.

Advanced cancer and the treatments prescribed are associated with impaired neutrophil and lymphocyte function, depressed cell-mediated and humoral immunity, and damage to skin and mucous membranes which allows organisms to enter the bloodstream more easily. *Escherischia coli*, pseudomonas, staphylococci and streptococci are the most frequent bacterial pathogens. Viruses such as herpes simplex and zoster (shingles), fungi, particularly candida, and protozoal infection of the lungs with pneumocystis are important non-bacterial causes of infection requiring specific treatment. Most of the infecting organisms come from within the patient, for example gut bacteria, and, providing sensible precautions are taken, infections transmitted from family or health care staff are of relatively minor importance.

If patients are infected while neutropenic, urgent admission to hospital and treatment with broad-spectrum intravenous antibiotics are required, as untreated septicaemia can be rapidly fatal. Occasionally, even in specialist cancer centres and despite efficient and aggressive treatment of infection, patients still die from overwhelming infection following chemotherapy.

PARANEOPLASTIC SYNDROMES

Neurological

Cancers, particularly of the bronchus, are associated with a number of neurological syndromes which are unrelated to direct compression or infiltration of neural tissue. The mechanisms which give rise to these problems are poorly understood. They are uncommon and usually are possible to diagnose only by excluding the presence of malignant disease in the central nervous system or around nerve roots. The syndromes include numbness and weakness due to sensory and motor peripheral neuropathies respectively, paralysis from spinal cord damage, unsteadiness from cerebellar degeneration, dementia from cerebral damage and a form of muscle weakness which resembles myasthenia gravis. These neurological conditions may be the first manifestation of cancer. Sadly, treatment for the underlying cancer frequently fails to produce much neurological improvement.

Hypertrophic pulmonary osteoarthropathy

Lung cancer is the principal cause of this condition in which the bones of the forearms and shins become inflamed and painful. Plain radiographs show characteristic appearances and usually the patient has a deformity of the nails known as clubbing. Anti-inflammatory drugs relieve many of the symptoms and the condition may improve if the underlying tumour can be removed or destroyed.

Other paraneoplastic syndromes

A variety of general effects of cancer are sometimes described as paraneoplastic phenomena, and almost every organ in the body can be affected by one of these syndromes. Fever, cachexia and anaemia are relatively common and may be the presenting symptoms of malignancy. In addition, thrombophlebitis and clotting disorders, arthritis, skin rashes, itching, muscle inflammation and renal impairment are uncommon but well-recognised complications of malignant disease.

Bibliography

PART 1

REFERENCES

Administration of Radioactive Substances Advisory Committee (ARSAC) 1998 Notes for guidance on the clinical administration of radiopharmaceuticals and use of sealed radioactive sources. HMSO, London

British Journal of Radiology (BJR) 1983 Central axis depth dose data for use in radiotherapy. Supplement 17. British Institute of Radiology, London

British Journal of Radiology (BJR) 1996 Central axis depth dose data for use in radiotherapy. Supplement 25. British Institute of Radiology, London

Bomford C K 1969 Computers in radiation dosimetry. MPhil Thesis, University of London

Bomford C K 1976 Reduced output of orthovoltage radiotherapy units. Medical Physics 3: 120–121

Bomford C K, Dawes P J D K, Lillicrap S C, Young J 1989 Treatment simulators. Supplement 23. British Journal of Radiology, London

Burns J E, Dale J W G, DuSautoy A R, Owen B, Pritchard D H 1988 New calibration service for high energy X radiation at NPL. Proceedings of a symposium on dosimetry in radiotherapy, Vienna. Vienna IAEA 2: 125–132

Conway J 1998 Treatment planning and computer systems. In: Cherry P, Duxbury A (eds) Practical radiotherapy, physics and equipment. Greenwich Medical Media, London

Cohen M 1966. The classification of treatment plans. 1st International Conference on the Use of Computers in Therapeutic Radiology, Cambridge

Davy T J, Johnson P H, Redford R, Williams J R 1975 Conformation therapy using the tracking cobalt unit. British Journal of Radiology 48: 122–130

EC 1997 Radiation Protection 91: criteria for acceptability of radiological (including radiotherapy) and nuclear medicine installations. Office for Official Publications of the European Communities, Luxembourg

Erianson M, Franzen L, Henriksson R, Littbrand B, Lofroth P O 1991 Planning of radiotherapy for patients with hip prosthesis. International Journal of Radiation Oncology, Biology, Physics 20(5): 1093–1098

Essapen S, Knowles C, Tait D 2001 Variation in size and position of the planning target volume in the transverse plane owing to respiratory movement to the lung. British Journal of Radiology 74: 73–76

Fleming J S, Perkins A C 2001 Targeted radiotherapy. Report No. 83. IPEM, York

Haywood J K, Bomford C K, Hatton J 1979 A less empirical method of representing megavoltage beams for use in rapid radiotherapy calculations. British Journal of Radiology 52: 709–718

Heales J C, Harrett A, Blake S 1998 Timer error and beam quality variation during 'ramp up' of a superficial X-ray therapy unit. British Journal of Radiology 71: 1306–1309

HMSO 1996 Radioactive Material (Road Transport) (Great Britain) Regulations 1996. HMSO, London

Hope C S, Laurie J, Orr J S, Halnan K E 1967 Optimisation of X-ray treatment planning by computer judgement. Physics in Medicine and Biology 12: 531–542

HSE 1985a Approved code of practice: the protection of persons against ionising radiation arising from any work activity. Health and Safety Commission, HMSO, London

HSE 1985b The ionising radiations regulations. (SI 1985 No. 1333). Health and Safety Executive, HMSO, London

HSE 1988a Ionising Radiations (Protection of Persons Undergoing Medical Examination or Treatment) Regulations (Statutory Instrument No. 778). HMSO, London

HSE 1988b Guidance notes for the protection of persons against ionising radiations arising from medical and dental use. Health and Safety Executive, HMSO, London

HSE 1993 Ionising Radiations (Outside Workers) Regulations. HMSO, London

HSE 1998a Fitness of equipment used for medical exposure to ionising radiation. Guidance Note PM77, 2nd edn. Health and Safety Executive, 1998

HSE 1998b Proposals for revised Ionising Radiations Regulations and Approved Code of Practice. Health and Safety Executive, London

HSE 1999 The ionising radiations regulations 1999. (SI 1999 No. 3232). Health and Safety Executive, The Stationery Office, London

HSE 2000 Ionising Radiation (Medical Exposure) Regulations 2000. HMSO, London

IAEA 1985 Regulations for the safe transport of radioactive material, No. 6 Safety Standards. International Atomic Energy Agency, Vienna (ISBN 92-0-123890-8)

IAEA 1986 Regulations for the safe transport of radioactive material, No. 6 Suppl Safety Standards. International Atomic Energy Agency, Vienna

ICRP 1977a International Commission on Radiological Protection. The handling, storage, use and disposal of unsealed radionuclides in hospitals and medical research establishments. Publication 25. Pergamon Press, Oxford

ICRP 1977b Recommendations of the International Commission on Radiological Protection. Publication 26. Pergamon Press, Oxford

ICRP 1982 General principles of monitoring for radiation protection of workers. Publication 35. International Commission on Radiological Protection, Pergamon Press, Oxford

ICRP 1987 Radiation dose to patients from pharmaceuticals. Publication 53. International Commission on Radiological Protection, Pergamon Press, Oxford

ICRP 1991 1990 recommendations of the International Commission on Radiological Protection. Annals of the ICRP. Publication 60. Pergamon Press, Oxford

ICRU 1979 Methods of assessment of absorbed dose in clinical use of radionuclides. Report 32. International Commission on Radiation Units and Measurements, Washington

ICRU 1979 Methods of assessment of absorbed dose in clinical use of radionuclides. Report 32. International Commission on Radiation Units and Measurements, Washington

ICRU 1980 Radiation quantities and units. Report 33. International Commission on Radiation Units and Measurements, Bethesda

ICRU 1985 Dose and volume specification for reporting intracavitary therapy in gynaecology. Report 38. International Commission on Radiation Units and Measurements, Bethesda

ICRU 1993 Prescribing, recording and reporting photon beam therapy. Report 50. International Commission on Radiation Units and Measurements, Bethesda

ICRU 1999 Prescribing, recording and reporting photon beam therapy. Report 62. International Commission on Radiation Units and Measurements, Bethesda

IEC 1998 International Standard 1508. Functional safety of electrical/electronic/programmable electronic safety related systems. International Electrotechnical Commission, London

IPEM/CoR/NRPB 1997 Recommended standards for routine performance testing of diagnostic X-ray imaging systems. IPEM Report 77. IPEM, York

IPEMB 1996a The IPEMB code of practice for electron dosimetry for radiotherapy beams of initial energy from 2 to 50 MeV based on an air kerma calibration. Physics in Medicine and Biology 41: 2557–2603

IPEMB 1996b The IPEMB code of practice for the determination of absorbed dose for X-rays below 300 kV generating potential (0.035 mm Al – 4 mm Cu HVL; 10–300 kV generating potential). Physics in Medicine and Biology 41: 2605–2625

IPEMB 1996c A guide to commissioning and quality control of treatment planning systems. Report 68. IPEMB Publications, York

IPSM 1988a Commissioning and quality assurance of linear accelerators. Report 54. Institute of Physical Sciences in Medicine, York

IPSM 1988b Are X-rays safe enough? Patient doses and risk in diagnostic radiology. IPSM Report 55. IPSM, York

IPSM 1990 Code of practice for high energy photon therapy dosimetry based on the NPL absorbed dose calibration service. Physics in Medicine and Biology 35: 1355–1360

IPSM 1992 Procedures for the definitive calibration of external beam radiotherapy equipment. Scope 1(1): 33–36

Jani S K, Pennington E C 1990 Tissue compensators using vinyl lead sheets for head and neck portals on 4 MV X-rays. Medical Physics 17: 481–482

Jones D, Rieke J W, Madsen B L, Hafferman M D 2000 An isocentrically mounted stand for total body irradiation. British Journal of Radiology 73: 776–779

Khoo V S 2000 MRI – 'Magic radiotherapy imaging' for treatment planning? British Journal of Radiology 73: 229–233

Klevenhagen S C, Thwaites D I 1993 In: Williams J R, Thwaites D I (eds) Kilovoltage X-rays in radiotherapy in practice. Oxford University Press, Oxford

Leksell L 1968 Cerebral radiosurgery. Acta Chirurgica Scandinavica 134: 585–595

McKenzie A L 2001 When two and two make three. IPEM. Scope 10(1): 21–23

Meredith W J 1967 Radium dosage: the Manchester system. E & S Livingstone, London

MIRD Medical Internal Radiation Dose Committee Pamphlets 5, 10 and 11. Society of Nuclear Medicine Publications, Reston

Moores B M, Henshaw E T, Watkinson S A, Pearcy B J 1987 Practical guide to quality assurance in medical imaging. John Wiley, Chichester

NRPB 1990 Patient dose reduction in diagnostic radiology. National Radiological Protection Board, Didcot

NRPB 1996 Doses to patients from medical X-ray examinations in the UK—1995 Review. R289. National Radiological Protection Board, Didcot

Nutting C, Dearnaley D P, Webb S 2000 Intensity modulated radiation therapy: a clinical review. British Journal of Radiology 73: 459–469

Partridge M, Donovan E, Fenton N, Reise S, Blane S 1999 Clinical implementation of a computer-controlled milling machine for compensating filter production. British Journal of Radiology 72: 1099–1103

Pierquin B, Wilson J-F, Chassagne D 1987 Modern brachytherapy. Masson, New York

Poynter A J 2000 Direct measurement of air kerma rate in air from CDCS J-type caesium therapy sources using a Farmer ionisation chamber. British Journal of Radiology 73: 425–428

RSA 1993 The Radioactive Substances Act, 1993. HMSO, London

RSEO 1985 The Radioactive Substances (Testing Instruments) Exemption Order, 1985. HMSO, London

Shrimpton P C, Wall B F, Jones D G et al 1986 A national survey of doses to patients undergoing a selection of routine X-ray examinations in English hospitals. NRPB-R2000. HMSO, London

Sievert R 1932 Eine Methode zur Messung von Roentgen-, Radium- und Ultra-Strahlung nebst einigen Untersuchungen ueber die Anwendbarweit derselben in der Physik und der Medizin. Acta Radiologica (Suppl 14)

Stedeford B, Morgan H M, Mayles W P (eds) 1997 The design of radiotherapy treatment room facilities. Report 75. IPEM, York

Thomas S J 1985 A computer-controlled difference compensator system. British Journal of Radiology 58: 665

Thomas S J 1999 Relative electron density calibration of CT scanners for radiotherapy treatment planning. British Journal of Radiology 72: 781–786

Thwaites D I et al 1992 A dosimetric intercomparison of megavoltage beams in UK radiotherapy centres. Physics in Medicine and Biology 37: 445–461

Tsalafoutas I A; Xenofos S; Papalexopoulos A, Nikoletopoulos S 2000 Dose calculations for asymmetric fields defined by independent collimators using symmetric field data. British Journal of Radiology 73: 403–409

Vollans S E, Wilkinson J M 2000 Calibration of pre-cut iridium–192 wires for low dose rate interstitial brachytherapy using a Farmer-type ionisation chamber. British Journal of Radiology 73: 201–205

Walton L, Bomford C K, Ramsden D 1987 The Sheffield stereotactic radiosurgery unit: physical characteristics and principles of operation. British Journal of Radiology 60: 897–906

Whilde N J, Conway J, Bomford C K 1993 The development of quality assurance for Sheffield's radiotherapy treatment planning systems. British Journal of Radiology 66: 1182–1185

WHO 1988 Quality assurance in radiotherapy. World Health Organization, Geneva

Young M E J, Batho H F 1964 Dose tables for linear radium sources calculated by electronic computer. British Journal of Radiology 37: 38–44

FURTHER READING

Alderson A R (ed) 1986 Dosimetry and clinical uses of afterloading systems. Report 45. Institute of Physical Sciences in Medicine, York

American Association of Physicists in Medicine 1983 A protocol for the determination of absorbed dose from high energy photon and electron beams. Medical Physics 10: 741–771

Ball J E, Moore A D 1986 Essential physics for radiographers. Blackwell, Oxford

Bird N J, Old S E, Barber R W 2001 Gamma camera positron emission tomography. British Institute of Radiology 74: 303–306

Bomford C K, Dawes P J D K, Lillicrap S C, Young J 1989 Treatment simulators. Supplement 23. British Institute of Radiology, London

Cohen M, Mitchell J S 1984 Cobalt–60 teletherapy: a compendium of international practice. International Atomic Energy Agency, Vienna

Conway J, Robinson M H 1997 CT virtual simulation, in the radiological sciences present and future. British Journal of Radiology Special Issue 70: S106–S118

Dobbs J, Barrett A, Ash D 1999 Practical radiotherapy planning, 3rd edn. Arnold, London

Frier M, Hardy J G, Hesslewood S R, Lawreance R 1988 Hospital radiopharmacy principles and practice. Report No. 57. IPSM, York

Gambhir S S, Czernin J, Schwimmer J 2001 A tabulated summary of the FDG PET literature. A Supplement to The Journal of Nuclear Medicine. Society of Nuclear Medicine Publications, Reston

Gifford D 1984 A handbook of physics for radiologists and radiographers. John Wiley, Chichester

Godden T J 1988 Physical aspects of brachytherapy. Adam Hilger, Bristol

Greene D 1986 Linear accelerators for radiation therapy. Medical Physics Handbooks 17. Adam Hilger, Bristol

Greening J R 1985 Fundamentals of radiation dosimetry. Adam Hilger, Bristol

ICRP 1982 Protection against ionising radiation from external sources used in medicine. Publication 33. International Commission on Radiological Protection. Pergamon Press, Oxford

ICRP 1985 Protection of the patient in radiation therapy. Publication 44. International Commission on Radiological Protection, Pergamon Press, Oxford

ICRP 1987 Data for use in protection against external radiation. Publication 51. International Commission on Radiological Protection, Pergamon Press, Oxford

ICRP 1987 Protection of the patient in nuclear medicine. Publication 52. International Commission on Radiological Protection, Pergamon Press, Oxford

ICRU 1976 Determination of absorbed dose in a patient irradiated by beams of X-or gamma rays in radiotherapy procedures. Report 24. International Commission on Radiation Units and Measurements, Bethesda

ICRU 1984 Radiation dosimetry: electron beams with energies between 1 and 50 MeV. Report 35. International Commission on Radiation Units and Measurements, Bethesda

ICRU 1988 Use of computers in external beam radiotherapy procedures with high energy photons and electrons. Report 42. International Commission on Radiation Units and Measurements, Bethesda

ICRU 1989 Tissue substitutes in radiation dosimetry and measurement. Report 44. International Commission on Radiation Units and Measurements, Bethesda

IPEM 1997 The design of radiotherapy treatment room facilities, Report No. 75. Institute of Physics and Engineering in Medicine, York

IPSM 1989 Radiation protection in nuclear medicine and pathology. Report 64. Institute of Physical Sciences in Medicine, London

Johns H E, Cunningham J R 1983 The physics of radiology. Thomas, Illinois

Kathren R L 1986 Radiation protection. Adam Hilger, Bristol

Khalkhali I, Maublant J C, Goldsmith S J 2000 Nuclear oncology. Lippincott Williams & Wilkins, Philadelphia

Klevenhagen S C 1985 Physics of electron beam therapy. Adam Hilger, Bristol

Lillicrap S C, Higson G R, O'Connor A J 1998 Radiotherapy equipment standards from the International Electrotechnical Commission. British Journal of Radiology 71: 1225–1228

Lillicrap S C, Owen B, Williams J R, Williams P C 1990 Code of practice for high energy photon therapy dosimetry based on the NPL absorbed dose calibration service. Physics in Medicine and Biology 35: 1355–1360

Lombardi M H 1999 Radiation protection in nuclear medicine. CRC Press, London

Mackenzie A L, Shaw J E, Stephenson S K, Turner P C R (eds) 1986 Radiation protection in radiotherapy. Report 46. IPSM, London

Mason J S, Elliott K M, Mitro AC 1997 The nuclear medicine handbook for achieving compliance with NRC Regulations. Society of Nuclear Medicine Publications, Reston

Massey J-B 1970 Manual of dosimetry in radiotherapy. IAEA Technical Report Series 110. IAEA, Vienna
Mayles W P M, Lake R A, McKenzie A L, Macauley E M, Morgan H M, Powley S K. 1999 Physics aspects of quality control in radiotherapy. Report 81. Institute of Physics and Engineering in Medicine, York
Mould R F 1985 Radiotherapy treatment planning. Adam Hilger, Bristol
Norwood H M, Stubbs B 1984. Patient movements during radiotherapy. British Journal of Radiology 57: 155–158
RCR/NRPB 1990 Patient dose reduction in diagnostic radiology. Documents of the NRPB 1(3) 1–46
Saha G B 2000 Physics and radiobiology of nuclear medicine. Springer, Berlin
Sandler A (ed) 1996 Diagnostic nuclear medicine. Lippincott Williams & Wilkins, Philadelphia
Schiepers C (ed) 2000 Diagnostic nuclear medicine. Springer, Berlin
Sutton D G, Williams J R (eds) 2000 Radiation shielding for diagnostic X-rays. Joint BIR/IPEM Working Party Report. British Journal of Radiology, London
Taylor A, Schuster D M, Alzaraki N 2000 A clinician's guide to nuclear medicine. Society of Nuclear Medicine Publications, Reston
Thrall J H, Ziessman H A 2001 Nuclear medicine: the requisites, 2nd edn. Mosby, St Louis
Trott N G (ed) 1987 Radionuclides in brachytherapy: radium and after. Supplement 21. British Journal of Radiology, London
Tsien K C, Cunningham J R, Wright D J, Jones D E A, Pfalzner P M 1967 Atlas of radiation dose distributions. IAEA, Vienna
von Schultess GK 2000 Clinical positron-emission tomography. Lippincott Williams & Wilkins, Philadelphia
Webb S 1997 The physics of conformal radiotherapy—advances in technology. IOP Publishing, Bristol
Webb S 2000 Conformal intensity-modulated radiotherapy (IMRT) delivered by robotic linac—conformality versus efficiency of dose delivery. Physics in Medicine and Biology 45(7): 1715–1730
Wilks R 1987 Principles of radiological physics. Churchill Livingstone, Edinburgh
Wilson M A 1998 Textbook of nuclear medicine. Lippincott Williams & Wilkins, Philadelphia
Wolters E Ch, Tolosa E (eds) 2001 New tools in the diagnosis of Parkinsonism. Current Issues in Neurodegenerative Diseases Volume 13. Academic Pharmaceutical Productions, Utrecht

PART 2

FURTHER READING

Brown J M 1989 Hypoxic cell radiosensitisers: where next? International Journal of Radiation Oncology, Biology, Physics 16: 987–993
Burnet N G, Nyman J, Turesson I, Wurm R, Yarnold J R, Peacock J H 1992 Prediction of normal-tissue tolerance to radiotherapy from in-vitro cellular radiation sensitivity. Lancet 339: 1570–1571
Caplin M E, Buscombe J R, Hilson A J, Jones A L, Watkinson A, Burroughs A K 1998 Carcinoid tumour. Lancet 352: 799–805
Cavalli F, Hansen H H, Kaye S B 2000 Textbook of medical oncology, 2nd edn. Martin Dunitz, London
Chaplin D J, Durand R E, Olive P L 1986 Acute hypoxia in tumors: implications for modifiers of radiation effects. International Journal of Radiation Oncology, Biology, Physics 12: 1279–1282
Coleman C N 1993 Beneficial liaisons: radiobiology meets cellular and molecular biology. Radiotherapy and Oncology 28: 1–15
D'Amico A V, Hanks G (eds) 1999 Radiotherapeutic management of prostate adenocarcinoma. Arnold, London.
Dachs G U, Dougherty G J, Stratford I J, Chaplin D J 1997 Targeting gene therapy to cancer: a review. *Oncology Research* 9: 313–325
Deacon J, Peckham M J, Steel G G 1984 The radioresponsiveness of human tumours and the initial slope of the cell survival curve. Radiotherapy and Oncology 2: 317–323
Dixon J M 2000 ABC of breast diseases, 2nd edn. BMJ Publishing Group, London
Dobbs J, Barrett A, Ash D 1999 Practical radiotherapy planning, 3rd edn. Arnold, London.
Halperin E C, Constine L S, Tarbell N J, Kun L E 1999 Pediatric radiation oncology, 3rd edn. Raven Press, New York
Hancock B W, Selby P J, MacLennan K, Armitage J O (eds) 2000 Malignant lymphoma. Arnold, London
Holland J F, Frei E, Bast R C, Morton D L, Kufe D W, Weichelsbaum R R 1997 Cancer medicine, 4th edn. Williams & Wilkins, Philadelphia
Horsman M R, Khalil A A, Siemann D W, Grau C, Hill S A, Lynch E M, Chaplin D J, Overgaard J 1994 Relationship between radiobiological hypoxia in tumors and electrode measurements of tumor oxygenation. International Journal of Radiation Oncology, Biology, Physics 29: 439–442
Kaisary A V, Murphy G P, Denis L, Griffiths K (eds) 1999 Textbook of prostate cancer, pathology, diagnosis and treatment. Martin Dunitz, London.
Kanaar R, Hoeijmakers J H J, van Gent D C 1998 Molecular mechanisms of DNA double-strand break repair. Trends in Cell Biology 8: 483–489
Lakhani S R, Dilly S A, Finlayson C J 1998 Basic pathology, 2nd edn. Arnold, London
Lenhard R E, Osteen R T, Gansler E 2001 Clinical oncology. American Cancer Society, Atlanta
Malpas J (ed) 1996 Cancer in children. British Medical Bulletin 52(4)
Marcus R, Cunningham D, Miles A (eds) 2001 The effective management of non-Hodgkin's lymphoma. Aesculapius Medical Press, London

Mauch P M, Armitage J O, Diehl V, Hoppe R T, Weiss L M (eds) 1999 Hodgkin's disease. Lippincott Williams & Wilkins, Philadelphia

McMillan T J, Peacock J H 1994 Molecular determinants of radiosensitivity in mammalian cells. International Journal of Radiation Biology 65: 49–55

O'Neill P, Fielden E M 1993 Primary free radical processes in DNA. Advances in Radiation Biology 17: 53–120

Peckham M, Pinedo H M, Veronesi U (eds) 1995 Oxford textbook of oncology. Oxford Medical Publications, Oxford

Perez C A, Brady L W 1997 Principles and practice of radiation oncology, 3rd edn. J B Lippincott, Philadelphia

Pinkerton C R, Plowman P N 1997 Paediatric oncology—clinical practice and controversies, 2nd edn. Chapman & Hall, London

Pizzo P A, Poplack D G 1996 Principles and practice of pediatric oncology, 3rd edn. Lippincott, Williams & Wilkins, Philadelphia

Plowman P N, McElwain T, Meadow A 1992 Complications of cancer management. Butterworth-Heinemann, Oxford

Pointon R C S 1991 The radiotherapy of malignant disease, 2nd edn. Springer-Verlag, Berlin

Potten C S, Merritt A, Hickman J, Hall P, Faranda A 1994 The characterisation of radiation-induced apoptosis in the small intestine and its biological implications. International Journal of Radiation Biology 65 71–78

Powell S N, Whitaker S J, Edwards S M, McMillan T J A 1992 DNA repair defect in a radiation-sensitive clone of a human bladder carcinoma cell line. British Journal of Cancer 65: 798–802

Price P, Sikora K (eds) 1995 Treatment of cancer, 3rd edn. Chapman and Hall, London

Royal College of Paediatrics and Child Health 1997 Guidance for services for children and young people with brain and spinal tumours. Royal College of Paediatrics and Child Health, London

Souhami R, Tobias J 1998 Cancer and its management, 3rd edn. Blackwell Science, Oxford

Tucker S L, Chan K S 1990 The selection of patients for radiotherapy on the basis of tumor growth kinetics and intrinsic radiosensitivity. Radiotherapy and Oncology 18: 197–211

Underwood J C E (ed) 2000 General and systematic pathology, 3rd edn. Churchill Livingstone, Edinburgh

Ward J F 1986 Mechanisms of DNA repair and their potential modification for radiotherapy. International Journal of Radiation Oncology, Biology, Physics 12: 1027–1032

Weichselbaum R, Fuks Z, Hallahan D, Haimovitz-Friedman A, Kufe D 1993 Radiation-induced cytokines and growth factors: cellular and molecular basis of modification of radiation damage. In: Yarnold J, Stratton M, McMillan T (eds) Molecular biology for oncologists. Elsevier, Amsterdam, pp 213–221

West C M L, Davidson S E, Roberts S A, Hunter R D 1993 Intrinsic radiosensitivity and prediction of patient response to radiotherapy for carcinoma of the cervix. British Journal of Cancer 68: 819–823.

Whitaker S J, Ung Y C, McMillan T J. 1995 DNA double-strand break induction and rejoining as determinants of human tumour cell radiosensitivity. A pulsed-field gel electrophoresis study. International Journal of Radiation Biology 67(1): 7–18

Withers H R, Taylor J M G, Maciejewski B 1988 The hazard of accelerated tumour clonogen repopulation during radiotherapy. Acta Oncologica 27: 131–137

Index

A

B

C

F

G

H

I

J

K

L

M

N

O

S

T

U